Pulseless Electrical Activity (PEA) Algorithm

(Electromechanical Dissociation [EMD]

Includes
- Electromechanical dissociation (EMD)
- Pseudo-EMD
- Idioventricular rhythms
- Ventricular escape rhythms
- Bradyasystolic rhythms
- Postdefibrillation idioventricular rhythms

- Continue CPR
- Intubate at once
- Obtain IV access
- Assess blood flow using Doppler ultrasound, end-tidal CO_2, echocardiography, or arterial line

↓

Consider possible causes

(Parentheses=possible therapies and treatments)

- Hypovolemia (volume infusion)
- Hypoxia (ventiiation)
- Cardiac tamponade (pericardiocentesis)
- Tension pneumothorax (needle decompression)
- Hypothermia
- Massive pulmonary embolism (surgery, ***thrombolytics***)
- Drug overdoses such as tricyclics, digitalis, β-blockers, calcium channel blockers
- Hyperkalemia[a]
- Acidosis[b]
- Massive acute myocardial infarction

↓

- Epinephrine 1 mg IV push, a,c repeat every 3-5 min

↓

- If absolute bradycardia (<60 BPM) or relative bradycardia, give ***atropine*** 1 mg IV
- Repeat every 3-5 min to a total of 0.03-0.04 mg/kg[d]

Class I:	definitely helpful
Class IIa:	acceptable, probably helpful
Class IIb:	acceptable, possibly helpful
Class III:	not indicated, may be harmful

a. *Sodium bicarbonate* 1 mEq/kg is Class I if patient has known preexisting hyperkalemia.

b. Sodium bicarbonate 1 mEq/kg:

Class IIa
- If known preexisting bicarbonate-responsive acidosis
- If overdose with tricyclic antidepressants
- To alkalinize the urine in drug overdoses

Class IIb
- If intubated and continued long arrest interval
- Upon return of spntaneous circulation after long arrest interval

Class III
- Hypoxic lactic acidosis

c. The recommended dose of ***epinephrine*** is 1 mg IV push every 3-5 min. If this approach fails, several Class IIb dosing regimens can be considered:
- Intermediate: ***epinephrine*** 2-5 mg IV push, every 3-5 min
- Escalating: ***epinephrine*** 1 mg-3 mg-5 mg IV push, 3 min apart
- High: ***epinephrine*** 0.1 mg/kg IV push, every 3-5 min

d. The shorter atropine dosing interval (3 min) is possibly helpful in cardiac arrest (Class IIb)

Asystole Treatment Algorithm

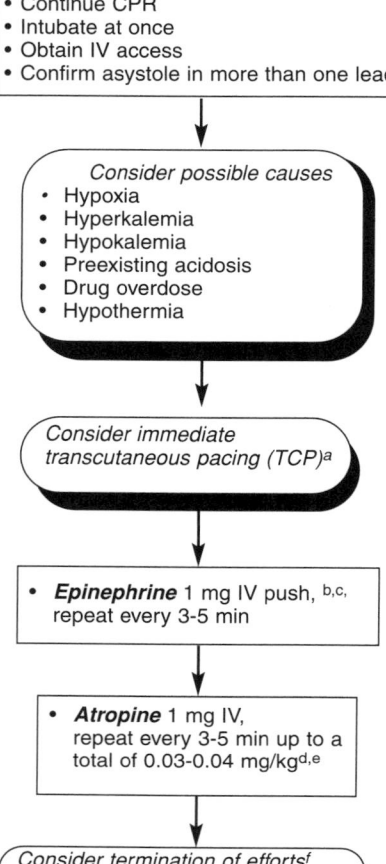

- Continue CPR
- Intubate at once
- Obtain IV access
- Confirm asystole in more than one lead

↓

Consider possible causes
- Hypoxia
- Hyperkalemia
- Hypokalemia
- Preexisting acidosis
- Drug overdose
- Hypothermia

↓

Consider immediate transcutaneous pacing (TCP)[a]

↓

- ***Epinephrine*** 1 mg IV push, [b,c] repeat every 3-5 min

↓

- ***Atropine*** 1 mg IV, repeat every 3-5 min up to a total of 0.03-0.04 mg/kg[d,e]

↓

Consider termination of efforts[f]

Class I:	definitely helpful
Class IIa:	acceptable, probably helpful
Class IIb:	acceptable, possibly helpful
Class III:	not indicated, may be harmful

a. TCP is a Class IIb intervention. Lack of success may be due to delays in pacing. To be effective TCP must be performed early, simultaneously with drugs. Evidence does not support routine use of TCP for asystole.

b. The recommended dose of ***epinephrine*** is 1 mg IV push every 3-5 min. If this approach fails, several Class IIb dosing regimens can be considered:
- Intermediate: ***epinephrine*** 2-5 mg IV push, every 3-5 min
- Escalating: ***epinephrine*** 1 mg-3mg-5 mg IV push, 3 min apart
- High: ***epinephrine*** 0.1 mg/kg IV push, every 3-5 min

c. ***Sodium bicarbonate*** 1 mEq/kg is Class I if patient has known preexisting hyperkalemia.

d. The shorter ***atropine*** dosing interval (3 min) is Class IIb in asystolic arrest.

e. ***Sodium bicarbonate*** 1 mEq/kg:

Class IIa
- If known preexisting bicarbonate-responive acidosis
- If overdose with tricyclic antidepressants
- To alkalinize the urine in drug overdoses

Class IIb
- If intubated and continued long arrest interval
- Upon return of spontaneous circulation after long arrest interval

Class III
- Hypoxic lactic acidosis

f. If patient remains in asystole or other agonal rhythm after successful intubation and initial medications and no reversible causes are identified, consider termination of resuscitative efforts by a physician. Consider interval since arrest.

The 5 Minute Emergency Medicine Consult

PETER ROSEN, M.D.

DIRECTOR, EM RESIDENCY PROGRAM

PROFESSOR, CLINICAL MEDICINE AND SURGERY

DEPARTMENT OF EMERGENCY MEDICINE

UNIVERSITY OF CALIFORNIA SAN DIEGO MEDICAL CENTER

SAN DIEGO, CALIFORNIA

ROGER M. BARKIN, M.D.

VICE-PRESIDENT FOR PEDIATRIC AND NEWBORN PROGRAMS

HEALTHONE

PROFESSOR OF SURGERY

DIVISION OF EMERGENCY MEDICINE

UNIVERSITY OF COLORADO HEALTH SCIENCES CENTER

DENVER, COLORADO

STEPHEN R. HAYDEN, M.D.

ASSISTANT CLINICAL PROFESSOR OF MEDICINE

ASSOCIATE DIRECTOR EM RESIDENCY PROGRAM

UNIVERSITY OF CALIFORNIA SAN DIEGO MEDICAL CENTER

SAN DIEGO, CALIFORNIA

JEFFREY J. SCHAIDER, M.D.

ASSOCIATE CHAIRMAN

DEPARTMENT OF EMERGENCY MEDICINE

COOK COUNTY HOSPITAL

ASSISTANT PROFESSOR OF EMERGENCY MEDICINE

RUSH MEDICAL COLLEGE

RICHARD WOLFE, M.D.

RESIDENCY DIRECTOR

DEPARTMENT OF EMERGENCY MEDICINE

HARVARD MEDICAL SCHOOL

BRIGHAM AND WOMEN'S HOSPITAL

BOSTON, MASSACHUSETTS

The 5 Minute Emergency Medicine Consult

LIPPINCOTT WILLIAMS & WILKINS
A **Wolters Kluwer** Company
Philadelphia • Baltimore • New York • London
Buenos Aires • Hong Kong • Sydney • Tokyo

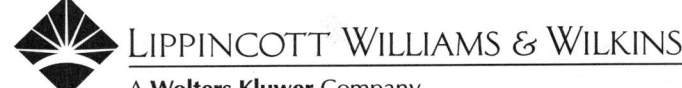

Editor: Elizabeth Greenspan
Managing Editor: Tanya Lazar
Marketing Manager: Kate Rubin
Production Editor: Jeffrey S. Myers

351 West Camden Street
Baltimore, Maryland 21201-2436

530 Walnut Street
Philadelphia, PA 19106

Printed in the United States of America

Library of Congress Cataloging-in-Publication Data

5 minute emergency medicine consult / edited by Peter Rosen . . . [et al.].
p. cm.
Includes bibliographical references and index.
ISBN 0-683-30177-2
1. Emergency medicine Handbooks, manuals, etc. 2. Medical emergencies Handbooks, manuals, etc. I. Rosen, Peter, 1935- II. Title: Five minute emergency medicine consult.
[DNLM: 1. Emergency Medical Services Handbooks. 2. Emergency Medicine Hand books. 3. Emergency Treatment Hand books. WB 39 Z9995 1999]
RC86.8.A14 1999
616.02'5—dc21
DNLM/DLC
for Library of Congress 99-22602
CIP

00 01 02 03
2 3 4 5 6 7 8 9 10

Dedication

This book is dedicated to the emergency medicine clinician who works in an environment where time is of the essence and rapid intervention is often essential. The 5 Minute Emergency Medicine Consult is ideal for this setting. It is our hope that the format and information will find its way to the bedside in our care of patients.

Preface

The purpose of this book is to give a terse, focused, and useful summary of the topic of emergency medicine. No human mind can retain all the facts, appropriate drugs and dosages, and management principles of a field that every day grows more complex.

The book is not intended to provide a description of research topics, controversies, changing styles, or theoretical management. Rather, where there is controversy, the authors have been asked to supply their best management principles. "Consider" is not a useful verb in medicine, especially in an arena where a decision must not only be made, but must be made under the pressure of a time constraint.

The authors have also been asked to discuss each topic as if they were in the middle of a busy ED, trying to give a precise summary to a resident who had queried them on the topic, or with whom they might be seeing a patient with that particular problem.

Not only is human memory incapable of recalling all useful facts in clinical emergency medicine, it is impossible for any emergency physician to be current on all phases of a modern practice. There are not enough hours in the day to read all the available literature, not only within the field of emergency medicine, but in all the pertinent related fields. It is our goal to supplement this data bank, and to help the practicing clinician to have a quick resource to turn for immediate information.

The book is not intended to replace clinical judgment, for after all, it is the clinician who must interpret the presenting signs and symptoms to judge which topic needs to be consulted. It is not a diagnostic engine, but rather a place to turn to confirm a diagnosis that has been suggested by a real clinical presentation.

There are many textbooks that can give a lengthy and complete, almost encyclopedic discussion of a given topic. This is often not useful in the middle of a busy ED, when you need a drug name or dosage and do not have the time to peruse a 50-page text. The 5 Minute Emergency Medical Consult is intended to be accurate, pointed, and readily encompassed, rather than being definitive.

The book is intended to be used, not only by the novice in emergency medicine practice, but by the experienced clinician as well. It is our hope that this will be the place to turn for any practicing emergency physician, and that our information will be found useful in the middle of the busiest practice. It is also our hope that the material represents the synthesis of the best styles and most immediate current thought on any topic; what do you need to know about a subject as opposed to what it would be nice to know. As a consequence, we feel it will be extremely helpful to the beginning student on his or her first rotation in the ED, as well as to the experienced attending.

The book is not intended as a substitute for thought, clinical acumen, or for other forms of education or training, but it is our goal to make it practical and aimed at the point of impact in a functioning emergency department.

This is not a book to read from cover to cover except over the time of a busy emergency medicine practice. We hope that it will be useful in your care of the patients that you are responsible for, and that it represents the distillation of the vast body of knowledge that has come to define the practice of emergency medicine.

To have good outcomes in emergency medicine, one must be prudent. It is our hope that these facts, presented in an easily accessible form will help that goal of safety.

It was enjoyable to attempt to meet this challenge, and we hope that this book will increase the fulfillment of practicing emergency medicine.

Peter Rosen, MD
Roger M. Barkin, MD
Steven R. Hayden, MD
Jeffrey J. Schaider, MD
Richard Wolfe, MD

Acknowledgment

We are tremendously appreciative to the innumerable contributors who have done a superb job in conceptualizing and implementing this reference. Special thanks are also due to the editorial and production staff of Lippincott Williams & Wilkins in helping to make it a reality. Special thanks are owed to Tanya Lazar and Jeff Myers. Our staffs and our families provided invaluable support during the many hours of its completion.

Contributors

JAMES ADAMS, MD
Department of Emergency Medicine
Brigham and Women's Hospital
Boston, Massachusetts

JONATHAN ADLER, MD
Department of Emergency Medicine
Massachusetts General Hospital
Boston, Massachusetts

STEVEN AKS, DO
Division of Toxicology
Cook County Hospital
Chicago, Illinois

MARILYN ALTHOFF, MD
Department of Emergency Medicine
Morristown Memorial Hospital
Morristown, New Jersey

THOMAS AMOROSO, MD
Division of Emergency Medicine
Beth Israel Hospital
Boston, Massachusetts

ANGELA C. ANDERSON, MD
Department of Emergency Medicine
Rhode Island Hospital
Providence, Rhode Island

ALTAF ANSARI, MD
Department of Emergency Medicine
Beth Israel Medical Center
New York, New York

KRIS ARNOLD, MD
Department of Emergency Medicine
Boston Medical Center
Boston, Massachusetts

PAUL ARNOLD, MD
Department of Emergency Medicine
The Toronto Hospital
Toronto, Ontario

ADAM BARKIN
Vanderbilt University
School of Medicine
Nashville, Tennessee

DAVID BARLAS, MD
Department of Emergency Medicine
North Shore University Hospital
Manhasset, New York

S. BRENT BARNES, MD
Section of Emergency Medicine
University of Oklahoma Health Sciences Center
Oklahoma City, Oklahoma

JOEL BARTFIELD, MD
Department of Emergency Medicine
Albany Medical Center
Albany, New York

ERIK BARTON, MD
Department of Emergency Medicine
Brigham and Women's Hospital
Boston, Massachusetts

KATHLENE BASSETT, MD
Department of Emergency Medicine
Children's Hospital
Denver, Colorado

CARL BAUM, MD
Division of Emergency Medicine
Children's Memorial Hospital
Chicago, Illinois

BARBARA J. BECK, MD
Acute Psychiatry Service
Massachusetts General Hospital
Boston, Massachusetts

BERNARD BECKERMAN, MD
Department of Emergency Medicine
North Shore University Hospital
Manhasset, New York

WALTER BELLEZA, MD
Division of Emergency Medicine
University of Maryland
Baltimore, Maryland

KYAN J. BERGER, MD
Department of Emergency Medicine
University of California - San Diego Medical Center
San Diego, California

SCOTT BERNS, MD
Department of Emergency Medicine
Rhode Island Hospital
Providence, Rhode Island

TONY BEST, MD
King Faisal Specialist Hospital and Research Center
Riyadh, Kingdom of Saudi Arabia

WILLIAM BINDER, MD
Department of Emergency Medicine
Massachusetts General Hospital
Boston, Massachusetts

HERBERT BIVINS, MD
Department of Emergency Medicine
University Medical Center
Fresno, California

ADAM BLACK, MD
Department of Emergency Medicine
University of Illinois
Chicago, Illinois

PAUL BLACKBURN, DO
Department of Emergency Medicine
Maricopa Medical Center
Phoenix, Arizona

JANICE BLANCHARD, MD
Department of Emergency Medicine
George Washington University
Washington, DC

JACQUES H. BLANCHET, MD
Department of Emergency Medicine
Baystate Medical Center
Springfield, Massachusetts

HOWARD BLUMSTEIN, MD
Department of Emergency Medicine
Alleghaney University Hospital East Falls
Philadelphia, Pennsylvania

KELLY BOOKMAN, MD
Department of Emergency Medicine
Aurora Humana Hospital
Aurora, Colorado

JOAN BOTHNER, MD
Department of Emergency Medicine
Children's Hospital
Denver, Colorado

JOSHUA BOVERMAN, MD
Acute Psychiatry Service
Massachusetts General Hospital
Boston, Massachusetts

JEFFERSON BRACEY, DO
Department of Emergency Medicine
University Medical Center
Las Vegas, Nevada

KENNETH BRAMWELL, MD
Department of Emergency Medicine
University of California - San Diego Medical Center
San Diego, California

PATRICIA BREEDEN, MD
Department of Emergency Medicine
University of Mississippi Medical Center
Jackson, Mississippi

JUDITH BRILLMAN, MD
Department of Emergency Medicine
University of New Mexico
Albuquerque, New Mexico

KATHRYN BRINSFIELD, MD
Department of Emergency Medicine
Boston City Hospital
Boston, Massachusetts

MELISSA BROKAW, MD
Department of Emergency Medicine
University of Rochester / Strong Memorial Hospital
Rochester, New York

DAVID BROWN, MD
Department of Emergency Medicine
Massachusetts General Hospital
Boston, Massachusetts

LANCE BROWN, MD, MPH
Department of Emergency Medicine
Los Angeles County / University of Southern California Medical Center
Los Angeles, California

RANDEL BROWN, MD
Department of Emergency Medicine
University of Arkansas
Little Rock, Arkansas

G. RICHARD BRUNO, MD
Department of Emergency Medicine
New York University/Bellevue Hospital Center
New York City, New York

ROBERT BUCKLEY, MD
Department of Emergency Medicine
US Naval Hospital
Rota, Spain

KENNETH H. BUTLER, DO
Division of Emergency Medicine
University of Maryland
Baltimore, Maryland

YVETTE CALDERON, MD
Department of Emergency Medicine
Albert Einstein Residency in Emergency Medicine
Bronx, New York

MARTIN J. CAREY, MB, BCH, MPH
Department of Emergency Medicine
University of Arkansas
Little Rock, Arkansas

TERESA CARLIN, MD
Department of Emergency Medicine
Johns Hopkins Hospital
Baltimore, Maryland

WALLACE CARTER, MD
Department of Emergency Medicine
New York University / Bellevue Hospital Center
New York, New York

MICHAEL CHAMALES, MD
Section of Emergency Medicine
University of Oklahoma Health Sciences Center
Oklahoma City, Oklahoma

LISA CHAN, MD
Department of Emergency Medicine
Albany Medical Center
Albany, New York

THEODORE C. CHAN, MD
Department of Emergency Medicine
University of California - San Diego Medical Center
San Diego, California

ANDREW CHANG, MD
Department of Emergency Medicine
Brigham and Women's Hospital
Boston, Massachusetts

ROBERT CHANG, MD
Department of Emergency Medicine
New York University / Bellevue Hospital Center
New York, New York

GORDON CHEW, MD
Department of Emergency Medicine
University of California - San Diego Medical Center
San Diego, California

KARLENE CHIN, MD
Department of Emergency Medicine
Beth Israel Medical Center
New York, New York

GREGORY CHRISTIANSEN, DO
Department of Emergency Medicine
Buffalo General Hospital
Buffalo, New York

LYDIA CIARALLO, MD
Department of Emergency Medicine
Rhode Island Hospital
Providence, Rhode Island

KATHRYN CLARK, MD
Department of Emergency Medicine
Children's Hospital
Denver, Colorado

RICK CLARK, MD
San Diego Regional Poison Center
San Diego, California

KATHY CLEM, MD
Department of Emergency Medicine
Loma Linda University Medical Center
Loma Linda, California

STEWART COFFMAN, MD
Division of Emergency Medicine
University of Texas Southwestern Dallas
Dallas, Texas

KARYN COLE, MD
Department of Emergency Medicine
Howard University Hospital
Washington, DC

JAMES COMES, MD
Department of Emergency Medicine
University Medical Center
Fresno, California

MARCO COPPOLA, DO
Department of Emergency Medicine
Darnall Army Community Hospital
Fort Hood, Texas

MARCO CORDERO, MD
Department of Emergency Medicine
Palos Hospital
Palos, Illinois

CHRISTY CORVER, MD
Bethesda, Maryland

KAREN COSBY, MD
Department of Emergency Medicine
Cook County Hospital
Chicago, Illinois

FRANCIS COUNSELMAN, MD
Department of Emergency Medicine
Eastern Virginia Medical School
Norfolk, Virginia

LINDA COWELL, MD
Department of Emergency Medicine
Rhode Island Hospital
Providence, Rhode Island

HILARIE CRANMER, MD
Department of Emergency Medicine
Brigham and Women's Hospital
Boston, Massachusetts

RICHARD A. CRAVEN, MD
Virginia Beach, Virginia

M. CORNELIA CREMENS, MD
Acute Psychiatry Service
Massachusetts General Hospital
Boston, Massachusetts

STEVEN CRESPO, MD
Department of Emergency Medicine
Boston Medical Center
Boston, Massachusetts

JOSEPH CRISANTHI, MD
Division of Emergency Medicine
University of Maryland
Baltimore, Maryland

MARK CROCKETT, MD
Division of Toxicology
Cook County Hospital
Chicago, Illinois

KEVIN CURTIS, MD
Department of Emergency Medicine
George Washington University
Washington, DC

LIESL CURTIS, MD
Department of Emergency Medicine
George Washington University
Washington, DC

RITA CYDULKA, MD
Department of Emergency Medicine
Metro Health Medical Center
Cleveland, Ohio

ROB DART, MD
Department of Emergency Medicine
Boston Medical Center
Boston, Massachusetts

PAUL DAVID, MD
Department of Emergency Medicine
Stanford University Medical Center
Stanford, California

DANIEL DAVIS, MD
Department of Emergency Medicine
University of California - San Diego Medical Center
San Diego, California

MARK DAVIS, MD
Division of Emergency Medicine
Beth Israel Hospital
Boston, Massachusetts

ROBERT DAVIS, MD
Department of Emergency Medicine
Rhode Island Hospital
Providence, Rhode Island

BEVERLY DAVISON, MD
Department of Emergency Medicine
Long Island Jewish Medical Center
New Hyde Park, New York

PETER DEBLIEUX, MD
Section of Emergency Medicine
Louisiana State University Medical Center
New Orleans, Louisiana

MAURICE DEFINA, MD
Department of EMS / Trauma
Hartford Hospital
Hartford, Connecticut

BETH ANNE DEGENNARO, MD
Department of Emergency Medicine
Hartford Hospital
Hartford, Connecticut

DAVID DELLA-GIUSTINA, MD
Department of Emergency Medicine
Madigan Army Medical Center
Tacoma, Washington

KIMBERLY DENT, MD
Department of Emergency Medicine
Rhode Island Hospital
Providence, Rhode Island

PAUL DESAN, MD
Acute Psychiatry Service
Massachusetts General Hospital
Boston, Massachusetts

PAUL L. DESANDRE, DO
Department of Emergency Medicine
Beth Israel Medical Center
New York, New York

JOSE DIAZ, MD
Department of Emergency Medicine
Cooper Hospital
Blue Bell, Pennsylvania

ISSER DUBINSKY, MD
Department of Emergency Medicine
The Toronto Hospital
Toronto, Ontario

SUSAN DUFEL, MD
Department of Emergency Medicine
Hartford Hospital
Hartford, Connecticut

EILEEN DUFFY, MD
LaGrange, Illinois

SUSAN J. DUFFY, MD
Department of Emergency Medicine
Rhode Island Hospital
Providence, Rhode Island

KIRK DUFTY, MD
Department of Emergency Medicine
Cook County Hospital
Chicago, Illinois

JOHN DUTTON, MD
Department of Emergency Medicine
Brigham and Women's Hospital
Boston, Massachusetts

NICOLE DUVAL, MD
Department of Emergency Medicine
Baystate Medical Center
Springfield, Massachusetts

JONATHAN EDLOW, MD
Division of Emergency Medicine
Beth Israel Hospital
Boston, Massachusetts

JEFFREY ELLIS, MD
Department of Emergency Medicine
University Medical Center
Las Vegas, Nevada

NORBERT ELSNER, MD
Department of Emergency Medicine
Albert Einstein Residency in Emergency Medicine
Bronx, New York

JANET ENG, DO
Holt, Michigan

TIMOTHY ERICKSON, MD
Department of Emergency Medicine
University of Illinois
Chicago, Illinois

CHRISTOPHER ERVIN, MD
Department of Emergency Medicine
Prince Georges Medical Center
Prince Georges, Maryland

MICHELLE ERVIN, MD
Department of Emergency Medicine
Howard University Hospital
Washington, DC

BARNET ESKIN, MD
Department of Emergency Medicine
Morristown Memorial Hospital
Morristown, New Jersey

BRIAN EUERLE, MD
Division of Emergency Medicine
University of Maryland
Baltimore, Maryland

SHAWN EVANS, MD
Department of Emergency Medicine
University of California - San Diego Medical Center
San Diego, California

CHARLES EVERLY, MD
Department of Emergency Medicine
Cook County Hospital
Chicago, Illinois

JAMAL FARRAN, MD
Department of Emergency Medicine
George Washington University
Washington, DC

SUSAN FARRELL, MD
Division of Emergency Medicine
Beth Israel Deaconess Medical Center
Boston, Massachusetts

JAMES FELDMAN, MD
Department of Emergency Medicine
Boston Medical Center
Boston, Massachusetts

IAN GLEN FERGUSON, DO
Department of Emergency Medicine
Kern Medical Center
Bakersfield, California

PETER FERRERA, MD
Department of Emergency Medicine
Albany Medical Center
Albany, New York

PAUL FILE, MD
Carmel Valley, California

MICHELLE FINKEL, MD
Department of Emergency Medicine
Brigham and Women's Hospital
Boston, Massachusetts

KELLY ANNE FOLEY, MD
Department of Emergency Medicine
Eastern Virginia Medical School
Norfolk, Virginia

JAMES FOSTER, MD
Department of Emergency Medicine
Stanford University Medical Center
Stanford, California

STEVEN FRIEDMAN, MD, MPH, CCFP(EM)
Department of Emergency Medicine
The Toronto Hospital
Toronto, Ontario

MARY ANNE FUCHS, MD
Department of Emergency Medicine
University of California - San Diego Medical Center
San Diego, California

STEVEN FURER, MD
Department of Emergency Medicine
New York Medical Center
Bronx, New York

MURTAZA GALAMHUSSEIN, MD
Department of Emergency Medicine
The Toronto Hospital
Toronto, Ontario

ROBERT GALLI, MD
Department of Emergency Medicine
University of Mississippi
Jackson, Mississippi

TAMI GASH-KIM, MD
Department of Emergency Medicine
University of California - San Diego Medical Center
San Diego, California

MARC GELMAN, MD
Department of Emergency Medicine
The Toronto Hospital
Toronto, Ontario

PAUL GENNIS, MD
Department of Emergency Medicine
Albert Einstein Residency in Emergency Medicine
Bronx, New York

DELARAM GHADISHAH, MD
Department of Emergency Medicine
University of California - Irvine Medical Center
Orange, California

MELISSA GILLESPIE, MD
Department of Emergency Medicine
Illinois Masonic Medical Center
Chicago, Illinois

BRET GINTHER, MD
Department of Emergency Medicine
University of California - Irvine Medical Center
Orange, California

ERIC GLASSER, MD
Department of Emergency Medicine
George Washington University
Washington, DC

DON GOFF, MD
Acute Psychiatry Service
Massachusetts General Hospital
Boston, Massachusetts

WILLIAM GOLDBERG, MD
Department of Emergency Medicine
New York University / Bellevue Hospital Center
New York, New York

JEFFREY GORDON, MD
Department of Emergency Medicine
Resurrection Hospital
Chicago, Illinois

DEEPI GOYAL, MD
Department of Emergency Medicine
University of Pittsburgh
Pittsburgh, Pennsylvania

KIMBERLIE GRAEME, MD
Department of Medical Toxicology
Good Samaritan Regional Medical Center
Phoenix, Arizona

CHARLES GRAFFEO, MD
Department of Emergency Medicine
Eastern Virginia Medical School
Norfolk, Virginia

STEVEN GREEN, MD
Department of Emergency Medicine
Loma Linda University Medical Center
Loma Linda, California

MYLES GREENBERG, MD
Division of Emergency Medicine
Beth Israel Hospital
Boston, Massachusetts

CONSTANCE S. GREENE, MD
Department of Emergency Medicine
Cook County Hospital
Chicago, Illinois

JILL GRIFFIN, MD
Department of Emergency Medicine
Baystate Medical Center
Springfield, Massachusetts

GEORGINA GROLEAU, MD
Division of Emergency Medicine
University of Maryland
Baltimore, Maryland

LAUREN GROSSMAN, MD
Department of Emergency Medicine
Cook County Hospital
Chicago, Illinois

PETER GRUBER, MD
Department of Emergency Medicine
Albert Einstein Residency in Emergency Medicine
Bronx, New York

JOHN GUISTO, MD
Department of Emergency Medicine
University of Arizona College of Medicine
Tucson, Arizona

LEON GUSSOW, MD
Department of Emergency Medicine
Cook County Hospital
Chicago, Illinois

DAVID HALE, MD, PHD
Ramsey Emergency Center
St. Paul, Minnesota

GREGORY S. HALL, MD
Department of Emergency Medicine
University of Arkansas
Little Rock, Arkansas

ROBERT HAMILTON, MD
Department of Emergency Medicine
University of California - San Diego Medical Center
San Diego, California

NICHOLAS HAN, MD
Department of Emergency Medicine
Beth Israel Medical Center
New York, New York

STEPHEN R. HAYDEN, MD
Department of Emergency Medicine
University of California - San Diego Medical Center
San Diego, California

GLENN HEBEL, MD
Middletown, Rhode Island

LAWRENCE HEISKELL, MD
Department of Emergency Medicine
University Medical Center
Las Vegas, Nevada

ROBIN HEMPHILL, MD, MCHE-EM
San Antonio, Texas

SEAN O. HENDERSON, MD
Department of Emergency Medicine
Los Angeles County / University of Southern California Medical Center
Los Angeles, California

GREGORY HENDEY, MD
Department of Emergency Medicine
University Medical Center
Fresno, California

DAVID HERZOG, MD
Acute Psychiatry Service
Massachusetts General Hospital
Boston, Massachusetts

RA'ED HIJAZI, MD
Department of Emergency Medicine
George Washington University
Washington, DC

JOHN HIPSKIND, MD
Emergency Department
Selma District Hospital
Selma, California

ROBERT HITCHCOCK, MD
Department of Emergency Medicine
New York Medical Center
Bronx, New York

CHRIS HO, MD
Department of Emergency Medicine
University of California - San Diego Medical Center
San Diego, California

LAURA HOEY, MD
Department of Emergency Medicine
George Washington University,
Washington, DC

MARTIN HORAK, MD
Department of Emergency Medicine
Brigham and Women's Hospital
Boston, Massachusetts

JEFFREY HORTON, MD
Department of Emergency Medicine
Kern Medical Center
Bakersfield, California

CARL HSU, MD
Department of Emergency Medicine
Beth Israel Medical Center
New York, New York

CATHERINE HURT, MD
Department of Emergency Medicine
University of California - San Diego Medical Center
San Diego, California

LISANDRO IRIZARRY, MD
Department of Emergency Medicine
Brooklyn Hospital Center
North Woodmere, New York

KENNETH V. ISERSON, MD
Department of Emergency Medicine
University of Arizona College of Medicine
Tucson, Arizona

PAUL ISHIMINE, MD
Department of Emergency Medicine
University of Pittsburgh
Pittsburgh, Pennsylvania

HAGOP ISNAR, MD
Department of Emergency Medicine
Hartford Hospital
Hartford, Connecticut

DAVID ISTVAN, MD
Department of Emergency Medicine
University of Pittsburgh
Pittsburgh, Pennsylvania

KENNETH JACKIMCZYK, MD
Department of Emergency Medicine
Maricopa Medical Center
Phoenix, Arizona

LIUDVIKAS JAGMINAS, MD
Department of Emergency Medicine
Rhode Island Hospital
Providence, Rhode Island

THEA JAMES, MD
Department of Emergency Medicine
Boston Medical Center
Boston, Massachusetts

GREGORY JAY, MD
Department of Emergency Medicine
Rhode Island Hospital
Providence, Rhode Island

ANDREW JENIS, MD
Department of Emergency Medicine
Buffalo General Hospital
Buffalo, New York

DAVID JERRARD, MD
Division of Emergency Medicine
University of Maryland
Baltimore, Maryland

DEAN JOHNSON, MD
Division of Emergency Medicine
University of Maryland
Baltimore, Maryland

GARY JOHNSON, MD
Department of Emergency Medicine
State University of New York Health Science Center
Syracuse, New York

NICHOLAS J. JOURILES, MD
Department of Emergency Medicine
Metro Health Medical Center
Cleveland, Ohio

PASCAL JUANG, MD
Department of Emergency Medicine
Brigham and Women's Hospital
Boston, Massachusetts

ROBERT JUNE, MD
Department of Emergency Medicine
Mt. Sinai Hospital
Chicago, Illinois

JOSEPH KAHN, MD
Department of Emergency Medicine
Boston Medical Center
Boston, Massachusetts

SUSAN G. KAMEN, MD
Division of Emergency Medicine
University of Maryland
Baltimore, Maryland

MICHELE KANTER, MD
Division of Toxicology
Cook County Hospital
Chicago, Illinois

LAWRENCE E. KASS, MD
Department of Emergency Medicine
University Hospital at Stony Brook
Stony Brook, New York

A. ANTOINE KAZZI, MD
Department of Emergency Medicine
University of California - Irvine Medical Center
Orange, California

ZIAD KAZZI, BS, MS IV
Faculty of Medicine
American University of Beirut
Beirut, Lebanon

SAMUEL KEIM, MD
Department of Emergency Medicine
University of Arizona College of Medicine
Tucson, Arizona

AILEEN KENNEDY, MD
Department of Emergency Medicine
New York University / Bellevue Hospital Center
New York, New York

ELICIA S. KENNEDY, MD
Department of Emergency Medicine
University of Arkansas
Little Rock, Arkansas

SIG KHARASCH, MD
Department of Pediatrics and Emergency Medicine
Boston Medical Center
Boston, Massachusetts

TAMAKI KIMBRO, MD
Department of Emergency Medicine
University of California - San Diego Medical Center
San Diego, California

JEFFREY KING, MD
Department of Emergency Medicine
Wayne State University
Detroit, Michigan

JOHN KING, DO
Department of Emergency Medicine
New York Medical Center
Bronx, New York

CARLYN KO, MD
Honolulu, Hawaii

PAUL KOLECKI, MD
Department of Surgery
Division of Emergency Medicine
University of Texas Southwestern Medical Center
Dallas, Texas

GEORGE KONDYLIS, MD
Department of Emergency Medicine
State University of New York Health Science Center
Syracuse, New York

E. KOVAL, MD
Department of Emergency Medicine
University of Rochester / Strong Memorial Hospital
Rochester, New York

RICHARD KRAUSE, MD
Department of Emergency Medicine
State University of New York Health Science Center
Buffalo, New York

DICK KUO, MD
Division of Emergency Medicine
University of Maryland
Baltimore, Maryland

MARY BETH KURZ, MD
Department of Emergency Medicine
George Washington University, Washington, DC

NANCY KWON, MD
Department of Emergency Medicine
New York University / Bellevue Hospital Center
New York, New York

JOHN LAFLEUR, MD
Department of Emergency Medicine
New York Medical Center
Bronx, New York

JOSEPH LAMANTIA, MD
Department of Emergency Medicine
North Shore University Hospital
Manhasset, New York

MICHAEL G. LAMAR, MD
San Diego, California

GREG LAMPE, MD
Department of Emergency Medicine
University of California - San Diego Medical Center
San Diego, California

MARK I. LANGDORF, MD, MHPE
Department of Emergency Medicine
University of California - Irvine Medical Center
Orange, California

JAMES L. LARSON, MD
Department of Emergency Medicine
University of North Carolina
Chapel Hill, North Carolina

LAURIE LAWRENCE, MD
Emergency Department
Vanderbilt University Hospital
Nashville, Tennessee

LEE V. LEAK, MD
Department of Emergency Medicine
New York Medical Center
Bronx, New York

JAMES LEAMING, MD
Department of Emergency Medicine
State University of New York Health Science Center
Syracuse, New York

CAROL LEDWITH, MD
Department of Emergency Medicine
Children's Hospital
Denver, Colorado

DAVID LEE, MD
Department of Emergency Medicine
North Shore University Hospital
Manhasset, New York

MOSES LEE, MD
Department of Emergency Medicine
Cook County Hospital
Chicago, Illinois

SHIRLEY LEE, MD
Department of Emergency Medicine
The Toronto Hospital
Toronto, Ontario

THOMAS LEE, MD
Department of Emergency Medicine
University of California - Davis Medical Center
Sacramento, California

ERIC LEGOME, MD
Department of Emergency Medicine
Massachusetts General Hospital
Boston, Massachusetts

THOMAS LEMKE, MD
Department of Emergency Medicine
Rhode Island Hospital
Providence, Rhode Island

RICHARD LENHARDT, MD
Department of Emergency Medicine
Brigham and Women's Hospital
Boston, Massachusetts

YAT LEUNG, MD
Department of Emergency Medicine
Brooklyn Hospital Center
North Woodmere, New York

DAVID LEVINE, MD
Department of Emergency Medicine
Cook County Hospital
Chicago, Illinois

TREVOR LEWIS, MD
Department of Emergency Medicine
Cook County Hospital
Chicago, Illinois

RICHARD LICHENSTEIN, MD
Division of Emergency Medicine
University of Maryland
Baltimore, Maryland

J. BRIAN LIDDY, MD
Department of Emergency Medicine
Baystate Medical Center
Springfield, Massachusetts

HARTWILL LIN, MD
Department of Emergency Medicine
University of Pittsburgh
Pittsburgh, Pennsylvania

CHRISTOPHER LIPINSKI, MD
Department of Emergency Medicine
University of Pittsburgh
Pittsburgh, Pennsylvania

EVAN LIU, MD
Department of Emergency Medicine
Allegheny University Hospital, Hahnemann Division
Philadelphia, Pennsylvania

GREGORY LOCKHART, MD
Department of Emergency Medicine
Rhode Island Hospital
Providence, Rhode Island

FRANK LOVECCHIO, DO
Department of Medical Toxicology
Good Samaritan Regional Medical Center
Phoenix, Arizona

BORIS VLADIMIR LUBAVIN, BS
Irvine, California

THOMAS LUKENS, MD
Department of Emergency Medicine
MetroHealth Medical Center
Cleveland, Ohio

ELIZABETH LYNCH, MD
Department of Emergency Medicine
Loma Linda University Medical Center
Loma Linda, California

GENE MA, MD
Department of Emergency Medicine
University of California - San Diego Medical Center
San Diego, California

CHARLES G. MACIAS, MD
Department of Emergency Medicine
Children's Hospital
Denver, Colorado

JOHN MACKAY, MD
Department of Emergency Medicine
Texas Tech University
El Paso, Texas

LAURA MACNOW, MD
Department of Emergency Medicine
Brigham and Women's Hospital
Boston, Massachusetts

MARK MADENWALD, MD
Department of Emergency Medicine
Naval Medical Center
Portsmouth, Virginia

TIMOTHY J. MADER, MD
Department of Emergency Medicine
Baystate Medical Center
Springfield, Massachusetts

DAVID MAGILNER, MD
Department of Emergency Medicine
Children's Hospital
Denver, Colorado

JOHN MAHONEY, MD
Department of Emergency Medicine
University of Pittsburgh Medical Center
Wexford, Pennsylvania

WILLIAM MALLON, MD
Department of Emergency Medicine
Los Angeles County / University of Southern California Medical Center
Los Angeles, California

MARK MANDELL, MD
Department of Emergency Medicine
Morristown Memorial Hospital
Morristown, New Jersey

JEFFREY MANKO, MD
Department of Emergency Medicine
New York University / Bellevue Hospital Center
New York, New York

DAVID MARBY, MD
Department of Emergency Medicine
Rhode Island Hospital
Providence, Rhode Island

ALLEN MARINO, MD
Department of Emergency Medicine
University of California - San Diego Medical Center
San Diego, California

ANDREW MCAFEE, MD
Department of Emergency Medicine
Brigham and Women's Hospital
Boston, Massachusetts

ROBERT MCCORMACK, MD
Department of Emergency Medicine
State University of New York at Buffalo
Buffalo, New York

ROBERT MCCORMACK, MD
Department of Emergency Medicine
Buffalo General Hospital
Buffalo, New York

JOHN MCCOURT, MD
Department of Emergency Medicine
University Medical Center
Las Vegas, Nevada

MARA MCERLEAN, MD
Department of Emergency Medicine
Albany Medical Center
Albany, New York

MARY PATRICIA MCKAY, MD
Department of Emergency Medicine
George Washington University
Washington, DC

BONNIE MCMANUS, MD
Department of Emergency Medicine
Michael Reese Hospital
Chicago, Illinois

SAUL MELMAN, MD
Department of Emergency Medicine
Cook County Hospital
Chicago, Illinois

MOSS MENDELSON, MD
Chesapeake, Virginia

ED MICHELSON, MD
Division of Emergency Medicine
Northwestern Memorial Hospital
Chicago, Illinois

SHAYLE MILLER, MD
Department of Emergency Medicine
Cook County Hospital
Chicago, Illinois

TREVOR MILLS, MD
Section of Emergency Medicine
Louisiana State University Medical Center
New Orleans, Louisiana

LESLIE MILNE, MD
Department of Emergency Medicine
Massachusetts General Hospital
Boston, Massachusetts

ANDREW MILSTEN, MD
Department of Emergency Medicine
New York Medical Center
Bronx, New York

MICHAEL MINOGUE, MD
Department of Emergency Medicine
Brigham and Women's Hospital
Boston, Massachusetts

ELIZABETH MITCHELL, MD
Department of Emergency Medicine
Boston Medical Center
Boston, Massachusetts

THOMAS MOATS, MD
Department of Emergency Medicine
University of California - San Diego Medical Center
San Diego, California

CHRIS MOORE, MD
Department of Emergency Medicine
Brigham and Women's Hospital
Boston, Massachusetts

PETER MOYER, MD
Department of Emergency Medicine
Boston Medical Center
Boston, Massachusetts

LINDA MUELLER, MD
Department of Emergency Medicine
Resurrection Medical Center
Chicago, Illinois

ASIF MUHAMMAD, MD
Department of Emergency Medicine
Beth Israel Medical Center
New York, New York

DAVID W. MUNTER, MD, MBA
Department of Emergency Medicine
Naval Medical Center
Portsmouth, Virginia

JOHN MUNYAK, MD
Department of Emergency Medicine
New York Medical Center
Bronx, New York

MICHAEL MURPHY, MD
Department of Emergency Medicine
Boston Medical Center
Boston, Massachusetts

ANTHONY MUSIELEWICZ, MD
Department of Emergency Medicine
United States Naval Hospital
Guam

ERIC NADEL, MD
Department of Emergency Medicine
Brigham and Women's Hospital
Boston, Massachusetts

ISAM NASR, MD
Department of Emergency Medicine
Cook County Hospital
Chicago, Illinois

SEAN-XAVIER NEATH, MD
Department of Emergency Medicine
University of California - San Diego Medical Center
San Diego, California

DAVID NELSON, MD
Department of Emergency Medicine
Rhode Island Hospital
Providence, Rhode Island

ROSCOE NELSON, MD
Department of Emergency Medicine
University of California - San Diego Medical Center
San Diego, California

ED NEWTON, MD
Department of Emergency Medicine
Los Angeles County / University of Southern California Medical Center
Los Angles, California

SEAN PATRICK NORDT, PHARMD
San Diego Regional Poison Center
San Diego, California

DANIELLE NOTEBAERT, MD
Lackawanna, New York

STACY NUNBERG, MD
Department of Emergency Medicine
Long Island Jewish Medical Center
New Hyde Park, New York

CHARLES ORSAY, MD
Division of Colorectal Surgery
Cook County Hospital
Chicago, Illinois

ALEXANDER OSTROW, MD
Department of Emergency Medicine
Monmouth Medical Center
Long Branch, New Jersey

FRANK PALOUCEK, PHARMD
Department of Pharmacology
University of Illinois
Chicago, Illinois

PARAS PANDYA, MD
Department of Emergency Medicine
Buffalo General Hospital
Buffalo, New York

BING PAO, MD
Atlanta, Georgia

ROBERT PARTRIDGE, MD
Department of Emergency Medicine
Rhode Island Hospital
Providence, Rhode Island

JOEL PASTERNACK, MD
Department of Emergency Medicine
University of Rochester / Strong Memorial Hospital
Rochester, New York

CHARLES PATTAVINA, MD
Department of Emergency Medicine
Rhode Island Hospital
Providence, Rhode Island

SUCHARITA PAUL, MD
Department of Emergency Medicine
Buffalo General Hospital
Buffalo, New York

TIMOTHY PAVEK, MD
Department of Emergency Medicine
University Medical Center
Las Vegas, Nevada

BRADLEY PECKLER, MD
Department of Emergency Medicine
Beth Israel Medical Center
New York, New York

TAMAS PEREDY, MD
Department of Emergency Medicine
Hartford Hospital
Hartford, Connecticut

NORVIN PEREZ, MD
Department of Emergency Medicine
New York Medical Center
Bronx, New York

ARTHUR PERPALL, MD
Division of Emergency Medicine
University of Maryland
Baltimore, Maryland

ARYEH J. PESSAH, MD
Division of Emergency Medicine
University of Maryland
Baltimore, Maryland

CHARLES POLLACK, MD
Department of Emergency Medicine
Maricopa Medical Center
Phoenix, Arizona

JANET POPONICK, MD
Department of Emergency Medicine
MetroHealth Medical Center
Cleveland, Ohio

ROBERT POWERS, MD
Department of EMS / Trauma
Hartford Hospital
Hartford, Connecticut

THOMAS PURCELL, MD
Department of Emergency Medicine
Kern Medical Center
Bakersfield, California

JOSEPH RABINOVICH, MD
Department of Emergency Medicine
Long Island Jewish Medical Center
New Hyde Park, New York

KATHLEEN RAFTERY, MD
Department of Emergency Medicine
Brigham and Women's Hospital
Boston, Massachusetts

SHYAMBHAI RAO, MD
Department of Emergency Medicine
North Shore University Hospital
Manhasset, New York

NIELS RATHLEV, MD
Department of Emergency Medicine
Boston Medical Center
Boston, Massachusetts

USHA P. REDDY, MD
Department of Emergency Medicine
Albany Medical College
Albany, New York

KRISTINE M. REID, MD
Department of Emergency Medicine
University of Pittsburgh
Pittsburgh, Pennsylvania

KEVIN REILLY, MD
Department of Emergency Medicine
Albany Medical Center
Albany, New York

CHRISTOPHER F. RICHARDS, MD
Department of Emergency Medicine
Brigham and Women's Hospital
Boston, Massachusetts

ANA RICHARDS, MD
Acute Psychiatry Service
Massachusetts General Hospital
Boston, Massachusetts

MARK RICHMOND, MD
Department of Emergency Medicine
Loma Linda University Medical Center
Loma Linda, California

KRISTINE RITTICHIER, MD
Department of Emergency Medicine
Children's Hospital
Denver, Colorado

JAIME RIVAS, MD
Department of Emergency Medicine
Palomar Hospital
Escondido, California

E. JEDD ROE, MD
Department of Emergency Medicine
Denver Health and Hospitals
Denver, Colorado

MICHAEL ROLNICK, MD
Division of Emergency Medicine
University of Maryland
Baltimore, Maryland

CHRISTY ROSA, MD
Department of Emergency Medicine
University of California - San Diego Medical Center
San Diego, California

CARLO ROSEN, MD
Department of Emergency Medicine
Massachusetts General Hospital
Boston, Massachusetts

LARRY ROSENTHAL, MD
Department of Emergency Medicine
University of Massachusetts Medical Center
Boston, Massachusetts

CHRISTOPHER ROSS, MD
Department of Emergency Medicine
Cook County Hospital
Chicago, Illinois

NATE RUDMAN, MD
Department of Emergency Medicine
Madigan Army Medical Center
Steilacoom, Washington

DINO RUMORO, DO
Department of Emergency Medicine
Resurrection Hospital
Chicago, Illinois

WILLIAM SABINA, MD
Department of Emergency Medicine
Rhode Island Hospital
Providence, Rhode Island

GARY SACHS, MD
Acute Psychiatry Service
Massachusetts General Hospital
Boston, Massachusetts

ANNIE T. SADOSTY, MD
Division of Emergency Medicine
University of Maryland
Baltimore, Maryland

MARK SAGARIN, MD
Department of Emergency Medicine
Brigham and Women's Hospital
Boston, Massachusetts

JOHN SAKLES, MD
Department of Emergency Medicine
University of California - Davis Medical Center
Sacramento, California

BONNIE SAMUELSON, MD
Emergency Department
Vanderbilt University Hospital
Nashville, Tennessee

ARTHUR SANDERS, MD
Department of Emergency Medicine
University of Arizona
Tucson, Arizona

DEBORAH SANDERS, MD
Department of Emergency Medicine
University of Mississippi Medical Center
Jackson, Mississippi

MARCELO SANDOVAL, MD
Department of Emergency Medicine
Beth Israel Medical Center
New York, New York

SALLY SANTEN, MD
Emergency Department
Vanderbilt University Hospital
Nashville, Tennessee

ADAM SAPERSTON, MD
Department of Emergency Medicine
Naval Medical Center
Portsmouth, Virginia

DANIEL SAVITT, MD
Department of Emergency Medicine
Rhode Island Hospital
Providence, Rhode Island

ASSAAD SAYAH, MD
Department of Emergency Medicine
Brigham and Women's Hospital
Boston, Massachusetts

SHARI SCHABOWSKI, MD
Department of Emergency Medicine
Cook County Hospital
Chicago, Illinois

JEFFREY J. SCHAIDER, MD
Department of Emergency Medicine
Cook County Hospital
Chicago, Illinois

JEFFREY SCHLAB, MD
Department of Emergency Medicine
Cook County Hospital
Chicago, Illinois

JAMES SCHMITT, MD
Department of Emergency Medicine
University of California - San Diego Medical Center
San Diego, California

HUGH SCHUCKMAN, MD
Department of Emergency Medicine
Akron City Hospital, Summa Health System
Akron, Ohio

THERESA SCHWAB, MD
Department of Emergency Medicine
Cook County Hospital
Chicago, Illinois

LIESE SCHWARZ, MD
Department of Emergency Medicine
Rhode Island Hospital
Providence, Rhode Island

NICK SCHWARTZ, MD
Department of Emergency Medicine
University of Pittsburgh
Pittsburgh, Pennsylvania

JAMES SCOTT, MD
Department of Emergency Medicine
George Washington University
Washington, DC

CHUCK SEAMENS, MD
Emergency Department
Vanderbilt University Hospital
Nashville, Tennessee

MARC SHAPIRO, MD
Department of Emergency Medicine
Rhode Island Hospital
Providence, Rhode Island

NATHAN SHAPIRO, MD
Department of Emergency Medicine
Brigham and Women's Hospital
Boston, Massachusetts

PHILIP SHAYNE, MD
Department of Emergency Medicine
Emory University School of Medicine
Atlanta, Georgia

LORNE SHERMAN, MD
Department of Emergency Medicine
North Shore University Hospital
Manhasset, New York

LEE W. SHOCKLEY, MD
Department of Emergency Medicine
Denver Health and Hospitals
Denver, Colorado

LORI SHORE, MD
Department of Emergency Medicine
University of California - San Diego Medical Center
San Diego, California

ROBERT SIDMAN, MD
Department of Emergency Medicine
Rhode Island Hospital
Providence, Rhode Island

JULIO SILVA, MD
Department of Emergency Medicine
Resurrection Hospital
Chicago, Illinois

C. MICHAEL SIMMONS, MD
Department of Emergency Medicine
Baystate Medical Center
Springfield, Massachusetts

KIM SING, MD
Department of Emergency Medicine
Medical College of Wisconsin
Milwaukee, Wisconsin

CHRISTIAN SLOANE, MD
Department of Emergency Medicine
University of California - San Diego Medical Center
San Diego, California

JAMES R. SMITH, MD
Department of Emergency Medicine
Hartford Hospital
Hartford, Connecticut

PAMELA SMITH, MD
Department of Emergency Medicine
Baystate Medical Center
Springfield, Massachusetts

REBECCA SMITH-COGGINS, MD
Department of Emergency Services
Stanford University Medical Center
Stanford, California

BRIAN SNYDER, MD
Department of Emergency Medicine
University of California - San Diego Medical Center
San Diego, California

LAURA J. SNYDER, MD
Department of Emergency Medicine
Rhode Island Hospital
Providence, Rhode Island

LINDA SPILLANE, MD
Department of Emergency Medicine
University of Rochester / Strong Memorial Hospital
Rochester, New York

BLAKE SPIRKO, MD
Department of Emergency Medicine
Hartford Hospital
Hartford, Connecticut

STUART SPITALNIC, MD
Department of Emergency Medicine
Rhode Island Hospital
Providence, Rhode Island

THOMAS OSBORNE STAIR, MD
Division of Emergency Medicine
University of Maryland
Baltimore, Maryland

MARA STANKOVICH, MD
Department of Emergency Medicine
Rhode Island Hospital
Providence, Rhode Island

DALE STEELE, MD
Department of Emergency Medicine
Rhode Island Hospital
Providence, Rhode Island

THEODORE STERN, MD
Acute Psychiatry Service
Massachusetts General Hospital
Boston, Massachusetts

MARY STEWART, MD
Emergency Medicine
MetroHealth Medical Center
Cleveland, Ohio

HELEN STRAUS, MD
Department of Emergency Medicine
Cook County Hospital
Chicago, Illinois

KAI STURMANN, MD
Department of Emergency Medicine
Beth Israel Medical Center
New York, New York

LOICE SWISHER, MD
Department of Emergency Medicine
Allegany University Hospital East Falls
Philadelphia, Pennsylvania

PAUL A. SZUCS, MD
Department of Emergency Medicine
Morristown Memorial Hospital
Morristown, New Jersey

NOUSHA TALEGHANI, MD, PHD
Department of Emergency Services
Stanford University Medical Center
Stanford, California

ROSS TANNENBAUM, MD
Department of Emergency Medicine
Silver Cross Hospital
Joliet, Illinois

GUY TARLETON, MD
Santa Barbara, California

CHERIE TERRY, MD
Department of Emergency Medicine
Howard University
Washington, DC

IRENE TIEN, MD
Department of Emergency Medicine
Hartford Hospital
Hartford, Connecticut

FRED TILDEN, MD
Department of Emergency Medicine
Hartford Hospital
Hartford, Connecticut

THEODORE TOERNE, MD
Division of Toxicology
Cook County Hospital
Chicago, Illinois

SAM TORBATI, MD
Department of Emergency Medicine
University of California - San Diego Medical Center
San Diego, California

SUSAN TORREY, MD
Department of Emergency Medicine
Baystate Medical Center
Springfield, Massachusetts

OWEN T. TRAYNOR, MD
Department of Emergency Medicine
University of Pittsburgh Medical Center
Wexford, Pennsylvania

ELIZABETH TSO, MD
Division of Emergency Medicine
University of Maryland
Baltimore, Maryland

TONI TUBB, MD
Department of Emergency Medicine
University of Mississippi Medical Center
Jackson, Mississippi

CLYDE TURNER, DO
Department of Emergency Medicine
Darnall Army Community Hospital
Fort Hood, Texas

ANDREW ULRICH, MD
Department of Emergency Medicine
Boston Medical Center
Boston, Massachusetts

GUY UPSHAW, MD
Department of Emergency Medicine
Children's Hospital
Denver, Colorado

THOMAS UTECHT, MD
Department of Emergency Medicine
University Medical Center
Fresno, California

FEDERICO E. VACA, MD
Department of Emergency Medicine
University of California - Irvine Medical Center
Orange, California

VERENA VALLEY, MD
Department of Emergency Medicine
University of Arkansas
Little Rock, Arkansas

KAREN VAN HOESEN, MD
Department of Emergency Medicine
University of California - San Diego Medical Center
San Diego, California

JAMES VANDENBERG, MD
Department of Emergency Medicine
Madigan Army Medical Center
Tacoma, Washington

TIMOTHY VANDUZER, MD
Emergency Medicine
Nellis Air Force Base, Nevada

VINCENT P. VERDILE, MD
Department of Emergency Medicine
Albany Medical Center
Albany, New York

SMEETA VERMA, MD
Deparment of Emergency Medicine
Albert Einstein Residency in Emergency Medicine
Bronx, New York

RAYMOND A. VIDUCICH, MD
University of Pittsburgh School of Medicine
Pittsburgh, Pennsylvania

GARY M. VILKE, MD
Department of Emergency Medicine
University of California - San Diego Medical Center
San Diego, California

ROBERT S. VISSERS, MD
Department of Emergency Medicine
University of North Carolina, University of North Carolina Hospitals
Chapel Hill, North Carolina

JAMES S. WALKER, DO
Section of Emergency Medicine
University of Oklahoma Health Sciences Center
Oklahoma City, Oklahoma

MATTHEW WALSH, MD
Department of Emergency Medicine
Texas Tech University Health Science Center
El Paso, Texas

PAULA WARD, MD
Division of Emergency Medicine
University of Texas Southwestern Medical School
Dallas, Texas

JOSEPH WATHERN, MD
Department of Emergency Medicine
Children's Hospital
Denver, Colorado

TIMOTHY WATT, MD
Department of Emergency Medicine
University of California - San Diego Medical Center
San Diego, California

JAY WEAVER, EMT-P
Boston Emergency Medical Services
Boston, Massachusetts

BRUCE WEBSTER, MD
Department of Emergency Medicine
Brigham and Women's Hospital
Boston, Massachusetts

KEN WILLIAMS, MD
Department of Emergency Medicine
Children's Hospital
Denver, Colorado

RICHARD WINTERS, MD
Department of Emergency Medicine
University Medical Center
Fresno, California

RUTH WOLD, MD
Department of Emergency Medicine
University of California - San Diego Medical Center
San Diego, California

LESLIE WOLF, MD, ABMT
Department of Emergency Medicine
Wright State University
Kettering, Ohio

JEANETTE WOLFE, MD
Department of Emergency Medicine
Baystate Medical Center
Springfield, Massachusetts

ROBERT WOOLARD, MD
Department of Emergency Medicine
Rhode Island Hospital
Providence, Rhode Island

KEITH WRENN, MD
Emergency Department
Vanderbilt University Hospital
Nashville, Tennessee

ELIZABETH WULFERT, MD
Department of Emergency Medicine
University of California - San Diego Medical Center
San Diego, California

JOEL YAPHE, MD
Department of Emergency Medicine
The Toronto Hospital
Toronto, Ontario

MICHAEL YARON, MD
Division of Emergency Medicine
University of Colorado
Health Sciences Center
Denver, Colorado

ABBAS ZAGNOON, MD
Department of Medicine
Wayne State University
Troy, Michigan

RICHARD ZANE, MD
Department of Emergency Medicine
Johns Hopkins Hospital
Baltimore, Maryland

AVIVA ZIGMAN, MD
La Jolla, California

Contents

ALPHABETICAL TABLE OF CONTENTS

TOPICAL TABLE OF CONTENTS

PRESENTING SIGNS/SYMPTOMS

ADMINISTRATIVE

CARDIAC EMERGENCIES

DERMATOLOGIC / SOFT TISSUE EMERGENCIES

ENDOCRINE EMERGENCIES34

ENVIRONMENTAL EMERGENCIES

GASTROINTESTINAL EMERGENCIES

GENITOURINARY EMERGENCIES

GYNECOLOGIC EMERGENCIES

HEAD AND NECK EMERGENCIES

HEMATOLOGIC EMERGENCIES

IMMUNE SYSTEM EMERGENCIES

INFECTIOUS DISEASE EMERGENCIES

METABOLIC EMERGENCIES

NERVOUS SYSTEM EMERGENCIES

NONTRAUMATIC MUSCULOSKELETAL EMERGENCIES

OBSTETRICAL EMERGENCIES

ONCOLOGIC EMERGENCIES

OPHTHALMOLOGIC EMERGENCIES

RENAL EMERGENCIES

TOXICOLOGIC EMERGENCIES

TRAUMATIC INJURIES

VASCULAR EMERGENCIES

The 5 Minute Emergency Medicine Consult

Abdominal Aortic Aneurysm

Clinical Presentation

SIGNS AND SYMPTOMS

- Unruptured
  - —Most often asymptomatic
  - —Abdominal pain
    - -Dull
    - -Constant, throbbing, or colicky
- Ruptured
  - —*Systemic*
    - -Syncope
    - -Hypotension
    - -Tachycardia
    - -Evidence of systemic embolization
  - —*Abdominal*
    - -Back pain
    - -Flank pain radiating to the groin in 10% of cases
    - -Abdominal pain
    - -Pulsatile abdominal mass
    - -Present in only 50% of patients
    - -Abdominal tenderness
    - -Abdominal bruit
    - -Gastrointestinal hemorrhage
  - —*Extremities*
    - -Lower extremity pain
    - -Diminished or asymmetric pulses in the lower extremities

MECHANISM/DESCRIPTION

- Focal dilation of the aortic wall with an increase in diameter by at least 50% (>3 cm)
- Gradual expansion and rupture
  - —Intraperitoneally
  - —Retroperitoneally
- Present in 2% of the elderly population
- Peak incidence
  - —Men 5.9% at the age of 80
  - —Women 4.5% at the age of 90
- 5-year risk of rupture
  - —Aneurysms <4 cm: 2%
  - —Aneurysms 4.0–5.0 cm: 3–12%
  - —Aneurysms >5 cm: 25–41%
- Intraperitoneal rupture is usually immediately fatal
- 50% of patients who reach the hospital alive survive
- Five-year survival after repair is 67%

ETIOLOGY

- Risk factors
  - —Male
  - —Age >65
  - —Cigarette smoking
  - —Atherosclerosis
  - —Hypertension
  - —Chronic obstructive pulmonary disease
- Uncommon causes
  - —Blunt abdominal trauma
  - —Infections of the aorta
    - -Mycotic aneurysm secondary to endocarditis

Pre-Hospital

- Establish 2 large-bore intravenous lines
- Rapid transport to the nearest facility with surgical backup
- Alert ED staff as soon as possible to prepare the following
  - —Operating room
  - —Universal donor blood
  - —Surgical consultation

Diagnosis

ESSENTIAL WORKUP

- Unstable patients
  - —Explorative surgery without further ancillary studies
  - —Bedside abdominal ultrasound
- Stable symptomatic patients
  - —Abdominal CT with intravenous contrast only

LABORATORY

- CBC
- Type and crossmatch blood
- Creatinine
- Urinalysis
- Coagulation studies

IMAGING/SPECIAL TESTS

- Abdominal ultrasonography
  - —Highly accurate for detecting AAA prior to rupture
  - —Sensitivity has been reported as low as 10% following rupture
  - —Indicated in the unstable patient
- Abdominal CT scan
  - —Intravenous contrast only
  - —Will demonstrate both aneurysm and site of rupture (intraperitoneal vs. retroperitoneal)
  - —Allows accurate measure of aortic diameter
  - —Indicated only in stable patients
- Aortography
  - —The presence of mural thrombi can lead to underestimation of the size of the aorta

DIFFERENTIAL DIAGNOSIS

- Other abdominal arterial aneurysms
- Renal colic
- Biliary colic
- Lumbosacral disc disease
- Pancreatitis
- Perforated viscus
- Mesenteric infarction
- Diverticulitis
- Gastrointestinal hemorrhage
- Aortic thromboembolism
- Myocardial infarction
- Addisonian crisis

Treatment

INITIAL STABILIZATION

- 2 large-bore intravenous lines
- Crystalloid infusion
- Cardiac monitor
- Early blood transfusion

ED TREATMENT

- Patients suspected of symptomatic AAA require
  - —Avoid overaggressive fluid resuscitation to limit blood loss
  - —Emergent surgical consult and operative intervention

MEDICATIONS

N/A

Disposition

ADMISSION CRITERIA

- All patients with symptomatic AAA require emergent surgical intervention

DISCHARGE CRITERIA

- Asymptomatic patients
- Close surgical follow-up
- Instructions to return immediately
  - —With any pain in the back, abdomen, or lower extremities
  - —With dizziness or syncope

Miscellaneous

ICD9: 441.3

CORE CONTENT CODE: 2.5.1.3

SUGGESTED READINGS

Ernst CB. Abdominal aortic aneurysm. N Engl J Med 1993;328:1167–1172.

Mabey BE. Abdominal aortic aneurysm. In: Rosen P, et al., eds. Emergency medicine: Concepts and clinical practice. 3rd ed. St. Louis: CV Mosby, 1992:1373–1383.

Walker JS, Dire DJ. Vascular abdominal emergencies. Emerg Med Clin North Am 1996;14:571–592.

Author: Carlo Rosen

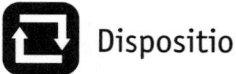

Abdominal Pain

Clinical Presentation

SIGNS AND SYMPTOMS

General

- Anorexia
- Malaise
- Tachycardia
- Hypotension
- Fever
- Nausea
- Vomiting
  - —Etiology requiring surgical intervention is less likely when vomiting precedes the onset of pain

Abdominal

- Diarrhea
- Constipation
- Distended abdomen
- Abnormal bowel sounds
  - —High pitched rushes with bowel obstruction
  - —Absence of sound with ileus or peritonitis
  - —Often unreliable
- Pulsatile abdominal mass
- Rovsing's sign
  - —Palpation of LLQ causes pain in RLQ
  - —Suggestive of appendicitis
- McBurney's point tenderness associated with appendicitis
  - —Palpation in RLQ two-thirds distance between umbilicus and right anterior superior iliac crest causes pain
- Murphy's sign
  - —Pause in inspiration while examiner is palpating under liver
  - —Suggestive of cholecystitis
- Psoas sign
  - —Pain on extension of the thigh
  - —Suggests inflammation around psoas muscle
- Obturator sign
  - —Pain on rotation of the flexed thigh, especially internal rotation
  - —Inflammation around internal obturator muscle
- Tender or discolored hernia site
- Rectal and pelvic examination
  - —Tenderness with pelvic peritoneal irritation
  - —Cervical motion tenderness
  - —Adnexal masses
  - —Rectal mass or tenderness

Genitourinary

- Flank pain
- Dysuria
- Hematuria
- Vaginal bleeding
- Tender adnexal mass on pelvis
- Testicular pain
  - —May be referred from renal or appendiceal pathology
- Testicular swelling
- High-riding testes
- Transverse lie of testis

Extremities

- Shoulder pain
  - —Referred pain from diaphragmatic involvement
- Pulse deficit or unequal femoral pulses

Skin

- Jaundice
- Herpes zoster
- Cellulitis

MECHANISM/DESCRIPTION

- Parietal pain
  - —Irritating material applied to the peritoneum
  - —Inflammation of the parietal peritoneum
  - —Pain transmitted by somatic nerves
  - —Exacerbated by changes in tension of the peritoneum
  - —Pain characteristics
    - -Sharp
    - -Well localized
    - -Abdominal tenderness
    - -Involuntary guarding
    - -Rebound tenderness
    - -Guarding
    - -Exacerbated by movement and coughing
- Visceral
  - —Distention of a viscous or organ capsule or spasm of intestinal muscularis fibers
    - -Pain is generally poorly localized
    - -Pain with intestinal distention is colicky
    - -Pain with a distended gall bladder or kidney is steady
  - —Inflammation
    - -Initially the pain is poorly localized
    - -Focal tenderness develops as the inflammation extends to the peritoneum or localizers
  - —Ischemia from vascular disturbances
    - -Pain is severe and diffuse with catastrophic vascular emergencies
    - -The pain is disproportional to the abdominal examination
- Referred
  - —Felt at distant location from diseased organ
  - —Due to an overlapping supply by the affected neurosegment to the perceived location of pain
- Abdominal wall pain
  - —Constant
  - —Aching
  - —Muscle spasm
  - —Involvement of other muscle groups

ETIOLOGY

- Peritoneal irritants
  - —Gastric juice
  - —Fecal material
  - —Pus
  - —Blood
  - —Bile
  - —Pancreatic enzymes
- Visceral obstruction
  - —Small intestines
  - —Large intestines
  - —Gall bladder
  - —Ureters and kidneys
  - —Visceral ischemia
  - —Intestinal
  - —Renal
  - —Splenic
- Visceral inflammation
  - —Appendicitis
  - —Inflammatory bowel disorders
    - -Gastroenteritis
    - -Lymphadenitis
    - -Crohn's disease
    - -Ulcerative colitis
  - —Cholecystitis
  - —Hepatitis
  - —Peptic ulcer disease
  - —Pancreatitis
  - —Pelvic inflammatory disease
  - —Pyelonephritis
- Abdominal wall pain
- Referred pain
  - —The possibility of intrathoracic disease must be considered in every patient with abdominal pain

Pre-Hospital

- Intravenous access and resuscitation if signs of hemodynamic instability
- In patients with epigastric pain who are at risk for coronary artery disease
  —Supplemental oxygen
  —Monitor

Diagnosis

ESSENTIAL WORKUP

- Historical characteristics define the type of pain and suggest underlying causes
  —Nature of onset of pain
  —Time of onset and duration of pain
  —Location of pain initially and at presentation
  —Extra-abdominal radiations
  —Quality of pain (sharp, dull, crampy)
  —Palliative or provocative factors
  —Relation of associated finding to onset of pain
  —Changes in bowel habits
  —History of trauma
  —Gynecological history
  —Visceral obstruction

LABORATORY

- CBC
  —WBC is unreliable in distinguishing surgical and nonsurgical disease
- Urinalysis
  —Pyuria
  —Hematuria
  —Glucosuria
  —Ketones
- Serum lipase
  —More accurate than a serum amylase in diagnosing pancreatic disorders
- Serum HCG
- Serum electrolytes and glucose
- Gonorrhea and chlamydia cultures should be obtained if a pelvic examination is performed

IMAGING/SPECIAL TESTS

EKG

- Indicated in patients with epigastric pain over the age of 40 or with risk factors for coronary artery disease

KUB and upright

- Indicated primarily if bowel obstruction is suspected
- Of little help in the evaluation of renal colic or gall bladder disease
- Air fluid levels and intestinal distention
  —Bowel obstruction
  —Ileus
  —Volvulus
  —Intussusception
- Intra-abdominal mass
- Aortic aneurysm

Upright chest radiograph

- Pneumoperitoneum
  —Perforated stomach, duodenum, or colon
- Extra-abdominal causes
  —Pneumonia
  —Pleural effusion

Ultrasound

- Biliary abnormalities
  —Cholelithiasis
  —Evidence of cholecystitis
  —Sonographic Murphy's sign
  —Wall thickening
  —Pericholecystic fluid
  —Ductal dilation
- Hydronephrosis
- Intraperitoneal fluid
  —Aneurysmal rupture
  —Ruptured ectopic pregnancy
  —Ascites
  —Ruptured ovarian cyst
- Aortic aneurysm
- Pelvic ultrasound
  —Intrauterine pregnancy
  —Adnexal mass
    -Ectopic pregnancy
    -Ovarian cyst
    -Ovarian torsion
    -Ovarian tumor
    -Tuboovarian abscess

Abdominal CT

- Spiral CT without contrast
  —Determines location and size of stone in patients with renal colic
- CT with intravenous contrast only
  —Vascular rupture suspected in a stable patient
- CT with intravenous and oral contrast
  —Indicated when there is a suspicion of a surgical etiology involving bowel or intraperitoneal hemorrhage
    -Ruptured spleen
    -Enlarged pancreas
    -Thickened colonic wall and streaking of the mesocolon is characteristic of diverticulitis
- CT with rectal contrast only
  —High accuracy reported in detecting appendicitis

IVP

- Indicated in patients with suspected ureteral calculi
- More time-consuming the spiral CT

Barium Enema

- Intussusception
- Volvulus

DIFFERENTIAL DIAGNOSIS

- Abdominal aortic aneurysm
- Abdominal epilepsy
- Abdominal migraine
- Abdominal wall hematoma or infection
- Adrenal crisis
- Appendicitis
- Black widow spider bite
- Bowel obstruction
- Cholecystitis
- Constipation
- Depression
- Diabetic ketoacidosis
- Diverticulitis

- Dysmenorrhea
- Ectopic pregnancy
- Esophagitis
- Fecal impaction
- Fitz-Hugh and Curtis syndrome
- Gastroenteritis
- Hirschsprung's disease
- Hepatitis
- Herpes zoster
- Incarcerated hernia
- Inflammatory bowel disease
- Intussusception
- Irritable bowel syndrome
- Ischemic bowel
- Lactose intolerance
- Lead poisoning
- Meckel's diverticulitis
- Myocardial infarction
- Neoplasm
- Ovarian cyst
- Ovarian torsion
- Pancreatitis
- Pelvic inflammatory disease
- Peptic ulcer disease
- Perforated viscous
- Pneumonia
- Renal/ureteral calculi
- Sickle cell crisis
- Splenic infarction
- Splenic rupture
- Spontaneous abortion
- Testicular torsion
- Urinary tract infection
- Volvulus

PEDIATRIC CONSIDERATIONS

- Under 2 years
  —Hirschsprung's disease
  —Incarcerated hernia
  —Intussusception
  —Neoplasm
  —Sickle cell crisis
  —Volvulus
- 2–5 years
  —Appendicitis
  —Incarcerated hernia
  —Meckel's diverticulitis
  —Neoplasm
  —Sickle cell crisis
- Over 5 years
  —Appendicitis
  —Ectopic pregnancy
  —Inflammatory bowel disease
  —PID

Treatment

INITIAL STABILIZATION

- Emergent laparotomy
  —Patients who are hemodynamically unstable with suspected vascular rupture
- IV fluids
- Nasogastric suction

ED TREATMENT

- Antiemetics are important for comfort
- Narcotics or analgesics should not be withheld as they do not impair decision-making
- Antibiotics are needed in potential perforation and in peritonitis
- Surgical consultation
  —Parietal pain
  —Suspicion of appendicitis
  —Hemodynamic instability
  —Bowel obstruction
  —Suspicion of bowel ischemic
  —Cholecystitis

MEDICATIONS

- Cefoxitin: 60 mg/kg IV
- Fentanyl: 1–2 μg/kg IV q hr
- Gentamycin: 2.5 mg/kg IV
- Prochlorperazine: 0.13 mg/kg IV/PO/IM q 6 PRN nausea; 25 mg PR q 6 in adults
- Promethazine: 1 mg/kg IM/PO/PR

Disposition

ADMISSION CRITERIA

- Surgical intervention
- Peritoneal signs
- Patient unable to keep down fluids
- Lack of pain control
- Medical cause necessitating in-house treatment (MI, DKA)
- IV antibiotics needed

DISCHARGE CRITERIA

- No surgical or severe medical etiology found in patient who is able to keep fluid down, has good pain control, and is able to follow detailed discharge instructions

Miscellaneous

ICD9: 789.0

CORE CONTENT CODE: N/A

SUGGESTED READINGS

Bugliosi TF, Meloy TD, Vukov LF. Acute abdominal pain in the elderly. Ann Emerg Med 1990;19:1383–1386.

Author: Michelle A. Finkel

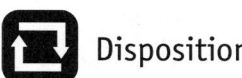

Abdominal Trauma, Blunt

Clinical Presentation

SIGNS AND SYMPTOMS

- Spectrum of presentation from abdominal pain with or without signs of peritoneal irritation to hypovolemic shock without physical exam findings
- Nausea or vomiting
- Labored respirations due to diaphragm irritation or upper abdominal injury
- Left shoulder pain with inspiration (Kehr's sign) from diaphragmatic irritation due to bleeding
- Delayed presentation possible with small bowel injury

MECHANISM/DESCRIPTION

- Injury results from a sudden increase of pressure to abdomen
- Solid organ injury usually manifests itself as hemorrhage
- Hollow viscous injuries result in bleeding and peritonitis from contamination with bowel contents

ETIOLOGY

- 60% of cases result from motor vehicle accidents
- Solid organs are injured more frequently that hollow viscous organs
- The spleen is the most frequently injured organ (25%), followed by the liver (15%), intestines (15%), retroperitoneal structures (13%), and kidney (12%)
- Less frequently injured are the mesentery, pancreas, diaphragm, urinary bladder, urethra, and vascular structures

PEDIATRIC CONSIDERATIONS

- Children tend to tolerate trauma better due to the more elastic nature of their tissues
- Due to the decreased size of the intrathoracic abdomen, the spleen and liver are more exposed to injury as they lie partially outside the bony rib cage

Pre-Hospital

CONTROVERSIES

- Aggressive fluid resuscitation is still considered standard of care
- Normal vital signs do not preclude significant intra-abdominal pathology

Diagnosis

ESSENTIAL WORKUP

- Evaluate and stabilize airway, breathing, and circulation
- Primary objective is to determine the need for operative intervention
- Examine the abdomen to determine presence of intra-abdominal bleeding or peritoneal irritation
- Injury in the retroperitoneal space or intrathoracic abdomen is difficult to assess by palpation
- Remember that the limits of the abdomen include the diaphragm superiorly and the intragluteal fold inferiorly and encompasses the entire circumference
- Abrasions or ecchymoses may be indicators of intra-abdominal injury; roll the patient to assess the back
- Bowel sounds may be absent secondary to peritoneal irritation, but this is usually a late finding
- Foley catheter (if no blood at the meatus, no perineal hematoma, and normal prostate exam) to obtain urine for urinalysis and record urinary output
- Plain film of the pelvis. Fracture of the pelvis and gross hematuria may indicate genitourinary injury and necessitate further evaluation of these structures with retrograde urethrogram, cystogram, and IVP. Microscopic hematuria in the presence of shock is an indication for genitourinary evaluation. CT is useful in renal injury diagnosis and should be performed on patients with abnormal IVP's
- Accomplish objective evaluation of the abdomen with either diagnostic peritoneal lavage (useful for picking up injuries in the intrathoracic abdomen, pelvic abdomen, and the true abdomen), ultrasonography for detection of fluid (although this is operator-dependent), or CT (useful for evaluating the retroperitoneal space and solid organs)
- Diagnostic peritoneal lavage (DPL) is considered positive in the context of blunt abdominal trauma with a RBC count of $> 100{,}000/mm^3$, WBC count of $500/mm^3$, or the presence of bile, feces, or food particles. These patients should proceed to laparotomy. A negative DPL necessitates an observation period with frequent examinations

LABORATORY

- Hgb/Hematocrit, which may be initially normal due to isovolemic blood loss
- Type and cross is essential
- Urinalysis for blood, creatinine
- ABG. The base deficit may aid in the diagnosis of hypovolemic shock and help guide the resuscitation

IMAGING

- Pelvic plain film
- Abdominal ultrasonography may be helpful to locate free fluid in the abdomen indicating hemorrhage
- CT with contrast useful in evaluating the retroperitoneum and solid organ injuries

DIFFERENTIAL DIAGNOSIS

- Lower thoracic injury may cause abdominal pain

Treatment

INITIAL STABILIZATION

- ABCs
- Ensure adequate airway; intubate if needed; O_2 100% by non re-breather face mask
- 2 large-bore IVs with crystalloid infusion
- Begin infusion of PRBCs if no response to 2 liters of crystalloid
- If in profound shock, consider transfusion of O-negative or type-specific blood on the way to the operating room

ED TREATMENT

- Continue stabilization begun in field
- NGT to evacuate stomach, decrease distension, and decrease risk of aspiration. This may relieve respiratory distress if caused by a herniated stomach through the diaphragm
- Placement of Foley catheter

MEDICATIONS

- Tetanus Toxoid booster: 0.5 cc IM for patients with open wounds
- Tetanus immune globulin: 250 Units IM for patients who have not had complete series
- IV Antibiotics: Unasyn 1 g IVPB or 2nd generation Cephalosporin

PEDIATRIC CONSIDERATIONS

- Crystalloid infusion for pediatrics is 20 cc/kg if patient is in shock
- Packed RBC dose is 1 cc/kg

Disposition

ADMISSION CRITERIA

Postoperative cases

Equivocal findings on DPL or CT

DISCHARGE CRITERIA

No patient in whom you suspect intra-abdominal injury should be discharged home without an appropriate period of observation despite negative exam or imaging studies

Miscellaneous

ICD9: 868.00

CORE CONTENT CODE: 18.4.11

SUGGESTED READING

Davis JJ, et al. Diagnosis and management of blunt abdominal trauma. Ann Surg 1976;183:672

Author: Stewart Coffman

Abdominal Trauma, Imaging

Clinical Presentation

SIGNS AND SYMPTOMS

- Abdominal trauma may present as an unstable patient with multiple associated injuries or as an isolated injury in a stable patient with no physical findings. In unstable patients, the management of the ABCs, treatment of hypovolemic shock, and control of major external hemorrhage initially take precedence
- Assessment of the abdomen will focus on the need for early surgical management. The diagnosis of specific organ injuries should come later

Pre-Hospital

CAUTIONS

- All patients with a significant mechanism of injury or suspicion of major trauma should be triaged to a facility equipped to manage trauma

PEDIATRIC CONSIDERATIONS

- Pediatric patients should be triaged to a pediatric trauma center or to an adult trauma center equipped to manage children

Diagnosis

ESSENTIAL WORKUP

- History including mechanism of injury, restraint, airbag or helmet use, pre-hospital vital signs, initial mental status and change in mental status, and any pre-hospital treatments performed and their effect on patient status
- AMPLE history (Allergies, especially to radiographic contrast agents, Medications, Past medical history, Last meal, Events leading up to the injury)
- Comprehensive physical exam including complete exposure and both a perineal and digital rectal exam
- Abdominal stab wounds should be locally explored after local anesthesia. Penetration of the abdominal wall fascia is considered a positive exploration and requires further evaluation
- Gunshot wounds to the abdomen require laparotomy
- Caution
  - —Physical exam is accurate in determining serious abdominal injury in only 45–50% of cases

IMAGING / SPECIAL TESTS

General APPROACH to imaging in blunt abdominal trauma

- The ideal abdominal imaging study is rapid, cheap, sensitive for operative injury, identifies nonoperative injuries requiring close observation and follow-up, requires minimal training to perform and interpret, and currently does not exist
- CT scan is ideal for many patients, especially children, but requires intravenous contrast material
  - —Unstable patients should not be transported to CT scan
  - —Ultrasound meets many of these criteria and is rapidly replacing CT and diagnostic peritoneal lavage (DPL) as the initial screening tool of choice
  - —Most patients require serial physical examinations and a period of observation after negative imaging studies

Diagnostic Peritoneal Lavage

- Advantages
  - —Rapid
  - —Easy to perform
  - —97.8 % accurate in diagnosing injury
- Disadvantages
  - —Invasive
  - —Does not identify specific organ injury
  - —1–2% complication rate
  - —May miss retroperitoneal injuries and intraperitoneal bladder rupture
- Indications
  - —Hemodynamically unstable patients

—Patients requiring emergent surgery for other conditions (e.g., craniotomy for epidural hematoma)
—Stab wounds that penetrate the abdominal fascia
- Contraindications
—Absolute: preexisting indication for exploratory laparotomy
—Relative: previous abdominal surgery, severe abdominal distention, pregnancy, pediatric patients
—Nasogastric tube and Foley catheter placement mandatory prior to procedure
—Positive test
-Aspiration of >10 cc of blood, bile, bowel contents, or urine
-DPL fluid in the urine or chest tube
-Blunt trauma >100,000 RBC/mm^3
-Penetrating trauma >1000 RBC/mm^3
—Considerations
-Favored in stab wound patients when local wound exploration is positive
-Favored in unstable blunt trauma patients as may be performed simultaneously with other emergent surgical interventions (e.g., craniotomy for epidural hematoma)
-Must always be accompanied by serial abdominal exams after procedure
-In the presence of pelvic fractures, use supraumbilical location
-In pregnancy, consider supraumbilical or open technique
-False-positive results may be obtained if performed more than 8 hours following injury

CT Scan
- Advantages
—Sensitive (85–98%)
—Provides specific-organ injury information
—Fosters nonoperative approach to certain liver and spleen injuries
—Detects retroperitoneal injuries
- Disadvantages
—Requires IV contrast (acute contrast reactions and renal failure)
—Isolated diaphragmatic, pancreatic, bowel injuries may be missed, especially if performed immediately after injury
- Indications
—Hemodynamically stable patients
- Contraindications
—Absolute: preexisting indication for exploratory laparotomy, hemodynamic instability, previous contrast reaction
—Relative: multiple allergies
- Considerations
—Modality of choice in children
—Many multiple-injury patients require CT imaging of the head, spine, chest, or pelvis. Modern equipment provides for rapid scanning of multiple anatomic regions in one session
—Monitoring must be continued in the CT suite. Patients should be accompanied by appropriate medical personnel
—Water may be substituted for oral contrast, but optimal detection of intestinal injury requires oral contrast and a 2–4 hour delay for intestinal transport

Ultrasound
- Advantages
—Rapid
—Noninvasive
—Sensitive for intraperitoneal fluid
—Can be performed at the bedside
—Does not require contrast agents or ionizing radiation
- Disadvantages
—Does not reliably identify specific organ injury
—Not well-suited for penetrating injuries as may miss significant bowel injuries not accompanied by hemoperitoneum
- Indications
—Blunt trauma, stable or unstable patients
- Contraindications
—Absolute: preexisting indication for exploratory laparotomy
—Relative: obesity, subcutaneous emphysema
- Positive test
—Demonstration of free fluid or obvious solid organ injury
- Adequate exam includes visualization of Morrison pouch, pericardium, both paracolic gutters, and the pelvis (Pouch of Douglas), and exam of the liver and spleen for parenchymal injuries
- Considerations
—Positive test should be followed by CT in a stable patient or laparotomy in an unstable patient
—Institutional factors will determine who performs the study. Trained sonographers with radiology backup are preferred

PEDIATRIC CONSIDERATIONS
- Because so many pediatric patients can be managed nonoperatively, CT scan, which provides the best anatomic information, is the study of choice in all but the most unstable pediatric patient

DIFFERENTIAL DIAGNOSIS
- See abdominal trauma chapter

Treatment

INITIAL STABILIZATION
- See abdominal trauma chapter

ED MANAGEMENT
- See abdominal trauma chapter

MEDICATIONS
- See abdominal trauma chapter

Disposition

ADMISSION CRITERIA
- See abdominal trauma chapter

DISCHARGE CRITERIA
- See abdominal trauma chapter

Miscellaneous

ICD9: 793.6

CORE CONTENT CODE: 23.3.6, 23.3.7.3, 18.2.3

SUGGESTED READINGS

Boulanger BR, McLellan BA. Blunt abdominal trauma. Emerg Med Clin North Am 1996;14(1):151–171

Chiquito PE. Blunt abdominal injuries. Diagnostic peritoneal lavage, ultrasonography and computed tomography scanning. Injury 1996;27(2):117–124

Colucciello SA. Blunt abdominal trauma. Emerg Med Clin North Am 1993;11(1):107–122

McKenney M, Lentz K, Nunez D, et al. Can ultrasound replace diagnostic peritoneal lavage in the assessment of blunt trauma? J Trauma 1994;37(3):439–441

Author: Chris Richards

Abdominal Trauma, Penetrating

Clinical Presentation

SIGNS AND SYMPTOMS

- Penetrating wound from knife, gun, or other foreign object
- Spectrum of presentation from localized pain to peritoneal signs
- Remember the borders of the abdomen: superior from the nipples (anteriorly) or inferior tip of scapula (posteriorly) to the inferior gluteal folds

MECHANISM/DESCRIPTION

- Solid organ injury usually results in hemorrhage
- Hollow viscous injury can lead to bowel content spillage and peritonitis

ETIOLOGY

- 80% of gunshot wounds and 20–30% of stab wounds to the abdomen result in significant intra-abdominal injury
- The most commonly injured structures are the liver (37%), small bowel (26%), stomach (19%), colon (17%), major vessel (13%), retroperitoneum (10%), mesentery/omentum (10%), and less often the spleen (7%), diaphragm (5%), kidney (5%), pancreas (4%), duodenum (2%), and biliary tract (1%)
- Injury to both thoracic structures and abdominal structures occurs 25% of the time

Pre-Hospital

CONTROVERSIES

- MAST trousers should not be used in the treatment of penetrating abdominal wounds
- The current standard of care in the treatment of hypovolemic shock is volume resuscitation with crystalloid solutions

CAUTIONS

- Apply sterile dressings to open wounds and eviscerated bowel
- Secure in place impaled foreign objects; do not remove them

Diagnosis

ESSENTIAL WORKUP

- Diagnosis of intra-abdominal injury from gunshot wounds to the abdomen are made by laparotomy in the OR
- Locally explore stab wounds to the abdomen
- If the wound penetrates the anterior fascial layer, the patient should receive a diagnostic peritoneal lavage
- If >1000 RBC/mm^3 are found in the lavage fluid, the patient should undergo laparotomy
- If <1000 RBC/mm^3 are present, the patient should be observed for 8–24 hours for the development of peritoneal signs

LABORATORY

- Hematocrit should be drawn initially and may be obtained serially to assess for ongoing hemorrhage
- Urinalysis for blood should be performed to assess for possible genitourinary injuries
- ABGs: The base deficit may be helpful in assessing degree of hypovolemia and guide volume resuscitation
- Type and cross should be performed in all patients with significant intra-abdominal injuries

IMAGING

- Plain films should be taken after placement of markers for localization of foreign bodies, missiles and associated fractures, and free air
- Bedside abdominal US may help in identifying intraperitoneal fluid or blood
- CT scan or IVP may be used if there is a suspicion of retroperitoneal injury

DIFFERENTIAL DIAGNOSIS

- Consider the possibility of accompanying intrathoracic injury with upper abdominal wounds
- Likewise, consider the possibility of intra-abdominal injury after penetrating wounds to the lower thoracic area

Treatment

INITIAL STABILIZATION

- ABCs
- Two large-bore IVs with crystalloid infusion
- 100% Oxygen by non-re-breather face mask
- Packed RBC infusion if no response to 2 L of crystalloid
  - —May use O-negative blood initially
  - —Type specific and crossmatched blood as it becomes available

ED TREATMENT

- A nasogastric tube (NGT) should be placed to decrease the chance of aspiration. This should be placed prior to diagnostic peritoneal lavage to decompress the stomach and decrease chances of iatrogenic injury
  - —A NGT may also relieve respiratory distress if there is a diaphragmatic injury with herniated abdominal contents in the thorax
- A Foley catheter should be placed to facilitate rapid assessment for genitourinary injury, as well as to assist the monitoring of urinary output
- Tetanus toxoid if appropriate; tetanus immune globulin if primary tetanus vaccination series not administered

MEDICATIONS

- Tetanus Toxoid 0.5 cc IM
- Tetanus Immunoglobulin 250 Units IM for patients who have not had complete series

PEDIATRIC CONSIDERATIONS

- Children in hypovolemic shock should receive 20 cc/kg boluses of crystalloid
- Children in severe hypovolemic shock should receive 1 cc/kg of packed RBCs
- Age less than 8 years is a relative contraindication for DPL

Disposition

ADMISSION CRITERIA

- Patients requiring abdominal surgery
- Observe all patients for at least 8 hours who had negative DPL after local exploration
  - —These patients should receive frequent abdominal exams
  - —Repeat hematocrits should be performed on these patients at regular intervals

DISCHARGE CRITERIA

- Patients with stab wounds who had no evidence of fascial involvement may be discharged after observation in the emergency department

Miscellaneous

ICD9: 868.00

CORE CONTENT CODE: 18.4.11.1

SUGGESTED READINGS

Thompson JS, Moore EE, Van Duzer-Moore S, et al. The evolution of abdominal stab wound management. J Trauma 1980;20:478

Thal ER. Evaluation of peritoneal lavage and local exploration in lower chest and abdominal stab wounds. J Trauma 1979;17:642

Author: Stewart Coffman

Abortion, Spontaneous

Clinical Presentation

SIGNS AND SYMPTOMS

- Lower abdominal pain, cramping
- Vaginal bleeding with or without the passage of clots or products of conception
- Dizziness or syncope
- Known positive pregnancy test or sexually active with a period of amenorrhea

DEFINITIONS

- *Threatened abortion:* vaginal bleeding, cervical os is closed, intrauterine pregnancy confirmed
- *Inevitable abortion:* vaginal bleeding, cervical os is open
- *Incomplete abortion:* vaginal bleeding, cervical os is open with partial passage of products of conception (POC) and some retained POC
- *Complete abortion:* vaginal bleeding, cervical os closed, complete passage of POC
- *Missed abortion:* nonviable fetus, os closed, +/− vaginal bleeding

MECHANISM/DESCRIPTION

- Spontaneous termination of a <20-week intrauterine pregnancy
- Vaginal bleeding in the first trimester of pregnancy is seen in 20–25% of pregnant patients; approximately 50% of these women will eventually miscarry

ETIOLOGY

- Risk factors include increased age of both the mother and father, increased parity
- Most early miscarriages are from abnormalities of the fetus

Pre-Hospital

CAUTIONS

- Patients with SAB/vaginal bleeding can have severe hemorrhage and present in shock

Diagnosis

ESSENTIAL WORKUP

- *History* including LMP, duration and amount of bleeding, passage of clots, presence of abdominal pain, fevers, dizziness or light-headedness
- *Physical examination*
  - —Determine hemodynamic status of patient. Pregnant patients beginning in the late first trimester have an increased blood volume and can lose substantial amount of blood before having abnormal vital signs. Pregnant patients also have a decreased blood pressure with an average of 110/70
  - —Pelvic exam to *determine whether the cervical os is opened or closed,* amount of bleeding, and the presence of any POC. The presence of adnexal tenderness or peritoneal irritation can be consistent with an ectopic pregnancy
  - —Bimanual exam to determine the size of the uterus
    - -Size of an orange: 6–8 weeks
    - -Fundus at the symphysis pubis: 12 weeks
    - -Fundus at the umbilicus: 16–20 weeks
  - —Gestations greater than 12 weeks should be referred to obstetrics
  - —Confirm pregnancy with urine or serum testing
  - —Rapid hemoglobin determination; type and Rh

LABORATORY

- Urine pregnancy test: most are positive at β-hCG levels of 50 mIU/ml approximately 1 week gestational age and remain positive 2–3 weeks after induced or spontaneous abortions
- Type and crossmatch for woman with low Hct or signs of active blood loss
- Quantitative β-hCG if indicated (see below)
- Any POC passed should be sent to pathology for confirmation

IMAGING/SPECIAL TESTS

- Vaginal ultrasound: gestational sac seen at 5 weeks; cardiac activity seen at 6.5 weeks
- Abdominal ultrasound: gestational sac at 6 weeks; cardiac activity seen at 8 weeks

DIFFERENTIAL DIAGNOSIS

- Cervicitis
- Ectopic pregnancy
- Trauma
- Septic abortions
- Molar pregnancy

Treatment

INITIAL STABILIZATION

- Oxygen, IV fluids via 2 large-bore IVs, cardiac monitor
- Transfuse PRBC if patient does not stabilize after 2–3 L of crystalloid
- Gynecologic consultation immediately
- Oxytocin or methergine may be necessary to control hemorrhage
- These patients are at high risk for having ruptured ectopic pregnancies and may need emergent operative intervention

ED TREATMENT

- Threatened abortion
  - —Pelvic rest, close follow-up with obstetrics
  - —Patients less than 6.5 weeks pregnant with no documented cardiac activity by vaginal ultrasound, need to be followed with serial β-hCG to assess the viability of the fetus and to rule out ectopic pregnancy
- Inevitable and incomplete abortions
  - —Dilation and curettage or evacuation, removal of POC at the cervical os to help decrease bleeding
  - —The confirmation of POC by pathology rules out ectopic pregnancy
- Complete abortion
  - —May treat with methylergonovine or oxytocin if bleeding is heavy
  - —If quantitative β-hCG is <1000 and the ultrasound is negative, may follow-up with obstetrics for serial β-hCG to confirm the levels are decreasing
- Missed abortion
  - —These patients are at risk for DIC especially if fetus is retained >4–6 weeks
  - —Obtain CBC, PT/PTT, FSP, and fibrinogen levels
  - —These patients may be followed closely as outpatients if stable and no evidence of DIC

MEDICATIONS

- Oxytocin: 20 IU in 1000 ml of NS at a rate of 20 mIU/min titrated to decrease bleeding
- Methylergonovine: 0.2 mg IM/PO qid PRN bleeding
- RHO immune globulin in Rh-negative women: 50 μg for women with threatened or complete abortion <12 weeks; 300 μg for women with threatened or complete abortion >12 weeks
- Patients need RhoGAM administration within 72 hours to prevent future isoimmunization

Disposition

ADMISSION CRITERIA

- Suspected ectopic pregnancy (see chapter: ectopic pregnancy)
- Any hemodynamically unstable patients with hypovolemia or anemia
- DIC
- Septic abortions
- Suspected gestational trophoblastic disease

DISCHARGE CRITERIA

- Many dilation and curettages are done in the emergency department for incomplete and inevitable abortions and may be discharged home if stable after 2–3 hours
- Patients with threatened abortions should be told to avoid strenuous activity
- Pelvic rest, i.e., no douching or sexual intercourse during active bleeding as this may increase the risk of infection
- Patients should be instructed to return to the emergency department for any increase in bleeding, dizziness or temperature >100.4°F

Miscellaneous

ICD9: 634.90

CORE CONTENT CODE: 12.3.3

SUGGESTED READINGS

Abbott J. Complications related to pregnancy. In: Rosen P, et al., eds. Emergency medicine: Concepts and clinical practice. 4th ed. St. Louis: CV Mosby, 1998: 2342–2364.

Hansen WF, Hansen AR. Problems in pregnancy. In: Tintinalli JE, ed. Emergency medicine: A comprehensive study guide. 4th ed. New York: McGraw Hill, 1996.

Turner LM. Vaginal bleeding during pregnancy. Emerg Med Clin North Am 1994;12:45.

Author: Aviva Zigman

Abruptio Placenta

Clinical Presentation

SIGNS AND SYMPTOMS

- Typically occur in second half of pregnancy
  - —*Painful vaginal bleeding* (may occur without trauma)
  - —*Abdominal pain*
  - —Signs of *hypotensive shock* may be present
  - —*Uterine cramps,* tenderness, tetany
  - —Back Pain
  - —Nausea, vomiting
  - —Decreased fetal heart tones and movement
  - —Petechiae, bleeding and other signs of disseminated intravascular coagulation (DIC)
  - —Nontender uterus may occur with complete abruption

MECHANISM/DESCRIPTION

- Separation of the placenta from the uterine wall. May occur from trauma or spontaneously during pregnancy. Dissection of blood into the decidua basalis or mechanical shearing between the placenta and uterus results in clot formation, bleeding, development of DIC, and maternal-fetal compromise

INCIDENCE/PREVALENCE

- Approximately 1% of all pregnancies
- 30% of bleeding episodes in the second half of pregnancy
- Accounts for 15% of all fetal deaths
- Risk of recurrence 15–20%

ETIOLOGY

- Unknown
- Blunt abdominal trauma
  - —Most common in second half of pregnancy
- Spontaneous dissection of blood into the decidua basalis
- Drugs especially sympathomimetics

RISK FACTORS

- Maternal hypertension
- Increased maternal age
- Increased parity
- Previous abruption
- Tobacco use
- African American
- Premature rupture of membranes with sudden decompression of uterus
- Precipitous first twin delivery endangers second twin
- Fibroids

Pre-Hospital

CAUTIONS

- Patients with abruption may be in shock and need full resuscitative measures
- In advanced pregnancy, transport in the left lateral recumbent position

Diagnosis

ESSENTIAL WORKUP

- Blood type, Rh, and crossmatch
- Rapid hemoglobin determination
- Ultrasound
  - —Ultrasound may demonstrate sonolucent clot or no abnormality
  - —False-negative with posterior abruptions (concealed hemorrhage)
- Determine fetal heart tones by Doppler (10 weeks gestation or later)
- Fetal monitoring sensitive for detecting early fetal distress
- Uterine tocographic monitoring may demonstrate frequent contractions, rarely tetany
- Assess for presence of amniotic fluid
  - —Nitrazine paper; pH >7 turns blue
  - —Ferning of fluid on glass slide

IMAGING/SPECIAL TESTS

- CBC, platelets
- PT/PTT (anticipate consumptive coagulopathy)
- Fibrinogen levels (level elevated with pregnancy), fibrin-split products
- Betke-Kleihauer
- Fibrinogen products (falsely elevated in pregnancy)
- MRI is most sensitive in detecting small or posterior abruption

DIFFERENTIAL DIAGNOSIS

- Placenta previa
- Vasa previa
- Bleeding during labor
- Vaginal lacerations
- Ovarian Torsion
- Uterine rupture
- Preterm Labor
- Pyelonephritis
- Gallstones
- Preeclampsia complications
- Other blunt abdominal injuries

Treatment

INITIAL STABILIZATION

- ABCs, oxygen, maternal cardiac and tocographic monitoring
- Fetal monitoring
- IV crystalloid resuscitation
- PRBCs, FFP, platelets as indicated
- Immediate OBGyn consultation

ED TREATMENT

- If abruption is suspected in the setting of trauma, maternal stabilization is of primary importance
  —C-spine, CXR, pelvic, and other indicated x-rays should be performed as needed

MEDICATIONS

- RhoGAM in Rh-negative women: 50 μg IM in women <12 weeks pregnant; 300 μg IM in women >12 weeks pregnant

Disposition

ADMISSION CRITERIA

- Patients with abruptio placenta must be admitted for maternal and fetal monitoring
- If DIC, amniotic fluid embolism, or significant hemorrhage occur, the patient should be admitted to an ICU setting
- Victims of multiple trauma with abruption should be admitted and managed in accordance with trauma protocols
- Transportation to higher trauma or obstetric level of care is appropriate if the patient is stable for transfer

DISCHARGE CRITERIA

- Patients with no evidence of abruption or other significant injury may be discharged after 4–6 hours of normal maternal and fetal monitoring
- Discharge instructions include pelvic rest, no intercourse, no heavy lifting, no prolonged standing

Miscellaneous

Expected course and prognosis

- Traumatic abruption: 1% maternal and 50% fetal mortality

Synonyms

- Placental abruption
- Ablatio placentae
- Accidental hemorrhage
- Premature separation of the placenta

ICD9: 641.20

CORE CONTENT CODE: 12.3.4

SUGGESTED READINGS

Charles D, Hurry D, eds. Obstetrics and gynecology. 6th ed. New York: Elsevier Science, 1986.

Cunningham FG, MacDonald PC, Grant NF, eds. Williams' obstetrics. 19th ed. Norwalk, CT: Appleton & Lange, 1993.

Dambro M, et. al. Griffith's 5 minute clinical consult. Baltimore: Williams & Wilkins, 1997.

Rosen P, ed. Emergency medicine. 3rd ed. St. Louis: CV Mosby, 1992.

Scott CJ, et al. Emergencies in pregnancy. Patient Care 1991;15:132–151.

Author: Shawn D. Evans

Abscess, Skin/Soft Tissue

Clinical Presentation

SIGNS AND SYMPTOMS

- Local: erythema, tenderness, pain, heat, swelling, fluctuantes
- Systemic: ranges from absent to fever, rigors, malaise, hypotension, and altered mentation
- Regional lymphadenopathy and lymphangitis may be present

MECHANISM/ DESCRIPTION

A localized collection of pus surrounded and walled off by inflamed tissue

- Bacterial: most abscesses are bacterial, with the microbiology reflective of the microflora of the body part involved
- Sterile: tend to be associated with drug abuse and injection of chemical irritants

ETIOLOGY

Conditions associated with soft tissue abscess formation include

- Soft tissue trauma
- Bacteremia with hematogenous seeding
- Obstruction of normal drainage (sweat glands)
- Tissue ischemia
- Intravenous drug abuse
- Endocarditis
- Lactation disease
- Crohn's disease

Specific abscesses and typical microbiology

- Orbital abscess: associated with paranasal sinusitis, hematogenous spread, or local skin trauma. Staphylococci, Streptococci, H. flu, E. coli, polymicrobial
- Breast abscess: microbiology is dependent on type of abscess
  —Puerperal: classically occurs during lactation, location is peripheral wedge and caused by Staphylococci
  —Duct ectasia: typically caused by ectatic ducts, location is periareolar, and is polymicrobial with a mix of Staphylococci, anaerobic Streptococci, bacteroides, and Enterococci
- Hidradenitis suppurativa: chronic abscesses of apocrine sweat glands, especially in the groin and axilla. S. aureus, S. viridans, E. coli and Proteus are common pathogens
- Pilonidal abscess: caused by epithelial disruption in gluteal fold over coccyx. S. species most common; also polymicrobial with bacteroides and E. coli
- Bartholin's abscess: obstruction of Bartholin duct. Composed of mixed vaginal flora and may include N. gonorrhea, C. trachomatis, and E. coli
- Perirectal abscess: originates in anal crypts and extends through ischiorectal space. Inflammatory bowel disease and diabetes are major predisposing factors. B. fragilis and E. coli are the most common pathogens. Requires treatment in the OR
- Pyomyositis: abscess in muscle, typically occurs in tropics. Increasingly common with HIV and diabetes. S. aureus most common
- Abscesses in association with IVDA: Staphylococci species, S. milleri, and anaerobes. Often isolates of oral origin. May be sterile
- Furuncle: arises from infected hair follicle. Most common on back, axilla, and lower extremities. Staphylococci species are most common
- Carbuncle: larger and more extensive than furuncle; often multiple in a honeycomb pattern on back of neck. More common in diabetics. Invariably caused by Staphylococci
- Paronychia: infection surrounding the nail fold. S. aureus
- Felon: closed space abscess in distal pulp of finger. S. aureus

Pre-Hospital

CAUTIONS

- Septic patients may require rapid transport with intravenous access and volume resuscitation

Diagnosis

ESSENTIAL WORKUP

- History and physical examination with special attention to identifying the presence subcutaneous air and involvement of deeper structures
- Gram stain is unnecessary for simple abscesses in healthy individuals. If indicated for more complicated situations, it may be helpful in differentiating sterile abscesses, those caused by mixed flora, or those due to S. aureus. S. aureus typically exists in pure culture
- Wound cultures are not indicated in simple abscesses in healthy patients. They are only needed with systemic involvement, a compromised host, abscesses of the central face or hand, and in treatment failures. They may help differentiate aerobic from anaerobic infections and help guide specific therapy

LABORATORY

- A glucose determination may be a useful screening test for diabetes given the association of abscess formations in diabetics
- Blood cultures are indicated if either endocarditis is suspected or patient is systemically ill, otherwise cultures are not indicated

IMAGING/SPECIAL TESTS

- Plain films may demonstrate the presence of gas in the tissue planes
- Ultrasound, CT, or MRI may be helpful when diagnosis is in question

DIFFERENTIAL DIAGNOSIS

- Cellulitis
- Aneurysm (especially with IV drug abusers)
- Cysts

Treatment

INITIAL STABILIZATION

- Immediate IV access, oxygen, crystalloid volume resuscitation, blood cultures, and antibiotic therapy are indicated for the septic patient with soft tissue abscesses

ED TREATMENT

- Incision and drainage is the mainstay of treatment
- Antibiotics are indicated for patients with sepsis, systemic illness, endocarditis, facial abscesses drained into the cavernous sinus, concurrent cellulitis (see medications below), and immunocompromised hosts

SPECIAL PEDIATRIC CONSIDERATIONS

- Incision and drainage is a painful procedure and may require sedation in the pediatric patient

MEDICATIONS

- Augmentin 250–500 mg po q8h (peds: 40 mg/kg/day divided into 3 doses)
- Cephalexin 250–500 mg po q8h; or 500 mg po q12h (peds: 25–50mg/kg/day po in 4 doses)
- Clindamycin 150–450mg po q6h (peds: 10–20 mg/kg/day po or IV in 3–4 divided doses)
- Dicloxacillin 250–500 mg po q6h (peds: 50–100 mg/kg/day in 4 divided doses)
- Erythromycin 500 mg–1 g po or IV q6h (peds: 40 mg/kg/day po divided q6h)
- Gentamycin 5mg/kg/day IV q24h (peds: 7.5 • mg/kg/day IV divided q8h)
- Vancomycin 500 mg IV q6h (peds: 40 mg/kg/day IV divided q6h)

Disposition

ADMISSION CRITERIA

- Sepsis, endocarditis, systemic illness, perirectal involvement, abscesses so extensive that it requires incision and debridement in the OR

DISCHARGE CRITERIA

- The majority of patients with uncomplicated abscesses can be treated with I&D and close follow-up

Miscellaneous

ICD9: 682.9

CORE CONTENT CODE: 3.2.1.1

SUGGESTED READINGS

Benson EA. Management of breast abscesses, World J Surg 1989;13:753–756

Canales FL, Newmeyer WL, Kilgore ES. The treatment of felons and paronychias. Hand Clinics 1989;5(4):515–522

Chiedozi LC. Pyomyositis: Review of 205 cases in 112 patients. Am J Surg 1979;137:255–259

Loyer EM, DuBrow RA, David CL, et al. Imaging of superficial soft-tissue infections: Sonographic findings in cases of cellulitis and abscess. AJR 1995;166:149–152

Meislin HW. Pathogen identification of abscesses and cellulitis. Ann Emerg Med 1986;15(3):329–332

Summanen PH, Talan DA, Strong C, et al. Bacteriology of skin and soft-tissue infections in intravenous drug users and individuals with no history of intravenous drug use. Clin Infect Dis 1995;20(Suppl 2):S279–282

Author: Nate Rudman

Abuse, Elder

Clinical Presentation

SIGNS AND SYMPTOMS

- Inconsistent history or physical findings
- Unexplained injuries
- Multiple visits to doctor or hospital
- Vague explanations
- Delay in obtaining medical care/previously untreated medical condition
- Medication difficulties
  - —Incorrect doses
  - —Lost medications
  - —Unfilled prescriptions
- Altered interpersonal interactions
  - —Withdrawn
  - —Indifferent
  - —Demoralized
  - —Fearful
- Caregiver with
  - —Financial dependence upon patient
  - —Substance abuse, psychiatric, or violence history
  - —Controlling behavior or poor knowledge of patient's condition

ETIOLOGY

- Caregiver stress, dependency, or psychopathology
- Victim dependency, or diminishment of ability to perform activities of daily living have been proposed

MECHANISM/DESCRIPTION

- Emotional abuse
  - —Insults
  - —Humiliation
  - —Threats to institutionalize or abandon the patient
- Physical abuse
  - —Physical or sexual assault
- Financial abuse
  - —Stealing or coercion involving patient monies or properties
- Neglect
  - —Behaviors by a patient or caregiver that compromise the patient's health or safety

Pre-Hospital

CAUTIONS

- Observe details of the patient's environment that will not be immediately available to the hospital care team
  - —Conditions and interpersonal interactions at the scene
  - —Physical environment to determine potential areas of danger

Diagnosis

ESSENTIAL WORKUP

- Perform any examination, laboratory, or x-ray indicated by the patient's condition
- Obtain history without family members/caregivers present
  - —Abused elders may fear institutionalization if they report caregivers
  - —Abused elders may feel embarrassment and responsibility for the abuse
  - —Frequently will not volunteer information to the health care team
- Document a clear and detailed description of the patient's findings including
  - —Skin findings
  - —Statements of the patient as they pertain to the abuse
- Safety assessment

DIFFERENTIAL DIAGNOSIS

- Patient may present with any chief complaint
  - —Potential differential diagnosis nonspecific
  - —Abuse best addressed by asking the patient about it directly in a setting apart from caregivers/family

Treatment

INITIAL STABILIZATION

- ABC's
- Treat life-threatening medical/traumatic condition as appropriate

ED TREATMENT

- May require separation of the patient and the caregiver or family member
- Competent elder patients are free to accept or decline any treatments or dispositions they wish despite the risks they may incur
- Many states have mandatory reporting requirements

Disposition

ADMISSION CRITERIA

- Medical condition calling for admission
- Abuse or neglect renders home conditions unsafe

DISCHARGE CRITERIA

- Medical conditions addressed
- Safe environment available
- Abuse or neglect successfully countered by social services or law enforcement

Miscellaneous

ICD9: N/A

CORE CONTENT CODE: N/A

SUGGESTED READINGS

Kleinschmidt K. Elder abuse: A review. Ann Emerg Med 1997;30(4):463–472

Lynch SH. Elder abuse: What to look for, how to intervene. Am J Nurs 1997;97(1):26–32

Vernon MJ, Bennett GC. Elder abuse. Br J Hosp Med 1996:56(5):234–237

Author: Helen Straus

Abuse, Pediatric

Clinical Presentation

SIGNS AND SYMPTOMS

- History and mechanism of causation does not fit the injury or illness
  - —Unexplained or poorly explained death of an infant
  - —Unexplained apnea, especially if recurrent
  - —Ingestion or toxin exposure with suspicious history
  - —Repeat toxin or drug exposure
- Mechanism and force of the causative agent consistent for the degree of injury
  - —Severe head injury explained by routine falling
- Discrepancy in the history between caregivers and the child's presentation
- Delay in seeking medical care
- History of injuries in the past
- History of violence or substance abuse in the home enhances potential of setting for abuse
- Unexplained or suspicious oral, facial, or dental trauma (occurs in 50% of abuse)
- Bruises
  - —Bruises sustained disciplining a child
  - —Patterned bruises (e.g., loop, strap, buckle, or cord marks, bites, finger impressions)
  - —Bruises in suspicious locations (e.g., pinna of the ear, genitalia, inaccessible locations)
  - —Bilateral black eyes without nasal injury
  - —Circumferential injuries of extremities
  - —Multiple bruises without explanation; multiple bruises of different ages
  - —Bruises that suggest use of a weapon or instrument
- Burns
  - —Unexplained, suspicious, or patterned burns
  - —Burns in the shape of an object
  - —Cigarette burns, especially multiple or in different stages of healing
  - —Glove- and sock-patterned liquid burns
  - —Burns in suspicious locations
    - -Back of the hand
    - -Buttocks
    - -Back
  - —Diaper area or doughnut distribution burns
  - —Bilateral burns
  - —Neglectful burns
- Near drowning of infant

Physical Injuries Suspicious for Maltreatment

- Head injury
- Unexplained CNS injury resulting in coma or obtundation
- Shaken baby syndrome
  - —Altered consciousness
  - —Closed head injury most often subdural or subarachnoid
  - —Intraparenchymal hemorrhage
- Retinal hemorrhages
- Subdural hematoma without history of significant trauma
- Fractures
  - —Rupture of the costovertebral junction
  - —Posterior rib fractures
  - —Metaphyseal avulsion fractures (bucket handle or corner fracture)
  - —Two or more fractures in different stages of healing
  - —Long-bone fracture in a preambulatory child
  - —Spiral fracture in a preambulatory child
  - —Uncommon fractures without a history of a *significant trauma* (vertebrae, sternum, scapula, pelvis)
  - —Unexplained fractures

Emotional Abuse and Neglect

- Suicidal gestures in children with no known psychiatric history
- Anorexia nervosa in patients less than 10 years
- Drug use in children less than 12 years
- Runaways, especially recurrent
- Failure to thrive without medical explanation
- Abandonment
- Delay in seeking care for a serious injury
- Serious noncompliance with medical care or parental refusal of necessary care

Munchausen by Proxy

- Recurrent illnesses without medical explanation
- Unexplained metabolic disorders suspicious for poisoning

Sexual Abuse

- Credible disclosure of sexual abuse by a child
- Suspicious genital or anal injuries: hymeneal or vaginal tears, hymeneal scars (especially between 3 and 9 o'clock), anal tears or anal dilation in absence of stool in antrum
- Presence of STD in child <12 years of age (exclude neonatal infection, HPV in child >2 years)
- Presence of sperm or seminal fluid
- Pregnancy in a child <12 years of age

MECHANISM/DESCRIPTION

- Child abuse effects approximately 14 million or 2–3% of US children each year
- Approximately 2000 children are known to die from maltreatment per year, 80% are less than 5 years of age and 40% are less than 1 year of age
- Infants and young children are the most vulnerable and at greatest risk of death and serious morbidity from maltreatment
- The homicide rate for children 4 years and under has reached a 40-year high
- It is estimated that 85% of childhood deaths from maltreatment are misidentified as accidental or due to other causes
- Misdiagnosis occurs because witnesses to injury are rare as most deaths occur in the home
- Many mandated reporters, including physicians fail to recognize the signs and symptoms of maltreatment
- Child maltreatment occurs in all strata of society
- Sexual abuse is consistent among all income groups
- Physical abuse and neglect increases with the stresses that coincide with poverty
- The diagnosis of child abuse and neglect depends on the medical provider's willingness to acknowledge its potential existence when developing a differential diagnosis for a medical problem

Pre-Hospital

- In young children, the diagnosis of abuse or neglect relies heavily on physical evidence
- Pre-hospital personnel are often the first and only persons outside of the family to witness the scene of an abusive situation
- To assist child abuse investigations, carefully document:
  - —The surroundings at the scene of an injury
    - -General appearance of the home
    - -Measure or estimate the height, weight, and/or size of any object reported responsible for an injury
  - —The statements of caregivers and witnesses, and the interactions between the caregivers and the child at the scene
  - —The statement of the child and/or other children at the scene (spontaneous utterances are powerful evidence)
- If the caregiver refuses treatment for the child and there is concern of maltreatment, call the police, followed by the local child welfare authorities
- Convey concerns and findings to hospital personnel both by word and with documentation

Diagnosis

- Complete physical examination, including inspection of genitalia in knee-to-chest and prone positions

LABORATORY

- If bruising is evident, evaluate blood for a coagulopathy or bleeding disorder
  —Send CBC, platelets, PT/PTT, and bleeding time
- If suspicious of possible blunt trauma, rib, or spinal fractures, send LFTs and amylase to assess for occult abdominal injury
- Obtain toxicologic and metabolic screens in all children with unexplained coma, obtundation, or change in mental status

IMAGING/SPECIAL TESTS

- Radiographic "skeletal series"
  —Any child <5 years of age with evidence of suspicious injury
  —Look for old fractures and occult injuries
- Bone scans
  —Occasionally helpful at diagnosing new fractures not yet visible on plain radiographs, especially in infants
  —May miss metaphyseal, spinal, or skull fractures
- Abdominal CT scan with oral and IV contrast
  —Evaluate liver, spleen, and other intra-abdominal injury
- Traumatic injuries
  —Blunt trauma injuries to the chest or abdomen without a history of significant trauma (may not be bruises or fractures due to compliance of chest wall), especially duodenal hematomas, pancreatic pseudocysts, bowel, spleen, or liver lacerations, and mesenteric or retroperitoneal hematomas
- CT Scan with bone windows to assess for acute intracranial injury and skull fractures
  —Skull fractures with suspicious or no history of significant trauma, especially depressed skull fractures, diastatic skull fractures, complex or multiple skull fractures, bilateral skull fractures, and fractures with intracranial injuries
- MRI
  —Helpful diagnosing and dating old intracranial hemorrhages
  —More sensitive than CT scan diagnosing shearing and diffuse axonal injuries seen in Shaken Baby Syndrome
  —If suspect closed head injury, obtain ophthalmologic consultation to evaluate for retinal hemorrhages
- Photographs
  —Provide powerful evidence and should be included in the medical record whenever possible
  —Photographs should include standard measures (e.g., include a coin in the picture), be signed and dated by the photographer, and include at least one shot of the child's face
  —Carefully document all physical findings

DIFFERENTIAL DIAGNOSIS

- Accidental injury
- Birth trauma
- Osteogenesis imperfecta
- Metabolic bone disease
- Accidental burns
- Infection with skin involvement (e.g., staphylococcal scalded skin syndrome)
- Dermatological disease (e.g., Ichthyosis, Incontinentia pigmenti, Epidermolysis bullosa, severe eczema)
- Cultural healing practices (e.g., coining or cupping of the skin in Southeast Asian cultures)
- Idiopathic thrombocytopenic purpura
- Henoch Schönlein purpura
- Leukemia
- Bleeding disorder (e.g., von Willebrand's disease, hemophilia)
- Infant deaths
  —SIDS
  —Neonatal sepsis
  —Congenital heart disease
  —Accidental poisoning
  —Inhalation or accidental toxin exposure (e.g., carbon monoxide, lead, mercury)
  —Hypoglycemia
- Seizure disorder
- Atypical migraine

Treatment

INITIAL STABILIZATION

N/A

ED TREATMENT

- Mandatory reporting of cases of suspected child abuse or neglect
  —Report your concerns to the local child welfare agency
  —Inform the family when the child welfare agency is notified
    -Emphasize your ongoing concern for the welfare of the child
- Consult the social worker
- Protect the child from further harm

MEDICATIONS

N/A

Disposition

ADMISSION CRITERIA

- The child requires observation for possible morbidity from occult injuries
- Any concern for the child's safety at home
- Access the local police or hospital security whenever necessary to protect the child

DISCHARGE CRITERIA

- Arrange for any siblings to be examined immediately or within 24 hours

Miscellaneous

ICD9: 995.5

CORE CONTENT CODE: 18.1.11.2.1.3

SUGGESTED READINGS

American Academy of Pediatrics, Section on Child Abuse and Neglect. A guide to references and resources in child abuse and neglect. Elk Grove Village, IL: American Academy of Pediatrics, 1992–93

Brodeur AE, Monteleone JA. Child maltreatment: A clinical guide and reference. St Louis: CV Mosby, 1994

Author: Susan Duffy

Acetaminophen, Poisoning

Clinical Presentation

SIGNS AND SYMPTOMS

Phase 1: 0.5–24 hours postingestion

- Occurs within the first few hours of ingestion
- Nausea, vomiting, and malaise
- Occurs with massive overdoses
- May not be present with smaller toxic doses

Phase 2: 24–72 hours postingestion

- "Quiescent period"
- Decreased GI symptoms
- Hepatic damage is occurring
  —Right upper quadrant pain and tenderness
  —Increases in liver enzymes, PT, bilirubin
  —Oliguria
  —An increase in acetaminophen (APAP) half-life implies hepatic toxicity

Phase 3: 72–96 hours postingestion

- Critical time period in the prognosis
- Peak liver function abnormalities
- Anorexia, nausea, vomiting
- If the PT continues to rise beyond the third day postingestion, there is high likelihood that the patient will require hepatic transplantation

Phase 4: 4–10 days postingestion

- Resolution of hepatic injury or progression to complete hepatic failure

MECHANISM/DESCRIPTION

- Liver failure caused by a toxic metabolite of APAP, which is created by cytochrome P450
  —Metabolite (NAPQI) normally detoxified by glutathione
  —In the overdose setting, glutathione is quickly depleted, resulting in toxicity to the liver
  —N-acetyl cysteine (NAC), antidote for APAP toxicity, is the central portion of the glutathione molecule, and provides replenishment of the liver's glutathione store
- APAP metabolized by cytochrome P450
  —5% in adults
  —Lower percentage in children (due to relatively high activity of the sulfonation enzyme system in children)
    -Children are relatively less likely to suffer toxicity from APAP than adults
- Increased risk of toxicity
  —Increased activity of the cytochrome P450 enzyme system
    -Patients taking antiseizure medications
    -Chronic alcoholics
  —Patients with poor nutrition have decreased glutathione stores
  —Consider treatment with NAC at a lower serum level of APAP (70%)—controversial

Pharmacokinetics

- Half-life is 4 hours in overdose setting; 1–3 hours in a nonoverdose setting
- Toxic dose >150 mg/kg
- Probable toxic level is 140 μg/ml at 4 hours postingestion (see nomogram for acute intoxication)
- Therapeutic plasma concentration is 5–20 μg/ml

Pre-Hospital

CAUTIONS

- Transport all pill bottles/pills involved in overdose for identification in ED

Diagnosis

ESSENTIAL WORKUP

- APAP level
  —Obtain 4-hour postingestion level or immediately on presentation if >4 hours postingestion
    -Use Rumack-Matthew nomogram as guide for the single acute overdose
    -Do not use nomogram in chronic ingestions or very late ingestions
  —Level <10 μg/ml between 2–4 hours postingestion rules out toxicity

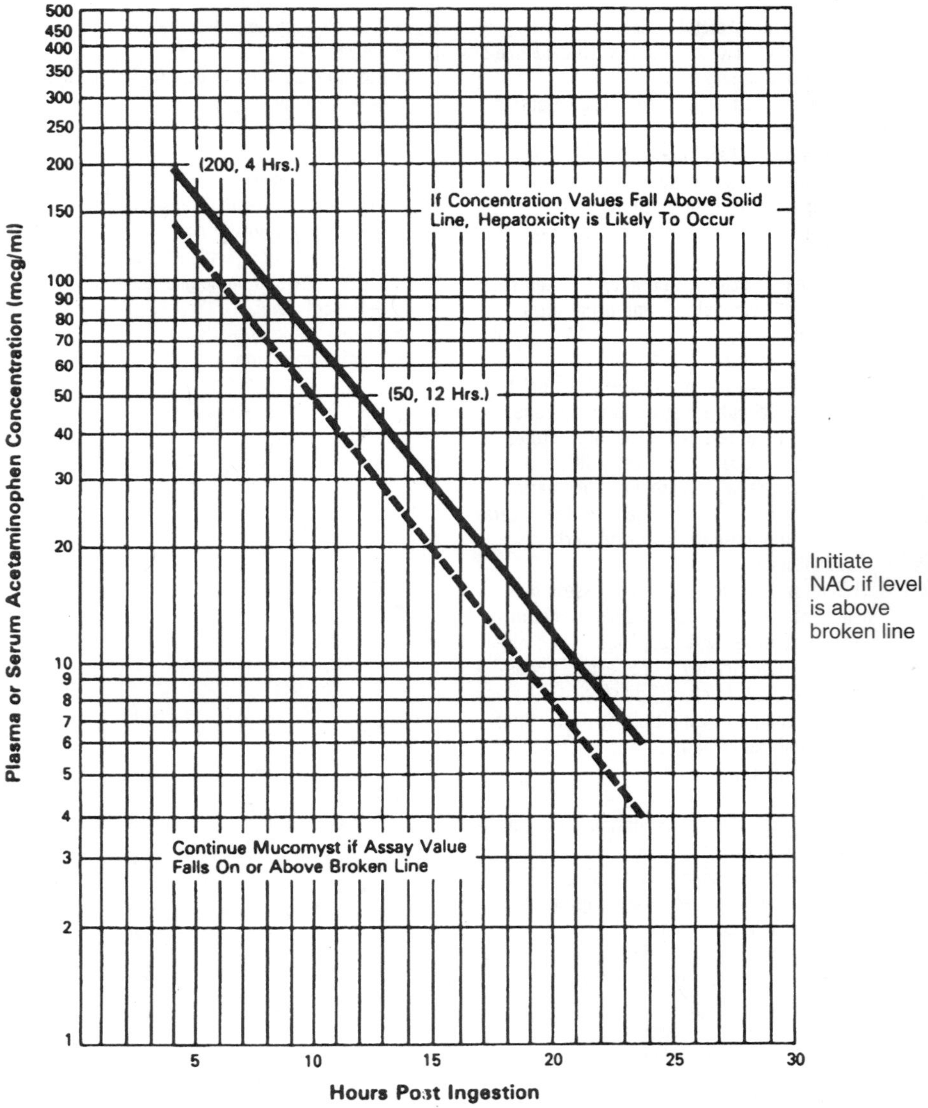

Figure 1.1. Rumack-Matthew nomogram. (Adapted from Rumack BH, Matthew H: Acetaminophen poisoning and toxicity. *Pediatrics* 55:871–876, 1975.

—Obtain two APAP levels drawn 4 hours apart if intial level is above broken line on nomogram
-Shows whether the half-life is prolonged (implying hepatic injury)

LABORATORY

- Electrolytes, BUN, Cr, glucose
- Liver enzymes
  —Baseline value in toxic ingestions
  —Elevated AST—first abnormality detected
  —AST/ALT levels may rise >10,000 in stage III of toxicity
- PT
- Bilirubin

DIFFERENTIAL DIAGNOSIS

- Suspect APAP as coingestant with other drugs in overdose
- Causes of acute onset hepatotoxicity
  —Reye's syndrome
  —Infectious hepatitis
  —Amanita sp. mushrooms toxicity
  —Other drug ingestions

Treatment

INITIAL STABILIZATION

- ABCs
- Narcan, thiamine, D50 (or Accucheck) for altered mental status

ED TREATMENT

Gastric Decontamination

- Gastric lavage if toxic ingestion and seen within 1 hour
- Administer activated charcoal immediately
  —Does not interfere with initial oral loading dose of NAC
  -The dose of NAC so high that absorption of up to 1/3 of NAC does not decrease the effectiveness of NAC
  —Very effective in APAP ingestion
- Avoid syrup of ipecac—will delay NAC/charcoal administration

NAC Administraton

- Administer if toxic level detected as defined by Rumack-Matthew nomogram
- <8 hours postingestion
  —Check APAP level
  —Initiate NAC if APAP level will not be available within 8 hours of ingestion and toxic ingestion suspected
  —NAC most effective if given within 8 hours of APAP ingestion
  —Discontinue NAC if APAP level nontoxic
- 8–15 hours postingestion
  —Initiate NAC immediately if possibility of >150 mg/kg APAP ingested
  —Check APAP level
  —Discontinue if APAP level is nontoxic
- 15–24 hours postingestion
  —Initiate NAC immediately if possibility of >150 mg/kg APAP ingested
  —Check APAP level and hepatic screening tests
  —Discontinue NAC if blood screening normal and patient asymptomatic
- >24 hours postingestion/chronic or repeated APAP ingestions
  —Initiate NAC if
  -Ingestion >150 mg/kg APAP
  -Symptomatic
  -Abnormal hepatic screening panel
  —Discontinue NAC if APAP falls to nondetectable level and no AST elevation occurs by 36 hours postingestion
- Pregnancy
  —No teratogenicity with NAC
  —NAC may be ineffective in protecting fetal liver
- Forms
  —Oral NAC
  -Poor taste/smells
  -Emesis after PO administration is common—repeat full dose if within 1 hour
  -Mix with fruit juice or noncarbonated drink to increase palatability
  -Use antiemetics (droperidol, metoclopramide, ondansetron) to promote PO administraton
  -Administer as a drip through NG if vomiting continues
  —IV NAC
  -Used in Europe
  -Not FDA approved
  -Used where vomiting prevents effective administration of NAC
  -Contact regional poison control center for recommendations

Other Measures

- Transplantation for fulminant hepatic failure
- Hemodialysis for renal failure

MEDICATIONS

- Activated charcoal slurry: 1–2g/kg up to 90 g PO
- Dextrose: D50W 1 amp (50 ml or 25 g) (peds: D25W 2–4 ml/kg) IV
- Droperidol 2.5–5 mg (peds: 0.05–0.06 mg/kg) IV
- Metoclopramide 10 mg (peds: 1 mg/kg) IV
- N-acetyl-cysteine (NAC): 140 mg/kg po loading (adult and pediatric) followed by 70 mg/kg q4 for 17 total doses
- Naloxone (Narcan): 2 mg (peds: 0.1 mg/kg) IV or IM initial dose
- Ondansetron: >80 kg 12 mg; 45–80kg 8mg (peds 0.15 mg/kg) IV
- Sorbitol: 1–2 g/kg to a max of 150 g (peds: >1-year-old: 1–1.5 g/kg as a 35% solution to a max of 50 g) PO mixed in the activated charcoal slurry
- Thiamine (Vitamin B_1): 100 mg (peds: 50 mg) IV or IM

Disposition

ADMISSION CRITERIA

- Hepatotoxic level of APAP requiring full course of NAC therapy (see treatment)

DISCHARGE CRITERIA

- Asymptomatic patients with nontoxic ingestions not requiring full course of NAC therapy

Miscellaneous

ICD9: 965.4

CORE CONTENT CODE: 17.2.1

SUGGESTED READINGS

Anker AL, Smilkstein MJ. Acetaminophen concepts and controversies. Emerg Med Clinic North Am 1994;12:335–349

Ellenhorn MJ, Schoonwald S, Ordog G, Wasserberger J. Acetaminophen. In: Ellenhorn's medical toxicology, 2d ed. Baltimore: Williams & Wilkins, 1997:180–195

Linden CH, Rumack BH. Acetaminophen overdose. Emerg Med Clin North Am 1984;2:103

Rumack BH, Peterson RC, Koch GG, et al. Acetaminophen overdose: 662 cases with evaluation of oral acetylcysteine treatment. Arch Intern Med 1981;141:380

Smilkstein MJ, Knapp GL, Kulig KW, et al. Efficacy of oral n-acetylcysteine in treatment of acetaminophen overdose. Analysis of the national multicenter study. New Eng J Med 1988;319:1557

Author: Mark Crockett

Acidosis

Clinical Presentation

SIGNS AND SYMPTOMS

- Nonspecific
- Vital signs
  - —Tachypnea or Kussmaul respirations with metabolic acidosis
  - —Hypoventilation with respiratory acidosis
- Somnolence
- Confusion
- CO_2 narcosis
- Myocardial conduction and contraction disturbances

MECHANISM/DESCRIPTION

Respiratory Acidosis

- Results from hypoventilation
- Reduced pH due to increased $PaCO_2$
- Defined as $PaCO_2 > 45$ mm Hg
- Classified into 3 broad categories
  - —Primary failure in CNS drive to ventilate
    - -Sleep apnea
    - -Anesthesia
    - -Sedative overdose
  - —Primary failure in transport of CO_2 from alveolar space
    - -COPD
    - -Myasthenic crisis
    - -Severe hypokalemia
    - -Guillain-Barré
  - —Primary failure in transport of CO_2 from tissue to alveoli
    - -Severe heart failure

Metabolic Acidosis

- Results from reduction in plasma bicarbonate decreasing the pH
- Divided into 2 groups
  - —Normal anion gap due to abnormally high net bicarbonate losses
    - -Kidneys fail to reabsorb or regenerate bicarbonate
    - -Extrarenal losses of bicarbonate (diarrhea)
    - -Excessive amounts of substances releasing hydrochloric acid have been given
  - —Increased anion gap due to
    - -Kidneys fail to excrete inorganic acids (phosphate, sulfates)
    - -Net accumulation of organic acids
    - -Inborn errors of metabolism in pediatric patients

ETIOLOGY

Nonanion Gap Metabolic Acidosis

- Gastrointestinal losses of bicarbonate
  - —Diarrhea
  - —Small bowel/pancreatic fistula
  - —Ileal loop (obstructed or too long)
  - —Anion exchange resins
  - —Ingestion of $CaCl_2$, $MgCl_2$
- Renal loss of bicarbonate—
  - —Renal tubular acidosis
    - -Type I—serum $HCO_3^- > 15$ MEq/L, low K^+, normal BUN, renal stone common
    - -Type II—serum $HCO_3^- < 5$ MEq/L, low K^+, normal BUN, renal stone rare
    - -Type IV—serum $HCO_3^- > 15$ MEq/L, normal/elevated K^+, elevated BUN, renal stone uncommon
  - —Carbonic anhydrase inhibitors
  - —Tubulointerstitial renal disease
  - —Hypoaldosteronism
    - -Deficiency
    - -Drug inhibition
- Addition of hydrochloric acid
  - —Ammonium chloride
  - —Arginine HCL

Anion Gap Acidosis: Pneumonic—ACAT MUD PILES

- Alcohol ketoacidosis
- Carbon monoxide /cyanide
- Aspirin
- Toluene
- Methanol
- Uremia
- Diabetic ketoacidosis
- Paraldehyde
- Iron/isoniazid
- Lactic acidosis
- Ethylene glycol
- Starvation

Increased Osmolar Gap: Pneumonic—ME DIE

- Methanol
- Ethylene glycol
- Diuretics (mannitol)
- Isopropyl alcohol
- Ethanol

Pre-Hospital

N/A

Diagnosis

ESSENTIAL WORKUP

- Electrolytes, BUN, Cr, glucose
  - —Decreased bicarbonate with metabolic acidosis
  - —Hyperkalemia and hypercalcemia with severe metabolic acidosis
- ABG
  - —pH
  - —CO_2 retention in respiratory acidosis
  - —Carbon monoxide level
  - —Correction factors
    - -Increase/decrease pH by 0.08 for each 10 mmHg decrease/increase in pCO_2
- Calculate anion gap = $Na^+ - (HCO_3^- + Cl^-)$
  - —Normal = 8–15

LABORATORY

- Urinalysis
  - —For glucose/ketones
- Measured serum osmolality
  - —Calculate serum osmolality = 2 Na^+ + glucose/18 + BUN/2.8
  - —Osmolal gap = difference between calculated and measured osmolality >
    - - ≤ 10 normal
- Toxicology screen
  - —Methanol/ethylene glycol/ethanol/isopropyl alcohol levels if increase osmol gap
  - —Aspirin/iron levels for suspected ingestion
- Serum ketones
- Serum lactate

Treatment

INITIAL STABILIZATION

- ABCs
  - —Early intubation for severe metabolic acidosis with progressive/potential weakening of respiratory compensation
- Naloxone, D50W (or Accucheck) and thiamine if altered mental status

ED TREATMENT

Respiratory Acidosis

- Treat underlying disorder
- Provide ventilatory support for worsening hypercapnia
- In chronic hypercapnia, identify and correct aggravating factors (e.g., pneumonia)

Metabolic Acidosis

- Identify if concurrent osmolal gap
- Treat underlying disorder
  - —Diabetic ketoacidosis
  - —Lactic acidosis
  - —Alcohol ketoacidosis
  - —Ingestion
- Rehydrate with 0.9% NS if hypovolemic
- Correct electrolyte abnormalities

MEDICATIONS

- Dextrose: D50W 1 amp (50 ml or 25 g) (peds: D25W 2–4 ml/kg) IV
- Naloxone (Narcan): 2 mg (peds: 0.1 mg/kg) IV or IM initial dose
- Thiamine (Vitamin B_1): 100 mg (peds: 50 mg) IV or IM

Disposition

ADMISSION CRITERIA

- Worsening metabolic acidosis
- ICU admission if pH <7.1 or altered mental status
- Respiratory acidosis

DISCHARGE CRITERIA

- Resolving anion gap metabolic acidosis

Miscellaneous

ICD9: 276.2

CORE CONTENT CODE: 4.1.1.1, 4.1.3.1

SUGGESTED READINGS

Hana JD, Scheinman JI, Chan JC. The kidney in acid-base balance. Pediatr Clin North Am 1995;42(6):1365–1395.

Kurtzman N. Acid-base disorders. Medicine Diseases of the North. February 1996 pp 67–125.

Author: Michelle Ervin

Acromioclavicular Joint Injury

Clinical Presentation

SIGNS AND SYMPTOMS

- Examine in standing or sitting position
- Acromioclavicular joint is painful and tender to palpation
- Pain is worsened by any motion of the upper extremity
- Ipsilateral arm is held in adduction supported by the contralateral arm
- Extreme adduction worsens the symptoms
- In more severe injuries the clavicle appears free floating

MECHANISM

- *Most common:* direct force from a fall on the lateral aspect of the shoulder
- *Less common:* indirect force from a fall on the outstretched hand

PEDIATRIC CONSIDERATIONS

- *Seldom* occurs in isolation in the pediatric population
- In children, there is tight approximation of the coracoclavicular and acromioclavicular ligaments to the periosteal tube which protects the AC joint from dislocation
- Distal clavicular fractures are more common than AC joint dislocations in children

Pre-Hospital

- Ice packs
- Sling immobilization
- Cervical spine immobilization if appropriate

Diagnosis

ESSENTIAL WORKUP

- Physical exam
- Radiographic evaluation as outlined below

CLASSIFICATION

Type 1

- Painful and tender but AC joint is stable
- Stretching but *incomplete rupture* of the coracoclavicular ligament
- X-rays are normal except for mild swelling

Type 2

- Pain, swelling, and tenderness are greater than Type 1
- Distal clavicle may appear prominent and mildly unstable
- Acromioclavicular ligament *completely torn*
- Coracoclavicular ligament remains intact
- Slight widening of the AC joint on x-ray

Type 3

- Localized symptoms are greater and the distal end of the clavicle is prominent and unstable
- *Disruption of both* the acromioclavicular and coracoclavicular ligament
- Distal end if the clavicle is noted to be displaced above the acromion on x-ray
- Widening of the coracoclavicular interspace by 25–100%

Type 4

- Rare
- Clavicle is displaced posteriorly into or through the trapezius muscle

Type 5

- Rare
- Severe vertical separation of the clavicle from the scapula

Type 6

- Clavicle is dislocated inferiorly into either a subacromial or subcoracoid position
- Usually associated with severe trauma

RADIOGRAPHY

- Minimum of two views most commonly the AP and lateral view
- The distal clavicle and acromion may be superimposed on the spine of the scapula so a slight angulation of the beam 15–30 ° will project the scapular spine out of view
- Additional views: apical oblique and axillary lateral can be used if joint dislocation suspected but not illustrated by routine radiography
- Stress films (holding weights) are not useful in the acute setting as they have low diagnostic yield, require additional patient radiation and are painful

SPECIAL TESTS

- Ultrasonography may demonstrate instability of the distal clavicle, hematoma formation or ligament remnant

DIFFERENTIAL DIAGNOSIS

- Clavicular fractures
- Shoulder dislocation
- In the atraumatic patient, consider osteoarthritis, osteomyelitis

PEDIATRIC CONSIDERATIONS

- True acromioclavicular separations are rare
- Most likely there is a clavicle fracture through the distal physis

Treatment

INITIAL STABILIZATION

- Sling immobilization
- Ice
- Analgesia (NSAIDs, Narcotics)

ED TREATMENT

Types 1 and 2

- Sling immobilization for 10–12 days
- Resume normal range of motion after 14 days

Type 3

- Controversial
- Conservative management vs. operative management
- Consider operative repair for athletes, heavy laborers and severe cosmetic deformities

Types 4, 5, and 6

- Immediate operative repair

SPECIAL CIRCUMSTANCES

- Operative repair may be considered for those with simultaneous distal clavicle fracture
- Late surgery for those with continuous pain

PEDIATRIC CONSIDERATIONS

Types 1 and 2

- Conservative management
- Should heal without major sequelae

Type 3

- Age <15 conservative management
- Age >15 may require more aggressive treatment

Types 4, 5, and 6

- Operative repair

Disposition

ADMISSION CRITERIA

- Open injury
- Types 4, 5, and 6 require admission for operative repair

DISCHARGE CRITERIA

- Types 1 and 2 can be discharged with orthopedic referral
- Type 3 should have urgent orthopedic referral
- Analgesics (NSAIDs)

Miscellaneous

ICD9: 810.03

CORE CONTENT: 18.4.12.2.1.1

SUGGESTED READINGS

Bossart PJ, Joyce SM, et al. Lack of efficacy of weighted radiographs in diagnosing acute acromioclavicular separation. Ann Emerg Med 1988;17:47–51

Gustilo RB, Kyle RF, Templeman DC. Fractures and dislocations. St. Louis: CV Mosby, 1993:303–315

Rockwood CA, Wilke KE, King RE, eds. Fractures in adults. Philadelphia: JB Lippincott, 1991:1181–1248

Rockwood CA, Wilke KE, King RE, eds. Fractures in children. Philadelphia: JB Lippincott, 1991:874–884

Ruiz E, Cicero J. Emergency management of skeletal injuries. St. Louis: CV Mosby, 1995:155–165

Authors: Aileen Kennedy, Wallace Carter

Acute Necrotizing Ulcerative Gingivitis (ANUG)

Clinical Presentation

SIGNS AND SYMPTOMS

- Sudden onset of generalized mouth pain
- Malaise
- Low grade fever is uncommon
- Foul breath
- Increased pain with chewing
- Generalized gingival inflammation with varying degrees of erythema
- Spontaneously bleeding gums
- Necrotic tissue in and about the gingival crest
- Gray-white pseudomembrane
  —Covers ulcerative lesions
  —Leaves a bleeding surface when removed
- Loss of gingival tissue especially interdental papillae
  —Pathognomic for ANUG
- Lesions generally located in the anterior incisor and posterior molar regions
- Painful regional lymphadenopathy

MECHANISM/DESCRIPTION

- Periodontal disease
- Bacteria invade nonnecrotic tissue
  —Cause inflamed gingiva with ulcerated and necrotic lesions
- Also known as trench mouth
- Not contagious
- Occurs in the young to middle aged
- Both sexes affected equally
- Predisposing factors
  —Poor oral hygiene
  —Local traumas
  —Motional and physical stress
  —Smoking
  —Immunodeficiencies
  —Vincent's angina—extension of ANUG to the tonsils and fauces
- Cancrum oris—extension of ANUG to the lips and buccal mucosa

ETIOLOGY

- An overgrowth of normal oral flora
  —Anaerobic fusiform bacilli
  —Spirochetes

Pre-Hospital

N/A

Diagnosis

ESSENTIAL WORKUP

- Clinical diagnosis
- Rule out systemic diseases when lesions have extended beyond the gingival tissue to
  —Buccal mucosa
  —Tongue
  —Palate
  —Pharynx

LABORATORY

- Laboratory tests not helpful
  —Gram stains show only normal flora

DIFFERENTIAL DIAGNOSIS

- Acute gingivitis
- Aphthous ulcers
- Traumatic ulcers
- Herpetic gingivostomatitis
- Squamos cell carcinoma
- Syphilis
- HIV
- Ulcers secondary to systemic disease
  —Diabetes mellitus
  —Uremia
  —Sickle cell disease
  —Blood dyscrasias
  —Connective tissue disorders

Treatment

INITIAL STABILIZATION

- 0.9%NS 500 cc (20 cc/kg) IV bolus for dehydration

ED TREATMENT

- Administer systemic and topical pain management
  - —Narcotics
  - —Viscous lidocaine
- Débride pseudomembrane
  - —Use gauze or cotton-tip applicator soaked in H_2O_2
  - —Removal of this membrane will leave a raw bleeding surface at ulcer base
  - —Removal imperative for tissue healing
- Dilute hydrogen peroxide rinses
  - —3% solution (dilute commercial solution)
- Indications for antibiotics (metronidazole or penicillin)
  - —Extensive gingival involvement
  - —Lymphadenopathy
  - —Systemic signs

Outpatient Therapy

- Improve oral hygiene with daily brushing and flossing of teeth
- Perform dilute hydrogen peroxide rinses up to 12 times daily
- Use analgesics for pain control
- Remove predisposing factors
- Avoid irritants (spicy foods, hot beverages)
- Adequate nutrition
- Relief should occur 24 hours after start of antibiotics
- Follow-up with a dentist to avoid recurrence

Complications

- Periodontal disease from soft tissue
- Alveolar bone destruction

MEDICATIONS

- Hydrogen peroxide (50% solution of 3%)
- Lidocaine (viscous 2%): adult: 15 ml po q 3 hrs PRN; peds: 5 ml po q 3 hrs for a 20-kg child
- Metronidazole: 250–750 mg po tid
- Penicillin VK: adult: 250–500 mg po qid × 5 days; peds: 25–50mg/kg/day divided tid qid
- Tylenol with codeine #3: 1–2 tabs po q 4 hrs PRN
  - —If 3–6 years old: acetaminophen 120 mg + codeine 12 mg/5ml; 5 ml po q 4 hrs PRN
  - —If 7–12 years old: 10 ml po q 4 hrs PRN

Disposition

ADMISSION CRITERIA

- Extensive disease with systemic signs
- Severely immunocompromised patient requiring IV antibiotic treatment
- Severe dehydration

DISCHARGE CRITERIA

- Able to maintain hydration

Miscellaneous

ICD9: 523.0

CORE CONTENT CODE: 6.3.2

SUGGESTED READINGS

Comer RW, Caughman WF, Fitchie JG, Gilbert BO. Dental emergencies. Management by the primary care physician. Postgrad Med 1989;85(3):63–77.

Laskaris G. Oral manifestations of infectious diseases. Dent Clin North Am 1996;40(2):395–423.

Robinson HBG, Miller AS. Colby, Kerr and Robinson's color atlas of oral pathology. 5th ed. Philadelphia: JB Lippincott, 1990:74.

Author: Susan Ferrel

Adnexal Mass

Clinical Presentation

SIGNS AND SYMPTOMS

- Signs and symptoms are highly variable
- Some of the common presentations include
  —Abdominal or pelvic fullness or pain
  —Vaginal bleeding +/− pelvic/abdominal pain
  —Tender adnexal mass
  —Fever with pelvic/abdominal pain in inflammatory adnexal disorders
  —Dysmenorrhea
  —Dyspareunia
  —Ascites with ovarian cancer
  —Urinary symptoms (e.g., retention, frequency, urgency, dysuria)
  —GI symptoms (e.g., nausea, vomiting, constipation)

ETIOLOGY

- Broad categories
  —Ovarian (cyst, cancer)
  —Tubal (abscess, ectopic pregnancy)
  —Uterine (fibroid, cancer)
  —Cervical origin
  —Gastrointestinal (cancer, diverticula)
  —Renal/urologic origin

Pre-Hospital

- IV access and fluid resuscitation may be necessary with hemorrhage (e.g., ruptured ectopic pregnancy) or septic shock (e.g., PID or ruptured tubo-ovarian abscess) associated with adnexal mass

Diagnosis

- Workup variable depending on patient's age, presentation, and differential diagnoses

ESSENTIAL WORKUP

- Pregnancy test
- Pelvic/intravaginal ultrasound is considered imaging modality of choice for locating pregnancy, identifying pelvic anatomy/pathology
- Rapid hemoglobin test, type, and Rh/crossmatch if hemodynamically unstable or pregnant

LABORATORY

- CBC, ESR if inflammatory etiology of adnexal mass is suspected
- Gram stain and cultures of cervical discharge helpful if PID is suspected
- BUN, creatinine if renal pathology is suspected
- Rectal guaiac
- Urinalysis and culture if UTI is suspected

IMAGING/SPECIAL TESTS

- CT of abdomen may be indicated if GI or renal etiology of mass is suspected

DIFFERENTIAL DIAGNOSIS

Prepubertal Age Group

- Ovarian neoplasms, benign or malignant
  —Germ cell tumors common
  —May present with ovarian torsion
- Functional, follicular ovarian cyst
- Wilms' tumor
- Neuroblastoma

Adolescent Age Group

- Pregnancy
  —Ectopic pregnancy
- Inflammatory masses
  —Adolescents have highest PID rates of any age group
  —Tubo-ovarian complex (inflammatory mass with matted bowel, tube, and ovary)
  —Tubo-ovarian abscess
  —Pyosalpinx
  —Hydrosalpinx
- Ovarian masses
  —Functional cysts common in adolescence
  —May present with pain caused by torsion, leakage or rupture
  —Neoplastic tumors (epithelial neoplasms, germ cell tumors, teratomas)
  —Endometriosis less common during adolescence
  —Obstructive genital anomalies (may give rise to hematocolpos or hematometrium)
  —Cystic masses derived from mesonephric elements (e.g., paraovarian or paratubal cysts)
- Uterine masses
  —Uterine abnormalities such as leiomyomas rare in adolescents
  —Obstructive uterovaginal anomalies present during adolescents

Reproductive Age Group

- Pregnancy
  —Ectopic pregnancy
  —Trophoblastic disease
- Ovarian/tubal
  —Functional cysts (follicular cysts, corpus luteum cysts, theca lutein cysts)
    -May present with rupture and hemoperitoneum requiring surgical management
  —Neoplastic tumors, benign or malignant
    -May present with torsion due to elongation of ovarian ligament
  —Endometriosis, ovarian endometriomas
  —Paraovarian or paratubal cysts
- Inflammatory masses
  —Same as adolescent group
  —Diverticular abscess
  —Appendiceal abscess
- Uterine
  —Leiomyomas (fibroids) most common benign uterine tumor
  —Leiomyosarcoma
  —Endometrial lesions, carcinoma or hyperplasia
- Renal/urologic
  —Pelvic kidney
- GI
  —Stool in sigmoid
  —GI malignancies
  —Matted bowel or omentum

Postmenopausal Age Group

- New adnexal mass in postmenopausal woman worrisome as incidence of ovarian cancer increases with age
- Masses from other organ systems more common in this age group (e.g., diverticulitis, bowel tumors, renal tumors, musculoskeletal tumors, lymphomas)
- Otherwise, similar differential as in reproductive age group

Treatment

INITIAL STABILIZATION

- ABCs if patient unstable, e.g., from hemorrhage

ED TREATMENT

- Dependent on etiology
- Emergent gynecologic consultation for hemodynamically unstable pregnant woman
- Evaluate for and treat etiologies of adnexal mass requiring emergent care: pregnancy, inflammatory diseases, ovarian/adnexal torsion, ruptured cysts, abscesses
- Arrange for referral to gynecologist and additional work up of nonemergent etiologies (e.g., ovarian cysts, etc.)

MEDICATIONS

- See PID chapter for treatment of inflammatory/infectious causes of adnexal masses
- NSAIDs adequate for most patients with pelvic/abdominal pain/cramping

Disposition

ADMISSION CRITERIA

- Hemodynamic instability, ectopic pregnancy, inability to tolerate oral liquids, severe pain
- Need for operative intervention

DISCHARGE CRITERIA

- Stable patients may have further workup and treatment as outpatients

Miscellaneous

ICD9: 625.8

CORE CONTENT CODE: 19.1.1, 19.1.3, 19.1.4

SUGGESTED READINGS

Gallup DG, Talledo E. Management of the adnexal mass in the 1990's. Southern Med J. 1997 Oct; 90(10):972–81.

Rapkin AJ. Benign diseases of the female reproductive tract: Signs and symptoms. In: Berek JS, et al., eds. Novak's gynecology. 12th ed. Baltimore: Williams & Wilkins, 1996:352–377.

Stenchever MA. Differential diagnosis of major gynecologic problems by age groups. In: Mishell DR, et al., eds: Comprehensive gynecology. 3rd ed. St. Louis: Mosby-Year Book, 1997:159–168.

Wheeler JE, Woodruff JD. Benign disorders of the ovaries and oviducts. In: DeCherney AH, Pernoll ML, eds. Current obstetric and gynecologic diagnosis and treatment. 8th ed. E. Norwalk, CT: Appleton & Lange 1994:744–753.

Author: Sam S. Torbati

Adrenal Insufficiency

Clinical Presentation

SIGNS AND SYMPTOMS

Symptoms

- Anorexia
- Nausea
- Vomiting
- Lethargy
- Abdominal pain
- Malaise
- Myalgias
- Dehydration (Primary adrenal insufficiency only)

Signs

- Sodium depletion
- Orthostatic blood pressure changes or frank shock
- Hyperkalemia
- Mental status changes
- Tachycardia
- Hyperpigmentation (primary adrenal insufficiency only)
- Vitiligo
- Muscle wasting
- Fever

Addisonian Crisis:

- Hypotension and shock
- Hyponatremia
- Hyperkalemia
- Hypoglycemia

MECHANISM/DESCRIPTION

- Inadequate hydrocortisone secretion to meet the body's needs during stress

Addisonian crisis (acute adrenal insufficiency)

- Life-threatening emergency
- Precipitated by intensification of
  - —Chronic adrenal insufficiency
  - —Acute adrenal hemorrhage
  - —Rapid steroid withdrawal
  - —Steroid dependant patient under stress due to pregnancy, surgery, trauma, infection, or dehydration.

ETIOLOGY

Primary Adrenal Failure

- Idiopathic: autoimmune
- Infectious
  - —Granulomatous: tuberculosis
  - —Protozoal and fungi: histoplasmosis, coccidioidomycosis, candidiasis
  - —Viral: CMV, herpes simplex
- Infiltration:
  - —Sarcoid
  - —Neoplasm
  - —Hemochromatosis
  - —Amyloidosis
  - —Iron depletion
- Postadrenalectomy
- Hemorrhage
  - —Sepsis
  - —Birth trauma
  - —Pregnancy
  - —Seizures
  - —Anticoagulants
- Congenital adrenal hyperplasia
- Congenital unresponsiveness to ACTH

Secondary Adrenal Failure

- Pituitary insufficiency:
  - —Infarction (Sheehan's syndrome)
  - —Hemorrhage
  - —Pituitary tumor
  - —ACTH deficiency
  - —Infiltration
- Hypothalamic insufficiency
- Head trauma
- Glucocorticoid administration

Pre-Hospital

N/A

Diagnosis

ESSENTIAL WORKUP

- Laboratory confirmation of the diagnosis not possible in the ED
- Adrenal crisis—life-threatening condition
  - —High degree of suspicion should prompt the initiation of therapy before definitive diagnosis;
- Plasma cortisol
  - —Level <20 μg/dl in the setting of shock suggests adrenal insufficiency.
- Electrolytes
  - —K^+
  - —Na^+
- BUN, Cr
  - —Elevated 2^0 dehydration
- Serum glucose
  - —May be low

LABORATORY

- CBC with differential
  - —Anemia
- Arterial blood gases
  - —Hypoxemia
  - —Acidosis
- Cosyntropin stimulation test
- Search for underlying infection

IMAGING/SPECIAL TESTS

- ECG
- CXR

DIFFERENTIAL DIAGNOSIS

- Sepsis
- Shock from any etiology
- Acute abdominal emergency

Treatment

INITIAL STABILIZATION

- ABCs
- Cardiac monitor
- Blood pressure support for hypotension
  - —0.9%NS IVF 500 cc–1 L (peds: 20 cc/kg) bolus
  - —Avoid pressors (if possible)
    - -May precipitate arrhythmias
- Supplemental oxygen to meet metabolic needs
- Correct hyperthermia
  - —Initiate cooling measures

ED TREATMENT

- Glucocorticoid replacement
  - —IV hydrocortisone or dexamethasone
  - —Dexamethasone will not interfere with the results of the cosyntropin stimulation tests
- Volume expansion
  - —D5W 0.9% NS at a rate of 500–1000 ml/hr for the first 3–4 hours
  - —Care should be taken to note the patient's age, volume, and cardiac and renal function
- For hypoglycemia
  - —Dextrose—D50W
- Treat life-threatening dysrhythmias secondary to hyperkalemia with calcium, bicarbonate, insulin/glucose
- Identification and correction of the underlying precipitant

MEDICATIONS

- Dexamethasone: 4 mg (peds: 0.15 mg/kg/dose) q 12 hrs
- Dextrose: 50–100cc D50 (peds: 2cc/kg of D10 over 1 min) IV
- Hydrocortisone: 100 mg (peds: 1–2 mg/kg/dose) IV q 6 hrs
- Insulin (regular): 10 units IVP
- Sodium bicarbonate: 1–2 mEq/kg IV

Disposition

ADMISSION CRITERIA:

- Admit all patients with acute adrenal insufficiency
- ICU admission for unstable or potentially unstable

DISCHARGE CRITERIA

- Normal laboratory evaluation with treated adrenal insufficiency

Miscellaneous

ICD9: 255.4

CORE CONTENT CODE: 4.2.2

SUGGESTED READINGS

Holmes L, Lakshmanan M. The patient with chronic endocrine disease. In: Herr RD, Cydulka RK, eds. Emergency care of the compromised patient. Philadelphia: JB Lippincott, 1994:123–133

Oelkers W. Adrenal insufficiency. N Engl J Med 1996;355;1206–1212

Wogan JM. Endocrine disorders. In: Rosen P, et al. Emergency medicine concepts and clinical practice. 4th ed. St. Louis: CV Mosby, 1998:2488–2503

Author: Rita Cydulka

Advance Directives

Clinical Presentation

SIGNS AND SYMPTOMS

- Settings where advance directives may be useful to guide actions
  - —CPR
  - —Endotracheal intubation
  - —Defibrillation
  - —Emergency cardiac pacing
  - —Ventilator usage
  - —Invasive testing and procedures
  - —Tube feeding
  - —Antibiotics
  - —Organ donation
- Legal document
  - —Defines patient's wishes regarding medical interventions
- Identifier
  - —Verifies that a legal document exists
  - —Bracelet
  - —Necklace
  - —Wallet card
- May be verbally rescinded by the patient at any time

MECHANISM/DESCRIPTION

- A document expressing a patient's choice about medical care prior to the need for such care
  - —Allows the physician to be aware and respect the patient's wishes
  - —This document is applied once the patient becomes decisionally incapacitated
- Criteria for effective advance directives
  - —Clear
  - —Concise
  - —Available
- Legislation regarding advance directives varies
  - —From state to state
  - —Within states
  - —Within the health care systems
- Patients may rescind advance directives at any time

ETIOLOGY

N/A

DIFFERENTIAL DIAGNOSIS

N/A

Pre-Hospital

- Rapid identification of a valid advance directive
- Follow operational protocols if a well recognized document or identifier is not available

CAUTIONS

- Careful identification of the patient and paperwork
- Exercise situational judgment in honoring the advance directive
- Controversial decisions should be made in favor of resuscitation
  - —Initiate full resuscitation
    - -Base station contact for further guidance
    - -Care can be withdrawn later
- Ambulance transport is indicated even when advance directives are applied

Diagnosis

ESSENTIAL WORKUP

- Identification of the patient
- Identification of the document
  - —Jurisdiction of origin
  - —Date of execution
  - —A dated document from a remote jurisdiction may be the only evidence of patient's wishes
- Determination of the specific therapies covered
- Establish that there is no better way to determine the patient's wishes
- Document lack of decisional capacity
- Honor life-sustaining procedures until all relevant issues are resolved
- Determine who assumes decisional capacity for the incapacitated patient
  - —This may be complex in certain settings
    - -Multiple care providers
    - -Multiple family members
    - -Divorced parents
    - -Court-appointed guardians
  - —Consult preferentially with the person named as the proxy

LABORATORY

N/A

IMAGING/SPECIAL TESTS

N/A

DIFFERENTIAL DIAGNOSIS

N/A

Treatment

INITIAL STABILIZATION

- Withhold specified care in incapacitated patients if given a valid advance directive
- Continue resuscitation with advance directives in certain cases
  - —Easily reversible condition
  - —Hypoglycemia
  - —Narcotic overdose
  - —A controversy with the advance directives is unresolved

ED TREATMENT

- Provide reasonable care short of that declined through advance directive
- Discuss choices and actions
  - —With the family and other concerned parties
  - —In understandable terms

MEDICATIONS

N/A

Disposition

ADMISSION CRITERIA

- Communicate the directive and surrounding conversations and actions to subsequent caregivers
  - —This information should be part of the medical record

DISCHARGE CRITERIA

N/A

Miscellaneous

ICD9: N/A

CORE CONTENT CODE: 20.8.2.6.7.3

SUGGESTED READINGS

Iserson KV, Saunders AB, Mathieu D. Ethics in emergency medicine. 2d ed. Tucson, Az: Galen Press, 1995.

Williams A. Advance directives. In: Harwood-Nuss A, ed. Emergency medicine. 2d ed. Philadelphia: Lippincott-Raven, 1996;1531–1534.

Authors: Ken Williams; Abigail R. Williams

Advanced Trauma Life Support

- Standardized approach for rapid assessment of the trauma patient
- While presented here as a sequential method for gathering information, it is important to understand that many of the steps can be performed simultaneously and life-threatening injuries must be immediately addressed and treated prior to going on to the next level

Clinical Presentation

SIGNS AND SYMPTOMS

Primary Survey

Airway/C-spine

- Look, listen and feel from nose/mouth to trachea/bronchial tree to assess patency
- Evaluate gag reflex
- The C-spine must be immobilized
- Ability to speak or the effective movement of air with respiration indicates patency
- Gurgling, stridor, wheezing, snoring, choking, gagging, or absence of air movement require immediate intervention
- Manage airway compromise prior to next step in primary survey

Breathing

- An awake, alert patient with normal speech and good air movement suggest effective breathing
- Symmetric chest wall rise/fall, equal breath sounds, normal respiratory rate and oxygen saturation >95% suggest effective breathing
- Asymmetric chest movement, unequal breath sounds, abnormal respiratory rate, decreased oxygen saturation, inadequate air movement, or an obtunded patient suggest ineffective breathing
- Decreased unilateral breath sounds, tracheal shift, hyperexpansion, hyperresonance to percussion, subcutaneous air, hypoxia, and hemodynamic compromise suggest tension pneumothorax
  —Manage immediately with needle thoracostomy
- Decreased breath sounds with dullness to percussion suggest hemothorax

Circulation

- Adequate circulating blood volume must be maintained
- Primary assessment includes blood pressure, heart rate, pulse quality, and end organ function (mentation, urine output, capillary refill)
- Tachycardia and oliguria indicate early shock; hypotension is a late finding
- Classes of hemorrhagic shock (see chapter: Hemorrhagic Shock)

Disability

- Assess level of consciousness, gross motor function, pupil size/reactivity
- Glasgow Coma Scale (GCS) is most commonly used; 8 or less indicates severe head injury/coma

Glasgow Coma Scale

EYE OPENING	VERBAL RESPONSE	MOTOR RESPONSE
Spontaneous = 4	Full sentences, oriented × 3 = 5	Follows commands = 6
Require verbal stimuli = 3	Full sentences, confused = 4	Localizes pain = 5
Require painful stimuli = 2	Understandable words = 3	Withdraws to pain = 4
Never open = 1	Garbled speech, moans = 2	Flexion/decorticate posture = 3
	No vocalizations = 1	Extensor/decerebrate posture = 2
		Flaccid = 1

- Spinal cord injuries are grossly assessed by observing movement of all extremities
- Pupil size and reactivity to light is a measure of brainstem function

Exposure

- Patient should be undressed completely

Secondary Survey

- Once the primary survey has been completed with the patient stabilized at each level, a complete physical exam from head-to-toe is completed
- "Tubes and fingers in every orifice"

PEDIATRIC CONSIDERATIONS

- See chapter on pediatric trauma

Pre-Hospital

- Triage to a major trauma center is dictated by local protocols
- Primary survey should be performed on scene and en route

Diagnosis

- Initial stabilization should begin simultaneously with essential work-up

ESSENTIAL WORKUP

- Primary and secondary survey
- Cervical spine, chest, and pelvis x-rays
- Hemoglobin/hematocrit, arterial blood gas, tube for blood typing
- Urine dip for blood (and subsequent urinalysis if positive)

LABORATORY

- Baseline coagulation and chemistry studies with massive injury or hemorrhage

IMAGING/SPECIAL TESTS

- Loss of consciousness, posttraumatic amnesia (anterograde or retrograde), or persistent altered level of consciousness is indication for head CT
- Significant blunt and penetrating chest trauma requires objective evaluation of the heart and great vessels with echocardiography, CT scan, angiography, or direct visualization
- Blunt abdominal trauma requires objective evaluation: Diagnostic Peritoneal Lavage, ultrasound, or CT depending on patient's condition
- Extremity injury
  —X-rays
  —Suspected vascular damage requires angiography or duplex ultrasound

Treatment

INITIAL STABILIZATION

The initial treatment should parallel the primary survey, with injuries treated prior to addressing the next assessment level

Airway with C-spine Control

- Jaw thrust, suctioning, and oropharyngeal or nasopharyngeal airways provide initial airway support
- Rapid sequence intubation is the airway management option of initial choice for multiple trauma patients
  - —Nasotracheal intubation, or cricothyroidotomy may be necessary

Breathing

- 100% oxygen and respiratory monitoring
- Tension pneumothorax should be diagnosed clinically and decompressed emergently with a needle thoracostomy below the axilla or above the second rib
  - —Tube thoracostomy should follow
- Open chest wounds should be covered with an adherent dressing and a tube thoracostomy performed
- Respiratory distress from flail segment or pulmonary contusion should prompt early intubation with mechanical ventilation and positive end-expiratory pressure

Circulation

- Two large-bore IVs with constant hemodynamic and cardiac monitoring
  - —Alternatives include central lines, venous cutdowns (saphenous or femoral), or pediatric intraosseous lines
- Aggressive fluid replacement with 3 parts fluid for every 1 part circulatory volume loss; adjust fluids based on ongoing assessment
  - —2 L initial bolus in adults, 20 cc/kg in children
- Whole blood, or autotransfused blood for Class III and Class IV hemorrhagic shock or uncontrolled bleeding
- Pericardial tamponade requires emergent pericardiocentesis/pericardial window
- External bleeding should be managed with direct pressure

Disability

- Head injury with GCS of 8 or less should initiate treatment for elevated ICP with mannitol; rapid sequence induction and intubation or surgical airway, oxygenation, and gentle hyperventilation (to a PCO_2 of 35 mmHg)
- Elevate head 20–30° maintaining spine immobilization

ED TREATMENT

- Definitive treatment is often surgical: prompt stabilization, early recognition of the need for operative intervention, and appropriate trauma surgical consultation is paramount

MEDICATIONS

- See chapter on rapid sequence intubation

PEDIATRIC CONSIDERATIONS

- Intraosseous lines are an alternative to IV lines for fluids and medications

Disposition

ADMISSION CRITERIA

- Most major trauma patients should be admitted for observation, monitoring, and further evaluation
- Patients with significant injuries or hemodynamic instability should be admitted to an ICU
- Patients requiring frequent assessments should be admitted to a monitored setting

DISCHARGE CRITERIA

- Minor trauma patients with negative objective workup may be observed in the emergency department for several hours and then discharged

Miscellaneous

ICD9: 959.80

CORE CONTENT CODE: 18.1.3

SUGGESTED READINGS

Committee on Trauma, American College of Surgeons. Advanced trauma life support instructor manual. 5th ed. Chicago: American College of Surgeons, 1993.

Jordan RC. Multiple trauma. In: Rosen P, et al., eds. Emergency medicine: Concepts and clinical practice. 4th ed. St. Louis: CV Mosby, 1998.

Krantz BE. Initial assessment. In: Feliciano DV, et al., eds. Trauma. Stamford, CT: Appleton & Lange, 1996:123.

Author: Daniel Davis

Air Embolism

Clinical Presentation

SIGNS AND SYMPTOMS

Cerebral

- Dive-related stroke
- Second leading cause of dive-related death (after drowning)
- Two main presentations
  - —Apnea and full cardiopulmonary arrest
  - —Any combination of neurologic deficits
- Presentation depends on the arterial distribution of the gas embolism
  - —Change in level of consciousness (40%)
  - —Sensory loss (20%)
  - —Motor deficit (20%)
  - —Paraplegia (10%)
  - —Seizure (4%)
  - —Visual changes
  - —Aphasia
  - —Paresthesias
- Rapid onset
  - —8.6% during the ascent
  - —83.6% <5 minutes after surfacing
  - —7.8% between 5–10 minutes after surfacing
- Spontaneous improvement minutes after the initial deficits may occur
  - —High incidence of relapse
  - —Improvement may be transiently related to postural changes that affect the distribution of the bubbles flowing to the brain

Pulmonary

- Shortness of breath
- Bloody, frothy sputum
- Subcutaneous air

Cardiac

- Myocardial infarction due to air in the coronary vessels
- Reduced cardiac output due to air trapped in ventricle
- Hamman's sign: crepitus on auscultation of the heart

Renal

- Renal infarction due to air embolism

MECHANISM/DESCRIPTION

- Extreme manifestation of pulmonary barotrauma
- Overpressurization of lung tissue causes pleural tear with air entering the vascular circulation
  - —Air bubbles tend to rise and enter the cerebral vessels where they can occlude vascular flow
  - —Boyles Law: pressure × volume = constant
  - —Trapped air (in lungs with closed glottis) expands on ascent
- Arterial embolism can also occur via pulmonary AV shunts, or as paradoxical embolism via a patent foramen ovale (up to 18% of the adult population)

ETIOLOGY

- Breath-holding during ascent
  - —Symptoms attributable to a shower of bubbles and multiple blood vessel involvement
- Iatrogenically during placement of CVP lines, cardiothoracic surgery, or hemodialysis
- Penetrating wounds to heart with emergent repair of cardiac wound

Pre-Hospital

CONTROVERSIES

- Trendelenburg positioning patients with cerebral arterial gas embolism (CAGE) is not effective
  - —Hypothesized that elevation of the legs could cause the air bubble to migrate away from the cerebral circulation and that increased hydrostatic pressure in brain will shrink bubbles
  - —Trendelenburg positioning may increase injury by increasing the intracerebral pressure

CAUTIONS

- Patients who experience sudden neurologic recovery can relapse quickly as bubble positions change

Diagnosis

ESSENTIAL WORKUP

- Recognize AGE as the diagnosis
  - —Altered mental status within 10 minutes of surfacing from compressed air dive
- Inquire as to unusual circumstances during ascent
  - —Breath-holding
  - —Panic/out of air situation
- Thorough neurologic exam must carefully document the extent of the deficits to the motor, sensory, cerebellar, and cranial nerves

LABORATORY

- Serum creatinine kinase activity has been shown to be a marker of the severity of CAGE
- CBC
- Electrolytes, BUN, Cr, glucose
- ABG when respiratory symptoms

IMAGING/SPECIAL TESTS

- CXR
  - —For evidence of pneumothorax or mediastinal emphysema (both rare)
- ECG
- CT head
  - —For altered mental status
  - —Do not delay recompression for CT when CAGE almost certain clinically

DIFFERENTIAL DIAGNOSIS

- CVA from causes unrelated to gas embolism
- Neurologic deficits due to decompression sickness

Treatment

INITIAL STABILIZATION

- ABCs
  - —100% oxygen by tight-fitting mask
  - —Intubation for ventilation/protection of airway required
  - —IV access with volume augmentation

ED TREATMENT

- Hyperbaric oxygen recompression therapy (see Hyperbaric Oxygen Therapy chapter)
  - —For all CAGE
  - —Arrange transportation to nearest hyperbaric facility
  - —Aircraft capable of full pressurization of flight below 1000 feet are best suited for transfers
  - —Prophylactic chest tube for simple pneumothorax to prevent conversion to tension pneumothorax during recompression
  - —Fill endotracheal and Foley catheter balloons with water or saline to avoid shrinkage/damage during recompression
- Divers Alert Network (DAN)
  - —Based at Duke University Medical Center
  - —Provides a 24-hour emergency hotline for medical consultation on the treatment of dive-related injuries and for referrals to hyperbaric chambers (telephone: (919) 684–8111)

Disposition

ADMISSION CRITERIA

- Admit all following initial hyperbaric therapy for observation and reexamination

DISCHARGE CRITERIA

- None should be discharged from the emergency department

Miscellaneous

ICD9: 958.0

CORE CONTENT CODE: 5.1

SUGGESTED READINGS

Edmonds C, Lowry C, Pennefather J. Diving and subaquatic medicine. Oxford: Butterworth-Heinemann, 1992

Jerrard DA. Diving medicine. Emerg Med Clin North Am 1992;10(2):329–338.

Smith RM, Neuman TS. Elevation of serum creatine kinase in divers with arterial gas embolism. N Engl J Med 1994;330:19–24

Author: Jeffrey Gordon

Airway Management

Clinical Presentation

SIGNS AND SYMPTOMS

Clinical Conditions Requiring Airway Management

- Failure to maintain or protect the airway
  - —Stridor
  - —Oropharyngeal swelling
  - —Absence of a gag reflex
  - —Inability to handle secretions
- Hypoxia or ventilatory failure
  - —Shortness of breath
  - —Cyanosis
  - —Altered mental status
  - —Status epilepticus

Recognition of a Difficult Airway

- Congenital
  - —Pierre Robin syndrome
  - —Treacher Collins' syndrome
  - —Goldenhar's syndrome
  - —Down's syndrome
  - —Klippel-Feil syndrome
  - —Goiter
- Anatomic
  - —Mallampati criteria
    - -Faucial pillars, soft palate visible only (Class II)
    - -Only soft palate visible (Class III)
    - -Rule of 3, 3, and 2
    - -Mouth can not be opened more than 3 finger breadths
    - -Horizontal length of the mandible >3 finger breadths
    - -Thyromental distance <2 finger breadths
- Acquired
  - —Infections
    - -Supraglottitis
    - -Croup
    - -Abscess (intraoral, retropharyngeal)
    - -Ludwig's angina
  - —Arthritis
    - -Rheumatoid arthritis
    - -Ankylosing spondylitis
  - —Benign tumor
    - -Cystic hygroma
    - -Lipoma
    - -Adenoma
    - -Goiter
    - -Malignant tumors
    - -Facial injury
    - -Cervical spine injury
    - -Laryngeal-tracheal trauma
    - -Obesity
    - -Acromegaly
    - -Acute burns

MECHANISM/DESCRIPTION

- Oral and nasopharyngeal airways
  - —Lift the base of the tongue off the hypopharynx
  - —Facilitate bag-valve-mask ventilation
  - —Inserted if a gag response is absent
- Oral rapid sequence intubation
  - —Induction of anesthesia and paralysis
  - —Minimize the risk of aspiration
  - —Method of choice for trauma patients with suspected head injury
  - —Contraindicated in patients who should not be paralyzed
- Oral awake intubation
  - —Oral intubation with sedation only
  - —Ketamine, a dissociative anesthetic, is ideal for this purpose
    - -Contraindicated in the head-injured patient due to intracranial pressure (ICP) elevation
  - —Indicated when paralysis is hazardous due to airway distortion (penetrating neck trauma)
- Blind nasotracheal intubation
  - —Indications
    - -Oral intubation is unsuccessful
    - -Neuromuscular blockade is dangerous
    - -Sitting or semi-reclined in patients who cannot tolerate the supine position: COPD; CHF; asthma
    - -Oral cavity is not accessible to allow oral intubation
    - -Limited cervical mobility: rheumatoid arthritis
  - —Contraindications
    - -Apnea
    - -Anticoagulation
    - -Massive facial trauma
    - -Nasal trauma
    - -Head trauma
    - -Upper airway abscess
    - -Acute epiglottitis
- Lighted stylet
  - —Light wand
  - —Transilluminate the neck
  - —Guide tube placement
  - —Alternative to laryngoscopic intubation
  - —Verifies ET tube placement
  - —Indications
    - -Blood in the oropharynx
    - -Failed airway
    - -Cricothyrotomy
  - —Surgical procedure
  - —Incision is made in the cricothyroid membrane
  - —Shiley tracheostomy tube is inserted in the airway
  - —Failed airway
  - —Massive facial trauma
  - —Total upper airway obstruction
  - —Contraindications
  - —Laryngeal crush injury
  - —Expanding zone II or III neck hematoma
- Percutaneous translaryngeal ventilation (PTV)
  - —A temporizing measure
  - —Percutaneous placement of a 12- or 14-gauge catheter through the cricothyroid membrane
  - —Intermittent ventilation via a high-pressure oxygen source
  - —Indications
    - -Failed oral or nasal intubation until cricothyrotomy is complete
  - —Contraindication
    - -Upper airway obstruction that prevents expiration
- Fiberoptic Intubation
    - -ET tube placed over the bronchoscope
    - -Performed via the nasotracheal or orotracheal approach
    - -Indications
    - -Anatomic limitations to visualization of the glottis
    - -Limited movement of the mandible or cervical spine
  - —Contraindications
    - -Patients who need immediate airway management
    - -Significant airway hemorrhage
- Retrograde tracheal intubation
  - —Another technique available when others have failed
  - —Retrograde advancement of a guidewire through a translaryngeal catheter
- Laryngeal mask airway
  - —A device that is inserted blindly into the oropharynx
  - —The patient is ventilated through a tube connected to a small inflatable mask
    - -The mask forms a low pressure seal around the laryngeal inlet
  - —Used to ventilate the patient *if* other airway methods have failed, until a definitive airway can be established

ETIOLOGY

N/A

PEDIATRIC CONSIDERATIONS

- An estimation of ET tube size is 16 + age/4
- Uncuffed ET tubes should be used in patients <8 years old
- For children <3 years old, the straight Miller blade is preferred
- For children <12 years old the preferred surgical airway is PTV

Pre-Hospital

CAUTIONS

- Indications for airway management and different methods are limited by available techniques
- Bag-mask ventilation only (COMMA) for basic life support providers
- Options for patients in cardiac and respiratory arrest for advanced life support providers
  - —Bag-mask ventilation and definitive airway management in the ED
  - —Oral intubation
  - —Pharyngotracheal lumen airway (PTLA)
    - -A device with two tubes and two balloons

–Blindly placed in either the trachea or the esophagus
–Functions as an ET tube or an esophageal obturator
–When endotracheal intubation is not available
—PTLA contraindications
–Pediatric patients
–Caustic ingestions
–Esophageal disease
–Presence of a gag reflex

CONTROVERSIES

- Rapid sequence intubation
  —Used in the field primarily by flight crews
  —Its use remains controversial for urban EMS systems in which transport times are short

Diagnosis

ESSENTIAL WORKUP

- Verification of correct tube placement
  —Auscultation over both axillae, the anterior lung fields, and the stomach
  —Observation of chest wall movement
  —Condensation on the tube during ventilation

LABORATORY

- End-tidal CO_2 colorimetric devices
  —In cardiac arrest, low CO_2 production may prevent color change with a correctly placed endotracheal tube
- Rise in pulse oximetry after intubation

IMAGING/SPECIAL TESTS

- Syringe aspiration technique
  —Detects esophageal intubation
  —A catheter-tipped 60-cc syringe is inserted through the adapter at the proximal end of the ET tube
  —Resistance to aspiration indicates occlusion from esophageal collapse
- Chest radiography
  —Indicated to exclude a main stem bronchus intubation
  —Esophageal intubation may incorrectly appear to be in the trachea

DIFFERENTIAL DIAGNOSIS

- Esophageal intubation
- Right mainstem intubation
- Extratracheal placement through a tear in a pyriform sinus or the trachea
- Pneumothorax

Treatment

INITIAL STABILIZATION

- Maintain line cervical immobilization
- Check all intubation equipment
  —Suction
  —Bag-valve-mask
  —Various sizes of ET tubes
  —Laryngoscope blades
  —Stylets
  —Oxygen
  —Medications
  —Monitoring equipment

ED TREATMENT

- Rapid sequence intubation
- Preoxygenation
  —100% FIO_2 for 5 minutes
- Premedication
  —Performed 2–3 minutes prior to administration of SCh
  —Minimize the rise in ICP
  -Defasciculating dose of vecuronium or pancuronium
  -Fentanyl
  -Lidocaine
  —Reactive airway disease
  -Lidocaine
  —Attenuate the vagal effect in children
  -Atropine
- Paralysis/Induction
  —Administration of an induction agent followed immediately by SCh
  —Thiopental
  -Contraindicated in the hypovolemic or hypotensive patient
  —Relative contraindications
  -Anticipated difficult oral intubation
  -Open globe injury
  -Organophosphate poisoning
  -Burns >3 days old
- Apply Sellick's maneuver
  —Digital cricoid pressure to occlude the esophagus and prevent regurgitation
- Mask ventilation should be avoided because it will increase the aspiration risk
- Intubation
  —45–60 seconds after SCh administration when the patient has lost muscle tone
  —Use a stylet with the endotracheal tube
  —Inflate the cuff once the tube is placed before bagging
  —Confirm correct placement of endotracheal tube
- For continued paralysis after intubation use vecuronium and a sedative agent

PEDIATRIC CONSIDERATIONS

- Atropine should be given with ketamine to decrease secretions
- A defasciculating dose of neuromuscular blocking agent is not needed for children ≤5 years old

MEDICATIONS

- Atracurium: 0.4–0.5 mg/kg IV
- Atropine: 0.02 mg/kg IV
- Diazepam: 2–10 mg IV (peds: 0.2–0.3 mg/kg)
- Etomidate: 0.3 mg/kg IV
- Fentanyl: 3 μg/kg IV
- Ketamine: 1–2 mg/kg IV or 4–7 mg/kg IM
- Lidocaine: 1.5 mg/kg IV
- Midazolam: 1–5 mg (0.07–0.3 mg/kg for induction) IV
- Propofol: 2–2.5 mg/kg IV
- Pancuronium: 0.01 mg/kg (defasciculating dose) IV; 0.1 mg/kg (paralyzing dose) IV
- Succinylcholine: 1.5 mg/kg (peds: 2 mg/kg) IV; 2.5 mg/kg IM or subcutaneous; 0.15 mg/kg (defasciculating pretreatment dose)
- Thiopental: 3 mg/kg IV
- Vecuronium: 0.01 mg/kg (defasciculating dose) IV; 0.1 mg/kg (paralyzing dose) IV

Disposition

ADMISSION CRITERIA

- All intubated patients should be admitted to an ICU

DISCHARGE CRITERIA

- Certain ED patients who have been intubated for airway protection or to facilitate diagnostic workup may be extubated in the ED after a period of observation, and then discharged

Miscellaneous

ICD9: N/A

CORE CONTENT CODE 23.1

SUGGESTED READINGS

Benumof JL, ed. Airway management. Principles and practice. St. Louis: CV Mosby, 1996.

Dailey RH, et al., eds. The airway: Emergency management. St. Louis: CV Mosby, 1992.

Walls RM. Airway management. In: Rosen P, et. al., eds. Emergency medicine: Concepts and clinical practice. 3rd ed. St. Louis: CV Mosby, 1992:2–24.

Walls RM. Rapid sequence intubation in head trauma. Ann Emerg Med 1993;22:1008.

Author: Carlo Rosen

Alcohol, Poisoning

Clinical Presentation

SIGNS AND SYMPTOMS

Acute Alcohol Intoxication

- Sedation
- Relaxation
- Euphoria
- Memory loss
- Poor judgement
- Ataxia/slurred speech
- Nausea/vomiting
- Obtundation/coma

Alcohol Withdrawal Syndrome

Early or Minor Withdrawal

- <8 hours after last drink (blood alcohol level becomes zero)
  —Symptoms of a hangover
  —Headache
  —Nausea/vomiting
- 12 hours after last drink
  —Mild tremors/anxiety
  —Anorexia, nausea, vomiting
  —Weakness
  —Myalgia
  —Vivid dreams/nightmares
- 12–36 hours after last drink
  —Irritable/agitated
  —Tachycardia/hypertension
  —Tremors in hands and tongue
- Alcohol hallucinosis
  —24 hours after last drink
  —Visual most common (bug crawling)
  —Auditory (buzz, clicks)
  —Present in minor and major withdrawal
- Alcoholic withdrawal seizures
  —8–12 hours after last drink
  —Brief, spontaneously abating tonic-clonic activity
  —Before delirium tremors (DT)

Late Alcohol Withdrawal or Major Withdrawal

- 48 hours after last drink
- Delirium tremors
  —Clouding of consciousness and delirium (hallmark)
  —Confusion, hyperactive, disoriented
  —Highly agitated
  —Systolic hypertension/tachycardia
  —Fever
  —Diaphoresis

MECHANISM/DESCRIPTION

Alcohol Intoxication

- Direct CNS depressant effect
- Blood alcohol levels drop by 15–45 mg/dl/hr depending on individual variables and chronicity of alcohol use

Alcohol Withdrawal

- Occurs after partial or complete alcohol abstinence in a chronic alcoholic
- CNS excitation
- Increased catecholamine levels
- Decrease in inhibitory activity of presynaptic α_2-receptors

PEDIATRIC CONSIDERATION

- Coma more common in adolescents at a lower alcohol level than adults
- Hypoglycemia occurs in acutely intoxicated children

Pre-Hospital

N/A

Diagnosis

ESSENTIAL WORKUP

- Investigate for life-threatening causes of seizures: hypoglycemia, intracranial hematoma, CNS infection, and electrolyte abnormalities
- Obtain accurate alcohol drinking/abstinence history
- Evaluate for major trauma

LABORATORY

- Electrolytes, BUN, creatinine, and glucose
- CBC
- Magnesium, calcium, and phosphate
  —With seizures
- PT if coagulopathy suspected
- Alcohol and toxicology screen
- Liver function test if liver disease suspected
- Ammonia level if hepatic encephalopathy suspected

IMAGING/ SPECIAL TESTS

- CT of head if
  —Altered mental status in greater proportion to intoxication
  —Suspect head trauma
  —Partial (focal) seizures
  —Signs of increase intracranial pressure or focal findings in neurologic exams
  —Acute head trauma and seizure
  —New onset seizure
  —Unimproved or deteriorating level of consciousness
- EEG differentiates alcohol withdrawal seizures from idiopathic epilepsy
- CXR if suspect pneumonia (fever, tachypnea, or abnormal lung exam)

DIFFERENTIAL DIAGNOSIS

Alcohol Withdrawal Related Seizures

- Withdrawal (Alcohol or drugs)
- Idiopathic or posttraumatic epilepsy exacerbations
- Acute intoxication or poisoning (carbon monoxide, isoniazid, amphetamine, anticholinergic, stimulant, phenothiazine)
- Infection (meningitis, encephalitis, brain abscess)
- Trauma (intracranial hemorrhage)
- CVA
- Tumor
- Noncompliance with anticonvulsant

Acute Alcohol Intoxication

- Hypoglycemia
- Carbon dioxide narcosis
- Mixed-drug overdoses
- Ethylene glycol and methanol poisoning
- Hepatic encephalopathy
- Psychosis
- Severe vertigo
- Psychomotor seizure

Treatment

INITIAL STABILIZATION

- ABCs
- Evaluate C-spine if associated trauma
- IV rehydration with D5.09% NS
- Administer narcan, thiamine, and glucose (or Accucheck) if altered mental status

ED TREATMENT

Alcohol Withdrawal Syndrome

- Benzodiazepine is drug of choice (lorazepam, diazepam, chlordiazepoxide)
  —Cross-tolerant to alcohol
  —Anticonvulsant effect
  —Large doses required with significant withdrawal
- Barbiturates (phenobarbital)
  —Cross-tolerant with alcohol
  —Anticonvulsant effect
  —Caution: narrow therapeutic index; high abuse potential; and its withdrawal can lead to seizures
- Butyrophenones (haloperidol)
  —Dopamine blocker, low anticholinergic, and fewer cardiovascular effects
  —Use with major withdrawal or DT with hallucinations that do not respond to benzodiazepines
- β-blocker (propranolol and atenolol)
  —Resolves symptoms secondary to noradrenergic activity: tremors, tachycardia
  —Consider as an adjunct in moderate withdrawal
- α-agonist (clonidine)
  —Centrally acting α_2-adrenergic agonist
  —Reduces the increased norepinephrine release in the brain causing sedation, lower blood pressure, and lower heart rate
  —No anticonvulsant effect
- Phenytoin
  —Not indicated in alcohol withdrawal seizures
  —Indicated if seizures secondary to idiopathic epilepsy, posttraumatic, or status epilepticus

Fluid and Electrolyte Disturbances

- Replete magnesium if
  —Hypomagnesemia
  —Clinical signs of ataxia, vertigo, hyperactive reflexes, tremors, athetoid and choreiform movements, Babinski sign, and hyperacusis
  —Hypokalemia
- Correct hyponatremia/hypokalemia
- Alcoholic ketoacidosis
  —Aggressive rehydration with D5.9% NS

MEDICATIONS

- Chlordiazepoxide (librium): 25–100 mg, PO or IV q 6h
- Dextrose: D50W 1 amp (50 ml or 25 g) (peds: D25W 2–4 ml/kg) IV
- Diazepam: 5 mg IV q 5–10 minutes until patient calm
- Haloperidol: 5–10 mg IV
- Lorazepam: 0.5–4 mg IV/IM q 5–10 minutes until patient calm
- Naloxone (Narcan): 2 mg (peds: 0.1 mg/kg) IV or IM initial dose
- Pentobarbital: 100 mg IV q 5–10 minutes until patient is calm or up to 600 mg
- Phenytoin: 15–18 mg/kg at 50 mg/min IV
- Thiamine (vitamin B_1): 100 mg (peds: 50 mg) IV or IM

Disposition

ADMISSION CRITERIA

- Hepatic failure, infection, dehydration, malnutrition, cardiovascular collapse, cardiac dysrhythmia, trauma
- Hallucinations, tachycardia >100/min, severe tremors, extreme agitation
- Wernicke's encephalopathy
- Confusion or delirium

DISCHARGE CRITERIA

- Clinically sober
- Able to ambulate
- Seizure free for 6 hours (with negative workup if first seizure)

Miscellaneous

ICD9 CODE: 980.0

CORE CONTENT CODE: 17.1.7, 17.2.2.1

SUGGESTED READINGS

Freedland ES, McMicken DB. Alcohol-related seizures, Part I: Pathophysiology, differential diagnosis, and evaluation. J Emerg Med 1993;11:463–473

Freedland ES, McMicken DB. Alcohol-related seizures, Part II: Clinical presentation and management. J Emerg Med 1993;11:605–618

Lamminpaa A. Alcohol intoxication in childhood and adolescence. Alcohol Alcohol 1995;30:5–12

Newman JP, Terris DJ, et al. Trends in the management of alcohol withdrawal syndrome. Laryngoscope 1995;105:1–7

Author: Karyn Cole

Alcoholic Ketoacidosis

Clinical Presentation

SIGNS AND SYMPTOMS

- Dehydration
- Fever absent unless there is an underlying infection
- Tachycardia due to
  - —Dehydration with associated orthostatic changes
  - —Concurrent alcohol withdrawal
- Tachypnea
  - —Common
  - —Deep, rapid, Kussmaul respirations frequently present
- Nausea and vomiting
- Abdominal pain
  - —Usually diffuse with nonspecific tenderness
  - —Rebound tenderness, abdominal distension, hypoactive bowel sounds uncommon
    - -Mandates a search for an alternative, coexistent illness
- Decreased urinary output from hypovolemia
- Mental status
  - —Minimally altered as a result of hypovolemia and possibly intoxication
  - —Altered mental status mandates a search for other associated conditions such as
    - -Head injury, CVA, intracranial hemorrhage
    - -Hypoglycemia
    - -Alcohol withdrawal

MECHANISM/DESCRIPTION

- Increased production of *ketone bodies* due to
  - —Malnourished and hypovolemic patient
  - —Depleted glycogen stores in the liver
  - —Elevated ratio of NADH/NAD due to ethanol metabolism
  - —Increased free fatty acid production
- Elevated NADH/NAD ratio leads to the predominate production of β-hydroxybutyrate (BHB) over acetoacetate (AcAc)

ETIOLOGY

- Malnourished, chronic alcohol abusers following a recent episode of heavy alcohol consumption
  - —Develop nausea/vomiting/abdominal pain
  - —Leading to the cessation of alcohol ingestion
  - —In combination with decreased caloric intake over the preceding several days
- Presentation usually occurs within 12–72 hours

Pre-Hospital

CAUTIONS

- Supportive measures including IV access with 0.9%NS, oxygen, and cardiac monitoring
- Search for historical clues that may suggest other etiologies such as toxic ingestions or diabetic history
- Attend to other possible coexistent illnesses such as GI bleeding

Diagnosis

ESSENTIAL WORKUP

- Presence of an increased anion gap metabolic acidosis secondary to the presence of ketones
- Recent history of alcohol consumption

LABORATORY

Acid Base Disturbance

- Increased anion gap metabolic acidosis hallmark
- Mixed acid base disturbance common
  - —Respiratory alkalosis
  - —Metabolic alkalosis secondary to vomiting and dehydration
  - —Hyperchloremic acidosis
- Mild lactic acidosis common
  - —Due to dehydration and the direct metabolic effects of ethanol
  - —Profound lactic acidosis should prompt a search for other disorders such as seizure, hypoxia, and shock
- Positive urine and serum nitroprusside reaction tests
  - —May not reflect the severity of the underlying ketoacidosis since BHB predominates and is not measured by this test
  - —May become misleadingly more positive during treatment as more AcAc is produced

Electrolytes

- Decreased serum bicarbonate
- Hypokalemia due to vomiting
- Hypocalcemia
- Hypophosphatemia
- Glucose
  - —Usually mildly elevated
  - —Hypoglycemia may be present
- BUN and creatinine mildly elevated due to dehydration

CBC

- Mild leukocytosis
- Thrombocytopenia and anemia commonly due to chronic alcoholism

Urinalysis

- Ketonuria without glucosuria

Amylase/Lipase

- Elevated with associated pancreatitis

Liver Function Tests

- Mildly elevated LFT

IMAGING/SPECIAL TESTS

- CXR if suspect associated pneumonia
- Abdominal films for free air if an acute abdomen is present
- CT scan of the head if associated trauma or unexplained altered mental status

DIFFERENTIAL DIAGNOSIS

- Increased anion gap metabolic acidosis
  - —Lactic acidosis
  - —Carbon monoxide poisoning
  - —Aspirin
  - —Methanol
  - —Ethylene glycol
  - —Paraldehyde
  - —Isoniazid
  - —Diabetic ketoacidosis—more severe hyperglycemia/diabetic history
- Hypovolemia
  - —GI bleeding
  - —Sepsis
- Abdominal pain
  - —Pancreatitis
  - —GI bleeding
  - —Gastritis
  - —Hepatitis
  - —Perforated ulcer
  - —Alcohol withdrawal

Treatment

INITIAL STABILIZATION

- Cardiac monitor and supplemental oxygen
- Narcan, thiamine, and dextrose if altered mental status
- IV: 0.9%NS
  - —500 cc–1 L bolus
  - —Promotes renal excretion of ketone bodies

ED TREATMENT

- Antiemetic for vomiting—promethazine or prochlorperazine
- Benzodiazepines for symptoms of alcohol withdrawal
- Start dextrose containing solutions (D5W0.9%NS)
  - —Avoid with significant hyperglycemia
  - —Repletes glycogen stores
  - —Decreases production of ketone bodies by stimulating the production of endogenous insulin
  - —More rapid resolution of the metabolic abnormalities than saline alone
- Thiamine repletion prior to glucose administration to avoid precipitating Wernicke's encephalopathy
- Sodium bicarbonate rarely indicated
  - —Consider in severe acidosis with associated cardiovascular dysfunction or irritability
- Electrolyte replacement
  - —Hypokalemia occurs with treatment and should be anticipated
  - —Hypophosphatemia may occur with treatment
  - —Magnesium replacement as indicated
- Insulin is not indicated and may precipitate hypoglycemia
- Treatment of associated disorders is usually indicated

MEDICATIONS

- D50W: one ampule of 50% dextrose (25 g) IVP
- Lorazepam (benzodiazepine): 2 mg IV and titrate to effect
- Narcan: 2 mg IVP
- Prochlorperazine: 5–10 mg IVP
- Promethazine: 12.5–25 mg IVP
- Thiamine: 100mg IVP

Disposition

ADMISSION CRITERIA

- Persistent metabolic acidosis
- Persistent orthostatic hypotension
- Persistent nausea and vomiting
- Abdominal pain of uncertain etiology
- Comorbid illness requiring admission for treatment
- Monitored bed due to electrolyte abnormalities requiring continued treatment

DISCHARGE CRITERIA

- Many patients can be managed in observation unit over 12 hours
- Tolerating oral fluids well
- Resolution of metabolic abnormalities
- No other associated illnesses requiring additional therapy

Miscellaneous

ICD9: 276.2

CORE CONTENT CODE: N/A

SUGGESTED READINGS

Adams SL. Alcoholic ketoacidosis. Emerg Med Clin North Am 1990;8(4):749–760

Adams SL, Matthews JJ, Flaherty JJ. Alcoholic ketoacidosis. Ann Emerg Med 1987;16(1):90–97

Duffens K, Marx JA. Alcoholic ketoacidosis—A review. J Emerg Med 1987;5(5):399–406

Wrenn KD, Slovis CM, et al. The syndrome of alcoholic ketoacidosis. Am J Med 1991;91(2):119–128

Author: Jefferson Bracey

Altered Mental Status

Clinical Presentation

SIGNS AND SYMPTOMS

Confusion

- Difficulty in maintaining a coherent stream of thinking and mental performance
  - —Remember to consider the level of education and language
- Inattention
- Memory deficit
  - —Inability to recall any of the following
    - -The date, inclusive of month, day, year, and day of week
    - -The precise place
    - -Items of generally acknowledged and universally known information
    - -Why the patient is in the hospital
    - -Address, zip code, telephone number, or social security number
- Impaired mental performance
  - —Difficulty retaining seven digits forward and four backward
  - —Serial calculations
    - -Holding the result of one calculation in a working memory in order to pursue the next step
    - -Serial 3-from-30 subtraction test
- Disorganized and rambling language
  - —May be mistaken for aphasia

Findings that Suggest an Underlying Cause

- Fever
  - —Infectious etiologies, drug toxicities, endocrine disorders, heat stroke
- Severe hypertension
  - —Suggestive of an intracranial structural lesion
- Hypotension
  - —Infectious and toxicological etiologies
- Eye resting position
  - —Dysconjugate gaze in the horizontal plane occurs with drowsiness
  - —Dysconjugate gaze in the vertical plane occurs with pontine or cerebellar lesions
  - —Sustained conjugate downward eye deviation occurs with a variety of neurologic disorders
  - —Sustained conjugate upward gaze occurs with hypoxic encephalopathy
  - —Ocular bobbing
    - -Cyclical brisk conjugate caudal jerks of the globes followed by a slow return to midposition
    - -Bilateral pontine damage, metabolic derangement, and brainstem compression
  - —Ocular dipping
    - -Slow, cyclical, conjugate, downward movement of the eyes followed by a rapid return to midposition
    - -Diffuse cortical anoxic damage
- Pupillary examination
  - —Normal size, shape, and response to light indicates intact midbrain function
  - —Nearly all toxic and metabolic causes of coma leave the pupillary reflexes sluggish but bilaterally intact
- Focal findings
  - —Hemiparesis
  - —Hemianopia
  - —Aphasia
  - —Myoclonus
  - —Convulsions
- Asterixis
  - —Arrhythmic flapping tremor
  - —Caused by metabolic encephalopathy
    - -Hepatic failure
    - -Anticonvulsant drug ingestion
- Myoclonic jerking and tremor
  - —Uremic encephalopathy
  - —Antipsychotic drug ingestion

MECHANISM/DESCRIPTION

- Dysfunction in either the reticular activating system in the upper brainstem or a large area of one of the cerebral hemispheres
- Definitions
  - —Clouding of consciousness
    - -Confusion: a behavioral state of reduced mental clarity, coherence, comprehension, and reasoning
  - —Diminished consciousness
    - -Drowsiness: the patient cannot be easily aroused by touch or noise and cannot maintain alertness for some time
    - -Stupor: the patient can be awakened only by vigorous stimuli, and an effort to avoid uncomfortable or aggravating stimulation is displayed
    - -Coma: the patient cannot be aroused by stimulation and no purposeful attempt is made to avoid painful stimuli

ETIOLOGY

- Hypoxic
  - —Severe pulmonary disease
  - —Anemia
  - —Shock
- Metabolic
  - —Hypoglycemia
  - —Diabetic ketoacidosis
  - —Nonketotic hyperosmolar coma
  - —Thiamine deficiency
  - —Hyperammonemia
  - —Uremia
  - —CO_2 narcosis
  - —Hyperglycemia
  - —Hyponatremia; hypernatremia
  - —Hypocalcemia; hypercalcemia
  - —Hypomagnesemia; hypermagnesemia
  - —Hypophosphatemia
  - —Acidosis; alkalosis
- Toxicologic
  - —Ethanol
  - —Isopropyl alcohol
  - —Methanol
  - —Ethylene glycol
  - —Salicylates
  - —Sedatives and narcotics
  - —Anticonvulsants
  - —Psychotropics
  - —Isoniazid
  - —Heavy metals
  - —Carbon monoxide
  - —Cyanide
- Endocrine
  - —Myxedema coma
  - —Thyrotoxicosis
  - —Addison's disease
  - —Cushing's disease
  - —Pheochromocytoma
- Environmental
  - —Hypothermia
  - —Heat stroke
  - —Neuroleptic malignant syndrome
  - —Malignant hyperthermia
- Intracranial hypertension
- Hypertensive encephalopathy
- Pseudotumor cerebri
- CNS Inflammation
- Meningitis
- Encephalitis
- Encephalopathy
- Cerebral vasculitis
  - —TTP
  - —Subarachnoid hemorrhage
  - —Carcinoid meningitis
  - —Traumatic axonal shear injury
  - —Primary neuronal or glial disorders
  - —Creutzfeldt-Jakob disease
  - —Marchiafava-Bignami disease
  - —Adrenoleukodystrophy
  - —Gliomatosis cerebri
  - —Progressive multifocal leukoencephalopathy
  - —Seizures and postictal state
  - —Supratentorial Lesions
  - —Hemorrhage
  - —Infarction
  - —Tumors
  - —Abscess
  - —Subtentorial Lesions
  - —Cerebellar hemorrhage
  - —Posterior fossa subdural or extradural hemorrhage
  - —Cerebellar infarct
  - —Cerebellar tumor
  - —Cerebellar abscess
  - —Basilar aneurysm
  - —Pontine hemorrhage
  - —Brainstem infarct
  - —Basilar migraine
  - —Brainstem demyelination

Pre-Hospital

CAUTIONS

- Airway management if loss of airway patency
- Supplemental oxygen
- Bag-mask ventilation with cricoid pressure
- Endotracheal intubation if no response to coma cocktail
- Intravenous access
- Coma cocktail
  —Dextrose
  —Naloxone
  —Thiamine
- Monitor patient
- Look for signs of an underlying cause
  —Medications
  —Medic alert bracelets
  —Document a basic neurologic examination
  —GCS
  —Pupils
  —Extremity movements

CONTROVERSIES

- Empirical dextrose should not be held or delayed if dextrostix is not available
  —Glucose can be safely administered before thiamine
  —Glucose does not worsen outcome in patients with stroke

Diagnosis

ESSENTIAL WORKUP

LABORATORY

- Dextrostix and glucose
- CBC
- Electrolytes
- BUN, creatinine
- Calcium
- Arterial blood gases
- Toxicologic screen
- Alcohol screen if toxic alcohols are suspected and serum osmolarity

IMAGING/SPECIAL TESTS

- Caloric stimulation of the vestibular apparatus
- Indicated to assess unresponsive patients
- Tympanic membrane perforation and cerumen impaction should be excluded
- Irrigate the external auditory canal with 10 cc of ice-cold water after elevating the head to 30°
- Bilateral tonic deviation of the eyes toward the stimulus indicates an intact brainstem
- Nystagmuslike quick corrective phases indicates intact cerebral hemispheres
- A normal response in an unresponsive patient raises the suspicion of psychogenic coma
- CT scan
  —Noncontrast only to rule out hemorrhage and mass effect
- Lumbar puncture
  —Indicated when the etiology remains unclear after laboratory and CT scan
  —Empiric antibiotics should be administered before the lumbar puncture to avoid any delay in therapy in patients with meningitis

DIFFERENTIAL DIAGNOSIS

- Locked in syndrome
  —Rare disorder caused by damage to the corticospinal, corticopontine, and corticobulbar tracts resulting in quadriplegia and mutism with preservation of consciousness
  —Communication may be established through eye movements
- Psychogenic unresponsiveness
  —Conversion reactions
  —Catatonia
- Malingering
- Akinetic mutism
- Dementia
  —The mental status waxes and wanes
  —Confusion due to poor recollection
  —Attention is preserved in the early stages

Treatment

INITIAL STABILIZATION

- Intravenous D_{50}
  —Empiric use when not administered in the field or dextrostix is unavailable
- Naloxone
- Thiamine

ED TREATMENT

- Consider empirical use of antibiotics for altered mental status of undetermined etiology
  —Broad spectrum with good CSF penetration such as ceftriaxone
- Empiric treatment if a toxic ingestion is suspected
  —Activated charcoal
  —Alcohol drip if methanol or ethylene glycol is suspected
- Correct body temperature
  —Warmed humidified O_2 if hypothermic
  —Ice packs and forced air movement over exposed wetted skin if severe hyperthermia
- Specific therapy directed at underlying cause once identified

MEDICATIONS

- Ceftriaxone: 100 mg/kg IV
- Dextrose: 1–2 ml/kg of $D_{50}W$ IV; neonate: 10 ml/kg $D_{10}W$ IV; peds: 4 ml/kg $D_{25}W$ IV
- Diazepam: 0.1–0.3 mg/kg slow IV (max 10 mg/dose) q 10–15 min × 3 doses
- Lorazepam: 0.05–0.1 mg/kg IV (max 4 mg/dose q 10–15 min)
- Naloxone: 0.01 mg/kg IV/IM/SC/ET
- Thiamine: 100 mg IM or 100 mg thiamine in 1000 ml of intravenous fluid wide open

Disposition

ADMISSION CRITERIA

All patients with acute changes in mental status require admission

DISCHARGE CRITERIA

Chronic altered mental status (e.g. dementia) without change from baseline

Miscellaneous

ICD9: 293.0, 293.81, 293.82, 294.1, 294.8

CORE CONTENT CODE: N/A

SUGGESTED READINGS

Hoffman RS, Goldfrank LR. The poisoned patient with altered consciousness. Controversies in the use of a "coma cocktail." JAMA 1995;274:562–69.

Samuels MA. The evaluation of comatose patients. Hosp Pract 1993;28:165–82.

Author: Richard Wolfe; David Brown

Amenorrhea

Clinical Presentation

SIGNS AND SYMPTOMS

- Absence of menstruation
- Low estrogen: atrophic vaginal mucosa, mood swings, and irritability
- High androgen: truncal obesity, hirsutism, acne, male-pattern baldness

MECHANISM/DESCRIPTION

- Primary: no spontaneous uterine bleeding by age 14 in the absence of the development of secondary sexual characteristics or by age 16 with otherwise normal development
- Secondary: absence of menstrual bleeding for 6 months in a woman with prior regular menses or for 12 months in a woman with prior oligomenorrhea

ETIOLOGY

- Pregnancy
- Menopause, ovarian failure
- Asherman's syndrome (intrauterine adhesions)
- Dysfunction of the hypothalamic-pituitary-ovarian axis
- Endocrinopathies
- Gonadal dysgenesis
- Obesity, starvation, intense exercise
- Drugs: oral contraceptives, antipsychotics, antidepressants, calcium channel blockers, chemotherapeutic agents, digitalis, marijuana
- Chromosomal abnormalities
- Autoimmune disorders

Pre-Hospital

- If amenorrhea is the result of pregnancy, stabilize patient according to specific abnormalities of pregnancy

Diagnosis

ESSENTIAL WORKUP

- Pregnancy test

LABORATORY

- If pregnancy test is negative, no further testing needed emergently
- May send TSH, prolactin, LH, FSH for follow-up by gynecology

IMAGING/SPECIAL TESTS

- None needed emergently

DIFFERENTIAL DIAGNOSIS

- Pregnancy

Treatment

INITIAL STABILIZATION

N/A

ED TREATMENT

- Reassurance and referral to gynecology

MEDICATIONS

- Defer for gynecology evaluation

Disposition

ADMISSION CRITERIA

- No need for admission

DISCHARGE CRITERIA

- All patients can be discharged with gynecology referral

Miscellaneous

ICD9: 626.0

CORE CONTENT CODE: 19.1.3.2

SUGGESTED READINGS

Kiningham RB, Apgar BS, Schwenk TL. Evaluation of amenorrhea. Am Fam Physician 1996;53(4):1185–1194.

Warren MP. Evaluation of secondary amenorrhea. J Clin Endocrinol Metab 1996;81(2):437–442.

Author: Christy Rosa

Clinical Presentation

SIGNS AND SYMPTOMS

Central Nervous System (CNS)

- Agitation
- Delirium
- Hyperactivity
- Tremors
- Dizziness
- Mydriasis
- Headache
- Choreoathetoid movements
- Hyperreflexia
- Cerebrovascular accident
- Seizures and status epilepticus
- Coma

Psychiatric

- Euphoria
- Increased aggressiveness
- Anxiety
- Hallucinations (visual, tactile)
- Compulsive repetitious actions

Cardiovascular

- Palpitations
- Hypertensive crisis
- Tachycardia or (reflex) bradycardia
- Dysrhythmias (usually tachydysrhythmias)
- Cardiovascular collapse

Other

- Rhabdomyolysis
- Myoglobinuria
- Acute renal failure
- Anorexia
- Diaphoresis
- Disseminated intravascular coagulation (DIC)

DESCRIPTION/MECHANISM

- Increased release of norepinephrine, dopamine, serotonin
- Decreased catecholamine reuptake
- Direct effect on α- and β-adrenergic receptors

ETIOLOGY

- Prescription drugs
  —Amphetamine (benzedrine)
  —Dextroamphetamine (Dexedrine)
  —Diethylpropion (Tenuate)
  —Fenfluramine (Pondimin)
  —Methamphetamine
  —Methylphenidate (Ritalin)
  —Phenmetrazine (Preludin)
  —Phentermine
- "Designer drugs"
  —Variants of illegal parent drugs
  —Often synthesized in "underground" laboratories
  —"Ice"
    -Crystalline methamphetamine hydrochloride
    -Smoked, insufflated, or injected
    -Rapid onset; duration several hours
  —"Crank"
  —"Ecstasy" (3,4,-methylenedioxymethamphetamine, MDMA, XTC)
    -Often used at dances and "rave" parties
    -Dehydration can lead to hyperthermia, fatality
  —MDA (3,4,-methylenedioxyamphetamine)
  —Methcathinone ("cat," "jeff," "mulka")
    -Derivative of cathinone, found in the evergreen tree *catha edulis*
    -Frequently synthesized in home laboratories
    -Does not show up on urine toxicology screens

Pre-Hospital

CAUTIONS

- Patient may be uncooperative or violent
- Secure IV access
- Protect from self-induced trauma

Diagnosis

ESSENTIAL WORKUP

- Vital signs
  —Temperature
    -Rectal temperature most reliable
    -Temperature >40 ° C indication for urgent cooling
  —Blood pressure
    -Severe hypertension can lead to cardiac and neurologic abnormalities
    -Late in course, hypotension may supervene
- ECG
  —Ventricular tachydysrhythmias
  —Reflex bradycardia

LABORATORY

- Urinalysis
  —Blood
  —Myoglobin
- Electrolytes, BUN/Cr, glucose
  —Hypoglycemia may contribute to altered mental status
  —Acidosis may accompany severe toxicity
  —Rhabdomyolysis may cause renal failure
  —Hyperkalemia—life-threatening consequence of acute renal failure
- Coagulation profile
  —PT, PTT, platelets
  —For DIC
- CPK
  —Markedly elevated in rhabdomyolysis
- Urine toxicology screen
  —For other toxins with similar effects (e.g., cocaine)
  —Some amphetamine-like substances (e.g., methcathinone) may not be detected
- ABG

IMAGING/SPECIAL TESTS

- CXR for
  —Adult respiratory distress syndrome
  —Noncardiogenic pulmonary edema
- CT (head)
  —Indications
    -Significant headache
    -Altered mental status
    -Focal neurologic signs
  —For subarachnoid hemorrhage, intracerebral bleed
- Lumbar puncture
  —Indications
    -Suspected meningitis (headache, altered mental status, hyperpyrexia)
    -Suspected subarachnoid hemorrhage
  —Indicated if subarachnoid hemorrhage suspected and CT normal

DIFFERENTIAL DIAGNOSIS

Drugs that Cause Delirium

- Anticholinergics
  —Belladonna alkaloids
  —Antihistamines
  —Tricyclic antidepressants
- Cocaine
- Ethanol withdrawal
- Sedative/hypnotic withdrawal
- Hallucinogens
- Phencyclidine

Drugs that Cause Hypertension and Tachycardia

- Sympathomimetics
- Anticholinergics
- Ethanol withdrawal
- Phencyclidine
- Caffeine
- Phenylpropanolamine
- Ephedrine
- Monoamine oxidase inhibitors
- Theophylline
- Nicotine

Drugs that Cause Seizures

- Carbon monoxide
- Carbamazepine
- Cyanide
- Cocaine
- Cholinergics (organophosphate insecticides)
- Camphor
- Chlorinated hydrocarbons

- Ethanol withdrawal
- Sedative/hypnotic withdrawal
- Isoniazid
- Theophylline
- Hypoglycemics
- Lead
- Lithium
- Local anesthetics
- Anticholinergics
- Phencyclidine
- Phenothiazines
- Phenytoin
- Propoxyphene
- Salicylates
- Strychnine

Treatment

INITIAL STABILIZATION

- ABCs
- Establish IV 0.9%NS access
- Cardiac monitor
- Naloxone, dextrose (or Accucheck) and thiamine if altered mental status

ED TREATMENT

Decontamination

- Gastric lavage
  - —Indicated for recent (1–2 hours) and life-threatening ingestions
  - —Instill activated charcoal through large-bore orogastric tube both before and after lavage
- Administer activated charcoal with sorbitol

Hypertensive Crisis

- Initially administer benzodiazepines if agitated
- α-Blocker (phentolamine) as second-line agent
- Nitroprusside for severe, unresponsive hypertension

Agitation, Acute Psychosis

- Administer benzodiazepines

Hyperthermia

- Benzodiazepines if agitated
- Emergent cooling if temperature >40°C
  - —Tepid water mist
  - —Evaporate with fan
  - —Paralysis
    - -Indicated if muscle rigidity and hyperactivity contributing to persistent hyperthermia
    - -Nondepolarizing agent (e.g., pancuronium)
    - -Intubation; mechanical ventilation
  - —Administer acetaminophen
  - —Apply cooling blankets

Rhabdomyolysis

- Administer benzodiazepines
- Hydrate with 0.9%NS
- Maintain urine output at 1–2 ml/min
- Hemodialysis (if acute renal failure and hyperkalemia occur)

Seizures

- Maintain airway
- Administer benzodiazepines
- Phenobarbital if unresponsive to benzodiazepines
- Phenytoin contraindicated

MEDICATIONS

- Activated charcoal slurry: 1–2 g/kg up to 90 g PO
- Dextrose: D50W 1 amp (50 ml or 25 g) (ped: D25W 2–4 ml/kg) IV
- Diazepam (benzodiazepine): 5–10 mg (ped: 0.2–0.5 mg/kg) IV
- Lorazepam (benzodiazepine): 2–6 mg (ped: 0.03–0.05 mg/kg) IV
- Nitroprusside: 1–8 μg/kg/min IV (titrated to blood pressure)
- Phenobarbital: 15–20 mg/kg at 25–50 mg/min until cessation of seizure activity
- Phentolamine: 1–5 mg IV over 5 minutes (titrated to blood pressure)
- Sorbitol: 1–2 g/kg to maximum 100 g po mixed in the activated charcoal slurry (ped: >1-year-old: 1–1.5 g/kg as a 35% solution to a max of 50 g)

Disposition

ADMISSION CRITERIA

- Hyperthermia
- Persistent altered mental status
- Hypertensive crisis
- Seizures
- Rhabdomyolysis
- Persistent tachycardia

DISCHARGE CRITERIA

- Asymptomatic after 6 hours observation
- Absence of above admission criteria

Miscellaneous

ICD9: 969.7

CORE CONTENT CODE: 17.2.43.1

SUGGESTED READINGS

Callaway CW, Clark RF. Hyperthermia in psychostimulant overdose. Ann Emerg Med 1994;24:68–75

Chan P, Chen JH, Lee MH, et al. Fatal and nonfatal methamphetamine intoxication in the intensive care unit. Clin Toxicol 1994;32:147–155

Derlet RW, Rice P, Horowitz BZ, et al. Amphetamine toxicity: Experience with 127 cases. J Emerg Med 1989;7:157–161

Emerson TS, Cisek JE. Methcathinone: A Russian designer amphetamine infiltrates the rural midwest. Ann Emerg Med 1993;22:1897–1903

Henry JA, Jeffreys KJ, Dawling S. Toxicity and deaths from 3,4-methylenedioxymethamphetamine ("ecstasy"). Lancet 1992;340:384–387

Author: Leon Gussow

Amputation, Traumatic/Reimplantation

Clinical Presentation

SIGNS AND SYMPTOMS

- The presentation of complete traumatic amputation is generally obvious
- Partial amputations may present with or without the vascular pedicle intact
  —Distal part may be dusky, and cyanotic
  —Decreased sensation, and 2-point discrimination
  —Delayed capillary refill, diminished or absent pulses
- Avoid being sidetracked by visually striking injuries. Evaluate for other relevant and perhaps life-threatening causes of shock

MECHANISM/DESCRIPTION

- Traumatic amputations result from motor vehicle accidents, crush injuries, injuries from heavy equipment or machinery, high speed tools, degloving injuries to digits, mammalian bites, and many other causes
- Warm ischemia time is approximately 4–6 hours
- Cold ischemia time: up to 12 hours for parts containing muscle; up to 30 hours for digits

Pre-Hospital

CAUTIONS

- Collect all amputated parts, including pieces of bone, tissue, skin
- For care of amputated parts, see Initial Stabilization principles below
- Transport to the nearest microvascular reimplantation center
- Time is of the essence and air transport from remote locations may be necessary

Diagnosis

ESSENTIAL WORKUP

- A general assessment of circulation, sensation, and function should be performed
  —Pulses, capillary refill (abnormal if delayed more than 2 seconds), and 2-point discrimination tests (abnormal if cannot distinguish between 1 and 2 points set apart by 5 mm on the hand)
  —Include Allen test for hand injuries
  -Compress radial artery firmly at the wrist while patient clenches fist tightly and then relaxes (hand in neutral position). Watch for return of pink color. Repeat maneuver while compressing ulnar artery. Persistence of pallor indicates occlusion of the opposite artery
- Pulse oximetry of a partially amputated part may be helpful in the assessment of vascular injury
- X-ray of the amputated part and amputation site to assess for bony injury

LABORATORY

- Laboratory tests are directed by a patient's condition, other medical issues, and amount of estimated blood loss
- CBC, PT/PTT, type and crossmatch, ECG, CXR is needed for preoperative evaluation

IMAGING/SPECIAL TESTS

- Radiographs to assess extent of fractures and presence of foreign body

DIFFERENTIAL DIAGNOSIS

- Near versus complete amputation
- Laceration of skin, muscle, or tendon

Treatment

INITIAL STABILIZATION

- Goals of ED treatment
  —Control hemorrhage
  —Avoid further damage to the injured part
  —Limit ischemia of the amputated part
  —Arrange expeditious consultation by appropriate surgical specialist
- Control hemorrhage
  —Apply direct pressure (bulky pressure dressing) and elevate the proximal stump
  —If above ineffective, apply pressure to pressure points
  —Use tourniquet as last resort (may damage blood vessels and nerves and possibly preclude reimplantation)
  —Tighten tourniquet (blood pressure cuff preferable) just tight enough to stop bleeding
  —Avoid hemostats, cautery, or vessel ligation
- Maintain normal blood volume with IV fluids. Treat shock and other injuries as appropriate
- Care of amputated part (same if complete or partial)
  —Gently irrigate with LR or NS (no soaps or betadine), avoid vigorous scrubbing
  —Wrap in gauze or cloth moistened with LR or NS
  —Place in clean, dry plastic bag
  —Place sealed bag in wet ice or refrigerator at 4°C
  —*Never place directly on ice*

ED TREATMENT

- In general, assume patient is a candidate for reimplantation until qualified surgical consultation is obtained
- Considerations in the decision to replant include
  —Age (younger patients have better outcomes)
  —Occupation
  —Patient motivation
  —General physical condition/other medical problems
  —Mechanism of injury (reimplantation more successful with clean laceration than with crush or avulsion)
  —Location of amputation (the more distal the better, upper extremity better than lower extremity)
  —Condition of the amputated part
  —Degree of contamination
  —Length of time from amputation
- General indications for reimplantation
  —Thumb
  —Multiple digits
  —Metacarpal amputation (palm)
  —Almost any body part in a child
  —Wrist and forearm
  —Elbow or proximal arm (only sharply or moderately avulsed, ischemia time critical)

—Individual digit distal to FDS insertion (functional and aesthetic limitations)
- Relative contraindications for reimplantation
  —Severely crushed or mangled parts
  —Amputations at multiple levels
  —Amputations in patients with other serious injuries or diseases
  —Arteriosclerotic vessels
  —Mentally unstable patients
  —Individual finger in adults proximal to FDS insertion
  —Ring avulsion
  —Prolonged warm ischemia
- Tetanus prophylaxis
- Antibiotics: the role of prophylactic antibiotics is unclear and depends on the amount of contamination. The antibiotic should have antistaphylococcal and Gram-negative coverage, e.g. cefazolin
- Keep patient NPO
- Pain medication

Fingertip Injuries

- Defined as distal to the insertion of the flexor and extensor tendons
- Primary goal is a painless fingertip with durable and sensate skin
- Soft-tissue loss without exposed bone: options include
  —Treat conservatively, cover with nonadherent dressing and allow the wound to heal by secondary intention (best for small or moderate-sized defects)
  —Apply a skin or composite graft
- Soft-tissue loss with exposed bone: Rarely is there sufficient local tissue to close primarily.
- Nonmicrovascular attachment of the fingertip as a composite graft is not recommended in adults.
- Options include
  —Shortening of the bone below the level of the skin with primary closure
  —Coverage by local or regional flaps
  —Microsurgical reimplantation for thumbs (because of functional importance) or fingers if at, or proximal to the distal interphalangeal (DIP) joint
- Traumatic ischemia is an accepted indication for hyperbaric oxygen therapy (HBO) after reimplantation or grafting has been performed
  —Prevent tissue reperfusion injury

MEDICATIONS

- Cefazolin: 0.5–1.5 g IV/IM q 6–8 hrs (peds: 25–50 mg/kg/day divided q 6–8 hrs)

PEDIATRIC CONSIDERATIONS

- Reimplantation is almost always attempted in children regardless of the severity of injury
- In fingertip injuries, conservative management is preferred
  —Children under 12 years: spontaneous regeneration of the fingertip occurs, usually with good cosmetic results
  —Nonmicrosurgical reattachment of the cleanly amputated fingertip as a composite graft can also be successful

Disposition

ADMISSION CRITERIA

- Hospitalization is required for all but trivial amputations and degloving injuries

DISCHARGE CRITERIA

- Minor injuries (e.g., fingertip amputations or mild degloving injuries closed primarily with stable vascular supply) can be discharged with orthopedic or surgical follow-up

Miscellaneous

ICD9: 886.0

CORE CONTENT CODE: 18.4.14.7

SUGGESTED READINGS

Fassler P. Fingertip injuries: Evaluation and treatment. J Am Acad Orthop Surg 1996;4:84–92.

Antosiare L. Hand. In: Rosen P, et al., eds. Emergency medicine: Concepts and clinical practice. 4th ed. St. Louis: CV Mosby, 1998:625–668.

Strauss M. Crush injury and other acute traumatic peripheral ischemias. In: Kindwall E, ed. Hyperbaric medicine practice. Flagstaff, AZ: Best Publishing, 1994.

Author: Mary Anne Fuchs

Amyotrophic Lateral Sclerosis

Clinical Presentation

SIGNS AND SYMPTOMS

- Bilateral weakness with muscle wasting is the most common presentation of amyotrophic lateral sclerosis (ALS)
- There are both lower motor neuron (weakness and wasting with fasciculation) and upper motor neuron signs (Babinski's sign with hyperreflexia)
- Either the arms or the legs may be affected first; late in the disease all of the limbs are affected
- Dysphagia or facial dysarthrias (drooling, dysphagia) occur, but are rarely the presenting symptoms
- Respiratory muscles and the vocal cords are affected late
- Muscle cramps and weight loss are common
- Muscle fasciculation is common but may not be apparent to the patient
- Extraocular muscles, sphincters, cognition, and sensation are spared
- 80% of cases begin between ages 40 and 70 years
- Death (usually from respiratory paralysis) is considered inevitable and most often occurs within 3–5 years of the diagnosis
- Musculoskeletal pain is common late in the disease and is related to complications, not the primary disease

DISEASE DESCRIPTION

- A progressive disease of adults usually manifests by muscle weakness, wasting, fasciculations, Babinski's sign and hyperreflexia. Partial or incomplete forms in which upper or lower motor neuron manifestations predominate also occur

ETIOLOGY

- The etiology of ALS is unknown. Pathologically, there is loss of both upper and lower motor neuron cells with a striking predilection for the motor system and sparing of other neurons

Pre-Hospital

CONTROVERSIES

- Most patients and families will have made a prior decision regarding respiratory support. Unless immediate intervention is essential, intubation should be avoided until these wishes have been ascertained. Noninvasive techniques such as application of oxygen, patient positioning, suctioning, and positive pressure mask ventilation are often alternatives to endotracheal intubation

Diagnosis

ESSENTIAL WORKUP

Previously Undiagnosed ALS

- The diagnosis of ALS is made clinically and rarely in the ED. Recognition of the possibility of this disease is sufficient and mandates referral for workup
- If ALS is suspected in the ED, forced vital capacity (FVC) should be performed

Known ALS Patient

- For patients with known disease who present with progressive symptoms, laboratory and imaging studies are used to evaluate potentially treatable complications
- FVC is a sensitive indicator of respiratory muscle weakness. FVC <50% of predicted is considered a sign of advanced disease. Comparisons with the patient's own previous baseline is useful
- Chest radiography may reveal evidence of aspiration or pneumonia or comorbid conditions such as CHF
- Pulse oximetry and blood gas analysis aid in the diagnosis of respiratory failure, changes tend to occur late in the course of the disease
- Electrolytes and other blood chemistry tests may reveal a treatable cause of increasing weakness
- Cervical spine, other skeletal radiography, or head CT may be needed in case of falls (common in ALS)

LABORATORY AND SPECIAL TESTING

- Electromyography (EMG) may help affirm the diagnosis. When the disease is suspected certain laboratory and imaging studies may be useful to help rule out treatable causes of weakness (see Differential Diagnosis)

DIFFERENTIAL DIAGNOSIS

- Cervical cord compression from tumor or spondylosis with osteophytes—similar clinical symptoms but usually acute onset with pain and sensory changes. Spinal MRI or myelography is used for diagnosis
- Thyrotoxicosis may mimic ALS—it is usually associated with marked systemic symptoms. TSH is best screening test
- Heavy metal (lead, mercury, arsenic) poisoning are suggested by the history. Blood levels are confirmatory
- Syphilis and Lyme disease may cause some of the signs and symptoms of ALS. Serologic tests are useful
- Lymphoma may have an associated lower motor neuron syndrome, which mimics ALS. A bone marrow biopsy is needed to rule this condition out

Treatment

- There is no specific therapy for ALS
- Treatment issues in the ED revolve around symptomatic therapy and identification and treatment of complications

INITIAL STABILIZATION

- Respiratory insufficiency or failure should be treated in the standard manner with the proviso that patient wishes regarding intubation and mechanical ventilation be ascertained and respected
- Weaning off the ventilator is very difficult. Average survival after institution of ventilation is 19 months (range: 1–61 months)

ED TREATMENT

- Sedation and pain control are appropriate for terminally ill patients in distress from respiratory insufficiency
- Joint pain may respond to NSAIDs
- Insomnia from pressure pain (due to immobility) may respond to diphenhydramine or amitriptyline
- Aspiration or drooling may be treated with amitriptyline (dries secretions)
- Muscle cramps may respond to baclofen
- Constipation is related to immobility and diet and is treated with laxatives, stool softeners, and dietary changes

MEDICATIONS

- Amitriptyline: 25–50 mg po qhs
- Baclofen: 10–25 mg po tid
- Diphenhydramine: 25–50 mg po qhs

Disposition

ADMISSION CRITERIA

- Need for respiratory support
- Dehydration, inanition
- Unable to be cared for at home due to progression of illness
- Complication (e.g., infection) that requires admission

DISCHARGE CRITERIA

- *Suspected ALS:* Refer for outpatient evaluation if general condition permits and other serious conditions requiring admission are ruled out
- *Complication of known ALS:* Discharge if effective outpatient treatment available

Miscellaneous

ICD9: 335.20

CORE CONTENT CODE: 11.5.3

SUGGESTED READINGS

Appel SH, Appel LV. Treatment of amyotrophic lateral sclerosis. In: Calne D, ed. Neurodegenerative diseases. 1st ed. Philadelphia: WB Saunders, 1994:523–542

Brooks BR. Natural history of ALS: Symptoms, strength, pulmonary function, and disability. Neurology 1996;47(Suppl 2);S71–S81

Caroscio JT. Amyotrophic lateral sclerosis: A guide to patient care. New York: Thieme Medical Publishers, 1986

Festoff BW. Amyotrophic lateral sclerosis: Current and future treatment strategies. Drugs 1996;51(1);28–44

Rowland LP. Natural history and clinical features of amyotrophic lateral sclerosis and related motor neuron diseases. In: Calne D, ed. Neurodegenerative diseases. 1st ed. Philadelphia: WB Saunders, 1994:507–521

Authors: Richard S. Krause, Paras Pandya

Anal Fissure

Clinical Presentation

SIGNS AND SYMPTOMS

- Sharp, cutting pain with or immediately following a bowel movement
- Bright red blood-streaked stool; small quantity; usually on toilet paper
- Pain and sphincter spasm severe enough to cause stool retention and avoidance of defecation
- Appearance
  - —Initially appears like a cut or break in lining of anal canal
  - —Then becomes more circumscribed and develops well-defined edges
  - —90% occur in the midline posteriorly

MECHANISM/DESCRIPTION

- Linear tear of the anal canal occurring at or just below the dentate line extending distally
- Associated swelling and hypertrophy of the surrounding tissues produce a sentinel pile distally

ETIOLOGY

- Traumatic event produced by the passage of a large hard stool causing a mechanical tear
- Chemical burn associated with an acute episode of diarrhea
- Anal intercourse/sexual abuse

PEDIATRIC CONSIDERATION

- Most common cause of rectal bleeding in infancy
- Fissures can be multiple involving anterior and lateral anal canal
- Often associated with constipation
- Always consider sexual abuse

Pre-Hospital

N/A

Diagnosis

ESSENTIAL WORKUP

- History
- Gentle gradual exposure of the perineum reveals fissure or sentinel pile
- Pain may be so severe that the patient will not allow digital examination
- If lesion is seen in the posterior midline position, rectal exam can be deferred until the patient is having less spasm and pain

LABORATORY

- Hct
  - —Indicated if history suggestive of significant bleeding

DIFFERENTIAL DIAGNOSIS

- If fissure is not found in the midline, it should arouse suspicion for other causes
- Crohn's disease
- Chronic ulcerative colitis
- Carcinomas
- Leukemia
- Lymphoma
- Syphilitic fissures
- Tuberculous ulcers
- Sexual abuse
- Hemorrhoid
- Perirectal abscess

PEDIATRIC CONSIDERATIONS

- Insertion of a clear test tube into the anus may aid visualization of internal fissures

Treatment

INITIAL STABILIZATION

N/A

ED TREATMENT

- Provide symptomatic relief of anal sphincter spasm and prevention of constipation
- Relief of anal sphincter spasm
  - —Warm sitz baths 3 times per day and after each bowel movement for at least 15 minutes at a time
  - —Nonconstipating analgesic (NSAID, acetaminophen)
  - —Benzodiazepine (diazepam) for several days
  - —Use of anesthetic and hydrocortisone containing ointments may delay healing
- Constipation prevention
  - —Add bran to the diet to create a bulky stool preventing constipation and stricture formation
  - —Adequate fluid intake
  - —Docusate sodium and psyllium seeds
  - —Karo syrup or mineral oil for children
- Surgical therapy indicated for fissures in chronic state or intensely painful fissures not responding to conservative measures

MEDICATIONS

- Diazepam (valium): 5 mg po TID PRN
- Docusate sodium (colace): 100 mg (peds: 20–60 mg/day q12–24h) po qd BID
- Psyllium seeds (metamucil): 1 tbs, max 30 g/day (peds: 0.5–1 tsp po qd) po qd TID
- Peds: Karo syrup or mineral oil 15 ml po qd

Disposition

ADMISSION CRITERIA

None

DISCHARGE CRITERIA

- Most anal fissures can be treated conservatively on an outpatient basis
- Presence of significant ulceration, hypertrophied tissue, epithelization, or a sentinel pile suggests chronicity
  - —Refer for operative treatment

Miscellaneous

ICD9: 565.0

CORE CONTENT CODE: 1.8.1.1

SUGGESTED READINGS

Alessandrini EA. Anorectal disease. In: Barkin R, et al., eds. Pediatric emergency medicine: Concepts and clinical practice. 2d ed. St. Louis: CV Mosby, 1997:826–828

Jensen SL. Treatment of first episodes of acute anal fissure: Prospective randomised study of lignocaine ointment versus hydrocortisone ointment or warm sitz baths plus bran. Br Med J 1986;292:1167–1169

Mazier WP. Hemorrhoids, fissures, and pruritus. Ann Surg Clin North Am 1994;74(6):1277–1291

Author: Anthony Best

Anaphylaxis

Clinical Presentation

SIGNS AND SYMPTOMS

- Symptoms begin within seconds to minutes after contact with an offending antigen
- Some patients may have an initial sensation of impending doom followed by more clearly definable symptomatology
- Respiratory: bronchospasm, laryngeal edema
- Cardiovascular: hypotension, dysrhythmias, myocardial ischemia
- Gastrointestinal: nausea, vomiting, diarrhea
- Cutaneous: urticaria, angioedema
- Hematological: activation of intrinsic coagulation pathway sometimes leading to DIC, thrombocytopenia
- Neurological: seizures
- Death can occur from airway obstruction or circulatory collapse

MECHANISM/DESCRIPTION

- An acute, widely distributed form of shock which occurs within minutes of exposure to antigen in a sensitized individual
- There are approximately 400–800 deaths annually in the United States attributed to anaphylaxis
- Release of bioactive molecules such as histamine, leukotrienes, and prostaglandins from inflammatory cells
  - —Mediator release results in increased vascular permeability, vasodilation, smooth-muscle contractions, and increased epithelial secretion
  - —Physiologically this is manifested in a decrease in total peripheral resistance, venous return and cardiac output, as well as intravascular volume depletion

ETIOLOGY

- IgE-mediated
  - —Antibiotics (especially penicillin family)
  - —Venom
  - —Latex
  - —Vaccines
  - —Foodstuffs (shellfish, soybeans, nuts, wheat, milk, eggs, nitrates/nitrites)
- Non-IgE mediated
  - —Iodine contrast media
  - —Opiates
  - —Vancomycin
  - —Quaternary ammonium muscle relaxants

Pre-Hospital

CAUTIONS

- Early intubation is paramount as laryngeal edema and spasm can progress rapidly
- Laryngeal edema can be managed with racemic epinephrine prior to intubation
- Subcutaneous epinephrine (0.5 mg of 1:1000 solution) can be administered en route even prior to establishment of an IV

Diagnosis

ESSENTIAL WORKUP

- Diagnosis is made based on clinical symptoms
  - —It is important not to underestimate the potential severity of an allergic reaction in its early stages
- EKG in patients with previous cardiac history or ischemic symptoms

LABORATORY

- While there are no specific tests necessary to make the diagnosis of anaphylaxis, an arterial blood gas may be helpful in evaluating ventilatory status
- These changes can be noted during anaphylaxis
  - —Elevation of plasma histamine
  - —Increase in hematocrit secondary to fluid extravasation

IMAGING/SPECIAL TESTS

- Hyperinflation on CXR
- EKG abnormalities including dysrhythmias, ischemic changes, infarction

DIFFERENTIAL DIAGNOSIS

- Pulmonary embolism
- Acute myocardial infarction
- Airway obstruction
- Asthma
- Tension pneumothorax
- NSAID reaction
- Vasovagal collapse
- Hereditary angioedema
- Serum sickness
- Systemic mastocytosis
- Pheochromocytoma
- Carcinoid syndrome

Treatment

INITIAL STABILIZATION

- ABCs
  - —Assure adequate ventilation
  - —Endotracheal intubation may be required but difficult because of laryngeal edema or spasm
  - —Transtracheal jet insufflation or cricothyrotomy may be necessary to control the airway
- Epinephrine IV/SQ or endotracheal administration
  - —Direct injection into the venous plexus at the base of the tongue is an option
- Volume resuscitation with crystalloids or colloids
- A tourniquet can be used to decrease venous return from the site of antigen entry

ED TREATMENT

- Continuous cardiac and vital sign monitoring until stable
- Persistent bronchospasm can be treated with β_2-agonist bronchodilators
- Hypotension should be treated with volume repletion
  - —Vasopressors, MAST garments and Trendelenburg positioning are useful adjuncts
- Antihistamines (both H_1 and H_2 blockers) have been shown to be helpful in preventing histamine interactions with target tissues
- Corticosteroids help prevent the progression or recurrence of anaphylaxis
- Glucagon is particularly useful in epinephrine-resistant anaphylaxis from β-adrenergic blocking agents

MEDICATIONS

- Diphenhydramine: adult: 50 mg IV; peds: 1–2 mg/kg slow IVP
- Epinephrine: 0.3–0.5 mg (use 1:1000 dilution for SQ route, and 1:10000 for IV route); peds: epinephrine 0.01 mg/kg SC/IV
- Glucagon: adult: 1 mg IV
- Hydrocortisone: adults: 500 mg IV; peds: 4–8 mg/kg/dose IV
- Methylprednisolone: adult: 125 mg IV; peds: 1–2 mg/kg IV
- Prednisone: adult: 60 mg po; peds: 1 mg/kg po
- Ranitidine: adult: 50 mg IV *or* cimetidine 300 mg IV

Disposition

ADMISSION CRITERIA

- Intubated patients, or patients in respiratory distress should be admitted to an ICU setting
- A monitored bed may be necessary for the patient who has not had substantial response to initial therapy
- Patients with significant generalized reactions and persistent symptoms should be admitted for observation for 24 hours

DISCHARGE CRITERIA

- Patients with complete resolution of symptoms may be discharged after several hours of ED observation
- Patients with allergic reactions should have follow-up within 48 hours of discharge to evaluate effectiveness of outpatient therapy
- A follow-up visit with an allergist is also recommended
- Patients should be advised to carry some type of treatment which can be self-administered in the event of future reactions such as the prefilled syringe *epi-pen*
- Patients with a known trigger should be counseled on strict avoidance of that trigger

Miscellaneous

ICD9: 995.0

CORE CONTENT CODE: 8.8.1

SUGGESTED READINGS

Barach EM, et al. Epinephrine for the treatment of anaphylactic shock. JAMA 1984;251:2118.

Bochner BS, Lichtenstein LM. Anaphylaxis. N Engl J Med 1991;324:1785–1790.

Muelleman RL, et al. Allergy, hypersensitivity and anaphylaxis. In: Rosen P, Barkin R, eds. Emergency medicine. St. Louis: CV Mosby, 1998:2759–2776.

Author: Sean-Xavier Neath

Anemia

Clinical Presentation

SIGNS AND SYMPTOMS

General

- Depends on
  —Rapidity of onset and underlying disease
  —Hemodynamic stability
  —Severity and type of anemia
- Asymptomatic if mild and chronic
- Fatigue
- Decreased exercise intolerance
- Tachypnea
- Heme-positive stool

Cardiovascular

- Dysnea on exertion
- Chest pain/angina
- Syncope
- Tachycardia, cardiomegaly, murmurs
- Postural hypotension

Dermatologic

- Skin
  —Cool (Vasoconstriction)
  —Pallor
  —Jaundice
  —Purpura
  —Telangiectasia
- Spoon-shaped nails (koilonychia)

CNS

- Neuropathy
- Altered mental status

Miscellaneous

- Bone or joint pain (with sickle cell disease)
- Hepatomegaly, splenomegaly
- Lymphadenopathy
- Findings reflect underlying disease

MECHANISM/DESCRIPTION

- Women: Hb <12 g/dl or Hct <37%
- Men: Hb <14 g/dl or Hct <42%
- Normal blood count values depend on age and ambient oxygen pressure
  —Increased Hb/Hct with neonates and people living above 4000 feet

AGE	*MEAN HGB (G/DL)*	*MEAN HCT (%)*
Birth	16.5	51
1 week	17.5	54
1 month	14.0	43
6 months	11.5	35
1 year	12.0	36
6 years	12.5	37
Adult male	14	42
Adult female	12	37

ETIOLOGY

- Excessive blood loss
  —Trauma
  —GI bleed
  —Menstruation
- Hemolysis (i.e. increased destruction)
  —Hypersplenism
  —Autoimmune hemolytic anemia
  —Mechanical trauma (prosthetic heart valves, vasculitis, TTP, HUS, DIC)
  —Toxins
  —Infections (malaria, Clostridia)
  —Membrane abnormalities
  —Intracellular RBC abnormalities (G6PD, sickle cell anemia, thalassemia)
- Decreased RBC synthesis
  —Hypochromic /microcytic
    -Iron deficiency
    -Thalassemia
    -Sideroblastic
    -Chronic disease
  —Normochromic/macrocytic
    -Hypothyroidism
    -Folic acid deficiency
    -B_{12} deficiency
    -Liver disease
    -Scurvy
  —Normochromic/normocytic
    -Aplastic anemia
    -Chronic renal failure
    -Malignancy
    -Adrenal insufficiency
    -Hyperparathyroidism
    -Alcohol abuse

Pre-Hospital

CAUTIONS

- Administer high flow oxygen
- Ongoing blood losses require close assessment and rapid transport
- Place multiple large bore IV catheters and infuse crystalloid if unstable

CONTROVERSIES

- Some current research suggests that rapid infusion of crystalloid may worsen hemorrhage in trauma

Diagnosis

ESSENTIAL WORKUP

- Bedside Hct
- Vital signs (including orthostatic)

LABORATORY

- CBC
- RBC indices
  —MCV (normal: 80–95 μm^3)
  —MCH (normal: 27–34)
  —MCHC (normal: 30–35%)
- Platelet count
- Reticulocyte count
  —Normal 0.5–1.5% (reticulocytes/1000 RBCs)
  —Falsely elevated in anemia if total RBC decreases
  —Corrected reticulocyte count = reticulocyte count × Hct/45
- Reticulocyte Index (RI) = [reticulocyte count (%) × Hct]/(2 × normal Hct)
  —RI <2% implies inadequate RBC production
  —RI >2% implies excessive RBC destruction or loss
- Stool for occult blood for GI bleed
- Electrolytes, BUN, Cr, glucose
  —For chronic renal failure
- Urinalysis
  —Hematuria
  —Hemoglobinuria in hemolytic anemia

Workup Strategy

- Hypochromic/microcytic anemias
  —Iron, transferrin, ferritin
- Macrocytic anemias
  —Folate
  —Vitamin B_{12}
  —Liver function tests
  —Thyroid function tests
- Hemolytic anemia
  —Coombs test
  —Serum bilirubin—increased unconjugated
  —Urinalysis for hemoglobinuria
  —Plasma for free hemoglobin
  —LDH

IMAGING/SPECIAL TESTS

- Peripheral smear
- Hb electrophoresis for sickle cell anemia/thalassemia
- Coomb's test—positive in autoimmune hemolytic anemia
- Iron, transferrin, ferritin

DISORDER	SERUM IRON	IRON-BINDING CAPACITY	FERRITIN
Iron deficiency	Decreased	Increased	Decreased
Chronic disease	Decreased	Decreased	Normal/ Increased
Thalassemia	Normal	Normal	Normal
Sideroblastic anemia	Increased	Normal	Increased

- Bone marrow biopsy to exclude
  —Leukemia, lymphomas, pancytopenia, agranulocytosis

DIFFERENTIAL DIAGNOSIS

- Dilutional anemia
- Increased plasma volume
- Fluid overload
- Congestive heart failure
- Acquired vs. inherited anemia
- Blood loss
- Nutritional deficiency/malabsorption
- Hemolysis
- Toxin causing bone marrow suppression
- Malignancy
- Chronic disease

PEDIATRIC CONSIDERATIONS

- Hemolytic anemia of the newborn due to Rh antibody crossing placenta when Rh-negative mother has Rh-positive child

Treatment

INITIAL STABILIZATION

- ABCs
- Oxygen
- IV fluid resuscitation with 0.9%NS if ongoing loss/hypotension

ED TREATMENT

- Depends on severity of anemia and acuteness of onset
- Transfusion for hemorrhage with unstable vital signs
- Most anemias seen in ED are chronic and do not require immediate intervention

Therapy for Specific Anemia

- Iron deficiency
  —$FeSO_4$ 300 mg po tid
  —Investigate underlying cause
  —Increase Hb expected in 2–3 weeks
- Renal failure
  —Recombinant erythropoietin when no endogenous erythropoietin produced
- Autoimmune hemolytic anemia
  —Corticosteroids (prednisone 60 mg/d until response)
  —Immunosuppressive agents
  —Plasmapheresis
  —Splenectomy if splenic sequestration
- Drug-induced hemolytic anemia: stop offending agent
- Anemia of chronic disease: treat underlying disease
- Vitamin B_{12} deficiency
  —B_{12} 1000 μg IM daily for 1 week, then weekly for 1 month, then monthly
  —Hematologic parameters normalize within 2 months
  —Neurologic symptoms present >6 months may be permanent
- Folate deficiency
  —Folic acid 1 mg po q day
- Aplastic anemia
  —Antithymocyte globulin
  —Bone marrow transplantation
- Sickle cell anemia
  —Supportive care with oxygen, rehydration, analgesia
  —Treat precipitating cause
- Marrow replacement for
  —Leukemia

Disposition

ADMISSION CRITERIA

- Unstable vital signs
- Ongoing blood losses
- Symptomatic anemia—worsening angina/dyspnea/syncope
- Pancytopenia
- Need for transfusion
- Need for aggressive evaluation

DISCHARGE CRITERIA

- Discharge vast majority of stable patient for outpatient workup

Miscellaneous

ICD9 CODE: 285.9

CORE CONTENT CODE: 7.5.1

SUGGESTED READINGS

Beutler E. The common anemias. JAMA 1988;259:2433–2437

Braunwald E, Isselbacher K, et al., eds. Harrison's principles of internal medicine. 13th ed. New York: McGraw-Hill, 1994

Colon-Otero G, Menke D, Hook CC. A practical approach to the differential diagnosis and evaluation of the adult patient with macrocytic anemia. Med Clin North Am 1992;76:581–597

Hoffman R, Benz E, Shattil S, et al., eds. Hematology: Basic principles and practice. New York: Churchill-Livingstone, 1991

Rosen P, Barkin R, eds. Emergency medicine: Concepts and clinical practice. 4th ed. St. Louis: CV Mosby, 1998

Scott R. Common blood disorders: A primary care approach. Geriatrics 1993;48:72–80

Author: Marc Gelman

Angina

Clinical Presentation

SIGNS AND SYMPTOMS

- Precordial discomfort that varies in severity and quality
  - —Tightness
  - —Heaviness
  - —Squeezing
  - —Pressure
  - —Strangulation
- Atypical locations
  - —Jaw
  - —Neck
  - —Teeth
  - —Ulnar aspect of left arm
  - —Both arms
  - —Wrist
  - —Epigastrium
- Occasionally only an anginal equivalent is present
  - —Shortness of breath
  - —Nausea
  - —Fatigue
  - —Diaphoresis
- Exacerbated by physical activity or anxiety
- Relieved by rest and nitrites

General

- Hypertension
  - —Chronically elevated
  - —Increased during an anginal attack

Cardiac

- Transient S3 or S4 gallop
- Mitral regurgitation murmur
- During an anginal attack
  - —Precordial lift
  - —Softening of S1
  - —Paradoxical splitting of S2

Extremities

- Assess for signs of peripheral vascular disease
  - —Bruits
  - —Pulse deficit

Skin

- Xanthomas

MECHANISM/DESCRIPTION

- Angina results from an imbalance between myocardial oxygen requirements and oxygen supply
- Presenting symptom of coronary artery disease in 38% of men and 61% of women
- Coronary artery disease is newly diagnosed in nearly 1.5 million persons annually
- The Canadian Cardiovascular Classification for angina
  - —Class I
    - -Ordinary physical activity does not cause angina
  - —Class II
    - -Slight limitation of normal activity
    - -Angina occurs with walking, climbing stairs, emotional stress, cold
  - —Class III
    - -Severe limitations of ordinary physical activity
    - -Angina on walking one or two blocks on a level surface
    - -Climbing one flight of stairs in normal conditions
  - —Class IV
    - -Inability to carry on any physical activity without discomfort
    - -Anginal symptoms may be present at rest
- Unstable angina
  - —Anginal symptoms occurring at rest for more than 20 minutes
  - —New onset angina
    - -Existing for 8 weeks or less
    - -Marked limitations of ordinary physical activity (class III)
  - —Acceleration of angina
    - -In frequency, duration, and severity
    - -To class III or more over the last 8 weeks
- Microvascular angina
  - —Changes in ST segment depression
  - —No coronary atherosclerosis
- Variant or Prinzmetal's angina
  - —Due to coronary spasm
  - —Reversible st segment elevation
  - —Angina at rest

ETIOLOGY

- Atherosclerosis
  - —Rupture of atherosclerotic plaque is the usual cause of decreased coronary blood flow
- Coronary vasospasm
  - —Prinzmetal's angina
  - —After nitroglycerin withdrawal
- Arteritis
  - —Disseminated lupus erythematosus
  - —Takayasu's disease
  - —Kawasaki's syndrome
  - —Rheumatoid arthritis
  - —Ankylosing spondylitis
  - —Hypertrophic cardiomyopathy
  - —Aortic valve disease
  - —Dissection of the coronary arteries

Pre-Hospital

CAUTIONS

- Intravenous access
- Oxygen
- Monitor
- Sublingual nitroglycerin
- Initiate treatment for reversible causes

Diagnosis

ESSENTIAL WORKUP

- Diagnosis of angina is clinical
- Ancillary studies are used to exclude other life threats and causes of chest pain

LABORATORY

- CBC
  - —Anemia may be an exacerbating factor
- Cardiac enzymes
  - —Normal
  - —Differentiates angina from myocardial infarction

IMAGING/SPECIAL TESTS

- Electrocardiogram
  - —Nonspecific ST-T wave changes
  - —Normal
  - —High likelihood of coronary artery disease
    - -ST segment elevation or depression $\geq$1 mm
    - -Deep symmetrical T wave inversions in precordial leads
    - -Any transient ECG changes during an anginal attack
  - —Intermediate likelihood of coronary artery disease
    - -ST segment depression $\geq$0.5 mm
    - -T wave inversion $\geq$1 mm in leads with dominant r waves
- Chest radiograph
  - —Detection of other causes of chest pain
    - -Pneumonia
    - -Pneumothorax
    - -Aortic dissection

DIFFERENTIAL DIAGNOSIS

- Aortic dissection
- Myocardial infarction
- Mitral valve prolapse
- Pericarditis
- Pulmonary embolus
- Pneumothorax
- Costochondritis
- Herpes zoster
- Thoracic outlet syndrome
- Esophageal spasm
- Esophageal reflux
- Peptic ulcer disease
- Pancreatitis
- Biliary colic
- Psychogenic

Treatment

INITIAL STABILIZATION

- Intravenous access
- Monitor
- Oxygen therapy
- Aspirin
- Nitroglycerin
- If symptoms persist after 3 sublingual nitroglycerins, assume myocardial infarction and switch to intrevenous nitroglycerin and intravenous morphine
- β-Blockers
  —Intravenous for high-risk unstable angina
  —Oral for intermediate and low-risk unstable angina
- Intravenous heparin for unstable angina
- Treat underlying cause of angina when present
  —Congestive heart failure
  —Dysrhythmia

MEDICATIONS

- Aspirin: 160–324 mg po
- Atenolol: 5 mg/min IV over 2 minutes (total 10 mg)
- Heparin: 80 IU/kg IV; maintenance infusion 18 IU/kg/hr IV
- Morphine: 2–4 mg IV every 5 min
- Nitroglycerin: 0.4 mg sublingual; 5–20 μg/min IV; titrate up by 10 μg/min every 5 min until relief; maximum 100–200 μg/min
- Propranolol: 0.5–1 mg IV

Disposition

ADMISSION CRITERIA

- New angina
- Accelerating angina
- Admit the patient to a monitored bed

DISCHARGE CRITERIA

- Stable angina

Miscellaneous

ICD9: 413

CORE CONTENT CODE: 2.2.3.1

SUGGESTED READINGS

Braunwald E, Mark DB, Jones RH. et al. Unstable angina: Diagnosis and management. Clinical practice guideline number 10. AHCPR Publication No 94-0602. Rockville, MD: Agency for Health Care Policy and Research and the National Heart, Lung, and Blood Institute, Public Health Service, US Department of Health and Human Services: May 1994 (amended).

Gersh BJ, Braunwald E, Rutherford JD. Chronic coronary artery disease. In: Braunwald E, ed. Heart disease: A textbook of cardiovascular medicine. 5th ed. Philadelphia: WB Saunders, 1997.

Katz DA, Griffith JL, Beshansky JR, et al. The use of empiric clinical data in the evaluation of practice guidelines for unstable angina. JAMA 1996;276:1568–1574.

National Heart Attack Alert Program Working Group. An evaluation of technologies for identifying acute ischemia in the emergency department: A report. Ann Emerg Med 1997;29:13–87.

Task Force of the European Society of Cardiology. Management of stable angina pectoris. Eur Heart J 1997;18:354–413.

Author: A. Perpall

Angioedema

Clinical Presentation

SIGNS AND SYMPTOMS

- Edema of the airway, face or extremities
- Abdominal pain associated with nausea, vomiting, and diarrhea
- Attacks of hereditary angioedema are not associated with hives
- Emotional stress or physical trauma can trigger attacks
- The lesions of angioedema are large swollen and nonpitting wheals
- The eyelids and lips are frequently involved
  —Involvement of the pharynx and larynx may cause airway obstruction

MECHANISM/DESCRIPTION

- Nonpruritic, well-demarcated, nonpitting edema of the dermis
- Primarily involves the periorbital and perioral regions
- Similar in pathological basis to urticaria except that affected tissue lies deeper
  —Urticaria affects superficial tissue and causes irritation to mast cells and nerves in the epidermis leading to intense itching
  —Angioedema occurs in deeper layers, which have fewer mast cells and nerves therefore causing less itching
- There are two types of angioedema: the classic hereditary form and the acquired forms
  —Hereditary angioedema is an autosomal dominant disorder caused by a deficiency of C1 esterase inhibitor (C1-INH) which leads to the formation of bradykinin resulting in angioedema
  —The acquired forms demonstrate normal quantities and function of C1-INH but it becomes bound to circulating antibodies that inactivate it
  —Absolute or functional deficiency of C1-INH from either type results in unopposed activity of the first component of the complement cascade resulting in higher levels of bradykinin which incites the formation of angioedema

ETIOLOGY

- Typical triggers include:
  —food additives
  —food allergies
  —drug allergies
  —insect stings
  —exposure to heat or cold
  —exercise
  —thyroid disease
  —diabetes
  —lupus
  —infections
  —contact allergies
  —ACE inhibitors

Pre-Hospital

- Early intubation may be necessary before airway edema becomes too severe

Diagnosis

ESSENTIAL WORKUP

- Diagnosis is made based on clinical presentation of large nonpitting, nonpruritic wheals
- A family history need not be present to diagnose the disease

LABORATORY

- CBC with differential, ESR, ANA, rheumatoid factor
- Skin biopsy if urticarial lesion is accessible

IMAGING/SPECIAL TESTS

- Measurement of C1-INH levels
  —Patients affected with hereditary angioedema have very low levels, carriers will have half-normal levels
- C4 and C2 levels are low during attacks in both hereditary and acquired forms
- These levels not routinely available in ED.

DIFFERENTIAL DIAGNOSIS

- Primary angioedema
  —IgE-mediated allergic reactions
  —Drug reactions
  —Food allergies
  —Inhalation, ingestion or contact with allergens
  —Panic attacks, globus hystericus
- Secondary angioedema
  —Physical urticaria such as cold, pressure, solar
  —Systemic mastocytosis
  —Familial cold urticaria
  —C3b inactivator deficiency
  —Amyloidosis
  —Exercise-induced anaphylaxis
  —Transfusion reaction
  —Collagen vascular disease
  —ACE-inhibitor reaction

PEDIATRIC CONSIDERATIONS

- Recurrent angioedema presenting around puberty should raise suspicion of hereditary angioedema
- The patient should be referred to an allergist/immunologist if there is a family history of angioedema, or if the angioedema is accompanied by abdominal pain, or triggered by trauma

Treatment

INITIAL STABILIZATION

- Active airway management and supportive measures are the primary goals of emergency treatment
- Early intubation may be necessary in severe cases
- Epinephrine, antihistamines, and steroids in obstructive airway swelling, though response is variable.

ED TREATMENT

- A C1-INH concentrate is available which is useful during acute attacks
- Fresh frozen plasma (which contains of C1 inhibitor) is also useful
- Plasmin inhibitors do not directly correct C2 and C4 deficiencies but appear to be clinically effective
- Angioedema associated with ACE inhibitors occurs in 0.1–0.2 % of cases and requires immediate withdrawal of the ACEI and replacement with another antihypertensive medication

MEDICATIONS

- C1-INH concentrate given in 5% dextrose over 10–45 minutes or fresh frozen plasma (if C1-INH is unavailable)
- Cimetidine 300 mg IV
- Diphenhydramine: adult: 50 mg IV; peds: 1–2 mg/kg slow IVP
- Epinephrine: 0.3–0.5 mg (use 1:1000 dilution for SQ route, and 1:10000 for IV route); peds: epinephrine 0.01 mg/kg SC/IV
- Glucagon: adult: 1 mg IV
- Hydrocortisone: adult: 500 mg IV; peds: hydrocortisone 4–8 mg/kg/dose IV
- Methylprednisolone: adult: 125 mg IV; peds: 1–2 mg/kg IV
- Prednisone: adult: 60 mg po; peds: 1 mg/kg po
- Ranitidine: adult: 50 mg IV

PEDIATRIC CONSIDERATIONS

- Because the prophylactic treatment currently available is anabolic steroids, careful consideration must be made before the use of danazol or stanozolol in children

Disposition

ADMISSION CRITERIA

- Patients with systemic symptoms that do not resolve completely will need to be hospitalized for observation
- A monitored bed is recommended for those with airway involvement

DISCHARGE CRITERIA

- Patients without systemic symptoms who are stable for discharge should been seen in outpatient follow-up in a few days
- Patients should be evaluated by an allergist/immunologist after the initial presentation

Miscellaneous

ICD9: 995.1

CORE CONTENT CODE: 8.8.2

SUGGESTED READINGS

Alsenz J, Bork K, Loos M. Autoantibody-mediated acquired deficiency of C1 inhibitor. N Engl J Med 1987;316:1360.

Kaplan AP. Urticaria and Angioedema. In: Kaplan AP Ed. *Allergy*. New York, NY: Churchill Livingstone. 1985:439–471.

Nadel ES, Brown DF. Angioedema. J Emer Med. 1988;16(3):477–9.

Sim TC, Grant JA. Hereditary angioedema: Its diagnostic and management perspectives. Am J Med 1990;88:656–664.

Author: Sean X. Neath

Ankle Fracture/Dislocation

Clinical Presentation

- Ankle fractures are intra-articular injuries, usually associated with significant ligamentous ruptures
- Ankle dislocations require a large degree of force and result from complete disruption of the articular elements of the ankle. Because of the bony anatomy of the ankle, dislocations are almost always associated with ankle fracture

SIGNS AND SYMPTOMS

- History of trauma; sounds of a snap or pop during the injury
- Local pain about the ankle, specifically at either or both malleoli (distal 6 cm), swelling, deformity, weakness
- Pain of the distal fibula
- Difficulty with ambulation, specifically inability to bear weight within one hour of the injury
- Soft tissue injury, ecchymosis, skin tenting or skin blanching about the ankle
- Neurovascular compromise, diminished capillary refill, diminished posterior tibial or dorsalis pedis pulses
- Diminished range of motion

MECHANISM/DESCRIPTION

Mechanism of injury

- There are three common mechanisms of ankle injury, each with a distinct injury pattern.
- These finding may occur singly, in combination, or not at all, depending on the forces involved
- *Inversion injury* (rotation inward)
  —Avulsion fracture of the lateral malleolus due to local distractive forces (unstable fracture if above the level of the mortise) or lateral ligamentous sprain
  —Oblique fracture of the medial malleolus as the talus is driven into the inferolateral tibia from below
- *Eversion injury* (rotation outward)
  —Avulsion fracture of the medial malleolus due to the local distractive force or deltoid ligament sprain
  —Oblique fracture of the fibula as the talus is driven into the lateral malleolus from below
- *External rotation injury*
  —Disruption of the syndesmosis between the tibia and fibula, or a fibular fracture above the plafond as the talus moves laterally
  —Anterior or posterior tibial fracture with separation of the distal tibia and fibula (unstable fracture)
- Tibial avulsion fracture or deltoid ligament sprain

PEDIATRIC CONSIDERATIONS

- Ankle fractures in children often involve the *physis* (growth plate), which may cause chronic deformity from growth plate injury
- Ligaments are strong, making the growth plate the structure most likely disrupted in children younger than 10 years of age
- *Tillaux fracture* is a Salter-Harris type III injury of the lateral tibial epiphysis caused by eversion and lateral rotation
- *Triplane fracture* is an unusual fracture of the distal tibia
  —Fracture lines traverse three distinct planes: coronal, transverse, sagittal

Pre-Hospital

- Goal of *immobilization* is aimed at reducing pain, bleeding, and further soft tissue injury
- *Soft splinting* is an effective, rapid method and is recommended for most patients
  —A pillow circumferentially wrapped and tapped or pinned makes and excellent splint

CAUTIONS

- Traction devices are contraindicated when an open injury exists
- Protruding bone should not be reduced and drawn back into the wound; the wound should be covered as early as possible with a clean, preferably sterile, dressing

Diagnosis

ESSENTIAL WORKUP

- Radiographic imaging as outlined below

IMAGING/SPECIAL TESTS

- Ankle injuries should be radiographed whenever there is concern for fracture
  - —Anteroposterior, lateral, and oblique (mortise) films
- *Ottawa Ankle Rules* are selective guidelines for ordering radiographs in patients 18–55 years of age with
  - —Bony tenderness at the posterior edge or tip of either malleoli (distal 6 cm)
  - —Inability to bear weight for four consecutive steps either immediately after the injury or in the ED
- Radiographs should also be considered in
  - —Patients with altered sensorium or diminished peripheral limb sensation
  - —Patients with multiple painful and distracting injuries
  - —Patients under 18 years of age
  - —Patients with injuries that occurred 10 days prior to evaluation
- Stress-testing the ligaments in a painful ankle is unnecessary in the ED if the patient will be re-examined in 3–5 days
- Stress radiographs of the ankle are usually unnecessary
- Axial tomography or CT scan may be useful to assess the degree of injury to the tibial plafond, intra-articular pathology, and pediatric epiphyseal injuries

DIFFERENTIAL DIAGNOSIS

- Ankle sprain
- Achilles tendon injury
- Maisonneuve fracture, proximal fracture at the fibular neck
- Os trigonum fracture
- Fifth metatarsal fracture (Jones Fracture)
- Peroneal tendon dislocation or injury
- Transchondral talar-dome fracture
- Ankle diastasis

SPECIAL PEDIATRIC CONSIDERATIONS

- In children under 10 years of age, the proximal fibula should be evaluated for possible fracture
- The physes (growth plates) should always be palpated to determine the likelihood of fracture

Treatment

INITIAL STABILIZATION

- Avoid weight bearing if painful
- RICE (rest, ice, compression, elevation)

ED TREATMENT

Ankle Fracture

- *All ankle fractures require orthopedic consultation or referral*
- Open ankle fractures and neurovascular compromise necessitate emergent orthopedic consultation
- *Stable injury* (injury to only one side of the ankle)
  - —Compression dressing, posterior splint with foot at a right angle, and elevation of the extremity
- *Unstable injury* (both sides of the ankle are injured)
  - —Orthopedic consultation to the ED
  - —Usually requires open reduction and internal fixation emergently before significant swelling develops

Ankle Dislocations

- Skin tenting and evidence of neurovascular compromise are indications for immediate reduction
- Most ankle dislocations, either anterior or posterior, require open reduction and internal fixation
- If closed reduction is performed, a posterior splint should be initially placed
  - —Always take postreduction roentgenograms in three planes

MEDICATIONS

- Primarily pain medications

Disposition

ADMISSION CRITERIA

- All unstable ankle fractures should be admitted following treatment
- Admit all ankle dislocations that are treated with either open or closed reduction

DISCHARGE CRITERIA

- Simple nondisplaced isolated fibular fractures may be discharged following casting if no neurovascular compromise is experienced

Miscellaneous

ICD9: 824.8, 837.0

CORE CONTENT CODE: 18.4.13.1.4

SUGGESTED READINGS

Martin DR, Villareal JM. Injuries of the ankle and foot. In: Harwood-Nuss AL, ed. Clinical practice of emergency medicine. 2d ed. Philadelphia: JB Lippincott, 1996

Moehring HD, Tan RT, Marder RA, et al. Ankle dislocation. J Orthop Trauma 1994;8:167–172

Reisdorff EJ, Cowling KM. The injured ankle: New twists to a familiar problem. EM Rep 1995:165(5):39–48

Stiell IG, McKnight RD, Greenberg GH, et al. Decision rules for use of radiography in acute ankle injuries: Refinement and prospective validation. JAMA 1993;269:1127–1132

Waeckerle JF, Steele MT. Ankle injuries. In: Tintinalli JE, Ruiz E, Krome RL, eds. Emergency medicine: A comprehensive study guide. 4th ed. New York: McGraw-Hill, 1996;1265–1271

Authors: Usha P. Reddy; Lawrence E. Kass

Ankle Sprain

Clinical Presentation

SIGNS AND SYMPTOMS

- Grade I (mild)
  —Pain
  —Minimal to no difficulty in ambulation
  —Localized edema absent to slight
  —No ligamentous instability (see Diagnosis below)
- Grade II (moderate)
  —Pain
  —Moderate difficulty with ambulation
  —Localized edema moderate to significant
  —Ecchymosis may be present
  —Ligamentous weakness (see Diagnosis below)
- Grade III (severe)
  —Pain
  —Unable to ambulate
  —Joint instability to exam (see Diagnosis below)
  —Marked edema
  —Ecchymosis usually present
  —Ligamentous weakness

MECHANISM/DESCRIPTION

- Ankle sprains are injuries to the ligamentous supports of the hinge (tenon-mortise) joint composed of the tibia, fibula, and talus. The injury may range from stretching with only microscopic damage (Grade I) to partial disruption (Grade II) to complete disruption (Grade III)
- 85–90% of all ankle sprains involve the lateral ligaments (anterior talofibular (ATFL), posterior talofibular (PTFL), and calcaneofibular (CFL)), and are usually the result of an inversion injury. The ATFL is the most commonly injured. If the ankle is injured in a neutral position, the CFL is often injured. In 20% of sprains, both the ATFL and the CFL are involved.
- The PTFL is rarely injured in the absence of disruption of both of the other lateral ligaments
- Injury to the deltoid ligament (connecting the medial malleolus to the talus and navicular bones) is usually the result of an eversion injury and is often associated with avulsion at the medial malleolus or talar insertion. It is rarely found as an isolated injury and, when found, one should suspect an associated lateral malleolus fracture, or fracture of the proximal fibula (Maisonneuve fracture)
- Syndesmosis sprains (injury to the tibiofibular ligaments and/or the interosseous ligament of the leg) occur during hyperdorsiflexion with eversion accompanied by axial loading. This mechanism forces the talar dome up and between the tibia and fibula. This is rarely an isolated injury and is usually accompanied by fracture of the lateral, medial, or posterior malleoli

PEDIATRIC CONSIDERATIONS

- Children under age 10 with traumatic ankle pain and no radiologic evidence of fracture most likely have a Salter-Harris I fracture, as the ligaments are actually stronger than the open epiphysis

Pre-Hospital

N/A

Diagnosis

ESSENTIAL WORKUP

- History may predict the type of injury found and should include
  —Time of injury
  —Mechanism
  —Whether a "pop" or "crack" was heard or felt at the time of injury
  —History of previous trauma
  —Relevant medical conditions (e.g., bone or joint disease)
  —Treatments attempted prior to arrival
  —Ability to bear weight subsequent to the injury
- Physical exam is aimed at detecting evidence of joint instability and evidence of other possible or associated injuries
  —Start exam at a site remote from the area of pain and include the proximal fibula and the base of the fifth metacarpal
  —Document neurovascular status distal to the injury
  —Range of motion should be determined and compared to the uninjured side. However, range of motion is often limited by pain and swelling
  —Stress testing is often limited by pain and may impair detection of ligament injury. Some authorities recommend infiltration with a local anesthetic to facilitate the exam, but this is rarely of use in the Emergency Department
  —Anterior drawer test is most useful for detecting ATFL (anterior talofibular ligament) injury. This is performed by holding the lower leg in position with one hand and grasping the underside of the heel with the other. With the ankle in a neutral position (0–10 ° of plantarflexion), an attempt is made to "pull" the foot anteriorly. Ligamentous laxity is described as mild, moderate, or marked
  —Talar tilt (inversion stress) test assesses the lateral collateral ligaments, especially the CFL (calcaneofibular ligament). With the ankle in a neutral position, one hand is used to immobilize the heel and distal tibia. With the other hand placed across the dorsum of the foot, an attempt is made to invert the midfoot. Laxity is described as mild, moderate, or marked
  —Disruption of the deltoid ligament will cause laxity with eversion. This test is performed in an identical fashion to the talar tilt test, except that eversion of the midfoot is attempted
  —Pain felt in the ankle when the distal tibia and fibula are compressed together ("squeeze test") suggests a syndesmosis injury
  —Thompson squeeze test assesses integrity of the Achilles tendon. This test is per-

formed by compressing the gastrocnemius muscle of the calf. An intact Achilles tendon will result in slight plantar flexion of the ankle

IMAGING/SPECIAL TESTS

- Ankle injuries should be radiographed whenever there is a concern for fracture. The *Ottawa Ankle Rules* describe a selective strategy for ankle x-rays in adults under age 55. The rules suggest that ankle x-rays are unnecessary except when the following are present
  - —Malleolar pain and either
    - -Bony tenderness along the distal 6 cm of either malleolus or
    - -Patient unable to take 4 unassisted steps both immediately after the injury and in the emergency department
  - —Though validated by the authors in the same hospital, other attempts at validation have yielded less than the anticipated 100% sensitivity. A large multicenter validation study is in progress. It is important to note that these studies specifically excluded individuals with other, potentially distracting, injuries and complicating medical diagnoses
- Stress radiographs are rarely useful in the emergency department

DIFFERENTIAL DIAGNOSIS

- Ankle fracture (lateral, medial, or posterior malleolus) or dislocation
- Achilles tendon injury
- Maisonneuve fracture
- Os trigonum fracture
- Fifth metatarsal fracture (Jones Fracture)
- Transchondral talar dome fracture
- Peroneal tendon dislocation or injury

Treatment

INITIAL STABILIZATION

- Prevent further injury. Avoid weight-bearing if painful
- RICE (Rest, Ice, Compression, Elevation)

ED TREATMENT

- Functional support (air splint, gel splint, etc.) for Grade I or II sprains
- Immobilization (sugar tong or posterior ankle splint) and early orthopedic consultation or referral for Grade III sprains
- Non-weight-bearing with crutches may be necessary initially if pain is severe, with early advancement as tolerated to protected weight-bearing
- Full sports activities may be resumed only when running and turning are pain-free
- Early passive range-of-motion exercises in dorsiflexion and plantar flexion (*not* inversion or eversion) are recommended by some authorities

Disposition

ADMISSION CRITERIA

- An isolated ankle sprain should not require admission

DISCHARGE CRITERIA

- Patients should be instructed to seek follow-up for pain that persists beyond 3–4 days

Miscellaneous

ICD9: 845.00

CORE CONTENT CODE: 18.4.14.2.1

SUGGESTED READINGS

Reisdorff EJ, Cowling KM. The injured ankle: New twists to a familiar problem. EM Rep 1995;16(5):39–48

Stiell IG, McKnight RD, Greenberg GH, et al. Decision rules for use of radiography in acute ankle injuries: Refinement and prospective validation. JAMA 1993;269:1127–1132

Waeckerle JF, Steele MT. Ankle injuries. In: Tintinalli JE, Ruiz E, Krome RL, eds. Emergency medicine: A comprehensive study guide. 4th ed. New York: McGraw-Hill, 1996:1265–1271

Authors: Lawrence E. Kass; Usha P. Reddy

Ankylosing Spondylitis

Clinical Presentation

SIGNS AND SYMPTOMS

- *Low back pain,* especially *sacroiliitis,* is the most common presentation. It is exacerbated by rest and improved with mild activity or stooping forward
- *Paralysis* from minor spinal trauma or manipulation
- May present with *cauda equina syndrome*
- Enthesitis (inflammation at tendon or ligament insertion) is common, especially *Achilles tendonitis* or *Plantar fasciitis*
- May have *asymmetric arthritis* of large joints of lower extremities
- *Uveitis* may precede onset of arthritis
- May have *aortic valve regurgitation*

ETIOLOGY

- Genetic predisposition in which prior significant trauma or infection may play a role
- HLA-B27 association

MECHANISM/DESCRIPTION

- Spinal predilection
- Onset before 40 years of age
- Male to Female ratio is 3:1
- Inflammation at the bony insertions of ligaments or tendons (entheses)
- May have systemic inflammatory manifestations such as uveitis
- The painful *spondylitis* of ankylosing spondylitis (AS) begins at the insertions of the outer fibers of the annulus fibrosis (enthesitis) of the vertebrae, which begin to ossify and may lead to complete fusion, *ankylosis,* of the vertebrae
- The fused spine is dangerously brittle when subjected to trauma, significantly increasing the risks for *fracture* and *paralysis*

PEDIATRIC CONSIDERATIONS

- Juvenile ankylosing spondylitis (JAS) has a much greater predilection for *extraspinal* joints and entheses of the lower extremities. Examine for
  - —*Asymmetrical arthritis* of the joints of the lower extremities, especially hip
  - —*Enthesitis* of the Achilles tendon attachment at the heel, the plantar fascia attachments to the sole of the foot, the patellar ligament attachment to the tibial tuberosity, and the quadriceps tendon attachments to the patella
- JAS may mimic a septic process with fever and systemic signs
- Onset of JAS is late childhood or adolescence (usually before age 16) primarily *boys*

Pre-Hospital

CAUTIONS

- There is an increased risk of traumatic spinal injury from even minor injuries

Diagnosis

ESSENTIAL WORKUP

- Exclude fracture or nerve injury in any new spinal pain of a patient suspected of AS
- Exclude sepsis or septic joint
- Evaluate for sacroiliitis with *pelvic rock* test (compression) or *Patrick test* (sacroiliac distraction)

LABORATORY

- ESR may be elevated
- CBC may show mild leukocytosis with slight to moderate anemia and thrombocytosis
- BUN, creatinine, and electrolytes may be useful to assess renal involvement

IMAGING/SPECIAL TESTS

- Pelvic x-ray: should be done in any adult patient who is believed to be an undiagnosed acute case of ankylosing spondylitis
  - —Sacroiliitis is essential to the diagnosis of AS. This is seen initially as subchondral bony erosions on the iliac side of the SI joint which later manifest as bony proliferation and sclerosis
- Lumbar, thoracic, and cervical spine x-rays to exclude fracture should be strongly considered in any patient thought to have AS and is complaining of *new pain to these areas with or without trauma*
- CT should be performed to further evaluate possible fractures on plain radiographs
- MRI should be performed emergently on any patient *neurologic deficit* to assess the integrity of the spinal cord
- Chest x-ray may show findings similar to TB with patchy inflammatory infiltrates

DIFFERENTIAL DIAGNOSIS

- *Mechanical* low back pain is generally improved with rest and exacerbated by exercise without signs of systemic inflammatory process
- *Infectious* low back pain is more constant unremitting and associated with fever
- *Neoplastic* low back pain is more typical in patients over the age of 40 and more constant and unremitting. Night pain is a characteristic symptom
- *Septic arthritis* should be excluded by arthrocentesis if single joint involvement, fever, and elevated WBC are present particularly in the absence of back pain
- *Psoriatic arthritis* usually presents in a patient with known psoriasis and has much greater predilection for the *hands and feet*

- *Reiter's disease:* the classic triad of arthritis, urethritis, and conjunctivitis is present in a minority of patients. Also called "reactive arthritis" due to appearance of arthritis (generally asymmetric large joints of lower extremities) about 1 month after an episode of urethritis or enteritis
- Arthritis associated with inflammatory bowel disease occurs in patients with Crohn's disease or ulcerative colitis. Primarily involves knee, elbow, ankle, or wrist, and usually exacerbated by flares of the bowel disease

PEDIATRIC CONSIDERATIONS

- Juvenile *rheumatoid* arthritis has a greater predilection for the small joints of the hands

Treatment

INITIAL STABILIZATION

- Trauma: ABCs while maintaining immobilization (including in-line spinal stabilization if intubation required)
- Acute paralysis: methylprednisolone IV and immediate neurosurgical evaluation

ED TREATMENT

- Control pain and inflammation with nonsteroidal anti-inflammatory drugs. Steroids may be useful in severe refractory cases
- Exclude infection by clinical presentation, laboratory analysis, and possibly arthrocentesis
- Exclude spinal fracture (use CT for equivocal findings on plain radiographs)

MEDICATIONS

- NSAIDs
  - —Ibuprofen: 35 mg/kg/day divided tid with food
  - —Indomethacin: 1–2 mg/kg/day divided tid with food
  - —Naproxen: 10–20 mg/kg/d divided bid with food
  - —Tolmetin sodium: 20–30 mg/kg/d divided tid with food
- Steroids
  - —Methylprednisolone: high-dose protocol for acute paralysis: 30 mg/kg bolus, then 5.4 mg/kg/hr for 24 hrs total; severe refractory pain: 1000 mg IV single dose (controversial)

PEDIATRIC CONSIDERATIONS

- Indomethacin is generally considered second-line therapy due to side effects

Disposition

ADMISSION CRITERIA

- Sepsis or septic joint cannot be excluded
- Pain is intractable
- Acute neurological impairment

DISCHARGE CRITERIA

- No serious injuries or neurologic deficit
- Pain controlled

SPECIAL PEDIATRIC DISPOSITION DECISIONS

- Referral for physiotherapy
- Resting splints for inflamed joints
- Orthoses for inflamed entheses (such as heel cushion inserts to rest Achilles tendon attachment)

Miscellaneous

ICD9: 720.0

CORE CONTENT CODE: 10.3.1

SUGGESTED READINGS

Burgos-Vargas R, Petty RE. Juvenile ankylosing spondylitis. Rheum Dis Clin North Am 1992;18:123–142.

El-Khoury GY, Kathol MH, Brandser EA. Seronegative spondyloarthropathies. Radiol Clin North Am 1996;34:343–345.

Fox MW, Onofrio BM, Kilgore JE. Neurological complications of ankylosing spondylitis. J Neurosurg 1993;78:871–878.

Author: Paul L. DeSandre

Anterior Cruciate Ligament Injury

Clinical Presentation

SIGNS AND SYMPTOMS

- Feeling of the knee "giving way," hearing a "pop," or feeling a tearing sensation at the time of injury
- Because of a paucity of pain fibers in the anterior cruciate ligament (ACL), acute injury may not be particularly painful
- May be able to ambulate despite a complete ACL rupture due to enough supporting stability of the dynamic stabilizers of the knee (semimembranosus, semitendinosus muscles)
- *Immediate effusion* (hemarthrosis within 2–3 hours) usually indicates a significant structural injury
  —About 70% of acute knee hemarthroses are due to ACL injury
  —Lack of hemarthrosis can occur: capsular disruption may allow extravasation of intra-articular blood
- Locking of the joint may occur due to interposition of the torn cruciate, or associated torn menisci, or loose body. Pseudolocking may be present from pain, effusion, or spasm
- Stress testing—*always compare the injured to the uninjured side*
  —*Lachman test* is most reliable
    -Knee flexed 20°, patient supine with thigh supported; tibia is brought forward on the femur, one hand holding proximal tibia, the other stabilizing the femur just above the patella
    -Pain with no motion is probable grade 1 injury
    -Pain with motion indicates partial tear or disruption
    -Firm endpoint of motion suggests partial tear
  —*Pivot shift test:* more specific for ACL injury but unreliable without anesthesia
    -Patient supine, knee in full extension
    -Internal rotation of tibia via a hand on foot is applied simultaneously with valgus stress form the other hand
    -With knee flexion to 20–30° the examiner experiences a jerk at the anterolateral corner of the proximal tibia
  —*Anterior drawer sign:* not as sensitive or specific as Lachman test
    -Knee flexed 90°, patient supine, hip flexed 45°, foot neutral and stabilized
    -Anterior motion is positive

ETIOLOGY

- The majority of injuries to the ACL are sports related. Noncontact injury is common
- Common mechanisms include a direct force to the anterior knee, a running patient who makes a sudden stop or cut with a planted foot, and a patient who is skiing and "catches a tip."

MECHANISM/DESCRIPTION

- The ACL inserts anterolaterally to the anterior tibial spine and to the posterior aspect of the lateral femoral condyle. Portions of the tendon are under tension (i.e., at risk) in both flexion and extension
- The ACL prevents excessive anterior movement, excessive internal rotation of the tibia on the femur, or hyperextension of the knee
- Mechanism of injury is often deceleration with flexion and rotation; also common is hyperextension

PEDIATRIC CONSIDERATIONS

- The ACL is the most frequently injured knee ligament in children

Pre-Hospital

CAUTIONS

- The knee must be adequately immobilized to prevent complete rupture of the ACL

Diagnosis

ESSENTIAL WORKUP

- Neurovascular evaluation, exclusion of fractures/dislocations, valgus/varus stress at 20° flexion, Lachman test, extensor mechanism function
- The Lachman test (as described above) is the most important and sensitive test for ACL injury
- Look for signs of associated ligament or meniscus injury

LABORATORY

- If the cause of a knee effusion is uncertain, synovial aspirate can be sent for cell count, Gram stain, and culture and crystals. This is usually not the case with an ACL injury

IMAGING/SPECIAL TESTS

- If minimal injury is detected by physical exam, plain films add very little to diagnosis or management
- With more severe injury, a knee series, including AP, lateral, oblique, and notch views, is obtained to rule out bony injury
- Plain films may reveal a lateral tibial plateau avulsion fracture, just below the joint line; this is diagnostic for an ACL rupture and is called the lateral capsular sign
- MRI is replacing arthroscopy for definitive images but is rarely indicated emergently

DIFFERENTIAL DIAGNOSIS

- Meniscal injury
- Collateral ligament injury
- Tibial plateau injury

PEDIATRIC CONSIDERATIONS

- Tears of the ACL in children often occur at the insertion site of the ligament

Treatment

INITIAL STABILIZATION

- Establish integrity of neurovascular function
- Immobilize the knee, ice, elevate

ED TREATMENT

- Injury is graded by severity
  - —Grade 3 is complete disruption of the ligament
  - —Grade 2 represents severe stretching with partial tear of the ligament
  - —Grade 1 is microscopic ligamentous damage with no clinical instability
- General care
  - —Immobilization/nonweight-bearing
  - —Ice for first 48 hours, elevation
  - —Analgesic
  - —First degree injury may be treated with compressive wrap and weight-bearing as tolerated
  - —Orthopedic referral within 1–2 weeks is necessary if significant ligamentous injury (grade 2 or 3) is present
  - —Reexamination is recommended at 48 hours if the ED exam is inconclusive or if history suggests a more significant injury than the initial exam demonstrates (i.e., severe symptoms, hearing a pop)
  - —Aspiration of a tense hemarthrosis may relieve pain
    - -Fat globules in the aspirate suggest a fracture

MEDICATIONS

- NSAIDs or narcotic pain medications are the mainstay

PEDIATRIC CONSIDERATIONS

- Surgical repair is generally recommended for adolescents with grade 3 injury

Disposition

ADMISSION CRITERIA

- Isolated ACL injury rarely requires emergent hospitalization. For suspected complete ruptures definitive therapy is often surgical, and orthopedic consultation is appropriate
- Controversy remains in the orthopedic literature as to whether conservative versus surgical treatment yields the best long-term results

DISCHARGE CRITERIA

- Most patients can be managed as outpatients with appropriate referral

Miscellaneous

ICD9: 959.7

CORE CONTENT CODE: 18.4.14.3

SUGGESTED READINGS

Gersoff WK, Clancy WG Jr. Diagnosis of acute and chronic anterior cruciate ligament tears. Clin Sports Med 1988;7(4):727.

Stiell IG, Greenberg GH, et al. Prospective validation of a decision rule for the use of radiography in acute knee injuries. JAMA 1996;275:611.

Swenson TM, Hamer CD. Knee ligament and meniscal injuries. Orthop Clin North Am 1995;26:529.

Zarins B, Adams M. Knee injuries in sports. N Engl J Med 1988;318(15):950.

Authors: Moss Mendelson; Francis Counselman

Anticholinergic, Poisoning

Clinical Presentation

SIGNS AND SYMPTOMS

Classic Toxidrome

- "Mad as a hatter"—altered mental status
- "Hot as a hare"—hyperthermia
- "Red as a beet"—flushed skin
- "Dry as a bone"—dry skin and mucous membranes
- "Blind as a bat"—blurred vision secondary to mydriasis

General

- Hyperthermia
- Altered mental status

HEENT

- Unreactive mydriasis
- Inability to accommodate

Cardiovascular

- Sinus tachycardia
- Dysrhythmias (Rare except in massive ingestions)
- Hypo- or hypertension
- Cardiogenic pulmonary edema

Pulmonary

- Tachypnea
- Respiratory failure

GI

- Decreased/absent bowel sounds
- Dysphagia
- Decreased GI motility
- Decreased salivation

GU

- Urinary retention

Integument

- Decreased sweating
- Flushed skin
- Dry, skin and mucous membranes

CNS

- Altered mental status
- Auditory or visual hallucinations
- Coma
- Seizures

MECHANISM

- Central and peripheral cholinergic blockade
- Depending on the drug involved, antagonism of muscarinic (most common), nicotinic, or both receptors

ETIOLOGY

- Many drugs contain *anticholinergic properties*
  —Mild at therapeutic doses
  —Life-threatening in overdose
- Anticholinergic substances
  —Antihistamines
  —Belladonna alkaloids, synthetic cogeners
  —Antiparkinsonian drugs
  —Cyclic antidepressants
  —Antipsychotics
  —Mydriatics
  —Skeletal muscle relaxants (orphenadrine, cyclobenzaprine)
  —Antispasmodics
  —Mushrooms—Amanita Muscaria, Amanita Pantherina
  —Plants—Deadly Nightshade, Mandrake
  —Jimson weed
    -Smoked or ingested
    -50–100 seeds contain the equivalent of 3–6 mg atropine
    -Mydriasis can persist for up to 1 week

Pre-Hospital

CAUTIONS

- Antiparkinsonian agent trihexyphenidyl (artane)
  —Commonly abused anticholinergic drugs because of its euphoric properties
- Scopoloamine eyedrops have been added to peoples beverages and to rob them
- Jimson weed
  —Common anticholinergic ingestion in adolescents
  —Young adult presents to the ED with blurred vision, dilated pupils, and delirium
- *Coingestion of alcohol with diphenhydramine* for the combined psychoactive effects

Diagnosis

ESSENTIAL WORKUP

- Diagnosis based on clinical presentation

LABORATORY

- Routine laboratory evaluation for altered mental status
  —Should be normal with pure anticholinergic toxicity
- Electrolytes, BUN, Cr, glucose
- CBC
- Acetaminophen level
  —Detects occult ingestion

IMAGING/SPECIAL TESTS

- ECG
  —Sinus tachycardia most common
  —QRS prolongation
  —AV dissociation
  —Bundle branch block
  —Dysrhythmias
- Abdominal radiograph
  —Some phenothiazines radiopaque

DIFFERENTIAL DIAGNOSIS

- Sympathomimetic toxidrome
  —Differentiated from anticholinergic toxicity by the presence of bowel sounds and moist skin
- Acute Psychiatric Disorders
  —Tachycardia/tachypnea present, but an otherwise normal physical exam

Treatment

INITIAL STABILIZATION

- ABCs
  - —IV/O_2/monitor/pulse ox
  - —Vitals including an oral/rectal temperature
  - —Oral/nasal tracheal intubation if indicated
- Naloxone, thiamine, D50 (or Accucheck) if altered mental status

ED TREATMENT

Decontamination

- Avoid ipecac
  - —Due to the risk of associated altered mental status/seizures
- Perform gastric lavage if <1 hour since oral ingestion of potentially toxic substance
- Administer activated charcoal and cathartic (sorbitol)
- Ocular lavage for eyedrop exposure
- Jimson weed considerations
  - —Gastric decontamination recommended up to 12–24 hours after the ingestion of seeds
  - —Administer polyethylene glycol electrolyte solution (Go-Litely) for seed ingestions

Physostigmine

- Reversible acetylcholinesterase inhibitor that crosses the blood brain barrier
- Reverses both central and peripheral anticholinergic effects
- Use with extreme caution due to risk of dysrhythmias (especially asystole), seizures, and cholinergic crises
  - —Place on cardiac monitor
  - —Observe for cholinergic symptoms
- Indications include the presence of peripheral anticholinergics signs and
  - —Seizures unresponsive to conventional therapy
  - —Uncontrollable agitation
  - —Hemodynamically unstable arrhythmias unresponsive to conventional therapy
  - —Hypertension uncontrolled by standard treatment
- Contraindications
  - —Cyclic antidepressant overdose (potentiates toxicity)
  - —Cardiovascular disease
  - —Bronchospasm
  - —Intestinal obstruction
  - —Heart block
  - —Peripheral vascular disease
  - —Bladder obstruction

Treat Complications

- Standard cooling measures for hyperthermia
- Treatment of hypertension usually unnecessary
  - —Conventional therapy for severely elevated BP
- Treat seizures with benzodiazepines and barbiturates
- Dysrhythmias
  - —Use standard antidysrhythmics
  - —Avoid class Ia antidysrhythmic due to the quinidine-like effect of many anticholinergic drugs
  - —Sodium bicarbonate may reverse the quinidine-like effects
- Use benzodiazepines for treatment of agitation
  - —Avoid phenothiazines due to anticholinergic effects and seizure threshold lowering properties

MEDICATIONS

- Activated charcoal slurry: 1–2 g/kg up to 90 g po
- Dextrose: D50W 1 amp (50 ml or 25 g) (peds: D25W 2–4 ml/kg) IV
- Diazepam (benzodiazepine): 5–10 mg (peds: 0.2–0.5 mg/kg) IV
- Phenobarbital: 15–18 mg/kg IV
- Polyethylene glycol-electrolyte solution (CoLyte, Golytely): 240 ml (peds: 25–40 ml/kg/hr) q 10 minutes until 4 L consumed or rectal effluent clear
- Naloxone (narcan): 2 mg (peds: 0.1 mg/kg) IV or IM initial dose
- Physostigmine: 0.5–2.0 mg (peds: 0.02 mg/kg) IV over 5 minutes
  - —Due to rapid elimination, repeat doses q 30–60 minutes
- Sorbitol: 1–2 g/kg to a max of 100 g (peds: >1-year-old: 1–1.5g/kg as a 35% solution to a max of 50 g) po mixed in the activated charcoal slurry
- Thiamine (vitamin B_1): 100 mg (peds: 50 mg) IV or IM

Disposition

ADMISSION CRITERIA

- ICU admission for moderate to severe anticholinergic symptoms (agitation control, temperature control, and observation for seizures or dysrhythmias)
- Any patient receiving physostigmine

DISCHARGE CRITERIA

- Mild and improving symptoms of anticholinergic toxicity after 6–8 hours of ED observation

Miscellaneous

ICD9: 971.1

CORE CONTENT CODE: 17.2.11.4

SUGGESTED READINGS

Amitai Y, Almog S, Singer R, et al. Atropine Poisoning in children during the Persian Gulf Crisis. JAMA 1992;268:630

Ellenhorn MJ, Schoonwald S, Ordog G, Wasserberger J. Antimuscarinic drugs. In: Ellenhorn's medical toxicology. 2d ed. Baltimore: Williams &Wilkins, 1997:840–860

Goldfrank L, Flomenbaum N, Lewin N. Anticholinergic poisoning. J Toxicol Clin Toxicol 1982;19(1):17

Hidalgo HA, Mowers RM. Anticholinergic drug abuse. Ann Pharmacother 1990;24:40

Hurlbut KM. Drug-induced psychoses. Emerg Med Clin North Am 1991;9(1):31–52

Savitt DL, Roberts JR, Seigel EG. Anisocoria from Jimson weed. JAMA 1986;255:1439

Wolf LR. Anticholinergic toxicity. In: Tintanelli J, et al., eds. Emergency medicine: A comprehensive study guide. 4th ed. New York: McGraw-Hill, 1996

Author: Leslie Wolf

Aortic Dissection, Thoracic

Clinical Presentation

SIGNS AND SYMPTOMS

GENERAL

- Hoarseness
- Syncope

CARDIOVASCULAR

- Thoracic pain (80–90%)
  - —Severe steady pain
  - —Sudden onset
  - —Retrosternal if type A dissection
  - —Interscapular if type B dissection
  - —Often migratory to chest, back, and epigastrium
- Hypertension (60–70%)
- Hypotension
- Diastolic murmur of aortic insufficiency
  - —50% of type A dissections
- Pericardial friction rub (5%)

GASTROINTESTINAL

- Abdominal or lumbar pain
- Nausea
- Vomiting

EXTREMITIES

- Extremity weakness or paralysis
- Peripheral pulse deficits (40–50%)

COMPLICATIONS

- Cardiac tamponade
- Myocardial infarction
- Congestive heart failure
- Hemothorax
  - —Predominantly left
- Hemoperitoneum
- Hemispherical stroke
  - —6% of cases
  - —Altered mental status
  - —Temporary blindness
- Ischemic myelopathy
- Intestinal ischemia
- Renal or lower limb ischemia

MECHANISM/DESCRIPTION

- Dissection of the layers of the aorta initiated by an intimal tear
  - —Blood, under the force of arterial pressure, goes through the intimal tear into the media
  - —Dissection of the layers of the vessel
  - —Development of a false lumen
- The dissection may extend both distally and proximally
  - —Blood flow may be limited in any of the branches of the aorta
  - —If the dissection extends proximally, the aortic valve may become incompetent
  - —Dissections through the adventitia lead to hemodynamic collapse
    - -Cardiac tamponade
    - -Pleural effusions
- Two major classifications
  - —Daily's classification
    - -Type A: dissection involving the ascending aorta
    - -Type B: dissections not involving the ascending aorta
  - —DeBakey's classification
    - -Type I: tear in the ascending aorta, extension beyond ascending aorta
    - -Type II: tear in ascending aorta, confined to the ascending aorta
    - -Type IIIA: tear in descending aorta, dissection not beyond the diaphragm
    - -Type IIIB: tear in descending aorta, dissection beyond the diaphragm
- Proximal dissections occur almost twice as often as distal dissections
- Incidence is 5 per million population per year
- Men are affected more commonly than women in a ratio of 2:1
- Most of the cases occur between the ages of 40 and 70
- In younger ages, it is usually associated with an underlying familial predisposition
  - —Marfan's syndrome
    - -33% of patients with Marfan's syndrome develop aortic dissection
    - -4–12% of individuals presenting with acute aortic dissection have Marfan's disease
  - —Congenital disorders of the aorta or aortic valve
- The overall mortality rate is 20–25%
  - —Most common causes of death are hemorrhage and acute heart failure
- The most common late complication in survivors is the rupture of a postdissection aneurysm
  - —10–20%
  - —more likely if uncontrolled hypertension

ETIOLOGY

Risk factors

- Hypertension
- Congenital diseases
  - —Bicuspid aortic valve
  - —Congenital aortic stenosis
  - —Coarctation of the aorta
- Cystic medial necrosis
- Congenital disorders of connective tissue
  - —Marfan's disease
  - —Ehlers-Danlos syndrome
- Inflammatory diseases of the aorta
  - —Syphilitic aortitis
  - —Polyarteritis nodosa
  - —Endocarditis
  - —Mycotic infections of the aorta
  - —Giant cell aortitis
  - —Systemic lupus
- Pregnancy
- Arteriosclerosis
- Cigarette use

Pre-Hospital

- Intravenous access
- Monitor

CAUTIONS

- Pre-hospital thrombolytics or heparin should not be administered if aortic dissection is suspected

Diagnosis

ESSENTIAL WORKUP

- EKG
  - —Changes compatible with MI are seen in 10–20% of patients
    - -A positive EKG does not rule out dissection
    - -ST-segment elevation is unusual
  - —A negative EKG
    - -Supports the diagnosis of dissection in patients with severe chest pain
  - —Signs of preexisting hypertension
    - -Left ventricular hypertrophy
    - -Left ventricular strain
    - -Pericarditic changes
    - -Diffuse ST elevation
    - -PR depression
    - -Electrical alternans

LABORATORY

- Nonspecific findings
- Hematuria
- Leukocytosis
- Elevated bun and creatinine due to hypertension or renal ischemia
- Anemia
- Normal SGOT
- Elevated LDH
- Elevated amylase
  - —Bowel ischemia
  - —Mild changes in coagulation panel
  - —Cardiac enzymes used to rule out myocardial infarction

IMAGING/SPECIAL TESTS

- Chest Radiograph
  - —Widened mediastinum
  - —Obliteration or blurring of the aortic knob
  - —Separation of the intimal calcification from the edge of the aortic contour
  - —Left pleural effusion
  - —Increases in the cardiothoracic ratio secondary to a pericardial effusion
- Transthoracic echocardiography
  - —Not indicated in the diagnosis of acute dissection
  - —Limited role in the evaluation of the complications of acute dissection

- Transesophageal echocardiography
  - —Performed at the bedside
  - —Provides information on the extent and type of dissection, aortic valve and coronary ostia
  - —Definitive investigation in severely ill patients
- Contrast-enhanced CT
  - —Indications for CT versus other studies depend on how quickly these can be performed
  - —Provides an accurate assessment of true and false lumina and the intimal flap
  - —Speed and ease of access often make this the study of choice
- MRI
  - —Allows an angled sagittal plane comparable to the aortogram
  - —Utility limited as significant time delays are required to perform this study
- Aortography
  - —Accuracy 95–99%
  - —Precise location of the intimal tear
  - —Delineation of the longitudinal extent of the false lumen

DIFFERENTIAL DIAGNOSIS

- Acute myocardial infarction
- Unstable angina
- Pneumothorax
- Pericarditis
- Pleuritis
- Intramural hematoma of the thoracic aorta
- Pulmonary embolus
- Musculoskeletal chest pain
- Chest pain of unknown origin

Treatment

INITIAL STABILIZATION

- Large-bore intravenous catheter access
- Supplemental oxygen
- Cardiac monitor
- Pulse oximetry
- Blood type and crossmatch
- Foley catheter

ED TREATMENT

- Intravenous β-blockers
  - —Reduction of the left ventricular contractility
  - —Decrease the heart rate down to 60 beats/min
  - —Propranolol or esmolol
  - —Labetalol may be used alone as it has both β_1- and β_2-receptor-blocking action
  - —Contraindications
    - -Bradycardia
    - -Bronchospasm
    - -Congestive heart failure
    - -Use of intravenous trimethaphan as a single agent
- Sodium nitroprusside
  - —Do not use before β-blockers because it may increase the heart rate and extend the dissection
- Pain management
  - —Intravenous morphine sulphate
- Emergent surgery
  - —Treatment of choice for patients with acute ascending aortic dissections (type A)
  - —Complicated type B cases
    - -Failure of medical management
    - -Expanding false lumens
    - -Intestinal, renal, and extremity ischemia
- Medical management
  - —Initial therapy for uncomplicated descending aortic dissections (type B)

MEDICATIONS

- Esmolol: 5 g in 500 cc (10 mg/ml) at 50–200 μg/kg/min
- Labetalol : 20 mg IV q 10 min up to 300 mg
- Morphine: 0.1mg/kg up to 2–4 mg IV q 5 min
- Nitroprusside: 50 mg in 250 ml D5W (200 μg/ml); start at 0.3 μg/kg/min (for 70-kg adult = 6 ml/hr); maximum 10 μg/kg/min
- Propranolol: 1 mg IV increments q 2 min
- Trimethaphan: 500 mg in 100 ml D5W (5 mg/ml); start at 1–10 mg/min (12–120 ml/hr)

Disposition

ADMISSION CRITERIA

- All patients should be admitted to the intensive care unit
- Emergent surgical consultation is indicated

DISCHARGE CRITERIA

N/A

Miscellaneous

ICD9: 441.01

CORE CONTENT CODE: 2.5.1.7

SUGGESTED READINGS

American College of Emergency Physicians. Clinical policy for the initial approach to adults presenting with a chief complaint of chest pain, with no history of trauma. Ann Emerg Med 1995;25:274–299.

Ergin MA, Griepp RB. Dissections of the aorta. In: Baue AE, et al., eds. Glenn's Thoracic and Cardiovascular Surgery. 6th ed. Stamford, CT: Appleton & Lange, 1996:2273–2298.

Howell JM, Hedges JR. Differential diagnosis of chest discomfort and general approach to myocardial ischemia decision making. Am J Emerg Med 1991;9:571–579.

Izzat MB, Jones AJ, Angelini GD. Acute aortic dissection. Br J Hosp Med 1994;52:523–528.

Najafi H. Thoracic aortic aneurysm: evaluation and surgical management. Comp Therapy 1994;20:282–288.

Sarasin FP, Louis-Simonet M, Gaspoz J-M, et al. Detecting acute thoracic aortic dissection in the emergency department: Time constraints and choice of the optimal diagnostic test. Ann Emerg Med 1996;28:278–288.

Van Shil P, Vanmaele R, De Maeseneer M, et al. Acute aortic dissection. Acta Chir Belg 1994;94:142–146.

Wolfson AB, Bessen HA. Thoracic aortic dissection: ruling in and ruling out. Ann Emerg Med 1996;28:349–351.

Author: Georgina Groleau

Aortic Rupture, Traumatic

Clinical Presentation

SIGNS AND SYMPTOMS

- Substernal chest pain, midscapular pain
- Shortness of breath, dyspnea, dysphagia, stridor, hoarseness (from expanding hematoma)
- Harsh precordial or midscapular systolic murmur
- *Acute coarctation syndrome:* hypertension of upper extremity; increased pulse amplitude of upper extremities, decreased in lower extremities; cyanosis of lower extremities
- Paraplegia, anuria, or ischemic extremity pain, due to impaired spinal blood supply
- Swelling of neck (extravasation of blood)
- Back pain with acute abdomen

MECHANISM/DESCRIPTION

- Several theories have been proposed
  —Shear forces created by unequal rates of horizontal deceleration of relatively fixed descending aorta and more mobile arch
  —"Bending" stress created by lateral impact leading to shear at fixed areas
  —Direct blast or compression forces causing twisting of the arch, forcing it superiorly and causing stretch
  —*Osseous pinch*—compression of thoracic cage causing tearing of major vessels between bony structures
  —*Water-hammer pulse wave*—sudden increase in intraluminal pressure in vessels when compressed causing disruption
- Most common location is the *isthmus* at the ligamentum arteriosum
  —Other: ascending aorta, descending aorta, arch, abdominal aorta
- Brachiocephalic vessels may also be injured
- Innominate artery most common branch of aorta injured
- Aortic tears described as involving the intima, intima and media, or transmural
- Most tears are transverse, not longitudinal
- Tears may be partially or completely circumferential

ETIOLOGY

- Most commonly due to motor vehicle accidents
- Other mechanisms: auto vs. pedestrian, airplane crashes, falls from heights, crush and blast injuries, direct blow to chest
- Cause of death in up to 20% of victims of lethal motor vehicle accidents
- Approximately 85% of patients with traumatic aortic injury (TAI) die before reaching the hospital
- Drivers are 50% more likely to sustain TAI than passengers
- Ejection doubles the risk of TAI

PEDIATRIC CONSIDERATIONS

- Rare in patients <15 years; range: 0.01–7.0% in recent studies
- Children may be protected by more compliant chest wall

Pre-Hospital

- Important information about the scene to convey to the emergency physician includes
  —Rate of speed, direction of impact
  —Damage to steering wheel
  —Ejection from vehicle
  —Restraints used
  —Driver or passenger
- Immediate transport of any patient with suspected TAI to trauma center

Diagnosis

ESSENTIAL WORKUP

- *Plain chest radiograph* is the primary screening tool

LABORATORY

- CBC
- Electrolytes
- PT/PTT
- Type and crossmatch

IMAGING/SPECIAL TESTS

- *Plain chest radiograph*—findings consistent with mediastinal hemorrhage, hematoma, or associated injuries, rather than direct evidence of TAI
  —Widened mediastinum (>8 cm AP supine, >6 cm PA upright, or >0.25 mediastinum-width to chest-width ratio)
  —Obliteration of aortic knob
  —Obscured descending aorta
  —Opacification of aortopulmonary window
  —Left apical capping
  —Deviation of trachea to right
  —Depression of left mainstem bronchus
  —Displacement of nasogastric tube to right
  —Widened left paraspinal stripe without spinal fracture
  —Left hemothorax, pneumomediastinum
  —Fracture of sternum, or first or second ribs
- *Aortography*—still considered the study of choice although other modalities are gaining favor (transesophageal echocardiography). Shows location and extent of injury. *Intra-arterial digital subtraction angiography,* if available, uses less contrast material and is faster
- Other
  —CT—may be considered in hemodynamically stable patients with low suspicion but equivocal chest film mediastinal hematoma indication for angiography
  —Spiral CT—recent studies have shown advantages over conventional CT but artifact and slice thickness may mask a small tear; aortography usually needed to confirm findings of normal study with near 100% sensitivity
  —Transesophageal echocardiography—can be done rapidly and in the ED. Demonstrates the isthmus well; may not visualize distal ascending aorta or arch well. Patients with cervical fractures, maxillofacial, or esophageal injuries are not suitable candidates
  —MRI—multiplanar capability allows entire aorta to be imaged but trauma patients often have support devices that cannot enter the magnetic field; not widely used in the diagnosis of TAI

DIFFERENTIAL DIAGNOSIS

- Mediastinal hematoma due to other causes
- Mediastinal lymphadenopathy
- Redundant aorta due to hypertension

PEDIATRIC CONSIDERATIONS

- Presence of thymus may make diagnosis of widened mediastinum difficult

Treatment

INITIAL STABILIZATION

- ABCs of trauma care
- In addition to usual resuscitative measures, avoid maneuvers that may result in Valsalva (e.g., gagging, straining)

ED TREATMENT

- *Emergent surgical consult*
- *Medical therapy of hypertensive patient* to lower risk of rupture of pseudoaneurysm
  - —Negative inotropics (e.g., esmolol) to target heart rate 60 +/−5 bpm, SBP 100–120 mm Hg, MAP 70–80
  - —Add vasodilators (e.g., nitroprusside sodium) as needed after β-blockade
- Central venous catheter
- Arterial pressure monitoring catheter
- *Acute coarctation syndrome* is a relative contraindication to antihypertensive therapy
- Peritoneal injuries take precedence. Patients with suspected intra-abdominal injuries should have diagnostic peritoneal lavage/ultrasound done in the ED
- Concommitment workup of other injuries
  - —Intraabdominal (see Abdominal Injury Chapter)
    - —Diagnostic Peritoneal Lavage (DPL)
    - —Ultrasound
    - —CT
  - —Pelvic (see Pelvic Trauma chapter)
    - —radiograph

MEDICATIONS

- Esmolol: 500–1000 μg/kg IV load; infusion 50-150 μg/kg/min; repeat load, increase drip 50 μg/kg/min q 5 min; max 300 μg/kg/min
- Nitroprusside: start at 0.3 μg/kg/min; maximum 10 μg/kg/min

Disposition

ADMISSION CRITERIA

- All patients with aortic injuries must be admitted to the *intensive care unit,* if not taken directly to the operating room

DISCHARGE CRITERIA

- None

Miscellaneous

ICD9: 901.0, 902.0

CORE CONTENT CODE: 18.4.10.6

SUGGESTED READINGS

Fabian TC, et al. Prospective study of blunt aortic injury: Multicenter trial of the American Association for the Surgery of Trauma. J Trauma 1997;42(3):374–380.

Feliciano DV. Trauma to the aorta and major vessels. Chest Surg Clin N Am 1997;7(2):305–323.

Lowe LH, et al. Traumatic aortic injury in children: Radiologic evaluation. AJR Am J Roentgenol 1998;170(1):39–42.

Weiss JP, et al. Traumatic rupture of the thoracic aorta. Emerg Med Clin North Am 1991;9(4):789–804.

White CS, et al. Pictorial review: Imaging of traumatic aortic injury. Clin Radiol 1995;50(5):281–287.

Author: Elizabeth Lynch

Aphthous Ulcer

Clinical Presentation

SIGNS AND SYMPTOMS

- Herpetiform
  - —Multiple pinpoint lesions along the lateral margin and tip of the tongue
- No regional lymphadenopathy

Minor Aphthae

- Burning sensation
- Shallow hyperemic ulcerations
  - —Smaller than 1 cm
  - —Exquisitely painful
  - —Single
  - —Multiple (aphthous stomatitis)
  - —Round to oval with
  - —Well-defined margins
  - —Covered by a thin exudate of yellowish-grayish fibrinous material
  - —Rimmed by a narrow zone of erythema
  - —Found on the anterior part of the oral cavity
    - -Unattached, nonkeratinized mucosa
    - -Lips
    - -Cheek
    - -Tongue
    - -Floor of mouth
  - —Spares other parts of the oral cavity
    - -The soft palate
    - -Pharynx
    - -Tonsillar fauces

Major Aphthae

- Lesions >1 cm
- Usually multiple
- Involves all areas of the oropharynx

MECHANISM/DESCRIPTION

- Most common disease of the oral mucosa
- Minor aphthae
  - —Last from 1–3 weeks
  - —Heals without scar formation
- Major aphthae (Sutton's disease)
  - —Lasts for several months
  - —Cause scar formation when they heal
  - —Often an underlying disease
  - —HIV
- Herpetiform
  - —The rarest clinical presentation
  - —Their course is similar to that of minor aphthae
  - —The name is a misnomer
    - -Herpes virus is not involved
    - -Little clinical resemblance to herpetic stomatitis
- Affects from 10–20% of the population
- No longer considered a single disease but several pathologic states with similar clinical manifestations
- Presents between the ages of 10–30
- Prevalent within families and affects women greater than men
- Nonsmokers greater than smokers

ETIOLOGY

- The etiology remains obscure and is probably multifactorial
  - —Heredity
  - —Inflammatory bowel disease
  - —Systemic lupus erythematous
  - —Behçet's syndrome
  - —Hypersensitivity to certain foods
  - —Emotional stress
  - —Hormonal (endocrine) influences
  - —Pregnancy
  - —Menstruation
  - —Nutritional deficiencies
  - —Mechanical trauma
  - —Autoimmune reactions
  - —Humoral antibodies active against oral mucosa
  - —Sensitized T lymphocytes
  - —Underlying infection

Pre-Hospital

N/A

Diagnosis

ESSENTIAL WORKUP

- Exclusion of other diseases with a detailed history and physical examination
  - —Signs and symptoms of blood dyscrasias
  - —Systemic complaints
  - —Associated skin, eye, genital or rectal lesions

LABORATORY

N/A

IMAGING/SPECIAL TESTS

N/A

DIFFERENTIAL DIAGNOSIS

- Acute necrotizing gingivitis
- Cancer
- Trauma
  - —Biting
  - —Dentures
- Immunocompromised host
  - —AIDS
  - —Agranulocytosis
- Underlying disease
  - —Systemic lupus erythematosus
  - —Crohn's disease
  - —Celiac disease
  - —Reiter's syndrome
  - —Behçet's syndrome
- Infection
  - —Syphilis
  - —Candidal infection
  - —Herpes stomatitis
    - -Many small lesions on fixed mucosa
    - -Cervical lymphadenopathy
    - -Fever
  - —Coxsackie virus (hand-foot-mouth disease)

Treatment

INITIAL STABILIZATION

N/A

ED TREATMENT

- Symptomatic treatment with analgesics
  - —Anesthetic lozenges and gels
- Apply the following therapies in stepwise fashion
  - —Topical steroids
    - -Triamcinolone acetonide in emollient
  - —Amlexanox
    - -Aphthasol
  - —Tetracycline oral suspension
  - —Intralesional steroid injection
    - -Kenalog 10
  - —Systemic steroids
  - —Thalidomide for HIV only

MEDICATIONS

- Amlexanox (aphthasol) 5% oral paste: apply topically qpc + qhs
- Tetracycline oral suspension: 250 mg/5 cc H_2O, S&S 2 min qpc + qhs
- Prednisone: 40 mg po qd for 7 days
- Thalidomide: 200 mg po qd for 4 weeks
- Triamcinolone acetonide: in emollient (kenalog in orabase): apply topically qpc + qhs; injection (kenalog 10): intralesional injection once

Disposition

ADMISSION CRITERIA

- Unable to eat or drink after appropriate analgesia

DISCHARGE CRITERIA

- Tolerating fluids
- Follow up with PCP if lesions have not resolved in 2 weeks
- Instruct patient to use good oral hygiene

Miscellaneous

ICD9: 528.2

CORE CONTENT CODE: 3.2.4.1

SUGGESTED READINGS

Damjanov I, Linder J. Anderson's pathology. 10th ed. St. Louis: Mosby-Year Book, 1996:1579–1580.

Jacobson JM, Greenspan JS, Spritzler J, et al. Thalidomide for the treatment of oral aphthous ulcers in patients with human immunodeficiency virus infection. N Engl J Med 1997;336(21):1487–1493.

Lynch MA, Brightman VJ, Greenberg MS. Burket's oral medicine, diagnosis and treatment. 9th ed. Philadelphia: JB Lippincott, 1994:26–30.

Petersen MJ, Baughman RA. Recurrent aphthous stomatitis: Primary care management. Nurse Pract 1996;21(5):36–47.

Ship JA. Recurrent aphthous stomatitis. An update. Oral Surg Oral Med Oral Pathol Oral Radiol Endod 1996;81(2):141–147.

Author: Jacques H. Blanchet

Apnea

Clinical Presentation

SIGNS AND SYMPTOMS

- Often patients look and act entirely normal following the event
- Some cases may require assisted ventilation
- The need for any resuscitative effort suggests a more serious event
- Apnea during sleep is more worrisome
- Fever or hypothermia are suggestive of an infectious etiology
- Tachypnea following an episode of apnea suggests a respiratory or a metabolic problem
- Shock suggests sepsis or hypovolemia

Pathologic Apnea

- Respiratory pause >20 seconds
- Cyanosis
- Marked pallor
- Hypotonia
- Bradycardia

Apparent Life-Threatening Event (ALTE)

- Frightens the observer
- Combination of any of the following
  —Apnea
  —Color change
  —Marked change in muscle tone

Apnea of Prematurity

- Periodic breathing in a premature infant
- Usually ceases by 37 weeks of gestational age

Apnea of Infancy

- Unexplained cessation of breathing for 20 seconds or longer
- Shorter respiratory pause associated with one of the following
  —Bradycardia
  —Cyanosis
  —Pallor
  —Marked hypotonia

MECHANISM/DESCRIPTION

- Cessation of airflow
  —Central or diaphragmatic (absence of respiratory effort)
  —Obstructive (usually upper airway)
  —Mixed
- Occurs in 0.5–6% of all infants
- Mean age of presentation between 8 and 14 weeks of age
- Male predominance

ETIOLOGY

- Central apnea
  —Seizure
  —Brain stem tumor
  —Increased intracranial pressure
  —CNS immaturity
- Obstructive apnea
  —Stridor
    -Vascular ring
    -Vascular cord paralysis
    -Foreign body
    -Croup
    -Epiglottitis
    -Laryngeal web
    -Tracheostomy plug
    -Subglottic stenosis
  —Premature infants
    -Positional
    -Laryngomalacia
    -Tracheomalacia
  —Abnormal airway
    -Choanal atresia/stenosis
    -Tracheoesophageal fistula
    -Craniofacial abnormalities
    -Enlarged tonsils
  —Mixed apnea
    -Dysrhythmias
    -QT prolongation
    -Pneumonia
    -Bronchopulmonary dysplasia
    -Sepsis
    -Pertussis
    -Meningitis
    -Encephalitis
    -Hypoglycemia
    -Seizure
    -Intracranial hypertension
    -Shock
    -Anemia
    -Poisoning
    -Neuromuscular disorders
- Suspected etiologies leading to near SIDS or ATLE
  —Suffocation
  —Electrolyte abnormality
  —Gastroesophageal reflux
  —Mineral deficiencies
  —Cardiac dysrhythmias
  —Amino acid deficiencies
  —Abnormal ventilatory response to hypoxia/hypercarbia
  —Occult trauma

Pre-Hospital

- All infants with an apneic event or ATLE should be transported to the ED
- Ventilatory support during apnea
- All cardiac arrests should be assumed to be secondary to respiratory arrest in children

Diagnosis

ESSENTIAL WORKUP

- Duration of apnea
- Position of sleep
  —Prone position is inadvisable
- Determine if the event occurred when the child was awake or asleep
- Presence and order of color changes
- Description of movements and muscle tone
- Assess for risk factors for SIDS
  —Term infant
  —Premature infant with low birth-weight
  —Male sex
  —Low socioeconomic class

LABORATORY

- Electrolytes
- Glucose
- BUN/creatinine
- Stool samples for clostridia and botulinum testing
- Suspicion of a serious infection
  —Pan cultures
  —Pertussis and chlamydia cultures

IMAGING/SPECIAL TESTS

- EKG
- CXR
  —Anteroposterior and lateral soft tissue neck films
  —Obstructive apnea
  —Stridor
- Lumbar puncture indicated with signs of infection

DIFFERENTIAL DIAGNOSIS

- Munchausen syndrome by proxy
- Breath-holding spell
- Gastroesophageal reflux
- Seizure

Treatment

INITIAL STABILIZATION

- Intubate and assist in ventilation as needed for persistent apnea
- Initiate CPR and PALS algorithms if arrest or near arrest
- Supplemental oxygen
- Intravenous access
- Cardiac monitoring
- Pulse oximetry

ED TREATMENT

- Theophylline or caffeine
  —Indicated for apnea of prematurity
  —Reduces periodic breathing

MEDICATIONS

- Caffeine 10mg/kg (loading dose) 2.5 mg/kg qd PO
- Theophylline: 6 mg/kg/d
- Dextrose 25: 2–4 ml/kg IV

Disposition

ADMISSION CRITERIA

- Pediatric ward with apnea/bradycardia monitor
  —Primary apnea
  —Any child with criteria for ALTE
- Pediatric intensive care unit
  —Any field or ED resuscitation

DISCHARGE CRITERIA

N/A

Miscellaneous

ICD9: 770.8

CORE CONTENT CODE: 16.14

SUGGESTED READINGS

Brooks JG. Apparent life-threatening events and apnea of infancy. Clin Perinatol 1992;19(4):809.

Steinschneider A, Richmond C, Ramaswamy V, Curns A. Clinical characteristics of an apparent life-threatening event (ALTE) and the subsequent occurrence of prolonged apnea or prolonged bradycardia. Clin Pediatr (Phila) 1998;37(4):223–229.

Torrey SB. Apnea. In: Fleisher GR et al., eds. Textbook of pediatric emergency medicine. 3rd ed. Baltimore: Williams & Wilkins, 1993:107–111.

Author: Hartwel Lin

Appendicitis

Clinical Presentation

SIGNS AND SYMPTOMS

- Abdominal pain—the prime symptom
  - —Classical Presentation
    - -Begins periumbilical and is poorly localized
    - -Constant; moderately severe
    - -After variable period (1–12 hours) localizes to the right lower quadrant
    - -Appendix located in "usual" position approximately 70% of the time
  - —Alternative pain locations
    - -One-third—pain localized *other than* in the RLQ
    - -Retrocecal appendix—back, flank, testicular pain
    - -Pelvic appendix—suprapubic pain
    - -Long appendix—the inflamed tip may cause pain in RUQ or LLQ
- Anorexia
  - —Initial symptom in 95%
  - —Almost always present
- Vomiting
  - —One to two episodes of vomiting common—generally not prolonged
  - —Usually *follows* the onset of pain (in gastroenteritis, vomiting *precedes* pain)
- Bowel habits: diarrhea (33%); constipation (9–33%)
- Vital signs
  - —Normal early
  - —Mild temperature elevation (less than 1°)—increases with perforation
  - —Evidence of toxicity with severe dehydration after perforation and sepsis occur
- Patient position
  - —Lie supine or on their side with legs (particularly the right) drawn up
  - —Prefer not to move
  - —"Appendicitis shuffle": walk with a limp, with right hip flexed, slightly bent over (children)
- Abdominal exam
  - —Tenderness usually located at McBurney's point (3.0—5.0 cm from the anterior-superior iliac spine on straight line drawn from that process to the umbilicus)
  - —Guarding
    - -Voluntary guarding early due to muscular resistance to palpation
    - -Involuntary guarding (rigidity) later as inflammation progresses and perforation occurs
  - —Rebound: pain with *any* rapid movement of the peritoneum—best assessed (particularly in children) by gently percussing the area
  - —Bowel sounds initially normal becoming decreased due to ileus
  - —Rectal exam—local tenderness in RLQ
- Specific findings
  - —*Rovsing's sign:* pain in the *right* lower quadrant when palpating the *left* lower quadrant
  - —*Psoas sign:* pain with extension of right hip
    - -Have patient lie on left side and slowly extend right hip, thus stretching the iliopsoas muscle
    - -Inflamed appendix touching iliopsoas muscle will cause pain
  - —*Obturator sign:* pain elicited by passive internal rotation of the flexed right thigh with the patient supine

Considerations in the Pregnant Patient

- Enlarging uterus displaces the appendix upwardly and laterally
- Hyperemesis gravidarum and other nonsurgical causes of vomiting should not cause abdominal *tenderness*

ETIOLOGY

- Inciting event: Luminal obstruction of the appendix, usually by a fecalith
- Appendiceal lumen becomes distended
- Appendix may rupture, spilling its contents into the peritoneal cavity; or it may wall off and form an abscess

MECHANISM/DESCRIPTION

Pain Migration

- Appendiceal distention stimulates stretch receptors, which relay pain via *visceral* afferent pain fibers to the 10th thoracic ganglion
  - —Vague pain sensed in periumbilical region
- As the inflammation extends to surrounding tissues, localized pain occurs due to stimulation of *parietal* nerve fibers
  - —Pain location dependent on the appendix position

SPECIAL PEDIATRIC CONSIDERATIONS

- Diagnosis much more difficult. Presentations often non-specific and difficult to localize
- 70–94% perforation rate in young children (< 2 yrs old) much higher due to delays in presentation and diagnosis
- Ask when the child last ate a good meal
  - —Not be able to complain of anorexia
  - —A half-eaten meal hours before complaints of pain may more accurately indicate the duration of symptoms
- Observe the child *before* the examination for subtle indications of local inflammation
  - —Limping gait
  - —Hesitation to move or climb
  - —Flexed right hip

Pre-Hospital

N/A

Diagnosis

ESSENTIAL WORKUP

- Suggestive history and physical exam sufficient to establish a preoperative diagnosis and warrant surgical consultation

LABORATORY

- CBC
  —WBC >10,000 present in 80%
  —Normal WBC does *not* exclude the diagnosis
- Electrolytes, BUN, Cr, glucose
  —For evidence of dehydration or toxicity
  —At the extremes of age
- Urinalysis
  —Generally normal
  —Abnormalities in 20–40% including mild pyuria, bacteriuria, and hematuria
    -Pyuria present if the inflamed appendix lies near the ureter or bladder
  —>30 RBC or >20 WBC—consider UTI as diagnosis
- Pregnancy test for females of child-bearing years
- Amylase/lipase
  —If risk factors for pancreatitis
  —Further observation/testing for patients in whom the history or physical exam is atypical or unclear

IMAGING/SPECIAL TESTS

- Not necessary unless the diagnosis is unclear
- CXR: to exclude RLL pneumonia that may have symptoms similar to appendicitis
- Plain films of the abdomen
  —May reveal a distended loop of small bowel in the right lower quadrant
  —Radiopaque fecalith (present in 10%) in RLQ—almost always associated with appendicitis
- Ultrasound: sensitivity 75–94%; specificity 84–94%
  —Study limited by
    -Obesity
    -Bowel gas
    -Retrocecal appendix
    -Operator dependent
  —Appendicitis findings
    -Noncompressible appendix 7 mm in AP diameter
    -Presence of appendicolith
  —Aids in diagnosis of other etiologies of abdominal pain
    -Tubo-ovarian abscess/PID
    -Ureteric stone
    -Appendiceal abscess
- CT: sensitivity 96%; specificity 89%
  —Oral *and* rectal contrast optimal
  —Defines appendiceal masses (i.e., phlegmon vs. abscess)
  —More likely to find alternative diagnoses than ultrasound
- Barium enema
  —Rarely performed—replaced by other modalities
  —Sensitivity/specificity—90% when optimal study
  —High incidence of technical failure
  —Risk of extravasation with perforated appendix
  —Findings consistent with appendicitis
    -Absent or incomplete filling of appendix
    -Irregularities of appendiceal lumen
    -Extrinsic mass effect on cecum or terminal ileum

DIFFERENTIAL DIAGNOSIS

- Pelvic inflammatory disease
- Gastroenteritis
- Tubo-ovarian abscess
- Ovarian cyst/torsion
- Renal stone
- Meckel's diverticulum
- Testicular torsion
- Bowel obstruction
- Diverticulitis (right-sided)
- Urinary tract infection
- Cholecystitis
- Pancreatitis

Treatment

INITIAL STABILIZATION

- ABCs
- Fluid resuscitation with LR or 0.9%NS
  —Observe tachycardia and urine output

ED TREATMENT

- Immediate surgical consult for convincing history and physical exam
- Preoperative antibiotics (cefoxitin or ampicillin sulbactam)
- NPO
- Order CT if a palpable mass is present in the RLQ to define phlegmon vs. abscess
- If diagnosis is uncertain, send labs and observe and reexamine
- Analgesics once diagnosis confirmed and patient to go for surgery

MEDICATIONS

- Ampicillin sulbactam (unasyn): 3 g (peds: 100–200 mg ampicillin/kg/24hrs) q 6 hrs IV
- Cefoxitin (mefoxin): 1–2 g (peds: 80–100 mg/kg/24hrs) q 6 hrs IV

Disposition

ADMISSION CRITERIA

- Surgical intervention of acute appendicitis
- Observation and/or further diagnostic workup if diagnosis is uncertain

DISCHARGE CRITERIA

- Patients with abdominal pain thought not to be appendicitis may be discharged if
  —Resolved or resolving symptoms
  —Minimal or no abdominal tenderness
  —Able to tolerate po intake
  —Adequate social support and able to return if symptoms worsen

Miscellaneous

ICD 9 CODE: 540.9, 540.0, 540.1

CORE CONTENT CODE: 1.6.3.1 APPENDICITIS

SUGGESTED READINGS

Calder JD, Gajraj H. Recent advances in the diagnosis and treatment of acute appendicitis. Br J Hosp Med 1995;54(4):129–133

Graffeo CS, Counjselman FL. Appendicitis. Emerg Med Clin North Am 1996;14:653–671

Martin LCF, Puente I, Sosa JL, et al. Open versus laparoscopic appendectomy. A prospective randomized comparison. Ann Surg 1995;222(3):256–261

Nitecki S, Assalia A, Schein M. Contemporary management of the appendiceal mass. Br J Surg 1993;80(1):18–20

Author: Paula Ward

Arsenic, Poisoning

Clinical Presentation

SIGNS AND SYMPTOMS

Gastrointestinal
- Garlicky odor
- Nausea, vomiting
- Abdominal pain
- Watery ("rice water")diarrhea
- Hemorrhagic gastroenteritis due to diffuse capillary damage

Cardiopulmonary
- Tachycardia
- Cardiogenic and noncardiogenic pulmonary edema
- Conduction abnormalities
  —QT interval prolongation
- Ventricular tachycardia/fibrillation
- Torsades de pointes

Neurologic
- Delirium
- Encephalopathy
- Seizures
- Coma
- Early painful dysesthesias
- Delayed sensorimotor peripheral neuropathy 2–6 weeks postacute exposure

Hematologic
- Pancytopenia
- Leukopenia reaches nadir 1–3 weeks
- Basophilic stippling
- Hemolytic anemia
- Eosinophilia

Dermatologic
- Hyperkeratosis
- Aldrich-Mees lines (5%) on nails 2–3 weeks postingestion
- Alopecia
- Toxic erythroderma

Hepatic
- Hepatic transaminase elevation
- Noncirrhotic portal hypertension

Oncologic
- Basal cell
- Squamous cell carcinoma
- Lung cancer
- Bowen's disease of the skin

MECHANISM
- Disrupts enzymatic reaction by binding to sulfhydryl groups (trivalent arsenic) or substituting for phosphate (pentavalent arsenic)
- Combines with globin chain of hemoglobin
- Trivalent arsenic 5–10 times more toxic than pentavalent arsenic
- Soluble arsenic compounds are well absorbed after inhalation or ingestion

ETIOLOGY
- Byproduct of copper, lead, zinc, and coal
- Pesticides and herbicides
- Food additive to poultry and livestock feed

Pre-Hospital

- Secure ABCs and remove from exposure

Diagnosis

ESSENTIAL WORKUP
- Urine arsenic level
- CBC

LABORATORY

Arsenic Level
- Spot urine arsenic level >1000 μg/l
  —Peak in 10–50 hours postexposure
  —May be elevated for up to 1–2 weeks postexposure
- Blood arsenic levels
  —Highly variable and of little use
  —Aresenic present in blood during first 2–4 hours postingestion
- Elevated arsenic levels in hair and nails persists for months

Other Tests
- CBC for
  —Anemia
  —Leukopenia
  —Leukocytosis
  —Basophilic stippling
- Electrolytes, BUN/Cr, glucose
- Urinalysis dipstick for occult blood (myoglobin)

IMAGING/SPECIAL TESTS
- Cranial CT/lumbar puncture for altered mental status as indicated

DIFFERENTIAL DIAGNOSIS
- Other heavy metal intoxications
- Cyclic antidepressants
- Encephalopathy
- Kosakoff's syndrome
- Shock
- Guillain-Barré syndrome
- Addison's disease
- Cholera

Treatment

INITIAL STABILIZATION

- Secure ABCs and monitoring
- D50W (or Accucheck), thiamine, narcan, and oxygen for altered mental status
- Avoid type Ia antiarrhythmics in treating dysrhythmias secondary to prolonged QT
- Administer 0.9%NS bolus followed by vasopressors for hypotension/shock

ED TREATMENT

Decontamination

- For acute oral ingestion
  - —Gastric lavage if recent (<1–2 hours) ingestion
  - —Activated charcoal
  - —Whole bowel irrigation (if lead containing material visible on x-ray after initial treatment)
- Dermal exposure
  - —If stable, decontaminate in the ED decontamination room prior to further evaluation

Chelation Therapy

- In symptomatic patients, administer BAL (dimercaprol) 3 mg/kg deep IM every 4–6 hours for 2 days then every 12 hours for 7–10 days
- In stable patients or those with chronic exposure, administer oral DMSA (succimer) 10 mg/kg every 8 hours or 5 days then same dose every 12 hours for 14 days

Hemodialysis

- For massive acute ingestions
- For hypotension in spite of fluid resuscitation
- For oliguria/progressive acidosis
- Administer BAL concurrently with hemodialysis

Alkalinization

- Administer sodium bicarbonate if evidence of acute hemolysis (positive urine dipstick for blood without urine RBCs on microscopy)
- Follow electrolytes/renal function closely

MEDICATIONS

- Dextrose: D50W 1 amp (50 ml or 25 g) (peds: D25W 2–4 ml/kg) IV
- Naloxone (Narcan): 2 mg (peds: 0.1 mg/kg) IV or IM initial dose
- Thiamine (vitamin B_1): 100 mg (peds: 50 mg) IV or IM
- Sodium bicarbonate: 1–2 mEq/kg added to 1 L of D5W

Disposition

ADMISSION CRITERIA

- Symptomatic patients

DISCHARGE CRITERIA

- Asymptomatic and urine level below 50 μg/L

Miscellaneous

ICD9: 985.1

CORE CONTENT CODE: 17.2.21

SUGGESTED READINGS

Ellenhorn MJ, Schoonwald S, Ordog G, Wasserberger J. Arsenic. In: Ellenhorn's medical toxicology. 2d ed. Baltimore: Williams & Wilkins, 1997:1538–1543

Ford M. Arsenic—Goldfrank's toxicologic emergencies. 5th ed. Norwalk, CT: Appleton & Lange, 1994:1011–1028

Trepka MJ, et al. Arsenic burden among children in industrial areas of Eastern Germany. Sci Total Environ 1996;180(2):95–105

Authors: Yat Leung; Lisandro Irizarry

Arterial Occlusion

Clinical Presentation

SIGNS AND SYMPTOMS

The 6 Ps

- Pain
- Pallor
- Paresthesias
- Paralysis
- Pulseless
- Poikilothermia

Chronic

- Claudication
- Decreased pulses after activity
- Hair-free atrophic skin
- Poorly healing wounds or ulcers
- Ankle-brachial index (ABI) measurements
  - —Use a Doppler probe
  - —Inflate a blood pressure cuff on the arm until the radial pulse is no longer heard
  - —Release the valve and note the pressure at which the radial pulse returns
  - —Repeat this procedure with the cuff around the calf and note the return of the dorsalis pedis and posterior tibialis pulse
  - —The ratio of the ankle pressure/radial pressure = ABI
    - -Normal: 1 or greater
    - -Typical claudicant: 0.5–0.8
    - -Rest pain/impending tissue injury: <0.3

ETIOLOGY

Thrombotic

- Low flow and hypercoagulable states

Embolic

- Atrial fibrillation
- Myocardial infarction
- Valvular disease
- Endocarditis
- Proximal arterial aneurysm
- Atherosclerotic plaques

Pre-Hospital

- Recognition of a potentially limb threatening emergency

CAUTIONS

- Do not elevate, ice, or warm the affected extremity

Diagnosis

ESSENTIAL WORKUP

- Acute arterial occlusion is a clinical diagnosis

LABORATORY

- Electrolytes
- BUN, creatinine
- CBC
- CPK
- Specimen for type and screen

IMAGING/SPECIAL TESTS

- EKG
- Angiography
- Duplex ultrasound

DIFFERENTIAL DIAGNOSIS

- Lumbar spine disorders
- Venous thrombosis
- Decreased cardiac output in the setting of advanced atherosclerotic disease
- Frostbite
- Peripheral neuropathy
- Fractures and sprains
- Muscle strains

Treatment

ED TREATMENT

- Prompt vascular surgery consultation
- Surgical options
- Fogarty catheter
- Thrombectomy
- Bypass grafting
- PTCA
- Intra-arterial agents
- Intravenous thrombolysis is not recommended
- Aspirin
- Heparin

MEDICATIONS

- Aspirin: 325 mg po; 4 chewable baby aspirin
- Heparin: 80 IU/kg loading bolus; 18 IU/kg/hr

Disposition

ADMISSION CRITERIA

- All patients with arterial occlusion should be admitted with an emergent vascular surgery consult

DISCHARGE CRITERIA

- Patients with chronic occlusive disease, resolved pain and stable ABI measurements
- No other acute medical issues (such as new atrial fibrillation)
- Vascular surgical followup can be assured
- Patients should be instructed to return for any recurrent or progressive symptoms

Miscellaneous

ICD9: N/A

CORE CONTENT CODE: 2.5.1.1, 2.5.1.4, 2.5.1.6

SUGGESTED READINGS

Bassiouny HS. Noninvasive evaluation of the lower extremity arterial tree and graft surveillance. Surg Clin North Am 1995;75:593–606.

Cooke JP, Ma AO. Medical therapy of peripheral artery occlusive disease. Surg Clin North Am 1995;75:569–579.

Spittell JA. Peripheral arterial disease. Dis Mon 1994;40:646–700.

Working party on thrombolysis in the management of limb ischemia. Thrombolysis in the management of limb ischemia. J Intern Med 1996;240:343–355.

Author: Stuart J. Spitalnic

Arthritis, Degenerative

Clinical Presentation

SIGNS AND SYMPTOMS

- Commonly found in patients over age 60
- Joint pain is progressive over months to years, exacerbated by weight bearing, and partially relieved by rest. Joint involvement is often asymmetric
- Joint stiffness after sedentary positioning
- Most commonly involved joints are knees, hips, spine, fingers, and metatarsophalangeals
- Finger joints may show classic Heberden's nodes—nodules located on the dorsal aspect of the distal interphalangeal joints
- Joint crepitus—particularly common in the patellofemoral joint
- Joint enlargement; varus or valgus deformity at the knee
- *Absence of systemic symptoms*

ETIOLOGY

- Trauma
- "Aging"
- Obesity
- Inflammation, or immune response

MECHANISM/DESCRIPTION

- Felt to be multifactorial with mechanical and rheumatological contributions. Final common pathway involves cartilage destruction, activation of chronic inflammatory response, and bony remodeling

SPECIAL PEDIATRIC CONSIDERATIONS

- Osteoarthritis is not seen in the pediatric population

Pre-Hospital

CAUTIONS

- Acute joint pain following trauma must be splinted as if fractured
- Patients with cervical arthritis may be difficult to fit with standard cervical collars. Tape and sandbags may be substituted

Diagnosis

ESSENTIAL WORKUP

- Careful joint examination with special attention to range of motion and functional ability (such as weight bearing)
- In the presence of effusion with warmth or erythema, aspiration of synovial fluid may help distinguish between osteoarthritis, gout, and septic arthritis

LABORATORY

- Not indicated in most cases
- Evaluation of synovial fluid for white blood cell count; crystal analysis, Gram stain, and culture if indicated

IMAGING/SPECIAL TESTS

- Radiographs not routinely necessary but may be obtained if the diagnosis is unclear or in the presence of trauma. Radiographs may show joint space narrowing, osteophyte formation, marginal erosions, or sclerosis of periarticular bone. The presence of degenerative changes may make radiographs, particularly of the cervical spine, difficult to interpret

DIFFERENTIAL DIAGNOSIS

- Rheumatoid arthritis
- Septic arthritis
- Gout

Treatment

INITIAL STABILIZATION

- Splint affected joints in the presence of acute trauma until fracture is ruled out

ED TREATMENT

- Goals of treatment are to maintain mobility, relieve pain, and prevent disability
- Avoid unnecessary joint immobilization
- Gentle stretching exercises and joint range of motion is recommended
- May need referral to physical therapy, which should generally be arranged by primary care physician
- Pain management with nonsteroidal anti-inflammatory medications or acetaminophen
- Intra-articular steroid injection is controversial but may be effective

MEDICATIONS

- Ibuprofen: 600 mg po q6h
- Enteric-coated aspirin: 325–650 mg po q6h
- Acetaminophen: 650–1000 mg po q4h
- Codeine (rarely): 30–60 mg po q4h

Disposition

ADMISSION CRITERIA

- Patients with osteoarthritis and no associated trauma should not require admission for this illness, except for elective surgery for joint replacement in the most severe cases

DISCHARGE CRITERIA

- Patients should be ambulatory and able to perform activities of daily living (ADL). The vast majority of patients will easily meet these criteria

Miscellaneous

ICD9: 715.90

CORE CONTENT CODE: 10.2.1

SUGGESTED READINGS

Blackburn WD. Management of osteoarthritis and rheumatoid arthritis: prospects and possibilities. Am J Med 1996;100(Supp 2A):24s–30s

Felson DT. The course of osteoarthritis and factors that affect it. Rheum Dis Clin North Am 1993;19(3):607–615

Spencer-Green G. Drug treatment of arthritis. Postgrad Med 1993;93(7):129–140

Author: E. Koval

Arthritis, Juvenile Rheumatoid

Clinical Presentation

SIGNS AND SYMPTOMS

Systemic Onset

- Fever
- Erythematous coalescing macular rash
  - —Spares the palms and soles
  - —Usually involves the trunk and proximal extremities
- Polyarthralgia
- Hepatosplenomegaly
- Enlarged lymph nodes
- Pleuritis
- Pericarditis
- Myocarditis
- Pulmonary edema

Pauciarticular Onset

- Asymmetrical arthritis
  - —Involves larger joints
  - —Joints are swollen, tender, and have a decreased range of motion
- Uveitis may be present

Polyarticular

- Arthritis is usually symmetrical
  - —Small or large joints
  - —Soft tissue swelling
  - —Decreased range of motion
    - -Cervical spine
    - -Lumbar spine
    - -Scoliosis
    - -Temporal mandibular joints

MECHANISM/DESCRIPTION

- Three major categories based on presentation
  - —Systemic, pauciarticular, polyarticular
- Group of syndromes characterized by chronic synovitis
  - —Persistent unexplained arthritis
  - —One or more joints
  - —Lasts over 6 weeks
  - —Children under the age of 16 years of age
- Affects approximately 60,000–250,000 children
- Most common childhood connective tissue disease
- Viral etiology is suspected
  - —Certain viruses attach to genetically altered HLA molecules
  - —Antigens stimulate T cells
  - —T cells produce inflammatory agents leading to joint irritation or destruction
- Systemic onset (Still's disease)
  - —10% of cases with equal male to female ratio
  - —High spiking fever
  - —Migratory rash
  - —Any number of joints may be involved
  - —Joint involvement may present weeks to months after other symptoms
- Pauciarticular onset
  - —50% of cases with 1:5 male to female ratio
  - —Four or less joints are involved at presentation with monoarticular involvement being common
    - -Type 1—Female predominance <6 years of age, associated with a 20% incidence of uveitis
    - -Type 2—Male predominance >9 years of age, many of whom will later develop a spondyloarthropathy such as Reiter's syndrome or ankylosing spondylitis
- Polyarticular
  - —40% of cases
  - —1:3 male to female ratio
  - —Five or more joints involved

ETIOLOGY

- Unknown

Pre-Hospital

CAUTIONS

- Splint the affected joint if trauma is a consideration

Diagnosis

ESSENTIAL WORKUP

- Clinical diagnosis after exclusion of other identifiable diseases that cause chronic synovitis

LABORATORY

- CBC
  - —WBC may be elevated
  - —Anemia of chronic disease
- Sedimentation rate may be elevated
- Rheumatoid factor only positive in 20% of cases
- ANA
  - —Positive in 30–40%% of children
  - —Most likely positive in pauciarticular disease I or polyarticular disease Rheumatoid-positive

IMAGING/SPECIAL TESTS

- Joint radiograph
  - —Early presentation
    - -Minimal findings of soft tissue swelling
    - -Joint effusion
  - —Late presentation
    - -Osteoporosis
    - -Joint destruction
    - -Early growth plate closure
- Arthrocentesis
  - —5000–8000 WBC/mm^3
  - —Negative Gram stain and culture
- HLA subtyping and specific allele identification
  - —Further defines subgroups and ultimate prognosis

DIFFERENTIAL DIAGNOSIS

- Septic arthritis
- Toxic viral synovitis
- Lyme disease
- Kawasaki's disease
- Rheumatic fever
- Tuberculosis
- Henoch-Schönlein purpura
- Systemic lupus erythematosus
- Trauma
- Fibromyalgia
- Drug reactions
- Neoplasia
- Sickle cell disease
- Hemophilia

Treatment

INITIAL STABILIZATION

- In toxic appearing children
  - —Intravenous access
  - —Supplemental oxygen

ED TREATMENT

- Aspirin
  - —The mainstay of therapy
  - —Goal of outpatient therapy is to acheive a serum salicylate level of 20–25 mg/dl
- NSAIDs
  - —May be used in the place of aspirin
  - —In the setting of aspirin toxicity
  - —After failure of an adequate trial of aspirin
- Slow-acting antirheumatic drug
  - —Gold compounds
  - —Hydroxychloroquine
- Steroids
  - —Cardiac, pulmonary, or ocular complications
  - —Intra-articular injections may be considered in patients with monoarticular arthritis
- Antibiotics
  - —Indicated for other causes of synovitis
    - -Empirical administration in toxic children for septic arthritis
    - -Coverage for Lyme disease while awaiting titers

MEDICATIONS

- Aspirin: 80–120 mg/kg divided qid po; titrate to achieve serum salicylate levels of 20–25 mg/dl
- Ibuprofen: 30–50 mg/kg divided qid up to 3200 mg
- Methylprednisone: 30 mg/kg qd IV up to 1 g for 1–5 days for high-dose pulse steroids
- Naprosyn: 10–20 mg/kg divided bid up to 1250 mg
- Prednisone: 0.5–2 mg/kg po
- Triamcinolone: up to 40 mg given intra-articular to large joints

Disposition

ADMISSION CRITERIA

- Unclear diagnosis
- Severe pain
- Ill-appearing child

DISCHARGE CRITERIA

- Septic joint has been ruled out
- Patient appears comfortable
- Appropriate follow-up has been arranged

Miscellaneous

ICD9: 714.3

CORE CONTENT CODE: 13.11.1

SUGGESTED READINGS

Christoph R. Musculoskeletal Disorders in Children. In: Tintinalli J, et al., eds. Emergency medicine: A comprehensive study guide. 4th ed. St Louis: McGraw-Hill, 1996:673–685.

Fink C, Fernadez-Vina M, et al. Clinical and genetic evidence that juvenile arthritis is not a single disease. Pediatr Clin North Am 1995;42:1155–1167.

Giannine E, Cawkwell G. Drug treatment in children with juvenile arthritis—past, present, and future. Pediatr Clin North Am 1995;42:1099–1121.

Simmons B, Nutting J, et al. Juvenile rheumatoid arthritis. Hand Clin 1996;12:573–588.

Tibbits G. Juvenile rheumatoid arthritis—old challenges, new insights. Postgrad Med 1994;96:75–87.

Author: Jeanette Wolfe

Arthritis, Monoarticular

Clinical Presentation

SIGNS AND SYMPTOMS

- Rapid onset of symptoms located to one joint
  —Local pain
  —Swelling
  —Warmth
  —Erythema
  —Decreased range of motion
- Infectious (septic) arthritis
  —Fever and chills
  —Large joints are affected more often
    -Adults: knee involvement > hip = shoulder > ankle > wrist
    -Pediatrics (rare): knee = hip
  —Arthritis of the axial skeleton (vertebrae, sternoclavicular, sacroiliac)
    -IV drug use
  —Abdominal pain and vaginal discharge
    -Gonorrhea
  —Lyme disease
    -Knees or shoulders are most commonly affected
    -Nonspecific constitutional symptoms
    -Centrally clearing, expanding, erythematous eruption
- Crystalline
  —Tissue extension may appear identical to cellulitis, septic arthritis
  —Gout
    -First metatarsophalangeal joint ("podagra") > ankle > tarsal joints > knee
  —Pseudogout
    -Knee > wrist > ankle = elbow.
  —Tophi: crystalline granulomas overlying affected joints
- Inflammatory
  —Regional enteritis, ulcerative colitis
    -Bloody diarrhea with mucous
    -Abdominal pain
    -Weight loss
  —Reiter's syndrome
    -Conjunctivitis
    -Urethritis
    -Balanitis
  —Psoriatic arthritis
    -Characteristic skin plaques
    -"Sausage digits"
  —Osteoarthritis
    -Prolonged morning stiffness
    -Pain relieved by rest

MECHANISM/DESCRIPTION

- Nonspecific, destructive process involving cartilage or bone
- Monoarticular arthritis predominately affects and remains localized to one joint
- The presence of one condition does not exclude another process of involvement
- Infection of the joint
  —Hematogenous spread
  —Contiguous extension (cellulitis, osteomyelitis)
  —Puncture wound
  —Inoculation during joint surgery
  —Increased risk
    -Extremes of age
    -Immunocompromised
    -IV drug users
    -Postjoint surgery
- Gout
  —Uric acid crystal deposition secondary to overproduction or underexcretion
  —Increased incidence with alcoholism, loop diuretics, renal failure, hypertriglyceridemia, obesity
  —Postmenopausal females
- Pseudogout
  —Calcium pyrophosphate dihydrate crystals
  —Increased incidence with elderly, trauma, surgery, hyperparathyroidism, hemochromatosis, hypothyroidism
- Osteoarthritis
  —Loss of articular cartilage with reactive changes at joint margins
  —Greater incidence with elderly men than with females until 60 years old, then ratio reverses
  —Morbidly obese individuals
  —Congenital dysplasia of the hip
  —Trauma, prior surgery, or inflammatory arthritis

ETIOLOGY

- Infectious
  —Bacterial
  —*Neisseria gonorrhea*
  —*Staphylococcus aureus:* Secondary to trauma; IV drug use
  —*Escherichia Coli:* Infants
  —*Hemophilus influenzae:* Children 6–24 months
  —Salmonella: Sickle cell disease
  —Gram-negative organisms, anaerobes: immunocompromised
- Spirochetal
  —Tuberculosis
  —Lyme disease
- Viral
  —More commonly polyarticular
- Fungal
  —More commonly chronic arthritis
- Crystalline
  —Gout
  —Pseudogout
- Inflammatory
  —Rheumatoid arthritis
  —Psoriatic
  —Inflammatory bowel disease
  —Reiter's syndrome
- Bone/cartilage disorders
- Osteoarthritis
- Loose body
- Tumor
- Trauma
  —Fracture
  —Internal derangement

Pre-Hospital

- Physical immobilization of the joint for pain control
- IV placement

Diagnosis

ESSENTIAL WORKUP

- A complete history is needed to determine the underlying cause
  - —Trauma
  - —Surgery
  - —Medications
  - —IVDA
  - —Intra-articular injections
  - —Immunosuppression

LABORATORY

- White blood cell count with differential
- Erythrocyte sedimentation rate (ESR)
- Blood cultures
- Panculture if suspicious for gonorrhea or patient septic
- Uric acid can be normal under all conditions and is not helpful

IMAGING/SPECIAL TESTS

- Plain films of the affected joint
  - —Infectious
    - -Soft tissue swelling
    - -Osteoporosis, erosion, or destruction at joint margins
  - —Crystalline
    - -Soft-tissue swelling
    - -Asymmetric bone erosions
    - -Reactive bone formation
    - -Soft-tissue calcification
  - —Bone and cartilage disorders
    - -Asymmetric joint narrowing
    - -Osteophytes
    - -Subchondral cyst formation
    - -Loose bodies
    - -Fracture
- Arthrocentesis and joint fluid analysis
  - —The definitive procedure
  - —Culture is the definitive study of the fluid
  - —White blood cell (WBC) count with differential, Gram stain, glucose, viscosity, crystal analysis
- MRI detects bone necrosis
- Synovial, bone biopsy
  - -Chronic, unexplained, monoarticular arthritis
  - -Gonococcal or mycobacterial disease is suspected and no fluid is available
  - —Technetium and gallium (more sensitive) scans detect infection in axial joints

DIFFERENTIAL DIAGNOSIS

See Etiology

Treatment

INITIAL STABILIZATION

- None required unless underlying illness or trauma mandates

ED TREATMENT

- Septic arthritis
  - —Empiric IV antibiotics for anticipated organism
    - -Gonorrhea: ceftriaxone
    - -IV drug use: penicillinase-resistant antibiotic + aminoglycoside
    - -Gram-negative: antipseudomonal β-lactam + aminoglycoside
  - —Surgery: open vs. closed (daily) drainage
- Crystalline
  - —NSAIDs
    - -Indomethacin
  - —Colchicine
    - -The first 24 hours of attack
    - -Local necrosis if extravasates
    - -Secondary choice to NSAIDs
  - —Prednisone when NSAIDs and colchicine are contraindicated
  - —ACTH
    - -Resistant cases
    - -Contraindication to NSAIDs
  - —Allopurinol: 200–600 mg q day
    - -Decreases uric acid production
    - -Avoid in acute therapy
  - —Probenecid
    - -Uricosuric
    - -Long-term use only
- Osteoarthritis
  - —NSAIDs
  - —Analgesics
  - —Physical support, rehabilitation (splints, braces)

APPEARANCE		WBC (PMN*)	GLUCOSE	GM STAIN	CRYSTALS	VISCOSITY
Septic	Turbid	>50,000	↓	(±)	(±)	↓
Gout	Turbid	25–100,000	↓ or normal	(neg)	**(+)	↑
Pseudogout	Turbid	200–100,000	↓	(neg)	***(+)	(±)
RA	Turbid	15–50,000	↑ or normal	(neg)	(neg)	↓
Osteoarthritis	Clear	200–4,000	normal	(neg)	(neg)	↑
Trauma	Bloody		normal	(neg)	(neg)	↓

*PMN: polymorphonucleocytes
** Negative birefringent crystals: yellow crystals against red background
*** Weakly positive birefringent crystals (rhomboidal)

MEDICATIONS

- ACTH: 40–80 IU IM then 40 IU IM q 6–12 hr until improvement
- Allopurinol: 200–600 mg q day
- Colchicine: 1–2 mg IV in 20 cc NS over 10 min
- Indomethacin: 75–200 mg per day, divided dosages
- Prednisone: 20–40 mg po q day × 3–4 days
- Probenecid: 250 mg bid starting; maximum 3 g q day

Disposition

ADMISSION CRITERIA

- All septic arthritis is admitted
  - —General medical/surgical bed
  - —ICU if generalized sepsis
- Crystalline
  - —Intractable pain
  - —Intractable nausea and vomiting (i.e., colchicine)
  - —Septic joint suspected in a patient with gout or pseudogout
- Traumatic joint injuries requiring surgical intervention

DISCHARGE CRITERIA

- Crystalline monoarthritis able to tolerate oral anti-inflammatory medication
- Inflammatory arthritis unless admission is required by overall disease manifestations
- Osteoarthritis
- Compliance with medications
- Timely close follow up is mandatory
- The patient should be instructed to return immediately if constitutional symptoms (fever, chills), or worsening joint symptoms (pain, swelling, erythema, warmth)

Miscellaneous

ICD9: 716.6

CORE CONTENT CODE: 10.2.1, 10.2.1.1, 10.2.1.2, 10.2.1.3, 10.2.1.4

SUGGESTED READINGS

Baker DG, Schumacher HR Jr. Acute monoarthritis. N Engl J Med 1993;329:1013–19.

Dearborn JT, Jergesen HE. The evaluation and initial management of arthritis. Prim Care 1996;23(2):215–39.

McCune WJ, Golbus J. Monoarticular arthritis. In: Kelly WN, Ruddy S, Harris ED, Sledge CB, eds. Textbook of rheumatology. Vol. 1. 5th ed. Philadelphia: WB Saunders, 1997:371–80.

Authors: Shari Dominguez; Paul Blackburn

Arthritis, Rheumatoid

Clinical Presentation

SIGNS AND SYMPTOMS

- Malaise, fatigue, generalized musculoskeletal pain
- After a period of weeks to months patients develop swollen, warm, painful joints, often worse in the morning
- Joint involvement is usually symmetric, starting in the small joints of the hands and feet, subsequently involving the wrists, elbow, and knees
- The DIP joints of the hand are generally not involved; presence of swelling in these joints should suggest another type of arthritis
- Synovitis usually develops gradually, though may be acute in presentation
- Extra-articular complications include subcutaneous nodules, vasculitis, pericarditis, myocarditis, pulmonary fibrosis, pneumonitis, Sjögren's syndrome, and mononeuritis multiplex
  —Evidence of pericarditis on echocardiogram is found in up to one-third of patients, though rarely of clinical significance
- In long-standing disease, there are classic joint findings, which may include MCP swelling with ulnar deviation, swan neck, and boutonniere deformities

Complications of Rheumatoid Arthritis (RA) that Precipitate Presentation to the ED

- Airway obstruction from cricoarytenoid arthritis or laryngeal nodules
- Heart block, constrictive pericarditis, or myocarditis
- Pulmonary fibrosis or pneumonitis
- Neurologic findings may result from cervical spine subluxation
- Patients can present with infectious complications of chronic steroid use or with fractures resulting from steroid induced osteopenia
- Patients may present with side effects related to chronic salicylate or NSAID use such as GI bleeding
- Drugs such as methotrexate, gold, or d-penicillamine also have toxic side effects, most commonly gastrointestinal

MECHANISM/DESCRIPTION

- Rheumatoid arthritis is a chronic systemic inflammatory disorder that attacks the joints. RA causes a nonsuppurative, proliferative synovitis, progressing to destruction of the articular cartilage and ankylosis of the joint
- Involvement of the knee is common; Baker's cysts may be seen in chronic disease
- Involvement of the spine is limited to the cervical region and may cause atlantoaxial subluxation, which rarely results in cord compression

ETIOLOGY

- Etiology is unknown. About 1% of the world's population is afflicted
  —Female to male ratio is 3:1
  —Typical age of onset is between 30 and 50
- Genetic predisposition is related to HLA-DR4 haplotype

Pre-Hospital

CAUTIONS

- Cervical spine immobilization and airway support for the rare cases in which patients develop respiratory or cervical spine problems related to rheumatoid arthritis

Diagnosis

ESSENTIAL WORKUP

- Diagnosis is based on careful clinical examination. Synovitis should be present for at least 6 weeks. A minimum of four of the following criteria is necessary
  —Stiffness of the involved joints in the morning for at least an hour
  —Arthritis in three or more joints with effusion or soft-tissue swelling
  —Arthritis of joint in hand (wrist, MCP, or PIP)
  —Symmetric arthritis
  —Rheumatoid nodules on extensor surfaces or juxta-articular surfaces
  —Significantly elevated rheumatoid factor
  —Characteristic x-ray changes include erosions and decalcification (not attributable to osteoarthritis)
- Initial workup should focus on demonstrating that other causes of arthritis are not present, especially septic arthritis, reactive arthritis, or gout
  —Arthrocentesis of a joint effusion may be required
- ECG, chest x-ray, C-spine or extremity x-ray, and hemoglobin testing are essential if the patient presents with complications of RA

LABORATORY

- CBC: mild anemia with leukocytosis and thrombocytosis
- ESR: often greater than 30
- Rheumatoid factor: elevated in about 70% of cases
- Joint fluid analysis: typically between 4000 and 50,000 white cells with 75% neutrophils; Gram stain of fluid should show no organisms
- ECG: conduction defects are rare but heart block may be seen

IMAGING/SPECIAL TESTS

- Joint x-ray typically shows joint effusion with juxta-articular erosions and decalcification, narrowing of joint space, and loss of cartilage
- Chest film may reveal pulmonary fibrosis, pleural changes, nodular lung disease, or pneumonitis. Cardiac silhouette may show changes related to myocarditis
- Cervical spine x-ray: atlantoaxial joint subluxation may occur

DIFFERENTIAL DIAGNOSIS

- Osteoarthritis
- Septic arthritis
- Reactive arthritis
- Gonococcal arthritis
- Lyme disease

- Gout
- Connective tissue disorders
  - —SLE, dermatomyositis, polymyositis, vasculitis, Reiter's syndrome, and sarcoid
- Rheumatic Fever
- Malignancy

PEDIATRIC CONSIDERATIONS

- *Juvenile rheumatoid arthritis* (JRA) is a distinct clinical entity affecting about 1 in 10,000 under age 15, with a female to male ratio of 2:1
  - —Peak age of onset is 1–3 years
  - —Large joints are more frequently involved than small joints
  - —Oligoarthritis is relatively frequent
  - —Diagnosis is based on clinical findings with characteristic joint symptoms for more than 6 weeks
  - —Three types of onset of JRA have been defined: oligoarthritis, polyarthritis, and systemic disease, each marked by a different symptom complex and prognosis

Treatment

INITIAL STABILIZATION

- ABCs
  - —Manage airway with attention to C-spine immobilization during intubation
  - —Treat complications of RA as appropriate

ED TREATMENT

- Salicylates or NSAIDs are first-line treatment for rheumatoid arthritis
  - —If one NSAID fails, another NSAID from a different chemical class may work better
  - —Adequate early treatment of rheumatoid arthritis is important as joint changes may be most progressive during the first 18 months if the inflammatory process is not arrested
- Glucocorticoids, methotrexate, and other second-line therapies should be initiated by a rheumatologist

MEDICATIONS

- Aspirin (ECASA): adult: 900 mg qid; peds: 100 mg/kg/day qid up to 3.6 g
- Auranofin: adult: 3–9 mg/d div bid; peds: 0.15 mg/kg/day up to 9 mg div bid
- Hydroxychloroquine: adult: 200–600 mg/d div bid; peds: 6 mg/kg/day up to 600 mg per day
- Ibuprofen: adult: 800 mg tid; peds: 20–40 mg/kg/day tid up to 2.4 g
- Sulfasalazine: adult: 500–1000 mg bid; peds: 30–60 mg/kg/day qid up to 2 g

Disposition

ADMISSION CRITERIA

- Patients with severe or life-threatening presentations of rheumatoid arthritis should be admitted to the hospital
- Admission is warranted when the diagnosis is unclear and serious illnesses such as septic joint or systemic vasculitis may be present
- Admission may be required for pain control or if the patient has inadequate social supports and self-care isn't likely
- Pediatric patients with fever and arthritis should be strongly considered for admission

DISCHARGE CRITERIA

- Patients without serious complications may be managed as outpatients with appropriate follow-up

Miscellaneous

ICD9: 714.0

CORE CONTENT CODE: 8.5.2.4

SUGGESTED READINGS

Anaya J, Diethelm L, Ortiz L, et al. Pulmonary involvement in rheumatoid arthritis. Semin Arthritis Rheum 1995;24(4):242–254.

Jain R, Lipsky P. Treatment of rheumatoid arthritis. Adv Rheum 1997;81(1):57–84.

Leicht M, Harrington T, Davis D. Cricoarytenoid arthritis: A cause of laryngeal obstruction. Ann Emerg Med 1987;16(8):885–888.

Weyand C, Goronzy J. Pathogenesis of rheumatoid arthritis. Adv Rheum 1997;81(1):29–55.

Authors: John King; John Lafleur

Arthritis, Septic

Clinical Presentation

SIGNS AND SYMPTOMS

- Septic arthritis (SA) presents abruptly as a single painful, swollen, warm, and tender joint
- Common findings include:
  —Fever
  —A separate source of infection (e.g., skin) (~50%)
  —Extremely painful joint motion in all planes
  —A joint effusion (least evident in sacroiliac, hip and shoulder)
- Any joint can be involved
- Most commonly knee more common than hip
- Commonly seen in intravenous drug abuse (IVDA): sacroiliac and sternoclavicular joints
- Polyarticular involvement in 10–20%
  —Patients with sepsis, or underlying systemic/connective tissue disorders)
- Gonococcal (GC) SA features
  —Commonly polyarticular
  —Migratory polyarthralgia, tenosynovitis, and dermatitis
  —Involvement of small joints (e.g., wrist, elbow, ankle)
  —Signs of urethral or vaginal GC infection may be present
  —Painless maculopapular lesions on the trunk, arms, and legs

ETIOLOGY

- Risk factors
  —Old age, infancy
  —IVDA, endocarditis
  —Females (GC)
  —Immunosuppression (AIDS, diabetes, chemotherapy)
  —Repeated intra-articular injections, preexisting joint diseases, trauma, or prosthesis
- No bacterial pathogen is identified in 10–20%
- Most common organisms
  —*Staphylococcus aureus* in adults and in patients with rheumatoid arthritis or diabetes
  —*Neisseria gonorrhea* (GC) in young, healthy, and sexually active
  —Other common pathogens: Group A β-hemolytic, B, C, and G Streptococci
  —Gram-negative rods (e.g., *H. influenzae, E. coli*) in old age, infancy, immunosuppression, and IVDA (e.g. *Pseudomonas*)
  —Anaerobes: diabetes, prosthetic joints
  —Mycobacterial and fungal etiologies (e.g., in HIV) have been isolated and produce a more indolent course

MECHANISM/DESCRIPTION

- Bacteria can be introduced into a joint by
  —Hematogenous spread (most common)
  —Invasive procedures
  —Contiguous infection (e.g., osteomyelitis, cellulitis)
- An acute inflammatory process results in WBC migration into the joint
- Synovial hyperplasia, cartilage damage, and formation of a purulent effusion
- Loss of function is irreversible in up to 50% of cases

PEDIATRIC CONSIDERATIONS

- Hip infections are most common
- Infants present with irritability, fever and loss of appetite
- Older children present with a limp, refusal to bear weight, or decreased joint function

Pre-Hospital

- No specific considerations

Diagnosis

ESSENTIAL WORKUP

Arthrocentesis

- Perform synovial fluid aspiration in any clinically suspected case of SA
- Send fluid for protein and glucose, cell count, gram stain and culture
- Typical findings in SA
  —A turbid, purulent or serosanguinous fluid
  —A leukocytosis (50,000–150,000/mm^3) with a polymorphonuclear predominance (>75%)
  —Lower cell counts reported in more recent literature
  —Often a depressed glucose level and an elevated protein
- The appearance of crystals does not rule out SA
- Use special stain or culture media when indicated (e.g., GC, anaerobes, fungus, mycobacterium)
- Intra-articular lidocaine reduces the sensitivity of subsequent cultures
- In non-GC SA, Gram stain and culture are positive in 50% and 90% of cases, respectively
  —Drops to nearly 10 % and 50 % in GC SA
- Fluoroscopic, sonographic, or CT guidance can be used in technically difficult aspirations
- If unsuccessful, surgical arthrotomy may be undertaken
- Arthrocentesis is contraindicated whenever there is an underlying joint prosthesis or an overlying skin infection
  —If cellulitis present, use an alternate approach through normal skin

LABORATORY

- Nonspecific serum leukocytosis, left shift, and ESR elevation are usually present
- Urinalysis and culture can reveal a urologic source for the pathogen
- Blood cultures may be useful: positive in 50–70% of non-GC SA; rarely positive in GC SA
- Culture any potential focus of infection (pharynx, urine, cervix or anus), particularly when suspecting GC

IMAGING/SPECIAL TESTS

- Plain radiographs to identify
  —Effusion
  —Baseline status of the joint
  —Contiguous osteomyelitis
  —Concurrent rheumatologic diseases
  —Fractures or foreign body
  —Joint loosening (a late and nonspecific sign)
- Ultrasound, CT, and MRI are more sensitive
  —Ultrasound may be used to guide aspiration of some joints (i.e. hip)

- Newer scintigraphic techniques are increasingly sensitive, specific and useful in diagnosis of SA
- Other Tests
  —Bacterial DNA amplification techniques are promising in early detection of pathogenic species

DIFFERENTIAL DIAGNOSIS

- Viral arthritis
- Rheumatoid arthritis
- Gout or pseudogout
- HIV-associated arthritis
- Reactive arthritis
- Lyme disease
- Osteomyelitis
- Endocarditis
- Trauma
- In children
  —Juvenile rheumatoid arthritis
  —Slipped capital femoral epiphysis
  —Legg-Calvé-Perthes
  —Metaphyseal osteomyelitis
  —Transient synovitis

PEDIATRIC CONSIDERATIONS

- Due to vaccine, *H. influenzae* is no longer most common
- *S. aureus* is most common
- Group B streptococcus, enterobacteria, and Gram-negative rods in the newborn
- Differentiating SA from metaphyseal osteomyelitis is challenging

Treatment

INITIAL STABILIZATION

- Patient may be septic and require IV fluid resuscitation
- If patient is toxic, do not delay antibiotic therapy for aspiration results

ED TREATMENT

- Promptly aspirate joint fluid
- Obtain necessary cultures
- Start empiric antibiotics: staphylococcal, streptococcal, and Gram-negative coverage
  —Combine β-lactamase-resistant penicillin (e.g., nafcillin) with an aminoglycoside (e.g., gentamycin) or a third-generation cephalosporin (e.g., ceftriaxone)
  —Initial guidance by Gram stain, patient's age, risk factors, and concurrent medical illness is appropriate
  —When suspecting GC, use a third-generation cephalosporin or a quinolone (e.g., ceftriaxone, ciprofloxacin)
  —Intra-articular antibiotics are contraindicated
- Early orthopedic consultation for drainage procedure
- Pain control: narcotics and moderately flexed splinting
- Immunological therapies are experimental at this point

MEDICATIONS

- Cefotaxime: 1 g IV q 8 hrs; peds: 50 mg/kg q 12 hrs
- Ceftriaxone: 1 g IV qd; peds: 50 mg/kg
- Ciprofloxacin: 400 mg IV q 12 hrs
- Gentamycin: 2–5 mg/kg IV load
- Piperacillin: 4 g IV q 6 hrs
- Nafcillin: 2 g IV q 4 hrs; peds: 25 mg/kg q 6 hrs
- Tobramycin: 1 mg/kg IV q 8 hrs; peds: 2.5 mg/kg q 8 hrs
- Vancomycin: 1 g IV q 12 hrs; peds: 10 mg/kg q 6 hrs

PEDIATRIC CONSIDERATIONS

- Open surgical drainage is the method of choice in pediatric hip SA
- Cover *H. influenzae* type B if prior immunization cannot be established

Disposition

ADMISSION CRITERIA

- All patients with suspected SA should be admitted
- Septic patients should be admitted to a monitored setting
  —May undergo drainage of their joint as indicated

DISCHARGE CRITERIA

- Cases where suspected SA has been adequately ruled out

Miscellaneous

ICD9: 711.00

CORE CONTENT CODE: 10.2.1.1

SUGGESTED READINGS

Baker D, Schumacher HR. Acute monoarthritis. N Engl J Med 1993;329(14):1013–1019.

Goldenberg D. Septic arthritis. Lancet 1998;35:197–202.

Malleson P. Management of childhood arthritis. Part 1: Acute arthritis. Arch Dis Child 1997;76:460–462.

Ryan M, Kavanagh R, Wall P, Hazleman B. Bacterial joint infections in England and Wales: Analysis of bacterial isolates over a four year period. Br J Rheum 1997;36:370–373.

Smith J, Piercy E. Infectious arthritis. Clin Infect Dis 1995;20:225–231.

Authors: Ziad Kazzi; A. Antoine Kazzi

Ascites

Clinical Presentation

SIGNS AND SYMPTOMS

- Abdominal distention and discomfort
- Weight gain; less frequently weight loss
- Shortness of breath and orthopnea
- Lower extremity edema
- Sacral, scrotal, and penile edema
- Abdominal wall hernias and muscle wasting
- Shifting dullness, flank fullness, fluid wave, and puddle sign
- Symptoms and signs of the underlying etiology

ETIOLOGY

- Parenchymal liver disease
  —Cirrhosis and alcoholic hepatitis
  —Fulminant hepatic failure
- Hepatic congestion
  —Congestive heart failure
  —Constrictive pericarditis
  —Tricuspid insufficiency or stenosis
  —Veno-occlusive disease and Budd-Chiari syndrome
- Malignancies
  —Peritoneal carcinomatosis
  —Hepatocellular carcinoma or metastatic disease
- Infections
  —Tuberculous or fungal peritonitis
  —Bacterial peritonitis
- Hypoalbuminemic states
  —Nephrotic syndrome
  —Severe malnutrition with serum albumin <2.0 g/dl
  —Protein-losing enteropathy
- Other conditions
  —Pancreatic ascites
  —Biliary ascites
  —Nephrogenous ascites
  —Benign ovarian tumors
  —Chylous ascites from lymphatic leak or obstruction
  —Connective tissue disease
  —Myxedema
  —Granulomatous peritonitis

MECHANISM

- Salt and water retention associated with *arterial vasodilation,* expansion of plasma volume, and *decreased effective plasma volume*
- Percolation of lymph from hepatic capsule due to disturbed Sterling's forces from sinusoidal portal hypertension >8 mm Hg
- Decreased plasma oncotic pressure from hypoalbunemia
- Peritoneal irritation due to an infectious, inflammatory or malignant process
- Damage to intra-abdominal lymphatics, veins, or arteries

PEDIATRIC CONSIDERATION

- Majority of pediatric cases due to
  —Malignancy (e.g., Burkitt lymphoma and rhabdomyosarcoma)
  —Nephrotic syndrome
- 80% of adult cases caused by
  —Cirrhosis
  —Alcoholic hepatitis

Pre-Hospital

CAUTION

- Sudden increase in abdominal girth, pain, or fever requires urgent evaluation for possible complicating factor such as
  —Infection
  —Development of hepatoma
  —Obstruction of hepatic outflow
  —Decompensated liver function
- Ambulance transport for extreme weakness, dizziness, or respiratory distress

Diagnosis

ESSENTIAL WORKUP

- Thorough search for liver disease, congestive heart failure, tuberculosis, malignancy, and other systemic disorders
- Abdominal paracentesis
  —Mandatory in new onset ascites, worsening encephalopathy, presence of fever, or abdominal pain/tenderness
  —Test ascitic fluid for
    -Cell count and differential
    -Albumin/total protein
    -Gram stain, and culture in blood culture bottles × 2
    -LDH, glucose, TB culture, amylase, triglyceride, cytology, and bilirubin useful

LABORATORY

- CBC
- Electrolytes, BUN, Cr, glucose
- Liver function tests/liver enzymes
- PT, PTT
- ABGs or pulse oximeter
- Urinalysis
- Spot urine for sodium
- Viral hepatitis serology
- Amylase/lipase
- α-Fetoprotein
- TSH

IMAGING/SPECIAL TESTS

- CXR: signs of CHF, pleural effusion, and cavitary or mass lesion
- Abdominal ultrasound
  —Confirmation of ascites, especially if <2 L, and evaluation of the liver, pancreas, spleen, and ovaries
  —May guide paracentesis
- Doppler study: evaluation of hepatic blood flow
- Abdominal CT scan
- Echocardiogram
- Peritoneoscopy: ascites of unknown etiology; especially TB

DIFFERENTIAL DIAGNOSIS

- Ascites is one of the five "F" causes of abdominal swelling;
  —Fluid (including cystic lesion in solid organ)
  —Fat
  —Flatus
  —Fetus
  —Feces
  —Other causes include massive organomegaly
- *Serum-ascites albumin gradient (SAAG)* = ascitic albumin minus serum albumin
  —Superior to ascitic fluid total protein in the differential diagnosis of ascites
  —SAAG ≥1.1 g/dl
    -97% accurate in predicting portal hypertension
    -Massive liver metastases
    -Spontaneous bacterial peritonitis
  —SAAG <1.1 g/dl
    -Peritoneal carcinomatosis
    -Tuberculosis
    -Pancreatic ascites
    -Nephrotic syndrome
    -Bowel obstruction or infarction
    -Vasculitis
  —Protein is high in CHF and low in Budd-Chiari

PEDIATRIC CONSIDERATION

- Malignancy and nephrotic syndrome most common etiology

Treatment

INITIAL STABILIZATION

- Symptomatic hypotension: administer volume expander (100 g albumin in 500 ml of 0.9%NS)

ED TREATMENT

- Early detection of the following complications is necessary
  —Spontaneous bacterial peritonitis
    -High degree of suspicion
    -Low threshold for paracentesis and prompt therapy
  —Tense ascites and hydrothorax
    -Provide supplemental oxygen
    -Perform therapeutic paracentesis (usually 1–2 L) or serial thoracocenteses (not chest tube) to relieve respiratory distress
  —Abdominal wall hernias
    -Watch for incarceration, ulceration, or rupture
    -Perform therapeutic paracentesis and obtain an emergent surgical consultation
  —Persistent leak at paracentesis site
    -Remove more fluid
    -If necessary, use stomal barrier device
  —*Meralgia parethetica*
    -Due to pressure on the lateral femoral cutaneous nerve
    -Relieve the pressure by paracentesis or diuresis
- Large volume paracentesis
  —5–10 L (100 ml/kg)
  —Can be performed safely in the ED in patients with stable hemodynamics
  —Replace with IV albumin (8 g/L fluid removed)
  —Monitor the patient for 8 hours prior to discharge
- Nonparacentesis reduction of acites
  —Strict sodium restriction
    -<1 g/day
    -Restrict water only if serum sodium <125 mEq/L
  —Spironolactone
    -Works best for cirrhotic ascites
    -Alternative agents: amilorideor triamterine
  —Furosemide
    -Works best for other causes of ascites
    -Add to spironolactone in cirrhotics at spironolactone/furosemide ratio of 100 mg/40 mg
    -Add metolazone for less responsive cases
  —Diuretic principles
    -Administer diuretics as a single morning dose for better effect and compliance
    -Obtain spot-urine sodium to evaluate response
    -Urinary Na >10 mEq/L are more responsive to diuretics
    -Diuretic-induced weight loss should not exceed 2 lbs/day in patients without edema and 5 lbs/day in patients with edema
    -Monitor electrolytes and renal function
  —*Refractory ascites*
    -Accounts for 10%
    -Assure compliance with diet and medications
    -NSAIDs diminish response to diuretics
    -Implement peritoneovenous shunt or surgical or transjugular intrahepatic portosystemic shunt *only if* program of therapeutic large volume paracentesis fails
    -Liver transplantation provides a cure
  —*Treatment of the underlying etiology* for ascites caused by conditions other than cirrhosis (e.g., antituberculous agents and treatments of CHF)

MEDICATIONS

- Amiloride: 10–40 mg/day po
- Furosemide: 40–160 mg/day (peds: 1–3 mg/kg) po
- Metolazone: 5 mg/day
- Spironolactone: 100–400 mg/day (peds: 1–6 mg/kg) po
- Triamterine: 100–300 mg/day po

Disposition

ADMISSION CRITERIA

- Decompensated CHF
- Fluminant liver failure
- Hepatic encephalopathy
- Spontaneous bacterial peritonitis
- Hepatorenal syndrome
- GI bleeding
- Refractory or tense ascites not responding to ED treatment

DISCHARGE CRITERIA:

- Patients responding to ED management

Miscellaneous

PATIENT CODE: 789.5

CORE CONTENT CODE: 1.9.3

SUGGESTED READINGS

Bataller R, Gines P. Practical recommendations for the treatment of acites and its complications. Drugs 1997:54:571

Gines P, Arroyo V, Vargas V, et al. Paracentesis with intravenous albumin as compared with peritoneovenous shunting in cirrhosis with refractory ascites. N Engl J Med 1991;325:829

Runyon BA. Treatment of patients with cirrhosis and acites. Sem Liver Dis. 1997;17:249

Runyon BA, Montano AA, Akriviadis EA, et al. The serum-ascites albumin gradient is superior to the exudate-transudate concept in the differential diagnosis of ascites. Ann Intern Med 1992;117:215

Runyon BA. Care of patient with ascites. N Engl J Med 1994;330:337

Author: Abbas Zagnoon

Asthma, Adult

Clinical Presentation

SIGNS AND SYMPTOMS

- Wheezing
- Dyspnea
- Chest tightness
- Cough
- Tachypnea
- Tachycardia
- Respiratory distress
  —Posture sitting upright or leaning forward
  —Use of accessory muscles
  —Inability to speak in full sentences
  —Diaphoresis
  —Poor air movement
  —Altered mental status

MECHANISM/DESCRIPTION

- Increased expiratory resistance
  —Bronchospasm
  —Airway inflammation
  —Mucosal edema
  —Mucous plugging
- Consequences
  —Air trapping
  —Increased dead space
  —Hyperinflation
- Risk factors for life-threatening disease
  —Prior intubations
  —Intensive care unit admissions
  —Chronic steroid use
  —Hospital admission for asthma during the past year
  —Inadequate medical management
  —Increasing age
  —Ethnicity (African Americans)
  —Lack of access to medical care

ETIOLOGY

- Pollen
- Dust mites
- Molds
- Animal dander
- Other environmental allergens
- Viral upper respiratory infections
- Occupational chemicals
- Tobacco smoke
- Environmental change
- Cold air
- Exercise
- Emotional factors
- Drugs
  —Aspirin
  —NSAIDs
  —β-Blockers

Pre-Hospital

- Recognize the "quiet chest" as respiratory distress
- Supplemental oxygen
- Continuous nebulized β-agonist
- Administration of subcutaneous epinephrine
  —Severe disease with decreased breath sounds
  —Limited inhalation of aerosolized medicine

Diagnosis

ESSENTIAL WORKUP

- Primarily a clinical diagnosis
- Measure and follow severity with peak expiratory flow rate (PEFR)
- Assess for underlying disease
  —Pneumonia
  —Pneumothorax

LABORATORY

- Arterial blood gas
  —Not helpful during the initial evaluation
  —The decision to intubate should be based on clinical criteria
  —Mild-moderate asthma: respiratory alkalosis
  —Severe airflow obstruction and fatigue: respiratory acidosis
- Pulse oximetry
  —Less than 90% is indicative of severe respiratory distress
  —Patients with impending respiratory compromise may still maintain a saturation above 90% until sudden collapse
- WBC
  —Leukocytosis is nonspecific
  —Pneumonia
  —Chronic steroid use
  —Stress of an asthma exacerbation
  —Demargination occurs after administration of epinephrine and steroids

IMAGING/SPECIAL TESTS

- Peak expiratory flow rate
  —Estimates the degree of airflow obstruction
  —Normal peak flow in an adult is 400–600
    -Between 100–300 indicates moderate airway obstruction
    -<100 is indicative of severe airway obstruction
    -Use serially as an objective measure of the response to therapy
- Forced expiratory volume (FEV)
  —More reliable measure of lung function than PEFR
  —More operator dependant
  —Difficult to use as a screening tool
  —Often unavailable in the ED
  —Severe airway obstruction: FEV1 less than 30–50 %
- Chest radiographs
  —Indications
    -Fever
    -Suspicion of pneumonia
    -Suspicion of pneumothorax or pneumomediastinum
    -Foreign body aspiration
    -First asthma attack
    -Comorbid illness
    -Diabetes
    -Renal failure
    -AIDS
    -Cancer
  —Findings
    -Hyperinflation
    -Scattered atelectasis
- EKG
  —Transient changes in severe asthma
    -Right axis deviation
    -Right bundle branch block
    -Abnormal p waves
    -Nonspecific ST-T wave changes
  —Indicated in patients at risk for cardiac disease
    -Dysrhythmias
    -Myocardial ischemia

DIFFERENTIAL DIAGNOSIS

- Congestive heart failure
- Myocardial ischemia
- Pulmonary embolus
- Pneumonia
- Bronchitis
- Bronchiolitis
- Croup
- Foreign body aspiration
- Upper airway obstruction
- Angioedema
- Allergic reaction
- Chronic obstructive pulmonary disease (COPD)
- Chronic cor pulmonale
- Chemical pneumonitis
- Carcinoid tumors
- Smoke inhalation
- Immersion injury
- Venous air embolus

Treatment

INITIAL STABILIZATION

- Immediate initiation of inhaled β-agonist treatment
- Intubate for fatigue
- Steroids

ED TREATMENT

β-Adrenergic Agonist

- Mild-moderate asthmatic
  —Administer every 20 minutes
- Severe asthmatic
  -Continuous nebulized treatment
- Nonselective β agonists (metaproterenol)
- Selective β_2 agonists (albuterol)
  —Fewer side effects than nonselective β agonists
- Subcutaneous β-agonist
  —Severe exacerbations
  —Limited inhalation of aerosolized medicine
  —More side effects because of systemic absorption
    -Tachycardia
    -Tremors
  —Relative contraindications: age >40 and coronary disease
- Corticosteroids
  —Reduce airway wall inflammation
  —Administered early
  —Onset of action may take 4–6 hours
  —Administer intravenously or orally
  —Intravenous solu-medrol in the treatment of severe asthma exacerbation
  —Mild-moderate exacerbations may be treated with oral prednisone
  —Inhaled corticosteroids are currently not recommended as initial therapy
- Oxygen
  —Maintain an oxygen saturation above 90%
- Aminophylline
  —Rare utility in acute flare-ups of disease
  —Toxicity
    -Nausea
    -Tremor
    -Anxiety
    -Palpitations
    -Tachycardia
- Anticholinergic agents
  —If minimal response to initial β-agonist treatment
  —Severe airflow obstruction
  —Inhaled anticholinergic agents should be used in conjunction with β-agonists
- Magnesium sulfate
  —No benefit in mild-moderate asthma
  —Benefit of magnesium remains unclear in severe asthma
- Heliox
  —Mixture of helium and oxygen (80:20, 70:30, 60:40)
  —Less dense than air
  —Decrease airway resistance
  —Decrease in respiratory exhaustion
  —Not currently recommended for routine use
- Ketamine
  —Bronchodilator and an anesthetic agent
  —Useful as an induction agent during intubation
  —Contraindications
    -Hypertension
    -Coronary disease
    -Preeclampsia
    -Increased intracranial pressure
- Halothane
  —Inhalation anesthetics are potent bronchodilators
  —Refractory asthma in intubated patients
- Intubation of the asthmatic patient
  —Rapid sequence intubation
    -Lidocaine to attenuate airway reflexes
    -Etomidate or ketamine as an induction agent
    -Succinylcholine should be administered to achieve paralysis
    -A large endotracheal tube >7 mm should be used to facilitate ventilation
    -May need to mechanically exhale for the patient

MEDICATIONS

- β Agonists
  —Albuterol: adult: 2.5 mg in 2.5 ml normal saline q 20 min inhaled; peds: 0.1–0.15 mg/kg/dose q 20 min (minimum dose 1.25 mg)
  —Metaproterenol: adult: 15 mg in 2.5 ml normal saline q 20 min inhaled; peds: 0.1–0.3 ml (5–15 mg)
  —Epinephrine: adult: 0.3 mg (1:1000) sc q 0.5–4.0 hrs x 3 doses; peds: 0.01 mg/kg up to 0.3 mg sc
  —Terbutaline: adult: 0.25 mg sc q 0.5 hrs x 2 doses; peds: 0.01 mg/kg up to 0.3 mg sc
- Corticosteroids
  —Methylprednisolone: adult: 60–125 mg IV; peds: 1–2 mg/kg/dose IV or po q 6 hrs x 24 hrs
  —Prednisone: adult: 40–60 mg po; peds: 1–2 mg/kg/day in single or divided doses
- Anticholinergics
  —Ipratropium bromide: 0.5 mg in 3 ml NS q 1 hr x 3 doses
  —Glycopyrrolate: 2 mg in NS q 1 hr x 3
- Magnesium: 2 g IV over 20 min
- Aminophylline: 0.6 mg/kg/hr IV infusion
- Rapid sequence intubation
  —Lidocaine: 1–1.5 mg/kg
  —Etomidate: 0.3 mg/kg *or*
  —Ketamine: 1–1.5 mg/kg
  —Succinylcholine: 1.5 mg/kg

Disposition

ADMISSION CRITERIA

Intensive Care Unit

- Persistent respiratory distress
- PEFR <100 and minimal air movement
- Intubated patients

Medical Wards

- PEFR <40% of predicted
- Patients without subjective improvement
- Patients with continued wheeze and diminished air movement
- Patients with moderate response to therapy and no respiratory distress
  —Factors which should favor admission
    -Prior intubation
    -Recent emergency department visit
    -Multiple emergency department visits or hospitalizations
    -Symptoms for more than 1 week
    -Failure of outpatient therapy
    -Use of steroids
    -Inadequate follow-up mechanisms
    -Psychiatric illness
- Complications
  —Pneumothorax
  —Pneumomediastinum
  —Pneumonia
  —Fatigue

DISCHARGE CRITERIA

- Patient reports subjective improvement
- Clear lungs with good air movement
- PEFR or FEV1 greater than 70% of predicted
- Peak flow should be greater than 300
- Adequate follow up within 48–72 hours

Miscellaneous

ICD9: 493

CORE CONTENT CODE: 16.6.1

SUGGESTED READINGS

Corbridge TC, Hall JB. The assessment and management of adults with status asthmaticus. Am J Respir Crit Care Med 1995;151:1296–1316.

Guidelines for the diagnosis and management of asthma: National Asthma Education Program Expert Panel Report. Bethesda, MD: Department of Health and Human Services. NIH publication no. 91-3042; 1991.

Jagoda A, Shepherd SM, Spevitz A, Joseph MM. Refractory asthma, part 1: Epidemiology, pathophysiology, pharmacologic interventions. Ann Emerg Med 1997;29:262–274.

Jagoda A, Shepherd SM, Spevitz A, Joseph MM. Refractory asthma, part 2. Airway interventions and management. Ann Emerg Med 1997;29:275–281.

Manthous CA. Management of severe exacerbations of asthma. Am J Med 1995;99:298–308.

Author: Eric S. Nadel

Asthma, Pediatric

Clinical Presentation

SIGNS AND SYMPTOMS

General

- Fatigue, somnolence
- Diaphoresis, agitation
- Hypoxia, cyanosis
- Tachycardia
- Dehydration
- Fever secondary to atelectasis
- Pulsus paradoxus

Respiratory

- Wheezing, rales, rhonchi
- Cough—acute or chronic
- Tachypnea
- "Tight chest"
- Dyspnea, shortness of breath with prolonged expiratory phase
- Retractions, accessory muscle use, nasal flaring
- Hyperinflation
- Often a history of recurrent episodes and chronic restrictions
- Complications
  —Recurrent pneumonia, bronchitis
  —Atelectasis
  —Pneumothorax, pneumomediastinum
  —Respiratory distress/failure/death

MECHANISM/DESCRIPTION

- 2.7 million children (<18 years) affected in the U.S.
- 850,000 ED visits per year in U.S.
- Inflammatory events lead to bronchoconstriction
  —Compounded by hyperreactivity of airways
  —Mediators of the inflammatory cascade exacerbate obstructive cycle
- Airway obstruction produces increased airway resistance and gas trapping
  —Mucosal edema
  —Bronchospasm
  —Mucous plugging
- Infants more vulnerable to respiratory failure
  —Increased peripheral airway resistance
  —Decreased elastic recoil with early airway closure
  —Unstable rib cage
  —Mechanically disadvantaged diaphragm
- Family history of allergy and asthma
- Medical history of early injury to airway (bronchopulmonary dysplasia, pneumonia, intubation, croup, reflux, passive exposure to smoking), reactions to foods and drugs, other allergic manifestations
- Environmental exposures such as pets, smoke, carpets, dusts

ETIOLOGY

Precipitating/Aggravating Factors

- Infection
  —Viral
  —Bacterial
- Allergic/irritant
  —Environment: pollens, grasses, mold, house dust mites, animal dander
  —Occupational chemicals: chlorine, ammonia
  —Irritants: smoke, pollutants, gases, aerosols
  —Food and additives
- Exercise
- Cold weather
- Emotional: stress phobia
- Intoxication: β-blockers, aspirin, nonsteroidal anti-inflammatory

Pre-Hospital

- Oxygen and oxygen saturation monitoring
- Nebulized β-adrenergic agonist: albuterol
- Intubate for impending respiratory failure
- Rapid transport and good communication with ED

Diagnosis

ESSENTIAL WORKUP

- Clinical diagnosis based primarily on physical examination and history
- Follow response to bronchodilator therapy with present illness and past episodes
- Exclude other differential considerations
- Pulse oximetry
  —Initial SaO_2 <91% (sea level) associated with significant illness: admission, relapse, prolonged course
  —Peak flow meters in cooperative patients (usually >5 years old)
  —<50% of best or predicted suggests severe obstruction
  —50–70% predicts moderate to severe obstruction
  —70–90% associated with mild to moderate obstruction
  —>90% considered normal

LABORATORY

- Arterial blood gas (ABG) adjunct to pulse oximetry and clinical examination to assess oxygenation and ventilation; rarely obtained
- CBC and electrolytes: nonspecific and indicated for specific issues
- Theophylline level: rarely needed unless patient on agent

IMAGING/SPECIAL TESTS

- Chest x-ray in the following patients
  —<1 year of age to exclude foreign body, atelectasis
  —First episode of wheezing (suggested)
  —Increasing respiratory distress or minimal response to therapy
  —Respiratory distress/failure

DIFFERENTIAL DIAGNOSIS

- Infection/inflammation
  —Bronchiolitis
  —Pneumonia: viral, bacterial, chemical, hypersensitivity
  —Aspiration
  —Lymphadenopathy
  —Anaphylactic reaction
- Trauma
  —Pneumothorax
  —Foreign body
- Vascular disorder
  —Compression of trachea by vascular anomaly
  —Pulmonary edema
  —Pulmonary embolism
  —Congestive heart failure
- Congenital disease
  —Cystic fibrosis
  —Tracheoesophageal fistula or tracheal anomaly
  —Bronchogenic cyst
- Intoxication: metabolic acidosis
- Neoplasm
- Vocal cord dysfunction

Treatment

INITIAL STABILIZATION

- Maintain SaO_2 >90–95%
- Beta adrenergic nebulizer(s): albuterol
- Intubate for respiratory failure

ED TREATMENT

- Assess for potential respiratory distress/failure
  —Cyanosis
  —Severe anxiety or irritability
  —Lethargy, somnolence, fatigue
  —Poor air entry, ventilation
  —Persistent tachypnea
  —Severe retractions
- Monitor oxygenation. Titrate oxygen saturation to SaO_2 >95% (sea level)
- β-Adrenergic nebulizer: albuterol
  —Frequent or continuous
  —Subcutaneous epinephrine/terbutaline in refractory asthma. Very rarely needed.
- Steroid therapy
  —Oral for moderate exacerbations if able to take oral medications
  —Intravenous for severe exacerbation and those unable to take orally
- Ipratropium bromide synergistic with beta adrenergic agent
- Intubate for respiratory failure
  —Ketamine, a bronchodilator, is useful induction agent

MEDICATIONS

- Albuterol (0.5% solution or 5 mg/ml)
  —Nebulizer 0.015 mg (0.03 ml)/kg/dose, up to 5 mg/dose q 10–20 min as needed
  —Metered-dose inhaler (with spacer) (90 μg/puff) 2 puffs q 5–10 min up to total of 10 puffs
- Terbutaline (0.01%): 0.01 ml/kg SQ q 15–20 min up to 0.25 ml/dose
- Epinephrine (1:1000)(1 mg/ml) 0.01 ml/kg SQ up to 0.35 ml/dose q 20 min
- Ipratropium bromide: nebulizer (0.02% inhaled solution 500 μg/2.5 ml) 250–500 μg/dose q 6 hrs in children >6 yrs
- Methylprednisolone: 1–2 mg/kg/dose IV q 6 hrs, max 125 mg/dose
- Prednisone: 1–2 mg/kg/dose po q 6–12 hrs, max 80 mg/dose
- Ketamine (for intubation): 1–2 mg/kg IV

Disposition

ADMISSION CRITERIA

- Persistent respiratory distress
  —Persistent wheezing
  —Increased respiratory rate/tachypnea
  —Retractions and use of accessory muscles
- SaO_2 <93% on room air (sea level)
- Peak expiratory flow rate (PEFR) <70–50% predicted levels
- Inability to take oral medicines, liquids
- Prior ED visit in last 24 hours
- Uncertain compliance, suboptimal environment
- Comorbidity
  —Congenital heart disease
  —Bronchopulmonary dysplasia
  —Cystic fibrosis
  —Neuromuscular disease

INTENSIVE CARE UNIT CRITERIA

- Severe respiratory distress
- SaO_2 <90% or PaO_2 <60 mm Hg on 40% oxygen (sea level)
- $PaCO_2$ >40 mm Hg
- Significant complications
  —Pneumothorax
  —Dysrhythmia
  —Theophylline toxicity

DISCHARGE CRITERIA

- Good response to therapy
  —Observe and monitor in ED for at least 60 minutes after last treatment
  —PEFR >70% predicted
  —SaO_2 >93% (sea level)
  —Relatively normal examination
- Treatment
  —Intensive β-adrenergic regimen for 3–5 days
  —Short course (3–5 days) of high dose steroids (2 mg/kg/day) for those presenting with moderate symptoms
  —Followup appointment in 24–72 hours
  —Instructions for worsening of signs and symptoms

Miscellaneous

ICD9: 493.9

CORE CONTENT CODE: 16.6.1, 13.9.5

SUGGESTED READINGS

Alario AJ, Lewander WJ, Dennhey P, et al. The relationship between oxygen saturation and clinical assessment of acutely wheezing infants and children. Pediatr Emerg Care 1995;11:331.

Mower WR, Sachs C, Nicklin EL, et al. Pulse oximetry as a fifth pediatric vital sign. Pediatrics 1997;99:681.

Schuh S, Johnson DW, Callahan S, et al. Efficacy of frequent nebulized ipratropium bromide added to frequent high-dose albuterol therapy in severe childhood asthma. J Pediatr 1995;126:639.

Wright AL, Holberg C, Martinez FD, et al. Relationship of parenteral smoking to wheezing and non-wheezing lower respiratory tract illnesses in infancy. J Pediatr 1991;118:207.

Author: N. Shapiro

Ataxia

Clinical Presentation

SIGNS AND SYMPTOMS

- Altered hand coordination
  —Abnormal finger-to-nose test with eyes closed
- Altered coordination in lower extremities
  —Abnormal heel-to-shin coordination
- Blurred vision
- Impaired balance
  —Dysfunction of two out of three of vision, vestibular sense, or proprioception
  —Evaluated by Romberg test and tandem gait
  —Swaying with eyes open and closed suggests a cerebellar lesion
- Impaired gait
- Slurred or explosive speech
- Intentional tremor
- Frontal lobe lesions
  —Wide based gait
  —Tendency to fall backwards
  —Motor perseveration
  —Grasp and suck reflexes
  —Urinary incontinence
  —Slowness in thinking
  —Headache
  —Altered mental status
- Subcortical lesions
  —Emotional lability
  —Brisk reflexes
  —Dysarthria
  —Dementia
- Brainstem lesions
  —Crossed motor or sensory findings
  —Internuclear ophthalmoplegia
  —Nystagmus
  —Dysarthria
- Cerebellar lesions
  —Truncal and gait ataxia if midline lesions
  —Limb ataxia if hemispheric lesions
  —Nystagmus
  —Hypotonia
  —Occipital headache
  —Occipital gaze palsy
- Posterior column dysfunction
  —Positive Romberg sign
  —Neck and arm pain
  —Positive Babinski sign
  —Loss of vibration and position sense
- Peripheral neuropathy
  —Loss of deep tendon reflexes
  —Decreased strength

MECHANISM/DESCRIPTION

- Disorder of coordination and rhythm
- May result from dysfunction at different levels of the cerebellar circuit
  —Cerebellum, spinocerebellar pathways, or vestibular sensory input, the integration of these inputs in the brainstem or cerebellum, or the motor output to the spinal neurons that control axial and proximal muscles
  —Sensory ataxia is caused by lesions that affect the peripheral sensory fibers, dorsal root ganglia cells, posterior columns of the spinal cord, lemniscal system in the brainstem, thalamus, or parietal cortex
- Different types of ataxia should be distinguished
  —Vertiginous ataxia due to dizziness
  —Cerebellar ataxia due to imbalance
  —Spinal cord and muscular ataxia due to weakness

ETIOLOGY

- Acute
  —Symmetrical
    -Toxicologic
      *Alcohol
      *Lithium
      *Diphenylhydantoin
      *Barbiturates
  —Acute viral cerebritis
  —Meningitis
  —Hydrocephalus
  —Postinfection syndrome
  —Hyponatremia
  —Hypothyroidism
  —Focal
    -Anterior cerebral artery syndrome
    -Cerebellar infarction
    -Cerebellar hemorrhage
    -Subdural hematoma of the posterior fossa
    -Cerebellar abscess
- Subacute
  —Symmetrical
    -Mercury
    -Hydrocarbons
    -Toluene
    -Vitamin B_1 or B_{12} deficiency
    -Lyme disease
    -AIDS
    -Toxoplasmosis
    -Mycoplasma
    -Legionella
    -Bacterial abscesses
    -Creutzfeldt-Jakob disease
  —Focal
    -Cerebellar glioma
    -Metastatic tumors
    -Paraneoplastic syndromes
      *Breast cancer
      *Hodgkin's Disease
      *Children with neuroblastomas
    -Multiple sclerosis
    -AIDS-related multifocal leukoencephalopathy
    -Lymphoma
    -Cervical spondylosis
    -Syringomyelia
    -Guillain-Barré syndrome
- Chronic
  —Stable gliosis
  —Inherited and developmental ataxias
    -Friedreich ataxia and other recessive ataxias
    -Ataxia-telangiectasia
    -Autosomal dominant cerebellar ataxia
    -Cerebellar hypoplasia
    -Hartnup disease
    -Niemann-Pick disease
    -Pyruvate decarboxylase deficiency
    -Dandy Walker and Arnold Chiari malformation
    -Joubert and Gillespie syndromes

Pre-Hospital

CAUTIONS

- Acute onset of ataxia may be due to stroke or hemorrhage
  —Monitor
  —Supplemental oxygen
  —Observe mental status carefully as deterioration may warrant field endotracheal intubation

Diagnosis

ESSENTIAL WORKUP

- A careful history and physical are essential to classify the ataxia and determine the etiology
  —Onset
    -Hours to days or acute
    -Weeks to months or subacute
    -Years or chronic
  —Bilateral, symmetrical, or focal involvement
  —Truncal or limb ataxia
  —Presence or absence of vertigo

LABORATORY

- Electrolytes
- Toxicological screen
- Anticonvulsant drug screen

IMAGING/SPECIAL TESTS

- Head CT scan
  —Identifies supratentorial masses, hemorrhage, or evidence of hydrocephalus
  —If MRI is unavailable, obtain both contrast and noncontrast studies
- MRI
  —Diagnostic study of choice to assess the posterior fossa
  —MR angiogram may be indicated if a vertebral basilar artery insufficiency is suspected
- Lumbar puncture
  —Rarely indicated unless fever or mental status changes suggest an infectious etiology
  —Indicated in the evaluation for possible Lyme disease although may be done in this setting as an outpatient
- Electromyography
  —Not indicated as part of the emergency workup
  —Assesses for denervation of peripheral nerves

DIFFERENTIAL DIAGNOSIS

- See etiology

Treatment

INITIAL STABILIZATION

- Empiric thiamine in chronic alcoholics and poorly nourished patients

ED TREATMENT

- Treatment should be determined by the underlying cause

MEDICATIONS

- Thiamine 100 mg IM or 100 mg thiamine in 1000 ml of intravenous fluid wide open

Disposition

ADMISSION CRITERIA

- Acute and subacute ataxia require admission if an underlying etiology cannot be established
- Patients who cannot ambulate safely without home support
- Patients with cerebellar hemorrhage should be admitted to the intensive care unit

DISCHARGE CRITERIA

- Reversible causes once the patient can ambulate without risk of injury
  —Alcohol, medications
- Cerebellar atrophy

Miscellaneous

ICD9: 334.0, 334.2, 334.3, 334.8

CORE CONTENT CODE: 11.13

SUGGESTED READINGS

Baloh RW. Approach to the dizzy patient. In: Baloh RW, ed. Neurotology. Baillieres Clin Neurol 1994;3:453.

Rosenberg RN. Ataxic disorders. In: Fauci AS, et al., eds. Harrison's principles of internal medicine. Philadelphia: McGraw-Hill, 1998:2363–368.

Author: Richard Wolfe

Atrial Fibrillation

Clinical Presentation

SIGNS AND SYMPTOMS

- Palpitations
- Dyspnea
- Weakness
- Lightheadedness
- Irregular pulse
- Intermittent failure of a QRS complex on the monitor to transmit a pulse
- S1 of variable density
- Loss of waves in the jugular pulse
- Signs of instability
  —Hypotension
  —Persistent angina
  —Pulmonary edema
  —Altered mental status
  —Acute neurologic injury

MECHANISM/DESCRIPTION

- Chronic atrial electrical activity
  —Rate of 350–600
  —No mechanical kick to atrial contraction
- AV node limits the number of impulses reaching the ventricles
  —Typical ventricular rate 160–200 if AV node is healthy
- Loss of organized atrial contractions and rapid ventricular rate
  —Decrease in stroke volume
  —Decrease in cardiac output
- Affects over 1 million Americans each year
- Most common dysrhythmia requiring intervention
- Rare in those less than 35 years of age
- Occurs in 5% of people over 70
- Spontaneously converts in 24 hours in patients with new onset atrial fibrillation
- Sinus rhythm is maintained in 30% without medical therapy
- Mortality is twice that of the general population
- Complications
  —CVA in 35% of patients
    -Embolic, especially on conversion
    -Hemorrhagic after anticoagulation
  —Mesenteric ischemia
  —Syncope
  —Angina

ETIOLOGY

- Predisposing conditions
  —Hypertension
  —Coronary artery disease
  —Hypothyroidism
  —Heavy alcohol intake
  —Mitral valve disease
  —Chronic pulmonary disease
  —Pulmonary embolus
  —Wolf-Parkinson-White syndrome
  —Hypoxia
  —Digoxin toxicity
  —Chronic pericarditis
  —Idiopathic atrial fibrillation

Pre-Hospital

CAUTIONS

- Monitor
- Oxygen

CONTROVERSIES

- Cardioversion
  —Unstable patients
    -Persistent ischemic pain
    -Hypotension
    -Confusion
  —Rarely required
  —Rarely successful

Diagnosis

ESSENTIAL WORKUP

- EKG to determine rhythm and suggest underlying cause
  —Slow the rate when in doubt of the underlying rhythm
- Ordering of ancillary studies should be based on the clinical examination to determine underlying causes

LABORATORY

- Pulse oximetry
- CBC
- Electrolytes
- Cardiac enzymes
- Thyroid function
  —Yield is very low without other signs of hypothyroidism

IMAGING/SPECIAL TESTS

- Echocardiogram
  —Transthoracic or transesophageal
  —Assess for atrial enlargement as an etiology
  —Assess for atrial thrombus and the need for immediate anticoagulation
  —Anticoagulation after 48 hours even if thrombus is absent

DIFFERENTIAL DIAGNOSIS

- Atrial flutter with variable AV block
- Multifocal atrial tachycardia
- Sinus rhythm with frequent premature atrial contractions
- Atrial tachycardia with variable AV block

Treatment

INITIAL STABILIZATION

- Oxygen
- Monitor
- Intravenous access
- Unstable patients
  —Immediate synchronized cardioversion starting at 100 J-min

EMERGENCY DEPARTMENT MANAGEMENT

- Stable patients with a narrow complex tachycardia
  —If pulse <120 beats/min no treatment is needed in the ED
  —Control rate if pulse >120 beats/min
    -Calcium channel blockers: verapamil and diltiazem are of equal value; parenteral or oral routes
    -β-Blockers
    -Procainamide if rate control is recalcitrant to other agents
  —Cardioversion
    -Should only be considered in patients who have been in A-Fib for less than 48 hours
    -Beyond 48 hours requires anticoagulation first
    -Ibutilide: requires correction of hypokalemia; posttreatment monitoring for at least 4 hours for possible Torsades des Pointes
- Wide complex irregular tachycardia
  —Wolf-Parkinson-White syndrome may be the underlying cause
  —Avoid all calcium channel blockers, β-blockers, and digoxin
  —Stable patients should be treated with procainamide
  —Unstable patients should be cardioverted

MEDICATIONS

- Diltiazem: 0.25 mg/kg IV over 2 min followed in 15 min by 0.35 mg/kg IV over 2 min
- Esmolol: 0.5 mg/kg over 1 min; maintenance infusion at 0.05 mg/kg/min over 4 min then 0.1–0.2 mg/kg/min continuously
- Metoprolol: 5–10 mg slow IV push at 5-min intervals to total of 15 mg
- Popranolol: 0.1 mg/kg divided into equal doses at 2–3-min intervals
- Verapamil: 2.5–5 mg IV bolus over 2 min; may repeat with 5–10 mg every 15–30 min to max of 20 mg
- Digoxin: 0.5 mg IV initially then 0.25 mg IV q 4 hrs until desired effect
- Procainamide: 6–13 mg/kg IV at 0.2–0.5 mg/kg/min until dysrhythmia controlled up to a total dose of 1000 mg, then 2–6 mg/min
- Quinidine gluconate: 324–648 mg po q 8–12 hrs
- Ibutilide (corvert): 1 mg IV for patients >60 kg; 0.01 mg/kg IV for patients <60 kg infused over 10 min; dose can be repeated once if NSR not restored within 10 min after infusion; patients must be monitored for 4 hrs afterward for QT prolongation and VT
- Heparin: load 80 IU/kg IV; infusion at 18 IU/kg/hr

Disposition

ADMISSION CRITERIA

- Hypotension
- Chest pain suggestive of cardiac ischemia or EKG evidence of myocardial injury
- New onset or worsening congestive heart failure
- Persistent or recurrent rapid ventricular rate
- Age over 65 years or significant concomitant medical problems
- Hemodynamic dependence on atrial contraction
  —Significant mitral or aortic stenosis
  Hypertrophic cardiomyopathy
- New onset atrial fibrillation

DISCHARGE CRITERIA

- Patients who convert to sinus rhythm
- Patients in chronic atrial fibrillation with adequate ventricular rate control

Miscellaneous

ICD9: 427.3

CORE CONTENT CODE: 2.4.1.1

SUGGESTED READINGS

Deantonio HJ, Movahed A. Atrial fibrillation: Current therapeutic approaches. Am Fam Physician 1992;45(6):2576–2584.

Golzari H, Cebul RD, Bahler RC. Atrial fibrillation: Restoration and maintenance of sinus rhythm and indications of anticoagulation therapy. Ann Intern Med 1996;125:311–323.

Havranek EP. The management of atrial fibrillation: Current perspectives. Am Fam Physician 1994;50(5):959–968.

The National Heart, Lung, and Blood Institute Working Group on Atrial Fibrillation. Current understanding and research imperatives. J Am Coll Cardiol 1993;22:1830–1834.

Zipes DP. Specific arrythmias: Diagnosis and treatment. In: Braunwald E, ed. Heart disease: A textbook of cardiovascular medicine. 5th ed. Philadelphia: WB Saunders, 1997:640–704.

Author: Kevin Curtis

Atrial Flutter

Clinical Presentation

SIGNS AND SYMPTOMS

- Palpitations
- Syncope/presyncope
- Fatigue
- Dyspnea
- Poor exercise capacity
- Tachycardia
  —Most often with a regular pulse
- Signs of instability
  —Hypotension
  —Chest pain
  —Heart failure
  —Heart rate >150 bpm

MECHANISM/DESCRIPTION

- Atrial dysrhythmia characterized by several electrocardiographic findings
  —Regular atrial rate between 250 and 350
  —Beat to beat uniformity
  —Sawtooth flutter waves
- A reentrant circuit in the right atrium is thought to be the underlying mechanism
- Most sensitive rhythm to cardioversion
  —More than 90% of cases with A-Flutter can be converted with 25–50 watt-sec
- Seldom occurs in absence of organic heart disease
- Less common than SVT or atrial fibrillation

PEDIATRIC CONSIDERATIONS

- Infants do not tolerate atrial flutter well
  —The AV node is capable of very rapid conduction
  —Extremely rapid ventricular rates can lead to shock or congestive heart failure
- Atrial flutter can occur in the fetus and young infant without associated cardiac defects
- Most older children have an underlying cardiac abnormality

ETIOLOGY

- Ischemic heart disease
- Valvular heart diseases
- Congestive heart failure
- Myocarditis
- Cardiomyopathies
- Pulmonary embolus
- Other Pulmonary disease
- Electrolyte abnormalities
- Postoperative following cardiac surgery

Pre-Hospital

CAUTIONS

- Intravenous access
- Supplemental oxygen
- Cardiac monitoring
- Transport to the nearest facility
- Unstable patients should be cardioverted in the field
  —Immediate synchronized cardioversion
  —Start with 50 J, then 100 J, 200 J, 300 J, and 360 J

CONTROVERSIES

- Adenosine
  —Used in some systems in the field for SVT
  —Unlikely to break atrial flutter
  —May aid in the diagnosis of atrial flutter by unmasking the flutter waves

Diagnosis

ESSENTIAL WORKUP

- EKG to determine rhythm and suggest underlying cause
  —Slow the rate when in doubt of the underlying rhythm
- Ancillary studies are based on the clinical examination to determine underlying causes

LABORATORY

- CBC
- Electrolytes
- Cardiac enzymes
- Thyroid function

IMAGING/SPECIAL TESTS

- EKG
  —Regular atrial rate between 250 and 350
  —Beat to beat uniformity of cycle length, polarity, and amplitude
  —Sawtooth flutter waves directed superiorly and most visible in leads II, III, aVF
  —AV block usually 2:1, but occasionally greater or irregular
  —If rhythm is equivocal, slow the rate to show the presence of flutter waves
    -Vagal maneuvers
    -Adenosine
- CXR
  —Left atrial enlargement
    -Straightening of left heart border
    -Double-density seen to the right of the spine
    -Elevation of left main stem bronchus
  —Cardiomegaly
  —Heart failure

DIFFERENTIAL DIAGNOSIS

- SVT
- Sinus tachycardia
- Atrial Fibrillation
- Multifocal atrial tachycardia
- Ventricular tachycardia

Treatment

INITIAL STABILIZATION

- Immediate synchronized cardioversion starting at 50 J-min if the patient is unstable
- Oxygen
- Monitor
- Intravenous access

ED TREATMENT

- Pharmacoconversion or cardioversion if the onset is within 48 hours
- Rate control prior to conversion to sinus rhythm if the onset is greater than 48 hours
- Anticoagulation
  - —Not currently recommended in all patients
    - -Atrial activity remains organized therefore risk of thrombus formation is low
  - —Patients who go back and forth between atrial fibrillation and flutter
    - -If symptom duration >48 hours
    - -Anticoagulation prior to cardioversion
- Rate control
  - —Rate control should be instituted prior to giving an antidysrhythmic
    - -Class I antidysrhythmic agents slow intra-atrial conduction without lengthening the refractory period
    - -Risk of a 1:1 AV conduction ratio and hemodynamic collapse
  - —ACLS recommendations for rate control (in order of preference)
    - -Diltiazem
    - -β-Blockers: atenolol; esmolol; metoprolol; popranolol
    - -Digoxin in congestive heart failure: the conversion rate parallels placebo for A-Flutter; may be useful for maintenance once the patient has been converted
  - —Adenosine
    - -Too short-lived to provide adequate rate control
    - -Primarily used for diagnostic purposes
- Pharmacoconversion
  - —Ibutilide
  - —Procainamide
  - —Oral alternatives
    - -Flecainide
    - -Propafenone
    - -Quinidine
    - -Sotalol
- Cardioversion
  - —50–360 J
  - —Sedation when possible
  - —Safest and most effective means of restoring sinus rhythm
  - —In most patients, it can be accomplished with 25–100 J

PEDIATRIC CONSIDERATIONS

- Verapamil is not recommended in infants as it is associated with a low cardiac output
- Digoxin is the first-line drug therapy for pediatric atrial flutter

MEDICATIONS

- Atenolol: 5–10 mg IV over 5 min
- Diltiazem: 0.25 mg/kg IV over 2 min followed in 15 min by 0.35 mg/kg IV over 2 min
- Esmolol: 0.5 mg/kg over 1 min; maintenance infusion at 0.05 mg/kg/min over 4 min then 0.1–0.2 mg/kg/min continuously
- Metoprolol: 5–10 mg slow IV push at 5-min intervals to total of 15 mg
- Popranolol: 0.1 mg/kg divided into equal doses at 2–3-min intervals
- Verapamil: 2.5–5.0 mg IV bolus over 2 min; may repeat with 5–10 mg every 15–30 min to max of 20 mg
- Digoxin: 0.5 mg IV initially then 0.25 mg IV q 4 hrs until desired effect
- Procainamide: 6–13 mg/kg IV at 0.2–0.5 mg/kg/min until arrhythmia controlled up to a total dose of 1000 mg, then 2–6 mg/min
- Quinidine gluconate: 324–648 mg po q 8–12 hrs
- Ibutilide (corvert): 1 mg IV for patients >60kg; 0.01mg/kg IV for patients <60kg infused over 10 min; dose can be repeated once if NSR not restored within 10 min after infusion; patients must be monitored for 4 hrs afterward for QT prolongation and VT

Disposition

ADMISSION CRITERIA

- New-onset atrial flutter requiring antidysrhythmics
- Symptomatic (i.e., chest pain that warrants a rule out or cardioversion)
- Congestive heart failure

DISCHARGE CRITERIA

- Chronic atrial flutter with good rate control

Miscellaneous

ICD9: 427.32

CORE CONTENT CODE: 2.4.1.1

SUGGESTED READINGS

Alpert MA, Hashimi MW, et al. Pathogenesis, recognition, and management of common cardiac arrhythmias. Part II: Supraventricular premature beats and tachyarrhythmias. South Med J 1995;88(2):153–174.

Anderson JL. Acute treatment of atrial fibrillation and flutter. Am J Cardiol 1996;78(8A):17–21.

Collier WW, Holt SE, et al. Narrow complex tachycardias. Emerg Med Clin 1995;13(4):925–954.

Olshansky B, Wilber DJ, et al. Atrial flutter—update on the mechanism and treatment. PACE 1992;15(12):2308–2335.

Waldo AL. An approach to therapy of supraventricular tachyarrhythmias: An algorithm versus individual therapy. Clin Cardiol 1994;17(Suppl II):II21–II26.

Author: Liesl Curtis

Atrioventricular Blocks

Clinical Presentation

SIGNS AND SYMPTOMS

- First degree AV block
  - —Asymptomatic
- Type I second degree block
  - —Regularly irregular pulse
- Type II second degree block and third degree block
  - —Dizziness
  - —Syncope
  - —Chest pain
  - —Dyspnea
  - —Irregular pulse
  - —Hypotension
  - —Rales
  - —Cyanosis
  - —Distended neck veins

MECHANISM/DESCRIPTION

- A disturbance in conduction from the atria to the ventricles
  - —SA node
  - —Internodal pathways
  - —AV node
  - —His bundle
  - —Bundle branches
  - —Purkinje network
- Multiple possible causes
  - —Organic lesion along the conduction pathway
  - —Increase in the inherent refractoriness of the conduction pathway
  - —Marked shortening of the supraventricular cycle
- First degree AV block
  - —Prolongation of the PR interval >0.20 sec
- Second degree AV block
  - —Type I (Wenckebach)
    - -Progressive prolongation of the PR interval until there is a nonconducted P wave and a dropped QRS complex
    - -Generally benign
    - -May be a complication of an inferior myocardial infarction
  - —Type II
    - -PR intervals are constant until a single or multiple beats are dropped
    - -Suggestive of a block below the AV node
    - -Often associated with acute anterior myocardial infarction or cardiomyopathy
    - -High likelihood of progressing to a complete AV block
- Third degree AV block
  - —Also known as complete heart block
  - —Complete AV dissociation
  - —Constant but independent PR and RR intervals
  - —Never a benign condition
  - —Associated with ischemic, structural or toxicological etiologies

ETIOLOGY

- Increased vagal tone
- Inferior myocardial infarction
  - —Type I second degree AV block
- Anterior myocardial infarction
  - —Type II second degree AV block
- Cardiomyopathy
- Medication
  - —Digoxin
  - —Calcium channel blockers
  - —β-Blockers
- Pediatric
  - —Congenital
  - —Congenital heart disease
  - —Myocarditis
  - —Endocarditis
  - —Rheumatic fever

Pre-Hospital

- Use a transcutaneous pacemaker for patients with AV block and hypotension

CAUTIONS

- Avoid atropine
  - —In type II second degree block, it may precipitate complete heart block
  - —Contraindicated in third degree heart block with a widened QRS complex

Diagnosis

ESSENTIAL WORKUP

- A 12-lead EKG to determine the type of block and identify evidence of infarction or drug toxicity
  - —First degree AV block
    - -Prolongation of the PR interval >0.20 sec
  - —Second degree AV block
    - -Type I (Wenckebach): progressive prolongation of the PR interval until there is a non-conducted P wave and a dropped QRS complex
    - -Type II: PR intervals are constant until a single or multiple beats are dropped
  - —Third degree AV block
    - -Constant but independent PR and RR intervals
- Question carefully for past cardiac history, risk factors for cardiac ischemia, and medications
- Identify underlying causes such as infarction or drug toxicity

LABORATORY

- Electrolytes
- Calcium
- Magnesium
- Digoxin level
- Cardiac enzymes
  - —Type II second and third degree block

IMAGING/SPECIAL TESTS

- Chest radiograph
  - —May identify a cardiomyopathy or congestive heart failure
- Echocardiogram
  - —Useful to identify regional wall motion abnormalities or valvular dysfunction

DIFFERENTIAL DIAGNOSIS

- Sinus bradycardia
- Atrioventricular dissociation
- Idioventricular rhythm

Treatment

INITIAL STABILIZATION

- Transcutaneous pacer
  —Profound bradycardia and chest pain
  —Shortness of breath
  —Hypotension
  —Mild sedation is recommended beforehand
- Atropine
  —Complete heart block and narrow QRS

ED TREATMENT

- First degree AV block
  —No treatment is required
  —Close monitoring
    -Associated with MI
    -Electrolyte abnormalities
- Type I second degree AV block
  —If symptomatic, atropine will enhance AV conduction
- Type II second degree AV block
  —Temporary transcutaneous or transvenous pacing
  —Atropine and isoproterenol are not effective
- Third degree AV block
  —Transient respond to atropine
  —Emergent pacemaking
  —Calcium
    -If calcium channel blocker overdose
  —Glucagon
    -If β-blocker or calcium channel blocker overdose
  —Digoxin-specific antibodies
    -Digoxin overdose with a complete heart block

MEDICATIONS

- Atropine: 0.5 mg IV repeat every 5 min as necessary; peds: 0.01–0.03 mg/kg IV/ET, maximum dose of 0.04 mg/kg
- Calcium chloride: 250–500 mg (2.5–5 ml) IV; peds: 20 mg/kg IV
- Glucagon: 5–10 mg IV over 5 min; 50 μg/kg IV over 5 min
- Isoproterenol: begin infusion at 2 μg/min and titrate to max 10 μg/min; peds: begin infusion at 0.1 μg/kg/min and titrate to max of 1.5 μg/kg/min

Disposition

ADMISSION CRITERIA

- Monitored bed
  —Type II second degree block
  —Complete AV block

DISCHARGE CRITERIA

- Asymptomatic first degree and type I second degree AV blocks
- Follow-up arranged for further evaluation as an outpatient

Miscellaneous

ICD9: 426.1

CORE CONTENT CODE: 2.4.2.3

SUGGESTED READINGS

Pelucio M, Jacoby RM. Dysrhythmias. In: Howell J, et al., eds. Emergency medicine. Philadelphia: WB Saunders, 1997:161–192.

Waller BF, Gering LE, Branyas NA, Slack JD. Anatomy, histology, and pathology of the cardiac conduction system: Part II. Clin Cardiol 1993;16:347–352.

Author(s): Jamal Farran; James Scott

Bacterial Tracheitis

Clinical Presentation

SIGNS AND SYMPTOMS

- Inspiratory stridor
- Barky or brassy cough
- Hoarseness
- Fever
- Respiratory distress
  - —Acute onset
  - —Follows insidious progression of symptoms
- Retractions
- Dyspnea
- Flaring
- Cyanosis
- Sore throat
- Dysphonia
- Usually no drooling or specific position of comfort

MECHANISM/DESCRIPTION

- Life-threatening disease
- Diffuse inflammatory process of larynx, trachea and bronchi
- Adherent or semiadherent mucopurulent membranes within the trachea
- Often predisposed by a preceding viral infection
- Rare disease of childhood that can occur in any age group
  - —Mean age is 4 years
  - —2% of children hospitalized for acute infectious upper airway obstruction
- More evident in the pediatric patient due to size and shape of subglottic airway
- Male:female ratio is 2:1
- Usually occurs in the fall or winter months mimicking croup
- Complications
  - —Pneumonia
  - —Septicemia
  - —Toxic shock
  - —ARDS
  - —Pulmonary edema
  - —Retropharyngeal cellulitis
  - —Subglottic stenosis
  - —Anoxic encephalopathy
    - -Prolonged hypoxia
    - -Respiratory arrest
  - —ETT complications including plugging and accidental extubation
  - —Cardiorespiratory arrest

ETIOLOGY

- *Staphylococcus aureus*
- *Hemophilus influenzae* type B
- Streptococcal species (usually β-hemolytic group A)
- Klebsiella
- Pseudomonas
- *Branhamella catarrhalis*
- Anaerobes

Pre-Hospital

- Maintenance of an adequate airway
- Avoid agitating children
- Racemic epinephrine
- Bag-valve-ventilation if respiratory status deteriorates
- Intubate if bag-valve-mask-ventilation is ineffective
- Rapid transport with ED notification

Diagnosis

ESSENTIAL WORKUP

- Avoid blood draws before initiating therapy

LABORATORY

- Diagnostic blood tests should never be done before definitive airway management
  - —WBC elevated but not specific
  - —Arterial blood gas
    - -Pulse oximetry is less invasive
- Blood cultures are rarely useful

IMAGING/SPECIAL TESTS

- Radiograph of lateral neck
  - —Not essential and should not be obtained if there is risk of acute airway obstruction
  - —Subglottic narrowing
  - —Clouding of tracheal air column
  - —Irregular tracheal margin
  - —Edema of subglottic trachea
  - —Concretions of epithelium inflammatory cells may appear as a foreign body
- Direct laryngoscopy
  - —Diagnostic study of chicle
  - —Should be performed in a setting where rapid surgical airway intervention can be performed
  - —Shaggy exudative membrane on the larynx
  - —Inflammation in the subglottic area
- Bronchoscopy
  - —Visualization of purulent tracheal secretions
  - —Culture of tracheal secretions

DIFFERENTIAL DIAGNOSIS

- Epiglottitis
- Croup
- Aspirated foreign body
- Diphtheria
- Intraluminal obstruction (cyst, tumor)
- Extrinsic compression (trauma, hematoma, vascular anomalies (rings and slings))
- Angioedema
- Peritonsillar abscess
- Retropharyngeal abscess
- Uvulitis
- Laryngeal candidiasis

Treatment

- Airway maintenance
  - —Most children will need eventual intubation
  - —When possible intubation should be attempted in the operating room and with a surgeon prepared to perform a tracheostomy
  - —ETT 1–2 sizes smaller than expected
  - —Frequent suctioning of secretions to maintain ETT patency
- IV access after the airway is stabilized
- Intravenous antibiotics
  - —Double coverage with cefuroxime and nafcillin or vancomycin
  - —Chloramphenicol and clindamycin for penicillin-allergic patients
- Hydration
- Bronchoscopy
  - —Complete stripping of membranes
  - —Tracheal toilet
  - —May prevent the need for a surgical airway

MEDICATIONS

- Cefuroxime: 50 mg/kg IV; max 3 g
- Chloramphenicol: 20 mg/kg IV loading dose
- Clindamycin: 10 mg/kg IV; max 1 g
- Nafcillin: 50 mg/kg IV; max 2 g
- Racemic epinephrine: 0.05 ml/kg/dose diluted to 3 ml with NS by nebulizer; max 0.5 ml
- Vancomycin: 10 mg/kg IV; max 1 g

Disposition

ADMISSION CRITERIA

- All children with suspected bacterial tracheitis
- Most should be admitted to an ICU setting

DISCHARGE CRITERIA

None

EXPECTED COURSE

- Most patients improve within 5 days and finish a 10-day course of antibiotics at home
- Mortality ranges from 4% to 20%

Miscellaneous

ICD9: 464.1

CORE CONTENT CODE: 6.3.3.2.1

SUGGESTED READINGS

Donnelly BW, McMillan JA, Weiner LB. Bacterial tracheitis: Report of eight new cases and review. Rev Infect Dis 1990;12:729–735.

Eckel HE, Widemann B, Damm M, Roth B. Airway endoscopy in the diagnosis and treatment of bacterial tracheitis in children. Int J Pediatr Otorhinolaryngol 1993;27(2):147–157.

Gallagher PG, Myer CM III. An approach to the diagnosis and treatment of membranous laryngotracheobronchitis in infants and children. Pediatr Emerg Care 1991;7:337–342.

Author: Kathryn Clark

Barbiturates, Poisoning

Clinical Presentation

SIGNS AND SYMPTOMS

CNS

- Lethargy
- Slurred speech
- Incoordination
- Ataxia
- Coma (mimicking death)
- Loss of reflexes

Cardiovascular

- Hypotension
- Bradycardia (direct myocardial depressant)

Ophthalmologic

- Miosis (generally associated with deep coma)
- Nystagmus
- Disconjugate gaze

Other

- Respiratory depression (inhibition of neurogenic respiratory drive)
- Hypothermia
- Bullae or "barb blisters" (not always present)

MECHANISM OF TOXICITY

- Increases γ-aminobutyric acid (GABA) activity
- Direct myocardial depression
- Inhibition of vascular smooth muscle

Pre-Hospital

CAUTIONS

- Moderate to severe poisonings require paramedic transport
- Intubation often necessary due to respiratory depression or loss of gag reflex
- Hypotension often requires intravenous fluids, inotropic support, and vasopressors

Diagnosis

ESSENTIAL WORKUP

- Obtain vital signs, check gag reflex, finger stick glucose
- Oxygen saturation monitor/ABG
- ECG/continuous cardiac monitoring
- Barbiturate poisoning can mimic death. Therefore cannot pronounce patient until barbiturate poisoning has been ruled out in patients in whom it is suspected

LABORATORY

- Electrolyte, BUN/Cr, glucose
  - —Patients down for a long period of time may be hyperkalemic from skeletal muscle breakdown and at-risk for rhabdomyolysis
  - —To assess renal function, potassium, bicarbonate, calcium, magnesium
  - —Calculate anion gap
- Urinalysis
  - —For myoglobin
  - —Toxic alcohols, primidone can cause crystalluria
- CPK for rhabdomyolysis
- Urine toxicology screen
- Obtain serum phenobarbital level (if known or suspected)
- Acetaminophen and salicylate levels if suspected suicide
- CBC for other etiologies for altered mental status

IMAGING/SPECIAL TESTS

- CT scan of head for altered mental status
- CXR for aspiration
- Lumbar puncture for altered mental status work up
- Thyroid function tests

DIFFERENTIAL DIAGNOSIS

- Sedative-hypnotic poisoning (including toxic alcohols)
- Carbon monoxide poisoning
- CNS infections
- Space-occupying lesions of the head
- Hypoglycemia
- Uremia
- Electrolyte imbalance (i.e., hypermagnesemia)
- Postictal state following seizure
- Hypothyroidism
- Liver failure
- Psychiatric illness

Treatment

INITIAL STABILIZATION

- ABCs
  - —Administer supplemental oxygen
  - —Severe poisonings usually require endotracheal intubation
- 0.9%NS
  - —Hypotensive patients require 1–2 L IV fluid resuscitation and other IV medications
- Activated charcoal effectively binds barbiturates and may decrease systemic absorption

ED TREATMENT

- Administer one dose of activated charcoal
  - —Initiate "gut dialysis" with repeat dose activated charcoal (without sorbitol) given every 2–4 hours (as long as bowel sounds are present)
- Rewarm patient if hypothermic (see hypothermia chapter)
- Treat hypotension resistant to IV fluid bolus with cardiac inotropy agents such as dopamine or dobutamine
- Trap phenobarbital ions in urine by administering sodium bicarbonate as an infusion to maintain blood pH 7.45
- Treat hyperkalemia (from muscle breakdown) with calcium, sodium bicarbonate, insulin and glucose, and/or potassium-binding agents
- Consider hemodialysis if patient has
  - —Decreased or no renal function
  - —Prolonged coma
  - —Serum phenobarbital level >100 mg/dl
- Repeat phenobarbital level 2–4 hours after initial level if the patient is symptomatic, or to identify if level is increasing

MEDICATIONS

- Activated charcoal: 1 g/kg po
- Dobutamine: begin with 10 μg /kg/min titrating to desired effect (to maximum of 20 μg/kg/min)
- Dopamine: begin with 5–10 μg /kg/min titrating to desired effect (to maximum of 20 μg/kg/min)
- Sodium bicarbonate
  - —Bolus: 1–3 ampules (44 mEq per ampule) IV over 20–30 minutes (peds: 1.0–2.0 mEq/kg/dose)
  - —1–2 ampules (45–50 mEq) in D5W 0.45% NS to achieve a blood pH of ~ 7.45 and maintain a good urine output (monitor serum potassium closely)

Disposition

ADMISSION CRITERIA

- ICU admission for
  - —Ataxia
  - —Drowsiness
  - —Coma
  - —Respiratory depression
  - —Hypotension
  - —Hypothermia
  - —Rhabdomyolysis

DISCHARGE CRITERIA

- Asymptomatic after minimum of 6 hours observation with two consecutive subtoxic phenobarbital levels (if applicable) prior to discharge

Miscellaneous

ICD9: 967.0

CORE CONTENT CODE: 17.2.42.1

SUGGESTED READINGS

Ellenhorn MJ, Schoonwald S, Ordog G, Wasserberger J. Sedative-hypnotic drugs. In: Ellenhorn's medical toxicology. 2d ed. Baltimore: Williams & Wilkins, 1997:684–687

Frenia ML, Schauben JL, Wears RL, Karlix JL, Tucker CA, Kunisaki TA. Multiple-dose activated charcoal compared to urinary alkalinization for the enhancement of phenobarbital elimination. J Toxicol Clin Toxicol 1996;34(2):169–175

Gröschel D, Gerstein AR, Rosenbaum JM. Skin lesions as a diagnostic aid in barbiturate poisoning. N Engl J Med 1970;283:409–411

Matthew H. Barbiturates. J Toxicol Clin Toxicol 1975;8:495–513

Pond SM, Olson KR, Osterloh J, Tong TG. Randomized study of the treatment of phenobarbital overdose with repeated doses of activated charcoal. JAMA 1984;251:3104–3108

Zawanda ET, Nappi J, Done G, Rollins D. Advances in the hemodialysis management of phenobarbital overdose. South Med J 1983;76:6–8

Authors: Sean P. Nordt; Rick Clark

Barotrauma

Clinical Presentation

SIGNS AND SYMPTOMS

- Middle ear (barotitis media)
- Begins as a clogged sensation
- Increasingly painful as the pressure differential across the tympanic membrane (TM) increases
- Progresses to rupture of the TM
  —Tympanic membrane appearance: TM congestion→TM edema→gross hemorrhage→TM rupture
- External ear
  —Canal mucosa becomes edematous, then hemorrhagic, and ultimately tears
- Inner ear
  —Sudden, severe vertigo
  —Tinnitus
  —Sensineural hearing loss in the affected ear
- Paranasal sinuses
  —Sinus congestion
  —Pain
  —Epistaxis
- External objects
  —Mask: conjunctival hemorrhage, facial edema and swelling
  —Tight fitting dive suit: edema and erythema of the skin
- Teeth (barodontalgia)
  —Severe tooth pain
- Gastrointestinal (aerogastralgia)
  —Excessive belching
  —Flatulence
  —Abdominal distention
- Pulmonary
  —Dyspnea
  —Cough with a frothy red sputum
  —Subcutaneous emphysema
  —Delayed symptoms including a bull neck appearance, dysphagia, and changes in voice character

DESCRIPTION/MECHANISM

- Injury to the body as a result of the expansion and contraction of gas in an enclosed space
- Boyle's law states that at a constant temperature, pressure (P) is inversely related to volume (V)
  —PV = K (constant) or $P_1V_1 = P_2V_2$
  —Increase of pressure mandates a reduction of volume by same factor
- Gas-filled cavities in the body are subject to expansion/contraction
  —Lung
  —Middle ear
  —Sinus
- Solid and liquid-filled spaces distribute the pressure equally
- Volume changes experienced during ascent are greatest in the few feet nearest the surface

ETIOLOGY

- Middle ear
  —Barotrauma of descent
  —Most common type of barotrauma
  —Seen in 30% of inexperienced divers and 10% of experienced divers
  —Results from inadequate equalization of pressure between the middle ear and the external ear canal
  —Eustachian tube provides the sole route of pressure equalization for the middle ear
- External ear
  —Barotrauma of descent
  —Due to the presence of a tight fitting hood, ear plugs, or a cerumen plug
  —Pressure cannot equalize throughout the canal and a relative intracanal vacuum is created as the pressure differential across the obstruction increases
- Inner ear
  —Barotrauma of descent
  —Results from forceful attempts at equalizing middle ear pressure
  —Increased middle ear pressure can raise intracranial pressure and cause rupture of the round or labyrinth windows allowing perilymph to enter the middle ear
- Paranasal sinus
  —Barotrauma of descent
  —Nasal ostia act as a valve to regulate sinus pressure
  —If the ostia fail to allow pressure equalization, congestion, edema, and hemorrhage can occur
- External Objects
  —Air pockets in dive suit/mask expand and contract
- Teeth
  —Air trapped inside a filling
- Gastrointestinal
  —Barotrauma of ascent
  —Swallowed air in the GI tract expands as external pressure decreases
- Pulmonary barotrauma (PBT or POPS—Pulmonary OverPressurization Syndrome)
  —Occurs with ascent
  —Lungs expand against a closed glottis
  —Cause for arterial gas embolism (see Embolism Chapter)
  —Divers with decrease lung compliance/increase lung volumes at increased risk (COPD, asthma)

Pre-Hospital

CAUTION

- For barotrauma of descent, unless an air-filled cavity has ruptured, no progression of the disease upon return to normal atmospheric pressure expected
- If patient transport requires air evacuation, maintain air cabin pressure at 1 atmosphere or fly below 1000 feet to avoid aggravating barotrauma

Diagnosis

ESSENTIAL WORKUP

- HEENT exam with particular attention paid to the TM to determine if rupture has occurred
- Pulmonary exam looking for signs of subcutaneous emphysema and pneumothorax
- Neurological exam looking for signs of inner ear pathology

LABORATORY

- ABG for pulmonary symptoms

IMAGING/SPECIAL TESTS

- Sinus imaging
  - —CT
  - —Plain films
- CXR for pneumothorax
- Abdominal series (upright, decubitus) for free air from a ruptured viscus

DIFFERENTIAL DIAGNOSIS

- Decompression sickness
- Otitis media
- Otitis externa
- Sinusitis

Treatment

INITIAL STABILIZATION

- ABCs
  - —100% oxygen for ill-appearing patients
  - —Intubation for in-patients with massive subcutaneous emphysema of the neck
  - —Immediate needle thoracostomy for evidence of tension pneumothorax

ED TREATMENT

- Establish IV access for unstable patients
- Control bleeding from the ear or nose
- Oral decongestants for middle ear or sinus congestion
- Antibiotics with TM or sinus rupture
- Analgesics

MEDICATIONS

- Amoxicillin: 250–500 mg (peds: 40 mg/kg/24 hrs) po TID
- Bactrim DS 1 tablet (peds: 40/200 per 5 ml-5 ml/10kg/dose) po BID
- Pseudoephedrine (sudafed) 60 mg (peds: 6–12 yrs old, 30mg; 2–5 yrs old, 15mg/dose) po q4–6 hrs

Disposition

ADMISSION CRITERIA

- Pulmonary barotrauma

DISCHARGE CRITERIA

- Discharge nonpulmonary barotrauma
- ENT follow-up for severe TM or sinus pathology

Miscellaneous

PATIENT CODE: 993.2

CORE CONTENT CODE: 5.1

SUGGESTED READINGS

Bradley ME. Pulmonary barotrauma. In: Bove AA, Davis JC. Diving medicine. 2d ed. Philadelphia: WB Saunders, 1990:188–191

Edmonds C, Lowry C, Pennefather J. Diving and subaquatic medicine. Oxford: Butterworth-Heinemann, 1992

Jerrard DA. Diving medicine. Emerg Med Clin North Am 1992;10(2):329–338

Raymond LW. Pulmonary barotrauma and related events in divers. Chest 1995;107;1648–1652

Author: Jeffrey Gordon

Bartholin's Abscess

Clinical Presentation

SIGNS AND SYMPTOMS

- Swollen and painful labia
- Tender, fluctuant mass on posterior-lateral margin of vestibule of vagina
- Warmth and erythema

ETIOLOGY

- The majority of Bartholin's abscesses involve anaerobic and aerobic microflora normally found in the vagina. Infections are often polymicrobial and include Bacteroides species, Peptostreptococcus species, E. coli, and other Gram-negative organisms. There is a limited role for N. gonorrhea in these abscesses and less commonly C. trachomatis

DESCRIPTION OF DISEASE

- Bartholin's glands are located inferiorly on either side of the vaginal opening. The ducts open on the sides of the vestibule. When the duct of a Bartholin's gland becomes obstructed a simple cyst develops. This is due to retention of secretions and is usually painless. If the cyst becomes secondarily infected it becomes an abscess. This is more common in females aged 20–40 years

Pre-Hospital

N/A

Diagnosis

ESSENTIAL WORKUP

- The diagnosis of Bartholin's abscess is based on the physical findings of a tender, localized, fluctuant mass in the region of the Bartholin's gland

LABORATORY

- Material from the abscess should be sent for GC and Chlamydia culture
- Culture of the cervix may increase the likelihood of finding of sexually transmitted disease

DIFFERENTIAL DIAGNOSIS

- Bartholin's cyst
- Carcinoma of Bartholin's gland (rare)
- Perineal hernia

Treatment

ED MANAGEMENT

- Treat with prompt incision and drainage using local anesthesia. The procedure is performed with the patient in the lithotomy position. Narcotic analgesia may be administered for patient comfort. Alternative approaches include
  —Simple incision and drainage
  —Word catheter method
  —Marsupialization
- Antibiotics are not necessary after routine incision and drainage. If mild cellulitis is present or patient is immunocompromised, broad-spectrum coverage may be started. If there is a suspicion of a sexually transmitted disease, treatment with antibiotics is recommended
- Simple I&D
  —After satisfactory local anesthesia, palpate the abscess between the thumb and index fingers. Spread the vulva apart and make a stab incision on the *mucosal* surface of the abscess, parallel to the hymenal ring
  —When incising the abscess, two tissue layers must be penetrated; first the labial mucosa and then the abscess wall. Free flow of pus indicates penetration of the abscess wall
  —Pack the wound with iodoform gauze and have the patient follow-up in 24–48 hours for removal of packing
  —Start sitz baths after 24 hours
  —The patient may need referral for marsupialization because there is a significant recurrence rate

- Word Catheter Method
  - —Word described the use of a small, inflatable, bulb-tipped catheter to treat a Bartholin's gland abscess. This results in an epithelialized tract and may make marsupialization unnecessary
  - —A stab wound is made as with simple I&D; it should be just large enough to easily admit the catheter so that when the balloon is inflated, it does not fall out
  - —After inserting the bulb tip of the catheter, inflate the balloon by injecting 2–4 cc water using a 25-gauge needle (to minimize the size of the puncture). Overinflation may cause patient discomfort. This may be remedied by withdrawing some water from the balloon
  - —Sitz baths may be started after 24 hours. Have the patient follow-up in 2–4 days
  - —The catheter is left in place for 6–8 weeks until epithelialization is complete. After the device is removed the gland resumes normal function. It is not uncommon for the catheter to fall out prematurely. If this occurs, the catheter may be reinserted, or the abscess can heal as with a simple incision and drainage
- Marsupialization
  - —This procedure also allows for a permanent fistula by suturing the wound edges of the abscess cavity to the edges of the labial mucosa. This may be technically more challenging in the acute phase as the walls of the abscess cavity are often friable making suturing difficult. It may be more expedient in the ED setting to reserve this for the patient's follow-up visit
  - —Excise an ellipse of labial mucosa which overlays the cyst cavity
  - —Incise the cyst and drain the contents
  - —Evert the edges of the abscess and suture them to the labial epithelium using an absorbable suture such as polyglactin. This opening will shrink but remain patent. Packing is not needed
  - —Start sitz baths in 24–48 hours. Have the patient follow-up within 1 week

MEDICATIONS

Broad Spectrum Coverage

- Amoxicillin/clavulanic acid: 875 mg po BID for 5 days with Metronidazole 500 mg po BID for 5 days
- Ciprofloxacin 500 mg po BID for 5 days with Metronidazole 500 mg po BID for 5 days

Disposition

ADMISSION CRITERIA

- Sepsis
- Significant cellulitis
- Evidence of necrotizing infection

DISCHARGE CRITERIA

- Nontoxic patients may be discharged with a designated follow-up plan

Miscellaneous

ICD9: 616.3

CORE CONTENT CODE: 19.1.5.1

SUGGESTED READINGS

Aghajanian A. Bartholin's duct abscess and cyst: a case control study South Med J 1994;87:26–29

Brook I. Aerobic and anaerobic microbiology of Bartholin's abscess. Surg Gynecol Obstet 1989;169:32–34

Word B. Office treatment of cyst and abscess of Bartholin's gland duct. South Med J 1968;61:514–518

Authors: Marilyn Althoff, Mark Mandell

Basal Cell Carcinoma

Clinical Presentation

SIGNS AND SYMPTOMS

- Skin malignancy that usually presents as a cutaneous nodule, shiny or pearly colored, waxy appearing, with fine telangiectasias over the surface and a depressed center
- May be single or multiple
- Cystic form contains cystic spaces within the tumor and may sometimes grossly appear as a cyst
- Pigmented form contains melanin pigment
- Sclerosing form has indistinct borders and a relative lack of nodularity or waxy appearance
- Usually painless leading to prolonged neglect of a lesion
- Very rarely metastasize, but may be locally invasive
- Most appear on the *sun-exposed areas of the skin,* especially the face, head, and neck, but may appear on any part of the body
- Rare in blacks

MECHANISM/DESCRIPTION

- Arise from the epidermis and cytologically resemble normal basal cells
- Account for over 75% of all skin cancers
- Most important risk factor is sunlight exposure

Pre-Hospital

N/A

Diagnosis

ESSENTIAL WORKUP

- Diagnosis requires biopsy of a suspicious lesion although rarely done in ED

DIFFERENTIAL DIAGNOSIS

- Squamous cell carcinoma
- Bowen's disease
- Actinic keratosis
- Paget's disease
- Seborrheic keratosis
- Nevus
- Melanoma

Treatment

INITIAL STABILIZATION

- No specific considerations

ED TREATMENT

- Common treatments involve electrodesiccation and curettage, cryosurgery, simple surgical excision, Mohs' micrographic surgery, or radiation therapy
- The size, type, and site of the lesion, as well as the age and sex of the patient, determine method of treatment and should involve referral to a dermatologist or experienced primary care provider

Disposition

ADMISSION CRITERIA

- Rarely, if ever, do patients with basal cell carcinoma require admission, except for complications of extensive local invasion

DISCHARGE CRITERIA

- Patients with suspected basal cell carcinoma may be discharged with referral to a dermatologist or experienced primary care provider

Miscellaneous

ICD9: 173.9

CORE CONTENT CODE: 3.7.1

SUGGESTED READINGS

Fleming ID, Amonette R, Monaghan T, Fleming MD. Principles of management of basal and squamous cell carcinomas of the skin. Cancer 1995;75:699–704.

Goldberg LH. Basal cell carcinoma. Lancet 1996;347:663–667.

Pariser DM, Phillips PK. Basal cell carcinoma: When to treat it yourself, and when to refer. Geriatrics 1994;49:39–44.

Washington CV. Skin cancer. In: Isselbacher KJ, Braunwald E, Wilson JD et al., eds. Harrison's principles of internal medicine. New York: McGraw Hill, 1994:1866–1867.

Author: Glenn Hebel

Bell's Palsy

Clinical Presentation

SIGNS AND SYMPTOMS

- Sudden onset of unilateral facial droop, incomplete eyelid closure, and loss of forehead muscle tone. Maximal deficit by 5 days in almost all cases (2 days in 50%)
- If forehead muscle tone is *not* lost, a central lesion is strongly implied (i.e., this is *not* Bell's palsy)
- Tearing (68%) or dryness of the eye (16%) and less frequent blinking on the affected side
- Bell's phenomenon (upward rolling of the eyeball on attempted lid closure) may be seen
- Subjective "numbness" of the affected side, abnormal taste, drooling, hyperacusis (sensitivity to loud sounds)
- Fullness or pain behind mastoid
- Viral prodrome frequently reported

Pre-Hospital

DESCRIPTION

Bell's palsy refers to acute, idiopathic peripheral palsy of CN VII (facial nerve)

- Complete recovery in 85% of the cases without treatment
- Degree of deficit correlates with prognosis. Complete lesions have the poorest prognosis. Partial lesions almost always have excellent results
- Recovery usually begins within 2 weeks (often taste returns first) and is complete by 2–3 months. Advanced age and slow recovery are poor prognosticators

ETIOLOGY

- Innervation to each side of the forehead is from both motor cortices. Unilateral cortical processes do *NOT* disrupt motor activity of the forehead. Therefore, only a peripheral or brain stem lesion can interrupt motor function of just one side of the forehead
- Idiopathic by definition but a viral cause (particularly Herpes simplex) suspected
- Lyme disease may cause peripheral seventh nerve palsy, but strictly speaking it is not Bell's Palsy
- Mechanism: edema and nerve degeneration within the stylomastoid foramen

EPIDEMIOLOGY

- Affects males and females equally
- Age predominance between the third and fifth decade (may occur at any age)
- Incidence 15–40/100,000/year

Diagnosis

ESSENTIAL WORKUP

- Diagnosis is clinical and based on the history and physical exam
- Motor weakness isolated to the seventh nerve distribution and involves both the upper and lower face
- An otherwise *normal* neurologic exam including all cranial nerves and extremity motor function

LABORATORY

- Not helpful in the diagnosis of Bell's Palsy
- Serum or CSF Lyme titers are useful if Lyme disease is suspected, or in an endemic area

IMAGING/SPECIAL TESTS

- Not helpful in the diagnosis of Bell's Palsy. CNS imaging (CT, MRI) useful if CNS pathology is suspected

DIFFERENTIAL DIAGNOSIS

- Brain stem events (mass, bleed, infarct) affecting CN VII almost always involve CN VI (abnormal EOM) and may affect the long motor tracts
- Lyme disease: history of tick bite, erythema migrans rash, or endemic area
- Ramsay Hunt syndrome: look for herpetic vesicles, inquire about tinnitus or vertigo
- Tumors: look for parotid, bone or metastatic masses, acoustic neuroma (deafness)
- Trauma: skull fracture or penetrating facial injury may damage CN VII
- Middle ear or mastoid surgery or infection, cholesteatoma
- Meningeal infection
- Guillain Barré syndrome: other neurologic deficits (i.e., ascending motor weakness or diminished DTRs) present
- Basilar artery aneurysm. Other cranial nerve deficits should be present
- Bilateral Bell's palsy occurs (1%). Consider multiple sclerosis, sarcoid, leukemia, and Guillain Barré
- Bell's palsy may reoccur. Treatment is unchanged

Treatment

INITIAL STABILIZATION

- Patients with an isolated peripheral CN VII palsy are stable

ED TREATMENT

- High dose oral steroids may hasten recovery if started within 3 weeks of onset. Recommended unless contraindicated
- Corneal damage may result from incomplete eyelid closure. Lubricating and hydrating ophthalmic preparations and eyelid taping at night are *essential*
- Some authors advocate acyclovir but this treatment is controversial
- Suspected Lyme disease should be treated with doxycycline or amoxicillin. The duration of treatment is controversial
- Surgical decompression may be necessary for complete lesions that do not improve

MEDICATIONS

- Acyclovir: 400 mg 5×/day po × 7d. (ped: no data to support its use)
- Lacri-Lube: qhs and prn; dryness/irritation in the affected eye (or equivalent)
- Prednisone: 60 mg/day po × 10d. (ped: 2 mg/kg/day po (max 60 mg))

Disposition

ADMISSION CRITERIA

- Isolated peripheral CN VII palsy does not require admission

DISCHARGE CRITERIA

- Isolated peripheral CN VII palsy may be treated on an outpatient basis. Follow-up should be within 1 week

Miscellaneous

ICD9: 351.0

CORE CURRICULUM CODE: 11.2.1

SUGGESTED READINGS

Adour K, et al. Bell's palsy treatment with acyclovir and prednisone compared with prednisone alone. Ann Otol Rhinol Laryngol 1996;105:371–378

Jabor MA, Gianoli G. Management of Bell's palsy. J La State Med Soc 1996;148(7):279–283

Little N. Selected neurologic disorders. In: Rosen P, et al., eds. Emergency medicine: concepts and clinical practice. 4th ed. St. Louis: CV Mosby, 1998:2212.

Morgan M, Nathwani D. Facial palsy and infection: the unfolding story. Clin Inf Dis 1992;14(1):263–271

Papazian MR, Campbell JH, Nabi S. Management of Bell's palsy. J Oral Max Surg 1993;51(6):661–665

Authors: Robert F. McCormack; Richard S. Krause

Benzodiazepine, Poisoning

Clinical Presentation

SIGNS AND SYMPTOMS

- Incoordination
- Sedation
- Slurred speech
- Ataxia
- Coma
  - —Hypotonia
  - —Hyporeflexia/areflexia
  - —Midposition or small pupils
- Respiratory arrest
  - -More likely with short-acting benzodiazepine (BZ) in either oral or IV overdose
- Hypothermia
- Complications: cerebral hypoxia, rhabdomyolysis, and pressure-induced neuropathies
- After the acute phase has elapsed, no long-term organ system toxicity occurs

MECHANISM

- Enhancement of the CNS inhibitory neurotransmitter γ-aminobutyric acid results in depression of spinal reflexes and the reticular activating system
- Pharmacological profile
  - —Highly lipophilic and protein bound
  - —Large V_D
  - —Liver metabolized
- Duration of action is inversely proportional to the lipophilicity

Pre-Hospital

CAUTIONS

- Attention to airway
- Bring in pill bottles/pills in suspected overdose

Diagnosis

ESSENTIAL WORKUP

- Diagnosis based on
  - —History of ingestion or recent injection
  - —Clinical findings associated with CNS depression
- Coma and pinpointed pupils
  - —No response to naloxone
  - —Reverse with flumazenil (FZ) administration
- Lack of response to a maximal dose of FZ strongly suggests that BZ is not the major cause of sedation

LABORATORY TESTS

- Pulse oximetry/capnography monitoring
- Electrolytes, BUN, Cr, serum glucose
- UA for myoglobin when coma present
- Core body temperature (low/high reading thermometer)
- ABG
- Urine/blood BZ qualitative screen
  - —Confirms exposure but does not indicate or measure intoxication
  - —False-negative tests reported
- Benzodiazepine serum levels
  - —Limited value
  - —Do not correlate with the clinical state
  - —Clinical signs and symptoms more important than theoretical LD_{50} or serum levels
- Alcohol(s) level
- Barbiturate level
- Acetaminophen level
- Pregnancy test

SPECIAL/IMAGING TESTS

- EKG
- CXR for aspiration pneumonia

DIFFERENTIAL DIAGNOSIS

- Drugs and toxins causing decrease level of consciousness
  - —Hypoglycemic
  - —Sedative-hypnotic
  - —Antidepressant-antipsychotic
  - —Narcotic
  - —Anticonvulsant
  - —Carbon monoxide/cyanide
  - —Alcohol agents
- Nontoxic medical condition
  - —Hypoxemia
  - —Hypothermia
  - —Head trauma (intracranial bleeding)
  - —Infection (meningitis or encephalitis)
  - —Electrolytes and metabolic disturbances

Treatment

INITIAL STABILIZATION

- ABCs
  —Secure airway and assist ventilation with supplemental oxygen to prevent hypoxemia and shock
  —IV access with 0.9%NS
  —Cardiac monitor
- Administer naloxone, thiamine, and dextrose if altered mental status

ED TREATMENT

- *Gastric emptying* (i.e., emesis, lavage): not necessary in pure BZ ingestion if activated charcoal (AC) is given promptly
- Activated charcoal po or via NGT
- *Multiple-dose activated charcoal* (MDAC)
  —Could be beneficial due to the enterohepatic recirculation profile of most BZ active metabolites
  —Use in conjunction with whole bowel irrigation (WBI) with Golytely when the ingested agent is a slow-release formulation
- No role for diuresis, dialysis, or charcoal hemoperfusion
- Flumazenil (FZ)
  —Use with either iatrogenic or intentional pure BZ overdose with altered mental status/respiratory depression
  —Competitive BZ receptor inhibitor—rapidly reverses BZ-induced coma and respiratory depression
  —Efficacy dependent on the dose of BZ being antagonized and the dose of FZ used
  —Do not administer empirically as part of any standard protocol therapy or in unknown poisoned patient
  —Onset within 1–2 minutes; peak at 6–10 minutes; duration 1–2 hours (repeat dosing if resedation)
  —Complications due to loss of BZ effect
    -Precipitates seizures with seizure history or seizure-prone overdoses (e.g., cyclic antidepressant, isoniazid, cocaine, propoxyphene, theophylline)
    -Arrhythmias in proarrhythmic coingestions (e.g., chloral hydrate, chloroquine)
    -Acute withdrawal state
  —Contraindication: suspected elevation of intracranial pressure

MEDICATIONS

- Activated charcoal: 1–2 g/kg po initial dose; MDAC: 0.5–1 g/kg q 2–4 hr po or by slow continuous NG-tube infusion (do not use cathartic with every dose)
- Dextrose: D50W 1 amp (50 ml or 25 g) (peds: D25W 2–4 ml/kg) IV
- Flumazenil (Romazicon)
  —Initial: 0.2 mg IV over 30 sec
  —If no response: 0.3 mg IV after 30 sec
  —If still no response: 0.5 mg IV and repeat q 30–60 sec if needed, to maximum dose of 3–5 mg
  —Continuous infusion at 0.2–1.0 mg/hr if multiple repeated doses required to maintain response
  —peds: dosing not established, recommended starting dose is 0.01 mg/kg IV, titrate up to a maximum dose of 1 mg, continuous infusion at 0.005–0.01 mg/kg/hr
- GoLytely or CoLyte WBI: 2 L/hr po, or by NG-tube for 4–6 h, or until rectal effluent is clear (peds: 40 cc/kg/hr)
- Naloxone (Narcan): 2 mg (peds: 0.1 mg/kg) IV or IM initial dose
- Thiamine (Vitamin B_1): 100 mg (peds: 50 mg) IV or IM

Disposition

ADMISSION CRITERIA

- Signs or symptoms of BZ overdose and most mixed overdoses should be admitted for observation in an intensive (intermediate) care unit

DISCHARGE CRITERIA

- Discharge after 4–6-hour observation period if no signs or symptoms of BZ poisoning develop, and no FZ was administered

Miscellaneous

ICD9: 969.4

CORE CONTENT CODE: 17.2.42.2

SUGGESTED READINGS

Arnold J. Determinants of pharmacologic effects and toxicity of benzodiazepine hypnotics: Role of lipophilicity and plasma elimination rates. J Clin Psychiatry 1991;52(9):11–14

Hobbs WR, Rall TW, et al. Hypnotics and sedatives: Ethanol. In: Gilman AG, Goodman LS, Rall TW et al. Goodman & Gilman's: The pharmacological basis of therapeutics. 9th ed. MacMillan, New York 1996:361–373

Osborn H, Goldfrank LR, Howland MA. Sedative-hypnotic agents: flumazenil. In: Goldfrank LR, ed. Toxicologic emergencies. 5th ed. Appleton and Lange Norwalk, CT 1994:787–810

Spivey WH, Roberts JR, Derlet RW. A clinical trial of escalating doses of flumazenil for reversal of suspected benzodiazepine overdose in the emergency department. Ann Emerg Med 1993;22:1813–1821

Weinbroum A, Halpern P, et al. The use of flumazenil in the management of acute drug poisoning—a review. Intensive Care Med 1991;17:32–38

Author: Jose Diaz

Beta-Blocker, Poisoning

Clinical Presentation

SIGNS AND SYMPTOMS

- Cardiovascular
  - —Hypotension
  - —Bradycardia
  - —Cardiac conduction delays
  - —Heart block
  - —Heart failure
- Neurologic
  - —Coma
  - —Seizures
- Pulmonary
  - —Bronchospasm
  - —Pulmonary edema
- Metabolic
  - —Hypoglycemia

MECHANISM

- Normal Physiology
  - —Cardiovascular—β_1-receptors
    - -ATP converted to cAMP by adenyl cyclase with stimulation of β-receptors
    - -cAMP activates protein kinase which phosphorylates proteins of the sarcoplasmic reticulum
    - -Sarcoplasmic reticulum releases calcium
    - -Excitation-contraction coupling occurs
- Effects of β-blockers
  - —Cardiovascular
    - -Decreased excitation/contraction
    - -Sodium channel blockade causes a prolongation of the QRS (with some agents)
  - —Neurologic
    - -CNS effects with the lipophilic agents (propranolol, metoprolol, labetalol)

Pre-Hospital

CAUTIONS

- Transport pills and pill bottles when overdose suspected

Diagnosis

ESSENTIAL WORKUP

- With unknown ingestion: suspect Beta-blocker poisoning with bradycardia/hypotension
- EKG
  - —Conduction delays
  - —1st, 2nd, or 3rd degree heart block
  - —Bradycardia

LABORATORY

- CBC
- Electrolytes, BUN, creatinine, glucose

DIFFERENTIAL DIAGNOSIS

- Calcium channel blocker toxicity
- Clonidine toxicity
- Digoxin toxicity
- Acute myocardial infarction with heart block

Treatment

INITIAL STABILIZATION

- ABCs
  - —Airway protection as indicated by mental status
  - —Supplemental oxygen as needed
  - —0.9%NS IV access
  - —Close hemodynamic monitoring
- Naloxone and thiamine if altered mental status
- Accucheck and treat hypoglycemia with D50W
- Treat prolonged seizures with benzodiazepines

ED TREATMENT

Goals

- HR >60 beats per minute
- Systolic BP >90 mm Hg
- Adequate urine output
- Improving level of consciousness

GI Decontamination

- Syrup of ipecac is contraindicated in the emergency department
- Consider lavage with Ewald tube if ingestion in within 1 hour
  - —Propranolol may cause esophageal spasm producing difficulty with passage and removal of gastric lavage tube
- Activated charcoal helpful especially in the presence of coingestants

Bradycardia/Hypotension

- Atropine
  - —Initial agent
  - —Low success rate
- Glucagon
  - —Administer if atropine does not increase HR
  - —Promotes cAMP production through a receptor site other than the β-receptor
  - —May cause nausea and vomiting
  - —Mix with normal saline or 5% dextrose in water
    - -Do not use the Phenol diluent that comes with glucagon
- IV fluids
  - —Administer cautiously in the hypotensive patient
  - —Swan-Ganz catheter or CVP monitoring to help follow volume status
- Amrinone
  - —Use in conjunction with glucagon to treat symptomatic sustained bradycardia

- Pressor agents
  - —Initiate when symptomatic hypotension/bradycardia persists after atropine/glucagon
  - —Use invasive monitoring to help guide therapy
  - —Utility may be limited due to β blockage—higher doses may be required
  - —Isoproterenol (nonselective β-agonist)-titrate for blood pressure and heart rate
  - —Epinephrine (potent α- and β-receptor agonist)—BP increases due to direct myocardial stimulation, increase in heart rate, and vasoconstriction; use if no BP response with isoproterenol
  - —High-dose dopamine
- Sodium bicarbonate
  - —In theory, this is used if there is evidence of prolongation of QRS >100 msec due to some of the β-blockers also causing sodium channel blockade leading to a prolonged QRS
  - —Not routinely administered for all beta blocker toxicities
- Electrical pacing—when other treatment options have failed

Enhanced elimination

- Hemodialysis helpful with water-soluble β-blocking agents (nadolol, atenolol, and sotolol)

MEDICATIONS

- Activated charcoal: 1gm/kg po
- Amrinone: loading dose 0.75 mg/kg; maintenance drip 2–20 μg/kg/min; titrate for effect
- Atropine: 0.5 mg (peds: 0.02 mg/kg) IV; repeat 0.5–1.0 mg IV (peds: 0.04 mg/kg)
- Dopamine: 2–20 μg/kg/min IV
- Dextrose: D50W 1 amp (50 ml or 25 g) (peds: D25W 2–4 ml/kg) IV
- Epinephrine: 2 μg/min (peds: 0.1 μg/kg/min); titrate to effect
- Glucagon: 3.5–5 mg IV (peds: 0.03–0.1 mg/kg) bolus followed by 70 μg/kg/hr infusion
- Isoproterenol: 5 μg/min IV and titrate for heart rate effect
- Naloxone (Narcan): 2 mg (peds: 0.1 mg/kg) IV or IM initial dose
- Sodium bicarbonate: 1 mEq/kg IVP
- Thiamine (Vitamin B_1): 100 mg (peds: 50 mg) IV or IM

Disposition

ADMISSION CRITERIA

- ICU admission for decreased level of consciousness or hemodynamic instability (bradycardia, conduction delays, hypotension)
- Long-acting or sustained-release preparations require observation and monitoring for 24 hours due to the potential delay in symptoms

DISCHARGE CRITERIA

- Asymptomatic 8–10 hours after ingestion of short- or immediate-release preparation

Miscellaneous

ICD9: 977.9

CORE CONTENT CODE: 17.2.15

SUGGESTED READINGS

Agura ED, Wexler LF, Witzburg RA. Massive propranolol overdose. Successful treatment with high-dose isoproterenol and glucagon. Am J Med 1986;80:755–757

Browning RG, Merigian KS. Acute beta-blocker poisoning. Top Emerg Med 1993;15:1–14

Kerns W, Kline J, Ford MD. β-Blocker and calcium channel blocker toxicity. Emerg Med Clin North Am 1994;12:365–390

Author: Janet Eng

Bipolar Disorder

Clinical Presentation

SIGNS AND SYMPTOMS

- Appearance
  - —Hyperactive, if not agitated
  - —Talkative, often with loud, rapid or "pressured" speech
- Affect
  - —Irritable
  - —Argumentative
  - —Often multiple recent arguments or fights
  - —Less commonly euphoric or expansive
  - —Often labile with depressed or tearful intervals (may confound diagnosis)
  - —Patient likely to describe mood as depressed or tense
- Neurovegetative
  - —Increased energy
  - —Engaged in multiple goal-directed activities many hours per day
  - —Feelings of energy
  - —Racing thoughts
  - —Decreased sleep
- Thought process
  - —Rapid, distractible, may be incoherent, delirious
- Thought content
  - —Psychosis possible
  - —Mood-congruent (e.g., delusions of grandeur or power)
  - —Mood-incongruent (may be indistinguishable from schizophrenia)
- Judgment
  - —Inflated self-esteem, perhaps to grandiose or psychotic extent
  - —Uncharacteristic, irresponsible behavior, such as financial or sexual indiscretions, with inability to recognize negative consequences of actions
  - —Substance abuse frequent during mania
- Sensorium
  - —Typically normal
  - —Confusion or delirium possible

MECHANISM/DESCRIPTION

- Mania
- Presentation is diverse, from simple irritability or cheerfulness to psychosis, delirium or agitation (without specific symptoms of mania)
  - —Full extent of pathology often revealed only by outside informants
  - —Onset gradual or acute, duration several weeks or months, possibly chronic
- Hypomania
  - —Milder symptoms without marked impairment
- Mixed mood
  - —Simultaneous symptoms of mania and depression
  - —Treat in emergency department as for mania
- Bipolar (formerly manic-depressive) disorder
  - —One or more episodes of manic or mixed mood
  - —Possibly with episodes of depressed mood
  - —Typically beginning in the teens or twenties
  - —Episodes of abnormal mood may be mild or severe
  - —Brief or prolonged, infrequent or nearly chronic
  - —Treatment-responsive or nearly intractable
- Schizoaffective disorder
- Psychotic features present even beyond episodes of abnormal mood

Diagnosis

ESSENTIAL WORKUP

- Psychiatric history
  - —Recent manic symptoms (often collateral sources critical)
  - —Past mania or depression
  - —Recent initiation or discontinuation of antidepressant
  - —Noncompliance with mood stabilizer
  - —Recent substance abuse
  - —Bipolar family history
- Medical history
  - —Especially endocrine, metabolic, or neurological disorders
  - —Current or recent medications
- Physical and neurological exam; vital signs
- Mania may present as delirium, therefore consider full differential diagnosis of delirium; particularly likely to be secondary to medical condition if first episode, age over 40, atypical or mixed presentation, and abnormal sensorium

LABORATORY

- Toxicological screen
  - —Urine or serum
- Electrolytes
- Blood glucose
- CBC
- TSH
- Lithium, carbamazepine, valproate serum levels if relevant
- Other tests as suggested by history or exam
- Pretreatment labs for lithium
  - —BUN and creatinine
  - —LFTs
  - —CBC

IMAGING/ SPECIAL TESTS

- Pretreatment studies for valproate or carbamazepine
  - —EKG if over 40

DIFFERENTIAL DIAGNOSIS

- Primary Mania of Bipolar or Schizoaffective Disorder
- Psychosis
  - —Agitated depression
  - —Personality disorders (borderline, narcissistic, antisocial)
  - —Attention deficit disorder
  - —Conduct or intermittent explosive disorders
  - —Organic brain syndrome
  - —Others
- Intoxication or withdrawal from depressants
- Intoxication with psychostimulants
  - —Cocaine
  - —Amphetamines
  - —Phencyclidine
  - —Hallucinogens
  - —Opiates
  - —Accidental or deliberate toxic overdose
- Antidepressants
- ECT
- Corticosteroid or thyroid hormones
- Anticholinergics
- Sympathomimetics (antiasthma or decongestant)
- Treatments of Parkinsonism
- Cyclobenzaprine (Flexeril)
- Recent discontinuation of antidepressant medication
- Endocrine or metabolic disorders
  - —Thyroid
  - —Parathyroid
  - —Corticosteroid
  - —Electrolyte disorders
  - —Hypoglycemia
  - —Hypoxia
  - —Renal or hepatic disease
  - —Porphyria
- Neurological: acute infection, postictal states, multiple sclerosis, post-CVA, certain tumors, general paresis, CNS vasculitis, others
- Any etiology of delirium

Treatment

INITIAL STABILIZATION

- High violence potential: quiet environment, prompt evaluation, nonconfrontational manner, adequate security backup, physical restraint and sedation as needed
- For cooperative patient: po neuroleptics (e.g., haldol, preferably as elixir) or benzodiazepines (e.g., lorazepam)
- For severe agitation: synergistic combination of IM haloperidol and lorazepam, and benztropine for prevention of acute dystonic reaction to haloperidol (omit benztropine if anticholinergic delirium suspected, age >40, or 2 mg benztropine received in last 12 hours)

ED TREATMENT

Patient for Discharge

- Neuroleptic agent
  - —Haloperidol, or risperidone, or perphenazine
  - —Low-range dose for moderate hypomanic symptoms
  - —High-range dose for agitation and more intense symptoms
- Benztropine for prevention of dystonic reactions for first 10 days of neuroleptic treatment if patient under 40
- Clonazepam for sleep
- Initiate or restart mood stabilizer therapy per consultation with outpatient psychiatrist (note that action of mood stabilizing agents requires days or weeks, even after full serum level is attained)

Acute Treatment of Mania

- Parenteral neuroleptic agents
- Other forms of sedation
- ECT
- Patient requiring hospitalization: consider sedation or initiation of mood stabilizer per consultation with receiving hospital

MEDICATIONS

For Acute Agitation

- Lorazepam: 1–2 mg po; may repeat q 30 min, not to exceed 12 mg per 24 hrs
- Haloperidol: 1–5 mg po; may repeat q 30 min, not to exceed 20 mg per 24 hrs; (consider benztropine 1–2 mg po bid prophylaxis of dystonic reaction); 5–10 mg IM or IV plus lorazepam 1 mg IM plus benztropine 1 mg IM repeat q 20 min as required

Typical Outpatient Medications

- Benztropine: 1 mg po bid
- Carbamazepine: 400–2000 mg per day (often split bid or tid; in acute mania, initiate at 200 mg po bid)
- Clonazepam: 0.5–2 mg po qhs or 0.5–2 mg po bid
- Haloperidol: 0.5–5 mg po bid
- Lithium: 600–3,000 mg per day (often split bid; in acute mania, initiate at 300 mg po tid)
- Perphenazine: 4–16 mg po bid
- Risperidone: 0.5–3 mg po bid
- Valproate, e.g., Depakote: 750–3,000 mg per day (often split bid; in acute mania, initiate at 250 mg po tid)

Disposition

ADMISSION CRITERIA

- Involuntary hospitalization is required by any of the following
  - —Exact standards vary by state
  - —Danger to self
    - -Risky actions, suicidal risk especially if mixed or labile mood or psychotic, medically unstable, hospitalization diagnostically required
  - —Danger to others
    - -Dangerous behaviors, assaultiveness
  - —Inability to care for self
    - -Unable to obtain basic food, clothing, and shelter with resultant risk to self

DISCHARGE CRITERIA

- Patients with mild symptoms may be discharged on medications as above if
  - —Necessary supports to ensure safety
  - —Patient compliant with treatment plan
  - —Appointment within 1–3 days
- Some patients who are not legally committable may refuse treatment
  - —Explain availability of treatment in future to patient and any involved friends or family

Miscellaneous

ICD9: 296.4, 296.5, 296.6, 296.7, 296.8, 296.81, 296.82

CORE CONTENT CODE: 14.2.1

SUGGESTED READINGS

Goodwin FK, Jamison KR. Manic-depressive illness. New York: Oxford University Press, 1990.

Sachs GS. Bipolar mood disorders: practical strategies for acute and maintenance treatment. J Clin Psychopharmacol 1996;16 (2 Suppl 1):32S–47S.

Authors: Paul Desan, Gary Sachs

Black Widow Spider Bite

Clinical Presentation

SIGNS AND SYMPTOMS

Local

- Pain
  - —Sharp or burning at the site within minutes of the bite
  - —Usually resolves spontaneously after a few minutes or hours
  - —May become worse and spread proximally from the bite
- Skin
  - —Two pinpricks from the spider's fangs
  - —Tender and blanched skin with surrounding erythema ("target lesion")
  - —Urticaria
  - —Piloerection
  - —Swelling
  - —Local sweating
  - —Often there is nothing at all to see or palpate at the wound site

Systemic

- Onset within 20–30 minutes
  - —Painful muscle cramps and spasms, which can lead to tremors and tonic contractions.
  - —Entire body may become progressively involved or symptoms may be regional
  - —Arm bites may lead to arm and chest muscle tightness and dyspnea
  - —Leg bites tend to cause spasm and rigidity in the thighs and abdomen
    - -Can be confused with acute abdominal emergencies, particularly in children
- Cutaneous dysesthesia and hyperesthesia
- Autonomic instability with perspiration, nausea, vomiting, tachycardia
- Restlessness, headache, agitation, and a sense of impending death
- Less commonly, fever, accelerated or slowed pulse, hypertension, dyspnea, arrhythmias, pulmonary edema, convulsions, shock and acute toxic psychosis may occur

Course

- In untreated patients, symptoms peak after 2–3 hours and then begin to resolve, occasionally recurring episodically over the following few days
- In otherwise healthy adults, complete resolution of symptoms occurs within 2–3 days
- Persistent neurological symptoms lasting weeks to months are often reported, including fatigue, generalized weakness or myalgias, paresthesias, headache, insomnia, impotence and polyneuritis
- Rarely fatal
- Severity of envenomation dependent on
  - —Number of bites
  - —Location of bites
  - —Size and condition of the spider
  - —Age, size and health condition of the victim

MECHANISM/DESCRIPTION

- Venoms contain potent neurotoxins
  - —Presynaptic nerve terminal membranes disrupted causing neurotransmitter release at the neuromuscular junction (acetylcholine), and in autonomic and cortical tissues (norepinephrine)
  - —Initially, postsynaptic terminals overstimulated, then blockaded, and neurotransmitters rapidly become depleted
- Morbidity and mortality are dose-dependent
- Greatest risk from venom:
  - —Premorbid hypertension or cardiovascular disease
  - —Children are also at greater risk from a given dose of venom

Etiology

- The black widow is found throughout North America, except the far north and Alaska
- Black Widow spiders preference is for dark, cozy hideaways outdoors and close to the ground
- More bites are reported during the warmer months when spiders are defending their webs and egg clutches
- Females are responsible for human envenomations
- Appearance:
  - —Black in color with red ventral markings shaped like an hourglass or a pair of spots on the globular abdomen
  - —Females have 25-50-mm leg spans and 15-mm long bodies

Pre-Hospital

CONTROVERSIES

- Venom extraction devices (e.g., Sawyer Extractor) have been recommended anecdotally but are probably ineffective if more than 10 minutes has elapsed since bite

CAUTIONS

- Immobilize the wound site and apply cool compresses or ice for comfort during transport to hospital
- Supportive measures may be required for patients with systemic symptoms
- Every effort should be made by caregivers at the scene to find and bring in the responsible spider for identification

Diagnosis

ESSENTIAL WORKUP

- Diagnosis based upon the clinical presentation
- Careful inquiry to elicit the spider bite history
- Identification of the spider (if it has been caught)

LABORATORY

- No specific blood test for Black Widow spider venom
- CBC usually normal but WBC can be mildly elevated
- Electrolytes, creatinine kinase, glucose, calcium, BUN and creatinine, and PT/PTT
  - —Usually normal
  - —Appropriate baseline studies in symptomatic patients

IMAGING/SPECIAL TESTS

- Abdomen radiograph
  - —Normal
- CXR and ABGs
  - —Indicated in rare cases with pulmonary edema
- ECG and cardiac monitoring
  - —Elderly
  - —Presence of unstable vital signs or dysrhythmias
- Calcium gluconate infusion
  - —May provide dramatic, but temporary relief
  - —Considered by some to be a good diagnostic test

DIFFERENTIAL DIAGNOSIS

- Acute abdomen
  - —Appendicitis
  - —Pancreatitis
  - —Peptic ulcer
  - —Black Widow spider victims have restlessness instead of quiet posture favored by most patients with peritoneal irritation. The abdominal wall rigidity is also unexpectedly nontender
- Sympathomimetics
  - —Cocaine
  - —Amphetamines
- Myocardial infarction
- Hypertensive emergency
- A high fever and WBC should prompt consideration of alternatives to spider bites

Treatment

INITIAL STABILIZATION

- ABCs
  - —Support airway and respiration if pulmonary edema is present
- Control seizures
- Stabilize dysrhythmias

ED TREATMENT

- Cleanse the bite site thoroughly
- Tetanus prophylaxis
- Benzodiazepines for agitation and restlessness
- Antiemetics for nausea and vomiting
- Muscle cramps/spasm therapy—combinations work synergistically:
  - —Calcium gluconate
  - —Benzodiazepines
  - —Narcotics
- Calcium gluconate for muscle cramps
  - —Commonly advocated but consensus is lacking on its utility
  - —Effects may be transient and multiple doses may be required
- Antihypertensive agents for symptomatic hypertension
- Specific antivenin
  - —Indications
    - -<16 or >65 years old or premorbid compromised health status
    - -Intractable cramps or muscle contractions
    - -Significantly increased blood pressure
    - -Respiratory distress
    - -Symptomatic and pregnant
  - —Always perform a skin test for sensitivity to horse serum first (test kit included in the antivenin package)
  - —Due to the small quantity of antivenin used, if serum sickness reactions occur they are usually mild
  - —Effectiveness is usually apparent within 2 hours of the first treatment and repeat doses are rarely necessary
  - —Antivenin probably helps to prevent persistent neuropathic symptoms and may be worth considering for that indication even if the acute stage illness is mild

MEDICATIONS

- Antivenin: 1 ampule (2.5 ml) diluted into 50 ml normal saline IV over 20 minutes
- Calcium gluconate: 10–20 ml of 10% solution IV q2–4h prn

Disposition

ADMISSION CRITERIA

- Symptomatic young, elderly, and pregnant patients
- Significant cardiovascular symptoms and signs, or severe hypertension, particularly in presence of premorbid cardiac disease or chronic hypertension
- Respiratory distress or pulmonary edema
- Persistent symptoms not responding to aggressive management and specific antivenin

DISCHARGE CRITERIA

- Asymptomatic patients, with no positive identification of a black widow spider, can be released after observation for 1–2 hours
- Asymptomatic patients with no comorbid illness, with a positive identification of the black widow spider, should be observed for a minimum of 4–6 hours and discharged if their condition does not change
- All discharged patients must be instructed what to watch for in terms of symptoms and to seek appropriate follow-up if needed

Miscellaneous

ICD9: 989.5

CORE CONTENT CODE: 5.10.5

SUGGESTED READINGS

Allen C. Arachnid envenomations. Emerg Med Clin North Am 1992;10(2):288–291

Clark MD, et al. Clinical presentation and treatment of black widow spider envenomation: A review of 163 cases. Ann Emerg Med 1992;21(7):782–787

Miller TA.Latrodectism: Bite of the black widow spider. Am Fam Physician 1992;45(1):181–187

Author: Paul Arnold

Bladder Injury

Clinical Presentation

SIGNS AND SYMPTOMS

- Abdominal or pelvic pain, difficulty voiding
- Hypotension, low urine output, gross or microscopic hematuria

MECHANISM/DESCRIPTION

- Blunt and less frequently penetrating trauma are the most common causes
  - —10–15% of pelvic fractures have associated bladder injury
  - —95% of bladder ruptures have an associated pelvic fracture
- Iatrogenic manipulation
- Spontaneous injury from another process: neoplasm, urethral obstruction, tuberculosis, radiation damage, occult trauma

ETIOLOGY

- Bladder rupture
  - —Intraperitoneal rupture (60% of bladder ruptures) occur by hydraulic compression
    - -Compressive forces cause a tear in the bladder dome, the weakest portion *in situ*
    - -Occurs more frequently with a distended bladder
  - —Extraperitoneal bladder rupture (30% of bladder ruptures)
    - -Damage from fracture fragments
    - -Shearing forces from ligaments attached to the bladder
    - -Extraperitoneal bladder rupture can occur with rising blood pressure
  - —Combined extra- and intraperitoneal rupture occurs in 10% of bladder ruptures
  - —Bladder contusion is more common (50–65% of all bladder injuries)
    - -Damage to the endothelial lining or the muscularis layer with an intact bladder wall
    - -It is a diagnosis of exclusion and usually resolves without intervention

POTENTIAL COMPLICATIONS

- Peritonitis
- Sepsis
- Incontinence
- Infected pelvic hematoma
- Fistulae

PEDIATRIC CONSIDERATIONS

- Intraperitoneal rupture is more common than in adults, because the bladder is an abdominal organ in pediatric patients
- Bladder injury is more common than in adults, because the pediatric bony pelvis is less rigid and transmits more force to adjacent structures

Pre-Hospital

CAUTIONS

- Do not attempt bladder catheterization in the field

Diagnosis

ESSENTIAL WORKUP

- Meticulous physical examination of perineum and pelvis
- Radiographic evaluation (retrograde urethrogram (RUG), cystography, see below)

LABORATORY

- Urinalysis
  - —Gross hematuria is noted in approximately 90% of patients with significant bladder or urethral trauma
  - —Microscopic hematuria is noted in less than 2%
- BUN and creatinine
  - —The BUN can be elevated secondary to resorption of urine from an intraperitoneal rupture
- Electrolytes
  - —Hyperkalemia and hypernatremia may result from resorption of urine within the peritoneum

IMAGING/SPECIAL TESTS

- Excretory urethrography may demonstrate bladder rupture or urethral injury in 15% of cases
- *Cystography* is the criterion standard for bladder evaluation
  - —Performed immediately unless other surgical or medical emergencies have greater priority
  - —A scout film (KUB) is initially obtained
  - —The first 100 cc of water-soluble contrast are infused by a Foley catheter into the bladder
- The plain film is repeated to evaluate for early extravasation
  - —If normal, an additional 200–300 cc of contrast are infused
  - —Cystogram films are now taken in the AP, lateral, and oblique planes to rule out a bladder injury
  - —Outlining of bowel or contrast within the paracolic gutters is indicative of an intraperitoneal rupture
  - —A tear-drop or star-shaped form are noted with extraperitoneal ruptures
  - —After drainage of the contrast, a postdrainage film is taken, which will occasionally demonstrate extravasated contrast not visible with a distended bladder
- CT scan is not sensitive enough to evaluate bladder injuries

DIFFERENTIAL DIAGNOSIS

- Perineal trauma
- Urethral trauma
- Renal or ureteric trauma

PEDIATRIC CONSIDERATIONS

- When cystography occurs, 3–5 cc/kg of total contrast material should be used

Treatment

INITIAL STABILIZATION

- ABCs of trauma care
- Early urologic consultation

ED TREATMENT

- Immediate surgical exploration for intraperitoneal ruptures and many extraperitoneal ruptures
- Extraperitoneal ruptures may be managed solely by catheter drainage if contraindications to surgical repair exist
- No specific interventions are required for bladder contusions

Disposition

ADMISSION CRITERIA

- Concurrent closed head injury, blunt abdominal trauma, or pelvic fracture requiring admission and observation
- Need for operative management of bladder or other injuries

DISCHARGE CRITERIA

- After thorough urologic evaluation, patients without significant bladder injury may be considered for outpatient management
  —Patients that are unable to void may require urinary catheter and leg bag

Miscellaneous

ICD9: 867.0

CORE CONTENT CODE: 18.4.11.9

SUGGESTED READINGS

Corriere JN Jr. Diagnosis and management of lower urinary tract injuries. AUA Update Series. Lesson 16. Vol. VII. AUA Office of Education Houston, TX 1988:121–127.

Harwood-Nuss AL, Sandler CM. Genitourinary trauma. In: Rosen P, Doris PE, Barkin RM, Barkin SZ, Markovchick, eds. Diagnostic radiology in emergency medicine. St. Louis: Mosby-Year Book, 1992.

Thomas CL, McAninch JW. Bladder trauma. AUA Update Series. Lesson 31. Vol VIII. AUA Office of Education Houston, TX 1989:241–247.

Sandler CM, et al. Lower urinary tract Trauma. World J of Urol. 1988. 16(1):69–75.

Authors: Kenneth Bramwell; Roscoe Nelson

Blow Out Fracture

Clinical Presentation

SIGNS AND SYMPTOMS

- Periorbital tenderness, swelling, ecchymosis
- Impaired ocular mobility or diplopia
  - —Upward gaze due to inferior rectus entrapment
  - —Ipsilateral lateral gaze with medial rectus entrapment
- Infraorbital hypoesthesia
  - —Due to compression/contusion of infraorbital nerve
- Enophthalmos
  - —Due to herniation of orbital fat through fracture
- Periorbital emphysema
- Normal visual acuity (unless associated ocular injury)
- Epistaxis

Associated Injuries

- Ocular injuries
  - —Ruptured globe
    - -Incidence 5–10% of blow out fractures
    - -Ophthalmologic emergency
  - —Subconjunctival hemorrhage
  - —Corneal abrasion/laceration
  - —Hyphema
  - —Iridodialysis
  - —Traumatic iridocyclitis (uveitis)
  - —Traumatic mydriasis
  - —Retinal detachment
  - —Vitreous hemorrhage
  - —Compressive orbital emphysema
  - —Retrobulbar hemorrhage
  - —Optic nerve injury
- Facial fractures
  - —Nasal bones
  - —Zygomatic arch fracture
- Neck injuries
- Intracranial injury

Late Complications

- Sinusitis
- Orbital infection
- Permanent restriction of extraocular movement
- Enophthalmos

MECHANISM/DESCRIPTION

- Defined as an orbital floor fracture without orbital rim involvement due to blunt trauma to the orbit
- Caused by blunt trauma to the orbit
- Force transmitted through the orbital structures to the weakest structural point—the orbital floor
  - —Results in fracture of the orbital floor
- Orbital floor serves as roof to air filled maxillary and ethmoid sinuses
  - —Communication between the spaces results in orbital emphysema
- Orbit contains fat which holds the globe in place
  - —Orbital floor fracture may result in herniation of the fat on the inferior orbital surface into the maxillary or ethmoid sinuses
  - —Leads to enophthalmos due to orbital volume loss
  - —Sinus congestion and fluid collection occur secondary to edema
- Infraorbital nerve runs through the bony canal 3 mm below the orbital floor
  - —Injury results in hypoesthesia of the ipsilateral cheek
  - —Distinguished from hypoesthesia due to swelling by testing for decreased sensation on the ipsilateral gingiva which is within the infraorbital nerve distribution
- Inferior rectus and the inferior oblique muscle run along the orbital floor
  - —Restriction of these extraocular muscles occur due to entrapment within the fracture, contusion or cranial nerve dysfunction
  - —Diplopia on upward gaze
  - —Inability to elevate the affected eye normally on exam
- Medial rectus located above the ethmoid sinus
  - —Less commonly entrapped
  - —Diplopia on ipsilateral lateral gaze

ETIOLOGY

- Most commonly caused by handballs, baseballs or fists

PEDIATRIC CONSIDERATIONS

- Orbital floor fractures—extremely unlikely before 7 years of age
- Lack of pneumatization of the paranasal sinuses—orbital floor is not a weak point in the orbit
- Orbital roof fractures with associated CNS injuries more common

Pre-Hospital

- Metal protective eyeshield if possible globe injury
- Place in supine position

Diagnosis

ESSENTIAL WORKUP

- Thorough ophthalmologic examination
  - —Visual acuity (should not be affected)
  - —Test extraocular movements for disconjugate gaze or diplopia
  - —Palpate bony structures for evidence of step-off
  - —Test sensation in inferior orbital nerve distribution
  - —Examine lid and adnexa
  - —Careful attention not to place pressure on the globe until ruptured globe excluded
  - —Slitlamp and funduscopic examination to identify associated injuries

LABORATORY

- Preoperative laboratory studies if indicated

IMAGING/SPECIAL TESTS

- Plain radiographs
  - —Facial films
  - —Orbits
  - —Water's view and exaggerated Water's view
    - -Classic "teardrop sign" illustrates herniated mass of orbital contents in the ipsilateral maxillary sinus
    - -Opacification of or air fluid level in the ipsilateral maxillary sinus (less specific)
    - -Orbital floor bony fracture
    - -Lucency in orbits consistent with orbital emphysema
- Diagnostic in up to 97%
- 10% false-positives and false-negative rate
- Tomograms helpful when available
- CT orbits
  - —If diagnosis in question and for follow-up
  - —Defines involved anatomy
  - —Obtain 1.5-mm cuts
- Forced duction test
  - —Distinguishes nerve dysfunction from entrapment
  - —Topical anesthesia applied to the conjunctiva on the opposite side and the globe is pulled away from the expected point of entrapment. If the globe is not mobile, the test is positive

DIFFERENTIAL DIAGNOSIS

- Retrobulbar hemorrhage
- Periorbital contusion/ecchymosis
- Cranial nerve palsy
- Ruptured globe
- Orbital cellulitis
- Periorbital cellulitis

PEDIATRIC CONSIDERATION

- Immature facial skeleton with lack of pneumatization of the paranasal sinuses makes plain radiographs of limited value
- Orbital CT—study of choice

Treatment

INITIAL STABILIZATION

- Initial approach and immediate concerns
  - —Rule out ruptured globe
  - —Assess for associated intracranial or cervical spine injuries
  - —Test visual acuity
    - -Decreased visual acuity suggestive of associated ocular injury

ED TREATMENT

- Apply cool compresses for the first 24–48 hours to decrease swelling in order to minimize/reverse herniation and avoid surgical intervention
- Avoid Valsalva maneuvers and nose blowing to prevent compressive orbital emphysema
- Prophylactic antibiotics (amoxicillin, cephalexin, erythromycin) to prevent infection
- Nasal decongestants (phenylephrine nasal spray)
- Analgesics
- Tetanus prophylaxis

MEDICATIONS

- Phenylephrine nasal spray: BID for 10–14 days
- Amoxicillin: 250–500 mg po TID 10–14 days
- Cephalexin: 250–500 mg po QID 10–14 days
- Erythromycin: 250–500 mg po QID 10–14 days

Disposition

ADMISSION CRITERIA

- Rarely indicated except with
  - —Severe herniation of orbital contents threatening vision
  - —Cosmetically enophthalmos typically >5 mm
  - —Associated injuries which mandate admission

DISCHARGE CRITERIA

- Consultation with facial trauma service
  - —Arrange follow up evaluation within 1–2 weeks of injury and to determine need for surgery
- Immediate ophthalmology evaluation if patient has evidence of visual loss or within 24 hours for complete retinal evaluation
- Need for surgical intervention
  - —Rarely indicated immediately
  - —85% resolve without surgical intervention
  - —Typically observe for 10–14 days until swelling resolves
  - —Surgery indications
    - -Persistent diplopia
    - -Restricted extraocular movements
    - -Cosmetically significant enophthalmos

Miscellaneous

ICD9: 829.0

CORE CONTENT CODE: 18.4.4.1.5

SUGGESTED READINGS

Anderson PJ, Poole MD. Orbital floor fractures in young children (Rev). J Craniomaxillofac Surg 1995;23(3):151–154

Joondeph BC. Blunt ocular trauma. Emerg Med Clin North Am 1988;6(1):151

Koltai PJ, Amjad I, Meyer D. Orbital fractures in children. Arch Otolaryngol Head Neck Surg 1995;121(12):1375–1379

Linden JA, Renner GS. Trauma to the globe. Emerg Med Clin North Am 1995;13(3):581–605

Author: Shari Schabowski

Boerhaave's Syndrome

Clinical Presentation

SIGNS AND SYMPTOMS

- Retrosternal chest pain
  - —Often pleuritic
  - —Radiates to the back
  - —Worsened with swallowing
- Dyspnea with mediastinitis
- Diaphoresis
- Voice changes
- Subcutaneous emphysema in neck and chest wall
- Mediastinal crackling on auscultation (Hamman's crunch)
- Fever
- Shock in severe cases
- If untreated, mediastinitis with abscess formation
- Not usually associated with bleeding

MECHANISM / DESCRIPTION

- Spontaneous esophageal rupture
- Sudden increase in intra-abdominal pressure
  - —Causes complete, full thickness, longitudinal tear in the distal esophagus at the left posterolateral aspect
- Esophagus has no serosal layer (which normally contains collagen and elastic fibers)
  - —Results in a weak structure vulnerable to perforation and mediastinal contamination
- Significant morbidity/mortality
  - —Due to explosive nature of the tear
  - —Almost instant contamination of the mediastinum with intraesophageal contents

ETIOLOGY

- Associated with forceful vomiting and retching
- Reported with heavy lifting, seizures, childbirth, blunt trauma, and laughing
- Common in middle-aged males
- Alcohol consumption and ingesting large meals predisposing factors

PEDIATRICS

- Described but rare in neonates

Pre-Hospital

CAUTIONS

- Airway control if unresponsive or airway patency in jeopardy
- Establish one large bore intravenous catheter and treat hypotension with 0.9%NS solution
- Avoid analgesics until patient in the ED to avoid the complication of hypotension

Diagnosis

ESSENTIAL WORKUP

- Upright CXR (preferably posteroanterior and lateral views if tolerated) evaluating for
  - —Pneumomediastinum
  - —Subcutaneous emphysema
  - —Pleural effusion (left side)
  - —Pneumothorax
  - —Widened mediastinum
  - —Hydropneumothorax
  - —Empyema
- *Esophogram:* identifies leak in esophagus
  - —Initially use water-soluble contrast material
  - —If the esophagus is intact, use barium contrast for better detail

LABORATORY

- CBC
- PT/PTT
- Blood cultures
- Pleural effusion amylase content

IMAGING

- ECG
- Endoscopy
  - —Useful for diagnosis
  - —Operator-dependent
- CT chest
  - —Sensitive at identifying free air but can not isolate the lesion
  - —Indicated if esophogram can not be obtained
  - —Evaluates other intrathoracic structures

DIFFERENTIAL DIAGNOSIS

- Myocardial infarction
- Pancreatitis
- Ruptured abdominal viscus
- Aortic aneurysm
- Pulmonary thromboembolism
- Mesenteric thrombosis
- Cholecystitis
- Spontaneous pneumomediastinum (clinically benign)

Treatment

INITIAL STABILIZATION

- ABCs
  - —Airway control—100% oxygen or intubate if unresponsive or airway patency is in jeopardy
  - —Establish IV access with at least one large bore catheter or more if unstable
  - —Treat hypotension
    - -Administer 1 L (20 cc/kg) bolus with 0.9%NS (or LR)
    - -Initiate dopamine if BP does not respond to fluids
  - —Central catheter placement if unstable for more efficient delivery of fluids and monitoring of central venous pressure

ED TREATMENT

- NPO
- Careful placement of a nasogastric tube to decompress the stomach
- Bladder catheter to monitor urine output
- Expedient diagnosis to decrease incidence of morbidity/mortality
- Prompt surgical consultation
- Definitive treatment
  - —Surgical repair of the perforation
  - —Adequate drainage
- Initiate broad-spectrum antibiotics directed against oral microflora and gastrointestinal pathogens
  - —Ampicillin/sulbactam plus gentamicin

MEDICATIONS

- Ampicillin/sulbactam: 3.0 g IVPB q 6 hrs
- Dopamine: 2–20 μg/kg min IVPB
- Gentamicin: 2 mg/kg load then 1.7 mg/kg IVPB q8 hrs or 5.1 mg/kg IVPB q day (assuming normal renal function)

Disposition

ADMISSION CRITERIA

- All cases of Boerhaave's Syndrome must be admitted to the surgical intensive care unit after definitive surgical repair of the lesion is performed
- Surgery should be performed directly from the emergency department without delay

DISCHARGE CRITERIA

- None

Miscellaneous

ICD9: 520.4

CORE CONTENT CODE: 1.1.2.2

SUGGESTED READINGS

Jagminas L, et al. Boerhaave's syndrome presenting with abdominal pain and right hydropneumothorax. Am J Emerg Med 1996;14(1);53–55

Kanowitz A, et al. Esophageal and diaphragmatic trauma. In: Rosen P, et al., eds. Emergency medicine: Concepts and clinical practice 3rd ed. St. Louis: CV Mosby, 1992

Troum S, et al: Surviving Boerhaave's syndrome without thoracotomy Chest 1994;106(1);297–298

Author: Dino Rumero

Botulism

Clinical Presentation

SIGNS AND SYMPTOMS

Foodborne

- Most common
  —Diplopia
  —Blurred vision
  —Bulbar weakness: dysphagia, dysarthria, dysphonia
- Subsequent symmetrical, descending weakness or paralysis of the extremities
- No sensory deficits
- Remains alert and responsive
- Ventilatory insufficiency from weakness of respiratory muscles
- Autonomic dysfunction
  —Dry mouth
  —Blurred vision
  —Orthostatic hypotension
  —Constipation
  —Urinary retention
- Nausea and vomiting with foodborne botulism only
- Afebrile

Infantile

- Constipation
- Weakness
- Poor suck
- Lethargy
- Hypotonia
- Flaccid facial expression
- Respiratory difficulty

Wound

- Finding similar to foodborne
- May be febrile

MECHANISM/DESCRIPTION

- Caused by a polypeptide, heat-labile exotoxin produced by *Clostridium botulinum*
  —Most potent poison known
- Toxin blocks neuromuscular transmission in cholinergic nerve fibers
- Symptoms occur by inhibition of acetylcholine release from presynaptic nerve membranes
  —Damage is permanent
  —Recovery is by formation of new synapses through sprouting from the axon
- Onset: 12–36 hours after exposure
  —Death can occur in 24 hours
- Slow recovery; symptoms often persist for months
- Mortality
  —Untreated: 60–70%
  —With supportive care: 10–15%
- Three types: *foodborne botulism, wound botulism,* and *infantile botulism* (see pediatric considerations)
- Foodborne botulism
  —Occurs by ingestion of preformed toxin; improperly canned food facilitates the necessary anaerobic conditions
  —Conditions required for exposure
    -Food product contaminated with *C. botulinum* bacilli or spores
    -Proper conditions for germination of spores exist
    -Time and conditions permit production of toxin before eating
    -Food not heated sufficiently to destroy botulism toxin
    -Toxin containing food ingested by susceptible host
- Wound botulism
  —Clinical evidence of botulism following trauma with a resultant infected wound and no history suggestive of foodborne illness
  —*Botulinum* isolated in about 50%
  —Wounds usually contaminated with soil
  —Seen rarely in chronic drug abusers

ETIOLOGY

- *C. botulinum* is a large, spore-forming, usually Gram-positive, strictly anaerobic bacilli ubiquitous in nature
- Each strain produces antigenically distinct toxins, designated types A through G
  —Types A, B, and E are responsible for the majority of human cases

PEDIATRIC CONSIDERATION

- *Infantile botulism* occurs from the ingestion of *C. botulinum* spores which germinate in the gut and produce the toxin
- 90% occur in children <6 months
- Progresses for 1–2 weeks, then stabilizes for 2–3 weeks before receding
  —Usually subacute presentation with low mortality
- Slower onset is attributed to the toxin being produced locally, as opposed to being ingested in one dose
- *C. botulinum* spores found in honey
  —Honey not recommended for children <6 months

Pre-Hospital

CAUTIONS

- Death is invariably from progressive ventilatory failure
  —Intubate as soon as respiratory insufficiency noted

Diagnosis

ESSENTIAL WORKUP

- Clinical diagnosis
- Workup focuses on differentiation from other conditions causing general paralysis
- Notify public health officials of diagnosis

LABORATORY

- CBC
- Electrolytes, BUN/Cr, glucose
  —Check for hypokalemia
- ABG
  —For signs of respiratory insufficiency
- Toxin detection in
  —Blood
  —Feces
  —Gastric contents
  —Suspected food and containers
- Anaerobic blood cultures

SPECIAL TESTING

- CSF testing
  —Normal
  —Helps differentiate from Guillain-Barré syndrome
- Electrophysiologic studies—normal nerve conduction with diminished evoked muscle action potential
- Edrophonium testing may be positive, but not to the degree seen in myasthenia gravis

DIFFERENTIAL DIAGNOSIS

- Myasthenia gravis (less acute)
- Lambert-Eaton myasthenic syndrome (less acute)
- Polio (fever and asymmetrical)
- Guillain-Barré (simultaneous sensory findings and elevated spinal fluid protein)
- Tick paralysis
- Magnesium intoxication
- Hypokalemic periodic paralysis

PEDIATRIC CONSIDERATIONS

- Often misdiagnosed as dehydration, sepsis, or Reye's syndrome

Treatment

INITIAL STABILIZATION

- Early intubation and ventilatory support is the key to survival
- Respiratory difficulties occur rapidly

ED TREATMENT

- Trivalent ABE antitoxin
  - —IV administration as soon as the diagnosis is made, without waiting for laboratory confirmation
  - —Use should be preceded by testing for hypersensitivity to horse serum
- NG suctioning if ileus is profound
- If no ileus, enemas and cathartics help remove unabsorbed antitoxin
- With *wound botulism*—perform wound debridement even if it appears to be healing
- Antibiotics for specific infectious complications

MEDICATIONS

- Trivalent botulism antitoxin: 2 vials (approximately 10,000 IU each of Types A, B, and E) IV

PEDIATRIC CONSIDERATIONS

- Antitoxin is rarely indicated for *infantile botulism*
- Antibiotics
  - —Ineffective in eradicating organism from the intestine
  - —Release of toxin in the gut through bacterial cell lysis may worsen neurologic symptoms

Disposition

ADMISSION CRITERIA

- Admit suspected botulism poisoning to monitored bed
  - —ICU admission for any respiratory deficiency

DISCHARGE CRITERIA

- Clinical course of botulism poisoning is unpredictable; it can become rapidly progressive and fatal
  - —Discharge only patients with a prolonged period of progressive recovery from symptoms

Miscellaneous

ICD9: 005.1

CORE CONTENT CODE: 9.1.1

SUGGESTED READINGS

Bleck TP. Clostridium botulinum. In: Mandell Gl, Bennett JE, Dolin R, eds. Mandell, Douglas, and Bennett's principles and practice of infectious diseases. 4th ed. New York: Churchill-Livingstone, 1995

Hatheway CL. Botulism: The present status of the disease. Curr Top Microbiol Immunol 1995; 195:55–75

Mechem CC, Walter FG.Wound botulism. Vet Hum Toxicol 1994;36(3):233–237

Wigginton JM, Thill P. Infant botulism: A review of the literature. Clin Pediatr 1993;32(11):669–674

Author: Philip Shayne

Bowel Obstruction

Clinical Presentation

SIGNS AND SYMPTOMS

- Abdominal pain
  - —Intermittent early
  - —Constant with strangulated obstruction
- Vomiting
  - —Bile-stained emesis with proximal obstruction
  - —Feculent emesis with distal obstruction
- Obstipation
- Vital signs
  - —Usually normal
  - —Tachycardia;
  - —Hypotension with significant fluid loss
  - —Fever with strangulation or perforation
  - —Hypothermia with sepsis
- Hyperactive and high pitched bowel sounds
- Abdomen examination
  - —Diffuse tenderness
  - —Peritoneal signs (rebound/guarding) indicates strangulation or perforation
- Rectal exam
  - —Rectal mass
  - —Occult blood in stool
- Hernias
  - —Inguinal
  - —Femoral
  - —Ventral hernia

MECHANISM/DESCRIPTION

- Obstruction of normal flow of intestinal contents due to mechanical or nonmechanical causes
- Obstruction leads to rapid increase in both anaerobic and aerobic bacteria with resultant increase in methane and hydrogen production
- Distended bowel becomes progressively edematous and increased intestinal secretions causes further distension
- Retrograde peristalsis causes vomiting

ETIOLOGY

Small Bowel

- Adhesions—most common
- Hernias
- Neoplasms
- Stricture—inflammatory bowel disease
- Trauma—bowel wall hematoma

Large Bowel

- Carcinoma
- Volvulus
- Diverticular disease

PEDIATRIC CONSIDERATIONS

- Intussusception
  - —Leading cause of intestinal obstruction in infants
  - —Most common between 3 and 12 months of age
- Incarcerated inguinal/umbilical hernia
- Malrotation with volvulus
  - —Double-bubble often seen on upright abdominal radiograph due to partial obstruction of duodenum resulting in air in stomach and in first part of duodenum
- Pyloric stenosis
  - —Progressive, projectile nonbilious vomiting often after feeding
  - —Male:female—5:1 incidence
  - —Onset usually 2–5 weeks of age

Pre-Hospital

CAUTIONS

- Abdominal pain, nausea/vomiting—very common symptoms in elderly patients with acute myocardial infarctions
  - —Abdominal distention, obstipation, and colicky pain suggests a gastrointestinal etiology

Diagnosis

ESSENTIAL WORKUP

- Plain radiographs of chest and abdomen
  - —Upright CXR
    - -Evaluate lung for pathology
    - -Check for free air beneath diaphragm
  - —Upright and supine abdomen—obstructive findings
    - -Distended loops of bowel (normal small bowel <3 cm in diameter)
    - -Air fluid levels
    - -Nearly completely fluid filled small bowel loops may produce "string of pearls" sign
- Careful examination for hernias
- Heme test stool

LABORATORY

- CBC
  - —Leukocytosis common
- Electrolytes, BUN/Cr, glucose
  - —Hypochloremia and hypokalemia with vomiting in proximal obstructions
  - —Prerenal azotemia with significant dehydration
- Amylase/lipase
- Urinalysis

IMAGING/SPECIAL TESTS

- CT abdomen, barium enema or upper GI
  - —If carcinoma or other mass lesion suspected as cause for obstruction

DIFFERENTIAL DIAGNOSIS

- Perforated ulcer
- Pancreatitis
- Cholecystitis
- Colitis
- Paralytic ileus
- Mesenteric ischemia
- Uremia

Treatment

INITIAL STABILIZATION

- ABCs
- 0.9%NS IV fluid resuscitation when
  —Significant volume depletion
  —Strangulated or perforated bowel

ED TREATMENT

- Nasogastric tube suction
- Foley catheter to monitor urine output
- Surgical consultation
- Administer antibiotics (cefoxitin) for suspected strangulated/perforated bowel
- Administer analgesic as needed after surgical consultation

MEDICATIONS

- Cefoxitin: 1–2 g q 6–8 hrs (peds: 0–7 days 40 mg/kg/24hrs q 12 hrs; >7 days 80–160 mg/kg/24hrs q 6 hrs) IVPB
- Demerol: 25 mg increments (peds: 1 mg/kg) IV PRN
- Morphine sulfate: 2–4 mg increments (peds: 0.1 mg/kg) IV PRN

Disposition

ADMISSION CRITERIA

- All patients with suspected/confirmed intestinal obstruction should be admitted with early surgical consultation obtained

DISCHARGE CRITERIA

- None

Miscellaneous

ICD9: 560.9

CORE CONTENT CODE: 1.6.1.1

SUGGESTED READINGS

Holder W. Intestinal obstruction. Gastroenterol Clin North Am 1988;17(2):317

Sanson TG, O'Keefe KP. Evaluation of abdominal pain in the elderly. Emerg Med Clin North Am 1996;14(3):615–627

Sivit C. Gastrointestinal emergencies in older infants and children. Radiol Clin North Am 1997;35(4):865

Author: Julio Silva

Bradyarrhythmias

Clinical Presentation

SIGNS AND SYMPTOMS

- Asymptomatic
- Syncope
- Near syncope
- Dizziness
- Bradycardia
- Low blood pressure

MECHANISM/DESCRIPTION

- Pulse less than 60 beats per minute
- Two possible mechanisms cause bradyarrhythmias
  —Depression of the predominate pacemaker in the sinus node
    -Results in sinus bradycardia if the sinus node remains the dominant pacemaker
  —Conduction system block antegrade to the AV node
- The dominant role may be assumed by a subsidiary pacemaker
  —AV node that sends 45–60 impulses/minute
  —Bundle branch and Purkinje network that send 30–40 impulses/minute
  —The resultant escape rhythms define the bradyarrhythmia

ETIOLOGY

- Sinus bradycardia
  —Overstimulation of the vagus nerve
  —Prolongation of sinus node refractory period
  —Acute inferior wall ischemia
  —β- or calcium channel blocker toxicity
  —Amiodarone toxicity
  —Clonidine toxicity
  —Myxedema
  —Hypoglycemia
  —Organophosphate toxicity
  —Carotid sinus oversensitivity
  —Eye manipulation
  —Increased intracranial pressure
  —Hypothermia
  —Drugs
    -Cimetidine
    -Ranitidine
    -Nitrates
    -Guanethidine
    -Acetylcholine
- Junctional bradycardia
  —Loss of normal atrial rhythm
  —β-Blocker or calcium channel blocker toxicity
  —Digitalis toxicity
  —Cardiac ischemia
- Idioventricular bradycardia
  —Loss of both SA and AV nodal activity
  —Myocardial infarction
  —Cardiac tamponade
  —Exsanguinating hemorrhage
  —Preterminal rhythm
- Second degree heart block: Mobitz type I (Wenckebach)
  —Increased refractory period in the AV node
  —β-Blocker or calcium channel blocker toxicity
  —Digitalis
  —Inferior wall ischemia
  —Other states with increased vagal tone
  —Normal variant
  —May be present during sleep in normal individuals
- Second degree heart block: Mobitz type II
  —Prolongation of refractory period in His-Purkinje system
  —Anteroseptal ischemia
  —Sclero-degenerative disease
- Third degree heart block
  —Complete loss of AV node and His-Purkinje conduction
  —Cardiac ischemia
  —Severe β- or calcium channel blocker toxicity
  —Digitalis toxicity
- Sick sinus syndrome (tachy/brady rhythm)
  —Impaired supraventricular impulse generation or conduction leading to intermittent bradycardia (sinus bradycardia, prolonged sinus arrest, or sinoatrial block) and intermittent tachycardias (SVT, junctional tachycardia, A-Fib, and A-Flutter)
  —Autonomic dysfunction
  —Medications given to limit the fast rate may exacerbate bradyarrhythmias
- Other causes
  —Medication
    -Quinidine
    -Procainamide
    -Disopyramide
    -Sotalol
  —Infection
    -Viral myocarditis
    -Acute rheumatic fever
    -EBV
    -Lyme myocarditis
    -Infiltrating myocardiopathies
    -Sarcoidosis
    -Amyloidosis
    -Neoplasm

Pre-Hospital

CAUTIONS

- Epinephrine
  —May be given to improve cardiac contractility and SVR
  —Avoid in patients suspected of cardiac ischemia
- External pacing
  —Initiated for poor perfusion that cannot be corrected by other means
  —Care must be taken to obtain ventricular capture as demonstrated by a pulse
  —Avoid medication or pacing in hypothermic patients
- Pediatrics
  —Correct hypoxemia before attempting to increase the heart rate

CONTROVERSIES

- Treat the patient not the rate
- Atropine
  —Will often increase the rate but may lead to increased ischemia
  —Should only be used for patients with evidence of hypoperfusion
  —Does not affect the rate in third degree heart block

Diagnosis

ESSENTIAL WORKUP

- 12-lead EKG and continuous cardiac monitoring

LABORATORY

- Serum glucose
- Serum potassium
- BUN and Creatinine
- Renal failure may potentiate drug toxicity inducing bradyarrhythmias
- Cardiac enzymes
- Detection of ischemia as an underlying cause
- Digoxin level if relevant
- Thyroid function tests

IMAGING/SPECIAL TESTS

- EKG
  - —Sinus bradycardia
    - -Normal P waves and intervals with narrow QRS
    - -Sinus arrhythmia is likely to be present
  - —Junctional bradycardia
    - -Narrow complex QRS arising from the AV node
    - -No normal P waves but retrograde P waves may be visible
  - —Idioventricular bradycardia
    - -Slow ventricular escape rhythm
    - -Wide QRS >0.16 sec
    - -Rate less than 40
    - -No P waves visible
  - —Second degree heart block: Mobitz type I (Wenckebach)
    - -Progressive prolongation of the PR interval unless a P goes unconducted
    - -The pause is less than fully compensatory
    - -The PR interval resets after the dropped systole
    - -QRS duration is normal
    - -Progression to complete heart block is rare
    - -The escape rhythm is often adequate for perfusion
  - —Second degree heart block: Mobitz type II
    - -Sudden failure of AV conduction without preceding prolongation of the PR
    - -Often associated with prolonged QRS
    - -High incidence of progression to complete heart block
    - -Escape rhythm is unstable and slow
    - -Third degree heart block
    - -Normal P waves marching out but dissociated from wide ventricular beats
    - -Rate usually in the 40s
  - —Sick sinus syndrome
  - —Intermittent bradycardia
    - -Sinus bradycardia
    - -Prolonged sinus arrest
    - -Sinoatrial block
  - —Intermittent tachycardia
    - -SVT
    - -Junctional tachycardia
    - -A-Fib
    - -A-Flutter
  - —Prolonged sinus recovery results in episodes of prolonged asystole
    - -Sinus pause
    - -Greater than 3 seconds

DIFFERENTIAL DIAGNOSIS

- Atrial fibrillation with slow ventricular response or depolarization without effective contraction

Treatment

INITIAL STABILIZATION

- IV access
- Supplemental oxygen
- Cardiac monitoring
- Pulse oximetry
- Airway control as needed
- External pacing in third degree heart block or idioventricular rhythms
- Follow with early placement of a transvenous pacemaker
- Atropine and epinephrine may combat bradyarrhythmias caused by overstimulation of the vagal nerve
- Isoproterenol may be required for continuous rate and blood pressure support
- If ischemia is the cause of the bradyarrhythmia, initiate appropriate treatment for ischemia
- Digitalis toxicity
  - —Treat hypo- and hyperkalemia
  - —Use atropine and pace if no response or transient response
  - —If no improvement, treat with digoxin-specific antibodies
- β-Blocker toxicity
  - —Glucagon
  - —Wean the infusion as the beta-blockade wears off
- Calcium channel toxicity
  - —Calcium chloride until the bradyarrhythmia resolves or normal perfusion is restored

ED TREATMENT

MEDICATIONS

- Atropine: adult: 0.5 mg IV; repeat every 5 min as necessary; maximum dose of 0.04 mg/kg; peds: 0.02 mg/kg, minimum 0.1 mg
- Calcium chloride: adult: 10–20 ml IV 10% solution bolus; peds: 20 mg/kg IV
- Dopamine: 2–5 μg/kg/min IV, maximum 20 μg/kg/min
- Epinephrine: adult: 2 μg/min, maximum 10 μg/min; peds: 0.01 mg/kg bolus; 0.2–2 μg/kg/min infusion
- Glucagon: 50 μg/kg bolus followed by 3–5 μg/min
- Isoproterenol: adult: 2–10 μg/min, titrate to heart rate; peds: 0.1–0.25 μg/kg/min infusion

Disposition

ADMISSION CRITERIA

- Admit patients with symptomatic bradycardia
  - —ICU
    - -New onset bradyarrhythmias with hypoperfusion
    - -Patients requiring transvenous pacemakers
    - -Patients requiring perfusion support
    - -Ongoing hypoperfusion
    - -Acute ischemic disease
    - -Emergent treatment with antidotes
  - —All others should be admitted to a telemetry unit

DISCHARGE CRITERIA

- Sinus bradycardia
  - —Asymptomatic
  - —Associated with dehydration that has been corrected
  - —Congenital asymptomatic third degree heart block

Miscellaneous

ICD9: 427.8

CORE CONTENT CODE: 2.4.1, 2.4.2

SUGGESTED READINGS

Gerwitz MH, Vetter VL. Cardiac emergencies. In: Fleisher GR, Ludwig S, eds. Textbook of pediatric emergency medicine. Baltimore: Williams & Wilkins, 1993;533–572.

Gibler WB. Arrhythmias and antiarrhythmic therapy. In: Gibler WB, Aufderheide TP, eds. Emergency cardiac care. St. Louis: Mosby-Year Book, 1994:345–384.

Author: Mary Patricia McKay

Bronchiolitis

Clinical Presentation

SIGNS AND SYMPTOMS

- Nasal congestion
- Cough
- Wheezing
- Retractions
- Grunting
- Crackles
- Fever that is usually ≤39.5°C

MECHANISM/DESCRIPTION

- Lower respiratory tract infection typified by
  —Bronchoconstriction with wheezes
  —Tachypnea
  —Upper respiratory prodrome

ETIOLOGY

- Respiratory syncytial virus in 85–90% of cases
- Influenza
- Parainfluenza
- Adenovirus

Pre-Hospital

CAUTIONS

- Monitor airway and breathing
- Supportive oxygen
- Apneic pauses
  —Suction
  —Tactile stimulation
  —Bag-mask ventilation

CONTROVERSIES

- Intubation, which is rarely warranted

Diagnosis

ESSENTIAL WORKUP

- The diagnosis is clinical
- Proof of a viral etiology is not necessary
- Pulse oximetry
  —Confirms proper oxygenation
  —Follows trends over the course of the illness

LABORATORY

- Nasal washes
  —Viral cultures
  —Fluorescent antibodies
    -Commercial kits are available
  —Indications
    -Clinical symptoms suggestive of pertussis or chlamydia
  —Conditions warranting antiviral therapy
    -Prematurity
    -Bronchopulmonary dysplasia
    -Chronic lung disease
    -Cardiac disease
    -Immunosuppression
  —Infants with apnea

IMAGING/SPECIAL TESTS

- Chest radiograph
  —Indicated only in special circumstances
    -Temperature >39.5°C
    -History of choking episode consistent with possible foreign body aspiration
    -Marked asymmetric chest exam
    -Illness does not resolve over 5–7 days
    -Respiratory distress
    -Sudden deterioration

DIFFERENTIAL DIAGNOSIS

- Reactive airway disease
  —History of atopy
  —Eczema
  —Prior episodes of wheezing
  —Strong family history of wheezing
  —Differentiated only by following the patient's course over time
- Bacterial pneumonia
- Pertussis
- Chlamydia
- Croup
- Foreign body aspiration
- Congestive heart failure
- Chronic lung disease
  —Cystic fibrosis

Treatment

INITIAL STABILIZATION

- Pediatric advanced life support
- Emergent intubation
  - —Apnea or respiratory failure in infants less than 3 months

ED TREATMENT

- Albuterol
  - —Indicated if severe or moderate respiratory distress
  - —Trial of 2 treatments of nebulized albuterol
  - —Only continue if clear response with decrease in the level of respiratory distress
  - —Children that respond can then receive oral albuterol solution
- Supplemental oxygen
- Parenteral hydration is needed to supplement oral fluids if dehydration from tachypnea
- Corticosteroids
  - —Use in children under 2 years of age in whom reactive airway is of concern
    - -Family history of asthma
    - -Recurrent wheezing
- Antibiotics are only indicated when a secondary bacterial pneumonia is present
- Ribavirin (virazole)
  - —Antiviral agent
  - —May be indicated to reduce the severity of the disease early in the course in children with severe underlying chronic disease
  - —Contraindicated in patients on ventilators

MEDICATIONS

- Albuterol: nebulized: 0.5 ml (2.5 mg/3 ml) in 2.5 ml saline q 20 min; oral: 0.1 mg/kg q 6 hrs
- Ribavirin: continuous inhalation 12–20hh/24hrs for 3–5 days; small particle aerosol generator

Disposition

ADMISSION CRITERIA

- Oxygen requirement
- Severe retractions
- Respiratory rate of 70 or greater
- Altered level of consciousness
- Inability to self-hydrate
- Apnea
- Severe underlying chronic lung disease or cardiac disease
- Patient less than 6 weeks of age
- Patient with a borderline oxygen saturation who lives at high altitude
- Immunodeficiency or immunosuppressive therapy

DISCHARGE CRITERIA

- Feeding well
- Acceptable room air saturation
- Absence of significant respiratory distress
- Follow-up should be arranged within 24 hours

Miscellaneous

ICD9: 466.1.9

CORE CONTENT CODE: 13.9.1

SUGGESTED READINGS

Dawson KP, Long A, Kennedy J, et al. The chest radiograph in acute bronchiolitis. J Paediatr Child Health 1990;26:290–211.

Gadomski AM, Lichensttein R, Horton L, et al. Efficacy of albuterol in the management of bronchiolitis. Pediatrics 1994;93:907–912.

Klassen TP, Rowe PC, Sutcliffe T, et al. Randomized trial of salbutamol in acute bronchiolitis. J Pediatrics 1991;118:807–811.

Menon K, Sutcliffe T, Klassen TP. A randomized trial comparing the efficacy of epinephrine with salbutamol in the treatment of acute bronchiolitis. J Pediatrics 1995;126:1004–1007.

Reijonen T, Korppi M, Pitkakangas S, et al. The clinical efficacy of nebulized racemic epinephrine and albuterol in acute bronchitis. Arch Pediatr Adol Med 1995;149:686–692.

Roosevelt G, Sheehan K, Grupp-Phelan J, et al. Dexamethasone ion bronchiolitis: A randomized controlled trial. Lancet 1996;348:292–295.

Author: Carol Ledwith

Bronchitis

Clinical Presentation

SIGNS AND SYMPTOMS

- Preceding URI symptoms
  - —Malaise
  - —Chills
  - —Fatigue
  - —Myalgias
  - —Coryza
  - —Sore throat
- Cough
  - —Initially dry and nonproductive
  - —Later becoming mucoid or mucopurulent
  - —Chest pain or burning
  - —Fever up to 102°F (38.5°C)
  - —Usually lasting 3–5 days
  - —Dyspnea may be present
  - —Hemoptysis
  - —Wheezing
  - —Scattered high or low pitched rhonchi
  - —Rales
  - —No evidence of consolidation

MECHANISM/DESCRIPTION

- Hyperemia of the mucus membranes
- Edema
- Production of mucopurulent exudate
- Impairment of the protective functions of the cilia, lymphatics, and phagocytes
- Airway obstruction
  - —Edema
  - —Secretions
  - —Bronchial muscle spasm
- Cigarette smoke may worsen the attacks

ETIOLOGY

- Viral infections
  - —Parainfluenza
  - —Respiratory syncytial virus (RSV)
  - —Adenovirus
  - —Coxsackie virus
  - —Common cold viruses
  - —Measles and herpes viruses
    - -Particularly severe bronchitis
- *Mycoplasma pneumoniae*
- *Chlamydia pneumoniae*
- *Bordetella pertussis*
- Other bacteria have not been conclusively proven to cause bronchitis
  - —*Streptococcus pneumoniae*
  - —*Haemophilus influenza*
  - —*Moraxella catarrhalis*

Pre-Hospital

CAUTIONS

- Oxygen
- Bronchodilators if wheezing

Diagnosis

ESSENTIAL WORKUP

- The diagnosis is clinical
- Pulse oximetry to confirm adequate oxygenation
- Exclude other respiratory disorders
- More involved workup if the symptoms last beyond the expected time frame

LABORATORY

- No specific test will help make the diagnosis immediately
- Viral cultures or bacterial cultures can be sent, but are rarely helpful
- An ABG may be drawn if there is concern of significant hypoxia
- CBC may show leukocytosis, but this is a nonspecific finding

IMAGING/SPECIAL TESTS

- Chest radiograph
  - —Indications
    - -Shortness of breath
    - -Hypoxia
    - -Chest pain
  - —Rules out other disorders, particularly pneumonia
  - —Helps confirm a benign process

DIFFERENTIAL DIAGNOSIS

- Influenza
- Pneumonia
- Reactive airway disease
- Aspiration
- Acute sinusitis
- Bronchiectasis
- Bacterial tracheitis
- Chronic bronchitis or COPD exacerbation in those with underlying chronic lung diseases
- Children
  - —Retained foreign body
  - —Cystic fibrosis
  - —Allergic respiratory disease

Treatment

INITIAL STABILIZATION

- There is rarely a need for aggressive initial management in these patients
- Administer oxygen if hypoxia is a concern
- Fluids may be given if there is accompanying dehydration

ED TREATMENT

- Treatment is symptomatic
- Cough suppressants
  —Use with caution for nonproductive exhaustive bouts of coughing
- β-Adrenergic inhaler for cough or wheeze
- Amantadine during known outbreaks of Influenza A
- Antibiotics
  —Generally not indicated
  —No improvement in symptoms
  —Return of fever
- Encourage patients to stop smoking
- Antipyretics for pain and fever

MEDICATIONS

- Albuterol: 0.5 ml in an 0.5% solution nebulized every 6 hrs
- Amantadine: 100 mg po bid

PEDIATRIC CONSIDERATIONS

- Use acetaminophen rather than aspirin for analgesia
- Ribavirin may be indicated for hospitalized children with RSV, parainfluenza, and influenza
- Repeated bouts in children should lead to referral for complete evaluation of the respiratory tract

Disposition

ADMISSION CRITERIA

- Underlying significant cardiopulmonary compromise
- Significant hypoxia

DISCHARGE CRITERIA

- No pulmonary compromise
- Instruct high risk patients to return if no improvement
  —Elderly
  —Debilitated
- Bedrest
- Fluids
- Aspirin or acetaminophen

Miscellaneous

ICD9: 466, 490

CORE CONTENT CODE: 1662

SUGGESTED READINGS

Hueston WJ. Albuterol delivered by metered-dose inhaler to treat acute bronchitis. J Fam Pract 1994;39:437–440.

King DE, Cameron W, Bishop L, et al. Effectiveness of erythromycin in the treatment of acute bronchitis. J Fam Pract 1996;42:601–605.

MacKay DN. Treatment of acute bronchitis in adults without underlying lung disease. J Gen Intern Med 1996;11:557–562.

Orr PH, Scherer K, Macdonald A, et al. Randomized placebo-controlled trials of antibiotics for acute bronchitis A critical review of the literature. J Fam Pract 1993;36:507–512.

Author: Robin Hemphill

Brown Recluse Spider Bite

Clinical Presentation

SIGNS AND SYMPTOMS

Initial Symptoms

- Asymptomatic or causes minor stinging and burning sensation

Clinical Course

- Local pain, with blanching, and induration over first 24 hours
- Blister may form in the center of the blanched area with circumferential erythema
  - —Enlarges and darkens gradually with the development of skin and subcutaneous fat necrosis over 3–4 days
  - —Most extensive necrosis develops where increased subcutaneous fat
  - —Lower extremity blisters spread distally under the influence of gravity
  - —Several weeks to months to heal by secondary intention
  - —Rarely evolves into ulcerative necrosis over the following days or weeks

Systemic Features

- General
  - —Rare
  - —Develop within 24–72 hours after the bite
  - —Larger amount of venom injected leads to more severe the systemic illness
  - —Local response is not dependent upon the extent of envenomation and cannot be used to predict the severity of subsequent systemic illness
- Fever, chills, malaise
- Nausea, vomiting, diarrhea
- Myalgias, arthralgias
- Petechial or urticarial rash
- Hemolysis leading to hemoglobinuria and acute renal failure
- Disseminated intravascular coagulopathy
- Shock

MECHANISM/DESCRIPTION

- Venom is a complex cocktail of enzymes and peptides
  - —Causing hemolysis and tissue necrosis
  - —Triggering complement cascades, platelet aggregation, and thrombosis, and release of inflammatory mediators
  - —Result is direct cytotoxic effects, coupled with indirect toxicity due to inflammation and vascular compromise
- Systemic toxicity due to an inflammatory or allergic phenomenon in response to antigenic properties of the venom

ETIOLOGY

- Found widely throughout the southern half of North America
- Spider not aggressive
- Humans bitten when they disturb a spider in its habitat, typically any warm and dry location in- or outdoors such as wood piles, bundles of rags, cellars, or attics
- Spider appearance
  - —Delicate body and legs spanning 10–25 mm
  - —Light-to-medium brown coloration with darker violin-shaped marking visible on the upper aspect of the head
  - —Three pairs of eyes

PEDIATRIC CONSIDERATIONS

- Toxicity proportional to the amount of venom and size of patient
- Children are more vulnerable to a given amount of venom than healthy adults

Pre-Hospital

CONTROVERSIES

- Venom extraction devices (e.g., Sawyer Extractor) have been recommended anecdotally but are probably ineffective if more than 10 minutes have elapsed since bite

CAUTIONS

- Immobilize wound site
- Cover with cool compresses
- Transport to hospital when patient experiences immediate onset of symptoms
- Find and bring in the responsible spider for identification
- Supportive measures for patients with systemic symptoms

Diagnosis

ESSENTIAL WORKUP

- Careful inquiry required to elicit the spider bite history
- Diagnosis based on the clinical presentation and the ruling out of other relevant possibilities

LABORATORY

- No specific tests available
- CBC, electrolytes, BUN, creatinine, PT/PTT should be taken for baseline monitoring
- Urinalysis for evidence of systemic hemolysis

IMAGING/SPECIAL TESTS

- Soft-tissue x-ray
  - —Useful if the differential includes suspected gas-forming organism, infection of ulcers

DIFFERENTIAL DIAGNOSIS

- Necrotic ulcers
- Other arachnid envenomations
- Soft-tissue infection
- Stevens-Johnson
- Erythema nodosum
- Diabetic ulcer
- Bed sore
- Vascular insufficiency with secondary ulcer in a lower limb
- Other etiologies of hemolytic anemia, DIC, anaphylactoid reactions

Treatment

INITIAL STABILIZATION

- IV fluids, oxygen, cardiac monitoring if the patient is experiencing systemic collapse

ED TREATMENT

Local Bite Care

- Supportive and expectant
- Clean/irrigate wound
- Tetanus prophylaxis
- Antibiotics
  - —Appropriate if the wound appears infected
  - —Do not use prophylactically
  - —Antistaphylococcal (first-generation cephalosporin or penicillinase-resistant penicillins)
- Topical steroids to the vesicular area around a bite are safe but of unknown benefit
- Systemic steroids
  - —Often recommended but usefulness controversial
  - —Administer within 24 hours of bite
- Dapsone/hyperbaric chamber therapy
  - —Used to treat or prevent local necrosis
  - —No consensus as to their value
  - —Before initiating Dapsone, screen for G6PD deficiency and monitor during therapy for methemoglobinemia, hemolysis, leukopenia
- Specific antivenin
  - —Being developed
  - —Unavailable in North America
- Excision of the necrotic wound may become necessary at a later date but is not indicated in the first 8 weeks as this may cause more severe ulcer formation

Systemic Problem Management

- Analgesics for pain control
- Hemoglobinuria
  - —Treated with intravenous fluids and alkalinization
  - —Monitor renal, fluid, and electrolyte status carefully
  - —PRBC for significant anemia
- Standard supportive care and interventions should be employed for shock, seizures, DIC, and coma
- Dialysis in the event of acute renal failure

MEDICATIONS

- Dapsone: adults—progressive dosage of 50–500 mg divided BID for 2 weeks (ped: 2 mg/kg/24hrs po for 2 weeks)
- Methylprednisolone: 125 mg IV single-dose in the Emergency Department, followed by prednisone 30–50 mg per day for 5 days (ped: methylprednisolone 1–2 mg/kg IV, prednisone 1–2 mg/kg po)

PEDIATRIC CONSIDERATIONS

- Use Dapsone only in severe cases due to potential for side effects such as hepatitis, methemoglobinemia, hemolytic anemia, and leukopenia

Disposition

ADMISSION CRITERIA

- Significant local reaction or signs of systemic toxicity
- Lower threshold for admission for
  - —Pediatric cases
  - —Compromised health status

DISCHARGE CRITERIA

- No evidence of systemic toxicity or severe progression of local wound necrosis postenvenomation
- Daily reassessment, including blood work, until 3–4 days postenvenomation to guard against the risk of systemic toxicity

PEDIATRIC CONSIDERATIONS

- Longer observation period before disposition of asymptomatic cases due to the higher mortality of spider bites in this population

Miscellaneous

ICD9: 989.5

CORE CONTENT CODE: 5.10.5

SUGGESTED READING

Allen C. Arachnid envenomations. Emerg Med Clin North Am 1992;10:2:288–291

Grendron BP. Loxosceles reclusa envenomation. Am J Emerg Med 1990;8(1):51

Mack RB. The bite of the spider woman. NC Med J 1992;53:5:200–203

Author: Paul Arnold

Bundle Branch Blocks

Clinical Presentation

SIGNS AND SYMPTOMS

- Asymptomatic
- Split-second heart sound
- Syncope
  - —Sustained monomorphic ventricular tachycardia is the underlying cause in 20–30% of patients

MECHANISM/DESCRIPTION

- Blockage of intraventricular electrical impulses through the bundle of His and the right and left bundles
- Right bundle branch block (RBBB)
  - —Delayed depolarization of the right ventricle
- Left bundle branch block (LBBB)
  - —Early activation of the right side of the septum and the right ventricular myocardium
  - —Last to be activated are the lateral wall and basal aspect of the left ventricle
  - —Two division of the left bundle branch
    - -The left anterior fascicular block (LAFB): initial septal activation proceeds inferiorly, anteriorly, and to the right
    - -The left posterior fascicular block (LPFB): rare finding; requires a previous EKG to make the diagnosis; activation begins in the midseptal areas and finishes in the inferior and posterior walls
- Complete bundle branch block
  - —The absence of conduction down the right or left bundle
  - —Conduction precedes down the unaffected bundle
  - —The affected ventricle depolarizes in a slower and less organized fashion
  - —Results in a wide QRS complex (>0.12 msec)
- Incomplete bundle branch block
  - —A delay in conduction down a particular bundle
  - —Results in an intermittently widened QRS
- Bifascicular block
  - —A right bundle branch block and a concomitant block of the LAF or LPF
- 80% of patients with an asymptomatic bundle branch block have associated heart disease

ETIOLOGY

- Myocardial infarction
- Cardiomyopathy
- Hypertension
- Congenital
- Exercise induced
- Postoperative following cardiac surgery
- Drugs
  - —β-Blockers
  - —Tricyclics
  - —Digitalis

Pre-Hospital

CAUTIONS

- Avoid confusing the EKG changes with ventricular tachycardia or ischemia
- Monitor

Diagnosis

ESSENTIAL WORKUP

- Bundle branch blocks are diagnosed by 12-lead EKG

LABORATORY

- Serum potassium
  - —Useful if hyperkalemia is suspected as the etiology of a widened QRS
- Cardiac enzymes
  - —New bundle branch block

IMAGING/SPECIAL TESTS

- EKG
  - —RBBB
    - -Complete: QRS ≥0.12 sec
    - -Incomplete: 0.10 sec <QRS <0.12 sec
    - -rsr′, rsR′ in V1 or V2 (an "M" shape)
  - —LBBB
    - -Complete: QRS ≥0.12 sec
    - -Incomplete: 0.10 sec <QRS <0.12 sec
    - -Broad slurred R waves in I, aVL, and V5-V6
    - -Absence of normal Q waves in I and V5-V6
    - -Criteria for diagnosing acute infarction: ST segment elevation ≥1 mm concordant with QRS complex; ST segment depression ≥1 mm in leads V1, V2, or V3; ST segment elevation ≥5 mm and discordant with QRS complex
  - —LAFB
    - -QRS duration <0.12 sec
    - -Dominant R wave in I
    - -Deep S wave in II, III, aVF
    - -QRS axis varies from −45 to −90
  - —LPFB
    - -QRS duration <0.12 sec
    - -R waves in I and V1
    - -Narrow Q wave in II, III, I and aVF
  - —Bifascicular block
    - -RBBB with left axis deviation
    - -RBBB with right axis deviation
- Electrophysiological testing
  - —Inpatient workup
  - —May predict complete heart block or the potential for ventricular tachycardia
  - —Indicated in patients with a bundle branch block presenting with syncope

DIFFERENTIAL DIAGNOSIS

- Ventricular tachycardia
- Left ventricular hypertrophy
- Hyperkalemia
- RBBB
  - —Anteroseptal myocardial infarction
  - —Inferior wall myocardial infarction
  - —Posterior wall myocardial infarction
- LAFB
  - —Anterolateral myocardial infarction
- LPFB
  - —Right ventricular hypertrophy
  - —Pulmonary disease
  - —Extensive lateral infarction
  - —Normal vertical heart

Treatment

INITIAL STABILIZATION

- Treat ischemic chest pain, shortness of breath, and syncope appropriately
- Complete heart block
- Apply external pacing electrodes to the back and chest
- Begin pacing by slowly increasing the stimulating current until capture is achieved
- Benzodiazepine sedation and narcotic analgesia are desirable

ED TREATMENT

- Asymptomatic patients require no specific treatment for BBB alone
- Temporary transvenous pacemaker insertion is emergently indicated in the setting of a bifascicular block with first or second degree heart block
- In the setting of an acute MI, rapid reperfusion reduces the incidence of permanent BBB
- Transvenous pacing is indicated in patients with an anterior MI and certain bundle branch blocks
  —Bifascicular block
  —Fascicular block with first or second degree heart block
- In patients with an inferior wall MI, a noninvasive external pacemaker will give ventricular capture

MEDICATIONS

N/A

Disposition

ADMISSION CRITERIA

- Acute MI
- Syncope due to high degree AV block
- Complete heart block
- Chest pain and new BBB

DISCHARGE CRITERIA

- Asymptomatic patients with BBB as an incidental or preexisting finding
- Refer for further evaluation of underlying cardiac disease

Miscellaneous

ICD9: 426

CORE CONTENT CODE: 2.4.2.4

SUGGESTED READINGS

Lamas GA, Muller JE, Turi ZG, et al. A simplified method to predict occurrence of complete heart block during acute myocardial infarction. Am J Cardiol 1986;57:1213–1218.

McAnulty JH, Rahimtoola SH, Murphy E, et al. Natural history of "high risk" bundle branch block. N Engl J Med 1982;307:137–143.

Newby KH, Pisano E, Krucoff MW, et al. Incidence and clinical relevance of the occurrence of bundle branch block in patients treated with thrombolytic therapy. Circulation 1996;94:2424–2428.

Willems JL, Robles EO, Bernard R, et al. Criteria for intraventricular conduction disturbances and pre-excitation. J Am Coll Cardiol 1985;5:1261–1275.

Author: Laura Hoey, James Scott

Burns

Clinical Presentation

SIGNS AND SYMPTOMS

- First degree burns: local erythema and pain
- Second degree burns: involve the epidermis and dermis and produces skin that is erythematous, moist, and swollen with blisters and bullae; sensation over the area is intact
- Third degree burns: full-thickness with destruction of the epidermis and dermis; thrombosed blood vessels may be seen under a firm translucent surface; skin charring may be seen in severe burns; the wounds are insensate
- Inhalation injury is associated with facial burns, carbonaceous sputum, pharyngeal injection, wheezing, hoarseness, smoke exposure in a closed space, and inhalation of toxic fumes
- Carbon monoxide poisoning should be suspected based on history of an exposure to combustion
- Cyanide poisoning should be suspected from burning wool, silk, nylon, and polyurethane found in furniture and paper

Pre-Hospital

CAUTIONS

- Frequent reevaluation of the airway due to possibility of inhalation injury and subsequent airway swelling
- Oxygen administration due to the possibility of carbon monoxide exposure
- Initiation of early intravenous fluid therapy

Diagnosis

ESSENTIAL WORKUP

ESTIMATE OF BURN PERCENTAGE		*TOTAL BODY SURFACE AREA (TBSA) PERCENT*		
ANATOMIC AREA		*INFANT*	*CHILD**	*ADULT*
Head and neck		20	20–10	9
Arms				
	Right	10	10	9
	Left	10	10	9
Legs				
	Right	10	10–15	18
	Left	10	10–15	18
Trunk				
	Front	20	20	18
	Back	20	20	18
Perineum		0	0	1
Total	100	100	100	

*With increasing age, the head contributes less to the percentage of TBSA and the legs contribute more. Adapted from Eliastam M. Manual of emergency medicine. St. Louis: Mosby Year-Book, 1989:406

- In adults, the "rule of nines" applies; the body can be divided into areas each a multiple of the number 9 (see table above)
- Arterial blood gas with CO level for closed space or inhalation exposures
- Fiber-optic bronchoscopy may be used to evaluate the degree of inhalation injury
- For severe burns, CBC, serum electrolytes, glucose, BUN, creatinine, and PT/PTT

IMAGING

- CXR may appear normal despite severe inhalation injury

DIFFERENTIAL DIAGNOSIS

- Electrical injury
- Chemical injury

Treatment

INITIAL STABILIZATION

- ABCs
  —Early intubation is necessary for patients with significant inhalation injury as marked airway edema can occur
- Intravenous access, supplemental oxygen
- Evaluation for concomitant trauma

ED MANAGEMENT

Fluid Resuscitation—Second and Third Degree Burns

- *Parkland formula:* 2–4 cc of lactated Ringer's or normal saline/kg/%BSA burn. One-half of this total is given in the first 8 hours and the remaining half over the next 16 hours
- For example: a 90-kg patient with a 40% TBSA (total body surface area) burn would require 2–4 cc × 90kg × 40% = 7200–14,400 cc over 24 hours, with 3600–7200 cc over the first 8 hours or 450–900 cc/hr
- For burns >20% TBSA, IV fluid therapy is guided using a bladder catheter. Urine output should be 0.5–1.0 cc/kg/hr for adults and 1.0 cc/kg/hr for children

Escharotomy

- Circumferentially burned extremities may develop cyanosis, decreased pulses or worsening neurologic status due to the tourniquet-like effect of the burn eschar
  —Elevate burned extremity
  —Escharotomy incisions on extremities should be made through the entire burn mid-medially and mid-laterally along the long axis of the limb to the subcutaneous layer
- A circumferential burn of the chest wall may prevent adequate ventilation unless escharotomy is performed
  —Make incision along the anterior axillary line from 2 cm below the clavicle to the tenth rib on each side of the chest
  —Make two more incisions across the body forming a square on the chest

Wound Care

- Sterile technique
- If admission to a burn unit is imminent, simple coverage of the wounds with sterile moist dressings is appropriate
- Do not delay transfer to burn unit for wound care
- Intravenous antibiotics are not indicated in the initial resuscitation

Outpatient Management of Minor Burns

- Use sterile technique for cleansing and debridement
- Loose necrotic skin should be removed. Broken, tense, or infected blisters should be débrided
- Topical antibacterial, such as sulfadiazine, agents in larger burns, deep partial thickness or full thickness burns, or those located in areas of apocrine sweat glands
- *Burn dressings* are made up of several layers to produce optimal healing
  - —Inner layer should be nonadherent porous mesh gauze that uses a nonpetroleum-based lubricant
  - —The next layer should be gauze capable of absorbing exudate
  - —The outer wrap should provide enough pressure to keep the dressing in place without constricting area affected
- Dressings should be changed at least daily
- Tetanus prophylaxis

PEDIATRIC CONSIDERATIONS

- Consider child abuse
- Children have a relatively greater body surface area to mass ratio and tend to lose heat more rapidly
- Hypoglycemia due to limited glycogen stores is more likely

MEDICATIONS

- Mafenide acetate cream: apply to wound 1–2 times/day, thickness of 1/16 inch (Sulfamylon)
- Morphine: 0.1–0.2 mg/kg titrated to effect for pain control after shock, trauma have been evaluated
- Povidone-iodine ointment: apply to wound 1–2 times/day to a thickness of 1/16 inch
- Silver sulfadiazine cream: apply to wound 1–2 times/day to a thickness of 1/16 inch

Disposition

ADMISSION CRITERIA

Injuries Requiring Transfer and Admission to a Burn Center

- Second and third-degree burns over more than 10% of the body surface area in patients under 10 or over 50 years of age
- Second and third-degree burns over more than 20% of the body surface area in any patient
- Second and third-degree burns with serious threat of functional or cosmetic impairment that involves the face, hands, feet, genitalia, perineum, or major joints
- Third degree burns over more than 5% of the total body surface area in any age group
- Electrical burns, including lightning injury
- Chemical burns with serious threat of functional or cosmetic impairment
- Any burn that is associated with a significant inhalation injury
- Immunosuppressed patients, diabetes, AIDS, cancer, or alcoholism

Burns That May Not Require a Burn Center, but May Require Admission

- Suspicion of child abuse in otherwise minor burns
- If patient is unable to care for wounds in outpatient setting (i.e., homeless)

DISCHARGE CRITERIA

- Adults with less than 15% TBSA partial thickness burns
- Children with less than 10% TBSA partial thickness burns
- Less than 2% TBSA full thickness burn in noncritical area (see below)
- No involvement of a critical area: eyes, ears, hands, feet, face, or perineum
- Ability to manage wounds as outpatient
- Absence of diabetes, AIDS, taking immunosuppressants
- Adequate follow-up for dressing change each day

Miscellaneous

ICD9: 949.0

CORE CONTENT CODE: 18.4.17.4, 18.6.6

SUGGESTED READING

Edlich RF. Thermal Burns. In: Rosen P, Barkin R, Danzyl D, eds. Emergency medicine: Concepts and clinical practice. 4th ed. St. Louis: CV Mosby, 1992:941

Dimrick AR. Burns. In: Schwartz GR, Safar P, Stone JH, eds. Principles and practice of emergency medicine. 3rd ed. Philadelphia: Lea & Febiger, 1992

Schwartz LR. Thermal burns. In: Tintinalli JE, Ruiz E, Krome R, eds. Emergency medicine: A comprehensive study guide. 4th ed. New York: McGraw-Hill, 1996:893

Author: Jim Larson

Bursitis

Clinical Presentation

SIGNS AND SYMPTOMS

- Localized pain that worsens with movement of structures adjacent to affected bursae
- Usually presents with acute onset, but may be chronic (especially in hip)
- May have low-grade temperature
- Localized swelling may be present with superficial bursal involvement
- Overlying erythema or skin trauma may be present with infectious bursitis
- Traumatic bursitis often follows specific traumatic event or recent overuse of related joints

MECHANISM/DESCRIPTION

- Bursae are sacs lined with synovial membrane. There are approximately 150 in the body located at sites of friction between bones, ligaments, tendons, muscles, and skin. They provide lubrication for movement
- Bursitis—inflammation of the bursae caused by trauma (acute or chronic), infection, crystal deposition, or systemic disease

ETIOLOGY

- Trauma (both acute and chronic)—most common cause
- Infection—may be obvious or microscopic
  - —Higher risk in diabetes, chronic alcohol abuse, uremia, and gout
  - —Staphylococci cause 90%
- Crystal deposition—calcium phosphate, urate
- Systemic disease—rheumatoid, gout, ankylosing spondylitis, psoriatic arthritis, Lupus, Rheumatic fever

Affected joints

- Potentially any bursa may be affected
- Commonly affected joints
  - —Shoulder
  - —Elbow—usually secondary to trauma; high incidence of infection
  - —Wrist and hand
  - —Hip—more common in older women
  - —Knee—often secondary to chronic trauma or arthritis
  - —Foot—calcaneal bursitis is almost always from improper shoes/high heels

Pre-Hospital

CAUTIONS

- May be difficult to distinguish from fractures. Suspicious joints should be immobilized, particularly in the setting of trauma

Diagnosis

ESSENTIAL WORKUP

- Full assessment of regional musculoskeletal function
- Any suspicion of infection warrants aspiration of bursae (especially olecranon and prepatellar bursae)
- Aspiration of hip and other deep bursae should be deferred to orthopedics or rheumatology, or may be guided in ED by ultrasound

LABORATORY TESTS

- For infection: CBC with differential
- Evaluation of related disease (e.g., uric acid level for gout)
- If joint aspiration is done, serum glucose should be sent
- Fluid analysis
  - —Analysis of bursa fluid: cell count with differential, glucose and total protein, crystal determination, Gram stain, culture
  - —Normal fluid is clear yellow and has 0–200 WBC; 0 RBC; low protein and glucose is same as serum
  - —Traumatic bursitis: fluid is bloody/xanthochromic and has <1200 WBC; many RBCs; low protein and normal glucose
  - —Infective bursitis: fluid is yellow, cloudy, and has 50,000–200,000 WBC; few RBCs; slightly increased protein and decreased glucose; bacteria on Gram stain
  - —Rheumatoid and microcrystalline inflammation: Fluid is yellow to cloudy and has 1000–40,000 WBC; few RBCs; slightly increased protein and variable glucose
  - —Because infection and inflammation may be difficult to differentiate, cultures must always be sent

IMAGING/SPECIAL TESTS

- X-rays may demonstrate chronic arthritic changes or calcium deposits
- Recommended when trauma is involved to rule out fracture

DIFFERENTIAL DIAGNOSIS

- Arthritis, gout
- Tendonitis
- Fracture, tendon/ligament tear, contusion, sprain
- Also in hips: neuritis, lumbar spine disease, sacroiliitis

Treatment

INITIAL STABILIZATION

- Immobilize joint if pain is severe

ED TREATMENT

- Shoulders should not be immobilized for more than 2–3 days due to the risk of adhesive capsulitis
- Ice affected areas for 10 minutes, 4 times a day until improved
- NSAIDs for at least 7 days; best if continued for 5 days after improvement to help prevent recurrence
- If no improvement within 5–7 days and infection has been ruled out (by culture) injection of lidocaine or steroids may be considered
  —Mix 2 ml of 2% lidocaine with 20–40 mg of depoglucocorticoid and inject 1–3 ml of this mixture into the bursae using sterile technique
  —Steroid injections should not be repeated until at least 2 weeks have passed and no more than two injections into one joint should be performed without rheumatologic or orthopedic consultation
- Treat associated diseases as needed (e.g., gout)
- Septic bursitis should be treated with antibiotics and drainage of bursae
  —Antibiotics treatment for septic bursitis should be based on the Gram stain
  —Penicillinase-resistant antistaphylococcal drug may be used if Gram stain is negative or shows Gram-positive cocci
  —If Gram-negative organisms are found, blood cultures should be done and another primary source for the infection should be sought
  —Antibiotics should be continued for 5–7 days beyond the sterilization of bursal fluid

MEDICATIONS

- Nonsteroidal anti-inflammatory agents (there are many choices, a few are listed below)
  —Diclofenac: 50 mg po bid tid
  —Ibuprofen: adult: 600 mg po q 6 hrs; pediatric: 5–10 mg/kg po q 6 hrs
  —Ketorolac: 30 mg IV/IM q 6 hrs or 10 mg po q 4–6 hrs
  —Piroxicam: 20 mg po qd

Disposition

- Most patients may be treated as an outpatient

ADMISSION CRITERIA FOR SEPTIC BURSITIS

- Patients with high fevers and chills/rigors, large surrounding cellulitis, unable to take oral antibiotics, failed outpatient therapy, or immunosuppressed
- Unusual organisms, extrabursal primary site or deep bursal involvement

FOLLOW-UP

- Most patients respond to therapy in 3–4 days and may follow-up with primary care provider within a week
- Septic bursitis requires repeated bursal aspiration every 3–5 days
- Rheumatology or orthopedic referral is recommended for patients who do not respond to intrabursal steroids or recurrent bursitis

Miscellaneous

ICD9: 727.3

CORE CONTENT CODE: 10.4.2

SUGGESTED READING

Butcher JD, et al. Lower extremity bursitis. Am Fam Physician 1996;53(7):2317–2324

Kopicky-Burd J. Nonarticular rheumatic disorders. In: Barker LR, ed. Principles of ambulatory medicine. 3rd ed. Baltimore: Williams & Wilkins, 1991:827–835

Talbot-Stern JK. Arthritis, tendonitis, and bursitis. In: Rosen P, ed. Emergency medicine. 3rd ed. St. Louis: Mosby-Yearbook, 1992:822–826

Author: Melissa Brokaw

Calcaneal Fracture

Clinical Presentation

SIGNS AND SYMPTOMS

- Foot and ankle pain
- Marked swelling of the foot and ankle
- Tenderness on palpation and movement of the foot and ankle
- Inability to bear weight
- Fracture blisters

MECHANISM

- Calcaneal fractures may be intra-articular or extra-articular depending on whether the fracture involves the posterior facet
- Twisting force is the usual mechanism for extra-articular calcaneal fractures
- Axial compression on the talocalcaneal joint as from a fall or motor vehicle accident is the usual mechanism for intra-articular calcaneal fractures. From the axial force, the posterolateral edge of the talus fractures the calcaneus obliquely

Pre-Hospital

CAUTIONS

- Pre-hospital care providers should remember that vertebral compression fractures and long bone fractures of the lower extremities are both associated with calcaneal fractures. Appropriate spinal precautions should be taken
- The calcaneus can be splinted with a pillow or air splint

Diagnosis

ESSENTIAL WORKUP

- Other associated injuries that are more life-threatening should be evaluated first
- Examine the pelvis, hip, knees, long bones of the lower extremities, and thoracolumbar spine for associated injuries
- Bilateral calcaneal fractures occur with falls, so both heels should be examined
- Evaluate for complication of compartment syndrome of the plantar muscles. The principal sign is severe, tense, swelling and pain unaffected by analgesics or immobilization. Compartment pressure should be obtained if there is concern of a compartment syndrome
- Evaluate neurovascular status

IMAGING

Plain Radiography

- *Lateral view,* which shows the height of the posterior facet, Bohler's angle and angle of Gissane
  - —Bohler's angle is made by connecting one line drawn from the superior margin of the posterior tuberosity of the calcaneus through the superior tip of the posterior facet and another line from superior tip of the posterior facet to the superior tip of the anterior process. This angle normally measures between 20–40°. An angle less than 20° indicates a depressed fracture
  - —The lateral process of the talus is wedge shaped in the lateral view. The apex of this wedge is the angle of Gissane. It normally measures approximately 135°
  - —These angles should be compared to those of the normal foot
  - —*Harris axial heel view* allows visualization of any lateral wall displacement, secondary sagittal fracture lines, angulation of the tuberosity, and shortening
  - —*Broden's view* allows visualization of the articular surface of the posterior facet
- The trabecular pattern should be closely examined for disruption which indicates fracture

Computed Tomography (CT)

- CT fully defines and classifies the fracture. Prognosis and the need for surgery are based on CT findings

DIFFERENTIAL DIAGNOSIS

- Ankle injuries
- Achilles tendon injuries
- Plantar fasciitis
- Other tarsal bone injuries

Treatment

INITIAL STABILIZATION

- While more severe injuries are being managed, the calcaneus should remain splinted, iced, and elevated

ED TREATMENT

- Search for and manage other injuries, especially spine and pelvis
- Keep limb splinted, elevated, and iced
- Consult with an orthopedic surgeon. The orthopedic surgeon will determine whether the patient is a surgical candidate based largely on the CT findings
- Nondisplaced fractures and extra-articular fractures are usually nonoperative. Patients are treated with nonweight-bearing immobilization with compressive dressing or cast for approximately 4–10 weeks depending upon the extent and location of the fracture
- Surgery in operative patients is not performed until swelling in the foot and ankle significantly decreases. This decrease may take 1–2 weeks. During this time, the patient is treated with bed rest, limb elevation, and use of a Jones dressing and posterior splint

MEDICATIONS

- Opioid analgesics
  —Calcaneal fractures usually cause severe pain and therefore, opioids need to be administered intravenously

Disposition

ADMISSION CRITERIA

- Pain management in patients with calcaneal fractures is usually very difficult. Patients with unbearable pain should be admitted for pain control
- Surgical candidates who may not be absolutely compliant with bed rest, limb elevation, and use of a Jones dressing and posterior splint should be admitted
- Open fracture
- Complication of compartment syndrome
- Associated spine, pelvic, or other injuries

DISCHARGE CRITERIA

- Patients with adequate pain control and nonoperative fracture can be discharged after consultation from an orthopedic surgeon
- Surgical candidates who will be totally compliant with treatment instructions and who have adequate pain control may be discharged. Again, discharge should be done after consultation with an orthopedic surgeon

SPECIAL PEDIATRIC CONSIDERATION

- Because of remodeling, children may not require the same aggressive surgical treatment as adults. The orthopedic surgeon may elect to treat the patient with nonweight-bearing immobilization. If this is the case, and pain management is adequate and parents are reliable, the patient may discharged

Miscellaneous

ICD9: 825.0

CORE CONTENT CODE: 18.4.13.1.3.1

SUGGESTED READINGS

Myerson MS. Primary subtalar arthrodesis for the treatment of comminuted fractures of the calcaneus. Orthop Clin North Am 1995;26(2);215–227

Sanders R, Fortin P, DiPasquale T, Walling A. Operative treatment in 120 displaced intra-articular calcaneal fractures. Clin Orthop 1993;290;87–95

Sanders R, Gregory P. Operative treatment of intra-articular fractures of the calcaneus. Orthop Clin North Am 1995;26(2);203–214

Author: Lisa Chan

Calcium Channel Blocker, Poisoning

Clinical Presentation

SIGNS AND SYMPTOMS

- Cardiovascular
  - —Hypotension
  - —Bradycardia
  - —Reflex tachycardia (dihydropyridine)
  - —Conduction abnormalities / heart blocks
- Neurologic
  - —CNS depression
  - —Coma
  - —Seizures
- Metabolic
  - —Hyperglycemia

MECHANISM/DESCRIPTION

Three Classes of Calcium Channel Blockers (CCB)

- Phenylalkylamines (Verapamil)
  - —Vasodilatation resulting in a decrease in BP
  - —Negative chronotropic and inotropic effects—reflex tachycardia not seen with a drop in BP
- Dihydropyridine (Nifedipine)
  - —Decrease vascular resistance resulting in a drop in BP
  - —Little negative inotropic effect—reflex tachycardia occurs
- Benzothiazepine (Diltiazem)
  - —Decrease peripheral vascular resistance leading to a decrease in BP
  - —HR and CO initially increased
  - —Direct negative chronotropic effect which leads to a fall in HR

Effects of Calcium Channel Blockade

- Calcium plays key role in cardiac and smooth muscle contractility
- Calcium channel blockers prevent
  - —The entry of calcium resulting in a lack of muscle contraction
  - —The normal release of insulin from pancreatic islet cells resulting in hyperglycemia

Pre-Hospital

CAUTIONS

- Transport pill/pill bottles to emergency department
- Calcium for bradycardic/unstable patient with confirmed CCB overdose

Diagnosis

ESSENTIAL WORKUP

- EKG
  - —Bradycardia (tachycardia with nifedipine)
  - —Conduction delays—QRS prolongation
  - —Heart blocks

LABORATORY

- Ionized calcium level when administering calcium
- Digoxin level if patient on digoxin (dictate safety of calcium administration)
- CBC
- Electrolytes, BUN, creatinine, glucose
  - —Hyperglycemia/metabolic acidosis may occur
- Toxicology screen if coingestants suspected

DIFFERENTIAL DIAGNOSIS

- β-blocker toxicity
- Clonidine toxicity
- Digitalis toxicity
- Acute myocardial infarction with heart block

Treatment

INITIAL STABILIZATION

- ABCs
  - —Airway protection as indicated
  - —Supplemental oxygen as needed
  - —0.9%NS IV access
  - —Hemodynamic monitoring

ED TREATMENT

Goals

- HR >60 beats per minute
- Systolic BP >90 mm Hg
- Adequate urine output
- Improving level of consciousness

GI Decontamination

- Syrup of ipecac—contraindicated in the emergency department
- Activated charcoal
  - —May be helpful especially in the presence of co-ingestants
- Whole bowel irrigation
  - —Beneficial with ingestion of sustained release preparations
  - —Contraindicated in hemodynamically unstable patients

Calcium

- First-line agent for calcium channel blocker toxicity
- Calcium chloride (10%)
- Contains 1.36 mEq Ca^{++}/ml (3× more calcium than calcium gluconate)
- Can cause tissue necrosis and sloughing with extravasation
- Very irritating to veins
- Calcium gluconate (10%)
  - —Contains 0.45 mEq Ca^{++}/ml
  - —Does not cause tissue necrosis like calcium chloride
  - —Calcium gluconate—preferred agent in an acidemic patient
- Follow serum calcium levels if repeated doses of calcium administered
- Contraindicated in digoxin toxicity because calcium can produce serious adverse effects in digoxin toxicity

Bradycardia/Hypotension

- IV fluids
  - —Administer cautiously in the hypotensive patient
  - —Swan-Ganz catheter or CVP monitoring to help follow volume status
- Atropine usually ineffective
- Pressor agents
  - —No clear evidence that one agent is more effective than another
  - —Institute invasive monitoring to help guide treatment
  - —Dopamine—β_1-receptor agonist at low doses which causes a positive inotropic effect on the myocardium and an α-receptor agonist at higher doses which leads to vasoconstriction
  - —Epinephrine—potent α- and β-receptor agonist
- Glucagon
  - —Promotes cAMP production through a receptor site other than the β-receptor
  - —May cause nausea and vomiting
  - —Mix with normal saline or 5% dextrose in water. Do not use the Phenol diluent that comes with glucagon
- Amrinone
  - —Selective phosphodiesterase III inhibitor
  - —Indirectly increases cAMP
- Electrical pacing—when other treatment options have failed
- Insulin
  - —Potential for treatment in the future

MEDICATIONS

- Amrinone: loading dose 0.75 mg/kg; maintenance drip 2–20 (g/kg/min; titrate for effect)
- Atropine: 0.5 mg (peds: 0.02 mg/kg) IV; repeat 0.5–1.0 mg IV (peds: 0.04 mg/kg)
- Calcium chloride: 10 cc of 10% solution slow IVP (peds: 0.2–0.25 cc/kg; repeat in 10 min if necessary) followed by infusion 20–50 mg/kg/hr
- Calcium gluconate: 10 cc of 10% solution slow IVP (peds: 1 cc/kg; may repeat in 10 min if necessary)
- Dopamine: 2–20 μg/kg/min; titrate to effect
- Epinephrine: 2 μg/min (peds: 0.1 μg/kg/min); titrate to effect
- Glucagon: 3.5–5 mg IV (peds: 0.03–0.1 mg/kg) bolus followed by 70 μg/kg/hr infusion
- Golytely WBI: 2 L/h po or by NG-tube for 4–6 hrs or until rectal effluent is clear (peds: 40 cc/kg/hr)

Disposition

ADMISSION CRITERIA

- Admit symptomatic patients to a monitored bed for hemodynamic monitoring
- Admit all ingestions of sustained-release calcium channel blockers for 24 hours of observation and monitoring due to the potential delay in symptoms

DISCHARGE CRITERIA

- Discharge asymptomatic patients 8 hours after ingestion of immediate-release preparation

Miscellaneous

ICD9: 977.9

CORE CONTENT CODE: 17.2.14.4

SUGGESTED READINGS

Clark RF, Hanna RC. Calcium channel blocker toxicity. Top Emerg Med 1993;15(3):15–26

Kerns W, Kline J, Ford MD. β-Blocker and calcium channel blocker toxicity. Emerg Med Clin North Am 1994;12:365–390

Kline JA, Leonova E, Raymond RM. Beneficial myocardial metabolic effects of insulin during verapamil toxicity in the anesthetized canine. Crit Care Med 1995;23:1251–1263

Author: Janet Eng

Candidiasis, Oral

Clinical Presentation

SIGNS AND SYMPTOMS

- Pseudomembranous candidiasis
  - —White mucosal plaques
  - —Adherent but removable
  - —Erythematous base
- Atrophic candidiasis
  - —Erythematous, painful stomatitis with few, if any, white patches
  - —Angular chelitis
    - -Cracking and erythema at the corners of the mouth
    - -Lesions are often asymptomatic
    - -Usually limited to the denture-bearing mucosa
- Hyperplastic candidiasis
  - —Immunosuppressed individuals
  - —Chronic, invasive ulcers
  - —Mucosal plaques that cannot be removed

MECHANISM/DESCRIPTION

- Overgrowth of candida albicans in the oral cavity
- Promoted by local alteration of protective factors
  - —The epithelial barrier
  - —Alteration in the microbial flora
  - —Changes in salivary flow
  - —Antimicrobial activity
- Candida organisms are normally present as oral flora in 20–60% of the population
- Varies in severity
  - —Superficial localized infection
  - —Severe systemic disease with a mortality of 50%
- Descriptive categories
  - —Acute pseudomembranous candidiasis (Thrush)
    - -Most commonly seen in infancy, old age, and with other serious underlying conditions (diabetes, leukemia, AIDS)
    - -Superficial confluent
  - —Acute and chronic atrophic candidiasis
    - -Has been described in up to 60% of denture-wearers
  - —Hyperplastic candidiasis
    - -Organism invades the buccal mucosa
    - -Immunosuppressed individuals
    - -High incidence with frequent malignant degeneration in tobacco users
- In immunocompetent individuals, a benign course is the norm
- Often recurrent in immunocompromised patients
- Early manifestation of AIDS in HIV-infected patients
- Pediatric considerations
  - —The prevalence of oral thrush in neonates is 5%
  - —It usually becomes evident at 5–8 days of age
  - —The source of infection is believed to be the maternal birth canal
  - —The susceptibility of infants is likely due to the immaturity of their immune system and lack of mature oral flora

ETIOLOGY

- Diabetes
- Immunosuppression
  - —AIDS
  - —Chemotherapy
  - —Use of immunosuppressive agents

Pre-Hospital

N/A

Diagnosis

ESSENTIAL WORKUP

- Determine if there is an etiology for a breakdown of host factors
- If no reason is found, evaluation for possible HIV infection or diabetes
- Exclude a systemic infection

LABORATORY

- CBC
  - —Exclude neutropenia in patients undergoing chemotherapy
  - —In the patient without predisposing conditions to assess immunocompetence
- Biopsy
- Fungal scrapings with Potassium Hydroxide preparation
- Culture on blood or Sabouraud's agar
  - —Positive may be due to normal flora

IMAGING/SPECIAL TESTS

N/A

DIFFERENTIAL DIAGNOSIS

- Hairy leukoplakia
- Hyperkeratosis
- Lichen planus
- Squamous cell carcinoma

Treatment

INITIAL STABILIZATION

N/A

ED TREATMENT

- Topical antifungal medications
- Systemic agents should be reserved for those with disease resistant to topical therapy
  —Fluconazole
  —Itraconazole
  —Ketoconazole
- Analgesia

MEDICATIONS

- Clotrimazole: 10 mg troche, dissolve in mouth over 20 min, 5 times per day
- Nystatin: 10 cc oral suspension, swish and swallow 4–5 times per day for 14 days; in infants, use 100,000 units and apply to affected areas with a cotton-tipped swab bid for 1–2 weeks
- Miconazole: 25 mg oral gel, use 4 times per day
- Ketaconazole: 200 mg once daily for 14–21 days
- Fluconazole: 100 mg once daily for 14–21 days (increasing resistance is developing)
- Itraconazole: 100 mg 1–2 times daily for 14–21 days (less hepatotoxicity than ketoconazole)

Disposition

ADMISSION CRITERIA

- Inability to tolerate oral intake due to discomfort
- Newly diagnosed immunocompromised state
- Systemic infection

DISCHARGE CRITERIA

- Candidiasis that does not threaten the hydration status of the patient may be discharged with close follow-up

Miscellaneous

ICD9: 112.0

CORE CONTENT CODE: 6.3.5

SUGGESTED READINGS

Fotos PG, Lilly JP. Clinical management of oral and perioral candidosis. Dermatol Clin 1996;14:273–280.

Greenspan D. Treatment of oropharyngeal candidiasis in HIV-positive patients. J Am Acad Dermatol 1994;31:S51–S55.

Hoppe JE. Treatment of oropharyngeal candidiasis in immunocompetent infants: a randomized multicenter study of miconazole gel vs. nystatin suspension. The Antifungals Study Group. Pediatr Infect Dis J 1997;16:288–293.

Lynch DP. Oral candidiasis. History, classification, and clinical presentation. Oral Surg Oral Med Oral Pathol 1994;78:189–193.

Mooney MA, Thomas I, Sirois D. Oral candidosis. Int J Dermatol 1995;34:759–765.

Author: Deepi Goyal

Carbamazepine, Poisoning

Clinical Presentation

SIGNS AND SYMPTOMS

- Neurologic manifestations common
- Cardiotoxicity rare, except in massive overdose

Central Nervous System (CNS)

- Ataxia
- Dizziness
- Drowsiness
- Nystagmus
- Hallucinations
- Combativeness
- Coma
- Seizures

Respiratory System

- Respiratory depression
- Aspiration pneumonia

Cardiovascular System

- Hypotension
- Conduction disturbances (mostly in elderly)
- Supraventricular tachycardia
- Sinus tachycardia or bradycardia
- ECG changes
  - —Prolongation of PR, QRS, and QTc intervals
  - —T wave changes

Miscellaneous

- Anticholinergic manifestations
  - —Decreased bowel sounds
  - —Mydriasis
  - —Flushing
  - —Urinary retention
- Neuromuscular changes
  - —Tremor
  - —Slurred speech
  - —Myoclonus
  - —Choreiform and choreoathetoid movements

DESCRIPTION/MECHANISM

- Anticholinergic
- Similarities to phenytoin and tricyclic antidepressants
- Sodium channel blocker
- Decreases synaptic transmission

Pre-Hospital

CAUTIONS

- Do *not* administer ipecac
- Intubate if significant respiratory depression or airway compromise
- Secure IV access
- Get complete information about all products potentially ingested

Diagnosis

ESSENTIAL WORKUP

- Continuous cardiac monitor
- Serum carbamazepine level
  - —Therapeutic = 6–12 mg/L
  - —Levels >25–40 μg/ml associated with serious toxicity
    - -Coma
    - -Seizures
    - -Respiratory failure
    - -Conduction defects
  - —Serum levels do not clearly predict clinical toxicity
    - -Active metabolite carbamazepine epoxide not measured

    Neurologic manifestations depend on CNS, not serum level
- ECG
  - —Conduction delays
    - -Increased QRS interval
    - -Increased PR interval
  - —Dysrhythmias
    - -Sinus tachycardia (massive carbamazepine overdose)
    - -Bradydysrhythmia (often seen in elderly with mild increase in carbamazepine level)
- Serum acetaminophen level

LABORATORY

- CBC
  - —Leukopenia or leukocytosis
- Electrolytes, BUN/Cr, glucose
  - —Hyperglycemia
  - —Hypokalemia
  - —Hyponatremia
- Arterial blood gas
- Urinalysis
  - —Glucosuria
  - —Ketonuria
- Pregnancy test
- SGOT, SGPT, bilirubin, alkaline phosphatase
  - —May be mildly elevated
  - —Usually not clinically significant

IMAGING/SPECIAL TESTS

- CXR for:
  - —Aspiration pneumonia
  - —Pulmonary edema

DIFFERENTIAL DIAGNOSIS

Drugs That Cause Decreased Mental Status:

- Alcohol
- Anticholinergics
- Barbiturates
- Benzodiazepines
- Lithium
- Opiates
- Phenothiazines

Drugs That Cause Seizures:
- Alcohol withdrawal
- Anticholinergics
- Camphor
- Isoniazid
- Lithium
- Phenothiazines
- Sympathomimetics
  - —Amphetamine
  - —Cocaine
- Tricyclic antidepressants

Drugs That Cause Abnormal Movement:
- Antihistamines
- Butyrophenones
- Caffeine
- Cocaine
- Ethylene glycol
- Levodopa
- Meperidine
- Phencyclidine
- Phenothiazines
- Phenytoin
- Tricyclic antidepressants

Treatment

INITIAL STABILIZATION
- ABCs
- Establish IV access with 0.9%NS
- Oxygen
- Cardiac monitor
- Naloxone, thiamine, D50W (or Accucheck) if altered mental status

ED TREATMENT

General Management
- Gastric lavage
  - —For recent ingestion (<1–2 hours) and significantly decreased mental status
  - —Most patients will not need gastric lavage
  - —If patient is lethargic, intubate before lavage
  - —Instill activated charcoal through orogastric tube both before and after lavage
- Activated charcoal
  - —Administer sorbitol with first dose (only) of activated charcoal
  - —Administer with caution if gastrointestinal activity is decreased
  - —Contraindicated if bowel sounds are absent
- Multidose activated charcoal
  - —Decreases mean half-life of carbamazepine
  - —Binds unabsorbed drug in gastrointestinal tract
  - —Interrupts enterohepatic circulation
  - —Do not give additional sorbitol
- Charcoal hemoperfusion
  - —Removes only small amount of ingested dose
  - —Patients usually do well with supportive care without hemoperfusion
  - —Indicated in cases of clinical deterioration or lack of improvement with good supportive care
- Psychiatric consultation

Respiratory Depression
- Intubation
- Ventilatory support

Hypotension
- 0.9%NS IV fluid resuscitation with 1 liter initial fluid bolus
- Norepinephrine if unresponsive to IV fluids

Seizures
- Diazepam (drug of choice)
- Phenobarbital (if diazepam ineffective)
- Phenytoin not effective in many toxic seizures

MEDICATIONS
- Activated charcoal (initial bolus): slurry 1–2 g/kg up to 100 g po mixed with sorbitol (below)
- Dextrose: D50W 1 amp (50 ml or 25 g) (peds: D25W 2–4 m/kg) IV
- Diazepam: 5–10 mg (peds: 0.2—0.5 mg/kg) IV
- Multidose activated charcoal: 25 g (peds: 0.25 g/kg) q 2 hrs po after bolus dose (above)
- Naloxone (Narcan): 2 mg (peds: 0.1 mg/kg) IV or IM initial dose
- Norepinephrine: 4–12 μg/min (peds: 0.05–0.1 μg/kg/min) IV titrated to effect
- Sorbitol: 1–2 g/kg to max 100 g (peds: >1-yr-old: 1–1.5 g/kg as a 35% solution to max 50 g) po mixed with activated charcoal slurry (first dose only)

Disposition

ADMISSION CRITERIA
- Decreased mental status at any time, even if resolving
  - —Observe at least 24 hours for late relapse
- Seizures
- Cardiac dysrhythmias
- Lack of psychiatric clearance after suicidal ingestion

DISCHARGE CRITERIA
- Asymptomatic after 6 hours observation
- Normal mental status
- Normal or baseline ECG
- Gastrointestinal motility present
- Psychiatric clearance (after suicidal ingestion)

Miscellaneous

ICD9: 966.3

CORE CONTENT CODE: 17.2.6

SUGGESTED READINGS

Hojer J, Malmlund H, Berg A. Clinical features in 28 consecutive cases of laboratory confirmed massive poisoning with carbamazepine alone. Clin Toxicol 1993;31:449–458

Kasarskis EJ, Juo C, Berger R, Nelson KR. Carbamazepine-induced cardiac dysfunction: Characterization of two distinct clinical syndromes. Arch Intern Med 1992;152:186–191

MacNab AJ, Birch P, MacReady J. Carbamazepine poisoning in children. Pediatr Emerg Care 1993;9:195–198

Seymour JF. Carbamazepine overdose: Features of 33 cases. Drug Safety 1993;8:81–88

Wason S, Baker RC, Carolan P, Seigel R, Druckenbrod RW. Carbamazepine overdose—the effects of multiple dose activated charcoal. Clin Toxicol 1992;30:39–48

Author: Leon Gussow

Carbon Monoxide, Poisoning

Clinical Presentation

SIGNS AND SYMPTOMS

Central Nervous System (CNS)

- Headache
- Dizziness
- Ataxia
- Confusion
- Acute encephalopathy
- Syncope
- Seizures
- Coma

Gastrointestinal

- Nausea
- Vomiting

Cardiovascular

- Chest pain
- Palpitations
- Tachycardia
- Premature ventricular contractions
- Dysrhythmias
- Myocardial ischemia/infarction

Respiratory

- Dyspnea
- Tachypnea
- Respiratory alkalosis
- Noncardiogenic pulmonary edema

Ophthalmologic

- Decreased vision
- Retinal hemorrhage

Other

- Rhabdomyolysis
- Lactic acidosis

DESCRIPTION/MECHANISM

- Formation of carboxyhemoglobin
  —Decreases oxygen-carrying capacity
  —Shifts oxyhemoglobin dissociation curve to left
- Binding to intracellular heme proteins (cytochrome oxidase, cytochrome P450)
  —Interrupts cellular respiration and oxygen utilization
  —Causes increased lactic acid
- Binding to myoglobin
  —Decreases oxygen extraction
  —Impairs function of skeletal and cardiac muscle

ETIOLOGY

- Endogenous (natural hemoglobin turnover)
- Incomplete combustion of carbon-containing compounds
  —Internal combustion engines
  —Natural gas
  —Space heaters
  —Kerosene heaters
  —Charcoal
  —Sterno
  —Indoor hibachis
  —Accidental fires
  —Fireplaces
  —Furnaces
  —Smoking (causes carboxyhemoglobin levels up to 10–15%)
- Methylene chloride
  —Found in some solvents and furniture-stripping compounds
  —Slowly released from tissues and metabolized by liver to carbon monoxide
  —Peak carboxyhemoglobin level delayed after exposure
  —Half-life approximately 2 times that of inhaled carbon monoxide

Pre-Hospital

CAUTION

- Remove patient from contaminated environment
- Assess for smoke inhalation or thermal injury
- Assess airway and ventilation to determine need for intubation
- Administer 100% oxygen to all patients suspected of having carbon monoxide toxicity

Diagnosis

ESSENTIAL WORKUP

- History
  —May present with mild, nonspecific symptoms
  —Question for
    -Similar symptoms in other household members
    -Malfunctioning furnaces
    -Use of space heaters or open ovens for supplemental heat
    -Ill pets
    -Women of childbearing age should be asked about possible pregnancy
- Arterial blood gas
  —Normal pO_2 and calculated oxygen saturation
  —Measured oxygen saturation will be low
  —Metabolic acidosis with severe exposure
- Carboxyhemoglobin level
  —*Caution:* patient may be critically ill from carbon monoxide despite an unimpressive carboxyhemoglobin level
  —Measure as soon as possible
  —Normal 0–3% (up to 10% in cigarette smokers)
  —Misleadingly low if a significant time has passed since exposure, or if supplemental oxygen administered
  —May not reflect clinical severity
  —Calibrate breathalyzers carefully
    -Less accurate than direct measurement

LABORATORY

- Electrolytes, BUN/Cr, glucose
  —Metabolic acidosis and increased anion gap associated with increased clinical severity
- Urinalysis
  —Myoglobin with rhabdomyolysis
- Cardiac enzymes
  —Draw serial enzymes if suspicion of myocardial ischemia or infarction
- Acetaminophen level
  —For suicidal exposures
- Salicylate level
  —For increased anion gap metabolic acidosis
- Pregnancy test

IMAGING/SPECIAL TESTS

- Pulse oximetry
  —Pulse oximeter reads carboxyhemoglobin as oxyhemoglobin
  —False elevated reading
- EKG
  —Carbon monoxide can precipitate myocardial ischemia or infarction
  —Dysrhythmias
  —Nonspecific ST-T changes
- CXR for aspiration, pulmonary edema
- CT head
  —White matter changes are typical of carbon monoxide poisoning, and associated with poor long-term neurologic outcome

—Low-density lesions in the globus pallidus may be clue to diagnosis in occult cases
—Rule out intracranial causes of altered mental status

DIFFERENTIAL DIAGNOSIS

- Viral illness
- Meningitis
- Encephalitis
- Intracranial bleed
- Influenza or viral syndrome
- Gastroenteritis
- Migraine
- Tension headache
- Ethanol intoxication
- Opiates
- Sedative/hypnotic overdose
- Cyanide poisoning
- Salicylate overdose
- Toxic alcohol exposure

Treatment

INITIAL STABILIZATION

- ABCs
- 0.9%NS IV
- Oxygen (100%)
- Cardiac monitor
- Naloxone, dextrose (or Accucheck), and thiamine if altered mental status

ED TREATMENT

Oxygen

- Administer 100% normobaric oxygen
  —Via mask or endotracheal tube
- Continue until carboxyhemoglobin level <5–10%
- Half-life of carboxyhemoglobin
  —Room air ~300 minutes
  —100% normobaric oxygen ~90 minutes
  —Hyperbaric oxygen (3 ATM) ~20 minutes

Hyperbaric oxygen

- Dose
  —100% at 3 ATM for 45 minutes
  —May be repeated
- Benefits
  —Decreases half-life of carboxyhemoglobin
  —Increases dissolved oxygen
  —May clear carbon monoxide from mitochondria and myoglobin
  —Decreases lipid peroxidation
  —Decreases incidence of cerebral edema
  —May decrease mortality and long-term neurologic morbidity in selected cases
- Potential adverse effects
  —Ear discomfort and tympanic membrane rupture
  —Pneumothorax
  —Seizure
  —Risk of transporting unstable patient
- Indications
  —History of coma at any time during or after exposure
  —Significant persistent neurologic deficits
  —Cardiac instability (must weigh potential benefit against risk of transfer)
  —Persistent metabolic acidosis
  —Carboxyhemoglobin level >40%
  —Carboxyhemoglobin level >15% in pregnant patient

Special Considerations in the Pregnant Carbon Monoxide Victim

- Fetal carboxyhemoglobin levels 10–15% higher than maternal
- Fetal carboxyhemoglobin clearance delayed compared to maternal
- Treat pregnant carbon monoxide victims with 100% oxygen for 5 times as long as it takes to get the maternal level <10%
- Hyperbaric oxygen if level >15%

MEDICATIONS

- Dextrose: D50W 1 amp (50 ml or 25 g) (peds: D25W 2–4 ml/kg) IV
- Naloxone (Narcan): 2 mg (peds: 0.1 mg/kg) IV or IM initial dose
- Thiamine (Vitamin B_1): 100 mg (peds: 50 mg) IV or IM

Disposition

ADMISSION CRITERIA

- Persistent symptoms after 4 hours of treatment
- Evidence of myocardial ischemia or cardiac instability
- Seizures
- Persistent metabolic acidosis
- Syncope
- Rhabdomyolysis

DISCHARGE CRITERIA

- Asymptomatic after 4 hours observation
- Absence of above admission criteria
- Psychiatric clearance (if suicidal exposure)

Miscellaneous

ICD9: 986

CORE CONTENT CODE: 17.2.13

SUGGESTED READINGS

Dolan MC. Carbon monoxide poisoning. Can Med Assoc J 1985;133:392

Olson KR. Carbon monoxide poisoning: Mechanisms, presentation, and controversies in management. J Emerg Med 1984:1:233

Raphael JC, Elkharrat D, Jars-Guincestre MC, et al. Trial of normobaric and hyperbaric oxygen for acute carbon monoxide intoxication. Lancet 1989;2:414

Sloan EP, Murphy DG, Hart R, et al. Complications and protocol considerations in carbon monoxide-poisoned patients who require hyperbaric oxygen therapy: Report from a ten-year experience. Ann Emerg Med 1989;18:629

Author: Leon Gussow

Cardiac Arrest

Clinical Presentation

SIGNS AND SYMPTOMS

- Loss of consciousness within 10 seconds
- Fixed and dilated pupils within 60 seconds
- Occasionally preceded by
  —Angina
  —Dyspnea
  —Palpitations
  —Fatigue
  —Other nonspecific complaints
- Immediately prior to arrest
  —Shock
  —Impaired mentation

MECHANISM/DESCRIPTION

- Sudden death
  —Death within 24 hours of symptom onset
  —Incidence of 0.26% in the United States
  —75% are due to cardiovascular disease
- 9–65% have return of spontaneous circulation (ROSC)
- 1–20% of patients survive to discharge
- No history of coronary heart disease prior to sudden death
  —50% of men
  —64% of women
- Factors affecting survival
  —Initial rhythm
  —Witnessed arrest
  —Etiology of the arrest
- Incidence of rearrest in neurologically intact survivors
  —30% at 1 year
  —60% at 5 years

ETIOLOGY

- Acute coronary ischemia
  —Underlying etiology in 50% of cardiac arrest
- Primary dysrhythmic event
- Myocardial hypertrophy
- Dilated cardiomyopathy
- Congenital and acquired electrical abnormalities
- Myocarditis
- Valvular heart disease
- Massive myocardial failure
- Cardiac rupture
- Metabolic abnormalities
  —Hypokalemia
  —Hyperkalemia
  —Hypermagnesemia
  —Hypomagnesemia
  —Hypocalcemia
- Noncardiogenic causes
  —Consider if pulseless electrical activity
  —Pericardial tamponade
  —Tension pneumothorax
  —Hemorrhage
  —Pulmonary embolus
  —Sepsis
  —Air embolism
  —Severe acidosis
- Drugs or toxins
  —Antidysrhythmics
  —Digoxin
  —β-Blockers
  —Calcium channel blockers
  —Tricyclic antidepressants
  —Cocaine
  —Heroin
  —Carbon monoxide
  —Cyanide

Pre-Hospital

- Prompt initiation of CPR
- Confirm underlying rhythm
- Early defibrillation with VT or VF
  —Automated external defibrillator
    -EMT basic or laymen
- Transport to the closest facility
  —If return of spontaneous circulation
    -Center equipped for interventional cardiac care
    -Pediatric critical care center for children
- Termination of resuscitative efforts
  —Persistent, confirmed asystole
  —Prolonged arrest

Diagnosis

ESSENTIAL WORKUP

- "Quick look"
  —Use the paddles of a cardiac defibrillator
- Assess underlying rhythm
- Investigation of the underlying etiology should occur after rosc

LABORATORY

- Indicated only when successful ROSC is achieved
  —Electrolytes
  —BUN
  —Creatinine
  —Creatinine kinase with isoenzymes
  —Arterial blood gas
  —Complete blood count
  —Therapeutic drug levels
  —Toxicological testing

IMAGING/SPECIAL TESTS

- Electrocardiogram
- Chest radiograph
- Echocardiogram

DIFFERENTIAL DIAGNOSIS

- Sudden loss of consciousness with a palpable pulse
  —Syncope
  —Seizure
  —Stroke
  —Hypoglycemia
  —Acute airway obstruction
  —Head trauma
  —Toxins

Treatment

INITIAL STABILIZATION

- Initiate advanced cardiac life support (ACLS)
- Continuous CPR as long as no pulse is palpable
  - —Interruptions must be kept to a minimum
    - -Stop CPR briefly to check the cardiac rhythm
    - -Endotracheal intubation
    - -Central venous line placement
- Secure the airway
- Obtain intravenous access
- Cardiac monitor
- Therapy based on the underlying rhythm according to ACLS protocols

ED TREATMENT

Pulseless VT or VF

- Immediate defibrillation with up to three countershocks
  - —200 J
  - —200–300 J
  - —360 J
- If defibrillation is unsuccessful
  - —Epinephrine
- If refractory to defibrillation and epinephrine
  - —Lidocaine
  - —Bretylium
- High-dose epinephrine
- Amiodarone
- Other adrenergic agents
  - —Methoxamine
  - —Phenylephrine
  - —Norepinephrine

Asystole

- Dismal prognosis if this is the presenting rhythm
- Epinephrine
- Atropine
- Confirmed in two or more leads
- Controversial adjunctive therapies
  - —High-dose epinephrine
  - —Alternative adrenergic agents
  - —Transcutaneous pacing

Torsades de Pointes

- Magnesium sulfate

Pulseless Electrical Activity (PEA)

- Epinephrine
- Atropine
- Treat for reversible cause of PEA
  - —Pneumothorax
  - —Cardiac tamponade
  - —Hypoxia
  - —Pulmonary embolus
  - —Hypovolemia (hemorrhage)

Sodium Bicarbonate

- Limited indications
  - —Hyperkalemia
  - —Tricyclic antidepressant overdose
  - —Rare instances of prolonged resuscitation

Postresuscitation

- Treat the underlying cause of the arrest
- EKG to search for potential coronary ischemia
- Ventilatory support
- Antidysrhythmic therapy
- Correcting electrolyte abnormalities
- Inotropic support

MEDICATIONS

- Epinephrine: 1 mg IV every 3–5 min
- Lidocaine: 100 mg IV 2–4 mg/min IV drip
- Bretylium: 5 mg/kg IV (repeat in 5 min with 10 mg/kg); 2 mg/min IV infusion
- Atropine: 1 mg IV every 3–5 min for a total of 0.04 mg/kg
- Procainamide: 20 mg/min slow IV to a total of 1 g or arrhythmia is suppressed; maintenance drip at 1–4 mg/min IV
- Magnesium: 1–2 g IV
- Sodium bicarbonate: 1 amp (44 mEq) IV

Disposition

ADMISSION CRITERIA

- Return of spontaneous circulation
  - —Coronary care unit or ICU
  - —Postresuscitation care

DISCHARGE CRITERIA

N/A

Miscellaneous

ICD9: 798

CORE CONTENT CODE: 22.1.8

SUGGESTED READINGS

Emergency Cardiac Care Committee and Subcommittees, American Heart Association. Guidelines for cardiopulmonary resuscitation and emergency cardiac care. JAMA 1992;268:2172–2295.

Gilman, JK, Jalal S, Naccurelli GV. Predicting and preventing sudden death from cardiac causes. Circulation 1994;90(2):1083–1092.

Heller RF, Steele PL, Fisher JD, et al. Success of cardiopulmonary resuscitation after heart attack in hospital and outside hospital. Br Med J 1995;311:1332–1336.

Author: Niels Rathlev

Cardiac Pacemakers

Clinical Presentation

SIGNS AND SYMPTOMS

- Permanent pacemaker failure
  - —Asymptomatic
  - —Complete cardiovascular collapse
  - —Dyspnea
  - —Bradycardia
  - —Tachycardia
  - —Diaphoresis
  - —Hypotension
  - —Fatigue
  - —Weakness
  - —Altered level of consciousness
- Conditions necessitating use of temporary pacing if secondary to significant dysrhythmia treatable by acute pacing
  - —Dyspnea
  - —Fatigue
  - —Weakness
  - —Diaphoresis
  - —Altered level of consciousness
  - —Hypotension
  - —Tachycardia
  - —Bradycardia
  - —Alternating tachycardia/bradycardia
  - —Irregular heart beat
  - —Peripheral edema
  - —Crackles on lung exam
  - —Symptomatic bradycardia
  - —Hemodynamic compromise in a patient with a permanent pacemaker
- Pacemaker syndrome
  - —Asynchronous atrioventricular contraction
    - -Lightheadedness
    - -Dyspnea
    - -Palpitations
    - -Syncope

MECHANISM/DESCRIPTION

- Permanent, implanted cardiac pacemakers
  - —A battery-powered energy source
  - —Used to stimulate myocardium
  - —Has two major parts
    - -The pulse generator, which provides the energy and is generally sewn into a pocket in the chest wall between pectoralis fascia and sub-q fat
    - -The electrical leads, which carry the energy from the pulse generator to electrodes and which stimulate the myocardium; lead tips must be embedded in myocardium to function properly
- Temporary pacemakers
  - —Transcutaneous pacer
    - -The electrodes are pads placed on the anterior and posterior aspects of the left chest wall
    - -Current from the external pulse generator moves between the electrodes and passes through the thorax and myocardium causing myocardial depolarization
  - —Transvenous pacer
    - -Transvenous electrodes are placed via central venous access into the right ventricle
    - -Direct contact with the endocardium
    - -Energy travels down the pacing wires and through the electrodes
    - -Direct depolarization of the myocardium
- Pacemaker magnet
  - —Donut-shaped magnet
  - —When placed over the pacemaker pulse generator, inhibits the pacemaker's capability to sense an event or to respond to an event
  - —The pacemaker stops operating in demand mode and begins operating in fixed mode
  - —Checks the pacing rate
  - —Possible complication: R-on-T phenomenon causing serious dysrhythmia

Pacemaker Terminology

- Fixed mode
  - —The pacemaker is set to fire at a set rate regardless of patient's underlying rhythm
  - —Commonly seen in very old pacers (early 1960s)
- Demand mode
  - —The pacemaker fires only when necessary
  - —It senses the underlying rhythm
  - —It will only pace the atria or ventricle if the intrinsic rhythm is absent
- Sensing
  - —Refers to the pacemakers ability to determine if the atria or ventricle are being intrinsically paced
- DDD
  - —An example of a three-letter designation that illustrates the type of pacemaker
  - —All pacemakers actually have a five-letter code to describe their function
  - —For emergency department purposes, only the first three letters of the code are necessary
  - —First letter in the code denotes chamber being sensed
    - -A = Atrium
    - -V = Ventricle
    - -D = Dual (senses both the atria and ventricle)
  - —Second letter in the code denotes chamber that may be paced
    - -A = Atria
    - -V = Ventricle
    - -D = Dual
  - —Third letter in the code lets you know what the pacer's capability is to respond to a sensed event
    - -I = Pacer is able to inhibit itself in response to a sensed event
    - -T = Pacer is able to trigger itself in response to a sensed event
    - -D = Dual response
    - -0 = No response
- Half a million people in the United States have permanent pacemakers
- Seven to 10% of permanent pacemakers malfunction annually in the United States

ETIOLOGY

- Pulse generator fails to provide the energy needed for myocardial contraction
  - —No spike on the EKG
- Pulse generator fires but the myocardium can not "capture" the energy
  - —No myocardial contraction
  - —Twiddler's syndrome
    - -Pacemaker failure caused by lead displacement
- The pacemaker does not sense an abnormal rhythm and therefore does not fire
- The pulse generator fires at an inappropriate rate and induces a tachycardia
  - —Pacemaker mediated tachycardia
    - -Reentrant tachycardia using the pacemaker as part of the loop
  - —Rapid, wide complex tachycardia with each ventricular beat initiated by a pacemaker spike
  - —Placement of a cardiac magnet should interrupt sensing and break the rhythm Responds to adenosine
  - —Runaway Pacemaker
    - -The pulse generator fires at a rate greater than the preprogrammed upper limit of the pacemaker; hemodynamic instability if 1 to 1 ventricular capture
    - -Does not respond to defibrillation or pharmacologic intervention
    - -Responds to overdrive pacing or by placing a magnet over the pulse generator
    - -May have to cut the electrodes at the pulse generator to stop the rhythm
    - -Urgent pacemaker replacement required

Pre-Hospital

CAUTIONS

- Resuscitate patients with pacemaker failure and signs of instability
- Oxygen administered via 100% nonrebreather
- Intubation as needed
- Placement of intravenous catheters
- Transcutaneous pacing
  - —Place negative electrode on left anterior chest wall
  - —Positive electrode on left posterior chest wall
  - —Turn the output dial to its maximum level; myocardial capture should occur
  - —Check for a femoral pulse
  - —Slowly drop the output level until you lose the capture; this voltage is the threshold necessary for myocardial capture
  - —Make sure the pacer is always functioning above threshold
  - —Set the pacer at a rate greater than the patient's intrinsic rhythm
  - —Administer intravenous pain medication or amnestics in the externally paced patient
- Perform CPR as needed
  - —There is no risk of electrical shock to the medical personnel
- It is safe to defibrillate a patient that has a permanent pacemaker

Diagnosis

ESSENTIAL WORKUP

- 12-Lead EKG to assess if there are any obvious evidence of pacemaker failure
- Metabolic workup to determine whether an acquired medical condition lead to an elevated myocardial threshold

LABORATORY

- Serum potassium
  —Hyperkalemia
- Arterial blood gas
  —Acidosis
  —Hypoxemia
- Serum levels of antidysrhythmic drugs

IMAGING/SPECIAL TESTS

- EKG
  —Diagnosis of conditions requiring temporary pacing
  —Any hemodynamically significant bradycardia
  —3rd degree AV block
    -Evidence of AV dissociation and ventricular complexes slower than atrial rate
  —Mobitz type II second degree heart block (PR interval prolongation with loss of QRS complex)
    -May be a warning of impending deterioration, especially in the setting of ischemia
  —Assess magnet rate
    -Particularly useful when the baseline EKG does not reveal pacer spikes
    -The magnet activates asynchronous pacing mode
    -Produces pacer spikes at a preprogrammed rate—regardless of the intrinsic rhythm
    -If the magnet rate equals the preprogrammed rate which was set at implantation, the pacer is OK
    -If the magnet rate is >10% slower than at implantation, the battery is depleted
    -If there are no pacer spikes there is *significant* pacemaker malfunction
- Chest Radiograph
  —Evaluate problem with pacer lead(s) and position
    -Fractured lead
    -Lead dislodgment
    -Perforation

DIFFERENTIAL DIAGNOSIS

N/A

Treatment

INITIAL STABILIZATION

- Resuscitate patients with pacemaker failure and signs of instability
- Oxygen administered via 100% nonrebreather
- Intubation as needed
- Intravenous access
- Transcutaneous pacing

ED TREATMENT

- Prepare for transvenous catheter placement
  —Candidates for thrombolytics
    -Place the central line in a compressible vessel
    -Femoral or brachial vein
  —Otherwise place cortiss in either the right internal jugular vein or the left subclavian
  —Perform the procedure under fluoroscopy if possible
  —Set the pulse generator to "asynchronous mode"
  —Turn the output dial all the way up
  —Advance the catheter through the central venous access cortiss until you see a QRS complex on the monitor
  —Check the femoral pulse
    -If you have a pulse and see a QRS complex, the pacer is "capturing"
  —Slowly turn the output dial down until your lose the QRS complex
    -This level defines the capture threshold
  —Turn the output dial up to 2 or 3 times the capture threshold
  —If the pacer is not capturing
    -Advance the catheter
    -Withdraw it
    -Twist it
  —Continuous EKG monitoring facilitates correct placement
    -Use a wire with an alligator clip at both ends
    -Hook one clip to V1 lead
    -Hook the other clip to the distal end (the negative electrode) of the pacing wire
    -As the catheter tip approaches the heart, the P wave amplitude increases
    -Once in the right atrium, the P wave becomes smaller than the QRS
    -At the tricuspid valve the deflection of the P wave changes from negative to positive
    -Once in the right ventricle, you should see pronounced ST elevation
- Following placement of the transvenous pacer, obtain a chest radiograph
  —Identify complications
    -Myocardial perforation
    -Pneumothorax
  —Check placement

MEDICATIONS

N/A

Disposition

ADMISSION CRITERIA

- All patients with permanent pacemaker failure
- CCU
- Signs of hemodynamic compromise
- All temporarily paced patients

DISCHARGE CRITERIA

- Asymptomatic pacemaker malfunction
- The pacemaker has been interrogated by a cardiologist
- The patient is not at risk for serious pacemaker failure

Miscellaneous

ICD9: 429.4

CORE CONTENT CODE: 2.11.3, 2.11.3.1, 2.11.3.2

SUGGESTED READINGS

Barold SS, Zipes DP. Cardiac pacemakers and antiarrhythmia devices. In: Braunwald E, ed. Heart disease: A textbook of cardiovascular medicine. 5th ed. Philadelphia: WB Saunders, 1997;705–731.

Ellenbogen KA, Mohanty PK, Thames MD. New insights into pacemaker syndrome gained from hemodynamic, humoral and vascular responses during ventriculo-atrial pacing. Am J Cardiol 1990;65(1):53.

Hayes DL, Vlietstra RE. Pacemaker malfunction. Ann Intern Med 1993;119:828–835.

Authors: Jill Griffin, Susan Torrey

Cardiac Transplantation Complications

Clinical Presentation

SIGNS AND SYMPTOMS

Acute rejection

- Nonspecific signs will predominate as hearts are usually denervated
  - —Fatigue
  - —Malaise
  - —Low-grade fever
  - —Nausea
  - —Vomiting
- Signs of heart failure
  - —Tachypnea
  - —Rales
  - —S3
  - —Murmur

Allograft Vasculopathy

- As early as 3 months posttransplant
- Insidious onset
  - —Fatigue
  - —Cough
- Acute onset
  - —Heart failure
  - —Sudden death
  - —Infarction
- Denervated hearts do not present with typical angina

Signs of infection

- Fever >37.5°C
- Skin lesions
- CMV
  - —Mild
    - -Fever
    - -Fatigue
    - -Vomiting
    - -Malaise
  - —Severe
    - -Pneumonitis
    - -Hepatitis
    - -Gastroenteritis
    - -Leukopenia

Pediatric Considerations

- Irritability
- Poor feeding
- Changes in sleep patterns

MECHANISM/DESCRIPTION

- Over 21,000 transplants done worldwide
- 5-year survival nationally is 67.8%
- Immunosuppression decreases rejection
- Frequent biopsies initially to evaluate rejection; echocardiography in children
- Substantial evidence indicates hearts eventually reinnervate
- Children are quickly weaned off steroids, whereas adults are left on
- Maintenance immunosuppression
- Cyclosporine or neoral (second-generation cyclosporine)
- Azathioprine or cell cept
- Complications occur most commonly in the first 6 weeks following cardiac transplant
  - —Period of heaviest immunosuppression

ETIOLOGY

- Acute rejection
  - —Most common in first 6 weeks
- Allograft vasculopathy
  - —Limits long-term survival
  - —Obliterative diffuse concentric lesions of small/medium arteries with superimposed focal plaques and thrombosis
  - —50% of hearts by 5 years
- Infection
  - —First month
    - -Nosocomial infections
    - -Pneumonia
    - -Mediastinitis
    - -UTI
  - —First year
  - —CMV
  - —HSV
  - —*Legionella*
  - —Fungal infections
  - —Pneumocystis carinii
  - —Pediatric Considerations
    - -Once off steroids, bacteremia risk similar to the general population
    - -High incidence of pneumonia
    - -Patients on steroids may not show meningeal signs
- Medication toxicity
  - —Cyclosporine
    - -Nephrotoxicity
    - -Hepatotoxicity
  - —Azathioprine
    - -Bone marrow suppression
    - -Leukopenia
  - —Steroids
    - -Osteoporosis
  - —Cushing's disease

Pre-Hospital

N/A

Diagnosis

ESSENTIAL WORKUP

- Assess for signs of rejection and cardiac dysfunction
  - —EKG
  - —Chest radiograph
  - —Echocardiography
- Blood and urine cultures if any sign of infection
- Electrolytes should be obtained to assess for cyclosporine toxicity

LABORATORY

- Electrolytes
  - —Cyclosporine effects
    - -Increased BUN, creatinine
    - -Hyperkalemia
    - -Metabolic acidosis
    - -Hyponatremia
- Fever
  - —Blood and urine culture
  - —LP if seizures, altered mental status, or severe headache
- CMV titers
- Buffy coat
- Urine antigen test
- Cyclosporine level trough
  - —Don't order random level

IMAGING/SPECIAL TESTS

- EKG
  - —New atrial arrhythmia
  - —Tachycardia
  - —20% decrease in total voltage (nonsensitive)
  - —Two P waves (native and donor heart); native p waves do not correspond to QRS
- CXR
  - —Cardiomegaly
  - —Pulmonary edema
  - —Pleural effusions
  - —Compare to previous (donor may be larger or smaller than recipient
- Echocardiography
  - —Decreased mitral deceleration time
  - —Initial diastolic dysfunction
  - —Biventricular enlargement
  - —Mitral/tricuspid regurgitation
  - —Echocardiography in pediatrics
- Possible rejection requires biopsy

DIFFERENTIAL DIAGNOSIS

- Rejection
- Cyclosporine toxicity
- Ischemia
- CMV
- Sepsis
- Viral illness
- Malignancy

PEDIATRIC CONSIDERATIONS

- Evaluate fever in standard manner *plus* chest x-ray and EKG
- If on steroids, then LP

Treatment

INITIAL STABILIZATION

- IV access
- Oxygen
- Monitor
- Intubation
- Defibrillation/pacing
- Vasopressors as required
- Arrhythmias
  —ACLS
  —Bradycardias don't respond to atropine—use isoproterenol

ED TREATMENT

- Hemodynamically significant rejection
  —Methylprednisolone
- Infarct/vasculopathy
  —Aspirin
  —Heparin
  —Possible angioplasty
  —Likely need retransplant
- CMV
  —Empiric IV ganciclovir
- HSV
  —Oral or IV acyclovir
- Diarrhea in pediatrics
  —Increase cyclosporine 25–50% in consultation with transplant team
- Fever in 3-36-month child without source
  —IM ceftriaxone after cultures
- Serious illness/trauma/operation
  —Steroid burst

MEDICATIONS

- Acyclovir: 5–10 mg/kg IV q 6 hrs (dose over 1 hr); genital herpes: 400 mg po tid × 7–10 days; varicella: 20 mg/kg up to 800 mg po qid for 5 days
- Ceftriaxone: 50 mg/kg IM
- Cyclosporine: based on *trough* levels, changed only by transplant team
- Neoral: per transplant team
- Imuran: per transplant team
- Cell cept: per transplant team
- Ganciclovir: 5 mg/kg bid for 2–3 weeks (adjust for renal function)
- Isoproterenol: 1–4 μg/min, titrate to effect max 10 μg/min
- Methylprednisolone: 1 g IV; peds: 10–20 mg/kg IV

Disposition

ADMISSION CRITERIA

- Hemodynamically significant rejection
- Vasculopathy/ischemia
- Fever in adult or child on steroids
- Suspected CMV
- Not tolerating oral medicines
- Syncope

DISCHARGE CRITERIA

- Only in consultation with transplant team
- Fever in nontoxic child
  —No steroid therapy after antibiotics
- Mild rejection

Miscellaneous

ICD9: N/A

CORE CONTENT CODE: 2.7

SUGGESTED READINGS

Chinnock R, Sherwin T, Robie S, et al. Emergency department presentation and management of pediatric heart transplant recipients. Pediatr Emerg Care 1995;11(5):355–360.

Conrad SA, Chhabra A, Vay D. Long-term follow-up and complications after cardiac transplantation. J La State Med Soc 1993;145(5):217–225.

Johnson MR. Clinical follow-up of the heart transplant recipient. Curr Opin Cardiol 1995;10:180–192.

Mill MR. Cardiac transplantation. In: Tintinalli JE, Ruiz E, Krome RL, eds. Emergency medicine: A comprehensive study guide. 4th ed. San Fransisco: McGraw-Hill, 1996: 399–404.

Authors: Virgil Davis; Samuel M. Keim

Cardiogenic Shock

Clinical Presentation

SIGNS AND SYMPTOMS

General

- Anxiety
- Hypotension
  - —Systolic blood pressure <90 mm Hg
  - —Decline by at least 30 mm Hg below baseline level
- Cyanosis
- Pallor
- Diaphoresis
- Dulled sensorium
- Decrease in body temperature
- Urine flow of less than 20 ml/hr

Neck

- Jugular venous distention

Respiratory

- Dyspnea
- Increased respiratory rate
- Rales

Cardiac

- Ischemic chest pain
- Tachycardia
- Weak, thready pulse
- Systolic apical blowing murmur
- Gallop rhythm
  - —S3 reflects severe myocardial dysfunction
  - —S4 is present in 80% patients in sinus rhythm with acute myocardial infarction
- Systolic click
  - —Suggests rupture of the chordae tendineae

Abdominal

- Epigastric pain
- Nausea and vomiting

Extremities

- Cold moist skin

Neurologic

- Obtundation

MECHANISM/DESCRIPTION

- Circulatory failure and shock due to a prior deficiency in the heart's ability to function as a pump
- Three possible underlying causes
  - —Necrosis of more than 40% of the left ventricular mass
  - —Right ventricular infarct
  - —Rupture of papillary muscles or the ventricular wall
- Patients presenting with hypotension and pulmonary edema have a 20% chance of survival
- 7–15% of patients hospitalized with AMI develop cardiogenic shock

ETIOLOGY

- Acute myocardial infarction
- Myocarditis
- Cardiomyopathy
- Valvular heart disease
- Dysrhythmias
- Drugs/toxins
  - —β-Blockers
  - —Calcium channel blockers
  - —Adriamycin

Pre-Hospital

CAUTIONS

- Supplemental oxygen
  - —100% O_2 by face mask
- Intravenous access
- Consider a small bolus of crystalloid if rales are absent
- Endotracheal intubation if loss of airway patency

CONTROVERSIES

- Transport only to a chest pain center capable of emergent catheterization

Diagnosis

ESSENTIAL WORKUP

- A careful history and physical examination is needed to exclude other causes of shock
- Ancillary studies further define the type and degree of cardiac injury and determine the indications for emergent catheterization or surgical intervention

LABORATORY

- CBC
  - —Leucocytosis is common
- ABG
  - —Used to help predict the need for airway management
  - —The patient's clinical status and the use of the pulse oximeter may be more timely
- Electrolytes
  - —Hyperkalemia is rarely associated with massive muscle destruction
- Cardiac enzymes

IMAGING/SPECIAL TESTS

- Electrocardiogram
  - —Similar findings to acute myocardial infarction
  - —Absence of EKG finding is the setting of shock makes the diagnosis very unlikely
  - —Obtain right-sided cardiac leads to determine if right ventricular infarction is present
- Echocardiography
  - —Akinetic ventricle
  - —Incompetent valve
  - —Ruptured septum, papillary muscle, or ventricular wall
- Swan-Ganz catheter
- Should be performed in the Intensive Care Unit

DIFFERENTIAL DIAGNOSIS

- Obstructive shock
  - —Myocardial infarction
  - —Right ventricular infarction
  - —Myocarditis
  - —Cardiomyopathy
  - —Drugs
    - -β-Blockers
    - -Calcium channel blockers
  - —Adriamycin
  - —Tension pneumothorax
  - —Cardiac tamponade
    - -Retrograde aortic dissection
    - -Constrictive pericarditis
  - —Pulmonary embolus
  - —Septal rupture
  - —Acute valvular incompetence
    - -Ischemia
    - -Endocarditis
  - —Spontaneous esophageal rupture
  - —"Cold" septic shock
  - —Air embolus
- Addisonian crisis
- Ruptured esophagus
- Hypovolemic shock
- Vasogenic Shock

Treatment

INITIAL STABILIZATION

- Intravenous access
- Monitor
- Endotracheal intubation
  - —Rapid sequence intubation using an induction agent with minimal cardiac effects
    - -Etomidate
    - -Fentanyl

ED TREATMENT

- Myocardial ischemia
  - —Aspirin
  - —Heparin
- Pulmonary edema
  - —Adequate blood pressure
    - -Vasodilators: nitroprusside; dobutamine; IV nitroglycerin
    - -Morphine
    - -Furosemide
    - -Amrinone if no improvement
  - —Hypotension
  - —Norepinephrine
- Right ventricular infarct
  - —Volume load
  - —Dobutamine
  - —Avoid diuretics
    - -Decreases preload, worsens already poor cardiac output
  - —Avoid dopamine
    - -Increases pulmonary vascular resistance
- Emergent cardiology consult for cardiac catheterization

MEDICATIONS

- Nitroprusside: 1–50 μg/kg/min
- Nitroglycerin: begin at 10 μg/min and increase 10 μg/min
- Furosemide: 20–100 mg IV
- Dobutamine: 2–10 μg/kg/min
- Morphine sulfate: 2–4 mg IV; may repeat q 5 min x 2
- Amrinone: 0.75 mg/kg then 5–10 μg/kg/min
- Norepinephrine: begin at 8–12 μg/min and increase infusion as needed

Disposition

ADMISSION CRITERIA

- All patients in cardiogenic shock require admission to a critical care unit

DISCHARGE CRITERIA

N/A

Miscellaneous

ICD9: 785.51

CORE CONTENT CODE: 2.2.3.3

SUGGESTED READINGS

Bengtson JR, Kaplan AJ, Pieper KS, et al. Prognosis after cardiogenic shock after acute myocardial infarction in the interventional era. J Am Coll Cardiol 1992;20:1482–1489.

Goldberg RJ, Gore JM, Alpert JS, et al. Cardiogenic shock after acute myocardial infarction: Incidence and mortality from a community-wide perspective, 1975–1988. N Engl J Med 1991;1117–1122.

Jorden RC. Cardiogenic shock. In: Harwood-Nuss A, et al., ed. The clinical practice of emergency medicine. 2d ed. Philadelphia: Lippincott-Raven, 1996. Harwood-Nuss A 591–593.

Author: Thomas Lemke

Cardiomyopathy

Clinical Presentation

SIGNS AND SYMPTOMS

Dilated Cardiomyopathy

- General
  - —Fatigue
  - —Weakness
- Respiratory
  - —Dyspnea on exertion
  - —Orthopnea
- Cardiac
  - —Chest pain
  - —S4 gallop is almost always present
  - —S3 gallop only after cardiac decompensation occurs
  - —JVD
  - —Dysrhythmias
  - —Mitral or tricuspid regurgitation
- Abdomen
  - —Enlarged, pulsatile liver
- Extremities
  - —Peripheral edema
  - —Systemic emboli

Hypertrophic Cardiomyopathy

- General
  - —Most often asymptomatic
  - —Presyncope or syncope on exertion
  - —Sudden death
- Respiratory
  - —Dyspnea
  - —Paroxysmal nocturnal dyspnea less common
- Cardiac
  - —Angina
  - —Congestive heart failure with severe outflow obstruction
  - —Ventricular arrhythmias are common
  - —Atrial fibrillation in 10% of patients
  - —Displaced LV impulse with palpable S4
  - —Systolic flow murmur at apex that increases with provocation
    - -Increases with standing
    - -Decreases with squatting

Restrictive Cardiomyopathy

- General
  - —Exercise intolerance
  - —Weakness
- Respiratory
  - —Dyspnea
  - —Pulmonary congestion
- Cardiac
  - —Exertional chest pain is usually absent
  - —JVD with Kussmaul's sign (rise with inspiration)
  - —Apex is usually easily palpated
  - —Mitral regurgitation
- Abdominal
  - —Increased abdominal girth
  - —Right upper-quadrant pain
  - —Ascites
  - —Hepatomegaly
- Extremities
  - —Edema
  - —Peripheral edema

Arrhythmogenic Right Ventricular Cardiomyopathy

- Dizziness
- Near syncope and syncope
- Palpitations
- Sudden death
- Ventricular arrhythmias

MECHANISM/DESCRIPTION

- Diseases of the myocardium associated with cardiac dysfunction
- Classification
  - —By dominant pathophysiology
  - —By specific disease with associated heart muscle abnormalities
  - —Dilated cardiomyopathy
    - -Dilated and impaired contraction of the left or both ventricles
    - -Idiopathic dilated cardiomyopathy accounts for 25% of all cases of heart failure
  - —Hypertrophic cardiomyopathy
    - -Left or right asymmetric ventricular hypertrophy
    - -Usually involves the interventricular septum
  - —Restrictive cardiomyopathy
    - -Restrictive filling and reduced volume of either or both ventricles
    - -Normal or near normal systolic function
  - —Arrhythmogenic right ventricular cardiomyopathy
    - -Progressive fibrofatty replacement of the right ventricular myocardium
    - -Relative sparing of the septum
  - —Unclassified cardiomyopathy
    - -Disorders such as fibroelastosis that do not fit into a dominant pattern
  - —Specific cardiomyopathy
    - -Heart muscle disease associated with a systemic disease or condition

ETIOLOGY

- Dilated
  - —Idiopathic
  - —Viral
  - —Genetic/toxic
  - —Immune
- Hypertrophic
  - —Familial disease with autosomal dominance
- Restrictive
  - —Idiopathic
  - —Amyloid
- Arrhythmogenic right ventricular
  - —Familial disease with dominant and recessive patterns
- Specific
  - —Infectious
    - -Lyme's disease
    - -Viral
    - -Chagas
    - -HIV
  - —Toxic agents
    - -Alcohol
    - -Chemotherapeutic agents
  - —Peripartum period
  - —Metabolic
    - -Hyperthyroidism
    - -Pheochromocytoma
  - —General systems diseases
    - -Lupus
    - -Scleroderma

Pre-Hospital

- Monitor
- Oxygen
- Avoid or use a lower dose of nitroglycerine
  - —History or suspicion of hypertrophic cardiomyopathy
- Cardioversion if with acute deterioration due to atrial fibrillation
- Left ventricular heart failure
  - —Oxygen
  - —Furosemide
  - —Morphine

Diagnosis

ESSENTIAL WORKUP

- Antecedent illness or exposure
  - —Chemotherapy
  - —HIV
  - —Lyme's disease
  - —Viral
- Underlying systemic condition
  - —Hemochromatosis
  - —Sarcoidosis
  - —Pregnancy
- Family history
  - —Familial sudden death
  - —Exertional complaints (syncope, dyspnea)

LABORATORY

- CBC
- ESR
- Cardiac enzymes
- Serologies
  - —Not useful in the emergency department

IMAGING/SPECIAL TESTS

- CXR
  - —Dilated cardiomyopathy
    - -Cardiomegaly
    - -Pulmonary congestion
    - -Pleural effusions
  - —Hypertrophic cardiomyopathy
    - -Normal to markedly increased cardiac silhouette
    - -Left atrial enlargement
  - —Restrictive cardiomyopathy
    - -Normal cardiac silhouette
    - -Pulmonary congestion
- ECG
  - —Hypertrophic cardiomyopathy
    - -LVH
    - -Abnormal septal Q waves
  - —Dilated, Lyme, Chagas, and toxic cardiomyopathies
    - -Atrial fibrillation
    - -Heart block
    - -Conduction abnormalities
- Emergency transthoracic 2D echocardiogram
  - —Indicated to confirm the diagnosis of cardiomyopathy
  - —Depressed left ventricular ejection fraction
  - —Excludes pericardial tamponade
- Formal transthoracic Doppler echocardiography
  - —Study of choice in patients with cardiomyopathy
  - —Defines morphological, functional and hemodynmiac features
  - —Identification of underlying disease
    - -Myocarditis
    - -Cardiac amyloidosis
- Nuclear scintigraphy
  - —Indicated when echocardiography is indeterminate
  - —Direct determination of the thickness of the septum and free wall
  - —Alternative assessment to echo of
    - -Ventricular volumes
    - -Ejection fraction
    - -Wall motion abnormalities
- CT and MRI distinguish between constrictive pericarditis and restrictive cardiomyopathy
- Cardiac catheterization
  - —Dilated cardiomyopathy
    - -Suspicion of ischemia
    - -Treatable systemic disease
  - —Hypertrophic cardiomyopathy
    - -Assessment of hemodynamic abnormalities

DIFFERENTIAL DIAGNOSIS

- Other causes of dyspnea
  - —COPD
  - —Asthma
  - —Interstitial lung disease
  - —Pulmonary embolism
  - —Pericardial tamponade
  - —Valvular heart disease
  - —Ischemic heart disease
  - —Hypothyroidism
  - —Constrictive pericarditis
- Other causes of syncope
  - —Hypovolemia
  - —Heat disorder
  - —Hypoglycemia

Treatment

- Inotropic and mechanical support with an intra-aortic balloon
  - —Indicated for fulminant dilated myopathy
- Anticoagulation
  - —Dilated cardiomyopathy
  - —Atrial fibrillation
  - —Systemic embolization
- Limited ED experience with agents effective in hypertrophic cardiomyopathy
  - —Disopyramide to reduce obstruction
  - —Amiodarone to convert and maintain sinus rhythm
- Standard treatment of CHF
- Standard treatment of atrial or ventricular dysrhythmias

MEDICATIONS

- Furosemide: 20–40 mg IV to a max of 200 mg on subsequent doses
- Morphine: 2–5 mg IV
- Nitroglycerine: 5 μg/min IV
- Heparin: IV push 150 IU/kg; maintenance drip 18 IU/kg/hr
- Disopyramide: 100–200 mg po q 6 hrs
- Amiodarone: 5 mg/kg over 10 min

Disposition

ADMISSION CRITERIA

- New or suspected cardiomyopathy
- Syncope where dysrhythmias or HCM are possible etiologies
- Familial history of premature sudden death
- Cardiogenic shock
  - —Consider transfer to a cardiac center capable of mechanical support and cardiac transplantation

DISCHARGE CRITERIA

- Diagnosed cardiomyopathy with mild CHF that improves with ED therapy
- Restrictive or hypertrophic cardiomyopathy
  - —Cardiology consultation for discharge planning

Miscellaneous

ICD9: 425.4

CORE CONTENT CODE: 2.2.2

SUGGESTED READINGS

Douglas WE, et al. Hypertrophic cardiomyopathy: Clinical spectrum and treatment. Circulation 1995;92:1680–1692.

Pisani B, Taylor DT, Mason JW. Inflammatory myocardial diseases and cardiomyopathies. Am J Med 1997;102:459–469.

Wynne J, Braunwald E. The cardiomyopathies and myocarditises. In: Braunwald E, ed. Heart disease: A textbook of cardiovascular medicine. 5th ed. Philadelphia: WB Saunders, 1997.

Author: James Feldman

Cardiomyopathy, Peripartum

Clinical Presentation

SIGNS AND SYMPTOMS

- Right- and left-sided symptoms from biventricular failure
- Dyspnea, orthopnea, cough, fatigue
- Cardiomegaly, pulmonary rales, S_3 gallop, peripheral edema usually present

DISEASE DESCRIPTION

- Onset of myocardial failure during last month of pregnancy or first 5 months after delivery
- Absence of a specific etiology
- Absence of a history of cardiac disease

ETIOLOGY

- Unknown, current theories favor postpartum volume overload, viral infection or immunologic response to an unknown maternal or fetal antigen
- Classified as a form of dilated cardiomyopathy

Pre-Hospital

CAUTIONS:

- It is important to differentiate an acute exacerbation of CHF from acute reactive airway disease. Both may present with shortness of breath and it may be difficult to distinguish rales, rhonchi, and wheezing in the field
- Historical clues that are useful in elderly patients (history of prior CHF or COPD; medicines appropriate for CHF or COPD) are frequently absent in pregnant patients
- Acute hypertension frequently accompanies CHF as well as other signs like peripheral edema and jugular venous distention

Diagnosis

ESSENTIAL WORKUP

- Chest x-ray—typically reveals pulmonary venous congestion, cardiomegaly
- Electrocardiogram—typically nonspecific
- Left ventricular hypertrophy, left atrial enlargement, T-wave flattening or inversion
- Arrhythmias common—ventricular ectopy (40%) and atrial fibrillation (20%)

LABORATORY

- Electrolytes, BUN, creatinine
- CK with MB fraction may be useful

IMAGING/SPECIAL TEST

- Echocardiography—demonstrates chamber enlargement and decreased ejection fraction

DIFFERENTIAL DIAGNOSIS

- Other causes of congestive heart failure and cardiomyopathy
- Pulmonary embolism
- Consider ischemia, anemia, hyperthyroidism

Treatment

INITIAL STABILIZATION

- ABCDE
  - —Prompt evaluation of respiratory and hemodynamic status
  - —Control airway as needed
  - —Supplemental oxygen
  - —Continuous positive airway pressure as needed

ED TREATMENT

- Lasix IV to control fluid retention and promote diuresis
- Digoxin IV po to control rate due to atrial fibrillation
- Anticoagulation therapy often recommended (30% cases complicated by systemic or pulmonary embolism)
- Refer to Congestive Heart Failure chapter for detailed management and medications

MEDICATION

- See Congestive Heart Failure chapter

Disposition

ADMISSION CRITERIA

- Patients with pulmonary edema, cardiogenic shock, or evidence of ischemia should be admitted to an ICU setting
- Patients with new onset CHF or symptoms not relieved by aggressive ED therapy should be admitted to a monitored setting

DISCHARGE CRITERIA

- Patients with new onset of peripartum cardiomyopathy should not be discharged

Miscellaneous

ICD9: 674.8

CORE CONTENT CODE: 2.2.2

SUGGESTED READING

Druelinger L. Postpartum emergencies. Emerg Med Clin North Am 1994;12(1):219–237

Authors: Clyde Turner; Marco Coppola

Carpal Fractures

Clinical Presentation

SIGNS AND SYMPTOMS

- Local pain
- Swelling
- Decreased range of motion of the wrist

MECHANISM

- Crush injury or direct blow
- Fall on an outstretched hand (FOOSH)

PEDIATRIC CONSIDERATIONS

- These injuries are rare in children, but the bones are poorly calcified in young children and fractures may be difficult to detect

Pre-Hospital

CAUTIONS

- Any patient with a wrist injury should be referred to a physician or ED as fractures may be easily missed on initial screening

Diagnosis

ESSENTIAL WORKUP

- A complete physical examination of the entire upper extremity and shoulder girdle is important so that associated injuries are not missed
- A set of wrist x-rays is essential

IMAGING/SPECIAL TESTS

- Special views may be obtained for most of the carpals if physical examination is suspicious
- This is one area where comparison with a good radiographic atlas may be very helpful to the less-experienced physician

DIFFERENTIAL DIAGNOSIS

- Scaphoid fracture
- Metacarpal fracture
- Distal radial or ulnar styloid fracture

PEDIATRIC CONSIDERATIONS

- Be wary of epiphyseal injuries of distal radius. Children rarely get simple sprains of the wrist

Treatment

INITIAL STABILIZATION

- Assess for other more serious injuries
- Immobilize the involved wrist pending definitive evaluation
- Intermittent ice application, elevation

ED TREATMENT

- Isolated fractures of the carpals (except the scaphoid) are very rare. If present, they should be treated with sugar-tong splinting of the wrist
- Chip fractures off the dorsal aspect of the triquetrum are treatable with simple sugar-tong splinting
- Associated injuries such as lunate or perilunate dislocation should be sought. Hamate fractures are rare, but may be associated with ulnar artery injury so an Allen test of hand circulation is imperative in a patient with this fracture
- Any open carpal fracture requires parenteral antibiotics and immediate orthopedic consultation

MEDICATIONS

- Mild oral analgesics and proper splinting should be sufficient for most of these injuries

Disposition

ADMISSION CRITERIA

- Open fractures are admitted for early operative irrigation and debridement
- Injuries requiring surgical management (open reduction) frequently are admitted for early intervention

DISCHARGE CRITERIA

- Closed nondisplaced carpal fractures treated with adequate splinting of wrist may be discharged to have orthopedic follow-up in several days

Miscellaneous

ICD9: 814.00

CORE CONTENT CODE: 18.4.12.1.3

SUGGESTED READINGS

American Society for Surgery of the Hand. The hand: Examination and diagnosis. 2d ed. New York: Churchill-Livingston, 1983

American Society for Surgery of the Hand. The hand: Primary care of common problems. 2d ed. New York: Churchill-Livingston, 1990

Chin HW, Propp DA, Orban DJ. In: Rosen P, et al. Emergency medicine: Concepts and clinical practice. 3rd ed. St. Louis: Mosby-Year Book, 1992:588–609

Uehara DT. The hand in emergency medicine. Emerg Clin North Am 1993;11(3)

Author: Matthew Walsh

Carpal Tunnel Syndrome

Clinical Presentation

SIGNS AND SYMPTOMS

- Pain
  - —Location: wrist or hand, sometimes radiating to the elbow
  - —Often worse at night—relieved by "shaking out" the hand
  - —Exacerbated by repetitive wrist movement and by activities in which the wrist is flexed (e.g., driving)
- Numbness/paresthesias in median nerve distribution (thumb, index, middle, and radial aspect of ring finger)
- Weakness of the abductor pollicis brevis and opponens muscles, which are innervated by the recurrent branch of the median nerve. Patient may complain of dropping things or having decreased fine motor control
- Atrophy of thenar muscles (a late finding)

ETIOLOGY

- Trauma
- Pregnancy, birth control pills
- Granulomatous disease: tuberculosis, sarcoidosis
- Mass lesions with median nerve compression
- Osteophytes
- Amyloid
- Multiple myeloma
- Rheumatoid arthritis
- Occupational/overuse syndromes—high impact/heavy repetition
- Endocrine disorders: hypothyroidism, diabetes mellitus, acromegaly
- Idiopathic

MECHANISM/DESCRIPTION

- The median nerve, flexor digitorum profundus, flexor digitorum superficialis, and flexor pollicis longus are located in the "carpal tunnel"—an area bound by the carpal bones and the transverse carpal ligament. Compression of the median nerve causes symptoms

SPECIAL PEDIATRIC CONSIDERATIONS

- Idiopathic carpal tunnel syndrome is rare in children. The majority have an underlying, correctable etiology including
- Trauma
- Mucolipidosis
- Hamartoma of the median nerve
- Anomalous flexor digitorum superficialis (FDS)
- Hemophilia with hematoma

Pre-Hospital

N/A

Diagnosis

ESSENTIAL WORKUP

- History of characteristic nocturnal pain and paresthesias in the median nerve distribution are essential to making the diagnosis. Muscle weakness and thenar wasting are later findings
- Provocative testing
  - —Tinel's sign: gentle tapping over the median nerve at the wrist produces tingling in the fingers in the median nerve distribution (sensitivity 64% and specificity 55%)
  - —Phalen's test: wrist flexion for 60 seconds produces numbness or tingling in the median nerve distribution (sensitivity ranges from 40% to 88%, with a specificity of 80–88%)
  - —Tourniquet test: BP cuff inflated to 200 mm Hg for 2 minutes produces paresthesias in the median nerve distribution

LABORATORY

- Not indicated in most cases
- Thyroid function studies; rheumatoid factor and immune panel if indicated by history and physical exam

IMAGING/SPECIAL TESTS

- Nerve conduction studies/electromyography = Gold Standard
- Wrist radiograph if trauma or degenerative arthritis suspected
- Computed tomography in select cases—may show encroachment of carpal tunnel
- MRI—displays the soft tissues well but has questionable value due to cost
- Ultrasound can be diagnostic

DIFFERENTIAL DIAGNOSIS

- Cervical nerve root compression—origin of median nerve is at the sixth and seventh cervical roots. Symptoms aggravated by erect posture and neck movement
- Hand-arm vibration syndrome—syndrome characterized by Raynaud's, numbness and tingling in ulnar and median nerve distributions when exposed to cold or vibration, weakened grip, and upper extremity myalgias. Associated with prolonged exposure to vibration
- Thoracic outlet obstruction
- Osteoarthritis of the first carpometacarpal joint

SPECIAL PEDIATRIC CONSIDERATIONS

None

Treatment

INITIAL STABILIZATION

- None necessary

ED TREATMENT

- Splint wrist in neutral or slightly extended position
- Aspirin or nonsteroidal anti-inflammatory medications
- Avoidance of repetitive wrist movement
- Referral to occupational medicine for ergometric testing if due to repetitive motion
- Wrist splint to be worn at night until follow up with hand surgeon
- May need referral to a hand surgeon for consideration of surgical release of transverse carpal ligament

MEDICATIONS

- Nonsteroidal anti-inflammatory agents (there are many choices, a few are listed below)
  —Diclofenac: 50 mg po bid tid
  —Ibuprofen
    -Adult: 600 mg po q 6 hrs
    -Pediatric: 5–10 mg/kg po q 6 hrs
  —Ketorolac: 30 mg IV/IM q 6 hrs or 10 mg po q 4–6 hrs
  —Piroxicam: 20 mg po qd
- Prednisolone suspension: 20–40 mg injected locally

Disposition

ADMISSION CRITERIA

None

DISCHARGE CRITERIA

- Discharge to home with appropriate follow-up with primary physician, occupational medicine, or hand surgeon

Miscellaneous

ICD9: 354.0

CORE CONTENT CODE: 10.4.5

SUGGESTED READINGS

Al-Qattan MM, Thompson HG, Clarke HM. Carpal tunnel syndrome in children and adolescents with no history of trauma. J Hand Surg 1996;21B(1):108–111

Hagberg M, Morgenstern H, Kelsh M. Impact of occupations and job tasks on the prevalence of carpal tunnel syndrome. Scand J Work Environ Health 1992;18:337–345

Pelmear P, Taylor W. Carpal tunnel syndrome and hand-arm vibration syndrome. Arch Neurol 1994;51:416–420

Whitley JM, McDonnell DE. Carpal tunnel syndrome a guide to prompt intervention. Postgrad Med 1995;97(1):89–96

Author: Linda Spillane

Cat Bite/Cat Scratch Disease

Clinical Presentation

SIGNS AND SYMPTOMS

Cat Bite Wounds

- Appearance
  - —Puncture wounds (most common)
  - —Superficial abrasions
  - —Lacerations
- Intense inflammatory response with prominent pain and swelling (due to *Pasteurella multocida*)
  - —70% within 24 hours
  - —90% within 48 hours
- Abscess formation
- Septic arthritis
- Osteomyelitis
- Sepsis

Cat Scratch Disease

- Small macule or vesicle that progresses to a papule
  - —Begins several days after inoculation
  - —Resolves within several days or weeks
- Regional lymphadenopathy occurs 3 weeks postinoculation
  - —Involves only one node
  - —Tender
  - —Nonsuppurative
  - —Resolves after 2–4 months
- Low-grade fever
- Malaise
- Headache
- Dermatologic changes (erythema nodosum)

MECHANISM/DESCRIPTION

Cat Bite Wounds

- Puncture wounds most frequent cause
- 30–50% infection rate in those seeking care

Cat Scratch Disease

- Three of the following four criteria
  - —Cat contact, with presence of scratch or inoculation lesion of the skin, eye, or mucous membrane
  - —Positive CSD skin test
  - —Characteristic lymph node histopathology
  - —Negative results of laboratory studies for other causes of lymphadenopathy

ETIOLOGY

Cat Bite Wounds

- *Pasteurella multocida*
  - —Gram-negative aerobe found in up to 80% of infections
  - —Infection appears <24 hours
- Infections developing >24 hours due to *Staphylococcus* or *Streptococcus*

Cat Scratch Disease

- Caused by *Rochalimaea henselae*

Pre-Hospital

N/A

Diagnosis

ESSENTIAL WORKUP

- Cat's behavior, provocation, location, ownership
- Time since attack

Cat Bite Wounds

- Status of tendon and nerve function
- Signs of infection

Cat Scratch Disease

- Inoculation papule or pustule at the scratch site
- Solitary or regional lymphadenopathy

LABORATORY

Cat Bite wounds

- Aerobic and anaerobic cultures from any infected bite wound

Cat Scratch Disease

- Presence of elevated titers of *Rochalimaea henselae* (newer), or
- Positive reaction to cat-scratch antigen (CSA)
  - —Inject 0.1 cc CSA intradermally
  - —Induration at the site 48–72 hours later equal to or exceeding 5 mm is positive

IMAGING/SPECIAL TESTS

- Plain radiographs
  - —If bony penetration or foreign bodies suspected

DIFFERENTIAL DIAGNOSIS

CSD-caused Lymphadenopathy

- Reactive hyperplasia (leading cause of lymphadenopathy in children under 16 years of age)
- Infection, chronic lymphadenitis, drug reaction, malignancy, and congenital conditions

Treatment

ED TREATMENT

Cat Bite wounds

- Wound irrigation
  - —Copious volumes of normal saline irrigation with an 18-gauge plastic catheter tip aimed in the direction of the puncture
  - —Avoid injection of saline through tissues planes due to force of irrigation
- Debridement
  - —Remove foreign material, necrotic skin tags, or devitalized tissues
  - —Do not debride puncture wounds
  - —Remove any eschar present so that underlying pus may be expressed and irrigated
- Primary closure of wounds
  - —Not recommended on
    - -Hand due to high morbidity associated with infection
    - -Wounds with extensive crush injury or those requiring extensive debridement
    - -Puncture wounds as these are more difficult to clean
    - -Wound older than 24 hours or infected at time of presentation
  - —Performed on other wounds after meticulous wound preparation
- Antibiotic agreed to be effective in the following
  - —Moderate or severe wounds
  - —Full-thickness puncture of hand, face, or lower extremity
  - —Wounds requiring surgical debridement
  - —Wounds involving joints, tendons, ligaments, or fractures
  - —Immunocompromised patients
  - —Wounds presenting more than 8 hours after the event
- Antibiotic choices
  - —Wound prophylaxis
    - -Amoxicillin, penicillin VK
    - -May give 1 dose of penicillin G prior to discharge
  - —Infections developing <24 hours (*P. Multocida*)—options
    - -Amoxicillin, augmentin, cefazolin, ceftriaxone, cephalexin, penicillin, tetracycline
    - -May give 1 dose of penicillin G in ED prior to discharge
  - —Infections developing >24 hours (*Staphylococcus* or *Streptococcus*)—options
    - -Dicloxacillin, cephalexin
  - —Initial empiric therapy for inpatient treatment for infections without sepsis—options
    - -Penicillin G, nafcillin
  - —Initial empiric therapy for inpatient treatment of suspected sepsis—options
    - -Imipenem/cilastatin; ampicillin/sulbactam
- Elevate injured extremity
- Tetanus prophylaxis

Rabies Immunoprophylaxis

- Not required if rabies not known or suspected
- Recommended in following situations
  - —Cat unable to be quarantined for 10 days in rabies known area
  - —Previously healthy cat becomes ill while being quarantined (and awaiting results of rabies fluorescent antibody test)
  - —An ill cat while awaiting rabies test results (to be continued or halted based on results of rabies test)
- Active Immunization
  - —Human diploid cell vaccine (HDCV): 1 cc IM on day 1, 3, 7, 14, and 28 following exposure
- Passive Immunization
  - —Human rabies immune globulin (HRIG): 20 IU/kg
  - —Up to one-half in area around wound with the rest IM

Cat Scratch Disease

- Analgesics
- Apply local heat to affected nodes
- Avoid lymph node trauma
- Antibiotics if severe disease is present as indicated by prolonged fever, systemic symptoms, and/or marked lymphadenopathy
  - —Ciprofloxacin
  - —Gentamycin
  - —Rifampin
  - —Trimethoprim-sulfamethoxazole

MEDICATIONS

- Amoxicillin (amoxil): 500 mg q 8 hrs (peds: 40 mg/kg/24hrs in 3 divided doses) po
- Amoxicillin/clavulanic acid (augmentin): 500 mg (40 mg/kg/24hrs) q 8 hrs po
- Ampicillin/sulbactam (unasyn): 1.5–3.0 g q 6 hrs IV
- Cefazolin (ancef): 1 g (peds: 25 mg/kg) IV
- Ceftriaxone (rocephin): 1 g (peds: 50 mg/kg) IM IV
- Cephalexin (keflex): 500 mg (peds: 50 mg/kg/24hrs) po q 6 hrs
- Ciprofloxacin (cipro): 500 mg q 12 hrs po or IV
- Dicloxacillin (pathocil): 500 mg q 6 hrs (peds: 50 mg/kg/24hrs) po
- Gentamycin (garamycin): 5 mg/kg/24hrs IV
- Imipenem/cilastatin (primaxin): 0.5–1.0 g (peds: 50 mg/kg/24hrs) q 6 hrs IV
- Nafcillin (unipen): 1–2 g (peds: 50–200 mg/kg/24hrs) q 4 hrs IV
- Penicillin G (pfizerpen): 1.2 million units (peds: 25,000 IU/kg) IM
- Penicillin VK (pen vee tabs): 500 mg (peds: 50 mg/kg/24hrs) q 6 hrs po
- Rifampin (rifadin): 10–20 mg/kg/24hrs q 12–24 hrs po
- Tetracycline (achromycin): 500 mg q 6 hrs po
- Trimethoprim-sulfamethoxazole (bactrim): 1 tablet (peds: 6–12 mg TMP, 30–60 mg SMX/kg/24hrs) po q 12 hrs

Disposition

ADMISSION CRITERIA

Cat Bite wounds

- Infected wounds at presentation
- Severe/advancing cellulitis/lymphangitis
- Signs of systemic infection
- Infected wounds that have failed to respond to outpatient (oral) antibiotics

Cat Scratch Disease

- Prolonged fever, systemic symptoms, and/or marked lymphadenopathy

DISCHARGE CRITERIA

- Healthy patient with localized wound infection—discharge on antibiotics with 24-hour follow-up
- 48-hour follow-up for noninfected wounds

Miscellaneous

ICD9: 879.8

CORE CONTENT CODE: 18.4.17.6

SUGGESTED READINGS

Chen SCA, Gilbert GL. Cat scratch disease: Past and present. J Paediatr Child Health 1994;30:467–469

Dire DJ. Emergency management of dog and cat bite wounds. Emerg Med Clin North Am 1992;10(4):719–734

Griego RD, et al. Dog, cat, and human bites: A review. J Am Acad Dermatol 1995;33:1019–1029

Klein JD. Cat scratch disease. Pediatr Rev 1994;15(9):348–353

Shinall EA. Cat-scratch disease: A review of the literature. Pediatr Dermatol 1990;7(1):11–18

Author: John Hipskind

Cauda Equina Syndrome

Clinical Presentation

SIGNS AND SYMPTOMS

- Back pain
- Radicular pain that may involve the buttocks, legs, perineal, and perianal regions
- Saddle anesthesia, other lower extremity sensory deficits
  —May be asymmetric
- Lower extremity motor deficits
  —Generally pure lower motor neuron deficits
- Urinary/fecal incontinence or retention
  —Often a late finding and may be mild

ETIOLOGY

- Compression of the lumbar and sacral nerve fibers in the cauda equina in the spinal canal, i.e., the nerve fibers below the conus medullaris which ends at the L1–L2 interspace
- Compression may be secondary to mass effect from a tumor, meningioma, neurofibroma, abscess, hematoma, or herniated disc, or result from blunt or penetrating trauma

Pre-Hospital

- Airway (and C-spine), breathing, and circulation
- If evidence of trauma, the patient should be transported with full spine immobilization

CAUTIONS

- Even in the nontrauma patient, spinal immobilization is important given the possibility of an unstable lesion

Diagnosis

ESSENTIAL WORKUP

- A thorough neurologic exam, including perianal sensation and rectal tone, is the most essential part of the workup
- Urinary catheterization for postvoid residual volume
  —Greater than 50–100 cc is considered abnormal

IMAGING/SPECIAL TESTS

- Plain film x-rays of the lumbosacral spine
- CT myelogram or MRI

DIFFERENTIAL DIAGNOSIS

- Conus medullaris or higher cord compression
- Osteoarthritis, sciatica, ankylosing spondylitis, spinal stenosis
- Radiculopathy from single nerve root compression
- Nonvertebral causes of leg pain (vascular claudication, hip pathology)
- Nonvertebral causes of back pain (muscular, abdominal pathology)

Treatment

INITIAL STABILIZATION

- ABCs
- Spine immobilization if trauma or unstable spine lesion is suspected
- Pain medication should be withheld, if possible, until after a neurosurgical evaluation
- NPO until evaluated by neurosurgery

ED TREATMENT

- Continuous monitoring of neurologic exam to detect progression of lesion
- When the compression is caused by an acutely herniated disc, abscess, or hematoma, decompression is urgent
- Immediate neurosurgical consultation is warranted in all cases
- If there is a suspicion of spinal cord trauma in the acute setting (<8 hours), high-dose methylprednisolone protocol should be administered

MEDICATIONS

- Morphine sulfate: adult: 2–4 mg IV q 5 min; peds: 0.1 mg/kg/dose q 5 min; max 15 mg
- Phenergan: adult: 25–50 mg IV q 4 hrs; peds: 0.25 mg/kg/dose q 4 hrs, max ½ adult dose
- High-dose steroid protocol
  —Methylprednisolone: 30 mg/kg IV bolus then 5.4 mg/kg/hr infusion over next 23 hrs

Disposition

ADMISSION CRITERIA

- All patients with acute cauda equina syndrome must be admitted to the neurosurgical service
- With rapid surgical decompression these patients have a good prognosis for recovery
- Patients presenting late (over 48 hours) have also been shown to benefit from surgical decompression

DISCHARGE CRITERIA

- Established cauda equina syndrome with prior complete evaluation and no new neurologic deficits may be discharged with close follow-up with their neurosurgeon

Miscellaneous

ICD9: 344.60

CORE CONTENT CODE: 10.3.4.5

SUGGESTED READINGS

Campana BA. Soft tissue spine injuries and back pain. In: Rosen P, et al., eds. Emergency medicine: Concepts and clinical practice. 4th ed. St. Louis: CV Mosby, 1998:878–905.

Green BA, et al. Spinal Cord Injury in Adults. In: Youmans JR, et al., eds. Neurological surgery. 4th ed. Philadelphia: WB Saunders, 1996, pp 1969–1940.

Miller DW, et al. General Methods of Clinical Examination. In: Youmans JR, et al., eds. Neurological surgery. 4th ed. Philadelphia: WB Saunders, 1996, pp 40.

Youmans, et al., eds. Neurological surgery. 4th ed. Philadelphia: WB Saunders, 1996.

Author: Kyan J. Berger

Caustic Ingestion

Clinical Presentation

SIGNS AND SYMPTOMS

Oropharyngeal

- Pain
- Erythema
- Burns
- Erosions
- Ulcers
- Drooling
- Hoarseness
- Stridor
- Aphonia
- Absence of visible lesions in the oropharynx does *not* exclude visceral injuries

Pulmonary

- Tachypnea
- Cough
- Pneumonitis if aspirated

Gastrointestinal

- Pain
- Emesis/hematemesis
- Melena, dysphagia
- Odynophagia
- Peritonitis due to perforation
- Esophageal or gastric perforation

Cardiovascular

- Tachycardia
- Hypotension
- Orthostatic changes

Hematologic

- Acid ingestion can cause RBC hemolysis

Dermatologic

- Pain
- Erythema
- First, second, or third degree burns

Ocular

- Pain
- Erythema
- Injection
- Corneal burns
- Full thickness corneal damage

Metabolic

- Metabolic acidosis

ETIOLOGY

- Direct chemical injuries
- Injuries occur secondarily to acid and alkali exposures
- Many caustic agents (Acids and alkalis) are found in common household and industrial products

Sources of Common Household and Industrial Caustics

CAUSTIC	HOUSEHOLD OR INDUSTRIAL PRODUCTS
Ammonia hydroxide	Jewelry cleaners, toilet bowl cleaners, glass cleaners, wax removers
Formaldehyde	Embalming agent
Hydrochloric acid	Toilet bowl cleaners
Hydrofluoric acid	Antirust agents, semiconductor industry
Iodines	Antiseptics
Phenol	Antiseptics, preservatives
Sodium hydroxide	Drain and oven cleaners, detergents, Clinitest tablets
Sodium borates, carbonates, phosphates, and silicates (builders)	Electric dishwasher detergent, washing machine detergent
Sodium hypochlorite	Bleach
Sulfuric acid	Automobile batteries

MECHANISM/DESCRIPTION

Alkalis

- Dissociate in the presence of H_2O to produce hydroxy (OH^-) ions which leads to liquefaction necrosis
- Postingestion—more commonly damages the esophagus than the stomach
- Esophageal damage (in the order of increasing damage) consists of
  - —Superficial hyperemia
  - —Mucosal edema
  - —Superficial blisters
  - —Exudative ulcerations
  - —Full-thickness necrosis
  - —Perforation
  - —Fibrosis with resulting esophageal strictures
- Do *not* directly produce systemic complications

Acids

- Dissociate in the presence of H_2O to produce hydrogen (H^+) ions which leads to a coagulation necrosis with eschar formation
- Postingestions—more commonly damage the stomach due to rapid transit time through esophagus
- Gastric damage (in the order of increasing damage) consists of
  - —Edema
  - —Inflammation
  - —Immediate or delayed hemorrhage
  - —Full-thickness necrosis
  - —Perforation
  - —Fibrosis with resulting gastric outlet obstruction
- Well-absorbed and can cause hemolysis of RBCs and a systemic metabolic acidosis

Pre-Hospital

CAUTIONS

- For oral burns or symptoms: rinse mouth liberally with water or milk
- Dilute stomach contents with oral fluids (5 cc/kg up to 250 cc)
- Copious irrigation for ocular/dermal exposure

Diagnosis

ESSENTIAL WORKUP

- History of or signs and symptoms of an exposure
- Absence of oropharyngeal lesions does *not* exclude visceral injury

LABORATORY

- CBC
- Electrolytes, BUN, Cr, glucose
- Arterial blood gas
- Blood cultures
  —If mediastinitis or peritonitis suspected
- Type and cross-match

IMAGING/SPECIAL TESTS

- CXR/abdominal radiographs for
  —Esophageal/gastric perforation
- Esophageal and gastric endoscopy
  —For symptomatic patients to determine the extent of injury
  —Perform within the first 12–24 hours after ingestion
  —Not recommended in the presence of respiratory distress without proper airway management
  —Not recommended in the presence of severe pharyngeal damage
- Radiographic contrast imaging not recommended acutely
  —May be used in follow-up for strictures

DIFFERENTIAL DIAGNOSIS

- Chemical injuries from corrosives, acids, alkalis, desiccants, vesicants, and oxidizing and reducing agents
- Foreign body ingestion
- Upper airway infection/angioedema

Treatment

INITIAL STABILIZATION

- ABCs
  —Prophylactic intubation if there is any evidence of respiratory compromise
  —Blind nasotracheal intubation contraindicated
- Treat hypotension with 0.9%NS IV fluid resuscitation

ED TREATMENT

Decontamination

- Dermal/ocular exposure
  —Immediate and thorough irrigation with water or 0.9%NS until physiologic pH attained
  —Alkalis require more irrigation than acids
- Ipecac, activated charcoal, gastroesophageal lavage, or a neutralizing acid or base contraindicated with caustic ingestions
- Dilution
  —250 cc (5 cc/kg) of water in the first 30 minutes of ingestion
  —Especially useful for solid caustic alkali ingestions
  —Excessive intake may induce vomiting and worsen esophageal damage
  —If respiratory distress, intubate prior to dilution
  —Contraindicated if esophageal/gastric perforation suspected

ADDITIONAL THERAPY

- NPO if oral exposure
- Broad spectrum antibiotics if mediastinitis or peritonitis suspected
- Antiemetics for nausea/vomiting
- Treat dermal exposures according to standard burn recommendations
- Detailed examination for ocular exposures
- Intravenous H_2 blockers for symptomatic relief
- Gastroenterology and surgical consultation
- Benefit of corticosteroids following esophageal damage is controversial
  —May prevent the formation of esophageal stricture
  —May promote bacterial invasion, immune suppression, and tissue softening
  —The decision to initiate corticosteroids requires input from entire team caring for patient
- Laparoscopy or laparotomy for perforation/full-thickness necrosis
- Topical hydrofluoric acid exposure (options depend on severity/location)
  —Intradermal injection of 10% calcium gluconate (0.5 ml/cm^2 of skin with 30-gauge needle)
  —Intra-arterial infusion of 10 ml of 20% calcium gluconate in 40 ml D5W over 4 hours

MEDICATIONS

- Methylprednisolone: 125 mg (peds: 2 mg/kg) IV
- Prochlorperazine (compazine): 5–10 mg IV (peds: 0.13 mg/kg/dose IM)
- Ranitidine (zantac): 50 mg IV q 6–8 hrs

Disposition

ADMISSION CRITERIA

- All symptomatic patients
- Nonaccidental ingestion

DISCHARGE CRITERIA

- Asymptomatic patients who accidentally ingested and are able to swallow without difficulty
- Minimal oropharyngeal pain with a corresponding visible lesion, no drooling, no respiratory compromise, no deep throat, chest, or abdominal pain, and able to swallow without difficulty can be discharged

Miscellaneous

ICD9: 983.2, 983.1

CORE CONTENT CODE: 17.2.15

SUGGESTED READINGS

Anderson KD, Rouse TM, Randolph JG. A controlled trial of corticosteroids in children with corrosive injury of the esophagus. N Engl J Med 1990;323:10:637–640

Hoffman RS. Caustics and batteries. In Goldfrank LR, Flomenbaum NE, Hoffman RS, et al., eds. Goldfrank's toxicologic emergencies. 5th ed. Norwalk, CT: Appleton and Lange 1994:1245–1263

Homan CS, Maitra SR, Lane BP, Geller ER. Effective treatment of acute alkali injury of the rat esophagus with early saline dilution therapy. Ann Emerg Med 1993;22:2:178–182

Author: Paul Kolecki

Cavernous Sinus Thrombosis

Clinical Presentation

SIGNS AND SYMPTOMS

Symptoms

- Headache
- Deep retrobulbar pain
- Fever
- Eyelid and facial swelling
- Dysesthesias of the forehead and cheek
- Diplopia/decreased visual acuity
- Progressive confusion and lethargy

Signs

- Ptosis
- Chemosis
- Periorbital and facial edema
- Ophthalmoplegia/unreactive pupil
- Retinal edema and hemorrhage/papilledema
- Confusion, lethargy, coma
- Cardiovascular collapse

MECHANISM/DESCRIPTION

Anatomy

- Cavernous sinuses lie superolateral to the sphenoid sinus and surround the sella
- Cranial nerves (CN) III, IV, V1, V2 traverse the lateral wall of the sinus
- CN VI and the internal carotid artery occupy the medial portion of the sinus

Pathophysiology

- Local head and neck infections seed the cavernous sinuses via the superior ophthalmic veins
- Static flow through the sinuses favors bacterial growth that incites an inflammatory response, leads to fibrin formation and platelet aggregation, and culminates in thrombosis
- Once thrombosed, the obstructive signs and symptoms that define the cavernous sinus syndrome rapidly evolve
- Fulminant infection may seed the meninges or spread systemically
- Obstruction of the superior ophthalmic, facial, and retinal veins gives rise to chemosis, periorbital and facial edema, and retinal engorgement and hemorrhage
- Inflammation of the cranial nerves leads to
  - -Ophthalmoplegia (CN III, VI, VI)
  - -Pupillary fixation (III)
  - -Dysesthesias of the forehead and cheek (V1, V2)
  - -Loss of the corneal reflex (V1)
- Local extension may cause pituitary necrosis and hypopituitarism
- Intracranial extension may cause meningitis, subdural empyema, intracerebral abscesses
- Extension to the internal carotid artery can cause thrombosis with hemiplegia, or erosive hemorrhage
- Blindness may result from
  - —Central retinal artery occlusion
  - —Central retinal vein occlusion
  - —Septic emboli
  - —Arteritis
  - —Ischemic optic neuritis
  - —Glaucomatous optic atrophy
  - —Corneal ulceration from loss of corneal reflex
- Septic emboli may cause distant abscesses, sepsis, death
- Mortality: 12–30%
- Morbidity: cranial neuropathies, blindness, seizures, vascular steal syndrome, hypopituitarism, and hemiparesis

ETIOLOGY

- *Septic* cavernous sinus thrombosis begins with
  - —Localized infection of the midface or sinuses (most common)
  - —Pharyngitis, otitis, odontogenic infections, head and neck surgery, and facial trauma
  - —Leading organism: *Staphylococcus aureus*
- *Aseptic* cavernous sinus thrombosis rare
  - —Granulomatous conditions (TB)
  - —Inflammatory disorders
  - —From mass effect (tumors at base of skull, aneurysms)
  - —Hypercoagulable states (postoperation, malignancy, pregnancy, oral contraceptives)

Pre-Hospital

N/A

Diagnosis

ESSENTIAL WORKUP

- Clinical diagnosis based on Eagleton's criteria
  - —Symptoms of venous obstruction
  - —Ophthalmoplegia
  - —Sepsis or meningitis
  - —Symptoms that begin unilateral and spread to become bilateral are diagnostic

LABORATORY

- CBC—leukocytosis, sometimes anemia
- Electrolytes, BUN, Cr, glucose
- PT, PTT, platelets
- Blood cultures—usually positive if septic
- CSF examination—may reveal a parameningeal infection or meningitis

IMAGING/SPECIAL TESTS

- MRI
  - —Leading modality for visualization of the dural venous sinuses
  - —Capable of visualizing thrombus at any stage
- Dynamic CT
  - —Bolus contrast infusion and rapid serial thin coronal sectioning has made CT competitive with MRI
  - —Findings include delayed filling of the involved sinus, a filling defect (thrombus), and a dilated superior ophthalmic vein
- Conventional CT
  - —Useful to detect cerebral hemorrhage or abscess
  - —Distinguishes between orbital cellulitis and early cavernous sinus thrombosis
- Orbital venography and carotid arteriography
  - —Replaced by less invasive technology
  - —Useful when CT is nondiagnostic and MRI is unavailable
- Two-Dimensional Time of Flight MR Angio (2D TOF MRA) flow studies and gadolinium-DTPA–enhanced MRI are promising modalities that may be of use in the future
- CXR
  - —Indicated as with all toxic patients
  - —May demonstrate septic pulmonary emboli or ARDS

DIFFERENTIAL DIAGNOSIS

- Should distinguish *septic* from *aseptic* thrombosis
- Early presentation of periorbital edema and chemosis may mimic *allergic blepharitis*
- *Orbital cellulitis:* unilateral and has a less toxic course
- Tolosa-Hunt syndrome (superior orbital fissure syndrome, idiopathic granulomatous inflammation of the cavernous sinus) has similar signs, but is slowly progressive and nontoxic

Treatment

INITIAL STABILIZATION

- IV fluids and empirical antibiotics as soon as diagnosis is suspected

ED TREATMENT

- Antibiotics
  —Nafcillin with metronidazole or chloramphenicol
  —If penicillin allergic, substitute vancomycin for nafcillin
- Anticoagulation
  —Significantly improves morbidity and may improve survival
  —Initiate only after CT shows absence of hemorrhage
- Drainage of any focal source of infection (sinus, mastoid) should be considered
  —Emergent consultation with a head and neck surgeon
- Eye protection to avoid corneal ulceration
- Steroids in aseptic thrombosis, or in septic thrombosis complicated by hypotension from pituitary insufficiency
- Fibrinolytics (urokinase, streptokinase) have been used anecdotally

MEDICATIONS

- Chloramphenicol: 1.0 g (peds: 50–100 mg/kg/24hrs) IV q 6 hrs
- Heparin: titrated to PTT 1.5–2.0 control
- Methylprednisolone: 125 mg (peds: 1–2 mg/kg) IV
- Metronidazole: 1.0 g (peds: 15 mg/kg) load, followed by 500 mg (7.5 mg/kg) IV q 6 hrs
- Nafcillin: 1.5 g (peds: 100 mg/kg/24hrs) IV q 4 hrs
- Vancomycin: 500 mg (peds: 10 mg/kg) IV q 6 hrs

Disposition

ADMISSION CRITERIA

- Admit all patients with suspected septic cavernous sinus thrombosis

DISCHARGE CRITERIA

None

Miscellaneous

ICD9: 607.2/325

CORE CONTENT CODE: N/A

SUGGESTED READINGS

DiNubile MJ. Septic thrombosis of the cavernous sinuses. Arch Neurol 1988;45:567–572

Karlin RJ, et al. Septic cavernous sinus thrombosis. Ann Emerg Med 1984;13(6):449–455

Southwick FS, et al. Septic thrombosis of the dural venous sinuses. Medicine (Baltimore) 1986;65(2):82–106

Tveteras K, et al. Septic cavernous and lateral sinus thrombosis. J Laryngol Otol 1988;102(10):877–882

Author: Karen Cosby

Cellulitis

Clinical Presentation

SIGNS AND SYMPTOMS

- Signs and symptoms common to the various cellulitis syndromes include
  - —Pain, tenderness, warmth
  - —Erythema
    - -Margin of erythema not sharply defined or elevated
  - —Edema/induration
  - —Fever/chills
  - —Tender regional lymphadenopathy
  - —Proximal lymphangitis
  - —Malaise
  - —Anorexia
  - —Accompanying subcutaneous abscess possible, with necrosis of overlying skin
  - —Superficial vesicles may develop
- Facial cellulitis in adults
  - —Milder cases with local erythema and swelling usually secondary to skin trauma
  - —Odontogenic cases more serious
    - -Presenting symptom may be toothache, sore throat or facial swelling
    - -Progressive extension into soft tissues of the neck accompanied by fever, erythema, neck swelling, and dysphagia

Pediatric Presentations

- Facial cellulitis in children
  - —Erythema and swelling of the cheek and eyelid
  - —Rapidly progressive
  - —Usually unilateral
  - —Upper respiratory tract symptoms
  - —Risk of cavernous sinus thrombosis and permanent optic nerve injury
- Perianal cellulitis
  - —Erythema and pruritus extending from the anus several centimeters onto adjacent skin
  - —Pain upon defecation
  - —Blood streaked stools

MECHANISM/DESCRIPTION

- Acute, spreading erythematous superficial infection of the skin and subcutaneous tissues
  - —Several specific types caused by a variety of pathogens
  - —Extension into deeper tissues can result in necrotizing soft tissue infection
- Progressive spread of erythema, warmth, pain and tenderness, usually with edema and induration
  - —Confluent or patchy
- Predisposing factors include
  - —Open wounds, including superficial abrasions, cracks, and traumatic wounds
  - —Preexisting skin lesion (furuncle)
  - —Prior surgery or trauma
  - —Vascular or immune compromise

ETIOLOGY

- Simple cellulitis
  - —*Staphylococcus aureus*
  - —Streptococcus groups A and B
- Extremity cellulitis after lymphatic disruption (saphenous venectomy, axillary node dissection, chronic lymphedema)
  - —Group A β-hemolytic Streptococci
- Facial cellulitis
  - —*Haemophilus influenzae* type B
  - —*S. pneumoniae*
  - —*Staphylococcus aureus,* associated with trauma
  - —Anaerobic oral flora, associated with intraoral laceration or dental abscess
- Facial cellulitis in children with no apparent portal of entry
  - —*Haemophilus influenzae* type B
  - —*S. pneumoniae*
- Less common causes
  - —Clostridia
  - —Anthrax
  - —*Pasteurella multocida*—common after cat and dog bites
  - —*Pseudomonas aeruginosa*
  - —*Erysipelothrix sp.*—raw fish or poultry handlers

PEDIATRIC CONSIDERATIONS

- Perianal cellulitis
- Group A Streptococcus
- Associated with antecedent pharyngitis

Pre-Hospital

- No specific considerations

Diagnosis

ESSENTIAL WORKUP

- Cellulitis is *a clinical diagnosis*
- Physical examination to reveal infection source

LABORATORY

- White blood count is not necessary
- If there is a source lesion, Gram's stain and culture may focus antimicrobial selection
  - —Aspiration and culture of the leading edge are not helpful
  - —Blood cultures usually negative
- Sedimentation rate mildly elevated

IMAGING/SPECIAL TESTS

- Plain radiographs may reveal abscess formation, subcutaneous gas, or foreign bodies
  - —*Extension to bone (osteomyelitis) not visualized early on plain radiographs*
- Extremity vascular imaging (Doppler ultrasound) can help rule out deep venous thrombosis

DIFFERENTIAL DIAGNOSIS

- Lymphangitis/lymphadenitis
- Thrombophlebitis/deep venous thrombosis
  - —Differentiation from cellulitis
    - -Absence of an initial traumatic or infectious focus
    - -No regional lymphadenopathy
    - -Presence of risk factors for DVT
- Insect bite
- Allergic reaction
- Acute gout/pseudogout
- Fasciitis/myositis
- Ruptured Baker's cyst
- Herpetic whitlow
- Cutaneous diphtheria

PEDIATRIC CONSIDERATIONS

- Differential diagnosis of *facial cellulitis*
  - —Allergic angioedema
  - —Conjunctivitis
  - —Contusion
- Differential diagnosis of *perianal cellulitis*
  - —Candida intertrigo
  - —Psoriasis
  - —Pin worm infection
  - —Child abuse
  - —Behavioral problem
  - —Inflammatory bowel disease

Treatment

INITIAL STABILIZATION

- Ensure adequate ABCs and hemodynamic stability
  - —*Airway compromise* possible with deep extension of facial cellulitis

ED TREATMENT

- Antibiotics by type of infection
  - —*Simple cellulitis*
    - -Oral first generation cephalosporins or dicloxacillin: 7–10 days
    - -IV cefazolin in the ED followed by one of the above at home, or by outpatient ceftriaxone for more severe cases
    - -IV first generation cephalosporin for inpatients, guided by culture results
  - —*Facial cellulitis in adults*
    - -Simple cases treated as for *simple cellulitis*
    - -If odontogenic source, drainage essential and airway compromise possible
    - -Include coverage for anaerobes: clindamycin, amoxicillin clavulanate, or erythromycin
  - —*Facial cellulitis in children*
    - -IV ceftriaxone, followed by amoxicillin clavulanate or cephalexin once improved
  - —*Perianal cellulitis*
    - -Penicillin
- Cool compresses for comfort
- Analgesics
- *Extremity elevation*

MEDICATIONS

- Amoxicillin clavulanate: adult: 500–875 mg po bid or 250–500 mg po tid; ped: 45 mg/kg/day po divided bid or 40 mg/kg/day po divided tid
- Azithromycin: adult and pediatric dosing: 10 mg/kg up to 500 mg po on day 1, followed by 5 mg/kg up to 250 mg po qd to complete 5 days
- Cefazolin: adult: 1–2 g IV q 6–8 hrs; ped: 50–100 mg/kg/day IV divided q 6–8 hrs
- Cephalexin: adult: 250–500 mg po qid; ped: 25–50 mg/kg/day po divided qid
- Clindamycin: adult: 450–900 mg IV q 8 hrs; ped: 20–40 mg/kg/day divided q 6–8 hrs
- Dicloxacillin: adult: 125–500 mg po qid; ped: 12.5–25 mg/kg/day po divided q 6 hrs
- Erythromycin base: adult: 250–500 mg po qid or 333 mg po tid; ped: Erythromycin ethyl succinate 30–50 mg/kg/day po divided qid
- Procaine Penicillin G: adult: 600,000 units IM bid initially, followed by Penicillin VK 250–500 mg po qid for those with mild illness. If toxic appearing, 600,000–2,000,000 units IV q 6 hrs; ped: 25–50,000 units/kg/day IM divided q 12 hrs, followed by Penicillin VK 25–50 mg/kg/day po divided qid. If toxic appearing, 100,000–400,000 units/kg/day IV divided q 6 hrs

Disposition

ADMISSION CRITERIA

- Toxic appearing
- Tissue necrosis
- History of immune suppression
- Concurrent chronic medical illnesses
- Unable to take oral medications
- Unreliable patients

DISCHARGE CRITERIA

- Mild infection in a nontoxic-appearing patient
- Able to take oral antibiotics
- No history of immune suppression or concurrent medical problems
- No hand or face involvement
- Has adequate follow-up within 24–48 hours

Miscellaneous

ICD9: 682.9

CORE CONTENT CODE: 3.2.1.2, 13.12.1.1

SUGGESTED READINGS

Abyad A. Cellulitis. In: Dambro M, ed. Griffith's 5-minute clinical consult [CD-ROM]. Baltimore: Williams & Wilkins, 1997

Magnussen CR. Skin and soft-tissue infections. In: Reese RE, Betts RF, eds. A practical approach to infectious diseases. 4th ed. Boston: Little, Brown and Co., 1996:96–132

O'Hanley P. Fungal, bacterial, and viral infections of the skin. In: Federman DD, ed. Scientific american medicine. New York: Scientific American, 1997;2(VII):1–23

Swartz MN. Cellulitis and subcutaneous tissue infections. In: Mandell GE, Bennett JE, Dolin R, eds. Mandell, Douglas and Bennett's principles and practice of infectious diseases. 4th ed. New York: Churchill-Livingstone, 1995:909–929

Author: John F. Mahoney

Cerebral Aneurysm

Clinical Presentation

SIGNS AND SYMPTOMS

- Commonly asymptomatic prior to rupture
- Sentinel headaches occur in 30–60% of patients prior to rupture; can be unilateral
- Seizures
- *Compression* of adjacent structures may cause neurologic symptoms
  —ACA aneurysms
    -Optic tract: altitudinal field cut or homonymous hemianopsia
    -Optic chiasm: bitemporal hemianopsia
    -Optic nerve: unilateral amblyopia
  —Aneurysms at the internal carotid-posterior communicating artery junction
    -Oculomotor nerve: fixed and dilated pupil, ptosis, diplopia, and temporal deviation of the eye with an inability to turn the eye upward, inward, or downward
  —Aneurysms in the cerebral cortex may produce focal deficits, including hemiparesis, hemisensory loss, visual disturbances, aphasia, and seizures
- *Rupture* results in *Subarachnoid Hemorrhage,* (SAH)
  —Headache; severe ("worst headache ever") with *sudden* onset ("thunderclap"); different from prior headaches; classically without focal deficits
  —Nuchal rigidity (most common sign)

DESCRIPTION

- An abnormal, localized dilation or outpouching of the wall of a cerebral artery occurring in 2–5% of the population
- Of those that rupture, 40% occur at the anterior communicating artery, 30% at the internal carotid, 20% in the middle cerebral artery, and 5–10% in the vertebrobasilar system

ETIOLOGY

- "Congenital" or Berry aneurysms, are the most common
  —Develop at weak points in the arterial wall and occur at bifurcations of major cerebral arteries
  —Incidence increases with age
  —Multiple in 20%
  —Increased incidence with polycystic kidney disease, cerebral AVM, type III collagen deficiency, fibromuscular dysplasia, Ehlers-Danlos syndrome, Marfan's syndrome, pseudoxanthoma elasticum, neurofibromatosis, moyamoya, coarctation of the aorta
- Arteriosclerotic (fusiform)
  —more common in peripheral arteries
- Inflammatory (mycotic)
  —10% of patients with bacterial endocarditis
- Traumatic, associated with severe closed head injury

PEDIATRIC CONSIDERATIONS

- Although rare in children, they are more likely to be giant (>25 mm) and occur in the posterior circulation
- Aneurysms in children have a high rate of hemorrhage and should be repaired early

Pre-Hospital

CAUTIONS

- Patients with SAH may need emergent intubation from rapidly deteriorating level of consciousness
- Patients must be transported to a hospital with emergent CT scanning and ICU-level treatment
- Neurological examination in the field can be extremely helpful. Assess level of consciousness, Glasgow Coma Scale score, gross motor deficits, speech abnormalities, gait disturbance, facial asymmetry, and other focal deficits

Diagnosis

ESSENTIAL WORKUP

- Emergent noncontrast head CT scan will diagnose >90% of SAHs
- Complete neurological examination
- Lumbar puncture with CSF analysis if CT scan is negative

LABORATORY

- Coagulation studies
- Baseline CBC, electrolytes, renal, and liver function tests

IMAGING/SPECIAL TESTS

- Chest x-ray—pulmonary edema
- 4-Vessel cerebral angiography remains the Gold Standard
- Transcranial Doppler ultrasound may be useful to detect vasospasm
- Magnetic resonance angiography (MRA)
- Helical CT scanning may be useful in detecting aneurysms >3 mm

DIFFERENTIAL DIAGNOSIS

- Neoplasm
- Arteriovenous malformation (AVM)
- Optic neuritis
- Migraine
- Meningitis
- Encephalitis
- Hypertensive encephalopathy
- Temporal arteritis
- Acute glaucoma
- Subdural hematoma
- Epidural hematoma
- Intracerebral hemorrhage
- Thromboembolic stroke
- Air embolism
- Sinusitis

Treatment

INITIAL STABILIZATION

- ABCs for patients with SAH
  —Supplemental oxygen
  —Continuous cardiac monitoring and pulse oximetry
  —Rapid sequence intubation may be required for airway protection, or for hyperventilation
- For altered mental status, give naloxone, D_{50} (or check blood glucose immediately), thiamine
- Management of acute hypertension is essential; this may be accomplished with labetalol, nitroprusside, or hydralazine
- Prevention of acute increases in intracranial pressure from vomiting should be accomplished with antiemetics
- Seizures should be managed acutely with intravenous benzodiazepines and phenytoin

ED TREATMENT

- Following initial stabilization, the major goals of early treatment of ruptured or leaking aneurysms are to prevent re-rupture, cerebral vasospasm, and hydrocephalus. See SAH chapter

Definitive Therapy of Aneurysm

- Optimal timing for angiography and surgery remain controversial, but there is a trend toward early surgery to decrease the incidence of rebleeding and cerebral vasospasm. Some patients may be candidates for interventional neuroradiologic treatment with detachable balloons or coils

MEDICATIONS

- Diazepam: 5–10 mg IV q 10–15 min, max 30 mg; peds: 0.2–0.3 mg/kg q 5–10 min, max 10 mg
- Docusate sodium: 100 mg po bid
- Hydralazine: 10–20 mg IV q 30 min
- Labetalol: 20 mg/min IV bolus, then 20–80 mg q 10 min, max 300 mg; follow with continuous infusion 0.5–2 mg/min
- Lorazepam: 2–4 mg IV q 15 min PRN; peds: 0.03–0.05 mg/kg/dose, max 4 mg/dose
- Nitroprusside: 0.25–10 μg/kg/min (adult and peds)
- Phenytoin: 20 mg/kg IV load at max 50 mg/min, max 1.5 g (adult and peds)
- Prochlorperazine: 5–10 g IV/IM q 6–8 hrs; peds: 0.2 mg/kg/d IM in 3–4 divided doses, max 40 mg/d

Disposition

ADMISSION CRITERIA

- Any patient with an acute aneurysmal subarachnoid hemorrhage should be admitted, preferably to an ICU
- Any patient with a symptomatic unruptured aneurysm should receive admission and urgent neurosurgical consultation given the high rate of rupture

DISCHARGE CRITERIA

- Patients with incidentally discovered asymptomatic intracranial aneurysms may be discharged with close neurosurgical follow-up
- Note that the overall risk of rupture is 1–2% per year, and that the critical size at which the risk of rupture outweighs the risk of surgery is controversial (classically 10 mm, but probably in the 4–8-mm range)

Miscellaneous

ICD9: 437.3

CORE CONTENT CODE: 11.1.1.1

SUGGESTED READINGS

Cerebrovascular diseases. In: Adams RD, Victor M, eds. Principles of neurology. 5th ed. New York: McGraw-Hill, 1993

Barrow DL, Reisner A. Natural history of intracranial aneurysms and vascular malformations. Clin Neurosurg 1993;40:3–39

Barsan WG, Kothari R. Stroke. In: Rosen P, et al., eds. Emergency medicine: Concepts and clinical practice. 4th ed. St. Louis: CV Mosby, 1997:2184–2197.

Linn FHH, Wijdicks EFM, van der Graaf Y, et al. Prospective study of sentinel headache in aneurysmal subarachnoid hemorrhage. Lancet 1994;344:590–593

Meyer FB, Morita A, Puumala MR, Nichols DA. Medical and surgical management of intracranial aneurysms. Mayo Clin Proc 1995;70(2):153–172

Authors: James D.R. Foster; Rebecca Smith-Coggins

Cerebral Vascular Accident

Clinical Presentation

SIGNS AND SYMPTOMS

- Aphasia
- Hemiparesis, hemiplegia
- Dysarthria, dysphagia
- Facial droop
- Ataxia, clumsiness
- Visual loss, photophobia, diplopia
- Headache
- Nausea, vomiting
- Vertigo, dizziness
- Altered level of consciousness, confusion, agitation
- Cardiac dysrhythmias, murmurs
- Cheyne-Stokes breathing, apnea
- Hypertension
- Transient ischemic attacks (TIA), focal neurological deficits that completely resolve in <24 hours, precede most thrombotic CVA

Anterior Cerebral Artery

- Contralateral hemiplegia (lower > upper), hemisensory loss, apraxia, confusion, impaired judgment

Middle Cerebral Artery

- Contralateral hemiplegia (upper > lower), hemisensory deficits, homonymous hemianopsia, dysphasia, dyslexia, agnosia
- Posterior cerebral artery
- Cortical blindness in half the visual field, visual agnosia, altered mental status, impaired memory, third nerve palsy, hemiballismus
- Vertebrobasilar System
- Impaired vision, visual field defects, nystagmus, diplopia
- Vertigo, dizziness
- Facial paresthesia, dysarthria, cranial nerve palsies, contralateral pain, and temperature deficits

DESCRIPTION

- A cerebrovascular accident (CVA), or stroke, is an interruption of the blood flow to a specific region of the brain, resulting in an array of neurologic findings determined by the specific area affected. The onset may be sudden and complete, or stuttering and intermittent

ETIOLOGY

- CVA may be ischemic (thrombotic or embolic) or hemorrhagic (intracranial or subarachnoid hemorrhage)
- Risk factors include diabetes, smoking, hypertension, coronary artery disease, peripheral vascular disease, oral contraceptive use, polycythemia vera, sickle cell anemia, and deficiencies of antithrombin III, protein C, or protein S
- *Thrombotic stroke* is caused by occlusion of blood vessels
  —Clot formation at an ulcerated atherosclerotic plaque is most common
  —Sludging (sickle cell anemia, polycythemia vera, protein C deficiency), arterial dissection, arteritis, or fibromuscular dysplasia
- *Embolic stroke* is caused by acute blockage of a cerebral artery by a piece of foreign material from outside the brain, including
  —Cardiac mural thrombi associated with mitral stenosis, atrial fibrillation, cardiomyopathy, congestive heart failure, or myocardial infarction
  —Prosthetic heart valves or abnormal native valves
  —Atherosclerotic plaques in the aortic arch or carotid arteries
  —Atrial myxoma
  —Ventricular aneurysms with ventricular thrombi

PEDIATRIC CONSIDERATIONS

- CVA in childhood are usually attributable to an underlying disease process such as sickle cell anemia, leukemia, or a blood dyscrasia

Pre-Hospital

CAUTIONS

- Patients may have difficulty moving or communicating following CVA
- Hyperglycemia may exacerbate an ischemic insult. Perform rapid blood glucose testing prior to administration of glucose containing fluids
- Neurological examination in the field is helpful and should include assessment of level of consciousness, Glasgow Coma Scale score, gross motor deficits, speech abnormalities, gait disturbance, facial asymmetry, and other focal deficits

Diagnosis

ESSENTIAL WORKUP

- Emergent noncontrast head CT scan to distinguish ischemic from hemorrhagic events; may be normal in the first 24–48 hours of ischemic stroke
- If CT normal and subarachnoid hemorrhage suspected, emergent lumbar puncture is indicated
- Electrocardiogram to evaluate for dysrhythmias and the presence of MI

LABORATORY

- Baseline CBC, electrolytes, renal function tests, LFT, PT/PTT
- Urinalysis—hematuria is seen in subacute bacterial endocarditis (SBE) with embolic stroke
- Sedimentation rate—elevated in SBE, vasculitis, hyperviscosity syndromes

IMAGING/SPECIAL TESTS

- Chest x-ray
- Echocardiography
- Carotid ultrasonography
- MRI can detect ischemia <2 hours after onset

DIFFERENTIAL DIAGNOSIS

- Intracranial bleeding
- Hypoglycemia
- Seizure disorder
- Panic attacks, depression
- Head trauma
- Meningitis
- Migraine
- Air embolism
- Transient ischemic attack (TIA)
- Hypertensive encephalopathy
- Neoplasm
- Subdural hematoma
- Giant cell arteritis

Treatment

INITIAL STABILIZATION

- ABCs
  - —Supplemental oxygen 2–4 L via nasal cannula
  - —IV access
  - —Cardiac monitoring and pulse oximetry
  - —Rapid sequence intubation may be required for airway protection or hyperventilation to decrease intracranial pressure (ICP)
- For altered mental status, give naloxone, thiamine, and check blood glucose

ED TREATMENT

- Treat elevated blood pressure if systolic BP >220 or diastolic BP >120 on repeated measurements, or if indicated for other concurrent problems (MI, aortic dissection, CHF, hypertensive encephalopathy)
- Control seizures with benzodiazepines then phenytoin
- Maintain euvolemia
- *Thrombolytics*
  - —Ischemic stroke only; administer within 3 hours of symptom onset
  - —Contraindications: hemorrhage on CT, recent stroke, severe head trauma, systolic BP >185, diastolic BP >110, active internal bleeding, bleeding diathesis, anticoagulation, intracranial neoplasm
  - —Avoid anticoagulants and antiplatelet drugs for 24 hours
- Treat increased ICP and cerebral edema
  - —Elevate head of bed 30°
  - —Hyperventilation to keep PCO_2 30 mm Hg
  - —Mannitol
- Urgent neurosurgical decompression may be required in the presence of brain stem compression
- Patients with completed or minor strokes, aspirin may prevent recurrence

MEDICATIONS

- Hydralazine: 10–20 mg IV q 30 min
- Labetalol: 20 mg/min IV bolus, then 20–80 mg q 10 min, max 300 mg; follow with continuous infusion 0.5–2 mg/min
- Mannitol: 1–2 g/kg IV over 5–10 min, then 0.5–1 g/kg q 4–6 hrs (adult and peds)
- Nitroprusside: 0.25–10 μg/kg/min (adult and peds)
- Trimethaphan: 1–4 mg/min
- Tissue plasminogen activator (TPA): 0.9 mg/kg IV, max 90 mg, with 10% of dose given as a bolus and the remainder infused over 60 min
- Aspirin: 81 mg po qd

Disposition

ADMISSION CRITERIA

- Patients with acute CVA should be admitted to the hospital; patients with severely decreased level of consciousness, hemodynamic instability, life-threatening cardiac dysrhythmias, or significantly increased intracranial pressure should be treated in an ICU

DISCHARGE CRITERIA

- Patients who present with completed strokes that are days to weeks old may be discharged if they are able to function independently or have adequate social support
- Patients with multiple prior strokes who experience relatively minor new episodes may also be treated on an outpatient basis if similar criteria are met and stroke completed

Miscellaneous

ICD9: 436

CORE CONTENT CODE: 11.1

SUGGESTED READINGS

Barsan WG, Kothari R. Stroke. In: Rosen P, et al., eds. Emergency medicine: Concepts and clinical practice. 4th ed. St. Louis: CV Mosby, 1997:2184–2197.

Hacke W, Kaste M, Fieschi C. et al. Intravenous thrombolysis with recombinant tissue plasminogen activator for acute hemispheric stroke: the European Cooperative Acute Stroke Study (ECASS). JAMA 1995;274:1017–1025.

Naradzay JFX, Gaasch WR. Acute stroke. Emerg Med Clin North Am 1995;14(1):197–216.

NINDS rt-PA Stroke Study Group. Tissue plasminogen activator for acute ischemic stroke. N Engl J Med 1995;333:1581–1587.

Authors: James D.R. Foster; Rebecca Smith-Coggins

Cervical Adenitis

Clinical Presentation

SIGNS AND SYMPTOMS

- Lymph node(s) in the cervical area
  - —Large
  - —Usually unilateral and solitary
  - —Tender
  - —Jugulodigastric node most commonly involved
  - —Submandibular nodes
  - —Anterior cervical nodes
  - —Posterior cervical nodes
- Fever
- Malaise
- Irritability
- Overlying cellulitis
  - —Warmth
  - —Erythema
  - —Suppuration
  - —Abscess
- Cellulitis-adenitis syndrome
  - —Anorexia
  - —Fever
  - —Irritability
  - —Facial or submandibular cellulitis
  - —Ipsilateral otitis media
- Concurrent illness
  - —URI
  - —Otitis media
  - —Pharyngitis
  - —Impetigo
  - —Dental infection

MECHANISM/DESCRIPTION

- Acute bacterial infection of one or more lymph nodes in the neck is the most common cause of a neck mass in a child
- The causative bacteria colonize regional areas of the head and neck
- Swelling of the affected lymph nodes
  - —Hyperplasia of sinusoidal cells
  - —Infiltration of leukocytes
    - -Lymphadenopathy
- If the reaction is not contained, the bacteria proliferate
  - —Lymphadenitis
- Pus forms when bacteria incite infiltration with neutrophils
- Abscess forms when host defenses are unable to clear infection
- 70–80% of cases are in the 1–4-year-old age group
- No sex difference

ETIOLOGY

- Group A β-hemolytic streptococcus and *Staphylococcus aureus*
  - —53–89% of all cases
- Group B streptococcus
  - —Newborns
  - —Cellulitis-adenitis syndrome with a 94% incidence of concurrent bacteremia
- Mixed aerobic/anaerobic infections
  - —20% of positive aspirate cultures
- *Staphylococcus aureus*
  - —Newborns
  - —More indolent course
  - —Higher frequency of suppuration
- Rare organisms
  - —*H. Influenza*
  - —Yersinia pestis
  - —Actinomyces
  - —Mycobacteria
  - —Nocardia species,
  - —Francisella tularensis
  - —Gram-negative bacilli

Pre-Hospital

N/A

Diagnosis

ESSENTIAL WORKUP

- Clinical diagnosis
- Identify source of infection
- Signs of systemic disease

LABORATORY

- Unnecessary if there is
  - —An obvious source of primary infection
  - —Cervical adenitis without suppuration
- If the etiology is unclear
  - —WBC count
  - —Tuberculin skin test
  - —Monospot
  - —Throat cultures
- Blood cultures in toxic patients only
- Generalized lymphadenopathy
- CBC
- ESR
- LFTs
- Antibody titers for specific etiologies if suggested by history or exam
  - —Toxoplasmosis
  - —EBV
  - —HIV
  - —CMV
  - —Intradermal skin testing
    - -Cat-scratch disease
    - -Mycobacteria

IMAGING/SPECIAL TESTS

- Needle aspiration
  - —Gram stain
  - —Acid-fast stains
  - —Cultures for aerobic and anaerobic bacteria
  - —Mycobacteria
  - —Fungi
- When source of infection is unclear, based on presentation
  - —Chest x-ray
  - —Lateral neck
  - —Panorex
- Ultrasound
  - —Differentiates cystic and sold structures
  - —Usually not required emergently

DIFFERENTIAL DIAGNOSIS

- Lymphadenopathy
  - —Reaction without bacterial infection of nodes
  - —Viral infection
    - -EBV, HSV, VSV, CMV
  - —Malignancy
  - —Infected congenital cysts
  - —Noninfectious inflammatory disorders
- Cat-scratch disease
- Atypical mycobacterial infection (scrofula)
- Tuberculous lymphadenitis
- Toxoplasmosis
- Tularemia
- Congenital cysts
- Malignancies
  - —Leukemia
  - —Lymphoma (Hodgkin's and non-Hodgkin's)
  - —Rhabdomyosarcoma
  - —Thyroid carcinoma

Treatment

INITIAL STABILIZATION

- Airway management
  - —Rare cases of airway compromise

ED TREATMENT

- Aspirate all fluctuant nodes
  - —If no material obtained, inject 1–2 ml of sterile saline and reaspirate
- Many oral antibiotics are effective
  - —Cephalexin
  - —Clindamycin
  - —Dicloxacillin
  - —Erythromycin
  - —Continue for 10-day course even if resolution of symptoms noted earlier
- Patients with suspected dental or periodontal disease
  - —Penicillin V or clindamycin
- Intravenous antibiotics if toxic
  - —Cefazolin or nafcillin
  - —Continue until clinical improvement is noted
- If anaerobes are suspected, penicillin G or clindamycin
- Apply warm, moist compresses
- Analgesics as needed

MEDICATIONS

- Cephalexin: 25–50 mg/kg/day q 6 hrs
- Cefazolin: 150 mg/kg/day IV q 8 hrs
- Clindamycin: 15–40 mg/kg/day IV q 6–8 hrs
- Dicloxacillin: 25–50 mg/kg/day q 6 hrs
- Erythromycin: 40 mg/kg/day q 6 hrs
- Nafcillin: 150 mg/kg/day IV q 4–6 hrs
- Penicillin G: 100,000–200,000 IU/kg/day divided q 4–6 hrs IV
- Penicillin V: 50 mg/kg/day q 6 hrs

Disposition

ADMISSION CRITERIA

- Toxic children
- Inability to take po
- Adenitis not improving on oral antibiotics
- Neonates

DISCHARGE CRITERIA

- Vast majority of children can be discharged on oral antibiotics
- Close follow-up with a primary care physician in 2–4 days
- Return to the ED if
  - —Worsening of local symptoms
  - —Development of systemic symptoms
  - —Inability to take po

Miscellaneous

ICD9: 289.3

CORE CONTENT CODE: 13.7.16

SUGGESTED READINGS

Bellet J, Klein B. Acute cervical lymphadenitis. In: Harwood-Nuss A, et al., eds. The Clinical practice of emergency medicine. 2d ed. Philadelphia: Lippincott-Raven, 1996:1078–1079.

Brook I. The swollen neck: Cervical lymphadenitis, parotitis, thyroiditis, and infected cysts. Infect Dis Clin North Am 1988;2(1):221–236.

Chesney P. Cervical adenopathy. Pediatr Rev 1994;15(7):276–284.

Author: Kristine M. Reid

Cervical Spine Injury, Adult

Clinical Presentation

SIGNS AND SYMPTOMS

- Neck pain, tenderness on palpation
- Numbness, weakness, paresthesias of upper or lower extremities
- Always assume a C-spine injury in any patient with
  - —Altered mental status (unconscious, intoxicated, drugs, or hypoxia) following trauma or if preceding history/events unknown
  - —Inability to communicate (mentally retarded, language barrier, or intubated) following trauma or if preceding history/events unknown
  - —Distracting injury
  - —Blunt trauma involving head or neck

ETIOLOGY

- Blunt trauma is the major cause of neck injuries
  - —Automobile accidents account for >50% of neck injuries from blunt trauma
  - —Falls account for approximately 20%
  - —Sporting accidents account for 15%
  - —Minor trauma in patients with severe arthritis may result in cervical injuries
- Penetrating trauma

MECHANISM/DESCRIPTION

- May have more than one mechanism concurrently

Flexion Injuries

- Simple *compression fracture:* this is usually a stable fracture
- *Anterior subluxation:* disruption of the posterior ligament complex without bony injury. This may be an unstable injury
- *Clay shoveler fracture:* avulsion fracture of the spinous process of C7, C6, or T1. This is usually a stable fracture
- Flexion *teardrop fracture:* this is an extremely unstable fracture and may be associated with acute anterior cervical cord syndrome
- *Bilateral facet dislocation:* this can occur from C2 to C7. This is an unstable injury

Hyperflexion/Rotation

- Unilateral facet dislocation "locked" vertebra: this is often a stable injury

Hyperextension

- Hyperextension dislocation: described as the syndrome of the paralyzed patient with a radiographically normal appearing C-spine
- *Extension teardrop fracture:* this is an avulsion fracture of the anterior inferior corner of the involved vertebral body. This is unstable in extension and stable in flexion
- *Posterior arch of the atlas fracture:* arch is compressed between the occiput and the spinous process of the axis during hyperextension
- *Avulsion fracture of the anterior arch of the atlas:* horizontal fracture of C1 and prevertebral soft tissue swelling on the lateral C-spine
  - —*Hangman's fracture* (traumatic spondylolisthesis of the axis): unstable fracture that involves the pedicles of C2

Extension-Rotation

- Pillar fracture: this is usually a stable fracture

Vertical Compression (Axial Loading)

- Jefferson fracture: burst fracture of both the anterior and posterior arches of C1. This is an extremely unstable fracture
- *Burst fracture:* This is a comminuted fracture of the vertebral body with variable retropulsion of the posterior body fragments into the spinal canal

PEDIATRIC CONSIDERATIONS

- Only 2% of all C-spine fractures or dislocations occur in patients less than 16 years of age
- Spinal cord injury without radiographic abnormality (SCIWORA) occurs in approximately 55–65% of pediatric spinal cord injuries. May present with only paresthesias
- The majority of C-spine injuries occur in the upper cervical region because the fulcrum of the C-spine in children is between C1 and C3
- Pseudosubluxation (apparent subluxation of C2 on C3 with normal spinous process alignment) can be seen in 30% of radiographs in children <8 years of age

Pre-Hospital

CAUTIONS

- If a C-spine injury is suspected, immobilize with a hard collar and backboard
- Immobilized patients require constant observation to avoid vomiting

CONTROVERSIES

- Immobilize the C-spine in patients with penetrating neck wounds only if a neurologic deficit is present. If the weapon is still embedded, immobilize the neck to avoid further injury

PEDIATRIC CONSIDERATIONS

- Infants and young children have a disproportionately large head and positioning a young child on a standard backboard may flex the neck, possibly aggravating a C-spine injury
- The standard backboard may be modified to accommodate the child's larger head size by using a board with a cutout for the occiput or by placing a thin cushion under the back at the level of the chest

Diagnosis

ESSENTIAL WORKUP

- Standard x-rays include three separate views: lateral, AP, and open-mouth view of the odontoid while still immobilized
- The lateral x-ray must include C1–T1; a swimmers view may be necessary
- Supine oblique views may help in identifying subtle rotational injuries
- CT should be obtained when C-spine fractures or dislocations are seen on plain films or unexplained neck pain/deficit with normal x-ray
- MRI has become a valuable tool in evaluation of patients with neurologic deficits

DIFFERENTIAL DIAGNOSIS

- Cervical muscle strain injury (whiplash)
- C-spine dislocation
- Cervical fracture-dislocation
- Complex or simple cervical fractures

Treatment

INITIAL STABILIZATION

- Immobilize the spine using a rigid collar and backboard, plus tape/towels or IV bags along the side of the neck
- ABCs: stabilize the airway, establish IV access and support circulation
  —The preferred method is careful orotracheal rapid sequence intubation with in-line spinal immobilization

ED TREATMENT

- Assess patient for other injuries. Remember that the abdominal examination in a C-spine injured patient is unreliable and further objective testing is indicated
- If a neurologic deficit is present, consult neurosurgery
- If the x-rays are abnormal, consult neurosurgery or the orthopedic spine service
- If the x-rays are normal, but the patient is having severe neck pain, obtain flexion-extension films. If abnormal, consult neurosurgery
- High-dose steroid protocol should be initiated for patients with neurologic deficits due to fractures or dislocations

MEDICATIONS

- High-dose steroid protocol
  —Methylprednisolone: 30 mg/kg IV bolus then 5.4 mg/kg/hr over the next 23 hours; begin within 8 hours of injury

Disposition

ADMISSION CRITERIA

- C-spine fractures or dislocations associated with a neurologic deficit or any unstable fracture or dislocation should be admitted to the ICU or monitored setting
- Stable C-spine fractures or dislocations should be admitted
- Because of the high incidence of SCIWORA, children with suspected C-spine injuries should be admitted
- Isolated spinous process fractures which are not associated with any neurologic deficit or instability on plain films
- Simple cervical wedge fractures with no neurologic deficit

DISCHARGE CRITERIA

- Patients with acute cervical strain "whiplash"
- Musculoskeletal injuries which are associated with mild-moderate pain, no neurologic deficit, and normal radiographs
- Patients with radiographically normal C-spine but continuous pain should be discharged with a hard collar and appropriate orthopedic follow-up

Miscellaneous

ICD9: 952.9

CORE CONTENT CODE: 18.4.3

SUGGESTED READINGS

Bonadio WA. C-spine trauma in children: Part II. Mechanisms and manifestations of injury, therapeutic considerations. Am J Emerg Med 1993;11(3):256–278.

Harris J, Mirvis S. The radiology of acute C-spine trauma. 3rd ed. Baltimore: Williams & Wilkins, 1996.

Hockberger R, Kirshenbaum K, Doris P. Spinal trauma. In: Rosen P, et al., eds: Emergency medicine: Concepts and clinical practice. 4th ed. St. Louis: CV Mosby, 1998:462–504.

Kathol MH. C-spine trauma. What is new? Radiol Clin North Am 1997;11(3):256–278.

Author: Elizabeth Wulfert

Cervical Spine Injury, Pediatric

Clinical Presentation

SIGNS AND SYMPTOMS

- Major or consistent mechanism of injury
- Child abuse
- Occasionally asymptomatic
  - —However, it is very rare to have a normal neurological examination in a children under 2 years of age because of the laxity of the spine
- Masked by altered mental status
- Signs of associated spinal cord injury
  - —These may be transient

General

- Generalized weakness
- Hypotension
- Normal or slowed heart rate
- Flushing
- Diaphoresis

Neck

- Pain
- Torticollis
- Decreased range of motion
- Muscle spasm
- Tenderness to palpation

Respiratory

- Diaphragmatic breathing

Abdominal

- Ileus
- Fecal retention
- Fecal incontinence
- Loss of rectal tone

Genitourinary

- Priapism
- Urinary retention

Neurologic

- Pain
- Paresthesias
- Paresis
- Localized weakness
- Paralysis
  - —Partial cord syndromes
  - —Quadriplegia
- Clonus
- Loss of reflexes

MECHANISM/DESCRIPTION

- Children <8 years old
  - —Anatomic differences lead to less fractures in the lower cervical spine
    - -Relatively larger head
    - -Ligamentous laxity
    - -Nearly horizontal facet joints
  - —Common injuries
    - -Upper cervical spine injuries (C1-C2)
    - -Subluxation
- Children between 8 and 12 years of age
  - —Increased incidence of pancervical injuries
- After 12 years of age
  - —Injuries occur more frequently in the lower cervical spine
    - -Evident radiographically
    - -Associated with immediate neurological deficit if a spinal cord injury coexists
- In the United States
  - —1–3% of all pediatric trauma hospital admissions
  - —Approximately 1000 children have resulting significant neurological deficits per year
- Spinal cord injury without radiographic abnormality (SCIWORA)
  - —Occurs in 5–50% of pediatric cervical spine injury
  - —Occurs more frequently, although not exclusively, in children <8 years old
  - —May have transient sensory symptoms
    - -Paresthesias
    - -Weakness
    - -Lightning/burning sensation down the spine
  - —Often occurs immediately following the injury
  - —May resolve by the time of evaluation
  - —Delayed onset of neurological deficit ranging from 30 minutes to 4 days

ETIOLOGY

- Motor vehicle and pedestrian accidents
- Falls
- Sports injuries
- Nonaccidental trauma

Pre-Hospital

CAUTIONS

- Immobilize all infants and children with potential CSI
  - —Appropriate size cervical collar
  - —Towels
  - —Padding
- Tape in combination with a car seat or spine board
  - —Infants and younger children
    - -The relatively larger occiput creates greater cervical flexion
    - -Use an occiput padding placed under the child's neck, shoulders and back
  - —Align the external auditory meatus with the shoulder

Diagnosis

ESSENTIAL WORKUP

- Detect transient or permanent signs of spinal cord injury
- Obtain cervical spine radiographs based on mechanism and either neck pain, altered mental status, or the lack of ability to cooperate
- Additional imaging studies are needed to define the extent of fracture (CT scan) or ligamentous injury

LABORATORY

N/A

IMAGING/SPECIAL TESTS

Cervical Spine Films

- Need to visualize all 7 cervical vertebrae
- Identifies >75% of fractures, dislocations, and subluxations
- Standard initial views: AP, lateral, and odontoid views
- Indications
  - —High-risk mechanism
  - —Altered mental status
  - —Neck pain
  - —Tenderness to palpation
  - —Neurological deficit
  - —History of transient symptoms
  - —Decreased mobility in the neck
  - —Distracting injuries
- Thickening of the prevertebral soft tissue
  - —Suggests underlying fracture or ligamentous injury
  - —Also thickened by expiration, swallowing, and neck flexion
  - —Normal predental spaces
    - -Space between the posterior arch of C1 and the anterior aspect of the odontoid process
    - -≤5 mm in children
    - -≤3 mm in adults
  - —Normal prevertebral spaces
    - -Anterior to C2; ≤7 mm
    - -Anterior to C3-C4; ≤5 mm or 40% of the AP diameter of the vertebral bodies
    - -Between C6 and the trachea: ≤14 mm under 15 years of age and ≤22 mm in adults
    - -However much variability exists
  - —Soft tissue below the glottis should be approximately twice as thick as above the glottis
- Pseudosubluxation of C2
  - —C2 anteriorly displaced on C3
  - —Often due to normal ligamentous laxity in children
  - —Maximum normal: 2.7 mm
  - —Draw a line from the anterior cortices of the spinous processes of C1 to C3
  - —If that line misses C2 by more than 2 mm
    - -True subluxation is present

- –An underlying hangman's fracture must be suspected
- —This posterior cervical line can be applied only at C2-C3
- —It does not exclude underlying ligamentous injury
- Epiphyseal growth plates may resemble fractures
  - –Posterior arch of C1 fuses at 4 years of age
  - –Anterior arch of C1 fuses at 7–10 years of age
  - –Base of odontoid fuses with body of C1 at 3–7 years of age

Flexion and Extension Views

- Indicated when occult ligamentous injury is suspected
  - —Negative cervical spine films
  - —No neurological abnormalities

CT Scan

- Fracture still suspected despite negative plain films
- In children <8 years old, CT is a useful tool to assess the occiput through C2
- Fractured areas
- Areas in which differentiating between a fracture and synchondrosis is difficult

DIFFERENTIAL DIAGNOSIS

- Cervical muscle strain
- Torticollis
- Cervical adenitis
- Retropharyngeal abscess
- Meningitis
- Guillain-Barré syndrome

Treatment

INITIAL STABILIZATION

- Maintain cervical spine immobilization
- During intubation
  - —One person should be devoted to in-line cervical immobilization

ED TREATMENT

- Methylprednisolone
  - —Any trauma patient with a neurological deficit consistent with spinal cord injury
- Neurosurgical evaluation
  - —True subluxation
  - —Fracture
  - —Transient or persistent neurological deficit

MEDICATIONS

- Methylprednisolone: loading dose 30 mg/kg over 15 min; maintenance infusion 5.4 mg/kg/hr over 23 hrs

Disposition

ADMISSION CRITERIA

- Altered mental status
- Signs/symptoms of spinal cord injury
- Cervical spine fracture
- Obtain appropriate consultation
  - —Neurosurgery
  - —Orthopedics

DISCHARGE CRITERIA

- Completely normal mental status
- No radiographic abnormalities
- No transient or persistent neurological deficit
- Educate parents
  - —SCIWORA can present with delayed onset of symptom
  - —Return if paresthesias, weakness, or paralysis

Miscellaneous

ICD9: 952.00, 952.05

CORE CONTENT CODE: 18.4.3.1

SUGGESTED READINGS

Fesmire FM, Luten RC. Evaluation of the pediatric cervical spine. In: Harwood-Nuss AL, Linden CH, Luten RC, Shepherd SM, Wolfson AB, eds. The clinical practice of emergency medicine. 2d ed. Philadelphia: Lippincott-Raven, 1996:1197–1202.

Proudfoot J. Pediatric cervical spine injury: Navigating the nuances and minimizing complications. Pediatr Emerg Med Rep 1996;1:83–94.

Swischuk LE. Emergency imaging of the acutely ill or injured child. 3rd ed. Baltimore: Williams & Wilkins, 1994:653–718.

Author: Steven Riley, Gary Schwartz

Cesarean Section, Emergency

Alert

The indication for a perimortem cesarean section to be performed by the emergency physician is a gravid female (>24 weeks gestation) in cardiopulmonary arrest who has not responded to initial resuscitative measures, regardless of the etiology. Cesarean delivery should begin within 4 minutes after maternal cardiac arrest.

Clinical Presentation

SIGNS AND SYMPTOMS

- Gravid female (>24 weeks gestation by fundal height) who is pulseless and apneic

ETIOLOGY

- Trauma (blunt or penetrating) is a leading cause of maternal mortality
- Cerebral vascular accident
- Pulmonary embolus
  —Thromboembolism is the number one cause of maternal mortality
- Amniotic fluid embolus
- DIC
- Placenta previa
- Miscellaneous medical disorders
  —Asthma
  —Congestive heart failure
  —Infection

Pre-Hospital

CAUTIONS

- "Scoop and Run"—time is of the essence!
- Place the patient in the left lateral decubitus position to avoid the uterus compressing the inferior vena cava (Supine Hypotension syndrome)
- In trauma cases where immobilization of the spine is important and placement in the left lateral decubitus position is not possible, manually displace the uterus to the patient's left or "wedge" the backboard so the right hip is elevated 45°

Diagnosis

ESSENTIAL WORKUP

- Physical examination for apnea and the absence of pulses in an obviously pregnant woman
- Quickly evaluate for reversible causes of cardiopulmonary arrest
  - —Tension pneumothorax, pericardial tamponade, Supine Hypotension syndrome, etc
- Assess gestational age by using fundal height
  - —Distance from pubis to fundus (in centimeters)
  - —Ultrasonography is beneficial if *immediately* available to assess the fetus

LABORATORY

- None immediately indicated

IMAGING/SPECIAL TESTS

- None are necessary to establish the diagnosis of cardiopulmonary arrest
- Do *NOT* waste time by attempting to determine fetal heart tones (FHT)

DIFFERENTIAL DIAGNOSIS

- Maternal cardiopulmonary arrest is a "final" common pathway. Evaluate for underlying cause or etiology

Treatment

INITIAL STABILIZATION

- ABCs
  - —Emergency intubation, high-flow oxygen, cardiac and blood pressure monitoring, two large-bore peripheral IVs, crystalloids, or O-negative blood as indicated
  - —Displace the uterus from the inferior vena cava
- The best way to ensure fetal survival is to ensure maternal survival
- If <24 weeks gestation, use ACLS and ATLS protocols directed at maternal resuscitation
  - —Do *not* perform emergent cesarean section
- If >24 weeks gestation, use "4 Minute Rule."
  - —Perform ACLS or ATLS for 4 minutes; if no response, then do an immediate emergent cesarean section

ED TREATMENT

- Call for STAT obstetrics, surgery, and pediatric consultations; but do *not* delay performing the procedure until the consultants arrive
- Ensure a Foley catheter is inserted to decompress the bladder
- Perform a Cesarean section
  - —Use linea nigra as a landmark for vertical midline incision
  - —Incise the abdominal wall with a scalpel starting at the pubic symphysis and extending all the way up to the umbilicus. This incision should be extended down through the fascial and peritoneal layers
  - —Retract the urinary bladder inferiorly against the pubic symphysis
  - —Make a small short vertical incision in the lower segment of the uterus just cephalad to the bladder
  - —This incision is extended cephalad with scissors
  - —Insert free hand into the uterus to avoid harming the fetus as the incision is extended to the uterine fundus
  - —Deliver the fetus, clamp the umbilical cord in two places and cut the umbilical cord between the two clamps
  - —Manually deliver the placenta
  - —Perform neonatal resuscitation as indicated
  - —Occasionally, maternal vital signs will return after delivery of the neonate
  - —Continue maternal resuscitation efforts as appropriate, suture the uterus

Disposition

ADMISSION CRITERIA

- Infant should be admitted to neonatal ICU
- If maternal resuscitation is successful, patient should be admitted to SICU

DISCHARGE CRITERIA

- Neither infant nor mother should be discharged

Miscellaneous

ICD9: 669.73

CORE CONTENT CODE: 12.7.8, 18.5.2.3, 23.4.2.3

SUGGESTED READINGS

Katz VL, Dotters DJ, Droegemueller W. Perimortem cesarean delivery. Obstet Gynecol 1986;68:571–575

Lanoix R, Akkapedd V, Goldfeder B. Perimortem cesarean section: Case reports and recommendations. Acad Emerg Med 1995;2:1063–1067

Strong TH, Lowe RA. Perimortem cesarean section. Am J Emerg Med 1989;7:489–493

Authors: Michael Chamales; James S. Walker

Chalazion

Clinical Presentation

SIGNS AND SYMPTOMS

- Firm circumscribed nodule along the lid margin
- Physically obstructed vision
- Pressure on the globe
- Typically long-standing
- Nontender
- No erythema or swelling

ETIOLOGY

- Chronic granulomatous inflammation in the Meibomian gland
  - —May evolve from internal hordeolum or obstructed Meibomian gland with inspissated secretions

Pre-Hospital

N/A

Diagnosis

ESSENTIAL WORKUP

- Ophthalmologic examination

DIFFERENTIAL DIAGNOSIS

- Hordeolum
- Meibomian gland carcinoma
- Pyogenic granuloma

Treatment

INITIAL STABILIZATION

N/A

ED TREATMENT

- Warm compresses
- Antibiotic ointment
- Referral to ophthalmology for incision and curettage or steroid injection

MEDICATIONS

- Erythromycin ophthalmic ointment in cul de sac and massage along lid margins qid

Disposition

ADMISSION CRITERIA

None

DISCHARGE CRITERIA

- Discharge all patients

Miscellaneous

ICD9: 373.2

CORE CONTENT CODE: 6.4.1.2

SUGGESTED READINGS

Cullom R. The Wills eye manual: Office and emergency room diagnosis and treatment of eye disease. Philadelphia: JB Lippincott, 1994:133–134

Lavrich JB, Nelson LB. Disorders of the lacrimal system apparatus. Pediatr Clin North Am 1993;40:767–804

Rubin S, Hallagan L. Lids, lacrimals and lashes. Emerg Med North Am 1995;13(3):631–647

Author: Shari Schabowski

Chancroid

Clinical Presentation

SIGNS AND SYMPTOMS

- Single erythematous pustule or papule
  - —Quickly breaks down into 1–3 soft painful chancres
  - —Soft and friable with ragged irregular borders
- Primary lesion usually excavated
- Moist, yellow to gray base
- Purulent and hemorrhagic secretion
- Location
  - —Male—penile shaft, glans, internal surface of foreskin, anus
  - —Female—cervix, vagina, vulva, perineum, anus
- Occurs 2–12 days postexposure
- Inguinal adenopathy
  - —In 50% cases
  - —Appears 3–14 days after initial ulcer
  - —Unilateral
  - —Painful
  - —Suppurative large nodes (buboes)
    - -Common
    - -May rupture
- Pain on urination secondary to contact with lesion
- Variants
  - —Phagedenic type—ulcer with secondary superinfection and rapid tissue destruction
  - —Giant chancroid—very large single ulcer
  - —Serpiginous ulcer—rapidly spreading, indolent, shallow ulcers in groin or thigh
  - —Follicular type—multiple small ulcers in perifollicular distribution

MECHANISM/DESCRIPTION

- Sexually transmitted disease
- Increased risk for HIV infection

ETIOLOGY

- Causative agent: *hemophilus ducreyi*

Pre-Hospital

N/A

Diagnosis

ESSENTIAL WORKUP

- Clinical diagnosis based on appearance

LABORATORY

- Confirm diagnosis with gram stain or culture
  - —Obtain specimen from
    - -Base/edge of ulcer
    - -Needle aspiration of inguinal node by placing needle through normal skin to avoid formation of fistula
    - -Do not incise node
  - —Gram stain positive 50–80%
    - -Gram-negative bacillus with a linear or school of fish pattern
  - —Culture positive in >80%
- UA for dysuria
- RPR for associated syphillis
- HIV
  - —Recommend follow-up HIV testing
- Test for other sexually transmitted diseases

DIFFERENTIAL DIAGNOSIS

- Syphilitic chancre
  - —Usually painless, indurated, clean
- Herpes genitalis
  - —Vesicles
- Lymphogranuloma venereum
- Granuloma inguinale

Treatment

INITIAL STABILIZATION

- Wear gloves to examine suspicious lesions

ED TREATMENT

- Antibiotic choices
  —Ceftriaxone: single IM dose
  —Azithromycin: single po dose
  —Erythromycin
    -Recommended for HIV positive patients
  —Ciprofloxcin
  —Amoxicillin/clavulanic acid
- Needle aspiration of suppurative nodes
  —To prevent chronic sinus drainage from spontaneous rupture
  —Use 18-gauge needle through lateral intact skin
- Sexual abstinence or condom use till lesion healed
- Examine/treat sexual partner
- Recommend follow up HIV testing
- Clinical course
  —Symptoms improve within 3 days of treatment
  —Ulcers improve within 7 days

MEDICATIONS

- Amoxicillin/clavulanic acid: 500 mg/125 mg po tid × 7 days
- Azithromycin: 1 g po
- Ceftriaxone: 250 mg IM
- Ciprofloxicin: 500 mg po bid × 7 days
- Erythromycin: 500 mg po × 7 days

Disposition

ADMISSION CRITERIA

None

DISCHARGE CRITERIA

- All patients

Miscellaneous

ICD9: 099.0

CORE CONTENT CODE: 19.4

SUGGESTED READINGS

Currie BP. Chancroid. In: Borchardt KA, ed. Sexually transmitted diseases: Epidemiology, pathology, diagnosis and treatment. CRC Press, Boca Raton, 1997

Marrazzo JD, Handsfield HH. Chancroid: New developments in an old disease. Curr Clin Top Infect Dis 1995;15:129–152

Orle KA, Gates CA, Martin DH, et al. Simultaneous PCR detection of Haemophilus ducreyi, Treponema pallidum and Herpes simplex virus types 1 and 2 from genital ulcers. J Clin Microbiol 1996;34:49–54

Authors: Norbert Elsner; Paul Gennis; David Levine

Chemical Weapons Poisoning

Clinical Presentation

SIGNS AND SYMPTOMS

Blood Agents (Cyanide and Cyanogens)

Vital Signs

- Tachypnea and hyperpnea (early); respiratory depression (late)
- Hypertension and tachycardia (early); hypotension and bradycardia (late)
- Death within seconds to minutes

CNS

- Headache
- Mental status changes
- Seizures
- Paralysis

Pulmonary

- Dyspnea
- Noncardiogenic pulmonary edema
- Cyanosis uncommon

GI

- Odor of bitter almonds
- Burning in mouth and throat
- Nausea, vomiting

Blister Agents (Mustards)

Dermatologic

- Skin erythema and edema (early)
- Necrosis and vesiculation (late)

HEENT

- Sore throat
- Sinusitis
- Eye pain
- Photophobia
- Lacrimation
- Blurred vision
- Blepharospasm
- Periorbital edema
- Conjunctival edema
- Corneal ulceration

Pulmonary

- Bronchospasm
- Tracheobronchitis
- Respiratory failure
- Hacking cough

GI

- Nausea, vomiting

Choking Agents/Lacrimators/Riot Control Agents (Chlorine, Phosgenes, Chloropicrin, "Tear Gases")

HEENT

- Eye pain
- Lacrimation
- Blepharospasm
- Temporary blindness

Dermatologic

- Skin irritation
- Papulovesicular dermatitis
- Superficial burns

Pulmonary

- Cough
- Chest tightness
- Dry throat
- Sensation of suffocation

Delayed toxicity (2–24 hours)

- Severe dyspnea
- Pulmonary edema
- Foaming white or bloody sputum
- Cyanosis
- Nephrotoxicity

Nerve Agents (Sarin, Tabun, Soman, VX)

HEENT

- Miosis
- Hypersecretion by salivary, sweat, lacrimal, and bronchial glands

CNS

- Irritability
- Nervousness
- Giddiness
- Fatigue
- Lethargy
- Memory impairment
- Depression
- Ataxia
- Convulsions
- Coma
- Respiratory failure

Pulmonary

- Bronchoconstriction

GI

- Nausea, vomiting
- Diarrhea
- Crampy abdominal pains
- Urinary and fecal incontinence

Musculoskeletal

- Fasciculations
- Skeletal muscle twitching
- Weakness
- Flaccid paralysis

MECHANISM

Blood Agents

- Inhibition of cellular respiration by binding to ferric ion in cytochrome oxidase

Blister Agents

- Alkylation and cross-linking of purine bases of DNA as well as alkylation of cysteine in proteins

Choking Agents/Lacrimators/Riot Control Agents

- Mainly irritants secondary to hydrolysis, alkylation, or other chemical inhibition

Nerve Agents

- Anticholinesterase organophosphate which cause cholinergic overstimulation at muscarinic, nicotinic and CNS sites
- *S.L.U.D.G.E. syndrome*
  - —Salivation
  - —Lacrimation
  - —Urination
  - —Defecation
  - —GI cramps
  - —Emesis

Pre-Hospital

CAUTIONS

- Avoid contamination
  - —Use chemical protective overgarment (CPOG) with charcoal layer to absorb penetrating mustard
- Decontamination
  - —Irrigate eyes copiously
  - —Wash skin
    - -Soap and water
    - -Chloramine powder or hypochlorite solution (household bleach diluted 1:10)
    - -2–4% sodium thiosulfate or phenol for mustards

Diagnosis

ESSENTIAL WORKUP

- History and symptomatology key to type of agent exposure
- PE
  - —Cyanide (bitter almonds)
  - —Mustard (faint, sweet odor of mustard or garlic)
  - —Check for S.L.U.D.G.E

LABORATORY

- ABG
  - —Cyanide—decreased AV oxygen saturation; lactic acidemia with anion gap
- CBC
  - —Leukopenia, thrombocytopenia, anemia with significant mustard exposure
- Electrolytes, BUN/Cr, glucose
- Urinalysis

IMAGING/SPECIAL TESTS

- CXR for pulmonary edema
- Erythrocyte cholinesterase activity for nerve agents

DIFFERENTIAL DIAGNOSIS

- Asthma / COPD exacerbations
- Stevens-Johnson syndrome
- Toxic epidermal necrolysis
- Pemphigus vulgaris
- Scalded skin syndrome
- Organophosphate / carbamate pesticide poisoning
- Botulism
- Radiation poisoning

Treatment

INITIAL STABILIZATION

- ABCs
- Early airway intervention for significant respiratory symptoms
- *Patient decontamination*
  - —Brush off powder chemical
  - —Irrigate skin / eyes with copious amounts of water or saline
  - —Remove and dispose of clothing in double bags
- Protection for health care workers
  - —Protective mask containing a charcoal filter
  - —Chemical-resistant suit
  - —Heavy rubber gloves / boots
  - —Establish IV access with 0.9%NS

ED TREATMENT

Blood Agents

- 100% Oxygen
- Sodium bicarbonate for acidosis
- Standard anticonvulsants PRN
- Lilly cyanide antidote kit
- Hydroxocobalamin/sodium thiosulfate
- Dicobalt-EDTA

Blister Agents

- Supportive care
- N-acetylcysteine in patients with respiratory complaints
- Standard burn management
- Atropine to relieve eye pain
- Monitor fluids, electrolytes, CBC
- Experimental antidotes: sodium thiosulfate, vitamin E, dexamethasone

Choking Agents/Lacrimators/Riot Control Agents

- Supportive care
- Chloropicrin and phosgenes require CXR and careful monitoring for respiratory complications
  - —Blurring of hila at 4–8 hours
  - —High dose steroids for pulmonary edema
- Phosgenes require monitoring of
  - —CBC for polycythemia
  - —Electrolytes, BUN/Cr, and urinalysis for nephrotoxicity

Nerve Agents

- Supportive care
  - —100% oxygen prior to atropine to minimize ventricular fibrillation
  - —Frequent airway suctioning
- Atropine
  - —Antagonizes muscarinic effects and some CNS but no effect on skeletal muscle weakness or respiratory failure
  - —Pupillary response and heart rate are not useful measures of adequate "atropinization"
  - —Stop atropine after patient regains consciousness and spontaneous ventilation (may need for periodic relapses)
- Pralidoxime chloride (2-PAM or protopam chloride)
  - —Regenerates cholinesterase by reversing phosphorylation (unless aging has occurred)
  - —Reduces abnormal skeletal muscle movements, improves skeletal muscle weakness, and reverses flaccid paralysis
  - —May repeat first dose immediately if no response, but >2 g qh may cause hypotension
  - —If improvement from first dose, repeat 60–90 minutes later
- Diazepam—given for seizures PRN if not relieved by above measures

MEDICATIONS

- Atropine: 2 mg IM or IV (6 mg in severely intoxicated patients) (peds: 0.02–0.08 mg/kg) then q 5–10 min
- Dexamethasone: 8 mg/kg IM
- Diazepam: 5–10 mg IV over 3–5 min (peds: 0.2–0.4 mg/kg up to 10 mg over 2–3 min)
- Hydroxocobalamin/sodium thiosulfate: 5 g IV (available in France)
- Lilly Kit
  - —Inhale amyl nitrite ampule for 30 seconds q min until sodium nitrite given
  - —Sodium nitrite: 10 ml IV over 3–5 min (peds: 0.15–0.33 ml/kg)
  - —Monitor methemoglobin and stay below 30%
  - —Sodium thiosulfate: 50 ml IV of 25% solution (peds: 1.65 ml/kg)
- Pralidoxime chloride (2-PAM, protopam chloride): 1–2 g IV over 20–30 min or 600 mg IM (diluted with water or saline to concentration of 300 mg/ml) given with first 3 atropine doses (peds: 15–25mg/kg IV)
- Vitamin E: 20 mg/kg IM

Disposition

ADMISSION CRITERIA

- ICU admission for
  - —Blood agents
  - —Nerve agents
- Admit to watch for developing respiratory complications
  - —Blister / choking /lacrimating agents

DISCHARGE CRITERIA

- Riot control exposures observe in ED for 6 hours and discharge if symptoms resolve

Miscellaneous

ICD9: 987.9

CORE CONTENT CODE: 17.2.26

SUGGESTED READINGS

Borak J, Sidell FR. Agents of chemical warfare: Sulfur mustard. Ann Emerg Med 1992;21(3):303–308

Dunn MA, Sidell FR. Progress in medical defense against nerve agents. JAMA 1989;262(5):649–652

Howard H, et al. Tear gas—harassing agent or toxic chemical weapon? JAMA 1989;262(5):660–663

Sidell FR, Borak J. Chemical warfare agents: II. Nerve agents. Ann Emerg Med 1992;21(7):128–134

Author: Kelly Bookman

Chest Pain

Clinical Presentation

SIGNS AND SYMPTOMS

Coronary Artery Disease

- Risk factors
  - —Male >35
  - —Female >45
  - —Postmenopausal
  - —Hypercholesterolemia
  - —Hypertension
  - —Family history
  - —Diabetes
  - —Smoking
- Anxiety
- Shortness of breath
- Pressure
- Squeezing pain
- Radiation to arm/jaw
- Tachycardia or bradycardia
- Diaphoresis
- Nausea
- Vomiting
- Signs of CHF

Aortic Dissection

- Risk factors
  - —Hypertension
  - —Connective tissue disorder
  - —Pregnancy
  - —Family history
  - —Coarctation of aorta
  - —Valvular disease
  - —Increasing age
- Sudden onset of pain with maximal intensity early
- Tearing pain
- Radiation to back
- Hypertension
- Differential pulses
- Associated neurologic changes

Pulmonary Embolism

- Risk factors
  - —Cancer
  - —Pregnancy/postpartum
  - —Oral contraceptives
  - —Postoperative
  - —Invalid
  - —Increasing age
  - —Trauma
- Pleuritic pain
- Shortness of breath
- Anxiety
- Diaphoresis
- Tachypnea
- Tachycardia
- Low-grade fever
- Localized rales
- Wheezes

Acute Pericarditis

- Risk factors
  - —Trauma
  - —Cancer
  - —Collagen vascular disease
  - —Anticoagulants
  - —Recent MI or surgery
  - —Drugs
  - —Recent viral infection
  - —Uremia
- Substernal pain
- Varies with respiration
- Increased with recumbency
- Relieved by leaning forward
- Anxiety
- Anorexia
- Fever
- Pericardial friction rub

MECHANISM/DESCRIPTION

- One of the most frequent chief complaints in the emergency department
- The primary consideration diagnosis and treatment of life threatening etiologies
- The identification of nonlethal causes can often be investigated in an outpatient setting

ETIOLOGY

- Cardiac/vascular
  - —Acute ischemic coronary disease
  - —Acute pericarditis
  - —Aortic dissection
  - —Valvular disease
- Gastrointestinal
  - —Esophageal reflux
  - —Biliary colic
  - —Gastritis/peptic ulcer disease
  - —Esophageal rupture
- Pulmonary
  - —Pulmonary embolus
  - —Pleurisy
  - —Pulmonary hypertension
  - —Pneumothorax
  - —Pneumonia
- Other
  - —Musculoskeletal
  - —Herpes zoster (Shingles)
  - —Functional/psychogenic

Pre-Hospital

- Intravenous access
- Cardiac monitoring
- Oxygen
- Pain control
  - —Nitrates
  - —Morphine
- All chest pain should be treated and transported as a possible life-threatening emergency

Diagnosis

ESSENTIAL WORKUP

- The history is the most important tool to distinguish between the various etiologies
- Have the patient define the key features
  - —Duration
  - —Location
    - -Retrosternal
    - -Subxiphoid
    - -Diffuse
  - —Frequency
    - -Constant
    - -Intermittent
    - -Sudden vs. Delayed onset
  - —Precipitating factors
    - -Exertion
    - -Stress
    - -Food
    - -Respiration
    - -Movement
  - —Quality
    - -Burning
    - -Squeezing
    - -Dull
    - -Sharp
    - -Tearing
    - -Heavy
  - —Associated symptoms
    - -SOB
    - -Diaphoresis
    - -Nausea
    - -Vomiting
    - -Jaw pain
    - -Back pain
    - -Radiation
    - -Palpitations
    - -Weakness
    - -Fatigue

Electrocardiogram

- Inexpensive and available
- Cardiac ischemia
  - —Sensitivity on initial tracing is less than 40%
  - —Certain signs increase suspicion
    - -T-wave inversion
    - -ST abnormalities
  - —Comparison with old tracings is often helpful and may be diagnostic
  - —Serial EKG
    - -Initial nondiagnostic pattern
    - -Change in symptoms
- Pulmonary embolism
  - —Classically associated with the S1, Q3, T3 pattern
    - -Sensitivity of this is less than 20%
    - -Sinus tachycardia is seen in less than 50%
- Aortic dissection
  - —May present with a ECG consistent with AMI due to dissection into the coronary artery
- Acute pericarditis
  - —Consistent although not universal pattern of ECG changes

-Diffuse ST elevations followed by T-wave inversions; not coexistent except in V1
-PR depression is seen in 80% of acute pericarditis
- Noncardiac causes of chest pain
  —Not usually associated with new abnormalities except sinus tachycardia

Treatment

Chest X-ray

- Pneumothorax
- Pneumonia
  —A complication of ischemic heart disease such as congestive heart failure
- Aortic dissection
  —Widened mediastinum seen in approximately 80% of patients
  —A normal chest x-ray does *not* rule it out
- Acute pericarditis
  —Usually normal unless massive effusion enlarges cardiac silhouette
- Esophageal rupture
  —Usually will show mediastinal air
  —May have left pleural effusion

LABORATORY

- CK-MB and Troponin T or I
  —They have a high positive predictive value
  —If negative initially, they cannot be used to rule out myocardial ischemia
- D-dimer
  —Sensitive but poor specificity for PE
  —Increased sensitivity with ELISA methods
- CBC/SMA-7
  —Screening labs for patients who present with chest pain
- Liver function tests/amylase
  —GI cause is suspected for the pain
- Toxicologic screen
  —Cocaine as suspected cause of chest pain if unable to confirm by history

IMAGING/SPECIAL TESTS

- Ultrasound
  —Test of choice for pericardial and valvular disease
  —May be helpful in acute ischemic coronary artery disease by showing wall motion abnormalities
  —Transesophageal echocardiography can be used in diagnosis of aortic dissection, especially in the unstable patient or those unable to tolerate contrast
  —Right ventricular dilation and hypokinesia may suggest pulmonary embolus
- Stress echocardiogram
  —Chest pain centers
  —Stable patients who have been ruled out for infarction
- CT scan
  —Sensitive for aortic dissection
  —Useful in stable patient
  —Some centers are using currently in diagnosis of pulmonary embolus and in stable cardiac effusion
- V/Q scan
  —Useful in pulmonary embolus
  —Can rule in or out based on high probability or normal scan
  —Otherwise, further testing based on clinical suspicion
- Angiography
  —Useful in dissection, especially in stable patients

Treatment

INITIAL STABILIZATION

- Intravenous access
- Oxygen
- Cardiac monitoring
- Oxygen saturation
- Pain and severe hypertension or hypotension should be controlled
- Acute myocardial infarction patients who meet criteria should have thrombolysis or catheterization as soon as possible (preferably <60 minutes) after arrival

MEDICATIONS

- Nitroglycerin: 0.4 mg sublingual, or 1–2 inches of nitropaste, or drip at 5–10 μg/min and titrate to effect
- Aspirin: 160–325 mg po
- Morphine sulfate: 2–4 mg every 5 min
- Propranolol: 1–2 mg IV every 2 min
- Metoprolol: 5 mg IV every 2 hrs up to 15 mg
- Esmolol: 50 μg/kg bolus then 50–200 μg/min drip
- Labetolol: 20 mg IV every 10 min up to 300 mg
- Nitroprusside: 0.3–10 μg/kg/min drip
- Aluminum and magnesium hydroxide: 15–30 ml po q 2–4 hrs
- Cimetidine: 300 mg IV/po q 6 hrs
- Donnatal: 5–10 ml po q 6 hrs

Disposition

- Dependent on the etiology of the pain. In general, there is usually a higher admission rate with negative evaluations due to the potential for adverse outcomes with the incorrect diagnosis. Recently, there has been an increase in the use of specialized chest pain centers to rule out and work up low-risk chest pain in the ED. In the future, increased use of markers and diagnostic tools such as sestamibi perfusion imaging and continuous 12-lead ECG may become more important
- Most patients may be admitted to a floor bed with telemetry if low-risk chest pain. High-risk patients are better served by an intensive care unit

ADMISSION CRITERIA

- There are no definite criteria for admission, although several protocols and practice guidelines exist or are being developed to deal with this situation. Decisions are usually complex based on risk factors, symptoms, combinations of diagnostic interventions, and patient preference. In general, if a cardiopulmonary risk for chest pain is the diagnosis or a high probability, it is often prudent to admit the patient

DISCHARGE CRITERIA

- Important to classify patient as very low risk for untoward event if discharge is planned

Miscellaneous

ICD9: 786.5

CORE CONTENT CODE: N/A

SUGGESTED READINGS

Braunwald E, Jones RH, Mark DB, et al. Diagnosing and managing unstable angina. Agency for Health Care Policy and Research. Circulation 1994;90(1):613–622.

Gibler WB, Runyon JP, Levy R, et al. A rapid diagnostic and treatment center for patients with chest pain in the emergency department. Ann Emerg Med 1995;25:1–8.

Goldman L, Cook EF, Brand DA, et al. A computer protocol to predict myocardial infarction in emergency department patients with chest pain. N Engl J Med 1988;318:797–803.

O'Gara PT, DeSanctis RW. Acute aortic dissection and its variants: toward a common diagnostic and therapeutic approach. Circulation 1995;92:1376–1378.

Selker, HP, Zalenski RJ, Antman EM, et al. An evaluation of technologies for identifying acute cardiac ischemia in the emergency department: executive summary of a National Heart Attack Alert Program Working Group Report. Ann Emerg Med 1997;29:1–12.

Pioped Investigators. Value of the ventilation perfusion scan in acute pulmonary embolism. Results of the prospective investigation of pulmonary embolism diagnosis (PIOPED). JAMA 1990;263:2753–2759.

The Global Utilization of Streptokinase and t-PA for Occluded Coronary Arteries (GUSTO) Angiographic Investigators. The effects of tissue plasminogen activator, streptokinase, or both on coronary artery patency, ventricular function, and survival after acute myocardial infarction. N Engl J Med 1993;329:1615–1622.

Authors: Eric Legome; Howard Weinberg

Chest Trauma, Blunt

Clinical Presentation

SIGNS AND SYMPTOMS

- Common mechanisms include MVA, MCA, auto versus pedestrian, auto versus bike, falls, and assaults
- Obvious contusion, wound, or other defect in the chest wall
- Crepitus or subcutaneous air in the chest wall
- Decreased or absent breath sounds
- Chest pain
- Tenderness to palpation
- Pain with deep inspiration or cough
- Dyspnea
- Usually occurs in combination with other injuries
- Hypotension

Pre-Hospital

CAUTIONS

- All patients with any signs of life in the field per EMS evaluation should be transported to a trauma center
- Full spinal precautions should be maintained due to the risk of concomitant cervical or thoracolumbar spine injury
- Needle decompression may be necessary if tension pneumothorax exists (unilaterally absent breath sounds, hypotension, jugular venous distention) and EMS protocols allow
- If large open pneumothorax exists, tape the dressing on three sides as a totally occlusive dressing can result in a tension pneumothorax

CONTROVERSIES

- Do not delay transport to hospital in order to obtain IV access, obtain en route

Diagnosis

ESSENTIAL WORKUP

- Rapid examination focusing on breath sounds, BP, pulses, heart sounds, and the chest wall
- Obtain immediate supine CXR; avoid upright CXR due to the potential for other injuries that may be exacerbated (especially spinal fractures)
- ECG and monitor to detect myocardial injury or dysrhythmias
- Baseline hemoglobin
- Pulse oximetry or arterial blood gas
- Type and screen

LABORATORY, IMAGING/SPECIAL TESTS

- If CXR reveals widened mediastinum and patient is hemodynamically stable, repeat CXR in upright position when it is safe to do so. If patient is unstable, emergent thoracotomy may be necessary to repair traumatic aortic disruption
- Chest CT with contrast, or arch arteriogram, is useful in identifying aortic and other large vessel injuries
- If there are signs of pericardial tamponade and patient is unstable, proceed to OR for a pericardial window
- If there are signs of tamponade and patient is stable, perform an urgent echocardiogram
- Gastrografin swallow for possible esophageal injury (e.g., pneumomediastinum)
- Bronchoscopy for possible upper airway injuries (e.g., large persistent air leak after chest tube)
- EKG if sternal tenderness is present or abnormalities on cardiac monitor

DIFFERENTIAL DIAGNOSIS

- Simple pneumothorax
- Tension pneumothorax
- Open pneumothorax
- Hemothorax
- Rib fractures
- Flail chest
- Pulmonary contusion
- Myocardial contusion
- Myocardial rupture
- Pericardial tamponade
- Traumatic aortic disruption
- Esophageal injury
- Large vascular injury (subclavian, pulmonary artery)
- Tracheobronchial injury
- Diaphragmatic injury

SPECIAL PEDIATRIC CONSIDERATIONS

- Rib cage is very elastic in children and can withstand significant forces without overt signs of external trauma, but may have major internal injuries

Treatment

INITIAL STABILIZATION

- Resuscitation attempts should only be initiated in patients who arrive in the ED with vital signs
- Any patient that presents in blunt traumatic arrest is not likely to survive an emergency department thoracotomy, and therefore it is not indicated in this group
- ABCs; intubate early if signs of respiratory insufficiency, shock or altered mental status exist
- If the patient is unstable and clinically has signs of a tension pneumothorax, perform a needle thoracostomy and place a chest tube immediately; do not wait to get a CXR. Place chest tube on the affected side or bilaterally if injury site is unclear
- Oxygen by face mask for stable patients
- Obtain vascular access, preferably 2 large IVs (>18-gauge)
- Maintain spinal immobilization

ED TREATMENT

- Notify trauma surgeon early of patients with significant injuries requiring surgical intervention or admission
- Tube thoracostomy if pneumothorax or hemothorax is identified (use at least a 36-French chest tube in an adult, largest that is practical for a pediatric patient)
- Fluid resuscitation as necessary. Note that aggressive fluid resuscitation may be harmful if severe pulmonary contusions exist
- Work-up for associated intra-abdominal injuries (e.g., with DPL, abdominal ultrasound, abdominal CT scan) because patients with chest trauma frequently have additional intra-abdominal injuries (liver or spleen lacerations, diaphragm injury)

MEDICATIONS

- Small doses of short-acting analgesics such as fentanyl (1–2 μg/kg) as needed for pain control, but must monitor patient closely to avoid respiratory depression. Longer acting analgesics when the patient is stable
- Tetanus booster if indicated
- IV antibiotics if wounds are grossly contaminated
- Methylprednisolone: 30 mg/kg IV over 1 hour, followed by a continuous drip of 5.4 mg/kg/hr for next 23 hours for signs of spinal cord injury

Disposition

ADMISSION CRITERIA

- Patients with conduction blocks, frequent ectopy, or ischemic changes on EKG should be admitted to a monitored bed for possible myocardial contusion
- Hemodynamically unstable patients should go to the operating room emergently for a thoracotomy or laparotomy
- More than 1000–1500 ml of blood out of the chest tube upon initial insertion indicates probable need for thoracotomy. Also more than 200 ml of blood per hour from chest tube for several hours suggests the need for surgical intervention to control hemorrhage
- Patients with significant rib fractures should be admitted for pain control, ideally with an epidural catheter
- Patients who lose their BP in the ED should undergo rapid open thoracotomy

DISCHARGE CRITERIA

- Patients with clinically insignificant chest wall contusions and an initial negative CXR can be observed for 6 hours in the ED and have a repeat CXR done. If the repeat CXR reveals no pneumothorax, hemothorax, or pulmonary contusion, and the patient is able to deep breathe and cough, they can be discharged home

Miscellaneous

ICD9: 862.8

CORE CURRICULUM CODE: 18.4.10

SUGGESTED READINGS

Bodai BI, Smith JP, Blaidell FW. The role of emergency thoracotomy in blunt trauma. J Trauma 1982;22(6):487

Calhoon JH, Grover FL, Trinkle JK. Chest trauma: Approach and management. Clin Chest Med 1992;13:55

Feliciano DV. The diagnostic and therapeutic approach to chest trauma. Semin Thorac Cardiovasc Surg 1992;4:156

Mansour KA, ed. Trauma of the chest. Chest Surg Clin North Am 1997;7

Sheikh AA, Culbertson CB. Emergency department thoracotomy in children: Rationale for selective application. J Trauma 1993;34(3):323

Author: John C. Sakles

Chest Trauma, Penetrating

Clinical Presentation

SIGNS AND SYMPTOMS

- Impaled object in the chest wall
- Obvious wound in the chest wall
- Chest pain
- Dyspnea
- Respiratory distress
- Altered mental status from hypoxemia
- Absent or altered breath sounds on one or both sides
- Hypotension

Pre-Hospital

CAUTIONS

- All patients with any signs of life in the field per EMS evaluation should be transported to a trauma center
- Full spinal precautions should be maintained due to the risk of concomitant thoracolumbar spinal cord injury
- Never remove impaled objects in the chest as exsanguination may follow
- Needle decompression may be necessary if tension pneumothorax exists (unilaterally absent breath sounds, hypotension, jugular venous distention) and EMS protocols allow
- If large open pneumothorax exists, tape the dressing on three sides as a totally occlusive dressing can result in a tension pneumothorax

CONTROVERSIES

- Do not delay transport to hospital in order to obtain IV access; obtain en route

Diagnosis

ESSENTIAL WORKUP

- Rapid examination focusing on breath sounds, BP, pulses, heart sounds, and the chest wall
- Upright CXR is preferred for identifying a pneumothorax, but a supine CXR should be taken first if spinal precautions are maintained
- Baseline hemoglobin
- Pulse oximetry or arterial blood gas
- Type and screen

LABORATORY, IMAGING/SPECIAL TESTS

- With GSWs, other areas (abdomen, pelvis, etc.) should be imaged (the total number of wounds and bullets must equal an even number)
- Echocardiogram if signs of tamponade or if wound is close to the heart
- Based on the location of wound, consider arteriogram of aortic arch, carotid arteries, or subclavian artery
- Esophageal gastrografin swallow or endoscopy to identify esophageal perforation
- Bronchoscopy to identify tracheobronchial injuries

DIFFERENTIAL DIAGNOSIS

- Simple pneumothorax
- Tension pneumothorax
- Open pneumothorax
- Hemothorax
- Rib fractures
- Flail chest
- Pulmonary contusion
- Myocardial contusion
- Myocardial rupture
- Pericardial tamponade
- Traumatic aortic disruption
- Esophageal injury
- Large vascular injury (subclavian, pulmonary artery)
- Tracheobronchial injury
- Diaphragmatic injury
- Intra-abdominal injury
- Spinal cord injury

Treatment

INITIAL STABILIZATION

- ABCs; intubate early if there are signs of serious chest injury, obvious respiratory distress, or hypotension
- 100% Oxygen by nonrebreathing face mask for stable patients
- Obtain vascular access, 2 peripheral large bore IVs (>18-guage), and fluid resuscitation as needed
- If the patient is unstable and clinically has signs of a tension pneumothorax, perform a needle thoracostomy and place a chest tube immediately; do not wait to get a CXR
- If the patient is unstable and has signs of pericardial tamponade, perform an emergent pericardiocentesis
- Maintain spinal immobilization if indicated

ED TREATMENT

- Notify trauma surgeon of patient
- Tube thoracostomy if a pneumothorax or hemothorax is identified (use at least a 36-French chest tube in an adult)
- Fluid resuscitation as necessary. Note that contused lung parenchyma will have leaky capillary beds and aggressive crystalloid resuscitation may aggravate pulmonary dysfunction
- Any wound with an entry or exit site inferior to the nipple or posterior tip of the scapula should be considered to have a concomitant intra-abdominal injury until proven otherwise. These patients should be worked up for penetrating abdominal trauma with a DPL, US, CT scan, exploratory laparotomy or laparoscopy
- Describe the nature of the wounds as accurately as possible, and retain any bullet fragments, clothes, or tissue removed from the wound
- Probing a chest wound is contraindicated as it potentially can create a pneumothorax or worsen hemorrhage rates
- Impaled objects should only be removed in the OR, not in the ED

MEDICATIONS

- Small doses of short-acting analgesics such fentanyl (1–2 μg/kg) or sedative agents such as midazolam (0.05 mg/kg) as needed for pain control and sedation. Monitor closely to avoid respiratory depression
- Tetanus booster if indicated
- IV antibiotics if wound grossly contaminated
- For spinal cord injury, methylprednisolone 30 mg/kg over 1 hour, followed by a continuous drip of 5.4 mg/kg/hr for 23 hours

Disposition

ADMISSION CRITERIA

- All patients with penetrating chest trauma should be admitted
- Any patient that has signs of life in the field but no blood pressure on ED arrival should have an emergent thoracotomy performed by the most experienced person present. If the source of bleeding is controlled and there are signs of cardiac activity, the patient should go to the OR for formal operative repair
- Hemodynamically unstable patients should go immediately to the operating room
- Any patient with intrathoracic penetration should have a chest tube placed and admitted for observation
- More than 1000–1500 ml of blood out of the chest tube upon initial insertion indicates the need for thoracotomy. Also more than 200 ml of blood per hour from chest tube for several hours suggests the need for surgical intervention
- Patients with large, persistent air leaks usually require surgery
- Patients with significant rib fractures should be admitted and have an epidural catheter placed for pain control, and pulmonary toilet

DISCHARGE CRITERIA

- Patients with isolated minor chest wounds and an initial negative CXR can be observed for 6 hours in the ED and have a repeat CXR performed. If repeat CXR reveals no intrathoracic penetration, the patient can be discharged home

Miscellaneous

ICD9: 862.9

CORE CURRICULUM CODE: 18.4.10.1

SUGGESTED READINGS

Baillot R, Dontigny L, Verdant A, et al. Penetrating chest trauma: A 20-year experience. J Trauma 1987;27(9):994

Baxter BT, et al. Emergency department thoracotomy following injury: Critical determinants for patient salvage. World J Surg 1988;12:671

Calhoon JH, Grover FL, Trinkle JK. Chest trauma: Approach and management. Clin Chest Med 1992;13:55

Feliciano DV. The diagnostic and therapeutic approach to chest trauma. Semin Thorac Cardiovasc Surg 1992;4:156

Ivatury RR, Cayten CG, eds. The textbook of penetrating trauma. Baltimore: Williams & Wilkins, 1996

Ivatury RR, Rohman M. Emergency department thoracotomy for trauma: A collective review. Resuscitation 1987;15:23

Mansour KA, ed. Trauma of the chest. Chest Surg Clin North Am 1997;7

Milham FH, Grindlinger GA. Survival determinants in patients undergoing emergency room thoracotomy for penetrating chest injury. J Trauma 1993;34(3):332

Author: John C. Sakles

Chlamydia

Clinical Presentation

SIGNS AND SYMPTOMS

Female

- 3–5% Asymptomatic carriers
- Cervicitis
  - —Yellow, mucopurulent endocervical discharge
  - —Cervical edema and friability
  - —Vaginal bleeding
- Vaginal itching
- Bartholin cyst
- Pelvic inflammatory disease
  - —Lower abdominal pain/tenderness
  - —Vaginal discharge
  - —Fever
  - —Nausea/vomiting
- Pregnancy related
  - —Preterm labor
  - —Postpartum endometritis

Male

- Urethritis
  - —Yellow-white thin discharge
  - —Urinary tract infection symptoms
    - -Dysuria
    - -Urgency
- Lymphogranuloma venereum
  - —Small, shallow, painless vesicles or ulcer in genital region
  - —May have rectal discharge or papule or stricture
  - —Massive inguinal adenopathy (buboes) 2–12 weeks after symptoms start
  - —Usually affects young males 20–40 years old
- Prostatitis
- Epididymitis
  - —Unilateral scrotal pain/tenderness
- Proctitis
- Reiter's Syndrome
  - —Reactive arthritis
  - —Urethritis
  - —Conjunctivitis

Other

- Pharyngitis
- Pneumonia
- Conjunctivitis
  - —Erythematous conjunctiva
  - —Mucopurulent discharge
  - —Photophobia
  - —Pseudoptosis
  - —Punctate keratitis

MECHANISM/DESCRIPTION

- Obligate intracellular parasite with features of both a virus and bacteria
  - —Growth cycle alternates between two morphological forms
- Produce intracellular infection
  - —Macrophage or nonmacrophage host cells support replication depending on species

ETIOLOGY

- Most common sexually transmitted disease in the United States
- Prevalence 3–5 times more than gonorrhea
- Major single cause of nongonococcal urethritis in heterosexual males
- Principal cause of infertility in females
- Number one cause of infectious blindness worldwide

PEDIATRIC CONSIDERATIONS

- Ophthalmia neonatorum—*Chlamydia trachoma*
  - —Bilateral conjunctivitis 5–13 days postbirth
  - —Corneal damage results in blindness if not treated
- Neonatal pneumonia
  - —Subacute onset
  - —Infants 1–4 months
  - —Staccato cough
  - —Eosinophilia
  - —Hypergammaglobulinemia

Pre-Hospital

N/A

Diagnosis

ESSENTIAL WORKUP

- Clinical diagnosis for chlamydia-related male sexually transmitted diseases (STD)
- Vaginal examination for chlamydia-related female STD

LABORATORY

- Gram stain of penile/vaginal discharge
  - —10 or more PMN at 1000 power without any gram negative diplococci
  - —Not sensitive/specific
- Identification of *Chlamydia trachomatis* by
  - —Monoclonal antibodies
  - —Antibody-antigen reaction
  - —DNA detection by polymerase chain reaction
  - —Plasmid DNA by direct probing
- UA for dysuria
  - —WBC in males
- RPR for syphilis with STD
- Pulse oximetry/ABG for pneumonia

IMAGING /SPECIAL TESTS

- CXR for pneumonia

DIFFERENTIAL DIAGNOSIS

- Gonorrhea
- Trichomonas
- Syphilis

Treatment

INITIAL STABILIZATION

- ABCs—supplemental oxygen for pneumonia

ED TREATMENT

Urethritis/Cervicitis

- Antibiotic options
  - —Doxycycline × 7 days
  - —Azithromycin 1 dose
  - —Ofloxacin × 7 days
  - —Erythromycin × 7 days
- Treat for concurrent gonorrhea
  - —3rd generation cephalosporin (cefixime/ceftriaxone)
- Recommend follow up RPR for syphilis/HIV
- Condom use until symptoms resolve and partner treated

Conjunctivitis

- Antibiotic options
  - —Doxycycline × 7 days
  - —Tetracycline × 7 days

Ophthalmia Neonatorum

- Erythromycin or tetracycline ophthalmic ointment for 21–60 days

Pneumonia

- Antibiotic options
  - —Doxycycline × 14 days
  - —Tetracycline × 14 days
  - —Erythromycin × 14 days

Lymphogranuloma Venereum

- Antibiotic options
  - —Doxycycline × 21 days
  - —Tetracycline × 21 days
  - —Erythromycin × 21 days

MEDICATIONS

- Azithromycin: 1 g po
- Cefixime (suprax) 400 mg po
- Ceftriaxone 250 mg IV
- Doxycycline: 100 mg po bid
- Erythromycin: 500 mg IV/po qid (peds: 20–40 mg/kg/24 hr)
- Ofloxacin: 300 mg po
- Tetracycline: 500 mg po qid

Disposition

ADMISSION CRITERIA

- Hypoxia with pneumonia

DISCHARGE CRITERIA

- Encourage treatment of partners with STD

Miscellaneous

ICD9: 78.88

CORE CONTENT CODE: 13.10.1

SUGGESTED READINGS

Adimora AA, Hamilton H, Holmes KK, Sparling PF. Sexually transmitted diseases—companion handbook. New York: McGraw Hill, 1994.

Berger RE. Sexually transmitted diseases. Adv Urol 1997;2:97.

Center for Disease Control and Prevention. 1993 Sexually transmitted disease treatment guidelines. MMWR 1993;42:1–102.

Author: David Levine

Chloral Hydrate, Poisoning

Clinical Presentation

SIGNS AND SYMPTOMS

- Central nervous system (CNS) depression from drowsiness to respiratory arrest
- Diminished sympathetic impulses
  - —Bradycardia
  - —Hypotension
- Nystagmus
- Miosis (early finding)
- Mydriasis (late finding)
- Hypotonia
- Rash
- Dysrhythmias
  - —Ventricular and supraventricular tachydysrhythmias
  - —Result from myocardial sensitization of trichloroethanol (TCE)
- Hemorrhagic gastritis after significant ingestions
- Pear-like breath odor

MECHANISM/DESCRIPTION

- Variable absorption and metabolism of chloral hydrate (CH)
  - —Difficult to determine a mg/kg dose for which toxicity will be exhibited
- CH and ethanol enhance the sedative effects of one another because their metabolism requires similar enzymes and cofactors
- CH is rapidly converted in liver to trichloroethanol (TCE), another CNS depressant
  - —Half-life of TCE = 9–40 hours

ETIOLOGY

- Hypnotic agent: used as an adult oral hypnotic, with doses ranging from 500 to 1000 mg
  - —Reciprocal potentiation of CH and ethanol led to term "slip 'em a Mickey"
    - -Reference to a late 19th-Century Chicago saloon proprietor, Mickey Finn, who used a concoction that probably contained CH and ethanol to render customers unconscious to rob them

PEDIATRIC CONSIDERATIONS

- Range of toxicity
  - —Significant toxicity found following ingestions of 1.5 g
  - —Survival reported in a child following a 38-g overdose
- Sedation
  - —Safe agent for sedation of children undergoing imaging studies
  - —Lack of analgesia limits use for medical and dental procedures
  - —Unsuitable for chronic dosing (ventilated patient) because active metabolites accumulate
- Dosage
  - —20–50 mg/kg/dose po to maximum 1 gm
  - —Onset in 15–60 minutes
  - —Duration 1–2 hours
  - —Rectal administration absorption erratic (not recommended)
- Increases the risk of hyperbilirubinemia and acidosis in newborns
  - —A highly protein bound metabolite, trichloroacetic acid (TCA), competes with bilirubin for albumin-binding sites

Pre-Hospital

CAUTIONS

- CH may increase release of catecholamines and sensitize the myocardium to catecholamines leading to ventricular dysrhythmia
- Chronic use of CH leads to physical dependence and tolerance
  - —Withdrawal syndrome occurs
- Sedation postingestion

Diagnosis

ESSENTIAL WORKUP

- History of CH administration

LABORATORY

- Levels of CH and TCE are not generally useful or available
- CBC
  - —Hct important with erosive gastritis
- Electrolytes, BUN/Cr, glucose
  - —If anion gap acidosis, search for concomitant ingestant
- ABG/pulse oximetry
  - —With respiratory depression
- Urinalysis
  - —Proteinuria found with significant overdose

IMAGING/SPECIAL TESTS

- Abdominal radiograph
  - —Undissolved capsules of CH radiopaque
  - —Unreliable due to the rapid dissolution time of CH
- ECG for dysrhythmias

DIFFERENTIAL DIAGNOSIS

- Consider other CNS depressants
  - —Alcohols
  - —Anticholinergics
  - —Antihistamines
  - —Barbiturates
  - —Benzodiazepines
  - —Other sedative-hypnotics

Treatment

INITIAL STABILIZATION

- Airway
  - —Maintain a patent airway
  - —Oxygen
  - —Provide respiratory support with intubation/ventilation

ED TREATMENT

- —Cardiac monitor
- —Pulse oximetry
- —IV access
- —Hypotension
- —0.9%NS fluid bolus 500 cc–1 L (peds: 20 cc/kg)
- —Pressor support for severe, persistent hypotension (dopamine)
- —Use β-adrenergic drugs carefully—may increase dysrhythmias
- Tachydysrhythmia therapy
  - —β Blockage (propranolol, esmolol)
  - —Lidocaine
- Gastric decontamination
  - —Gastric lavage if <1 hour has elapsed since an acute ingestion
  - —Activated charcoal is of limited use
- Hemodialysis for massive acute CH overdose

MEDICATIONS

- Dopamine: 2–20 μg/kg/min IV
- Esmolol: 50–200 μg/kg/min IVPB (onset in seconds, $T^1/_2$ = 9 minutes): load 500 μg/kg over 1 min, followed by 50 μg/kg/min. If adequate therapeutic effect not achieved within 5 min, repeat loading dose and increase infusion to 100 μg/kg/min. Titrate infusion rate upwards at 50 μg/kg/min q 4–5 min as needed. Omit further loading doses once nearing therapeutic target
- Lidocaine: 1 mg/kg IVP
- Propranolol: 1–2 mg slow IVP (peds: 0.01–0.02 mg/kg IV; maximum 1 mg IV) over 10–15 min while monitoring pulse and blood pressure

Disposition

ADMISSION CRITERIA

- Respiratory depression
- Hypotension
- Risk of injury from fall
- Cardiac dysrhythmia

DISCHARGE CRITERIA

- If no toxicity observed within 3 hours of a dose

PEDIATRIC CONSIDERATIONS

- CH effects may be prolonged in younger patients

Miscellaneous

ICD9: 967.1

CORE CONTENT CODE: 17.2.42

SUGGESTED READINGS

American Academy of Pediatrics Committee on Drugs and Committee on Environmental Health. Use of chloral hydrate for sedation in children. Pediatrics 1993;92(3):471–473.

Ellenhorn MJ, Schonwald S, Ordog G, Wasserberger J. Chloral hydrate. In: Ellenhorn's medical toxicology. Baltimore: Williams & Wilkins, 1997:695.

Hardman JG, Limbird LE, eds. Goodman & Gilman's the pharmacologic basis of therapeutics. 9th ed. New York: McGraw-Hill, 1996.

Krauss BS, Shannon MW, Damian FJ, Fleisher GR, eds. Guidelines for pediatric sedation. Dallas: American College of Emergency Physicians, 1995.

Osborn H, Goldfrank LR. Sedative-hypnotic agents. In: Goldfrank LR, ed. Goldfrank's toxicologic emergencies. 5th ed, Norwalk, CT: Appleton & Lange, 1994.

Salmon AG, Kizer KW, Zeise L, et al. Potential carcinogenicity of chloral hydrate—a review. Clin Toxicol 1995;33(2):115–121.

Wythe ET. Sedative-hypnotic agents. In: Olson KR, ed. Poisoning and drug overdose. 2d ed. Norwalk, CT: Appleton & Lange, 1994.

Author: Carl Baum

Cholangitis

Clinical Presentation

SIGNS AND SYMPTOMS

- Charcot's Triad
  - —Classic presentation of fever and chills; RUQ pain and jaundice found in only 50–70%
  - —Addition of shock and altered mental status denotes a more advanced form of biliary sepsis known as *Reynold's Pentad*
- Fever found in >90%
- Abdominal pain present in >70%—localizing to RUQ
- Peritoneal findings found in 30%
- Clinically apparent jaundice may be absent in up to 40%
- AIDS sclerosing cholangitis presents with similar symptoms but with more chronic indolent course

MECHANISM/DESCRIPTION

- Partial or complete obstruction of the common bile duct due to gallstones, tumor, cyst, or stricture
- Increased intraluminal pressure in biliary tree
- Bacterial multiplication results in bacteremia and sepsis
- Purulent infection of biliary tree which may involve the liver and gallbladder

ETIOLOGY

- Bacterial sources of infection include
  - —Ascending duodenal source
  - —Gallbladder infection
  - —Portal venous seeding
  - —Hematogenous spread with hepatic secretion
  - —Lymphatic spread
- Bacterial organisms include
  - —Anaerobes (*Bacteroides sp.* and *Clostridium sp.*)
  - —Intestinal coliforms (*E. coli*)
  - —Enterococcus
- AIDS sclerosing cholangitis characterized by
  - —Papillary stenosis
  - —Sclerosing cholangitis
  - —Extrahepatic biliary obstruction
  - —CMV, cryptosporidium, and microsporidia isolated but causal role not established

PEDIATRIC CONSIDERATIONS

- Extremely rare in childhood
- Clinical presentation similar
- Most commonly found following surgical correction for primary biliary atresia or choledochal cyst

Pre-Hospital

CAUTION

- Stabilize septic shock

Diagnosis

ESSENTIAL WORKUP

- EKG in patients at risk for coronary artery disease
- CBC, liver function test (LFT), amylase, lipase, U/A, blood cultures
- Gallbladder ultrasound or HIDA scan

LABORATORY

- CBC—leukocytosis with "left shift" unless immunocompromised or severe sepsis
- LFTs consistent with cholestasis
  - —Elevated direct bilirubin and alkaline phosphatase
  - —Minimal elevation of transaminases (<200 IU/ml)
  - —Changes may lag symptom onset by 24–48 hours
- Amylase/lipase normal or mildly elevated
- U/A: (+) Bilirubin

IMAGING /SPECIAL TESTS

- *Ultrasound* detects the level of ductal obstruction and the presence of gallstone etiology
- *Radionuclide scanning (HIDA)*
  - —Indicates obstruction when tracer not found in duodenum with 1 hour
  - —More sensitive than ultrasound in detecting obstruction in the first 24–48 hours before ductal dilation occurs
- *Abdominal Radiograph/CXR*
  - —Useful to rule out intestinal obstruction, perforation, or pneumonia
  - —20% gallstones radiopaque

DIFFERENTIAL DIAGNOSIS

- Acute cholecystitis
- Hepatitis or hepatic abscess
- Acute pancreatitis
- Right pyelonephritis
- Right lower lobe pneumonia or pulmonary embolism
- Perforated duodenal ulcer
- Appendicitis
- Sepsis with nonspecific elevation of liver function tests
- Fitz-Hugh-Curtis Syndrome

Treatment

INITIAL STABILIZATION

- Immediate IV fluid resuscitation for dehydration, hemodynamic compromise, and sepsis
- Vasopressors (dopamine) for hypotension refractory to volume replacement

ED TREATMENT

- Broad spectrum antibiotics for coliforms, anaerobes, and enterococcus such as
  —Ampicillin/sulbactam
  —Ticarcillin/clavulanic acid
  —Piperacillin/tazobactam plus aminoglycoside (gentamicin or tobramycin)
  —Substitute clindamycin in penicillin allergy
  —Substitute aztreonam for aminoglycoside in renal insufficiency
- NPO
- NG suctioning if protracted vomiting or ileus
- IV fluid (0.9%NS) replacement and maintenance
- Narcotic analgesia if hemodynamically stable and diagnosis reasonably established
- Immediate surgical consultation
- Emergency invasive biliary drainage procedure (surgical, percutaneous, or ERCP) if no response to medical treatment in 12–24 hours

MEDICATIONS

- Ampicillin/sulbactam: 3 g IVPB
- Aztreonam: 2 g IVPB
- Clindamycin: 600 mg IVPB
- Dopamine: 2–10 mcg/min IVPB titrate to maintain BP
- Gertamicin 5 mg/kg q 24° or 1.5–2 mg/kg and then 3–5 mg/kg/24 hr q 8 hr; follow levels
- Meperidine: 0.5 mg/kg IVP titrated up to 2.0 mg/kg for pain relief
- Promethazine (antiemetic): 12.5–25mg IVP
- Piperacillin/tazobactam: 3.375 mg IVPB
- Ticarcillin/clavulanic acid: 3.1 g IVPB
- Tobramycin 1.5–2 mg/kg load IV then 3–5 mg/kg/24hr q 8 hr; Follow levels

Disposition

ADMISSION CRITERIA

- All patients with acute cholangitis should be admitted with immediate surgical and gastroenterologic consultation
- Admit patients with signs of septic shock to the ICU

DISCHARGE CRITERIA

None

Miscellaneous

ICD9: 576.1

CORE CONTENT CODE: 1.3.2

SUGGESTED READINGS

Csendes A, Diaz JC, Malvenda F, et al. Risk factors and classification of acute suppurative cholangitis. Br J Surg 1992;79: 655–658.

Hanau LH, Steigbigel NH, Cholangitis: Pathogenesis, diagnosis and treatment. Curr Clin Top Infect Dis 1995;311:99–105.

Lai EC, Mok FP, Tan ES, et al. Endoscopic biliary drainage for severe acute cholangitis. N Engl J Med 1992;326:1582–1586.

Lipsett PA, Pitt HA. Acute cholangitis. Surg Clin North Am 1990;70:1297–1312.

Moscati RM. Cholelithiasis, cholecystitis and pancreatitis. In: Hunter DM, ed. Gastrointestinal emergencies, Part II. Emerg Med Clin North Am 1996;14:719–737.

Author: Robert Buckley

Cholecystitis

Clinical Presentation

SIGNS AND SYMPTOMS

Acute Calculous Cholecystitis

- Dull, aching, epigastric, or RUQ pain
  - —Radiation to tip of right scapula, acromion, or thoracic spine
  - —Duration >6 hours more suggestive of cholecystitis than uncomplicated biliary colic
- As inflammation progresses, parietal peritoneal irritation leads to sharp, localized pain
- *Murphy's sign*
  - —Inspiratory arrest with gentle palpation of RUQ due to increased pain
  - —Found in most cases
- Localized parietal peritoneal signs
  - —Percussion tenderness
  - —Rebound
  - —Found as the disease progresses
- Nausea, vomiting, fever, and chills often reported, but are absent in majority of cases
- Jaundice in 20%
- History of prior attacks of biliary colic or known gallstones favors diagnosis

Acalculous Cholecystitis

- Occurs in critically ill patients (burns, sepsis, trauma, or postoperative)
- Localized pain and tenderness frequently absent
- Often presents with symptoms of generalized sepsis of unknown source

MECHANISM/DESCRIPTION

- Cholecystitis is defined as inflammation of the gallbladder

ETIOLOGY

- Acute calculous cholecystitis
  - —Due to bile stasis secondary to prolonged obstruction by a gallstone in the gallbladder neck, cystic duct, or common bile duct
  - —Leads to increased intraluminal pressure and mucosal damage
  - —Release of inflammatory mediators result in distention, edema, and increased vascularity
  - —Coliforms and anaerobes lead to infection—primary causal role is controversial
- Acalculous cholecystitis
  - —10% of cases
  - —Underlying critical illness leads to biliary stasis and mucosal ischemia
  - —Subsequent mucosal inflammation and infection

PEDIATRIC CONSIDERATIONS

- *Acute calculous cholecystitis* extremely rare in childhood (see Cholelithiasis)
- *Acalculous cholecystitis* more common than calculous form in children.
  - —Associated with systemic bacterial infections, scarlet fever, Kawasaki disease, and parasitic infections

Pre-Hospital

N/A

Diagnosis

ESSENTIAL WORKUP

- EKG in patients at risk for coronary artery disease
- CBC, liver function tests (LFTs), amylase, lipase, U/A, and HCG
- Gallbladder US or HIDA scan

LABORATORY

- CBC
  - —WBC >12,000 cells/mm^3 supports diagnosis but may be normal in over half
- Liver function tests
  - —Transaminases, bilirubin, amylase, and lipase may be minimally elevated but are generally normal
  - —Disproportionate elevation of direct bilirubin and alkaline phosphatase compared to transaminases suspicious for common duct obstruction or cholangitis

IMAGING/SPECIAL TESTS

- Ultrasound
  - —Generally the first-line imaging procedure
  - —Positive findings include gallbladder wall thickening (>5 mm) or pericolic fluid—sensitivity 90%, specificity 80%
  - —Optimal if patient NPO >8 hours
- Radionuclide scanning *(HIDA)*
  - —Most useful when clinical suspicion remains high despite equivocal findings on ultrasound or when acalculous cholecystitis suspected
  - —Positive when inflamed gallbladder fails to visualize
  - —Sensitivity >95%, specificity 90%
  - —False-positives increase in nonfasting state
- Abdominal x-rays
  - —Excludes intestinal perforation or obstruction
  - —Air in the gallbladder wall consistent with emphysematous cholecystitis
  - —Gallstones radiopaque in up to 20%

DIFFERENTIAL DIAGNOSIS

- Biliary colic
- Hepatitis or hepatic abscess
- Cholangitis
- Pancreatitis
- Duodenal perforation
- Peptic ulcer disease
- Gastritis
- Duodenal perforation
- Right lower lobe pneumonia, pleurisy or pulmonary infarction
- Myocardial infarction
- Abdominal aortic aneurysm
- Appendicitis
- Fitz-Hugh-Curtis syndrome
- Pyelonephritis

Treatment

INITIAL STABILIZATION

- IV, oxygen, cardiac monitoring until myocardial ischemic cause excluded
- Initiate IV fluid therapy for dehydration, hemodynamic compromise or sepsis

ED TREATMENT

- Broad spectrum antibiotics for coliforms, anaerobes, and enterococcus
  —Ampicillin/sulbactam
  —Ticarcillin/ clavulanic acid
  —Piperacillin/ tazobactam
  —Alternate: clindamycin with gentamicin in penicillin allergic
- NPO
- IV fluid replacement and maintenance
- Antiemetics (promethazine) if vomiting
- NG suctioning if refractory vomiting or ileus
- Anticholinergics less useful than in simple biliary colic
- Narcotic analgesia (meperidine) once diagnosis firmly established
- Surgical consultation

MEDICATIONS

- Ampicillin/sulbactam: 3.0 g IVPB
- Clindamycin: 600 mg IVPB
- Gentamicin: 2.0 mg/kg IVPB
- Glycopyrrolate (anticholinergic): 0.2 mg IVP q 10 mins up to 3 doses PRN pain
- Meperidine: 0.5 mg/kg IVP titrated up to 2.0 mg/kg for pain relief
- Piperacillin/tazobactam: 3.375 mg IVPB
- Promethazine: 12.5–25 mg IVP
- Ticarcillin/clavulanic acid: 3.1 g IVPB

PEDIATRIC CONSIDERATIONS

- Therapy similar to adults

Disposition

ADMISSION CRITERIA

- All cases of cholecystitis should be admitted for parenteral antibiotics, analgesia, fluid replacement, and cholecystectomy in 24–72 hours
- Unstable patients (gallbladder perforation or sepsis) require immediate surgery

DISCHARGE CRITERIA

- Discharge should rarely be considered once the diagnosis of cholecystitis is confirmed

Miscellaneous

ICD9: 575.10

CORE CONTENT CODE: 1.3.1

SUGGESTED READINGS

Silen W. Cholecystitis and other causes of acute pain in the right upper quadrant of the abdomen. In: Silen W, ed. Cope's early diagnosis of the acute abdomen. 18th ed. Oxford: Oxford University Press, 1991:132–141.

Gruber PJ, Silverman RA, Gottesfeld S, Flaster E. Presence of fever and leukocytosis in acute cholecystitis. Ann Emerg Med 1996;28:273–277.

Moscati RM. Cholelithiasis, cholecystitis and pancreatitis. In: Hunter DM, ed. Gastrointestinal emergencies, Part II. Emerg Med Clin North Am 1996;14:719–737.

Singer AJ, McCracken G, Henry MC, et al. Correlation among clinical, laboratory, and hepatobiliary scanning findings in patients with suspected acute cholecystitis. Ann Emerg Med 1996;28:267–272.

Shea JA, Berlin JA, Escarce JJ, et al. Revised estimates of diagnostic test sensitivity and specificity in suspected biliary tract disease. Arch Intern Med 1994;154:2573–2581.

Author: Robert Buckley

Cholelithiasis

Clinical Presentation

SIGNS AND SYMPTOMS

- Dull, aching epigastric or RUQ pain
  - —Arising over 2–3 minutes, continuous (rather than "colicky") and lasting from 30 minutes to 6 hours before dissipating
  - —May radiate to the tip of right scapula, acromion, or thoracic spine
  - —Often correlated with ingestion of large fatty meal
  - —Tenderness to deep palpation but without rebound
  - —*Murphy's sign* (inspiratory arrest during deep palpation of the RUQ) may be present during the episode of colic, but should resolve when symptoms pass
- Anorexia
- Nausea/vomiting
- Afebrile
  - —Fever and chills suggest cholecystitis or cholangitis

MECHANISM

- Symptoms arise when gallstones pass through the cystic or common bile ducts leading to impedance of normal bile flow and gallbladder spasm
- Cholesterol stones
  - —Most common type of gallstone
  - —Form when its solubility exceeded
- Pigment stones
  - —20%
  - —Comprised of calcium bilirubinate
  - —Associated with clinical conditions such as hemolytic anemias which lead to increased concentration of unconjugated bilirubin

ETIOLOGY

- Incidence increases with age and favors females to males 2:1

PEDIATRIC CONSIDERATIONS

- Gallstones are exceedingly rare in childhood
- Most commonly associated with sickle cell disease, hereditary spherocytosis, or other hemolytic anemias that result in pigment stone formation

Pre-Hospital

N/A

Diagnosis

ESSENTIAL WORKUP

- Obtain EKG on those whose pain may be due to myocardial ischemia
- CBC, liver function tests (LFTs), amylase, lipase, U/A, and HCG

LABORATORY

- CBC
  - —WBC usually normal but may elevate after vomiting
  - —Leukocytosis suggestive of cholecystitis or cholangitis
- Liver function tests
  - —Usually normal
  - —Elevation suggests common duct obstruction, cholangitis, cholecystitis, or hepatitis
- Amylase/lipase
  - —Normal or minimally elevated with passage of gallstone
  - —Elevation in context of severe persistent epigastric pain suggests pancreatitis
- U/A
  - —Exclude nephrolithiasis or pyelonephritis
  - —Bilirubinuria suggests common duct obstruction or hepatitis

IMAGING/SPECIAL TESTS

- Ultrasound
  - —Detects gallstones with sensitivity and specificity >90%
  - —Dilation of common bile duct >10 mm indicates obstruction but may be normal with acute obstruction
  - —Gallbladder wall thickening >5 mm or pericolic fluid 90% sensitive and 80% specific for cholecystitis
  - —Accuracy enhanced in fasting patient with noncontracted gallbladder
- Radionuclide scanning (HIDA)
  - —Useful to exclude CBD obstruction or cholecystitis
  - —Cannot detect gallstones
- Plain x-rays
  - —Not helpful in diagnosing uncomplicated cholelithiasis
  - —Excludes intestinal perforation or intestinal obstruction
  - —Up to 20% of gallstones radiopaque
  - —Reveals rare complications such as air in gallbladder wall in emphysematous cholecystitis or air-filled gallbladder in biliary-enteric fistula
- CT scanning
  - —Less sensitive than ultrasound to detect gallstones
  - —Most useful to exclude other causes of upper abdominal pain such as aortic aneurysm, perihepatic abscess, or pancreatic pseudocyst

DIFFERENTIAL DIAGNOSIS

- Myocardial infarction
- Abdominal aortic aneurysm
- Acute cholecystitis, cholangitis, or choledocholithiasis
- Renal colic or pyelonephritis
- Duodenal ulcer perforation
- Acute pancreatitis
- Intestinal obstruction
- Peptic ulcer disease, gastritis, or gastroesophageal reflux
- Right lower lobe pneumonia, pleurisy, or pulmonary infarction
- Hepatic abscess
- Fitz-Hugh-Curtis syndrome

Treatment

INITIAL STABILIZATION

- IV access

ED TREATMENT

- IV hydration with 0.9%NS if vomiting
- NPO
- Anticholinergics (glycopyrrolate) commonly used despite lack of clinical trials proving benefit
- Parenteral NSAIDs (ketorolac) may lessen biliary spasm but may exacerbate peptic causes of pain
- Narcotic analgesics (meperidine) with antiemetic (promethazine)
  —Administer for refractory pain once diagnosis is reasonably established

MEDICATIONS

- Glycopyrrolate (anticholinergic): 0.2 mg IVP q 10 min up to 3 doses until pain relieved
- Ketorolac: 60mg IM or 30 mg IVP. In elderly: 30 mg IM or 15 mg IVP
- Meperidine: 0.5 mg/kg IVP titrated to pain relief up to 2.0 mg/kg IV
- Promethazine: 12.5–25 mg IVP

PEDIATRIC CONSIDERATIONS

- Initial treatment strategy similar to adults

Disposition

ADMISSION CRITERIA

- Admission and surgical or gastroenterologic consultation for evidence of
  —Acute cholecystitis
  —Acute cholangitis
  —Common duct obstruction
  —Gallstone pancreatitis

DISCHARGE CRITERIA

- Lack of clinical, laboratory, or radiographic evidence of cholecystitis, cholangitis, common duct obstruction, or pancreatitis
- Resolution of all pain and tenderness
- Ability to tolerate oral fluids

Miscellaneous

ICD9: 572.4

CORE CONTENT CODE: 1.3.3

SUGGESTED READINGS

Moscati RM. Cholelithiasis, cholecystitis and pancreatitis. In: Hunter DM, ed. Gastrointestinal emergencies, Part II. Emerg Med Clin North Am 1996;14:719–737.

Rothrock SG, Green SM, Gorton E. Atropine for the treatment of biliary tract pain: A double-blind, placebo-controlled trial. Ann Emerg Med 1993;23;1324–1327.

Shea JA, Berlin JA, Escarce JJ, et al. Revised estimates of diagnostic test sensitivity and specificity in suspected biliary tract disease. Arch Intern Med 1994;154:2573–2581.

Silen W. The colics. In: Silen W, ed. Cope's early diagnosis of the acute abdomen. 18th ed. Oxford: Oxford University Press, 1991:149–153.

Author: Robert Buckley

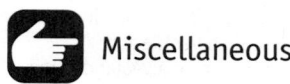

Chronic Obstructive Pulmonary Disease

Clinical Presentation

SIGNS AND SYMPTOMS

- Dyspnea on exertion
- Barrel chest
- Cough
- Wheezing
- Retractions
- Low I:E ratio
- Cyanosis
- Poor air movement
- Orthopnea
- Leg edema
- Jugular venous distention
- S_3 and S_4 gallops

MECHANISM/DESCRIPTION

- A variety of processes, often present in the same patient, that result in large airway obstruction and impaired ventilation
  - —Emphysema: irreversible alveolar destruction decreases large airway elastic recoil
  - —Chronic bronchitis: airway inflammation without alveolar destruction
  - —Reactive airway disease: reversible bronchospasm, mucous plugging, and mucosal edema
- Chronic obstructive pulmonary disease (COPD) affects 15% of the US population
- Prognosis depends on stage
- Poor prognosis for end-stage COPD (bedridden, baseline pCO_2 >60 mm Hg)
- Excellent prognosis for patients with early COPD (minor or no dyspnea on exertion, normal pCO_2) with aggressive treatment and smoking abstinence

ETIOLOGY

- Smoking is the overwhelming cause
- α-Antitrypsin deficiency
- Air pollution
- Other pulmonary diseases

Pre-Hospital

- Supplemental oxygenation
  - —100% via nonrebreather
  - —Do not withhold for fever of CO_2 retention as this will only occur over a period of hours
- Initiate nebulized bronchodilator therapy

Diagnosis

ESSENTIAL WORKUP

LABORATORY

- Pulse oximetry
- Arterial blood gas analysis
  - —Timed to influence decision-making
  - —Contemplating admission after maximal ED therapy
  - —Monitoring ventilatory response to oxygen therapy

IMAGING/SPECIAL TESTS

- Chest radiography
  - —Diagnosis of lobar collapse, pneumothorax, pneumonia, congestive heart failure (CHF)
- Spirometry
  - —Gold standard for diagnosing COPD
- Echocardiography
  - —Used to diagnose left-ventricular failure

DIFFERENTIAL DIAGNOSIS

- CHF
- Pneumonia
- Pulmonary embolus
- Upper airway obstruction
- Restrictive lung disease

Treatment

INITIAL STABILIZATION

- Oxygen therapy
  - —Alert hypoxic patients
  - —Suppression of ventilation is rare except in "blue bloaters" or end-stage COPD
  - —With mild altered mental status, an oxygen challenge is warranted
- Intubation for airway control
  - —Ineffective ventilation
  - —CO_2 narcosis with pulse oximetry below 85%
- Ventilator settings
  - —Allow sufficient expiratory time to minimize air trapping and subsequent barotrauma, despite hypercapnia
- Bronchodilator therapy
  - —Anticholinergic and β-agonist medications
- Subcutaneous terbutaline
  - —Poor air movement precludes nebulized absorption
- Empirical antibiotics for signs of infection
- Steroid therapy

MEDICATIONS

- Albuterol: 2.5 mg via nebulizer q 10–30 min
- Ipratroprium bromide: 0.5 mg via nebulizer q 6 hrs
- Methylprednisolone: 125 mg IV every q 6 hrs
- Prednisone: 40 mg po qd × 5 days
- Terbutaline: 0.25 mg SC q 30 min

Disposition

ADMISSION CRITERIA

- ICU admission
  - —Intubated patients
  - —CO_2 narcosis with oxygen saturation <90%
  - —Clinical tiring in the ED
  - —Severe ABG decompensation
  - —Severe cardiopulmonary disease
    - -Myocardial infarction
    - -Pneumonia
    - -Pulmonary edema
    - -Pulmonary embolism
- Admission to a regular hospital bed
  - —COPD patients with an additional pulmonary insult
    - -Pneumonia
    - -Lobar collapse
    - -CHF
  - —Outpatient failure after maximal ED therapy
  - —ABG decompensation
  - —Accessory muscle use
  - —RR >40 at rest
  - —Markedly decreased exercise tolerance

DISCHARGE CRITERIA

- Mild flare
- Complete resolution in the ED
- No underlying acute pulmonary disorders
- Outpatient course of steroids to prevent relapse

Miscellaneous

ICD9: 491.2

CORE CONTENT CODE: 16.6.3

SUGGESTED READINGS

Mandavia DP, Dailey RH. Chronic obstructive pulmonary disease. In: Rosen P, et al., eds. Emergency medicine: Concepts and clinical practice. 4th ed. St. Louis: CV Mosby, 1992:1494–1510.

Pinsky MR. Through the past darkly: ventilatory management of patients with chronic obstructive pulmonary disease. Crit Care Med 1994;22:1714–1717.

Author: Michael D. Witting

Cirrhosis

Clinical Presentation

SIGNS AND SYMPTOMS

- May be silent
- Insidious onset with nonspecific findings
  —Malaise
  —Fatigue
  —Anorexia
  —Nausea/vomiting
  —Weight loss
  —Pruritus
  —Hyperpigmentation
- Jaundice
- Spider telangiectasias
- Palmar erythema
- Dupuytren's contractures
- Parotid and lacrimal gland enlargement
- Testicular atrophy/impotence/loss of libido/gynecomastia
- Ascites
- Amenorrhea
- Abdominal collateral circulation including caput medusae, hepatosplenomegaly, or hepatic atrophy
- Abdominal discomfort or tenderness
- Signs of complications
  —Hepatic encephalopathy (HE)
  —GI bleeding from esophageal varices
  —Portal hypertensive gastropathy or peptic ulcer disease

MECHANISMS/DESCRIPTION

- Dynamic process of inflammation, cellular injury and necrosis, diffuse fibrosis, and formation of regenerative nodules
- Progressive liver failure and loss of lobular and vascular architecture
- Intrahepatic portal hypertension due to increased resistance at the sinusoid, compression of the central veins, as well as anastomosis between the arterial and portal systems

ETIOLOGY

- Chronic viral hepatitis, C/C-GB or B (with or without D)
- Alcohol abuse
- Autoimmune hepatitis/cirrhosis
- Biliary cirrhosis, primary (PBC) or secondary (sclerosing cholangitis)
- Metabolic (hemochematosis and Wilson's disease)
- Drugs (methotrexate, amiodarone and α-methyldopa, or toxins)
- Cardiac cirrhosis and hepatic venous outflow obstruction (Budd-Chiari Syndrome)
- Nonalcoholic steatohepatitis
- Sarcoidosis and amyloidosis
- Hepatocellular carcinoma, diffusely infiltrating

PEDIATRIC CONSIDERATIONS

- Etiology—*congenital anomaly* of the biliary system
  -Biliary atresia, and arteriohepatic dysplasia (Alagille syndrome)
  —*Metabolic* such as cystic fibrosis, α_1- antitrypsin deficiency, fructosemia, tyrosinemia, galactosemia, and glycogen storage disease (types III and IV)
- If acquired in infancy, hepatitis B could lead to cirrhosis during childhood

Pre-Hospital

CAUTIONS

- Attention to active GI bleeding, encephalopathy, or tense infected ascites

Diagnosis

ESSENTIAL WORKUP

- Detailed historical and physical exam search for clues to liver disease

LABORATORY

- CBC
  —Anemia
  —Macrocytosis
  —Leukopenia
  —Thrombocytopenia
- Impaired liver function
  —High bilirubin
  —Low albumin
  —Prolonged PT
  —Hypoglycemia
- Increased liver enzymes
  —AST, ALT—reflect injury
  —Alkaline phosphatase and 5'- nucleotidase reflect cholestasis
  —May be normal in inactive cirrhosis
- Electrolytes, BUN, and Cr
  —Renal dysfunction and hepatorenal syndrome
- ABG or pulse oximeter for
  —Suspected pneumonia
  —CHF
  —Hepatopulmonary syndrome: intrapulmonary vascular dilation, and hypoxia, in association with liver disease
- Search for etiology as appropriate
  —Hepatitis B surface antigen
  —Hepatitis C antibody
  —ANA and antismooth-muscle antibody (autoimmune hepatitis)
  —Antimitochondrial antibody (primary biliary cirrhosis)
  —Serum iron, transferrin saturation, and ferritin (hemochromatosis)
  —Ceruloplasmin (Wilson's disease)
  —Carbohydrate deficient transferrin (a marker for alcoholism)
  —α_1-Antitrypsin (deficiency)
  —Serum immune electrophoresis (high IgM in PBC)
  —Cholesterol (chronic cholestasis)
  —α-Fetoprotein (hepatocellular cancer)

IMAGING/SPECIAL TESTS

- CXR for pleural effusion, cardiomegaly, and CHF
- Abdominal ultrasound for biliary obstruction, liver architecture, ascites, splenomegaly
- CT scan or MRI to explore abnormal finding on US
- Cholangiogram (endoscopic or radiologic) for suspected biliary obstruction
- EGD indicated for UGI bleeding or variceal surveillance
- Liver biopsy to confirm diagnosis

DIFFERENTIAL DIAGNOSIS

- Ascites
  —Increased right heart pressure
  —Hepatic vein thrombosis
  —Peritoneal malignancy/infection
  —Pancreatic disease
  —Thyroid disease
  —Lymphatic obstruction
- Upper GI bleeding
  —PUD
  —Gastritis
- Encephalopathy
  —Metabolic
  —Toxic

Treatment

INITIAL STABILIZATION

- Treat complications such as active GI bleeding or HE
- Naloxone, dextrose (or Accucheck) and thiamine for altered mental status
- Reverse hypotension with IV fluids to prevent acute ischemic hepatic injury

ED TREATMENT

- For suspected variceal bleed
  —Octreotide
  —Reverse coagulopathy
    -Fresh-frozen plasma 1 IU/hr until bleeding is controlled
    -Desmopressin (DDAVP)—improves bleeding time, and prolonged PTT
  —Endoscopic sclerotherapy
- Initiate broad spectrum antibiotics in suspected sepsis
  —Cefotaxime
- Treat complicating conditions—ascites and HE—see Ascites and Hepatic Encephalopathy chapters
- Treat pruritus with
  —Cholestyramine, ursodeoxycholic acid, or rifampin
  —Naloxone infusion 0.2 µg/kg/min for temporary relief for extreme cases
- Consult gastroenterologist or transplant coordinator whenever postliver-transplant patient presents to the ED with liver dysfunction, suspected sepsis, or possible treatment-related complication
- For prolonged PT administer vitamin K 10 mg sq daily for 3 days
- Relieve biliary obstruction (e.g., stricture) by endoscopic, radiologic, or surgical means
- Provide nutritious diet; high in calorie and adequate in protein (1 g/kg), unless there is complicating HE
- β-Blockage (propranadol) for large esophageal varices
  —Titrated to pulse rate of 60 or 25% reduction of resting pulse

Specific Therapy

- Hemochromatosis: phlebotomy or deferoxamine (iron-chelating agent)
- Autoimmune hepatitis: prednisone with or without azathioprine (Imuran)
- Chronic hepatitis B or C: α-interferon (avoid in decompensated cirrhosis)
- Primary biliary cirrhosis: ursodeoxycholic acid
- Wilson's disease: penicillamine, trientine, or zinc oxide
- The only cure for most advanced cirrhosis is liver transplantation

MEDICATIONS

- Azathioprine: 1–2 mg/kg po
- Cefotaxime: 1–2 g q 6–8 hrs (peds: 50–180 mg/kg/24hrs q 6 hrs) IV
- Cholestyramine: 4 g po 1–6 times/day
- Desmopressin (DDAVP): 0.3 µg/kg in 50 ml saline infused over 15–30 min
- Dextrose: D50W 1 amp (50 ml or 25 g) (peds: D25W 2–4 ml/kg) IV
- Naloxone (Narcan): 2 mg (peds: 0.1 mg/kg) IV or IM initial dose
- Octreotide: 50–100 µg IV bolus followed by 50 µg IV infusion
- Prednisone: 40mg (peds: 1–2mg/Kg) po q day
- Propranadol: 40 (initial)–240 mg (peds: 1–5 mg/kg/24hrs) po tid
- Rifampin: 600 mg (peds: 10–20 mg/kg) po qd
- Thiamine: 100 mg (peds: 50 mg) IV or IM
- Ursodeoxycholic acid: 8–10 mg/kg/24hrs tid

Disposition

ADMISSION CRITERIA

- Acute decompensation or complicating conditions
- Advanced grades HE, sepsis, active GI bleed, and hepatorenal and hepatopulmonary syndromes require ICU
- First presentation with clinically evident cirrhosis, unless close outpatient work-up is possible

DISCHARGE CRITERIA

- The majority of patients with compensated cirrhosis could be treated as an outpatient

Miscellaneous

ICD9: 571.5

CORE CONTENT CODE: 1.2.2

SUGGESTED READINGS

McGuire BM, Bloomer JR: Complications of cirrhosis. Post Grad Med 1998;103(2):209.

Munoz SJ. Long-term management of liver transplant recipient. Med Clin North Am 1996;80:1103.

Rosen HR, Shackleton CR, Martin P. Indications for and timing of liver transplantation. Med Clin North Am 1996;80:1069.

Author: Abbas Zagnoon

Clavicle Fracture

Clinical Presentation

SIGNS AND SYMPTOMS

- Local pain, tenderness and swelling over the fracture site
- Crepitus is often present due to the clavicle's subcutaneous position
- Arm held in adduction against the chest wall with resistance to motion
- Shoulder displaced anteriorly and inferiorly

DESCRIPTION

- Clavicle fractures account for 5% of all fractures in all age groups
- 80% of clavicle fractures involve the middle third
- 15% occur in the distal third
- 5% occur in the medial third

Classification

- Group I: middle third fractures
- Group II: distal-third fractures
  - —Type I: coracoclavicular ligaments are intact (nondisplaced)
  - —Type II: severing of the coracoclavicular ligaments (conoid)
  - —Type III: articular surface involvement of the acromioclavicular joint
- Group III: medial (proximal)-third fractures

MECHANISM

- Direct trauma to the clavicle
- Fall on the lateral shoulder
- Fall on the outstretched hand
- Pediatric Considerations
- Most common of all pediatric fractures
- May occur in newborns secondary to birth trauma

Pre-Hospital

CAUTIONS

- Medial-third fractures are frequently accompanied by other injuries due to the severe force (intrathoracic injuries, sternal fractures, subluxation of the sternoclavicular joint)
  - —Consider spinal immobilization if appropriate
- Immobilize injured extremity

Diagnosis

ESSENTIAL WORKUP

- ABCs: look for other life-threatening injuries
- History: determine the mechanism of injury
- Physical exam
  - —Palpate the clavicle for tenderness, crepitus, and swelling
  - —Examine the humerus and shoulder joint for other fractures, dislocations, or subluxations
  - —Assess if the fracture is *open* or *closed*
- Evaluate for associated injuries (often serious and life-threatening) that must be excluded
  - —Skeletal injuries
    - -First rib fracture with underlying aortic injury
    - -Sternoclavicular joint separation/fracture-dislocation
    - -Acromioclavicular joint separation/fracture-dislocation
    - -Cervical spine injuries
  - —Vascular injuries
    - -Carefully check radial and ulnar pulses to assess for possible injury to the subclavian or internal jugular vessels
  - —Neurologic injuries
    - -A meticulous neurologic exam (both sensory and motor) is required to assess injury to the brachial plexus or any of its branches (including the ulnar, median, and radial nerves)
    - -The ulnar nerve is most frequently injured
  - —Pulmonary injuries
    - -Auscultate for equal bilateral breath sounds to rule out a concomitant pneumothorax or hemothorax

IMAGING/SPECIAL TESTS

- AP radiographs of both clavicles are mandatory and must include
  - -Upper third of the humerus
  - -Shoulder girdle (rule out other fractures)
  - -Upper lung fields (rule out pneumothorax)
- Oblique and apical lordotic views
  - —May be helpful, especially for medial and distal clavicle fractures that are not easily visualized on the AP view
- Stress views (weight-bearing) for *distal* clavicle fractures are no longer routinely recommended
- Angiography
  - —Should be performed if there is any evidence or suspicion of vascular injuries (most commonly *subclavian* vessels)

DIFFERENTIAL DIAGNOSIS

- Distal fractures: consider acromioclavicular separation
- Medial fractures: consider sternoclavicular separation
- Shoulder fracture/dislocation

Treatment

INITIAL STABILIZATION

- Ice packs to affected area
- Pain management using either narcotics or NSAIDs
- Immobilize affected side in a sling

ED TREATMENT

- Open fracture: uncommon occurrence, but usually requires open debridement and internal fixation (obtain immediate orthopedic referral)
- Closed fracture: if severely displaced, attempt closed reduction and immobilize depending on *type of fracture*
  - —Middle third
    - -If nondisplaced, a sling or shoulder immobilizer is enough to provide support
    - -Controversy exists as to whether closed reduction is necessary since the alignment is rarely maintained regardless of splinting technique
    - -To perform a closed reduction, 1% lidocaine should be injected into the fracture hematoma. The shoulders are pulled upward, outward, and backward, and the fracture is then manipulated into place
    - -Sedation may be given to alleviate pain or anxiety
    - -A figure-of-eight splint is then applied
    - -Ice should be applied for the first 24 hours
    - -Analgesia (narcotics or NSAIDs) for pain
  - —Distal third type I
    - -Ice for the first 24 hours
    - -Immobilization with a sling or shoulder immobilizer
    - -Orthopedic referral
    - -Analgesia (narcotics or NSAIDs) for pain
    - -Early range of motion
  - —Distal third type II
    - -Ice for the first 24 hours
    - -Immobilization with a sling or shoulder immobilizer
    - -Orthopedic referral (may require operative repair)
    - -Analgesia (narcotics or NSAIDs) for pain
  - —Distal third type III: same as type II
  - —Medial (proximal) third
    - -Ice for the first 24 hours
    - -Immobilization in a sling or shoulder immobilizer for support
    - -Analgesia (narcotics or NSAIDs) for pain
    - -Orthopedic follow-up
    - -Immediate referral if there are signs of neurovascular injury
- Reassess neurovascular status after all splints are applied

PEDIATRIC CONSIDERATIONS

- Children who do not cooperate with the figure-of-eight splint should be referred to an orthopedic surgeon for possible shoulder spica placement
- Most children will tolerate a shoulder immobilizer best

Disposition

ADMISSION CRITERIA

- Open fracture
- Associated injuries that are potentially life-threatening

DISCHARGE CRITERIA

- Isolated closed clavicle fracture without other injuries
- Appropriate support services at home (especially for elderly)
- Orthopedic follow-up
- Adequate pain management

MEDICATIONS

- Acetaminophen: 500–1000 mg po q 6 hrs PRN, peds: 15–20 mg/kg po q 6 hrs PRN
- Ibuprofen: 600–800mg po q 6 hrs PRN with meals, peds: 5–10 mg/kg po q 6 hrs PRN

Miscellaneous

ICD9: 810.00

CORE CONTENT CODE: 18.4.10.5

SUGGESTED READINGS

Allman FL. Fractures and ligamentous Injuries of the clavicle and its articulation

J Bone Joint Surg 1967;49A:774–784.

Heppenstall RB. Fractures and dislocations of the distal clavicle. Orthop Clin North Am 1975;6:477–486.

Neer CS.: Fractures of the distal third of the clavicle. Clin Orthop 1968;58:43–50.

Post M. Current concepts in the treatment of fractures of the clavicle. Clin Orthop 1989;245:89–101.

Rockwood CA. Rockwood and Green's fractures in adults. 4th ed. Philadelphia: Lippincott-Raven, 1996.

Rowe CR. An atlas of anatomy and treatment of midclavicular fractures. Clin Orthop 1968;58:29–42.

Simon RR. Emergency orthopedics: The extremities. Norwalk, CT: Appleton and Lange, 1987.

Author: Jeffrey Manko

Cluster Headache

Clinical Presentation

SIGNS AND SYMPTOMS

- Unilateral, excruciating, nonthrobbing, incapacitating headache
- Pain is ocular or retro-ocular
- Rarely lasts longer than 2 hours
- Associated with nasal congestion, lacrimation, rhinorrhea, conjunctival injection, or facial flushing on the same side
- Horner's syndrome may be seen
- Headaches occur in clusters; several times per day for weeks or months at a time
- Occurs predominantly in middle-aged males
- Attacks are more likely after ingestion of alcohol, nitroglycerine, or histamine-containing compounds
- Episodes are often nocturnal, and are more common in spring and fall
- More likely in times of stress, prolonged strain, overwork, and upsetting emotional experiences
- No prodrome or aura

MECHANISM/DESCRIPTION

- Not clearly understood, but may be the result of vasoactive substances released from mast cells

ETIOLOGY

- Etiology is unclear at present
- Affects 0.1% of the population

Pre-Hospital

CAUTIONS

- Recognize more severe life-threatening causes of headache
- Administration of oxygen by face mask may alleviate symptoms

Diagnosis

ESSENTIAL WORKUP

- An accurate history and physical examination should confirm the diagnosis

LABORATORY

- Lumbar puncture (if meningitis or subarachnoid hemorrhage is suspected)
- ESR (if temporal arteritis is suspected)

IMAGING/SPECIAL TESTS

- CT scan/MRI (to rule out hemorrhage, tumor)

DIFFERENTIAL DIAGNOSIS

- Migraine headache
- Trigeminal neuralgia
- Meningitis
- Temporal arteritis
- Intracerebral mass lesion
- Herpes zoster
- Intracerebral bleed
- Hypertension
- Dental causes
- Orbital/ocular disease (acute glaucoma)
- Temporal mandibular joint syndrome

Treatment

INITIAL STABILIZATION

- ABCs
- Rule out life-threatening causes of headache
- Administration of supplemental oxygen

ED TREATMENT

- Pain management

MEDICATIONS

- Ergots: DHE 1cc IM or IV; the repeat in 1 hour if necessary
- Fentanyl: 2–3 μg/kg IV
- NSAIDs: Ketorolac 15–30 mg IM or IV
- Meperidine: 50–75 mg IM or IV
- Morphine: 2–4 mg IV or IM, may repeat q 10 min
- Oxygen: 100% via face mask
- Prochlorperazine: 10 mg IM or IV
- Sumatriptan: 6 mg sq, may repeat in 1 hr (max of 2 doses in 24 hrs)

Disposition

ADMISSION CRITERIA

- Persistent headache unresponsive to usual measures
- Suicidal ideation associated with unremitting headache or severe depression

DISCHARGE CRITERIA

- Patients with moderate to complete pain relief and with a confident diagnosis of cluster headache
- Follow-up with a neurologist should be arranged

Miscellaneous

ICD9: 346.20

CORE CONTENT CODE: 11.10

SUGGESTED READINGS

Diamond S. The management of migraine and cluster headaches. Compr Ther 1995;21(9):492–498.

Kumar KL. Recent advances in the acute management of migraine and cluster headaches. J Gen Intern Med 1994;9(6):339–348.

Mathews NT. Cluster headaches. Neurology 1992;42(3):22–31.

Authors: Gary Johnson; George Kondylis

COBRA/Patient Transfer Issues

Clinical Presentation

SIGNS AND SYMPTOMS

Enforcement Procedures

- Following a violation
  - —MEDICARE participation of the physician or hospital is terminated in 23 days
  - —Notice of termination is published in newspapers at 19 days
  - —To prevent this a plan of correction must be submitted, implemented, and approved
    - -If corrective plan is accepted, reevaluation is made within 90 days
  - —Appeals take up to 3 years and funding is not reinstated during the process
  - —Hospitals that fail to report violations by other hospitals have been cited
  - —Application of standards vary in different regions of the country

OIG Enforcement

- Operates separately from HCFA
- Receives and uses HCFA and PRO findings
- If violation is found, it issues a civil monetary penalty (CMP)
  - —$50,000 per violation for both hospitals and physicians
  - —$25,000 for hospitals with under 100 beds
  - —CMP not covered by malpractice insurance

MECHANISM/DESCRIPTION

- Consolidated Omnibus Budget Reconciliation Act (COBRA)
  - —Also known as EMTALA (Emergency Medical Treatment and Labor Act)
  - —Federally mandated standards of practice for hospitals and physicians
  - —Passed in 1986; amended in 1988, 1989, and 1994
  - —Initially motivated by the issue of patient dumping
    - -Denial of care or transfer of patients based on inability to pay for care
- COBRA preempts state law
- 700 Hospitals or 1 in 6 hospitals have received COBRA enforcement actions from HCFA
- Few have received termination of funding; 1 did in 1996 for following an HMO procedure
- Costs for plans and actions to make corrections, for consultants, lawyers, equipment, and personnel
  - —Generally about $150,000 for small hospitals
  - —$1.8 million for one 400–500 bed hospital
  - —Several hundred civil suits have been filed with some verdicts and settlements of more than $3 million

ETIOLOGY

- COBRA duties of a hospital
  - —Provide a MSE (Medical Screen Examination) to all patients that present to its premises regardless of ability to pay
  - —Provide stabilizing care
  - —Not to transfer unstable patients
  - —Transfer only for medical necessity
  - —Maintain an on-call system for specialists
  - —Accept requests for in-coming transfers
- Medical screening exam
  - —Provide all necessary testing and on-call services
  - —Determine presence of an Emergency Medical Condition (EMC)
  - —Address affected and potentially affected areas and known chronic conditions
  - —Florida law requires all necessary treatment and surgery
  - —All necessary definitive treatment should be rendered
  - —Only true followup care may be referred to physicians offices or clinics
  - —Triage without an MSE is not acceptable
  - —Screening of psychiatric patients must rule out trauma, disease, or organic condition
  - —Screening of intoxicated patients must rule out trauma, toxic, psychological, and medical causes
  - —Use of nonphysician medical screening personnel is discouraged but not prohibited
- Emergency medical condition
  - —Broader under COBRA than typical medical usage
  - —Any condition that is a danger to the health and safety of the patient or unborn fetus
  - —Includes conditions that may result in risk of impairment or dysfunction of any body part
  - —Undiagnosed acute pain that is sufficient to impair normal function
  - —Pregnancy with contractions
  - —Symptoms of substance abuse
  - —Psychiatric disturbances, i.e., severe depression, inability to comprehend danger or care for one's self
- Managed care conflicts with COBRA
  - —Third-party payers do not have the authority to authorize treatment, only payment
  - —Hospitals that follow HMO and insurance company procedures do so at their own risk and will be held to COBRA compliance
  - —It's acceptable to obtain information during the routine registration process but the information must not be acted on
  - —No advance approval may be obtained from a third-party payer or employer
  - —Calls to insurance companies and employers have resulted in citations
  - —Handing a phone to the patient to speak to their insurance has resulted in citations
  - —Transfers may not be based on MCO direction or policy

Pre-Hospital

N/A

Diagnosis

ESSENTIAL WORKUP

- HCFA—responsible for investigation and partially responsible for enforcement
- Office of Inspector General (OIG) of the DHHS is responsible for other enforcement aspects
- Violations also may be reported to Office of Civil Rights, IRS, JCAHO
- Civil suits are heard in state and federal courts
- Possible violations must be reported by receiving hospitals within 72 hours
- Other sources of information regarding violations
  —Physician complaints
  —Patient complaints
  —EMS system complaints
  —Routine site visits
  —Newspaper articles
  —PRO screens
  —State reporting

LABORATORY

N/A

IMAGING/SPECIAL TESTS

N/A

DIFFERENTIAL DIAGNOSIS

N/A

Treatment

N/A

Disposition

ADMISSION CRITERIA

- HCFA conducts investigation

DISCHARGE CRITERIA

- Professional Review Organization (PRO)
  —Acts as a nonbinding advisor to OIG
  —Does not generally affect HCFA findings
  —Goes by standard medical practice rather than HCFA
  —Tension exists between PRO and HCFA offices
- State enforcement
  —Agencies have varying familiarity with HCFA
  —COBRA enforcement is increasing
  —State agencies are often required to comply with federal inspections, including COBRA
  —Actions under COBRA

Summary

- Evaluation of patients must not be based upon insurance status
- MCOs cannot refuse care, only payment
- MSE must be performed regardless of approval from patients' insurance company
- Transfers and acceptances of transfers must be based on medical needs
- Patients may refuse or request transfers

Miscellaneous

ICD9: N/A

CORE CONTENT CODE: 20.7.2.4

SUGGESTED READINGS

Bitterman RA. What is an "appropriate" medical screen examination under COBRA? ED Leg Lett 1997;8(3):35–44.

Bitterman RA. Dealing with managed care under COBRA. Emerg Phys Leg Bull 1997;7(4):1–8.

COBRA statute: 42 USC §1395.

COBRA regulations 48924—Special responsibilities of Medicare hospitals in emergency cases.

Frew Consulting Group. COBRA Online. www.medlaw.com/novnl.htm

Author: Steven Crespo

Clinical Presentation

SIGNS AND SYMPTOMS

- Sympathomimetic toxidrome

Cardiovascular

- Hypertension
- Tachycardia
- Chest pain (angina)

Respiratory

- Tachypnea
- Pleuritic chest pain
  - —Pneumomediastinum
  - —Pneumothorax
  - —Bronchitis
  - —Pulmonary infarction
- Cough

Central Nervous System

- Agitation
- Tremulousness
- Coma
- Seizures
- Stroke

Miscellaneous

- Hyperthermia (poor prognosis)
- Limb ischemia (inadvertent intra-arterial injection)
- Corneal ulcerations (heavy crack smokers)
- Due to local chemical and thermal irritation causing disruption in corneal epithelium
- Rhabdomyolysis

MECHANISM/DESCRIPTION

- Sympathomimetic
- Inhibits neurotransmitter reuptake at the nerve terminal
- Metabolism
  - —Hepatic degradation
  - —Nonenzymatic hydrolysis
  - —Cholinesterase metabolism

ETIOLOGY

- IV, nasal, oral administration
- Oral ingestion
  - —Body stuffers
    - -Ingest hastily wrapped packets in attempt to evade police
    - -Body packers
    - -Ingest cocaine packets in order to smuggle the drug
    - -Cocaine wrapped carefully in packets containing large amounts of drug
    - -Oral, rectal, vaginal routes

Pre-Hospital

CAUTIONS

- Establish IV access
- Cardiac monitor
  - —Chest pain may be ischemic
  - —Benzodiazepines to control agitation
  - —Used as "speedball" (combination of heroin and cocaine)—administer naloxone increments to reverse coma

Diagnosis

ESSENTIAL WORKUP

- Recognition of the sympathomimetic toxidrome caused by cocaine
  - —Distinguish from anticholinergic toxidrome

Toxidrome Recognition

SIGN	*SYMPATHOMIMETIC*	*ANTICHOLINERGIC*
Heart rate	Increased	Increased
Blood pressure	Increased	Increased
Skin	Moist	Dry
Bowel sounds	Present	Diminished
Hyperthermia	Present	Present
Urinary retention	Absent	Present

- History of route of drug ingestion
  - —If oral ingestion, inquire how the packets were wrapped due to leakage potential.

LABORATORY

- CBC
- Electrolytes, BUN/Cr, glucose
- Urinalysis dip for myoglobin
- CPK for
  - —Anginal chest pain
  - —Abnormal ECG
  - —Myoglobinuria

IMAGING/SPECIAL TESTS

- EKG
  - —For anginal chest pain
  - —Consider possibility of myocardial infarction with cocaine chest pain
- CXR
  - —For chest pain or shortness of breath
  - —Check for pneumomediastinum, pneumothorax, aortic rupture
- KUB
  - —For body packers/stuffers
  - —Usually negative for stuffers because drug is loosely packed in cellophane
  - —Positive for packers because drug is densely packed and usually radiopaque
- CT of the abdomen with contrast
  - —When unreliable history of body packers/stuffers and KUB negative
- CT brain: when altered mental status/severe headache
  - —Cerebral ischemia/hemorrhage occurs

DIFFERENTIAL DIAGNOSIS

- Other agents with sympathomimetic effects
- Theophylline
- Caffeine
- Amphetamines
- Albuterol
- Tricyclic antidepressants
- Antihistamines
- PCP
- Thyrotoxicosis
- Neuroleptic malignant syndrome
- Hallucinogens

Treatment

INITIAL STABILIZATION

- ABCs
- IV access
- Cardiac monitor
- Narcan, thiamine, dextrose (or Accucheck) for altered mental status

ED TREATMENT

- Supportive care for mildly symptomatic patients
- Benzodiazepines
  —For agitation and tremor
  —Initial agents for hypertension and tachycardia
- Cooling measures for hyperthermia
  —Evaporative-convective method
- Treat rhabdomyolysis
  —0.9%NS hydration
  —Alkalinization with IV bicarbonate in severe cases

Cardiac Chest Pain

- Aspirin
- Nitrates
- Oxygen
- Opiates
- Avoid β-blockage due to unopposed α stimulation
- Angiography/angioplasty/thrombolysis for acute myocardial infarction

Hypertension/Tachycardia

- Benzodiazepine initial agent
- Use α-blocking agent (phentolamine) as sole agent or combine with β-blocker (propranolol, esmolol) if unresponsive to benzodiazepine
  —Use labetalol cautiously (does not have equal α- and β-blocking properties)
- IV nitroglycerin/nitroprusside for severe unresponsive hypertension

Body Packer/Stuffers

- Treat asymptomatic or minimally symptomatic body packers and body stuffers
  —With oral activated charcoal,
  —Followed by whole-bowel irrigation with polyethylene glycol-electrolyte lavage solution (PEG-ELS)
- Surgical consultation for symptomatic body packers and stuffers
  —If toxicity is not easily managed with pharmacologic therapy (above), remove the packets intraoperatively

MEDICATIONS

- Diazepam: 5 mg incremental doses IV
- Lorazepam: 2 mg incremental doses IV
- Phentolamine: 5 mg IV q 15–20 min
- Nitroglycerin: 10–100 μg/min IV infusion
- Nitroprusside: 0.3 μg/kg/min IV (titrate to effect up to 10 μg/kg/min)
- Polyethylene glycol (Golytely): 4 L po over 4 hrs until complete bowel evacuation
- Activated charcoal slurry: 1–2 g/kg up to 90 g po
- Esmolol: 50–200 μg/kg/min IV infusion titrated to effect
- Dextrose: D50W 1 amp (50 ml or 25 g) (peds: D25W 2–4 ml/kg) IV
- Naloxone (narcan): 2 mg (peds: 0.1 mg/kg up to 2 mg) IV or IM initial dose
- Thiamine (vitamin B_1): 100 mg (peds: 50 mg) IV or IM

Disposition

ADMISSION CRITERIA

- Altered mental status
- Abnormal vital signs: HR >100, BP >120 diastolic, or hypotension
- Hyperthermia
- Cocaine-induced myocardial ischemia
- Body stuffers and body packers
- ICU admission for moderate to severe toxicity

DISCHARGE CRITERIA

- Mental status and vital signs normal after 6 hours of observation
- Body packers or stuffers with confirmed expulsion of packets and no clinical signs of toxicity after 12 hours of observation

Miscellaneous

ICD9: 968.5

CORE CONTENT CODE: 17.2.18

SUGGESTED READINGS

Ellenhorn MJ, Schoonwald S, Ordog G, Wasserberger J. Cocaine. In: Ellenhorn's medical toxicology. 2d ed. Baltimore: Williams & Wilkins, 1997:356–385.

Goldfrank LR, Hoffman RS. The cardiovascular effects of cocaine. Ann Emerg Med 1991;20:165–175.

Haim DY, Lippmann MI, Goldberg SK, et al. The pulmonary complications of crack cocaine. Chest 1995;107:233.

Hollander JE. The management of cocaine-associated myocardial ischemia. N Engl J Med 1995;33:1267.

Author: Steven Aks

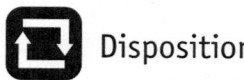

Coccyx Fractures

Clinical Presentation

SIGNS AND SYMPTOMS

- Tenderness localized to coccyx
- Low back pain, buttock pain, rectal bleeding (if associated rectal tear)
- Ecchymosis and localized tenderness along gluteal crease
- Pain when sitting or defecating

MECHANISM/DESCRIPTION

- Fall landing in sitting position is most common
- Also can occur during childbirth
- Surgical procedures performed in area of coccyx
- Fractures of the coccyx are usually transverse
- More common in women

Pre-Hospital

CAUTIONS

- Although the mechanism may be low impact, patients should be immobilized until other spine injuries are properly evaluated

Diagnosis

ESSENTIAL WORKUP

- History and examination
- Exam reveals ecchymosis and tenderness in the gluteal fold
- Rectal examination is diagnostic and reveals tenderness and crepitus of coccyx
- Anoscopy should be performed if gross blood is present to evaluate for possible rectal perforation (very rare)
- Examination of entire spine is necessary to evaluate for concomitant injury

IMAGING/SPECIAL TESTS

- Radiographs will identify other suspected spine injuries
- Displaced coccyx fractures can be seen on the lateral view
- Radiographs are not necessary if isolated coccyx fracture is apparent on rectal exam
- Nondisplaced fractures are difficult to see on x-ray

DIFFERENTIAL DIAGNOSIS

- Contusion, hematoma
- Pilonidal cyst

Treatment

INITIAL STABILIZATION

- Spine immobilization for suspected concomitant cervical, thoracic, or lumbar injuries
- Pain control with NSAID or narcotic analgesics

ED TREATMENT

- Symptomatic treatment
- Bedrest initially until ambulation can be tolerated
- Reduction of displaced coccygeal fractures is not necessary
- If associated rectal injury, surgical consult is required
  —Antibiotics to cover enterics; cefoxitin, cefotetan, metronidazole
- Cushions ("doughnuts")
- Sitz baths
- Stool Softeners

MEDICATIONS

- Cefotetan: adult: 2 g IV; peds: 80 mg/kg/day div q 6–8 hrs
- Cefoxitin: adult: 2 g IV; peds: 80–160 mg/kg/day div q 6 hrs
- Metronidazole: adult: 500 mg–1 g IV; peds: 30 mg/kg/day div q 12 hrs

Disposition

ADMISSION CRITERIA

- Virtually all patients can be managed as outpatients
- Only patients with severe pain, inability to walk or to take care of themselves, or other serious injury need admission

DISCHARGE CRITERIA

- Vast majority can be managed as outpatients with appropriate follow-up
- Healing is slow
- Pain may be chronic
- Orthopedic consultation and possible coccygectomy may be required in severe cases

Miscellaneous

ICD9: 805.6

CORE CONTENT CODE: 18.4.3.1.4

SUGGESTED READINGS

Cwinn AA. Pelvis and hip. In Rosen P, et al., eds. Emergency medicine: Concepts and clinical practice. 4th ed. St. Louis: CV Mosby, 1998:739–762.

Pollack C. Pelvic trauma. In: Harwood-Nuss, A, et al., eds. The clinical practice of emergency medicine. 2d ed. Philadelphia: Lippincott-Raven, 1996.

Simon R, Koenigsknecht SJ. Emergency orthopedics: The extremities. 4th ed. E. Norwalk, CT: Appleton & Lange, 1996.

Rockwood, Green. Fractures in adults. 4th ed. Philadelphia: Lippincott-Raven, 1996.

Authors: Jaime B. Rivas; Teresa Carlin

Collagen Vascular Disease

- The collagen vascular diseases are a heterogenous group of disorders, some with very distinct clinical features, but most sharing similar clinical and serological findings

Clinical Presentation

SIGNS AND SYMPTOMS

- The most common signs and symptoms of the group as a whole include
  - —Arthralgias
  - —Myalgias
  - —Raynaud's phenomenon
  - —Esophageal dysfunction
  - —Positive test for antinuclear antigen

MECHANISM/DESCRIPTION

These diseases may present in the emergency department as inflammatory or pain syndromes, cardiovascular, neurological, hematological emergencies, or acute renal failure

- American Rheumatism Association 1983 Classification
  - —Rheumatoid arthritis
  - —Juvenile arthritis
  - —Lupus erythematosus
  - —Scleroderma
  - —Diffuse fasciitis with or without eosinophilia
  - —Polymyositis(PM)—dermatomyositis
  - —Necrotizing vasculitis and other forms of vasculopathy
  - —Sjögren's syndrome
  - —Mixed connective tissue disease or overlap syndrome
  - —Others: polymyalgia rheumatica, relapsing polychondritis, erythema nodosum

ETIOLOGY

- Etiology is unclear but genetic factors, viral influences, and immunological and other host factors have all been implicated

PEDIATRIC CONSIDERATIONS

- Juvenile rheumatoid arthritis occurs in 0.16–0.43 per 1000 children in U.S.
- Kawasaki's disease
  - —Present as mucocutaneous lymph node syndrome or acute febrile disease in children under 5 years of age
  - —Skin changes include redness, induration, and edema of palms and soles that leads to desquamation of fingertips
  - —Oropharyngeal mucosa is also injected, giving a strawberry tongue appearance
- Henoch-Schönlein Purpura
  - —Onset at age 5–15 years
  - —Palpable purpura of the lower abdomen and buttocks
  - —Arthritis and arthralgias occur in 80% of the cases, abdominal cramps in 20–40%, and nephritis in 50%

Pre-Hospital

CAUTIONS

- Atlantooccipital instability or subluxation may occur with hyperextension of the neck during endotracheal intubation in a patient with chronic rheumatoid arthritis
- Neuromuscular disease associated with PM may lead to ventilatory failure necessitating endotracheal intubation

Diagnosis

ESSENTIAL WORKUP

- Thorough history including family history, medications, allergies, recent exposures
- Physical examination including skin and musculoskeletal system
- Most common tests are CBC, ESR that is elevated with inflammatory conditions, and C-reactive protein
  - —Upper limits of normal for ESR is age divided by 2 for males, and age plus 10 divided by 2 for females
  - —Increased ESR up to 80–100 mm is seen in 95% of the patients with giant cell arteritis and polymyalgia rheumatica (PM), and should be included in the emergency department evaluation of all older patients with headaches

LABORATORY

- Acute phase reactants
  - —Proteins that are rapidly synthesized in the liver in response to acute inflammation or tissue necrosis
  - —Fibrinogen, prothrombin, haptoglobin, transferrin, C-reactive protein
- Antinuclear antigen or ANA
  - —Positive in 95% patients with SLE; also seen in rheumatoid arthritis, Sjögren's syndrome, and systemic sclerosis
- Anti-Sm and anti-DNA
  - —Highly specific but not sensitive for SLE
- Rheumatoid or RH factor
  - —Positive in 75–90% of the patients with rheumatoid arthritis; also positive in Sjögren's syndrome, SLE, and cryoglobulinemia
- HLA-B27
  - —Seen in 95% of the cases of ankylosing spondylitis

IMAGING/SPECIAL TESTS

- Conventional radiography, computed tomography, magnetic resonance imaging, ultrasonography, and scintigraphy to evaluate the details of bones, joints, and soft tissue
- Synovial fluid analysis, synovial biopsy, and arthroscopy in specific circumstances

DIFFERENTIAL DIAGNOSIS

- Infectious arthritis
- Nonrheumatic conditions of bone and joints
- Psychogenic arthralgias
- Neoplastic diseases including leukemia
- Hematological disorders
- Miscellaneous diseases
  - —Sarcoidosis
  - —Hypertrophic osteo arthropathy
  - —Chronic active hepatitis
  - —Familial Mediterranean fever

Treatment

INITIAL STABILIZATION
- ABCs, IV, oxygen, monitoring

ED TREATMENT
Pharmacological Treatment
- NSAIDs
  —Aspirin and NSAIDs alleviate pain, decrease inflammation, and have antipyretic effect but do not prevent tissue injury due to the disease process
- Corticosteroids
  —High dose steroids produce a short-term decrease in the inflammatory process and often play a key role in these diseases
  —Used topically, intra-articularly, orally in high or low maintenance doses as well as intravenous high dose therapy
  —Antirheumatic and cytotoxic drugs
  —Antimalarial drugs: chloroquine and hydroxy chloroquine
  —Sulfasalazine, d-penicillamine, gold, methotrexate, azathioprine, cyclophosphamide, cyclosporin
  —These agents work through different mechanisms and the patients need to be very closely monitored for toxicities, thus they should not be prescribed in the ED
  —Biological agents and somatic gene therapy are also being actively considered

Surgical Treatment
- Specific severe musculoskeletal deformities may be corrected surgically
- These procedures include arthrodesis, synovectomy as well as joint replacement procedures
- Atlantooccipital subluxation requires prompt neurosurgical intervention, and upper airway obstruction from CA arthritis requires urgent tracheostomy

MEDICATIONS
- Ibuprofen: adult: 400–800 mg po q 6–8 hrs; peds: 5–10 mg/kg/dose po divided qid
- Methylprednisolone: adult: 125 mg IV in ED; peds: 1–2 mg/kg IV in ED
- Prednisone: adult: 60 mg po q day, taper; peds: 1–2 mg/kg/day po divided bid, taper

Disposition

ADMISSION CRITERIA
- Intractable pain or unremitting fever
- Coagulation disorder or new bleeding diathesis
- Hematological complications

ICU Admission
- Acute coronary or cerebral ischemia
- Acute renal failure
- Acute upper airway obstruction or ventilatory failure
- Acute cerebritis, carditis, or inflammatory cardiomyopathy
- Pulmonary hemorrhage
- Acute Atlantooccipital or subaxial subluxation

DISCHARGE CRITERIA
- No serious complications present
- Able to tolerate oral liquids and medication
- Appropriate followup with private MD or rheumatology can be arranged.

Miscellaneous

ICD9: 446.20

CORE CONTENT CODE: 8.5.2

SUGGESTED READINGS

Abramson SB, Weissmann G. The mechanism of action of nonsteroidal anti-inflammatory drugs. Arthritis Rheum 1989;32:1–9.

Boumpas DT, Chrousos GP, et al. Glucocorticoid therapy for immune mediated diseases: Basic and clinical correlates. Ann Intern Med 1993;119:1198–1208.

Desmet GD, Knockaert DC, Bobbaers HJ. Temporal arteritis: The silent presentation and delay in diagnosis. J Intern Med 1990;227(4):237–240.

Juby A, Johnston C, Davis P. Specificity, sensitivity and diagnostic predictive value of selected laboratory generated autoantibody profiles in patients with connective tissue diseases. J Rheumatol 1991;18:354–358.

Koopman WJ, ed. Arthritis and allied condition. 13th ed. Baltimore: Williams & Wilkins, 1997.

Sox HC Jr, Liaug MH. The erythrocyte sedimentation rate: Guidelines for rational use. Ann Intern Med 1986;104:515–223.

Authors: Altaf H. Ansari; Asif Muhammad

Colon Trauma

Clinical Presentation

SIGNS AND SYMPTOMS

- Colon trauma is generally associated with other intra and extra-abdominal injuries
- Injuries of significant severity may have *minimal early findings*
- It is not common to determine specific organ injury upon physical exam
- Retroperitoneal injuries are more likely to have a delayed presentation, but all colon injuries may present in a delayed manner
- On examination assess for the following
  - —Assess the abdomen for peritoneal signs
  - —Ecchymosis or hematoma on lower abdomen from lap belt compression
  - —Ecchymosis on epigastric region from steering wheel compression
  - —Grey-Turner sign from retroperitoneal hematoma
  - —Foreign bodies, blood, or heme-positive stool upon rectal examination
  - —Bowel sounds are not helpful

MECHANISM/ DESCRIPTION

- Trauma causing colon perforation will produce inflammation into the cavity in which it lies
- Peritoneal inflammation from hollow viscus perforation often requires hours to develop
- Mesenteric tears from blunt trauma cause hemorrhage and bowel ischemia
- Delayed perforation from ischemic or necrotic bowel may occur
- Peritonitis and sepsis may develop from the extravasated intraluminal flora
- Ascending and descending colon segments are retroperitoneal
- The left colon has a higher bacterial load than the right

ETIOLOGY

Penetrating Abdominal Trauma

- Much more common cause of colon trauma than blunt abdominal trauma
- Gunshot wounds have the highest incidence
- Transverse colon is most commonly injured

Blunt Abdominal Trauma

- Burst injury occurs from compression of a closed loop of bowel
- Direct compression as occurs when intestine is squeezed between a lap belt and the vertebral column
- Shearing forces may tear the bowel or its mesentery

Transanal Injury

- Iatrogenic endoscopic or barium enema injury
- Foreign bodies via sexual activities may reach and injure the colon
- Compressed air under high pressure such as at automobile repair facilities can perforate the colon even if the compressor is not inserted into the anus
- Swallowed sharp foreign bodies (i.e. toothpick) may penetrate the colon, particularly the cecum, appendix, and sigmoid. In general, however, foreign bodies tend to pass the colon without complications

SPECIAL PEDIATRIC CONSIDERATIONS

- In contrast to adults, children have an equal frequency of blunt and penetrating colon injuries

Pre-Hospital

CAUTIONS

- Follow standard pre-hospital guidelines for trauma (i.e., ABCs)
- Do not remove penetrating foreign bodies
- Do not attempt to replace eviscerated bowel; cover with moist saline dressings
- Obtain history of mechanism of injury, vehicle damage, and seat belt involvement

CONTROVERSIES

- Use of intravenous crystalloid resuscitation to prevent hypotension is still considered the standard of care.

Diagnosis

- The diagnosis of colon injury remains a medical challenge secondary to the lack of sensitivity of both physical exams and diagnostic tests. Colon trauma is most frequently diagnosed in the operating room
- Morbidity and mortality increase if the diagnosis of colon injury is delayed

ESSENTIAL WORKUP

- Hemodynamically unstable patients are diagnosed in the OR
- Both physical examinations and diagnostic studies are required to increase their individual limited sensitivity to colonic injury
- Serial abdominal examinations may be required as inflammation takes time to develop
- Abdominal CT with contrast is the best diagnostic study in stable patients
- Ultrasound and DPL are more helpful in the potentially unstable patient

IMAGING/SPECIAL TESTS

- CT scanning with triple contrast allows intraperitoneal and retroperitoneal visualization
- CT may miss colon injuries but the scans are usually not completely normal
- DPL or ultrasound in addition to CT will increase sensitivity
- Water-soluble enema with fluoroscopy is useful if above tests are inconclusive
- DPL will not detect retroperitoneal injuries
- Fecal or vegetable material on DPL analysis indicates hollow viscus injury
- Lavage white cell response may be negative secondary to delayed peritoneal inflammation
- In hollow viscus injuries, the lavage WBC count to RBC count ratio is higher than that typically seen with solid organ injuries (e.g., liver)
- Lavage amylase levels are not helpful in the detection of colon injuries but are helpful in small bowel injuries
- See general abdominal trauma chapter for further DPL interpretations
- Plain abdominal radiographs can show indirect signs such as intraperitoneal and retroperitoneal free air

DIFFERENTIAL DIAGNOSIS

- Any intra-abdominal organ injury should be entertained preoperatively
- A fractured pelvis may present similarly to intraperitoneal injuries in children

SPECIAL PEDIATRIC CONSIDERATIONS

- Children are often extremely frightened and may require rectal examination with anesthesia

Treatment

INITIAL STABILIZATION

- Refer to general abdominal trauma section
- Airway, breathing, and circulation management should precede abdominal or colon evaluation
- Aggressive management with crystalloid and blood replacement is required because shock increases the mortality rate from colon injury

ED TREATMENT

- Early surgical consultation is necessary as surgery is the definitive treatment
- Eviscerated bowel should be covered in saline soaked gauze in a nondependent position
- Administer broad-spectrum antibiotics to cover anaerobic and Gram-negative bacteria if colon injury is suspected
- Tetanus prophylaxis should be assured

MEDICATIONS

- Prophylactic antibiotic options (not exclusive)
  —Adult: aztreonam 2 g IV and clindamycin 900 mg IV; peds: aztreonam 90–120 mg/kg/24 hrs divided by q 6–8 hrs IV and clindamycin 25–40 mg/kg/24 hrs divided by q 6–8 hrs IV
  —Adult: cefoxitin 2 g IV; peds: 80–160 mg/kg/24 hrs divided by q 4–6 hrs IV
  —Adult: gentamicin 1.5 mg/kg IV and clindamycin 600 mg IV; peds: gentamicin 6–7.5 mg/kg/24 hrs divided by q 8 hrs and clindamycin 25–40 mg/kg/24 hrs divided by q 6–8 hrs IV

Disposition

ADMISSION CRITERIA

- Colon injuries require admission for surgical repair
- All foreign bodies that penetrate the colon require removal to prevent sepsis
- Patients with abdominal ecchymosis from seat belt compression require admission and observation because of potential for undiagnosed hollow viscus injury

DISCHARGE CRITERIA

- Patients with mechanism that is not suspicious for serious abdominal injury, completely normal abdominal exam, normal hemodynamic status, and no other injury may be considered for discharge with appropriate precautions
- If there is any doubt about the possibility of colon injury, the patient should be admitted and observed

Miscellaneous

ICD9: 863.40

CORE CONTENT CODE: 18.4.11.4

SUGGESTED READINGS

Asbun H, Irani H, Roe E, Bloch J. Intra-abdominal seatbelt injury. J Trauma 1990;30:189–193.

Carrillo EH, Somberg LB, Ceballos CE, et al. Blunt traumatic injuries to the colon and rectum. J Am Coll Surg 1996;183:548–552.

Stokes M, Jones D. ABC of colorectal diseases. Colorectal trauma. BMJ 1992;305:303–306.

Authors: Blake Spirko; Fred Tilden

Coma

Clinical Presentation

SIGNS AND SYMPTOMS

General

- No spontaneous eye opening
- Lack of response to painful stimuli
- No motor activity
- Regular cardiorespiratory function
- Glasgow Coma Scale (GCS) Scoring
  - —Eye opening
    - -Open
      - *Spontaneously 4
      - *To verbal command 3
      - *To pain 2
    - -No response 1
  - —Best motor response
    - -To verbal command
      - *Obeys 6
    - -To painful stimulus
      - *Localizes pain 5
      - *Flexion withdrawal 4
      - *Flexion-abnormal 3
      - *Extension-abnormal 2
      - *No response 1
  - —Best verbal response
    - -Oriented and converses 5
    - -Disoriented and converses 4
    - -Verbalizes 3
    - -Vocalizes 2
    - -No response 1
- Hypothermia
  - —Infection, hypoglycemia, myxedema coma, alcohol and sedative poisoning
- Fever
  - —Infection, thyrotoxicosis, anticholinergics, sympathomimetics, neuroleptic malignant syndrome, hypothalamic hemorrhage
- Hypertension
  - —Structural lesion, hypertensive encephalopathy
- Hypotension
  - —Systemic disease
  - —Sepsis should be highly considered

HEENT

- Mydriasis
  - —Organophosphates
- Miosis
  - —Narcotics
  - —Anticholinergics
  - —Pontine lesion
- Loss of pupillary reflexes or unequal pupils
  - —Structural lesions
- Evidence of head trauma
  - —Contusions
  - —Hematomas
  - —Lacerations
  - —Hemotympanum
- Neck
  - —Nuchal rigidity
    - -Meningitis
    - -Subarachnoid hemorrhage

Neurologic

- Decorticate posturing
  - —Flexion of elbows and wrists
  - —Adduction and internal rotation of shoulders
  - —Suppination of the forearms
  - —Suggests severe damage above the midbrain
- Decerebrate posturing
  - —Extension of elbows and wrists
  - —Adduction and internal rotation of shoulders
  - —Pronation of the forearms
  - —Suggests damage at the midbrain or diencephalon
- Asymmetrical movements
  - —Structural lesions
- Persistent twitching of an extremity
  - —Status epilepticus

MECHANISM/DESCRIPTION

- Unarousable unresponsiveness
- Light coma
  - Responds to noxious stimuli
- Deep coma
  - Does not respond to pain
- Loss of either arousal or cognition
  - Loss of arousal
    - Arousal is primarily a brain stem function
    - Impairment of the reticular activating system
  - Loss of cognition
    - Requires dysfunction of both cerebral hemispheres
- Stupor
  - Deep sleep though not unconsciousness
  - Exhibits little or no spontaneous activity
  - Awaken with stimuli
  - Little motor or verbal activity once aroused
- Obtundation
  - Mental blunting with mild or moderate reduction in alertness
- Delirium
  - Floridly abnormal mental status
    - Irritability
    - Motor restlessness
    - Transient hallucinations
    - Disorientation
    - Delusions
- Clouding of consciousness
  - A disturbance of consciousness
  - Impaired capacity
    - To think clearly
    - To perceive, respond to, and remember current stimuli

ETIOLOGY

- Diffuse brain dysfunction
  - Lack of nutrients
    - Hypoglycemia
    - Hypoxia
  - Poisoning
    - Ethanol
    - Isopropyl alcohol
    - Ethylene glycol
    - Methanol
    - Salicylates
    - Sedatives
    - Narcotics
    - Anticonvulsants
    - Isoniazid
    - Heavy metals
  - Infection
    - Bacterial meningitis
    - Encephalitis
    - Falciparum meningitis
    - Rabies
  - Hepatic encephalopathy
  - Endocrine Disorders
    - Myxedema coma
    - Thyrotoxicosis
    - Addison's disease
    - Cushing's disease
    - Pheochromocytoma
  - Electrolyte disorders
    - Hypernatremia, hyponatremia
    - Hypercalcemia, hypocalcemia
    - Hypermagnesemia, hypomagnesemia
    - Hypophosphatemia
    - Acidosis, alkalosis
  - Temperature regulation
    - Hypothermia
    - Heat stroke
    - Neuroleptic malignant syndrome
    - Malignant hyperthermia
  - Uremia
  - Postictal state, status epilepticus
  - Psychiatric
- Supratentorial 19%
  - Hemorrhage 15%
    - Intraparenchymal hemorrhage
    - Epidural hematoma
    - Subdural hematoma
    - Subarachnoid hemorrhage
  - Infarction 2%
    - Thrombotic arterial occlusion
    - Embolic arterial occlusion
    - Venous occlusion
  - Tumor or abscess 2%
    - Hydrocephalus
    - Herniation
    - Hemorrhage from erosion into adjacent blood vessels
- Subtentorial lesions 12%
  - Infarction
  - Hemorrhage
  - Tumor
  - Basilar migraine
  - Brain stem demyelination

Pre-Hospital

CAUTIONS

- Airway management if loss of airway patency
  - Supplemental oxygen
  - Bag-mask ventilation with cricoid pressure
  - Endotracheal intubation if no response to coma cocktail
- Intravenous access
- Coma cocktail
  - Dextrose
  - Narcan
- Monitor patient
- Look for signs of an underlying cause
  - Medications
  - Medic alert bracelets
  - Document a basic neurologic examination
  - GCS
  - Pupils
  - Extremity movements

CONTROVERSIES

- Empirical dextrose should not be held or delayed if dextrostik is not available
  - Glucose can safely be administered before thiamine
  - Glucose does not worsen outcome in patients with stroke
  - Hypoglycemia is a much more likely cause of coma than a CVA

Diagnosis

ESSENTIAL WORKUP

- Detect and treat reversible causes
- Determine the underlying cause
- Immediate exclusion of comalike states
  - —Noting resistance to passive opening of eyelids, fluttering of eyelids when stroked, abrupt eyelid closure, eye movement by saccadic jerks (rather than roving), or finding the eyes rolled back
  - —Provocation of nystagmus with ice-water caloric testing
  - —Before paralyzing a patient for intubation an attempt should be made to detect a locked-in syndrome
  - —Demonstrating that the patient is able to blink on verbal command will establish this diagnosis
  - —Intubation is still indicated to prevent aspiration

LABORATORY

- Dextrostick
- CBC
- Electrolytes

IMAGING/SPECIAL TESTS

- Head CT scan
  - —Diagnosis of hemorrhage and midline shift
- Lumbar puncture
  - —All patients with coma of unknown etiology, particularly if fever is present
  - —Antibiotics may be administered before lumbar puncture
    - -This will have little effect on CSF cell count, differential, glucose, and protein for as long as 68 hours
  - —Control seizures first
  - —Noninvasive diagnostic studies such as CT scan should be performed before lumbar puncture in adults and children if there is evidence of increased intracranial pressure, a mass lesion, preexisting trauma, or focal findings
    - -Risk of tonsillar herniation in patients with a mass lesion is very small
- Electroencephalography
  - —Performed to rule out suspected seizure activities
  - —Little use in the emergency evaluation
    - -Status epilepticus should be treated empirically
    - -Rarely necessary to distinguish seizures from myoclonic movements
    - -Unlike EEG studies performed in a laboratory, lighting will cause artifacts

DIFFERENTIAL DIAGNOSIS

- Locked-in syndrome
- Psychogenic unresponsiveness

Treatment

INITIAL STABILIZATION

- Oxygenation
  - —Nonrebreather face mask
  - —Augment breaths with bag-valve mask
  - —Endotracheal intubation
- Empiric use of naloxone

ED TREATMENT

- Consider empirical use of antibiotics for coma of undetermined etiology
  - —Broad spectrum with good CSF penetration such as ceftriaxone
- Administer mannitol if clinical or radiographic evidence of impending herniation
- Stop seizure activity with benzodiazepines
- Empiric treatment for a toxic ingestion
  - —Activated charcoal
  - —Alcohol drip if methanol or ethylene glycol suspected
- Correct body temperature
  - —Warmed humidified O_2 if hypothermic
  - —Ice packs and forced air movement over exposed wetted skin if severe hyperthermia
- Specific therapy directed at underlying cause once identified

MEDICATIONS

- Ceftriaxone: 100 mg/kg IV
- Dextrose: 1–2 ml/kg of $D_{50}W$ IV; neonate: 10 ml/kg $D_{10}W$ IV; peds: 4 ml/kg $D_{25}W$ IV
- Diazepam: 0.1–0.3 mg/kg slow IV (max: 10 mg/dose) q 10–15 min × 3 doses
- Lorazepam: 0.05–0.1 mg/kg IV (max: 4 mg/dose q 10–15 min)
- Mannitol: 0.25–1.0 g/kg IV over 20 min
- Naloxone: 0.01 mg/kg IV/IM/SC/ET
- Physostigmine: 0.06–0.08 mg/kg IV
- Thiamine: 100 mg IM or 100 mg thiamine in 1000 ml of intravenous fluid wide open

Disposition

ADMISSION CRITERIA

- All patients who do not have a readily identifiable and completely reversible cause should be admitted

DISCHARGE CRITERIA

- Comatose patients with correctable hypoglycemia and opiate toxicity who respond completely to aggressive ED treatment

Miscellaneous

ICD9: 780.01

CORE CONTENT CODE: N/A

SUGGESTED READINGS

Ellenhorn MJ, ed. Ellenhorn's medical toxicology: diagnosis and treatment of human poisoning. Philadelphia: Williams & Wilkins, 1997:16–19.

Ferrera PC, Chan L. Initial management of the patient with altered mental status. Am Fam Physician 1997;1773–1780.

Plum F, Posner J. The diagnosis of stupor and coma. 3rd ed. Philadelphia: FA Davis, 1986.

Wolfe R, Brown D. Coma in emergency medicine: concepts and clinical practice. 4th ed. Rosen P, ed. Mosby: St Louis 1998:2106–2118.

Authors: Gregory D. Jay; Linda C. Cowell

Compartment Syndrome

Clinical Presentation

SIGNS AND SYMPTOMS

- Severe, constant pain over the compartment which is disproportionate to extent of injury
- Pain increases with active contraction and passive stretching
- Muscle weakness
- Hypesthesia
- "6 P's": *pain, pressure, paresis, paresthesia, pulses present*

PATHOPHYSIOLOGY

- Elevated tissue pressure in closed spaces that compromises blood flow through capillaries supplying muscles and nerves
- Normal tissue pressure is less than 10 mm Hg
- Capillary blood flow in a compartment is compromised at pressures above 20 mm Hg
- Muscles and nerves can develop ischemic necrosis at pressures above 30 mm Hg
- When distal pulses are diminished on exam, muscle necrosis is probably present
- The four compartments of the leg are most frequently involved, but compartment syndrome can occur in the arm, forearm, hand, foot, shoulder, buttocks, and thigh

ETIOLOGY

- Compression: circumferential cast, burn eschar, or mast trousers
- Increased volume with the compartment from edema or hematoma caused by direct trauma, fracture, overexertion of muscles, or limb compression during prolonged recumbency

Pre-Hospital

CAUTIONS

- Keep the extremity at the level of the heart to promote arterial flow but not diminish venous return
- Do not use ice if compartment syndrome is suspected—it may compromise microcirculation

Diagnosis

ESSENTIAL WORKUP

- The diagnosis is suggested by the above signs and symptoms and the appropriate clinical situation
- Palpation may or may not reveal tenseness and swelling

IMAGING/SPECIAL TESTS

- X-rays should be performed if fracture is suspected
- Diagnosis is aided by measurement of compartment pressures with a portable pressure monitoring system such as the Stryker IC pressure monitor system (Stryker Surgical, 420 East Alcott Street, Kalamazoo, MI 49001), which allows for intermittent pressure measurements via an 18-gauge needle or continuous pressure monitoring with the attachment for an indwelling catheter
- The technique for using the pressure monitoring system is as follows
  —Prep overlying skin with antiseptic solution
  —Local anesthetic can be infiltrated into the *subcutaneous tissue only,* taking care not to inject intramuscularly which may artificially elevate intracompartmental tissue pressure measurements
  —The needle used for pressure measurements is advanced through the skin until a popping sensation is felt when the fascia is pierced
  —0.2 ml of saline is injected to clear the lumen of the needle, and the intracompartmental pressure measurement is then read
  —To ascertain correct placement of the needle within the compartment, external pressure may be applied over the muscle compartment or the muscles can be passively stretched to increase the intracompartmental pressure transiently. Once these maneuvers are discontinued, the pressure should drop to baseline and stabilize

DIFFERENTIAL DIAGNOSIS

- Chronic compartment syndrome
- Fascial hernia
- Stress fracture
- Arterial occlusion
- Neuropraxia
- Deep vein thrombosis
- Cellulitis
- Osteomyelitis
- Tenosynovitis
- Synovitis

Treatment

INITIAL STABILIZATION

- Acutely injured extremities that are casted should have the cast univalved and spread, and underlying cast padding should be cut
- Keep the extremity at the level of the heart

ED TREATMENT

- Acute compartment syndrome is a surgical emergency
- Mainstay of treatment is fasciotomy, particularly for compartment pressures over 30–40 mm Hg

MEDICATIONS

- There is no place for medications including steroids or vasodilators in the treatment of compartment syndrome
- Pain medication as indicated

Disposition

ADMISSION CRITERIA

- Emergent orthopedic or surgical consultation for compartment pressures over 30 mm Hg
- For compartment pressures over 20 mm Hg but less than 30 mmHg, surgical consultation should be sought and the patient admitted. For compartment pressures between 15 and 20 mm Hg, serial measurement of pressures should be taken; if the patient cannot be relied upon to return for repeat measurements, they should be admitted

DISCHARGE CRITERIA

- Compartment pressure less than 10–15 mm Hg—patients should be given symptomatic treatment and instructed to return for increased pain, swelling, development of paresthesias

Miscellaneous

ICD9: 958.8

CORE CONTENT CODE: 18.4.14.4

SUGGESTED READINGS

Mabee JR. Compartment syndrome: A complication of acute extremity trauma. J Emerg Med 1994;12(5):651–656.

Moore RE, Friedman RJ. Current concepts in pathophysiology and diagnosis of compartment syndromes. J Emerg Med 1989;7(6):657–662.

Mayeda DV. Knee and lower leg. In: Rosen P, et al., eds. Emergency medicine: Concepts and clinical practice. 3rd ed. St. Louis: CV Mosby, 1992.

Authors: Patricia Breeden; Robert Galli

Congenital Heart Disease

Clinical Presentation

SIGNS AND SYMPTOMS

Newborn

- Asymptomatic if ductus arteriosus is still patent
- Lethargy
- Poor feeding
- Dyspnea

Cyanotic Congenital Heart Disease

- Mucous membrane cyanosis that increases with agitation
- Hypercyanotic spells or "Tet spells"
  —Occurs in patients with Tetralogy of Fallot
  —Follows events that decrease the systemic vascular resistance
    -Wakening
    -Feeding
    -Following defecation
- Murmur
  —Absence does not preclude cardiac disease
  —Characteristics most suggestive of congenital heart disease
    -Grade >3
    -Pansystolic
    -Late systolic
    -Diastolic
- Single S2 heart sound
- Increased right ventricular impulse on precordial palpation
- Retractions and tachypnea
  —Less severe than those seen with primary pulmonary disease

Shock-Producing Congenital Heart Disease

- Hypotension
- Skin mottling
- Delayed capillary refill
- Diminished or absent femoral or dorsalis pedis pulses
- Cool and pale extremities
- Apical diastolic flow rumble
  —Significant left-to-right shunting
- Gallop
- Hepatomegaly
- Splenomegaly

Syncope and Sudden Death

- Syncope with exercise
  —Hypertrophic obstructive cardiomyopathy
    -Family history of sudden death before age 50
    -Systolic ejection murmur along the lower left sternal border
    -Prominent peripheral pulses
  —Anomalous coronary artery syndrome
    -Asymptomatic
    -Chest pain
    -Nonspecific findings in infants: unexplained intermittent irritability; dyspnea; diaphoresis

MECHANISM/DESCRIPTION

- Aberrant embryonic development of the heart or great vessels
- Complex multifactorial genetic and environmental causes
  —Chromosomal aberrations account for fewer than 10 percent
- Newborns with congenital heart disease (CHD)
  —A patent ductus arteriosus can compensate for the cardiac anomaly
    -Oxygenated pulmonary blood enters the systemic circulation
    -Systemic blood enters the pulmonary circulation
    -Closure of the ductus coincides with onset of symptoms
  —Symptoms usually present in the first 2 weeks of life
- Patients with CHD may present as older children and adults
  —Mild lesions
  —Multiple lesions counterbalance each other
  —Compensatory mechanisms
- Three basic structural abnormalities
  —Obstruction to flow through valves or the great vessels
  —Abnormal communication between chambers or great vessels
  —Transposition of the great vessels
- Four types of functional abnormalities
  —Ventricular or atrial hypertrophy
  —Systemic or pulmonary hypertension
  —Left-to-right shunt
  —Right-to-left shunt
    -Cyanotic CHD
    Fixed right-to-left shunt at any level
    -Certain conditions trigger cyanosis in older children and adults with CHD
    Cardiac shunt obstruction
    Pulmonary disease
    Decreased systemic vascular resistance: fever; dehydration
- CHD presenting as syncope or sudden death
  —Most causes of syncope are vasovagal in nature and are not life-threatening
  —Hypertrophic obstructive cardiomyopathy (HOC)
    -Syncope during exercise
  —Anomalous coronary artery anatomy
    -Aberrant left coronary artery (LCA)
    Anomaly most commonly associated with sudden death
    The LCA travels between the aorta and the pulmonary artery
    It becomes compressed between the two great vessels during exercise

ETIOLOGY

- Right-to-left shunt (cyanotic CHD)
  —Transposition of the great arteries
    -A parallel circulatory system
    -The aorta arises from the right ventricle (RV)
    -The pulmonary artery (PA) arises from the left ventricle (LV)
  —Tetralogy of Fallot
    -RV outflow stenosis, right ventricular hypertrophy (RVH), ventricular septal defect (VSD), overriding aorta
  —Tricuspid atresia
    -No direct communication between the right atrium (RA) and RV
    -The RV is not fully developed
  —Truncus arteriosus
  —A single great artery leaves the heart to provide systemic, pulmonary and coronary circulations
  —Total anomalous pulmonary venous return
    -Pulmonary venous blood enters the systemic venous system or RA
  —Ebstein's anomaly
    -Downward displacement of the tricuspid valve
  —Patent ductus arteriosus (PDA)
  —Eisenmenger's complex
    -Large ventricular septal defect with pulmonary hypertension
  —Eisenmenger's reaction
    -Atrial septal defect or PDA with pulmonary hypertension
- Left-to right shunt
  —Atrial septal defect
  —Ventricular septal defect
  —Ruptured sinus of Valsava aneurysm
  —Coronary arteriovenous fistula
  —Anomalous origin of the left coronary artery
  —Aortopulmonary window
  —Patent ductus arteriosus
- Obstructing lesions causing shock
  —Hypoplastic left heart syndrome
  —Critical aortic stenosis
  —Coarctation of the aorta and interrupted aortic arch
- Syncope producing CHD
  —Hypertrophic obstructive cardiomyopathy
  —Aortic stenosis
  —Anomalous coronary artery
  —Congenital heart block

Pre-Hospital

CAUTIONS

- Avoid 100% nonrebreathers in cyanotic newborns
  - —High oxygen tensions promote ductal closure

Diagnosis

ESSENTIAL WORKUP

- All children suspected of CHD require a chest radiograph and an EKG
- Exclude noncardiac causes of cyanosis, shock, and syncope in newborns

LABORATORY

- ABG
  - —Helps to distinguish pulmonary disease from cardiac disease in the cyanotic newborn
  - —Cyanotic patients with primary CHD commonly have a normal to low pCO_2
  - —Oxygen challenge test
    - -No response to 10 minutes of 100% oxygen by showing an increase in arterial pO_2
- CBC
  - —Erythrocytosis identifies chronically cyanotic patients

IMAGING/SPECIAL TESTS

- EKG
  - —Usually abnormal
  - —Left or right ventricular hypertrophy
  - —Absent left ventricular forces
  - —Absent anterior forces
  - —Dysrhythmias
  - —ST-T wave changes
- Chest radiograph
  - —Normal
  - —Abnormal heart size and shape
    - -Generalized cardiomegaly
    - -Egg-on-side: transposition of the great arteries
    - -Boot-shaped: Tetralogy of Fallot
    - -Box or funnel-shaped: Ebstein's anomaly
    - -Snowman: total anomalous pulmonary venous return to superior vena cava
  - —Pulmonary edema
  - —Abnormal position of the stomach bubble or liver
  - —A right aortic arch
- Echocardiogram
  - —Should be performed emergently in all infants with suspected and undiagnosed CHD
- Head CT
  - —Indicated in patients with known CHD who present with seizures or focal neurologic symptoms
  - —Assess for thromboembolic events or abscess formation
  - —Risk of stroke is increased in children with CHD below the age of 4

DIFFERENTIAL DIAGNOSIS

- Shock-producing CHD
  - —Sepsis
  - —Hypovolemia
  - —Cardiomyopathy
  - —Dysrhythmia
  - —Adrenal insufficiency
- Noncardiac causes of cyanosis
  - —Pulmonary abnormalities
  - —Pneumonia
  - —Pulmonary edema
  - —Pneumothorax
  - —Lung agenesis
  - —Bronchopulmonary dysplasia
  - —Chronic obstructive lung disease
- Restrictive lung disease
- Hypoventilation
- Central nervous system depression
  - —Trauma
  - —Drugs
  - —Infection
- Upper Airway Obstruction
  - —Tracheal rings
  - —Epiglottitis
- Hypotonia
  - —Spinal cord insults
  - —Neuromuscular disease
  - —Drugs
- Diaphragmatic hernia
- Abnormal hemoglobin
  - —Methemoglobin
  - —Sulfhemoglobin

Congenital Heart Disease

Treatment

INITIAL STABILIZATION

- Cyanosis or hypotension in the neonate
  - —Endotracheally intubate all symptomatic patients
  - —The FIO_2 delivered should be no higher than 0.40 with ductal-dependent CHD
  - —High oxygen tensions promote ductal closure
- Place air filters on the intravenous lines of all patients with CHD

ED TREATMENT

- Administer prostaglandin E1 (PGE1) to all symptomatic newborns
  - —Continuous intravenous infusion
  - —Promotes reopening of the ductus arteriosus
  - —Provides temporary compensation in most patients less than 2 weeks of age
  - —Side effects of PGE1
    - -Apnea
    - -Hypotension
    - -Fever
    - -Restlessness
  - —Not effective in managing total anomalous pulmonary venous return
  - —May exacerbate pulmonary and tricuspid valve regurgitation in patients with Ebstein's anomaly
  - —The overall benefits to the majority of patients presenting in distress far outweigh the potential risks or side effects
- Treat apnea with ventilation and hypotension with fluids
- Cyanosis in the child or adult with known CHD
  - —Administer 10–20 cc/kg NS IV if dehydration seems likely
  - —Provide supplemental oxygen if pulmonary disease is suspected
  - —Treat fever with antipyretics
  - —Administer antibiotics if pneumonia is suspected
- Patients with "Tet spells"
  - —Provide a calming environment
  - —Place patient in the knee-chest position to increase SVR and promote left-to-right shunting
  - —Provide supplemental oxygen if it does not agitate the patient
- Symptomatic patients with hypertrophic obstructive cardiomyopathy
  - —Give 10–20 cc/kg NS IV
  - —Administer propranolol IV
- Inotropic support for shock caused by CHD
  - —Dobutamine or dopamine
- Administer antibiotics if sepsis or pneumonia is suspected
  - —Ampicillin and gentamicin

MEDICATIONS

- Acetaminophen: 15 mg/kg po or PR
- Ampicillin: 50 mg/kg IV
- Dobutamine: 5–20 μg/kg/min IV
- Dopamine: 5–20 μg/kg/min IV
- Gentamycin: 2.5 mg/kg IV
- Ibuprofen: 10 mg/kg po
- Morphine sulfate: 0.1–0.2 mg/kg SQ or IV
- Phenylephrine: 0.5–5 μg/kg/min IV
- Propranolol: 0.1 mg/kg IV
- Prostaglandin E1: 0.05 μg/kg/min
- Sodium bicarbonate: 1–2 mEq/kg IV

Disposition

ADMISSION CRITERIA

- All newborns with suspected CHD
  - —Admit to PICU
  - —Surgical consultation for cardiac repair
- Children and adults with an acute worsening of cyanosis
- Known CHD with symptomatic or suspected respiratory syncytial virus
- Patients with worsening CHF

DISCHARGE CRITERIA

- Patients with Tetralogy of Fallot who respond to minimal intervention
  - —Calming and knee-chest positioning
  - —Close follow-up
- Cardiology referral for syncope
  - —Syncope during exercise
  - —Absence of prodromal symptoms just prior to syncopal episode
  - —Family history of sudden death
  - —Abnormal EKG findings

Miscellaneous

ICD9: 745.1, 745.2, 745.3, 746.2, 746.85

CORE CONTENT CODE: 13.2.2

SUGGESTED READINGS

Burton DA, Cabalka AK. Cardiac evaluation in infants. Pediatr Clin North Am 1994;41:991–1015.

Flynn PA, Engle MA, Ehlers KH. Cardiac issues in the pediatric emergency room. Pediatr Clin North Am 1992;39(5):995–996.

Friedman WF. Congenital heart disease in infancy and childhood. In: Braunwald E, ed. Heart disease. 5th ed. Philadelphia: WB Saunders, 1997:877–962.

Author: Angela Anderson

Congestive Heart Failure

Clinical Presentation

SIGNS AND SYMPTOMS

- General
  - —Fatigue
  - —Weakness
  - —Anxiety
- Left heart failure
  - —Dyspnea
  - —Orthopnea
  - —Paroxysmal nocturnal dyspnea
  - —Decreased exercise tolerance
  - —Rales
  - —Wheezes
  - —Dullness at lung bases
  - —S3 gallop
  - —S4 may be present
- Right heart failure
  - —Dyspnea on exertion
  - —Jugular venous distention
  - —Increased liver span
  - —A positive abdominojugular reflex
  - —Ascites
  - —Dependent edema
- Severe impairment
  - —Confusion
  - —Tachypnea
  - —Tachycardia
  - —Mild hypotension
  - —Cyanosis
  - —Pulsus alternans
  - —Frothy sputum
  - —Cheyne-Stokes respirations

MECHANISM/DESCRIPTION

- Failure of the heart to pump blood at a rate sufficient to satisfy tissue metabolism
  - —Low output failure
    - -Decreased cardiac output secondary to myocardial muscle failure
  - —High output failure
    - -Cardiac output is normal or high
    - -Output is insufficient to fulfill the requirement of metabolizing tissue
      Hyperthyroidism
      Severe asthma
- Acute CHF
  - —Rapidly progressive failure state
  - —Usually caused by a precipitating event
  - —The heart does not have the reserve to compensate for the added burden
- Chronic CHF
  - —Slowly progressive failure state
- Left-sided failure
  - —Hemodynamic burden placed on the left ventricle
  - —Results in back up of pressure and fluid behind the involved chamber
  - —Pulmonary congestion occurs
- CHF affects approximately 2% of the U.S. population
- Most common inpatient diagnosis over the age of 65
- The incidence of CHF increases twofold for each decade of life
- The presence of CHF increased the likelihood of mortality
  - —8 times for men
  - —5 times for women

ETIOLOGY

- Decreased myocardial contractility
  - —Ischemia
  - —Infarction
  - —Cardiomyopathy
  - —Myocarditis
  - —Decreased contractile efficiency
    - -Drug related
    - -Metabolic disorder
- Pressure overload states
  - —Hypertension
  - —Valvular abnormalities
  - —Congenital heart disease
- Restricted cardiac output
  - —Myocardial infiltrative disease
- Volume overload
- Thyrotoxicosis
- Severe anemia

Pre-Hospital

- Intravenous access
- Supplemental oxygen
  - —100% nonrebreather mask
- Cardiac monitor
- Pulse oximetry
- Sublingual nitrates
- Furosemide
- Endotracheal intubation may be required in severe cases

CAUTIONS

- Administration of morphine
  - —CHF may be difficult to distinguish from an acute exacerbation of COPD

Diagnosis

ESSENTIAL WORKUP

- The chest radiograph is essential in confirming the diagnosis and in assessing severity

LABORATORY

- Arterial blood gas
- Electrolytes
  - —Generally normal before treatment
  - —Hyperkalemia with severe low output states
- BUN and creatinine
  - —Elevation in severe CHF
- Cardiac enzymes
  - —May be useful if ischemia or infarction is presumed to be the underlying cause

IMAGING/SPECIAL TESTS

- Chest radiograph
  - —Cardiomegaly
  - —3 phases of pulmonary findings
    - -Pulmonary redistribution
      Cephalization of vessels
    - -Interstitial edema
      Effusions
      Kerley B lines
      Classic butterfly infiltrate
    - -Frank alveolar infiltrates
      May be asymmetric and mistaken for pneumonia
- ECG
  - —Assess for underlying cardiac ischemia
- Echocardiography
  - —Acute valvular pathology
  - —Pericardial tamponade

DIFFERENTIAL DIAGNOSIS

- Left-sided CHF
  - —Acute exacerbation of COPD
  - —Asthma exacerbation
  - —Acute respiratory distress syndrome
  - —Pneumonia
  - —Constrictive pericarditis
  - —Pericardial tamponade
- Right-sided CHF
  - —Nephrotic syndrome
  - —Cirrhosis

Treatment

INITIAL STABILIZATION

- Intravenous access
- Supplemental oxygen
- Place patient in a upright position
- Cardiac monitor
- Pulse oximetry
- Control airway as needed
  —Continuous positive airway pressure
    -CPAP
    -Nasal Bi-PAP
    -May decrease the need for intubation
  —Endotracheal intubation for impending respiratory failure

ED TREATMENT

- Normotensive or hypertensive patients
  —Rapid acting nitrates
    -Sublingual nitroglycerin
    -Nitro paste
    -IV nitroglycerin
    Pulmonary edema
    Failure of sublingual nitroglycerin and nitro paste to provide relief
  —Morphine sulfate
  —Intravenous diuretics
    -Lasix or bumex
    -Sodium nitroprusside for afterload reduction may be required for severe persistent hypertension
- Hypotensive patients
  —Avoid nitrates, morphine and diuretics
  —Agents that increase myocardial contractility
    -Dopamine
    -Dobutamine
    -Amrinone
    -Milrinone
- In less severe or chronic cases of low output CHF
  —ACE inhibitors such as enalapril improve hemodynamic and increase exercise capacity
  —Use in conjunction with other diuretics

MEDICATIONS

- Nitroglycerin: 0.4 mg sublingual; 1–2 inches of nitro paste; 5–20 μg/min, max of 100–200 μg/min
- Morphine sulfate: 2–4 mg IV q 5 min
- Lasix: 20–100 mg IV
- Bumex: 0.5–2.0 mg IV
- Nitroprusside: 0.5–10 μg/kg/min
- Dopamine: 2–20 μg/kg/min
- Dobutamine: 2–10 μg/kg/min
- Amrinone: 0.75 mg/kg IV load; 5–10 μg/kg/min
- Enalapril: 2.5–20 mg/day po
- Digoxin: 1 mg load over 1 day; 0.125–0.375 mg/day po

Disposition

ADMISSION CRITERIA

- Intensive care unit
  —Pulmonary edema
  —Cardiogenic shock
  —Concomitant myocardial infarction or ischemia
- Medical wards
  —New onset CHF
  —Symptoms not relieved by aggressive ED therapy

DISCHARGE CRITERIA

- Mild exacerbation of chronic CHF
  —Responds to treatment
- Close follow-up should be arranged with continuation of diuretic and vasodilator therapy

Miscellaneous

ICD9: 428.0

CORE CONTENT CODE: 2.2.1

SUGGESTED READINGS

Armstrong PW, Moe GW. Medical advances in the treatment of congestive heart failure. Circulation 1993;88(6):2941–2952.

Schamberger MS. Cardiac emergencies. Pediatr Ann 1996;25(6):339–344.

Smith TW, et al. Management of heart failure. In: Braunwald E, ed. Heart disease. 5th ed. Philadelphia: WB Saunders, 1997:492–514.

Authors: John F. Jardine, Robert Partridge

Conjunctivitis

Clinical Presentation

SIGNS AND SYMPTOMS

General

- Red eye (conjunctival irritation)
- Gritty, foreign body sensation
- Discharge
- Eyelid sticking (worse on arising)
- Conjunctival edema (chemosis) and eyelid edema
- Normal visual acuity, anterior chamber, and intraocular pressure

Bacterial—General

- Mucopurulent or purulent discharge
- Preauricular nodes

Gonococcal

- Hyperacute, copious purulent discharge—"pouring out" of the eye
- Severe chemosis and lid edema
- Inflammatory membranes
- Invade intact conjunctiva and cornea within 24 hours and cause ulcerations, scarring, and perforations leading to blindness

Chlamydia

- Lacrimation
- Mucopurulent discharge
- +/− Photophobia
- Concomitant genital infection (>50%)
  —Transmission occurs via autoinoculation from genital secretions

Viral—General

- Watery, mucous discharge, lacrimation
- Foreign body sensation
- Pinpoint subconjunctival hemorrhages
- Inflammatory membranes

Herpes Simplex Virus (HSV)

- Acute follicular conjunctival reaction
- Skin lesions or vesicles along eyelid margin or periocular skin
- Corneal involvement—dendritic lesion

Herpes Zoster Virus (HZV)

- Associated with pain or paresthesias of the skin
- Rash or vesicles involving the distribution of cranial nerve V_1
- Dendritic characters on cornea
- Rarely vesicles or ulcers form on the conjunctiva

Allergic

- Hallmark: itching
- Either hyperemic or pale conjunctiva
- Watery discharge
- Papillary hypertrophy
- Frequent history of allergy, atopy, nasal symptoms

Contact Related

- Acute symptoms result of corneal ulceration

MECHANISM/DESCRIPTION

- Inflammation of the conjunctiva arising from a broad group of clinical causes

ETIOLOGY

Bacterial

Gonococcal

- Ophthalmic emergency
  —*N. gonorrhoeae* can invade intact conjunctiva and cornea within 24 hours and cause ulcerations, scarring and perforations leading to blindness
  —Often occurs in newborns

Chlamydia

- Transmission occurs via autoinocculation from genital secretions

Viral

- Adenovirus most common
- Frequently associated with recent URI symptoms or exposure to someone with a red eye

Herpes Simplex Virus

- Recurrent ocular infection occurs in 25% patients within 2 years
- Use of steroids is *contraindicated*

Allergic

- Frequent history of allergy, atopy, nasal symptoms

Contact Related

- Most vision threatening cause of "red eye"
- May be due to chemical irritation, hypersensitivity from preservatives, medications
- *Pseudomonas* commonly implicated organism
- Anaerobes may be causative in patients using saliva to wet lenses

PEDIATRIC CONSIDERATIONS

- Often a manifestation of systemic disease in infants
- Neonates become infected during passage through the birth canal
  —Gonococcal, herpetic, chlamydial organisms most common
- *Ophthalmia Neonatorum* is conjunctivitis within the first 4 weeks of life
- *C. trachomatis* is
  —Not eradicated by silver nitrate
  —Substantial percentage of infants treated with erythromycin still develop conjunctivitis

Pre-Hospital

N/A

Diagnosis

ESSENTIAL WORKUP

- History for: onset of inflammation; environmental or work-related exposure; ill contacts; sexual activity, discharge, rash; use of over-the-counter medicines or cosmetics; systemic diseases
- Careful physical examination with slitlamp including fluorescein staining

LABORATORY

- Bacteriologic studies
  - —Not indicated in routine cases
  - —Indications
    - -Ophthalmia neonatorum (except chemical)
    - -Suspected gonococcal ophthalmia
    - -Compromised host
    - -Signs and symptoms of systemic disease
    - -Refractory to treatment within 48–72 hours (with good compliance)
- Positive Gram stain for Gram-negative intracellular diplococci
  - —Sufficient to initiate systemic and topical treatment for gonococcal disease
- RPR
  - —For suspected cases of STDs

DIFFERENTIAL DIAGNOSIS

- Dry eye
- Foreign body
- Corneal abrasion
- Allergies/hypersensitivity
- Nasolacrimal obstruction
- Anterior uveitis
- Acute angle-closure glaucoma (most serious cause)
- Scleritis/episcleritis
- Subconjunctival hemorrhage

PEDIATRIC CONSIDERATIONS

- Gram stain and culture all cases of ophthalmia neonatorum
- Giemsa stain of conjunctival scrapings reveals diagnostic basophilic epithelial cytoplasmic inclusions in a significant number of infants with chlamydial disease
- Rapid EIA test available for diagnosis of neonatal chlamydial conjunctivitis

Treatment

INITIAL STABILIZATION

- Initiate empiric antibiotic therapy with broad spectrum topical agent
- Systemic therapy for gonococcal, chlamydial, and meningococcal conjunctivitis, ophthalmia neonatorum, and all severe infections regardless of cause
- Manage herpetic eye infections in consultation with an ophthalmologist

ED TREATMENT

- Remove discharge from the eye(s)
- Antibiotics—topical
  - —Instill drops q 2 hrs with ointment at bedtime
  - —Continue therapy for 48 hrs after clearing of symptoms
  - —Discontinue therapy and obtain cultures if no improvement in 48–72 hrs (with good compliance)
- Antibiotics—systemic
  - —Parenteral therapy mandatory for gonococcal infection
  - —Chlamydia requires systemic treatment of sexual partners and parents of neonates
- Eye irrigation
  - —Indicated at least hourly in gonococcal ophthalmia
  - —Symptomatic relief in allergic or viral cases
  - —Use saline or buffered solutions, preferably without preservatives
- Personal hygiene—frequent handwashing and use of separate towels and washcloths
- Isolation—use precautions at work or school
- Allergic conjunctivitis
  - —Antihistamine drops (naphcon A)
  - —Cromolyn sodium ophthalmic solution
- Do not use steroids in the initial management

MEDICATIONS

General

- Bacitracin ophthalmologic ointment
- Ciprofloxin: 0.35% 1-drop q 1–6 hrs
- Erythromycin: 0.5% ointment
- Gentamicin: 0.3% ointment q 3–4 hrs or drops q 1–4 hrs
- Sulfacetamide: 10% 1-drop q 1–6 hrs
- Tobramycin: 0.3% ointment q 3–4 hrs or drops q 1–6 hrs

Chlamydia

- Adults
  - —Doxycycline: 100 mg po bid for 3 weeks
  - —Erythromycin: 500 mg po qid for 3 weeks
  - —Tetracycline: 250–500 mg po qid for 3 weeks
- Neonates
  - —Erythromycin: 50 mg/kg/d po in 4 divided doses for 14 days

Gonococcal

- Adults
  - —Ceftriaxone: 1 g IV or IM daily for 3–5 days or as needed
  - —Erythromycin: 500 mg po qid for 2–3 weeks or doxycycline 100 mg po bid for 2–3 weeks
  - —PLUS topical antibiotics as above
- Neonates: aq. penicillin G 100,000 IU/kg/d in 4 divided doses for 7 days or ceftriaxone 25–50 mg/kg IV daily for 7 days

Viral

- Artificial tears

HSV or HZV

- Trifluorothymidine: 1% 5 times per day or
- Vidarabine: 3% ointment 5 times per day

Allergic

- Naphazoline (naphcon A): 1 drop bid-qid
- Cromolyn sodium (crolom): 1 drop q 4–6 hrs

Disposition

ADMISSION CRITERIA

- Known or suspected gonococcal infection (any age group)

DISCHARGE CRITERIA

- Close follow-up for all cases

Miscellaneous

ICD9: 372.30

CORE CONTENT CODE: 6.4.1.3

SUGGESTED READINGS

Bertolini J, Pelucio M. The red eye. Emerg Med Clin North Am 1995;13(3):561–579.

Cullom RD, Chang B. Conjunctiva/sclera/external disease. In: The Wills eye manual: Office and emergency room diagnosis and treatment of eye diseases. 2d ed. Philadelphia: JB Lippincott, 1994:109–115.

Jackson WB. Differentiating conjunctivitis of diverse origins. Surv Ophthalmol 1993;38(Suppl):S91–S104.

Author: Mary Stewart

Conscious Sedation/Rapid Sequence Intubation

Clinical Presentation

N/A

Pre-Hospital

N/A

Diagnosis

N/A

Treatment:

INITIAL STABILIZATION:

Conscious Sedation

- Preparation
  - —Apply cardiorespiratory monitor, pulse oximeter, and blood pressure monitor
  - —Secure functioning IV line
  - —Administer 2–4 L oxygen via nasal cannula
  - —At bedside have:
    - -Bag and mask
    - -Suction with Yankauer tip
    - -Reversal agents (flumazenil and naloxone)
  - —Immediately available in emergency department
    - -Laryngoscopes
    - -Endotracheal tubes
    - -Defibrillator equipment
    - -Medications for intubation
- Medication administration
  - —Start at the lower end of the drug dosage and titrate upwards to effect
  - —End point
    - -Drowsy patient that frequently falls asleep when not stimulated

Rapid Sequence Intubation

- Preparation
  - —Assemble appropriate medicines
  - —Apply cardiorespiratory monitor, pulse oximeter, and blood pressure monitor
  - —Test laryngoscope blade
  - —Test endotracheal tube balloon
    - -Adult male: 7.5–8.5-French
    - -Adult female: 7.0–8.0-French
    - -Child: size = (age × 4)/4
  - —At bedside have
    - -Bag and mask
    - -Functioning suction with Yankauer tip
  - —Establish two intravenous lines
  - —Apply 100% oxygen via nonrebreather

ED TREATMENT

Conscious Sedation

- Anxiolysis
  - —For imaging procedures in children
  - —Medication alternatives
    - -Chloral hydrate po
    - -Midazolam IV/intranasal
    - -Ketamine IM
- Mild-to-moderately painful procedure
  - —For laceration repair, minor procedures, or gynecological exam in children
  - —Medication alternatives
    - -Fentanyl and midazolam IV
    - -Ketamine IV/IM
- Severely painful procedure
  - —For fracture/dislocation reduction
  - —Medication alternatives
    - -Fentanyl and midazolam IV
    - -Ketamine IV

Rapid Sequence Intubation

Steps

- Preoxygenation with 100% for 5 minutes
  - —Allow 3–5 minutes before desaturation below 90% occurs
  - —Do not bag as inflation of the stomach increases aspiration risk
- Pretreatment (3 minutes prior to succinylcholine)
  - —Administer pretreament dose: vecuronium or pancuronium 1 mg (peds: 0.01 mg/kg) or rocuronium 0.06 mg/kg for
    - -Patient comfort
    - -Increase intracranial pressure
    - -Ocular trauma
  - —Administer lidocaine 100 mg (peds: 1 mg/kg) for
    - -Hypertension
    - -Increased intracranial pressure
    - -Status asthmaticus
  - —Administer fentanyl (1–3 μg/kg) for
    - -Increased intracranial pressure
  - —Administer atropine (0.02 mg/kg)
    - -For children <5 years old
    - -Prior to ketamine administration
- Administer sedative agent immediately prior to succinylcholine
  - —Etomidate 0.3 mg/kg
    - -Minimal hemodynamic effects
    - -Best for hypotensive patients
  - —Thiopental 3–5 mg/kg
    - -For increased intracranial pressure
    - -May cause hypotension
  - —Ketamine 1.5–2 mg/kg for status asthmaticus
- Administer succinylcholine
  - —Dose = 1–1.5 mg/kg
  - —Apply cricoid pressure (release after intubation successful)
  - —Use alternative agent in ocular trauma, hyperkalemia, 2 days after severe crush injury or burn
  - —Alternative agents
    - -Rocuronium 0.6–1.2 mg/kg
    - -Vecuronium 0.15–0.25 mg/kg
- Attempt intubation in 30–45 seconds when patient flaccid
- Confirm tube placement

MEDICATIONS

- Chloral hydrate: 50–100 mg/kg (max 2 g) po
  - —Onset: 15–60 minutes
  - —Duration: 1–2 hours
  - —Cautions
    - -Contraindicated in hepatic and renal failure
- Etomidate: 0.3 mg/kg IV
  - —Onset: <60 seconds
  - —Duration: 3–5 minutes
- Fentanyl: 1–4 μg/kg IVP titrated in increments of 1 μg/kg
  - —Analgesia: 90 seconds
  - —Duration: 20–30 minutes
  - —Cautions
    - -Respiratory depression
    - -Truncal rigidity and seizures if large doses
    - -Hypotension in hypovolemia
- Flumazenil: 0.2 mg (peds: <20 kg: 0.01 mg/kg initial then 0.005 mg/kg; >20 kg: 0.2 mg initial then 0.005 mg/kg) over 15 sec repeated q 1 min to maximum of 1 mg IV
- Ketamine: 1.5–2 mg IV for intubation; 3–4 mg/kg IM for sedation
  - —Onset: 60 seconds IV with peak at 5 minutes
  - —Duration: 15 minutes IV
  - —Cautions
    - -Contraindicated in hypertension and ischemic heart disease
    - -Elevation of both intracranial and ocular pressures
    - -Emergence phenomenon
    - -Stimulation of secretions
- Midazolam (sedation)
  - —Adults: 0.02–0.1 mg/kg IV
  - —Peds: 0.05–0.15 mg/kg IV/IM; 0.2–0.5 mg/kg of 5 mg/ml preparation (max 6 mg) intranasal
  - —Onset: 1–3 minutes IV; 10–20 minutes IM; 10–15 minutes intranasal
  - —Duration: 30–120 minutes IV; 1–2 hours IM; 25–60 minutes intranasal
  - —Cautions
    - -Respiratory depression
    - -Hypotension
- Midazolam (induction): 0.1–0.3 mg/kg IV
  - —Onset: 35 seconds
  - —Dosage: 0.1–0.3 mg/kg
  - —Cautions
    - -Hypotension
- Naloxone (narcan): 2 mg (peds: 0.1 mg/kg) IV or IM initial dose
- Succinylcholine: 1–1.5 mg/kg IV
  - —Onset: within 60 seconds
  - —Duration: 6–10 minutes
  - —Cautions
    - -Fasciculations
    - -Hyperkalemia
    - -Increased intraocular pressure
    - -Malignant hyperthermia
- Thiopental: 3–5 mg/kg IV
  - —Onset <30 seconds IV
  - —Duration: 5–8 minutes
  - —Cautions
    - -Hypotension
    - -Histamine release (avoid in asthmatics)

Disposition

ADMISSION CRITERIA

- ICU admission for intubation
- Postconscious sedation
- Inability to ambulate
- No responsible adult to accompany home

DISCHARGE CRITERIA

- Stable cardiovascular and airway
- Baseline cognitive and motor functions with normal mental status
- Responsible adult accompanying patient
- No driving or participating in activities requiring optimal mental functioning for 24 hours

Miscellaneous

ICD9: N/A

CORE CONTENT CODE: 21.1.3.3.1, 23/2 ANESTHESIA

SUGGESTED READINGS

Chung D, Lam A. Essentials of anesthesiology. 3rd ed. Philadelphia: WB Saunders, 1997.

Kraus, Shannon M, Damian FJ, et al. Guidelines for pediatric sedation. Dallas: American College of Emergency Physicians, 1995.

Scaletta T, Schaider J. Emergent management of trauma. New York: McGraw-Hill, 1996.

Author: Chris Ross

Constipation

Clinical Presentation

SIGNS AND SYMPTOMS

- Infrequent passage of dry, hard stools or straining at defecation
- Change of stool pattern
- Poorly localized abdominal pain, often spasmodic
- Abdominal distention/fullness
- Vomiting or decreased passage of flatus
- Firm hard stool on digital exam
  —May have empty rectum
- Tenesmus
- Encopresis in children
- Signs of peritonitis are not seen with constipation

MECHANISM/DESCRIPTION

- Perceived as a decrease in the frequency of bowel movements or as increased straining/pain with defecation
- 99% of normal population have a bowel frequency ranging from 3 bowel movements per day to 3 per week

ETIOLOGY

- Due to muscle disorders that affect the sphincter mechanism or may be secondary to delayed transit time in the colon
- Associated with
  —Immobility
  —Deficiency of dietary fiber
  —Dehydration
  —Depression
  —Degenerative neurologic diseases
- Decrease colonic motility due to medications (anticholinergics, opiates)
- Impaired colonic motor function (Hirschsprung's disease)
- Laxative abuse may damage the colonic myenteric plexus
- Pain produced by fissures or thrombosed hemorrhoids may cause avoidance of defecation
- Electrolyte abnormalities
  —Hypercalcemia
  —Hypokalemia
- Hormonal abnormalities
  —Hypothyroidism
  —Diabetes mellitus

PEDIATRIC CONSIDERATIONS

- Normal bowel habits different in children
  —First 2–3 months 1 bowel movement per feeding to 1 every other day is normal
  —2 months to 1 year: 2–3/day is normal
  —1–5 years: 1–2/day is normal
- In infancy consider
  —Effect of maternal drugs
  —Congenital gastrointestinal anomalies
  —Cystic fibrosis
  —Hirschsprung's disease
  —Poor intake
  —Anal fissures

Pre-Hospital

N/A

Diagnosis

ESSENTIAL WORKUP

- Thorough history and physical examination; note abdominal distention, presence of bowel sounds and masses
- Digital examination for
  —Rectal tone
  —Stool consistency
  —Masses
  —Occult blood

LABORATORY

- Only necessary when considering underlying disorders
- CBC may show
  —Leukocytosis with inflammatory processes
  —Anemia with colon neoplasm
- Electrolytes and calcium indicated if at risk for
  —Hypokalemia
  —Hypercalcemia
- Thyroid function tests indicated if patient appears to be hypothyroid

IMAGING/SPECIAL TESTS

- Rarely indicated unless suspect underlying process
- Abdominal radiograph—large amount of stool in the colon
- Barium enema examination for anatomical defects (tumor)

DIFFERENTIAL DIAGNOSIS

- Colonic disorders
  —Tumors
  —Intussusception
  —Inflammatory strictures
  —Diverticular disease
  —Irritable bowel syndrome
  —Bowel obstruction
- Metabolic/endocrine disorders
  —Hypothyroidism
  —Addison's disease
  —Cushing's syndrome
  —Diabetes mellitus
  —Hypercalcemia
- Anorectal disorders
  —Anal stenosis
  —Rectal prolapse
  —Anal fissure
  —Perianal abscess
- Drugs
  —Aluminum-containing antacids
  —Iron supplements
  —Opiates
  —Anticholinergics
  —Antiparkinson drugs
  —Antispasmodics

PEDIATRIC CONSIDERATIONS

- In differential diagnosis, consider breast feeding, effect of maternal drugs, meconium ileus/plug, GI anomalies, and sepsis
- Often occurs during period of toilet training

Treatment

INITIAL STABILIZATION
N/A

ED TREATMENT
- Requires stepwise management
  - —Initial clean out
  - —Maintenance
  - —Behavior modification
- Clean out can be "from above and below"
  - —Enemas
  - —Suppositories
  - —Manual disimpaction
  - —Laxatives
- Maintenance
  - —Increase oral fluids and dietary fibers
  - —Stool softeners
  - —Bulk-forming agents
- Behavior modification
  - —Dietary changes
  - —Toilet training—place elderly and young on the toilet at regular intervals
- Change medications causing constipation

MEDICATIONS

Bulk Agents
- Bran/fiber
- Psyllium seeds (metamucil): 30 g/day (peds: 0.5–1 tsp/day)

Enemas
- Fleet: 120 ml (peds: 60–120 ml) PR
- Tap water: 100–500 ml PR

Osmotic agents
- Milk of magnesia: 15–30 ml (peds: 1 tsp–2 tbs) po
- Lactulose: 15–30 ml (peds: 1 tsp–2 tbs) po bid
- Polyethylene glycol (Golytely): 2–6 L (peds: 150 ml/kg) po

Stool Softeners
- Docusate sodium (colace): 60–360 mg/day (peds: 3–5 mg/kg/24hrs tid) po
- Karo syrup (for infants): 1–2 tsp to each bottle
- Senna extract (senekot): 1–2 tabs (peds: 0.5–1 tsp) po

Disposition

ADMISSION CRITERIA
- Severely constipated patients experiencing severe abdominal pain that cannot be relieved
- Neurologically impaired/elderly who cannot be cleaned out in the emergency department or at home
- Bowel obstruction or surgical emergencies

DISCHARGE CRITERIA
- No comorbid illness requiring admission
- Pain-free
- Adequately cleaned out

Miscellaneous

ICD9: 564.0

CORE CONTENT CODE: 22.4.5

SUGGESTED READINGS

Donatelle EP. Constipation: Pathophysiology and treatment. Am Fam Physician 1990;1335–1342.

Orenstein JB. Constipation. In: Barkin R, et al., eds. Pediatric emergency medicine: Concepts and clinical practice. 2d ed. St. Louis: CV Mosby, 1997:804–807.

Read NW, Celik AF, Katsinelos P. Constipation and incontinence in the elderly. J Clin Gastroenterol 1995;20(1):61–70.

Author: Anthony Best

Contact Dermatitis

Clinical Presentation

SIGNS AND SYMPTOMS

- *Acute lesions:* Skin erythema and pruritus. May see edema, papules, vesicles, bullae, serous discharge or crusting
- *Subacute:* Vesiculation less pronounced
- *Chronic lesions:* May see scaling, lichenification, pigmentation, or fissuring with little to no vesiculation. May have a characteristic distribution pattern

MECHANISM/DESCRIPTION

- An *eczematous eruption* (superficial inflammatory process primarily in the epidermis)
- Irritant
  —Direct injury to the skin resulting in nonimmunologic inflammatory reaction
  —Usually gradual onset with indistinct borders
- Allergic
  —Delayed hypersensitivity reaction (requires prior sensitization)
  —Usually rapid onset (12–48 hours), may correspond to exact distribution of contact (e.g., watchband)

ETIOLOGY

- Irritant
  —Strong soaps, solvents, chemicals, certain foods, urine, feces, continuous exposure to moisture (diaper rash), etc
- Allergic
  —Common allergens include plants, cement (prolonged exposure may result in severe alkali burn), metals (especially nickel), solvents, epoxy, chemicals in rubber (e.g., elastic waistbands) or leather, lotions, cosmetics, topical medications (e.g., neomycin, benzocaine, parabens), some foods, etc
  —Poison ivy, oak, sumac (rhus dermatitis)
  —Common form of allergic contact dermatitis
    -Direct: Reaction to oleoresin from plant
    -Indirect: Contact with pet or clothes with oleoresin on surface or fur, or in smoke from burning leaves
    -Lesions may appear up to 3 days after exposure and may persist up to 3 weeks
    -Fluid from vesicles is not contagious and does not produce new lesions
- Shoe dermatitis
  —Common; identify by lesions limited to distal dorsal surface of foot usually sparing the interdigital spaces
- Photodermatitis
  —Inflammatory reaction from exposure to an irritant (frequently plant sap) and sunlight

PEDIATRIC CONSIDERATIONS

- Allergic contact dermatitis is less frequent in children, especially infants, than adults
- Major sources of pediatric contact allergy
  —Metals, shoes, preservatives or fragrances in cosmetics and topical medications, and plants
- Circumoral dermatitis: seen in infants and small children, may result from certain foods (irritant or allergic reaction)

Pre-Hospital

N/A

Diagnosis

ESSENTIAL WORKUP

- Medical history
  —Include date of onset, time course, pattern of lesions, relationship to work, exposures (home and at work), new products (lotions, cosmetics, etc.), medications, and jewelry
- Physical examination
  —Special attention to character and distribution of the rash

LABORATORY

- No specific tests in the ED are helpful

IMAGING/SPECIAL TESTS

- Patch testing
  —Generally not done in the ED, refer to subspecialist
- When tinea is suspected consider evaluating for fluorescence with a Wood's lamp

DIFFERENTIAL DIAGNOSIS

- Atopic dermatitis: associated with family history of atopy
- Seborrheic dermatitis: scaly or crusting "greasy" lesions
- Nummular dermatitis: "coin-like" lesions
- Intertrigo: dermatitis where skin is in apposition
- Infectious eczematous dermatitis: dermatitis with secondary bacterial infection, usually *Staphylococcus aureus*
- Cellulitis: warm, blanching, painful lesion
- Impetigo: yellow crusting
- Scabies: intensely pruritic, frequently interdigital with "tracks."
- Psoriasis: silvery adherent, scaling, lesions well delineated, affecting extensor surfaces, scalp and genital region
- Herpes simplex: groups of vesicles, painful, burning
- Herpes zoster: painful, follows dermatomal pattern
- Bullous pemphigoid: diffuse bullous lesions
- Tinea: maximum involvement at margins, fluoresces under Wood's lamp
- Pityriasis alba: discrete, asymptomatic, hypopigmented lesions
- Urticaria: pruritic raised lesions (wheal) frequently with surrounding erythema (flare)
- Acrodermatitis enteropathica: vesiculobullous lesion of hands and feet, associated with failure to thrive, diarrhea, and alopecia
- Letterer-Siwe tumor (Langerhans cell histiocytosis)
  —Associated with hepatosplenomegaly and adenopathy

Treatment

INITIAL STABILIZATION

- Rarely required in absence of concomitant pathology

ED TREATMENT

General

- Primarily symptomatic
- Wash area with mild soap and water
- Remove or avoid offending agent (including washing clothes)
- Cool, wet compresses, especially effective during acute blistering phase
- Antipruritic agents
  - —Topical: calamine lotion, corticosteroids (does not penetrate blisters)
  - —Systemic: Antihistamines, corticosteroids
- Aluminum acetate (Burrows) solution: weeping surfaces
- Avoid benzocaine-containing products—may further sensitize skin

Rhus Dermatitis

- Follow general measures plus
  - —Aseptic aspiration of bullae may relieve discomfort
  - —Severe reaction: systemic corticosteroids for 2–3 weeks with gradual taper. Premature termination of corticosteroid therapy may result in rapid rebound of symptoms

Shoe Dermatitis

- Follow general measures plus
  - —Wear open toe, canvas, or vinyl shoes
  - —Control perspiration—change socks, absorbent powder

MEDICATIONS

Systemic

- Antihistamine (H_1-receptor antagonist, 1st and 2nd generation)
- Diphenhydramine hydrochloride (benadryl): Adult: 25–50 mg IV/IM/PO q 6 hr PRN; peds: 5 mg/kg/24hrs divided q 6 hr PRN
- Hydroxyzine hydrochloride (atarax): Adult: 25–50 mg po IM up to qid PRN; peds: 2 mg/kg/24hrs po divided qid or 0.5 mg/kg IM q 4–6 hr PRN
- Loratadine (claritin): Adult: 10 mg po bid
- Corticosteroid
  - —Prednisone: Adult: 40–60 mg po qd; peds: 1–2 mg/kg/24hrs (max 80 mg/24hrs) divided qd/bid

Topical

- Aluminum acetate (Burrows) solution: apply topically for 20 min tid until skin is dry
- Calamine lotion: qid PRN
- Corticosteroid
  - —Hydrocortisone: cream 1%; ointment 0.5 or 1%; lotion 0.25, 0.5, or 1%; gel 0.5%; aerosol 0.5% tid qid
- Triamcinolone: ointment 0.025, 0.1%; cream 0.025, 0.1%; lotion 0.025, 0.1% tid qid

Disposition

ADMISSION CRITERIA

- Rarely indicated unless severe systemic reaction or significant secondary infection

DISCHARGE CRITERIA

- Symptomatic relief
- Adequate follow-up with primary care physician or dermatologic specialist

Miscellaneous

ICD9: 692.9

CORE CONTENT CODE: 3.1.3

SUGGESTED READINGS

Habif TP. Clinical dermatology. St Louis: CV Mosby, 1996:81–99.

Hurwitz S. Clinical pediatric dermatology. Philadelphia: WB Saunders, 1993:68–82.

Juckett G. Plant dermatitis. Post Grad Med 1996;100(3);159–171.

White IR. Occupational dermatitis. BMJ 1996;313:487–489.

Author: Jeffrey Horton

Conversion Disorder

Clinical Presentation

SIGNS AND SYMPTOMS

- Circumstances at the onset of symptoms
  - —Symptoms often begin during a time of stress or conflict
- Similar symptoms have been experienced in the past
- History of a previously diagnosed conversion episode
  - —Most reliable predictor of a conversion disorder
- Loss of voluntary motor or sensory function that can't be explained by pathophysiologic mechanisms
- Voluntary motor symptoms
- Abnormal movements
  - —Gait disturbances
  - —Incoordination
    - -Tremors
    - -Ticks
    - -Jerks
- Paralysis/paresis
  - —Mono, hemi, or paraplegia
- Aphonia
  - —Patients can still whisper or cough
- Urinary retention
- Pseudoseizures
  - —The most common expression of conversion disorder
  - —Usually disorganized thrashing motor movements rather than organized tonic-clonic activity
  - —Tongue biting, incontinence, postictal period are uncommon
- Sensory symptoms
  - —Anesthesia—commonly stocking-glove distribution
- Visual symptoms
  - —Blindness
  - —Tunnel vision
  - —Diplopia
- Deafness
- Anosmia
- Intractable vomiting
- Amnesia
- Pseudocyesis
- La belle indifference
  - —A calm acceptance of serious symptoms
  - —Once felt to be characteristic of conversion disorders
  - —It is not a reliable diagnostic indicator

MECHANISM/DESCRIPTION

- Involuntary loss or alteration of voluntary motor or sensory function not explained by a medical condition
- The symptoms tend to occur suddenly and are not consciously produced by the patient
- The symptoms usually simulate a neurologic disorder
- The conversion disorder represents an unconscious expression of a psychological conflict
  - —May provide the patient with both a primary and a secondary gain
  - —The primary gain allows the person to express repressed emotional pain via physical symptoms
  - —Secondary gain may also occur as the patient receives attention and sympathy for their problem
- Conversion disorders are rare
  - —Their peak occurrence is in adolescence and early adulthood
  - —They are extremely rare in patients less than 10 years of age or older than 35
  - —Diligently search for an organic problem if conversion symptoms appear in older patients
  - —One-third of patients diagnosed as a conversion disorder have an underlying medical condition
- 2–4 times more common in women than in men
- Groups of patients are more likely to manifest conflict as a conversion disorder
  - —Patients from rural communities
  - —Lower socioeconomic status
  - —Lower educational background
- Recurrence in 20–25% of patients

ETIOLOGY

N/A

Pre-Hospital

N/A

Diagnosis

ESSENTIAL WORKUP

- A detailed careful history and physical examination is the cornerstone for making a diagnosis
  - —The presence of certain psychological diagnostic criteria must be demonstrated
  - —Diagnostic criteria adapted from DSM IV, 1994
    - -The patient must have voluntary motor or sensory symptoms suggestive of a medical disorder
    - -The patient must demonstrate that psychologic factors are associated with the symptoms

      A temporal relationship between a conflict and the development of symptoms

      The symptoms allow the patient to avoid a stressful situation or activity

      The symptoms are not intentionally produced

      The symptoms are not caused by a medical condition or a substance

      The symptoms cause clinically significant distress or impairment of function
  - —The diagnosis can usually be made without ancillary testing
  - —Further testing should only be undertaken if the symptoms remain confusing
    - -Ancillary studies should be directed towards organic causes on the differential diagnosis
- Psychiatric consultation may be required to confirm the diagnosis

LABORATORY

- Serum glucose to exclude hypoglycemia
- Serum potassium for transient diffuse weakness during a crisis to exclude periodic paralysis
- Toxicologic screen
- Lyme titers if the patient is from endemic areas with a history of a rash or exposure to ticks

IMAGING/SPECIAL TESTS

- MRI
  - —Indicated if multiple sclerosis or CNS tumors are suspected
  - —This study can be performed as an outpatient
- EEG
  - —Atypical seizure is suspected

DIFFERENTIAL DIAGNOSIS

- Multiple sclerosis
- Seizure disorder
- Guillain-Barré
- Myasthenia gravis
- Malingering
  —This is a conscious deception rather than an unconscious psychologic process
- Factitious syndrome
  —These patients want to assume the "sick role"
  —They rarely present with neurologic symptoms
- Dystonic reaction
  —Involuntary muscle spasm cured with anticholinergic agents
- SLE
- Atypical migraine
- CNS tumors
- Periodic paralysis
- Lyme disease
- Hypoglycemia

Treatment

INITIAL STABILIZATION

- Search for serious reversible causes of the patient's symptoms
  —Hypoglycemia
  —Hypoxia
  —Drug ingestion
  —Trauma

ED TREATMENT

- The symptoms give the patient a mechanism to cope with a psychologic stress and are usually transient
  —Be supportive and treat the patient with respect
  —Do not be confrontational
  —Provide assurance that the problem is not serious
  —Explain that the symptoms will begin to improve shortly and will ultimately resolve completely
  —Attempt to reduce the underlying psychologic conflict by eliminating the precipitating pressure
- Psychiatric consultation
  —May be helpful in addressing the underlying psychological issues
  —Nonspecific supportive therapy
  —Medication
  —N/A

Disposition

ADMISSION CRITERIA

- If normal daily activities cannot be carried out because of persistent symptoms
- The presence of a dangerous underlying illness has not been excluded
- The psychiatrist feels that inpatient psychiatric evaluation and treatment is necessary

DISCHARGE CRITERIA

- Psychiatric follow-up
- Follow-up with a primary physician
  —More than one-third of patients eventually are diagnosed with an organic disorder

Miscellaneous

ICD9: 300.11

CORE CONTENT CODE: 14.4.1

SUGGESTED READINGS

American Psychiatric Association. Diagnostic and statistical manual of mental disorders. 4th ed. Washington, DC: American Psychiatric Association, 1994.

Hales RE, Somatoform disorders. In: Hales RE, ed. The American Psychiatric Press textbook of psychiatry. 2d ed. Washington, DC: American Psychiatric Press, 1994:605–611.

Lazarr A. Conversion symptoms. N Engl J Med 1981;305:745–748.

McCahill ME. Somatoform and related disorders: Delivery of diagnosis as first step. Am Fam Physician 1995;52:193–203.

Purcell TB. The somatic patient. Emerg Med Clin North Am 1991;9:137–159.

Author: Kenneth Jackimczyk

Cor Pulmonale

Clinical Presentation

SIGNS AND SYMPTOMS

- Exertional dyspnea
- Easy fatigability
- Weakness
- Syncope
- Cough
- Hemoptysis
- Wheezing
- Hoarseness
- Jugular venous distention
  —Prominent a- and v-waves
- Hepatomegaly
- Ascites
- Hepatojugular reflex
- Peripheral edema
- Left parasternal heave on cardiac palpation
- Pulmonic component of the second heart sound increases in intensity

MECHANISM/DESCRIPTION

- Ventricular failure confined to the right ventricle
  —Right ventricular hypertrophy or dilation is an adaptive response to pulmonary hypertension
- The pulmonary circulation is a low-resistance, low-pressure system
  —The pulmonary arteries are thin-walled and distensible
  —Mean pulmonary arterial pressure is usually 12–15 mm Hg
  —Normal left arterial pressure is 6–10 mm Hg
  —The resulting pressure difference driving the pulmonary circulation is only 6–9 mm Hg
- Three factors affect pulmonary arterial pressure
  —Cardiac output
  —Pulmonary venous pressure
  —Pulmonary vascular resistance
- Pulmonary hypertension can arise by a number of mechanisms
  —A marked increase in cardiac output
  —Left-to-right shunt secondary to congenital heart disease
  —Hypoxia
    -Most commonly causes pulmonary vascular resistance to increase
    -The resulting hypercapnia and acidosis induce vasoconstriction
  —Pulmonary venous pressure increase
    -A compensatory rise is seen in the pulmonary arterial system so that flow is maintained across the pulmonary vascular bed
    -Pulmonary embolus causes such a change by increasing resistance to pulmonary blood flow
    -Left ventricular failure achieves the same result by directly influencing pulmonary venous pressure
  —Dramatic rises in blood viscosity or intrathoracic pressure
    -Impedes blood flow
- Approximately 86,000 patients die from chronic obstructive pulmonary disease each year
  —Associated right ventricular failure is a significant factor in many of these cases
  —In those over the age of 50 with COPD, 50% develop pulmonary hypertension and are at risk for development of cor pulmonale
- The course of cor pulmonale is generally related to the progression of the underlying disease process
- Once biventricular failure is noted, life expectancy is usually less than five years

ETIOLOGY

- Chronic hypoxia
  —COPD
  —Chronic hypoxia at high altitude
  —Sleep apnea
- Primary pulmonary hypertension
- Cystic fibrosis
- Congenital heart disease
  —Left-to-right shunts
- Severe anemia
- Pulmonary embolism
- Collagen vascular diseases
- Thoracic deformities
  —Kyphoscoliosis
- Obesity
- Mitral stenosis
- Pulmonary veno-occlusive disease
- Increased blood viscosity
  —Polycythemia vera
  —Leukemia
- Increased intrathoracic pressure
  —COPD
  —Mechanical ventilation with positive end-expiratory pressure

Pre-Hospital

- Supportive therapy
  —Supplemental oxygen
  —Intravenous access
  —Cardiac monitoring
  —Pulse oximetry
- Treat bronchospasm from associated respiratory disease
  —β-Agonist nebulizers

CAUTIONS

- Vasodilators and diuretics do not have a role in the field
- Severely hypoxic patients may require endotracheal intubation

Diagnosis

LABORATORY

- Pulse oximetry or arterial blood gas
  - —Resting pO_2 40–60 mm Hg
- Hematocrit
  - —Frequently elevated
- Other laboratory tests are not generally useful

IMAGING/SPECIAL TESTS

- Chest radiograph
  - —Signs of pulmonary hypertension
    - -Large pulmonary arteries
    - -An enlarged right ventricular silhouette
    - -Does not indicate the severity of disease
- Electrocardiogram
  - —Right axis deviation
  - —Tall, peaked P waves (P pulmonale)
  - —Right ventricular hypertrophy
  - —Transient changes due to hypoxia
    - -Right precordial T wave flattening
    - -ST depression in II, III, and AVF
- Echocardiography
  - —Noninvasive
  - —Right ventricular dilation or hypertrophy in the setting of normal left ventricular dimensions
  - —Assessment of tricuspid regurgitation
  - —Doppler quantitation of pulmonary artery pressure
- Ventilation-perfusion scans or pulmonary angiography
  - —Useful in the setting of acute cor pulmonale
- Computed tomography or magnetic resonance imaging
  - —Delineates size and shape of the ventricles and pulmonary arteries
- Right heart catheterization
  - —The most precise estimate of pulmonary vascular hemodynamics
  - —Gives accurate measurements of pulmonary arterial pressure and pulmonary capillary wedge pressure

DIFFERENTIAL DIAGNOSIS

- Primary disease of the left side of the heart
- Congenital heart disease
- Hypothyroidism
- Cirrhosis

Treatment

INITIAL STABILIZATION

- Emergency Department therapy is directed at the underlying disease process and reducing pulmonary hypertension

ED TREATMENT

- Supplemental oxygen sufficient to raise arterial saturation to 90%
  - —Improving oxygenation reduces pulmonary arterial vasoconstriction and right ventricular afterload
  - —The improved cardiac output enhances diuresis of excess body water
  - —Care must be taken to monitor the patient's ventilatory status and pCO_2 as hypercapnia may reduce respiratory drive and cause an acidosis
- Diuretics, such as furosemide, may be added cautiously to reduce pulmonary artery pressure by contributing to the reduction of circulating blood volume
- Patients should be maintained on salt and fluid restriction
- There is no role for digoxin in the treatment of cor pulmonale
- Bronchodilator therapy is particularly helpful for those patients with COPD
- Selective β-adrenergic agents such as subcutaneous terbutaline 0.25 mg SQ
  - —Bronchodilator affects and reduces ventricular afterload
- Acutely decompensated COPD patients
  - —Early steroid therapy
  - —Antibiotic administration
- In general, improvement in the underlying respiratory disease results in improved right ventricular function

MEDICATIONS

- Furosemide: 20–60 mg IV
- Terbutaline: 0.25 mg SQ

Disposition

ADMISSION CRITERIA

- New onset hypoxia
- Anasarca
- Severe respiratory failure
- Admission criteria for the underlying disease process

DISCHARGE CRITERIA

- Patients without hypoxia or a stable oxygen requirement
- Close followup as long as the underlying etiology has responded to acute management

Miscellaneous

ICD9: 415.0, 415.1, 416, 416.0, 416.1, 416.8, 416.9,

CORE CONTENT CODE: 2.2.1.3

SUGGESTED READINGS

Alpert JS. Pulmonary hypertension. In: Bennett JC, et al., eds. Cecil's textbook of medicine. 20th ed. Philadelphia: WB Saunders, 1996:271–277.

Arroliga AC, Matthay MA, Matthay RA. Pulmonary thromboembolism and other pulmonary vascular diseases. In: George RB, et al., eds. Chest medicine: Essentials of pulmonary and critical care medicine. 3rd ed. Baltimore: Williams & Wilkins, 1995:271–302.

MacNee W. Pathophysiology of cor pulmonale in chronic obstructive pulmonary disease (Parts I and II). Am J Resp Crit Care Med 1994;150:833, 1158.

Author: E. Jedd Roe

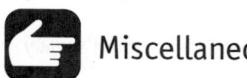

Corneal Abrasion

Clinical Presentation

SIGNS AND SYMPTOMS

- Severe ocular pain
- Tearing
- Blepharospasm
- Foreign-body sensation
- Photophobia
- Conjunctival injection
- Blurred vision
- Headache

MECHANISM/DESCRIPTION

- Traumatic desquamation of portions of the corneal epithelium
- Focal epithelial loss secondary to removal of corneal foreign body
- Previous corneal transplant, corneal surgery or radial keratotomy
  —Predispose patient to a more severe injury following minor trauma to eye

ETIOLOGY

- Contusive force
- Direct contact injury
  —Human fingernail
  —Branches
  —Fingers/toes
  —Hairbrushes/combs
  —Sand/stones
  —Metallic object
  —Snow
  —Pens/pencils
  —Toys
  —Activated charcoal
  —Airbag deployment
- Mechanical action of eyelid
  —Blinking or rubbing eye with loose foreign body
- Projectiles at high speeds
  —Carefully examine for globe perforation
- Poorly fitting contact lens or prolonged use

PEDIATRIC CONSIDERATIONS

- Signs and symptoms may differ
  —Excessive crying
  —Conjunctival erythema
  —Tearing
  —Eye rubbing
  —Lid edema
  —Grunting respiration
- Less than 12 months old
  —Frequently no history of eye trauma
  —Often no eye signs
- Greater than 12 months old
  —More often will have history of minor eye trauma
  —Positive eye signs
  —No excessive crying
- Compression injuries to cornea associated with birth
  —Localized edema
  —Corneal clouding
  —Clear within hours

Pre-Hospital

N/A

Diagnosis

ESSENTIAL WORKUP

- History
  —Past ocular trauma
  —Ocular/periocular surgery
  —Preexisting visual impairment
  —Glasses
  —Contact lens use (extended wear have increased risk of corneal ulcer)
  —Time of onset
  —Associated symptoms
  —Treatment prior to visit
  —Use of safety glasses
  —Systemic disease
- Complete eye exam
  —Visual acuity
  —Evert upper lids to check for retained foreign body (FB)
  —Bright white light for visual inspection of cornea to rule out infiltrate/edema/loss of corneal luster
  —Slitlamp to evaluate anterior segment
  —Fluorescein to identify area of damaged corneal epithelium

LABORATORY

N/A

IMAGING/SPECIAL TESTS

N/A

DIFFERENTIAL DIAGNOSIS

- Herpes simplex virus keratitis
- Recurrent corneal erosion syndrome
- Ultraviolet keratitis (snow blindness)
- Corneal ulcer
- Corneal dystrophy (inherited)
- More extensive injury than corneal abrasion
  —Laceration of cornea
  —Perforation of cornea
  —Hyphema
  —Iris prolapse
  —Lens disruption

PEDIATRIC CONSIDERATIONS

- Hand-held slitlamp and Wood's lamp—helpful in examination of pediatric eye

Treatment

INITIAL STABILIZATION

- Instill topical anesthetic (proparacaine)

ED TREATMENT

- Examination
- Removal of superficial FB
- Cycloplegic (optional)
  —Cyclopentolate (mydriasis 1–2 d)
  —Tropicamide (mydriasis 6 hrs)
- Antibiotic ointment/drop options
  —Ciprofloxacin
  —Erythromycin
  —Gentamicin
  —Sulfacetamide
  —Tobramycin
  —Contact lens wearers must be covered for Pseudomonas
    -Use aminoglycoside or quinolone
- Eye patch
  —Controversial regarding efficacy
  —No patch required for small abrasions
  —Never patch contact lens-related injury
  —Never patch infection prone injury
    -Fingernail
    -Vegetable matter
    -Removal of wood particles
  —Patch noncontact lens related abrasions greater than 10mm square
  —Disadvantages of patching
    -Removes binocular vision
    -Uncomfortable
    -Increases corneal temperature
    -Decreases corneal oxygenation
    -Decrease tear exchange
- Tetanus prophylaxis
  —When contaminants include dirt, fecal material, or saliva
  —Routine tetanus not necessary
- Or topical analgesics

MEDICATIONS

- Ciprofloxacin: 0.35% 1 gtt qid
- Cyclopentolate: 0.5, 1.0, or 2.0% drops (mydriasis 1–2 d) 1 gtt tid
- Diclofenac: 0.1% drops 1 gtt qid
- Erythromycin: 0.5% ointment qid
- Gentamicin: 0.3% ointment qid
- Gentamicin: 0.3% drops q 6 hrs
- Ketorolac: 0.5%, drops 1 gtt qid
- Proparacaine: 0.5% 1 gtt
- Sulfacetamide: drops 10% qid
- Sulfacetamide: ointment 10% qid
- Tobramycin: 0.3% drops q 6 hrs
- Tobramycin: 0.3% ointment q 6 hrs
- Tropicamide: 0.5, 1.0% drops (mydriasis 6 hrs) 1 gtt

PEDIATRIC CONSIDERATIONS

- Patching poorly tolerated

Disposition

ADMISSION CRITERIA

- Associated injuries requiring admission

DISCHARGE CRITERIA

- All simple corneal abrasions
- Follow-up in 24–48 hours with ophthalmologist for reexamination and ongoing care
- Follow-up with emergency department when access to specialist is limited

Miscellaneous

ICD9: 918.1

CORE CONTENT CODE: 6.4.1.4

SUGGESTED READINGS

Benson WH, et al. Tetanus prophylaxis following ocular injuries. J Emerg Med 1993;11:677–683.

Garcia GE. Management of ocular emergencies and urgent eye problems. Am Fam Physician 1996;53(2):565–574.

Kaiser PK, Pineda R, Corneal Abrasion Patching Study Group. A study of topical nonsteroidal anti-inflammatory drops and no pressure patching in the treatment of corneal abrasions. Ophthalmology 1997;104:1353–1359.

Kaiser PK, Pineda R, Corneal Abrasion Patching Study Group. A comparison of pressure patching versus no patching for corneal abrasions due to trauma or foreign body removal. Ophthalmology 1995;102:1936–1942.

Poole SR. Corneal abrasion in infants. Pediatr Emerg Care 1995;11(1):25–26.

Schein OD. Contact lens abrasions and the nonophthalmologist. Am J Emerg Med 1993;11(6):606–608.

Torok PG, Mader TH. Corneal abrasions: Diagnosis and management. Am Fam Physician 1996;53(8):2521–2529.

Author: Melissa Gillespie

Corneal Burn

Clinical Presentation

SIGNS AND SYMPTOMS

- Severe ocular pain
- Photophobia
- Lacrimation
- Foreign-body sensation
- Conjunctivae injection
- Corneal edema
- Corneal opacification
- Impaired visual acuity
- Limbal blanching
- Lens opacification
- Vesicles clear fluid (hypothermal injury)
- Vesicles hemorrhagic fluid
- Necrosis of iris, ciliary body

MECHANISM/DESCRIPTION

- Inappropriate exposure of cornea to chemicals, heat, cold, electrical, or radiant energy causing damage to the cornea and often extending to adjacent structures
- Severity of injury related to duration of exposure, type of agent, anion concentration, pH of solution
- Alkalis
  —Cause immediate rise in pH
  —Highly soluble in lipid, therefore rapidly penetrate the eye causing severe corneal injury
  —Penetration can occur in less than 1 minute
  —Exception: Calcium alkalis penetrate relatively poorly secondary to SOAP formation, can cause corneal opacification so may appear worse but actually have better prognosis than other alkali burns
- Acids
  —Immediately coagulate proteins of the corneal epithelium
  —Cause opacification
  —Coagulation often produces a barrier to deep penetration
  —Exception: The lipophilicity of HF acid causes it to act similar to a base with more rapid penetration
- Thermal burn
  —Causes direct injury to cornea
  —Damage primarily dependant on duration and intensity of heat
  —Globe often spared secondary to
    -Blinking
    -Bell's phenomenon
    -Tears
    -Protective bony structure of the orbit
- Electrical injury
  —Occurs with current flow through the head, with input at or near the eye

ETIOLOGY

- Alkalis
  —Ammonia
    -Fertilizer, refrigerant, household ammonia, cleansing agents
  —Potassium hydroxide
    -Caustic potash
  —Magnesium hydroxide
    -Sparklers, flares, fireworks
  —Lye—NaOH
    -Caustic soda, drain cleaners
  —Lime—$CaOH_2$
    -Fresh lime, quicklime, calcium hydrate, slaked lime, hydrated lime, plaster, mortar, cement, whitewash
  —Nonspecific alkali
    -Motor vehicle airbag upon inflation releases alkali
- Acids
  —Sulfuric acid—H_2SO_4
    -Car battery acid
  —Sulphurous acid—H_2SO_3
    -Preservatives (fruit and vegetable), bleach, refrigerants
  —Hydrofluoric acid—HF
    -Used in etching silicon/glass, cleaning brick, electropolishing metals, control of fermentation in breweries, commercial/household rust removal
- Thermal
  —Hot liquids, molten metal
  —Flames
  —Hot smoke/gases
  —Flash burn
  —Steam
  —Cigarette burns

PEDIATRIC CONSIDERATIONS

- Consider child neglect or abuse

Pre-Hospital

CAUTIONS

- Irrigate at scene 15–30 minutes, unless other coexisting life-threatening conditions require immediate transfer
- Continuous irrigation en route to hospital with normal saline

Diagnosis

ESSENTIAL WORKUP

- History
  —Type of exposure
  —Duration of exposure
  —Time of onset
  —Time irrigation initiated
  —Preexisting visual impairment
  —Protective eyewear
  —Contact lens use
  —Treatment prior to arrival
- Complete eye exam (after irrigation)
  —Visual acuity
  —Bright-white light for visual inspection of cornea/conjunctivae/limbus
  —Slitlamp to evaluate anterior segment inflammation
  —Fluorescein to identify damaged corneal epithelium
  —Check for lenticular clarity
  —Fundus exam
  —Measure intraocular pressure (especially in delayed presentation)
  —Lid/eyelash exam
  —Check pH with acid/alkali burns

LABORATORY

N/A

IMAGING/ SPECIAL TESTS

N/A

DIFFERENTIAL DIAGNOSIS

- Infection
  —Viral keratitis
  —Corneal ulcer
- Corneal erosion syndrome
  —Corneal foreign body
  —Corneal abrasion
  —Hypothermal injury

PEDIATRIC CONSIDERATIONS

- Handheld slitlamp and Wood's lamp helpful in examination of pediatric eye

Treatment

INITIAL STABILIZATION

- Chemical exposure
  —Irrigate with any available diluting substance but preferably water or normal saline
- Thermal exposure
  —Cool moist dressing with overlying icepacks

ED TREATMENT

Chemical Exposure—Alkalis/Acids/Mace

- Continuous irrigation until pH at fornices is neutral
- Remove all particulate matter
- Topical anesthetic (proparacaine)
- Examination
- Antibiotic prophylaxis for staph/pseudomonas until epithelialization is complete
  —Gentamicin ointment plus erythromycin or
  —Bacitracin
- Cycloplegics to minimize posterior synechiae formation
  —Cyclopentolate 1%
  —Atropine 1%
- Oral analgesics
- If increased intraocular pressure
  —Immediate ophthalmologic consultation
  —Administer acetazolamide 125 mg po qid and timolol 0.5% drops bid
- Topical steroids to control anterior uveitis (consult ophthalmology)
- Eye patch (consult ophthalmology)
- May require surgical intervention if frank corneal penetration
- Ophthalmologic consultation by phone in mild injuries
- Immediate ophthalmologic consultation in all moderate to severe injuries; if unavailable at your hospital, arrange transfer to closest eye center
- Hydrofluoric acid
  —Treat as above, plus 1% calcium gluconate eyedrops
  —Systemic analgesia × 24 hours

Thermal Exposure

- Frequent moist dressing changes
- Antibiotics drops qid
- Generous lubricant application
- Moisture chamber when extensive injury to eyelid
- Steroids (consult ophthalmologist; do not use for more than one week duration)

Electrical Injury

- Irrigation
- Wound care
- Antibiotic ointment
- Cycloplegic (if anterior uveitis)
- Analgesia

MEDICATIONS

- Artificial tears
- Atropine: 0.5, 1.0, 2.0% drops (cycloplegia 5–10 d, mydriasis 7–14 d) 1 gtt tid
- Bacitracin ointment: qid
- Ciprofloxacin: 0.35% 1 gtt qid
- Cyclopentolate: 0.5, 1.0, 2.0% drops (cycloplegia 1–2 d, mydriasis 1–2 d) 1 gtt TID
- Erythromycin: 0.5% ointment qid
- Gentamicin 0.3% ointment Qid
- Gentamicin: 0.3% drops 1gtt q 6 ointment qid
- Proparacaine: 0.5% drops 1 gtt
- Sulfacetamide: 10 % ointment qid
- Sulfacetamide: 10% drops qid
- Tobramycin: 0.3% ointment q 6 h
- Tobramycin: 0.3% drops q 6 h
- Tropicamide: 0.5, 1.0% drops (cycloplegia none; mydriasis 6 h) 1 gtt

PEDIATRIC CONSIDERATIONS

- Patching poorly tolerated
- May require systemic analgesia for complete examination

Disposition

ADMISSION CRITERIA

- Intractable pain
- Increased intraocular pressure
- Corneal penetration requiring immediate surgical intervention
- Hydrofluoric acid burn, admit for 24 hours of systemic analgesia
- Suspected child abuse

DISCHARGE CRITERIA

- All mild corneal burns
- Mandatory follow-up with ophthalmologist in 12–24 hours; arrange prior to patient discharge

Miscellaneous

ICD9: 940.4, 940.3, 940.2

CORE CONTENT CODE: 5.2

SUGGESTED READINGS

Beiran I, Miller B, Bentur Y. The efficacy of calcium gluconate in ocular hydrofluoric acid burns. Hum Exp Toxicol 1997;16(4):223–228.

Duma SM, et al. Airbag-induced eye injuries: A report of 25 cases. J Trauma 1996;41(1):114–119.

Guy PR, Taggart I, Adeniran A, Burd DA. Corneal burns with eyelid sparing and their treatment. Burns 1994;20(6):561–563.

Hammerton ME. Management of ocular burns. Aust Fam Phys 1995:24(6):1006–1010.

Lipshy KA, Wheeler WE, Denning DE. Ophthalmic thermal injuries. Amer Surg 1996;62(6):481–483.

Webster RG. Corneal trauma. In: Smolin G, Thoft RA, eds. The cornea: Scientific foundations and clinical practice. 3rd ed. Boston: Little, Brown and Company, 1994.

Author: Melissa Gillespie

Corneal Foreign Body

Clinical Presentation

SIGNS AND SYMPTOMS

- Foreign-body sensation
- Ocular pain
- Scleral injection (red eye); segmental injection may occur near the site
- Tearing
- Blurred or decreased vision
- Photophobia
- Visible foreign body or rust ring (slitlamp may be needed to visualize)
- Iritis
- Hypopyon (if there is severe inflammation in the anterior chamber)

MECHANISM/DESCRIPTION

- Common complaint: something fell, flew, or landed in the eye
- Hot, high-speed projectiles may not produce initial pain
- Corneal epithelium disrupted to a corneal abrasion
- Scar formation
  —None if only the epithelium affected
  —Occurs if Bowman's membrane or the stroma affected

ETIOLOGY

- Tolerated poorly
  —Organic material (wood chips, splinters, insect stingers, and tarantula hairs)
  —Oxidizing inorganic material (iron, copper)
- Tolerated well
  —Inert objects (paint chips, glass, plastic, fiberglass, precious metals)

Pre-Hospital

- Place a hard eyeshield in case corneal perforation has occurred

Diagnosis

ESSENTIAL WORKUP

- Injury history to assess
  —The likelihood of perforation (e.g., hammering metal, using lathes or grinders, high-speed projectiles, and the use of safety glasses)
  —The type of material—some more difficult to locate (e.g., fiberglass, glass)
- Visual acuity (mandatory)
- Inspection of the cornea for localization of the foreign body and exclude evidence of perforation
- Slitlamp examination
- Fluorescein evaluation after slitlamp examination so subtle cell and flare is not masked

IMAGING/SPECIAL TESTS

- Orbital radiographs—when suspicion for intraocular foreign body (high-velocity injury)
- Ocular CT/MRI or ultrasound—when suspect nonmetallic intraocular foreign body

DIFFERENTIAL DIAGNOSIS

- Conjunctival foreign body
- Corneal abrasion
- Corneal perforation with or without intraocular foreign body
- Corneal ulcer
- Keratitis

PEDIATRIC CONSIDERATIONS

- Unable to cooperate with the slitlamp examination and subsequent removal
  —Early referral to ophthalmologist

Treatment

INITIAL STABILIZATION

- Topical anesthetic to assist in examination, localization of the foreign body, and visual acuity determination

ED TREATMENT

Deep Foreign Bodies

- Refer those in the stoma to ophthalmology as perforation into the anterior chamber can occur with manipulation
- Small, inert, deeply embedded foreign bodies may be best left in place to avoid excessive scarring that can occur with the removal procedure

Removal Techniques

- Irrigation
  —Surrounding epithelium rapidly proliferates over the edges of the material making this method unlikely to succeed with embedded object
  —Direct the 0.9%NS solution at an oblique angle so as not to drive the object further into the cornea
- Moist cotton applicator
  —Brush unembedded foreign body off the corneal surface
  —Do not perform with an embedded foreign body—may drive it further into the cornea or cause excessive epithelial disruption
- 25-gauge needle
  —Using a slitlamp, hold the needle with the thumb and forefinger allowing the other fingers to be stabilized on the patient's nose or cheek
  —Lift the foreign body off the cornea
  —Keep the needle parallel to the corneal surface with the bevel directed towards the doctor
  —Use a tuberculin syringe to help with manipulation of the needle
- Corneal burr or spud
  —Employ similar to the needle

Removal Tips

- Slitlamp use recommended with instrumentation
- Keep patient's head and chin firmly against the head rest and his eyes fixated on a target
- Manual assistance to hold open the lids if the patient can not keep his eyes open
- Rest the instrumenting hand on the cheek of the patient to maintain stability and guard against sudden movements

Rust Rings

- Within a few hours, iron-containing foreign bodies will oxidize leaving a rust stain on adjacent epithelial cells
- Removal recommended as rust rings delay healing and are a continual irritative focus
- Remove with Alger brushes, drills, and needles
- Extraction may be difficult with fresh injuries
  - —Ring will soften over the next few days and may be more easily removed later by ophthalmologist

Postremoval Therapy

- Treat resultant corneal abrasion and possibly iritis with
  - —Antibiotics drops
  - —Cycloplegic agent
  - —Double patch not necessary
- Determine tetanus status
- Analgesics (acetaminophen with codeine/NSAID)

MEDICATIONS

- Cyclopentolate 1–2%: 1 drop tid (lasts up to 2 days)
- Gentamicin opthalmic: 2 drops q 6 h
- Homatropine 2 or 5%: 1 drop qd tid (lasts up to 3 days)
- Sulfacetamide 10%: 1 drop q 6 h
- Tobramycin opthalmic: 2 drops q 6 h

Disposition

ADMISSION CRITERIA

- Penetration into the globe
- Corneal ulcer
- Alkali substance causing a chemical burn

DISCHARGE CRITERIA

- All patients with corneal foreign bodies
- Follow-up with an ophthalmologist in 24 hours especially for
  - —Rust rings removal
  - —Removed vegetative material because of the risk of ulceration

Miscellaneous

ICD9: 930.9

CORE CONTENT CODE: 6.4.1.6

SUGGESTED READINGS

Augeri PA. Corneal foreign body removal and treatment. Optom Clin 1991;1:59–70.

Cakanac CJ, Ajamian PC. Cornea and conjunctiva: Clinical procedures. Boston: Butterworth-Heinemann, 1996.

Kaiser PK. A comparison of pressure patching versus no patching for corneal abrasions due to trauma or foreign body removal. Ophthalmology 1997;104:169.

Knoop K, Trott A. Ophthalmologic procedures in the emergency department—Part III: Slit lamp use and foreign bodies Acad Emerg Med 1995;2224–2230.

Author: Loice Swisher

Croup

Clinical Presentation

SIGNS AND SYMPTOMS

- Nonspecific upper respiratory prodrome
- Low-grade fever
- Barking cough
- Hoarse voice
- Stridor
  - —Inspiratory stridor suggests a supraglottic lesion
  - —Expiratory stridor suggests lower airway involvement
- Spasmodic croup
  - —Sudden onset at night
  - —Without prodrome
  - —Consistent response to mist
  - —Cool air alone
  - —Often recurrent
- Croup score
  - —Stridor
    - -0 = None
    - -1 = Audible with stethoscope at rest
    - -2 = Audible without stethoscope at rest
  - —Retractions
    - -0 = None
    - -1 = Mild
    - -2 = Moderate
    - -3 = Severe
  - —Air entry
    - -0 = Normal
    - -1 = Decreased
    - -2 = Severely decreased
  - —Cyanosis
    - -0 = None
    - -4 = With agitation
    - -5 = At rest
  - —Level of consciousness
    - -0 = Normal
    - -5 = Altered

MECHANISM/DESCRIPTION

- An infection of the upper and lower respiratory tract
  - —Laryngotracheitis
  - —Inflammatory edema of subglottic region
- Commonly presents in children 6 months to 3 years

ETIOLOGY

- Parainfluenza types 1 and 2
- Influenza A
- Adenoviruses
- Respiratory syncytial virus
- Measles
- Enteroviruses
- Mycoplasma pneumoniae
- Herpes simplex

Pre-Hospital

- Allow child to assume position of comfort
- Humidified oxygen

CAUTIONS

- Do not remove parent from child
- Avoid scary or painful procedures
  - —Intravenous access
  - —Mask oxygen

Diagnosis

ESSENTIAL WORKUP

- Mild symptoms
  - —History and physical examination only
- Respiratory distress
  - —Differentiate croup from epiglottitis after airway stabilized

LABORATORY

- Pulse oximetry
- Other tests are not routinely indicated

IMAGING/SPECIAL TESTS

- AP and lateral neck radiographs
  - —"Steeple sign" indicates narrowing of subglottic trachea
  - —Not routinely indicated for mild symptoms
  - —Should not delay definitive visualization and intubation in operating room in child with concern for epiglottis
  - —Subject to misinterpretation
  - —Not always diagnostic

DIFFERENTIAL DIAGNOSIS

- Epiglottitis
- Bacterial tracheitis
- Foreign body
- Peritonsillar abscess
- Retropharyngeal abscess
- Angioedema
- Congenital airway anomalies
- Acquired subglottic stenosis

Treatment

INITIAL STABILIZATION

- Allow child to maintain position of comfort
- Defer painful or scary procedures
- If respiratory failure
  - —Bag-valve-mask ventilation usually successful
  - —Tracheal intubation by most experienced person available
- Endotracheal tube 0.5–1.0 mm smaller than usual size

ED TREATMENT

- Pulse oximetry if tolerated
- Humidified O_2
- Nebulized epinephrine for croup score >3 after mist
- Steroids may reduce the severity of disease
  - —Indicated for patients requiring racemic epinephrine because of stridor at rest
- Oral or intravenous hydration
- Suspected epiglottitis or planned intubation
  - —Operating room for halothane/oxygen anesthesia
  - —Direct laryngoscopy and intubation
  - —Surgeon standing by for emergent tracheostomy

MEDICATIONS

- Racemic epinephrine: 0.25–0.5 cc nebulized
- Dexamethasone: 0.6 mg/kg IM/IV or po q 6 hours

Disposition

ADMISSION CRITERIA

- Need for more than one treatment with racemic epinephrine
- Persistent stridor at rest
- Recurrent stridor 3—4 hours after initial EPI/dexamethasone treatment
- PICU
  - —Persistent severe obstruction
  - —Need for frequent treatments with nebulized epinephrine

DISCHARGE CRITERIA

- Oxygenation normal on room air at the time of discharge
- Resolution of symptoms without repeated doses of racemic epinephrine
- The child remains asymptomatic for 4 to 6 hours
- Discharge on steroids with mandatory follow-up in 12 to 24 hours

Miscellaneous

ICD9: 464.4

CORE CONTENT CODE: 13.7.3

SUGGESTED READINGS

Cruz MN, Stewart G, Rosenberg N. Use of dexamethasone in the outpatient management of acute laryngotracheitis. Pediatrics 1995;96:220–23.

Geelhoed GC. Croup. Pediatr Pulmonol 1977;23:370–74.

Ledwith CA, Shea LM, Mauro RD. Safety and efficacy of nebulized racemic epinephrine in conjunction with oral dexamethasone and mist in the outpatient treatment of croup. Ann Emerg Med 1995;25:331–37.

Authors: David Marby; Dale Steele

Cushing's Syndrome

Clinical Presentation

SIGNS AND SYMPTOMS

- Cardiovascular
  - —Uncontrolled hypertension
  - —Myocardial infarction
- Neurologic
  - —Atherosclerotic or embolic stroke
  - —Pseudotumor cerebri (seen primarily with exogenous Cushing's from glucocorticoid administration)
  - —Spinal lipomatosis with cord or nerve-root compression
- Gastroenterologic
  - —Peptic ulcers
  - —GI hemorrhage
  - —Pancreatitis (seen primarily with exogenous Cushing's from glucocorticoid administration)
  - —Fatty liver
- Psychiatric
  - —Mood disorders (40%)
  - —Depression
  - —Bipolar disorder
  - —Memory impairment
  - —Euphoria
  - —Toxic psychosis
- Musculoskeletal
  - —Myopathy
  - —Pathologic fractures
  - —Osteoporosis
  - —Aseptic necrosis humeral or femoral heads (seen primarily with exogenous Cushing's from glucocorticoid administration)
  - —Delayed bone age
  - —Endocrine
  - —Glucose intolerance
  - —Hyperlipidemia
  - —Amenorrhea
- Hematologic
  - —Increased neutrophils, decreased lymphocytes and eosinophils, opportunistic infections
- Ophthalmologic
  - —Cataracts (seen primarily with exogenous Cushing's from glucocorticoid administration)
  - —Glaucoma (seen primarily with exogenous Cushing's from glucocorticoid administration)
- Dermatologic
  - —Pigmented striae
  - —Thin skin
  - —Impaired wound healing
  - —Ecchymoses
  - —Acne
  - —Female balding
  - —Round face
  - —Hirsutism
  - —Central obesity with buffalo hump and supraclavicular adipose deposition
  - —Hyperhidrosis

MECHANISM/DESCRIPTION

- Excessive glucocorticoid effects

ETIOLOGY

- Pituitary adenoma secreting ACTH
- Tumor-producing ectopic ACTH—usually neuroendocrine cells of the APUD type (*a*mine *p*recursor *u*ptake *d*ecarboxylase)
  - —Small cell lung carcinoma
  - —Uterine cervix
  - —Islet cell tumor of pancreas (MEA I-type syndrome)
  - —Medullary thyroid cancer
  - —Pheochromocytoma
  - —Ganglioneuroma
  - —Melanoma
  - —Prostate
  - —Carcinoid tumor (lung, pancreas, GI tract, thymus, or ovary)
- Adrenal production of cortisol from adenoma, carcinoma, or micronodular disease
- Exogenous administration of glucocorticoids either therapeutically or surreptitiously

PEDIATRIC CONSIDERATIONS

- Suspect if increasing in obesity while falling off in height on the growth chart

Pre-Hospital

CAUTIONS

- Acute Addisonian crisis under stress may develop with iatrogenic Cushing's syndrome
- Patients may have extremely labile behavior
- Cause of death in untreated Cushing's syndrome is
  - —Infection
  - —Stroke
  - —Myocardial infarction
  - —Suicide

Diagnosis

ESSENTIAL WORKUP

- Cannot confirm diagnosis in ED
- If suspicion of iatrogenic Cushing's exists, check for impending Addisonian crisis
- Search for life-threatening conditions
  - —Myocardial infarction
  - —Stroke
  - —Sepsis
  - —Pathologic fracture
  - —Uncontrolled DM
  - —Psychiatric emergency necessitating admission

LABORATORY

- Electrolytes, BUN, Cr, glucose
  - —Hypokalemia
  - —Metabolic acidosis (due to renal KCl loss)
  - —10% with metabolic alkalosis
  - —Diminished glucose tolerance (75%) (50% have glycosuria, 20% overt DM)
- CBC
  - —Increased WBC
  - —Decreased eosinophils

IMAGING/SPECIAL TESTS

- ECG for myocardial ischemia
- CXR for tumor-causing ectopic ACTH
- MRI for pituitary tumor
- CT for adrenal carcinoma, adenoma, or hyperplasia
- Plain films for possible pathologic fractures
- Dexamethasone suppression test (follow-up study with primary physician)
  - —If suspicion of endogenous Cushing's syndrome exists
  - —Screening test—1 mg at 11:00 PM with an 8 AM cortisol level drawn
    - -Low specificity
  - —Decrease false-positives by stopping alcohol, estrogens, spironolactone, phenytoin, and barbiturates
  - —High dose dexamethasone suppression test needed to confirm the diagnosis
    - -2 mg qid of dexamethasone with cortisol level 6 hours later
    - -Compare day 2 urine-free cortisol and 17-hydroxyketosteroids with baseline levels

DIFFERENTIAL DIAGNOSIS

- Alcohol-induced pseudo-Cushing's syndrome
- Obesity
- Psychiatric states
  - —Depression
  - —Obsessive compulsive disorder
  - —Chronic alcoholism
  - —Panic disorder
- Physiologic states
  - —Chronic stress
  - —3rd trimester pregnancy
  - —Chronic strenuous exercise
- Malnutrition

Treatment

INITIAL STABILIZATION

- Initiate treatment for associated complications
  - —MI
  - —Stroke

ED TREATMENT

- IV rehydration/glucose-lowering agents for hyperglycemia
- Culture and antibiotics for suspected infection
- Antihypertensive agents for uncontrolled blood pressure
- Administer steroids with iatrogenic Cushing's if patient under stress to prevent Addisonian crisis
- Medications to lower cortisol levels (bromocriptine, ketoconazole, aminoglutamide, metapyrone)
  - —Used rarely with severe symptoms in patients awaiting surgery
  - —Institute under the direction of an endocrinologist

Definitive Therapy

- Iatrogenic
  - —Taper steroids as rapidly as possible
  - —Calcium, vitamin D, and estrogen supplementation if possible
- Pituitary Cushing's
  - —Transsphenoidal surgery (radiation for surgical failures and a few select patients)
- Adrenal adenoma/carcinoma
  - —Adrenal resection with medical therapy for metastatic lesions not resectable
- Ectopic ACTH
  - —Tumor resection (if possible) with medical therapy for metastatic lesions not resectable

MEDICATIONS

- Hydrocortisone: 100–200 mg (peds: 1–2 mg/kg) IVP

Disposition

ADMISSION CRITERIA

- Complications which require admission such as
  - —Myocardial infarction
  - —Stroke
  - —Sepsis
  - —Pathologic fracture
  - —Uncontrolled DM
  - —Psychiatric emergency
- Impending Addisonian crisis

DISCHARGE CRITERIA

- Well-appearing, stable patient without admission criteria (above)

Miscellaneous

ICD9: 255.0

CORE CONTENT CODE: 4.2.1

SUGGESTED READINGS

Jeffcoate W. Alcohol-induced pseudo-Cushing's syndrome. Lancet 1993;341:676–677.

Noble J, ed. Textbook of primary care medicine. 2d ed. St. Louis: CV Mosby, 1996.

Tsigos C, Crousos G. Differential diagnosis and management of Cushing's syndrome. Ann Rev Med 1996;47:443–461.

Wallach J, ed. Interpretation of diagnostic tests. 6th ed. Boston: Little, Brown and Company, 1996:588–594.

Yanovski J, Cutler G. Glucocorticoid action and the clinical features of Cushing's syndrome. Endocrinol Metab Clin North Am 1994;3:487–509.

Author: Hugh Schuckman

Cyanide, Poisoning

Clinical Presentation

SIGNS AND SYMPTOMS

- Heart and brain—most sensitive organs—first to show manifestation of toxicity

CNS

- Headache
- Confusion
- Syncope
- Seizures
- Coma

Cardiovascular

- Dyspnea
- Chest pain
- Cardiorespiratory collapse and death

Other

- Nausea/vomiting

MECHANISM/DESCRIPTION

- Toxicity through inhalation, dermal, or GI tract absorption
- Intracellular toxin that inhibits aerobic metabolism through interruption of oxidative phosphorylation
  —Leads to decreased O_2 utilization and ATP production
- Inhibits antioxidant defense enzymes contributes to oxidative damage
- Stimulates neurotransmitter release in CNS/PNS

Cyanide (CN) Detoxification

- Rhodanese—a hepatic mitochondrial enzyme responsible for the metabolism
  —Combines CN with sulfur (rate-limiting step) covalently (irreversible) to form a less toxic and water soluble thiocyanate (T-CN)
  —Forms less toxic reversible cyanhemoglobin when combined with Hgb (Fe^{+2})
  —Forms nontoxic cyanocobalamin (B_{12}) when combined with hydroxocobalamin (B_{12a})
  —Rate of CN removal requires adequate bioavailability of sulfur compounds (thiosulfate)

ETIOLOGY

- Fires (combustion by product of natural and synthetic products)
- Vehicle exhaust
- Industry (metal plating, chemical synthesis, plastic manufacturing, laboratory analysis, pesticides)
- Solvents (nail polish remover, metal polishes)
- Byproduct of nitroprusside metabolism (nonenzymatic)
- Byproduct of *P. Aeruginosa* and *pyocyaneus* infections
- Amygdalin (converted by intestinal flora to CN) containing plants (apricot and peach pits, apple and pear seeds, and cassava)

Pre-Hospital

CAUTIONS

- Remove the source of CN
- Prevent others from becoming contaminated
- Remove and bag all contaminated clothing and wash affected areas copiously with soap and water

Diagnosis

ESSENTIAL WORKUP

- History of exposure (not routinely available)
- Clinical clues (frequently absent)
  —Peculiar odor of bitter almonds
  —Bright red (arterialization) retinal vessels
  —Cherry red skin color in an apneic noncyanotic patient
- Significant CN poisoning
  —Abrupt onset and/or deteriorating toxic effects
  —Lactic acidosis
  —High venous O_2 saturation (due to blocked O_2 consumption)—arterialization of venous blood gases

LABORATORY TESTS

- CBC
- Electrolytes, BUN, Cr, glucose
  —Anion gap acidosis
- Liver profile
- CPK
- Carboxyhemoglobin (CO) level
- Methemoglobin (MH) level
- Cyanide level
  —Support the clinical diagnosis if performed in a timely fashion
  —Analyze sample immediately after venipuncture since CN in vitro production and transformation are both time and temperature dependent
  —Levels >0.5–1 mg/L—toxic
  —Levels 2.5–3.0 mg/L—fatal
- Thiocyanate level
- Blood gas determinations
  —Increased arterial saturation gap [calculated − direct (measure) O_2 saturation (co-oximeter)]
  —Elevated mixed venous O_2: MvO_2 [normal ~ 35–40]
  —Elevated mixed venous O_2 saturation (co-oximeter): $S_{mv}O_2$ [normal ~ 75%]
  —Decreased arteriovenous O_2 difference: ${}_{AV}O_2D$ [normal ~ 3–4.8 ml/dl]
- Elevated lactate level

IMAGING/SPECIAL TESTS

- Cyanomethemoglobin level
- Acetoacetate level
- β-Hydroxybutyrate level [normal ~-0.3 μmol/l]
- Pyruvate level

DIFFERENTIAL DIAGNOSIS

- Carbon monoxide
- Hydrogen sulfide
- Methemoglobinemia
- Sulfhemoglobinemia
- Inert gases "asphyxiants"
- Causes of high anion gap metabolic acidosis

Treatment

INITIAL STABILIZATION

- ABCs
- Administer 100% oxygen
  - —Even in presence of normal PaO_2
  - —Acts synergistically with antidotes
- Gastric decontamination for oral ingestions
  - —Perform gastric lavage and administer activated charcoal (AC)
  - —Follow by repeat dose of AC
  - —Do not induce emesis

ED TREATMENT

CN Antidote Kit

- Administer if manifesting significant CN toxicity with persistent high anion gap metabolic acidosis and a narrow arterial-venous O_2 difference
- Administration often instituted empirically—CN levels not immediately available
- Contents: amyl nitrite pearls, sodium nitrite, and thiosulfate (TS)
- Nitrite action
  - —Induce a CN scavenging MH by oxidizing Hgb (Fe^{+2} to Fe^{+3}), which attracts extracellular CN away from the mitochondria forming CN-MH, which is less toxic
  - —Do not administer empirically or prophylactically
- TS action
  - —Substrate for the enzyme rhodanase
  - —Combines with CN to form a less toxic T-CN
  - —May administer empirically
- Use clinical response and not methemoglobin levels to guide nitrite administration
- Side effects
  - —Hypotension (nitrite-induced vasodilation)
  - —Methemoglobinemia
    - -Does not function as O_2 transporter
    - -Impairs oxygen delivery
    - -Elevated level leads to further tissue hypoxia

Hydroxocobalamin (B_{12a})

- Alternate safe antidote
- Binds to CN
  - —Forms nontoxic cyanocobalamin (B_{12}); renally excreted
- Advantages
  - —No MH induction
  - —Does not cause hypotension
- Limitations
  - —Large amount needed to successfully treat poisoned patients (50 g B_{12a}:1 g CN)
  - —Use of TS combined with B_{12a} may reduce the amount of B_{12a} required

Combined TS and B_{12a} Therapy

- Victims of smoke inhalation may have combination of
  - —CN toxicity
  - —Methemoglobinemia
  - —CO toxicity
- Avoid further reduction in oxygen transport—initially treat with TS and/or B_{12a} until the CO and MH levels known

Hyperbaric Oxygen (HBO) Therapy

- Maximizes tissue oxygenation despite toxic MH level
- Employ as adjunct to above antidotes in severe cases or when antidotes have failed

Antidote Alternatives

- Not yet FDA approved
- Do not institute empirically due to toxicity
- Dicobalt edetate
  - —Inactivates CN by chelation
  - —Associated with hypertension, dysrhythmias, and metabolic acidosis
- Dimethylaminophenol
  - —Induces a much faster scavenging MH
  - —Nephrotoxic

MEDICATIONS

- Activated charcoal: 1–2 g/kg po
- Hydroxocobalamin (B_{12a})
  - —Dose equivalent to 50 times the amount of CN exposure infused in 30 minutes
  - —Empiric single dose = 4–5 g (50 mg/kg) IV in D5W
  - —Prophylactic IV infusion at 25 mg/hr in nipride usage

CN Antidote Kit (Eli Lilly Antidote Kit)

- Amyl nitrite pearls
  - —Crush 1–2 ampules in gauze and hold close to the nose, in the lip of the face mask, or within the ambu-bag
  - —Inhale for 30 sec/min until IV access obtained
- N-nitrite ($NaNO_2$)
  - —10 ml (300 mg) (peds: 0.19–0.33 ml/kg) IV as 3% solution over 5–20 min
  - —May repeat once at one-half dose within 30–60 minutes
  - —Keep MH level $<30\%$
  - —Dilute; infuse slowly if hypotensive
- N-thiosulfate
  - —50 ml (12.5 g) (peds: 0.95–1.95 ml/kg) IV over 10–15 minutes of a 25% solution
  - —Half the initial dose may be given after 30–60 minutes

Disposition

ADMISSION CRITERIA

- ICU admission

DISCHARGE CRITERIA

None

Miscellaneous

ICD9: 989.0

CORE CONTENT CODE: 17.2.17

SUGGESTED READINGS

Houeto P, Borron SW, Sandouk P, et al. Pharmacokinetics of hydroxocobalamin in smoke inhalation victims. Clin Toxicol 1996;34(4):397–404.

Isom GE, Borowitz JL. Modification of cyanide toxicodynamics: Mechanistic based antidote development. Toxicol Lett 1995;82/83:795–799.

Kulig KW. Case studies in environmental medicine: Cyanide toxicity. Agency for Toxic Substances and Disease Registry 1991;15:1–17.

Nakatani T, Kosugi Y, Mori A, et al. Changes in the parameters of oxygen metabolism in a clinical course recovering from potassium cyanide. Am J Emerg Med 1993;11:213–217.

Yen D, Tsai J, Wang LE, et al. The clinical experience of acute cyanide poisoning. Am J Emerg Med 1995;13:524–528.

Author: Jose Diaz

Cyanosis

Clinical Presentation

SIGNS AND SYMPTOMS

- A bluish discoloration of the skin and mucous membranes
  - —Peripheral
    - -Nail beds
    - -Extremities
  - —Central
    - -Lips
    - -Trunk
    - -Face
- Clubbing of digits suggests certain pulmonary and congenital heart diseases
- Asymptomatic cyanosis
  - —Consider methemoglobin
- Duration
  - —Congenital heart disease is usually present since birth
  - —Chronic bronchitis may have baseline cyanosis
- Exposure to drugs or chemicals

MECHANISM/DESCRIPTION

- 5 g of reduced hemoglobin per 100 cc of capillary blood
  - —The bluish color results from the absolute amount of reduced hemoglobin
  - —Anemic patients are less likely to develop cyanosis
  - —Polycythemic patients more likely
  - —White-skinned patients detectable when hemoglobin saturation has fallen to 85%
  - —Dark-skinned patients detectable when the saturation falls below 75%
- Abnormal pigment methemoglobin
  - —More than 10% of the hemoglobin
  - —Asymptomatic (Smurf syndrome)
  - —Fatal at levels of 60–70%

ETIOLOGY

Central Cyanosis

- Respiratory
  - —Lower oxygen tensions seen at altitudes greater than 8000 ft
    - -Alveolar hypoventilation
    - -Intoxication
    - -Asthma
    - -COPD
    - -Upper airway obstruction
  - —Ventilation/perfusion mismatch
    - -Asthma
    - -Pulmonary embolism
    - -Pneumonia
- Decreased oxygen diffusion
  - —Pulmonary edema
- Pulmonary arteriovenous fistulas
  - —Hereditary telangectasia
- Cardiac
  - —Pulmonary edema
  - —Congenital heart disease with right-to-left shunt
    - -Tetralogy of Fallot in adults
- Methemoglobinemia
  - —Exposure to nitrates
    - -Nitroglycerin
    - -Contaminated well water
    - -Food additives
  - —Lidocaine
  - —Sulfonamides
  - —Dapsone
  - —PCP treatment
- Hereditary deficiency
  - —NADH
  - —Methemoglobin reductase

Peripheral Cyanosis

- Cold air or water exposure
- Arterial or venous obstruction
  - —Single extremity
- Superior vena cava obstruction
  - —Upper half of body
- Patent ductus arteriosus with pulmonary hypertension and right-to-left shunt
  - —Lower half of the body

Pediatric Cyanosis

- Respiratory
  - —Upper airway obstruction
    - -Croup
    - -Epiglotitis
    - -Bacterial tracheitis
    - -Retropharyngeal abscess
    - -Foreign body aspirations
  - —Lower airway and parenchymal disease
    - -Asthma
    - -Bronchiolitis
    - -Atelectasis
  - —Pneumonia
- Cardiac
  - —Congenital heart disease with right to left shunting
    - -Tetralogy of Fallot
    - -Pulmonary stenosis
    - -Transposition of great vessels
    - -Tricuspid atresia
    - -Ebstein's anomaly
    - -Truncus arteriosus
  - —Total anomalous pulmonary venous return
- Systemic infection
  - —Meningitis
  - —Sepsis
- Methemoglobinemia
- Cyanosis at birth secondary to excess hemoglobin M
- Breath holding

Pre-Hospital

- Intravenous line
  - —Caution in children with signs of upper airway obstruction
- 100% O_2 via nonrebreather
- Cardiac monitoring
- Pulse oximetry
- Intubation may be necessary if additional signs of respiratory distress
- Difficult airway if signs of upper airway obstruction are present
- Nebulized albuterol should be given for bronchospasm
- If signs of pulmonary edema
  - —Nitrates
  - —Furosemide
  - —Morphine
- Nebulized epinephrine may be given for croup

Diagnosis

ESSENTIAL WORKUP

- Assess stability and need for airway management
- Assess for methemoglobinemia
- Determine underlying cause of cyanosis secondary to respiratory or cardiac disorders

LABORATORY

- Transcutaneous measurement of oxygen saturation
- ABG
  - —Oxygen tension
  - —Measured hemoglobin oxygen saturation
    - -A low O_2 saturation with normal oxygen tension suggests methemoglobinemia
- Color of extracted blood
  - —Brown color suggests methemoglobinemia
- Methemoglobin level
- CBC
  - —Total hemoglobin
- Hyperoxia test
  - —In cyanotic infant
  - —Assists in distinguishing pulmonary from congenital cardiac disease
  - —Failure of the PAO_2 to increase above 100 mm Hg when exposed to an FiO_2 of 0.9
  - —Suggests heart disease

IMAGING/SPECIAL TESTS

- Chest x-ray may distinguish between respiratory and cardiac disease
  - —Inspiratory/expiratory chest films if a radiolucent foreign body is suspected
- EKG to assess for ischemia
- Bedside echocardiography
  - —Wall motion abnormalities
  - —Pericardial fluid
- Neck radiographs
  - —If upper airway pathology is suspected
  - —Subglottic narrowing (croup)
  - —Prevertebral swelling (retropharyngeal abscess)
  - —Epiglottic swelling
  - —Foreign bodies

DIFFERENTIAL DIAGNOSIS

- Florid skin discoloration of polycythemia
- Argyria
  - —Silver sulfide deposited on the skin by the action of light on ingested silver compounds
  - —Does not fade when pressure is applied

Treatment

INITIAL STABILIZATION

- Oxygen 100% nonrebreather
- Airway management if unstable

ED TREATMENT

- Management of underlying respiratory or cardiac disorders
- Methylene blue when methemoglobinemia is greater than 30% of hemoglobin

MEDICATIONS

- Albuterol: nebulized (5 mg/cc) 0.03 cc/kg
- Dexamethasone: IV/IM 0.2 mg/kg
- Furosemide: IV 20–80 mg
- Magnesium: IV 2 g over 10 min
- Methylene blue: IV 1–2 mg/kg of 1% solution over 5 min
- Methylprednisolone: IV 2 mg/kg
- Morphine: IV 2–4 mg every 5 min
- Nitroglycerin: sublingual or IV 0.4 mg
- Prostaglandin EI: IV 0.05–0.1 μg/kg/min
- Racemic epinephrine: nebulized 0.05 cc/kg

Disposition

ADMISSION CRITERIA

- The majority of patients presenting with cyanosis will require admission to the hospital
- Admission to the intensive care unit
  - —Determined by the underlying etiology and the ED course

DISCHARGE CRITERIA

- Reversible causes of hypoxia
  - —Reactive airway disease responding to Beta-agonists and steroids in the ED
  - —Pulmonary edema in a patient with known congestive heart failure with complete resolution after diuresis and observation

Miscellaneous

ICD9: 782.5

CORE CONTENT CODE: 22.1.14

SUGGESTED READINGS

Cline MS. Curing the "nitrate blues." Postgrad Med 1994;96(3):124–126.

DiMaio AM, Singh J. The infant with cyanosis in the emergency room. Pediatr Clin North Am 1992;39(5):987–1006.

Perloff JK. Systemic complications of cyanosis in adults with congenital heart disease. Hematologic derangements, renal function, and urate metabolism. Cardiol Clin 1993;11:689–699.

Authors: Peter Moyer; Sig Kharasch

Cystic Fibrosis

Clinical Presentation

SIGNS AND SYMPTOMS

- General
  - —Failure to thrive
  - —Poor weight gain
  - —Recurrent respiratory infections
  - —Frequent illness
  - —Anasarca in infancy
  - —Salty taste of skin
- HEENT
  - —Nasal polyps
  - —Severe headaches due to sinusitis
- Pulmonary
  - —Early onset of a persistent, dry hacking paroxysmal cough
  - —Frequent bouts of pneumonitis or bronchiolitis in the first years of life
  - —Wheezing
  - —Respiratory distress
  - —Hemoptysis
  - —Cor pulmonale
  - —Pneumonia
  - —Pneumothorax
  - —Congestive heart failure
  - —Pulmonary hypertension
- Gastrointestinal
  - —Abdominal pain
    - -Distal ileal obstructive syndrome or "meconium ileus equivalent"
    - -Cholelithiasis
    - -Pancreatitis
    - -Ileocecal intussusception
  - —Foul smelling, fatty stools
  - —Jaundice
    - -Cirrhosis or cholelithiasis
  - —Rectal prolapse
  - —Hematemesis
- Extremities
  - —Bone pain
  - —Edema
  - —Joint effusions

MECHANISM/DESCRIPTION

- Defects of the cystic fibrosis transmembrane conductance regulator (CFTR)
- CFTR functions as an ATP-regulated chloride channel
  - —Abnormal electrolyte transport in exocrine glands and secretory epithelia
  - —Thickened mucus,
  - —Recurrent pulmonary infections
  - —Progressive obstructive damage to the lungs
  - —Decreased exocrine pancreatic function
  - —Malabsorption
- Affects 1/2500 Caucasians
- Less prevalent in most non-Caucasian populations
- Diagnosed in the first decade of life in about 70% of cases
- Median life expectancy in the U.S. is close to 30 years
- Pulmonary complications are the most common reason for admission
- Cardiorespiratory failure is the most common cause of death

ETIOLOGY

- Recessively inherited genetic disease
- Involves the CFTR gene on the long arm of chromosome 7
- Different mutations results in differing disease phenotypes
- Classical disease in those homozygous for the DF508 mutation
- Common organisms in patients with pneumonia
  - —*Pseudomonas aeruginosa*
    - -Very common colonizer
    - -Often multiple drug resistances
  - —*Burkholderia cepacia*
    - -Prevalence 5%
    - -Often with multiple drug resistances
    - -Often bodes rapid clinical deterioration
  - —*Hemophilus influenza*
  - —*Staphylococcus aureus*
  - —*Aspergillus*

Pre-Hospital

CAUTIONS

- Supportive measures
- Determine DNR status

Diagnosis

ESSENTIAL WORKUP

- Test patients with chronic or unsual respiratory and gastrointestinal complaints for CF
- Obtain history of prior cultures in patients with known CF
- *Pseudomonas aeruginosa* often plays a recurrent role in CF lung disease
- Often multiply resistant organisms

LABORATORY

- Sweat chloride test
  - —Chloride concentration ≥80 mEq/L
  - —With classic signs and symptoms, a positive test confirms the diagnosis
- Stool sample
  - —Trypsin or chemotrypsin absent or diminished
  - —Increased fat in 72h fecal fat excretion
- Cytogenetic analysis
  - —Indicated if the symptoms are highly suggestive, but the sweat test is negative
  - —Positive if 2 abnormal genes are present
  - —Genotyping, however, cannot establish the diagnosis
  - —Detects only 70 of the 500 CTFR mutations
  - —There may be an ameliorating or neutralizing second mutation elsewhere
- ABG
  - —Hypoxemia
  - —Metabolic alkalosis
- Serum electrolytes
  - —Hyponatremic-hypochloremic alkalosis
- Serum glucose
  - —Hyperglycemia and new onset diabetes occurs primarily in adolescents and adults ketoacidosis is rare
- Sputum culture
  - —To determine if pseudomonas colonization is present
- CBC
  - —Thrombocytopenia
- Liver function tests and prothrombin time
  - —Indicated when CF is complicated by hematemesis or signs of liver failure

IMAGING/SPECIAL TESTS

- CXR
  - —Hyperaeration
  - —Peribronchial thickening
  - —Atelectasis
  - —Hilar lymphadenopathy
  - —Possible pneumothorax
  - —Bronchiectasis
  - —Blebs
  - —Comparison to previous CXR for acute pulmonary deterioration
- Abdominal radiographs
  - —Indicated if abdominal pain, vomiting, or abdominal distention
  - —Distal ileal obstruction syndrome
  - —Intussusception

- Barium enema
  —Indicated if suspicion of intussusception
- Sinus films
  —Of limited use as regular sinus films are always cloudy
  —Comparisons to previous x-rays and CT are needed
- Bronchoalveolar lavage
  —High percentage of neutrophils and absolute neutrophil count
  —Unnecessary in patients with obvious pulmonary symptoms
- Studies indicated in patients at high risk with a difficult diagnosis
  —Semen analysis
    -Azoospermia
  —Nasal potential-difference measurements
    -Complex and time-consuming study

DIFFERENTIAL DIAGNOSIS

- Respiratory presentations
  —Asthma
  —Recurrent pneumonias
  —Bronchiectasis
  —Pertussis
  —Immunodeficiency
- Gastrointestinal presentations
  —Chronic diarrhea
  —Gastroenteritis
  —Milk allergy
- Elevated electrolyte levels in sweat
  —Fucosidosis
  —Glycogen storage disease type I
  —Mucopolysaccharidosis
  —Hypothyroidism
  —Vasopressin-resistant diabetes insipidus
  —Adrenal insufficiency
  —Familial cholestasis
  —Familial hypoparathyroidism
  —Malnutrition
  —Ectodermal dysplasia
  —Atopic dermatitis
  —Infusion of prostaglandin E1

Treatment

INITIAL STABILIZATION

- Oxygen if hypoxemia if $PaO_2 < 50$
- Clarification of DNR status

ED TREATMENT

- Pneumothorax
  —Observation if <5–10%
- Thoracostomy
- Consultation with the primary CF physician or pulmonary specialist
- Right heart failure
  —Diuretics
- Hemoptysis
  —Blood products
  —Ventilatory support
- Distal ileal obstructive syndrome
  —Usually requires surgery
  —Blood products are used for the correction of coagulation abnormalities and red cells may be required for replacement in hematemesis
  —Early consultation with an endoscopist to find the cause and help with therapy of hematemesis is useful
  —Intussusception can be corrected with barium enema but at times requires surgery; an attempt at manual reduction of rectal prolapse should be made; a surgical consult may be required for difficult cases or for recurrences
- Replace electrolytes and fluids according to the abnormalities
- Hyperglycemia (bg >250) should be treated with insulin
- Antibiotics
- Based on culture and sensitivity
- Pneumonia
  —*Staphylococcus aureus*
    -Cephalothin
    -Nafcillin
  —*Hemophilus influenzae*
    -Ticarcillin and clavulanate
  —*Pseudomonas aeruginosa*
    -Tobramycin and ticarcillin
  —*Staphylococcus aureus pseudomonas aeruginosa*
    -Ticarcillin and tobramycin
  —*P. aeruginosa* and *Burkholderia cepacia*
    -Ceftazidime and ciprofloxacin
  —*Burkholderia cepacia*
    -Chloramphenicol
    -Trimethoprim azole
- Sinusitis
    -Antibiotic therapy may be needed for sinus problems
    -The choice should be based on cultures and sensitivities

MEDICATIONS

- Cephalothin: 25–50 mg/kg q 6 hrs
- Nafcillin: 25–50 mg/kg every q 6 hrs
- Ticarcillin: 100 mg/kg q 6 hrs
- Clavulanate: 3.3 mg /kg q 6 hrs
- Gentamycin: 3 mg/kg q 8 hrs
- Ceftazidime: 50–75 mg/kg q 8 hrs
- Chloramphenicol: 15–20 mg/kg q 6 hrs
- Trimethoprim-sulfamethoxazole: 5–25 mg/kg q 6 hrs

Disposition

ADMISSION CRITERIA

- Pulmonary exacerbation with significant deterioration from baseline
- Hemoptysis
- Hematemesis
- Intussusception
  —Not reduced with barium enema
  —Prolonged duration
- Hyperglycemia

DISCHARGE CRITERIA

- Close follow-up to verify the sensitivities of culture results and change therapy as needed
- Avoid hot weather
- Oral salt supplements during times of profuse sweating
- Chloride sweat test for siblings for new diagnosis of CF

Miscellaneous

ICD9: 277.0

CORE CONTENT CODE: 13.9.3

SUGGESTED READINGS

Nishioka GJ, Cook PR. Paranasal sinus disease in patients with cystic fibrosis. Otolaryngol Clin North Am 1996;29(1):193–205.

Ramsey BW. Management of pulmonary disease in patients with cystic fibrosis. N Engl J Med 1996;335(3):179–188.

Schindlow DV, Taussig LM, Knowles MR. Cystic Fibrosis Foundation consensus conference report on pulmonary complications of cystic fibrosis. Pediatr Pulmonol 1993;15(3):187–198.

Stern RC. The diagnosis of cystic fibrosis. N Engl J Med 1997;336(7):487–491.

Authors: Jacques H. Blanchet; Holley F. Allen

Dacryoadenitis

Clinical Presentation

SIGNS AND SYMPTOMS

- Sudden onset unilateral eyelid erythema
- Swelling and tenderness located in the temporal aspect of the upper lid under the orbital rim
- Ipsilateral conjunctival injection and chemosis
- Fever
- Tearing
- Discharge
- Moderately ill appearing, systemic toxicity
- Ipsilateral preauricular adenopathy
- Normal visual acuity, slitlamp and funduscopic exam

MECHANISM/DESCRIPTION

- Infection of lacrimal gland
- May occur secondary to contiguous spread from bacterial conjunctivitis or periorbital cellulitis

ETIOLOGY

- Uncommon infection, usually seen in children and young adults
- Acute suppurative
  - —In adults, bacteria most common cause
    - -*Staphylococcus aureus*
    - -*Streptococci*
    - -*Chlamydia trachomatis*
    - -*Neisseria gonorrhea*
- Chronic dacryoadenitis
  - —Slowly progressive painless swelling without systemic symptoms
  - —Viruses most common cause
    - -Mumps, measles (particularly in children)
    - -EBV
    - -CMV
    - -Coxsackie
    - -Varicella zoster
- Most diseases causing inflammation of the lacrimal gland are not infectious
  - —Autoimmune diseases
  - —Sjögren's syndrome
  - —Sarcoidosis
  - —Tumor
    - -25% of all lacrimal gland swelling

PEDIATRIC CONSIDERATIONS

- Viral—most common cause in children
  - —Mumps the most common
- Slowly enlarging mass may be a dermoid

Pre-Hospital

N/A

Diagnosis

ESSENTIAL WORKUP

- Complete eye exam including visual acuity, slitlamp, and funduscopic examination normal
- Determine the likelihood of Gonorrhea as the etiology
  - —High risk systemic illness and visual loss

LABS

- Gram stain/culture of drainage
  - —May identify the pathogen and guide therapy
- CBC
  - —WBC may be elevated

IMAGING/SPECIAL TESTS

- Radiographic studies not indicated for dacryoadenitis
- Orbital CT (if diagnosis unclear) to rule out orbital cellulitis, tumor or other etiology

DIFFERENTIAL DIAGNOSIS

- Autoimmune disease
- Lacrimal gland tumor
- Hordeolum
- Periorbital (preseptal) cellulitis
- Severe blepharitis
- Orbital cellulitis
- Acute conjunctivitis
- Acute dacryocystitis
- Insect bite
- Traumatic injury

Treatment

INITIAL STABILIZATION

- Rule out orbital cellulitis

ED TREATMENT

- Apply cool compresses to decrease inflammation and pain
- Antibiotics
  - —Oral (cephalexin, amoxicillin/clavulanate) for mild infection
  - —IV (cefazolin, Ticarcillin/clavulanate) for severe infection
- Analgesics
- Tetanus toxoid if necessary
- Incision and drainage rarely necessary except in very severe cases
  - —Perform with consultation to facial surgery service or ophthalmology

MEDICATIONS

- Amoxicillin/clavulanate (augmentin): 250–500 mg (peds: 20–40 mg of amoxicillin/kg/24hr) po q 8 hrs
- Cefazolin: 500–1000 mg (peds: 50–100 mg/kg/24hr) IV q 6–8 hrs
- Cephalexin: 250–500mg (peds: 25–100 gm/kg/24 hr) po qid
- Ticarcillin/clavulanate: 3.2 g (peds: 200–300 mg of ticarcillin/kg/24hrs) IV q 4–6 hrs

PEDIATRIC CONSIDERATIONS

- Viral most commonly etiology
  - —Treat with cold compresses and analgesics
- If etiology is unclear treat with antibiotics as with adults

Disposition

ADMISSION CRITERIA

- Acutely ill, toxic appearing
- Immunocompromised

DISCHARGE CRITERIA

- Well-appearing who can tolerate oral antibiotics

Miscellaneous

ICD9: 375.00

CORE CONTENT CODE: 6.4.1.5

SUGGESTED READINGS

Boruchoff SA, Boruchoff SE. Infections of the lacrimal system. Inf Dis Clin North Am 1992;6(4):925–933.

Cullom R. The Wills eye manual: Office and emergency room diagnosis and treatment of eye disease. Philadelphia: JB Lippincott, 1994:644.

Kanski JJ. Clinical ophthalmology. Oxford: Butterworth-Heinemann, 1994:66–69.

Rubin S, Hallagan L. Lids, lacrimals and lids. Emerg Med Clin North Am 1995;13(3):631–647.

Author: Shari Schabowski

Dacryocystitis

Clinical Presentation

SIGNS AND SYMPTOMS

- Unilateral, red, painful, swollen mass inferior and medial to the inner canthus
- Tearing or discharge
- Associated with cellulitis extending to the lower lid (may be extensive)
- Fever
- Nontoxic appearance

MECHANISM/DESCRIPTION

- Suppurative infection of the lacrimal sac which is located adjacent to the lacrimal duct near the inner canthus of the eye
- Under normal conditions, tears drain via pumping action at the lacrimal duct moving tears to the lacrimal sac and then to the middle turbinate into the sinuses
- Infection occurs when the duct becomes partially or completely obstructed
  —Resulting in stasis in this conduit and overgrowth of bacteria
- Infection may also occur secondary to trauma, a dacryolith or following nasal surgery or sinus surgery
- May be recurrent and may become chronic
- Complications include mucocele, fistula formation, corneal involvement, facial, periorbital or orbital cellulitis

ETIOLOGY

- Most common bacteria are ocular and sinus flora
- *Staphylococcus aureus*—most common organism in acquired acute dacryocystitis
- Most commonly occurs in infants and postmenopausal females

PEDIATRIC CONSIDERATIONS

- Congenital nasolacrimal obstruction due to stenosis occurs in approximately 2–4% of full term newborns and presents as acute dacryocystitis
- *Streptococcus pneumoniae* - most common organism in congenital dacryocystitis

Pre-Hospital

N/A

Diagnosis

ESSENTIAL WORKUP

- Expression of purulent material from the punctum when pressure is applied to the mass confirms the diagnosis
- Visual acuity, complete eye exam including; slitlamp and funduscopic exam

LABORATORY

- Gram stain, culture and sensitivity and chocolate agar plating of the expressed material
  —Helps direct specific antibiotic treatment
- Blood culture
  —For extensive cellulitis

IMAGING/SPECIAL TESTS

- Plain sinus radiographs when coexistent sinusitis suspected
- CT of orbit/sinus with recurrent cases where tumor may cause obstruction

DIFFERENTIAL DIAGNOSIS

- Periorbital (preseptal) cellulitis
- Acute ethmoid sinusitis
- Acute maxillary sinusitis
- Insect bite
- Traumatic injury
- Orbital cellulitis
- Acute conjunctivitis
- Acute blepharitis

Treatment

INITIAL STABILIZATION

Initial Approach and Immediate Concerns

- Confirm diagnosis by expressing purulent material
- Begin treatment to avoid extension of infection to adjacent structures
- Determine if symptoms are recurrent

ED TREATMENT

- Warm compresses and gentle massage to relieve the obstruction
- Facilitate outflow from the obstructed tract with nasal packing with local anesthetic and strong vasoconstrictor
- Topical ophthalmic antibiotic drops
- Systemic antibiotics to resolve infection and prevent spread to adjacent structures
  —Oral for mild infection
  —IV when febrile or severe infection
- Analgesics
- Incision and drainage in severe cases
- Duct instrumentation to facilitate drainage not indicated in acute setting (controversial)
  —Reserve instrumentation of the duct for the nonacute setting if necessary at all
  —Only 50% of adults show improvement after manipulation
  —Manipulation while the duct is inflamed may result in injury to the duct and permanent obstruction due to scarring and stenosis

MEDICATIONS

- Amoxicillin/clavulanate (augmentin): 250–500 mg (peds: 20–40 mg of amoxicillin /kg/24 hrs) po q 8 hrs
- Cefaclor: 20–40 mg/kg/24hr po q 8 hrs
- Cefazolin: 500–1000 mg (peds: 50–100 mg/kg/24hr) IV q 6–8 hrs
- Cefuroxime: 50–100 mg/kg/24 hrs IV q 8 hrs
- Cephalexin: 250–500mg (peds: 25–100 g/kg/24hrs) po qid
- Cocaine hydrochloride: 4% topical solution single-dose nasal spray
- Erythromycin ophthalmic ointment: 2 drops qid to affected eye
- Tetracaine and phenylephrine topical solution single-dose nasal spray
- Trimethaprim/polymyxin ointment: 2 drops qid to affected eye

PEDIATRIC CONSIDERATION

- Newborns respond well to massage and topical antibiotics in about 95% of cases
- If no resolution in the first year of life, may require probing of the duct by an ophthalmologist
- Children <4 years of age (particularly 6 months–2 years) who develop dacryocystitis
  —At increased risk for *Hemophilus influenza* infection (those who have not completed 2 HiB vaccinations)
  —*Hemophilus influenza B* carries a high risk of bacteremia, septicemia, and meningitis
  —Treat afebrile, well-appearing patient with a responsible parent with oral cefaclor or amoxicillin/clavulanate
  —Administer cefuroxime IV in acutely ill patient

Disposition

ADMISSION CRITERIA

- Adult
  —Febrile toxic appearing
  —Concomitant medical problems including diabetes or immunosuppression
  —Extensive cellulitis
  —Suspicion of adjacent spread with meningitis or orbital cellulitis
- Children
  —Acutely ill appearance
  —Concomitant medical problems
  —Extensive cellulitis
  —High risk of *Hemophilus influenza*
  —If reliable follow-up within 24 hours cannot be arranged

DISCHARGE CRITERIA

- Well-appearing healthy individual

Miscellaneous

ICD9: 375.30

CORE CONTENT CODE: 6.4.1.5

SUGGESTED READINGS

Boruchoff SA, Boruchoff SE. Infections of the lacrimal system. Infect Dis Clin North Am 1992;6(4):925–933.

Cullom R. The Wills eye manual: Office and emergency room diagnosis and treatment of eye disease. Philadelphia: JB Lippincott, 1994:644.

Kanski JJ. Clinical ophthalmology. Oxford: Butterworth-Heinemann, 1994:66–69.

Lueder GT. Neonatal dacryocystitis associated with nasolacrimal duct cysts. J Pediatr Ophthalmol Stabismus 1995;32(2):102–106.

Marx OL. Clinical bacteriology of dacryocystitis in adults. Ophthal Plast Reconstr Surg 1993;9(2):125–131.

Rubin S, Hallagan L. Lids, lacrimals and lids. Emerg Med Clin North Am 1995;13(3):631–647.

Author: Shari Schabowski

Decompression Sickness

Clinical Presentation

SIGNS AND SYMPTOMS

Cutaneous

- Scarlatiniform, erysipeloid or mottled rash
  —*Cutis marmorata*
- Peau d'orange appearance due to lymphatic obstruction

Musculoskeletal

- Pain
  —Classic "bends"
  —Dull, deep aching
  —Often in a joint (elbow and shoulder most common)
  —Not exacerbated by movement or reproduced with palpation
- No external physical signs

GI

- Nausea/vomiting
- Abdominal pain

Pulmonary

- Dyspnea
- "Chokes" = triad of
  —Substernal pressure
  —Cough
  —Dyspnea
  —Due to large bubbles in the pulmonary tree

CNS

- Weakness/fatigue
- Numbness/paresthesia
- Agitation
- Headache
- Dizzy
- Vertigo
- Convulsion
- Bowel/bladder incontinence
- Lethargy
- Visual disturbance
- "Staggers"
  —Vestibular system and the posterior column involvement

MECHANISM/DESCRIPTION

Henry's Law

- Amount of gas that will dissolve in a solution is directly proportional to the partial pressure of that gas
- Increases in partial pressure result in larger amount of gas dissolved in tissue
- Decreases in partial pressure result in gas coming out of solution

Dalton's Law

- Total pressure exerted by a mixture of gases is equal to the sum of the partial pressure of each of the component gases

Sequence

- Increases in ambient pressure cause an increase in partial pressure of nitrogen inspired
- Nitrogen accumulates in the tissues in higher and higher concentrations the longer pressures remain elevated
- Decompression Sickness (DCS) results when ambient pressure keeping nitrogen in solution decreases too rapidly on ascent, preventing gradual removal of the excess body burden of nitrogen
- As the nitrogen removal gradient is overwhelmed, tissues become supersaturated, and bubble formation occurs

ETIOLOGY

- Bubble location determines clinical effects
  —Blood flow obstruction and tissue ischemia from intravascular bubbles
  —Tissue distention and compression from interstitial bubbles
  —Compression of arterioles, nerves, and lymphatics
  —Endothelial damage leading to stimulation of coagulation and clotting cascades
  —Bubbles sensed as foreign by host defenses lead to the release of chemotactic and other factors
- Risk factors for DCS
  —Greater depth, longer bottom time, and quicker rate of ascent
  —Use of dive tables/computers does *not* eliminate DCS
  —Increased incidence with age and weight (body fat), hypothermia, dehydration, exercise, multiple dives in a day
- Airplane flight can precipitate DCS due to lower cabin pressure

Pre-Hospital

CONTROVERSIES

- "In water" recompression
  —Return injured diver/patient to a depth where symptoms are ameliorated
  —Extremely difficult
  —Need large amount of surface support
  —Use as last resort only

CAUTIONS

- Recognize DCS
  —Postdive extremity pain often attributed to a muscle strain
  —Serious neurological complaints often minimized because the diver does not consider DCS
- Time after surfacing to presentation of DCS
  —50%—symptoms within 1 hour
  —95%—symptoms within 12 hours
  —60% of neurologic DCS within 10 minutes

Diagnosis

ESSENTIAL WORKUP

- Clinical diagnosis: recognize risk factors and clinical presentation
- Trial of pressure
  - —Rapid relief of symptoms upon recompression in a hyperbaric chamber may be the only way to diagnose DCS

LABORATORY

- CBC
  - —Increased Hct due to hemoconcentration
- Electrolytes, BUN, Cr, glucose
- Urinalysis
- ABG/pulse oximetry
  - —Monitor oxygenation

IMAGING

- CXR
  - —Concomitant pulmonary barotrauma
  - —Aspiration pneumonia
- Head CT when altered mental status

DIFFERENTIAL DIAGNOSIS

- Musculoskelatal injury unrelated to bubble formation
- Inner or middle ear barotrauma
- Arterial gas embolism
- CVA

Treatment

INITIAL STABILIZATION

- ABCs
- Provide normobaric (100%) oxygen via mask or ETT
  - —Increases inert gas (nitrogen) elimination from the tissues reducing gas bubble size
  - —Increases oxygen delivery to the injured tissue
- Early recompression in hyperbaric chamber

ED TREATMENT

- IV rehydration with 0.9%NS
  - —Diver usually dehydrated due to diuretic effect of pressure, exercise, breathing dry compressed air
  - —Increased fluid assists with offgassing and dissolution of nitrogen
- Hyperbaric oxygen recompression therapy (see Hyperbaric Oxygen Therapy Chapter)
  - —For all DCS except for cutaneous
  - —Arrange transportation to nearest hyperbaric facility
  - —Aircraft capable of full pressurization of flight below 1000 feet are best suited for transfers
  - —Prophylactic chest tube for simple pneumothorax to prevent conversion to tension pneumothorax
  - —Fill endotracheal and Foley catheter balloons with water or saline to avoid shrinkage/damage during recompression
- Divers Alert Network (DAN)
  - —Based at Duke University Medical Center
  - —Provides a 24-hour emergency hotline for medical consultation on the treatment of dive-related injuries and for referrals to hyperbaric chambers
  - —Telephone 919-684-8111

Disposition

ADMISSION CRITERIA

- Refer all patients with suspected or diagnosis DCS for hyperbaric therapy

DISCHARGE CRITERIA

- Patients not requiring hyperbaric treatment
- Stable patients with mild symptoms may be discharged post-HBO treatment
- Air travel may exacerbate symptoms as ambient pressure decreases

Miscellaneous

ICD9: 993.3

CORE CONTENT CODE: N/A

SUGGESTED READINGS

Bartlett RB. Diving emergencies in critical decisions in emergency medicine. Vol 10. Num 10. Lesson 20. Dallas, TX, American College of Emergency Physicians, 1997.

Kizer KW. Scuba diving and dysbarism. In: Auerbach PA, ed. Wilderness medicine. 3rd ed. St. Louis: CV Mosby, 1995:1176–1208.

Madsen J, Hink J, Hyldegaard O. Diving physiology and pathophysiology. Clin Physiol 1994;14:597–626.

Moon RE, Vann RD, Bennett PB. The physiology of decompression illness. Sci Am 1995;(Aug) pg 70–77.

Author: Jeffrey Gordon

Deep Vein Thrombosis (DVT)

Clinical Presentation

SIGNS AND SYMPTOMS

- Gradual onset of pain
- Swelling and a sense of fullness of the involved extremity
- Swelling
  - —Greater than 1 cm circumferential difference in legs is significant
- Tenderness on compression of the calf
- Warmth
- Palpation of a "cord"
- Painful white leg
  - —Phlegmasia alba dolens
- Painful blue leg
  - —Phlegmasia cerulea dolens

MECHANISM/DESCRIPTION

- Clot formation in the deep veins of the extremities or pelvis
  - —Clot is formed when clot promoting forces overpower clot dissolving forces
  - —The clot may be septic or bland
- Increased interstitial pressure leads to hypoperfusion creating blanching and, ultimately, cyanosis, resulting in phlegmasia alba dolens or phlegmasia cerulea dolens
- Deep vein thrombosis (DVT) is part of a systemic process better known as venous thromboembolism
- The most significant complication: pulmonary embolism (PE) from which an estimated 60,000 Americans die annually
- 2 million cases of DVT occur in the USA annually
- Recurrence of either DVT or PE occurs in 5–8% of patients within 3 months and in 20% by 2 years
- Postthrombotic syndrome occurs in 30% of patients

ETIOLOGY

- Hypercoagulable states
  - —Cancer
  - —Nephrotic syndrome
  - —Sepsis
  - —Inflammatory conditions such as ulcerative colitis
  - —Increased estrogen (pregnancy, oral contraceptives)
  - —Various protein (S, C, and antithrombin 3) deficiencies
- Stasis
  - —Prolonged bedrest
  - —Immobility from a cast
  - —Long plane or train ride
  - —Neurologic disorders with paralysis
  - —Congestive heart failure
  - —Obesity
- Vascular damage
  - —Trauma
  - —Surgery
  - —Central lines
- Multifactorial issues
  - —Advancing age and prior thromboembolism

Pre-Hospital

- Immediate stabilization is not needed
- Intravenous access and supplemental oxygen if associated with chest pain or shortness of breath

Diagnosis

ESSENTIAL WORKUP

- No blood test confirms or excludes DVT with certainty. Because clinical examination is unreliable for diagnosing DVT, imaging studies are necessary

LABORATORY

- D-dimer
  - —Rarely indicated as imaging studies most often make the diagnosis
  - —Measured by the ELISA technique (and not by latex agglutination)
  - —The absence of D-dimer in the blood is strong, but not definitive, evidence against the presence of thromboembolism
  - —The presence of D-dimer is very nonspecific

IMAGING/SPECIAL TESTS

- Contrast venography
  - —Historic gold standard
  - —Accurate but invasive, expensive, associated with dye reactions and can precipitate phlebitis
- Impedance plethysmography is rarely used since the advent of duplex scanning
- Ultrasound (duplex scanning)
  - —The combination of color Doppler and B-mode ultrasound
  - —Rapid, inexpensive, and highly accurate in detecting proximal clot
  - —The initial procedure of choice

DIFFERENTIAL DIAGNOSIS

- Superficial DVT
- Cellulitis
- Torn muscles and ligaments
- Ruptured Baker's cyst
- Bilateral edema
  - —Heart, kidney, or liver disease
  - —Rarely caused by DVT
- Causes of unilateral edema that can lead to DVT
  - —Abdominal mass
    - -Gravid uterus or tumor
  - —Lymphedema
- Postphlebitic syndrome

Treatment

INITIAL STABILIZATION

- Most patients with DVT do not require immediate stabilization
- When phlegmasia alba dolens or phlegmasia cerulea dolens are present, rapid intervention is needed
  —Fluid resuscitation
  —Immediate anticoagulation
  —Thrombolysis or surgical thrombectomy

ED TREATMENT

Proximal DVT

- Anticoagulation
  —Intravenous heparin
  —Low molecular-weight heparin (LMWH)
    -Enoxapirin
    -Laboratory monitoring is unnecessary
- Caval interruption with a filter
  —Patients with an absolute contraindication to anticoagulation
    -Active internal bleeding, uncontrolled hypertension, significant recent trauma or surgery, and CNS tumor
  —Recurrent thromboembolism despite documented adequate anticoagulation
    -APTT of ≥1.5 times control for heparinized patients
    -INR of ≥2 for warfarinized patients
- Treatment of distal DVT remains controversial

MEDICATIONS

- Heparin: 80 IU/kg bolus followed by a drip of 18 IU/kg/hr; APTT should be checked in 6 hrs and the infusion rate adjusted accordingly
- Enoxaparin: 30 mg SQ bid
- Warfarin: 10 mg po can be started on the first day of heparin or LMWH

Disposition

ADMISSION CRITERIA

- Admit all patients for initiation of anticoagulation

DISCHARGE CRITERIA

- Patients with distal DVT and in patients with a very high clinical suspicion but with an initially negative ultrasound
  —Follow as an outpatient and restudy in 3–5 days

Miscellaneous

ICD9: 451, 451.0, 451.1, 451.2

CORE CONTENT CODE: 2.5.2.3

SUGGESTED READINGS

Hirsh J, Hoak J. Management of DVT and PE. Circulation 1996;93:2212–2245.

Levine M, et al. A comparison of LMWH administered primarily at home with unfractionated heparin administered in the hospital for proximal DVT. N Engl J Med 1996;334:677–681.

Pearson SP, et al. A critical pathway to evaluate suspected DVT. Arch Intern Med 1995;155:1773–1778.

Author: Jonathan Edlow

Defibrillators, Implantable

Clinical Presentation

SIGNS AND SYMPTOMS

Infectious

- Local infection
  - —Warmth
  - —Erythema
  - —Pain
  - —Fluctuance
- Spreading infection
  - —Fever
  - —Leukocytosis
  - —Elevated erythrocyte sedimentation rate (ESR)

Vascular

- Axillary or subclavian vein thrombosis, with unilateral upper extremity edema
- Rarely, *superior vena cava (SVC) syndrome*
- Tachypnea, tachycardia, hypoxia, and pleuritic chest pain due to *pulmonary emboli*

Lead/Device Related

- Premature battery depletion or mal-sensing by defibrillator due to erosion of lead insulation or lead fracture
- Undersensing by the internal cardiac defibrillators (ICD) observed with lead fracture or battery depletion may lead to untreated ventricular arrhythmias

Sensing Related

- Oversensing by ICDs of pacemaker spikes in patients with permanent pacemakers, supraventricular arrhythmias, and T waves as the QRS complex have all resulted in inappropriate delivery of shocks

Therapy (Shock) Related

- Shock or after multiple shocks
- Acute cardiac arrest

Implantation Site Related

- Pocket *seroma* and *hematoma*
  - —Noninfectious causes of swelling around the implantation site

MECHANISM/DESCRIPTION

- Cardiac defibrillators (ICDs) are being implanted in increasing numbers
  - —Low morbidity associated with implanting and testing
  - —Small size
  - —Ability to prevent death due to life-threatening arrhythmias
- Newer generations of ICDs are more complex and are beyond the scope of most emergency room personnel

ETIOLOGY

- Infection
  - —*Staphylococcus aureus* (most aggressive)
  - —*Staphylococcus epidermidis* (more indolent)
  - —*Escherichia coli*
  - —*Pseudomonas spp.* and *Streptococcal spp.* (less common) are found in 1–7% of cases
- Vascular related
  - —Venous thrombosis/embolism secondary to stenosis as a result of the ICD lead(s)
- Lead/device related
  - —ICD leads are subject to the same long-term problems that are associated with pacemaker leads (i.e., lead dislodgment, insulation breakdown)
  - —Newer generation ICDs generally last 5–8 years, depending on the frequency of delivered therapies, the need for back up pacing, and lead integrity
- Sensing related
  - —Erroneous sensing of supraventricular tachyarrhythmias as ventricular
  - —Lead fractures can result in body motion artifact to be sensed as ventricular arrhythmias
- Therapy (shock) related
  - —Patients with ICDs can have cardiac ischemic syndromes and present with unstable angina, MI, or intractable arrhythmias
  - —Antiarrhythmic drugs and electrolyte abnormalities can be proarrhythmic

Pre-Hospital

CAUTIONS

- Apply standard ACLS protocols during cardiac arrest situations
  - —External defibrillation may be necessary
- Deactivation of ICD
  - —Averts inappropriate firing of the unit
  - —All units may be temporarily inhibited from firing while a magnet is positioned over the pulse generator
- Avoid magnetic fields because they can deactivate ICDs
- Search for Medic-Alert tags

Diagnosis

ESSENTIAL WORKUP

Infection

- CBC
- Blood cultures
- Erythrocyte sedimentation rate (ESR)
- CXR
- ECG
- Seroma and hematoma are a diagnosis of exclusion
  - —Do not aspirate routinely ICD pockets
    - -May lead to infection

Vascular Related

- Vascular ultrasound with Doppler for suspected superior vena cava syndrome
- Ventilation/perfusion (V/Q) scan for pulmonary embolus

Lead/Device Related

- CXR for lead fracture
- *Interrogation* of the unit by a cardiologist/electrophysiologist
  - —Suspected battery depletion will also be confirmed by interrogation

Sensing/Therapy (Shock) Related

- Cardiac monitor
  - —Diagnosis of an inappropriately diagnosed and treated supraventricular tachyarrhythmia can be difficult unless the patient experiences an episode while being monitored
- Careful history to elicit whether the patient was experiencing symptoms related to arrhythmia or whether the therapy was received during normal physical activity (i.e., sinus tachycardia)
- Interrogation of the unit's stored memory (requires a cardiologist/electrophysiologist)
- Electrolytes
- Obtain antiarrhythmic drug history
  - —Potential drug interactions yielding an acquired long QT syndrome
- ECG/CPK
  - —Transient ST segment changes and elevations of the cardiac enzymes may be seen after shock delivery and does not necessarily indicate myocardial damage

DIFFERENTIAL DIAGNOSIS

- Infectious versus noninfectious

Treatment

INITIAL STABILIZATION

- ABCs
- Institute ACLS protocol for life-threatening dysrhythmia
- Place on monitor with defibrillator
- IV access
- Consult with a qualified cardiologist/electrophysiologist for ICD-related problems

ED TREATMENT

Infection

- After obtaining appropriate cultures (do not aspirate material from ICD pocket) administer parenteral antibiotics (vancomycin)
- Consult with a cardiologist regarding unit removal
- Seroma and hematoma—prophylactic therapy with antibiotics remains controversial

Vascular Related

- Venous thrombosis
  - —Rarely embolic to the upper extremities and does not require anticoagulation
  - —Conservative therapy with warm packs usually sufficient
  - —Some authorities institute therapy with heparin and coumadin to prevent further extension and possible embolic events

Lead/Device Related

- Suspected lead-related problems require consultation with a qualified cardiologist/electrophysiologist or surgeon with lead/device extraction experience
- Patients with nonfunctioning ICDs (lead- or device-related) need external defibrillator pads and close monitoring at all times

Therapy Related

- Repeated firing necessitates prompt interrogation of the unit by a cardiologist
  - —Appropriate ICD therapies
    - -Patients' arrhythmias need prompt intervention, i.e., treatment of ischemia, institution of antiarrhythmic therapy, and correction of electrolyte disturbances
  - —Inappropriate ICD therapies
    - -May warrant temporary deactivation with a magnet and close monitoring, until the unit can be reprogrammed

Other

- Magnetic resonance imaging (MRI) contraindicated
  - —Magnetic field may disable ICDs
- Electrocautery should generally be avoided

MEDICATIONS

- Cefazolin: 1g IV q 8 hrs
- Vancomycin: 1 g IV q 12 hrs

Disposition

ADMISSION CRITERIA

Infection

- Admission for intravenous antibiotics and hardware removal/revision

Noninfectious

- Expanding pocket hematoma with skin tension needs admission for pocket exploration and hemostasis to avoid pressure skin necrosis

Lead/Device Related

- Admission for lead and device interrogation

Sensing Related (Undersensing)

- Patients presenting with a symptomatic dysrhythmia not recognized/treated by the ICD need to be admitted

Therapy Related

- Defer to the cardiologist who interrogates the unit for disposition
- Patients experiencing ICD therapy and not feeling up to his or her baseline, should be admitted

DISCHARGE CRITERIA

Noninfectious

- Pocket seroma and hematoma need regular inspection but can be discharged

Sensing related (Oversensing)

- May discharge after cardiologist/electrophysiologist interrogates and reprograms the ICD

Therapy Related

- A patient who has experienced an appropriate ICD shock for symptomatic arrhythmia and who feels well may be discharged after consultation with patient's cardiologist/electrophysiologist

Miscellaneous

ICD9: N/A

CORE CONTENT CODE: 2.11.4

SUGGESTED READINGS

Davidson T, VanRiper S, Harper P, Wenk A. Implantable cardioverter defibrillators: a guide for clinicians. Heart Lung 1994;23(3):205–215.

Pfeiffer D, Jung W, Fehske W, et al. Complications of pacemaker-defibrillator devices: diagnosis and management. Am Heart J 1994;127(42):1073–1080.

Pinski S, Troman R. Implantable cardioverter-defibrillators: implications for the non-electrophysiologist. Ann Intern Med 1995;122(10):770–777.

White R, Feldman R. The automatic internal cardioverter defibrillator (AICD): description and guidelines for interaction during cardiac arrest. Ann Emerg Med 1989;18(5):586–588.

Authors: Robert Sidman; Larry Rosenthal

Delirium

Clinical Presentation

SIGNS AND SYMPTOMS

- Disturbed consciousness
- Reduced awareness of the environment
- Difficulties in focusing, shifting, and maintaining attention
  - —Restlessness
  - —Distractibility
  - —Lability
- From hyperactive to comatose
- Cognitive changes
  - —Disorientation
  - —Impaired memory
  - —Disorganized thinking and speech
  - —Misperceptions, illusions, delusions, and hallucinations
- Time course
  - —Hours to days
  - —Fluctuates daily
  - —Disturbed sleep/wake cycle

MECHANISM/DESCRIPTION

- Acute change in global cerebral functioning
  - —Diffuse derangements of cerebral acetylcholine
    - -Memory impairment and sedation
  - —Excess of dopamine neurotransmitter systems
    - -Hyperactivity, agitation, and delusional perceptions
- Waxing and waning arousal and attention
- Attendant hyperactivity or hypoactivity
- Delirium is caused by an underlying medical condition

ETIOLOGY

- Life threats
  - —Withdrawal from barbiturates
  - —Wernicke's encephalopathy
  - —Hypoxia and hypoperfusion of the brain
  - —Hypertensive crisis
  - —Hypoglycemia
  - —Hyper/hypothermia
  - —Intracranial bleed or mass
  - —Meningitis/encephalitis
  - —Poisoning/medications
  - —Status epilepticus
- General categories of disorders causing delirium
  - —Medications
  - —Drug abuse
    - -Intoxication
    - -Withdrawal
  - —Metabolic abnormalities
  - —CNS pathology
  - —Hypoxemia
  - —Vitamin deficiencies
  - —Endocrinopathies
  - —Infections
  - —Toxins
  - —Collagen vascular illnesses

Pre-Hospital

CAUTIONS

- Intravenous access
- Glucose measurement or empiric dextrose administration
- Narcan if associated respiratory insufficiency
- Monitor patient
- Look for signs of an underlying cause
  - —Medications
  - —Medic alert bracelets
- Document a basic neurologic examination
  - —GCS
  - —Pupils
  - —Extremity movements

Diagnosis

ESSENTIAL WORKUP

- Vital signs and physical examination
- Neurologic examination with careful attention to the changes in mental status
- Ancillary studies to determine the underlying cause

LABORATORY

- Electrolytes
- BUN and creatinine
- Glucose
- CBC
- Toxicology screens
- Further studies based on signs and symptoms
  - —Arterial blood gases
  - —Liver functions tests
  - —Calcium
  - —Magnesium

IMAGING/SPECIAL TESTS

- Electrocardiogram
- Head CT scan
- Lumbar puncture

DIFFERENTIAL DIAGNOSIS

- Psychiatric illness
  - —Dementia
  - —Mania
  - —Catatonic or severe undifferentiated schizophrenia
  - —Conversion reactions

Treatment

INITIAL STABILIZATION

- Chemical sedation in severely agitated patients
  - —Neuroleptics
    - -Haloperidol or droperidol
  - —Benzodiazepines
    - -If withdrawal is likely
    - -Lorazepam

ED TREATMENT

- Diagnosis and treatment of the underlying medical condition
- Thiamine should be administered in all alcoholic and malnourished patients
- Mildly agitated patients
  - —Oral neuroleptics or benzodiazepines
    - -Alprazolam, diazepam, or lorazepam orally
- Moderately agitated patients
  - —Parenteral haloperidol or droperidol with or without adjunctive lorazepam
  - —Intravenous use preferred if multiple doses are needed
- Severely agitated patients with life-threatening crises
  - —Parenteral use of anesthetic
  - —Consider paralytic agents

MEDICATIONS

- Alprazolam: 0.25–0.5 mg po
- Diazepam: 2.5–5 mg po
- Haloperidol: 5–10 mg IV/IM
- Droperidol: 2.5–5 mg IV/IM
- Lorazepam: 0.5–2 mg IV/IM/PO
- Naloxone: 0.01 mg/kg or 0.4–2.0 mg or more IV/IM/SC/ET
- Thiamine: 100 mg IV/IM/PO

Disposition

ADMISSION CRITERIA

- Based on the severity of the medical condition causing the delirium

DISCHARGE CRITERIA

- Treatable cause of the delirium reverses
- The patient's mental status clears while in the emergency department

Miscellaneous

ICD9: 780.09

CORE CONTENT CODE: 14.8.1

SUGGESTED READINGS

Levine RL. Pharmacology of intravenous sedatives and opioids in critically ill patients. Crit Care Clin 1994;10(4):709–731.

Lewis LM, Miller DK, Morley JE, Nork MJ, Lasater LC. Unrecognized delirium in ED geriatric patients. Am J Emerg Med 1995;13(2):142–145.

Lipowski ZJ. Update on delirium. Psychiatr Clin North Am 1992;15:335.

Murray GB. Confusion, delirium, and dementia. In: Cassem NH, ed. Handbook of general hospital psychiatry. 3rd ed. St. Louis: Mosby-Year Book, 1991:89–120.

Trzepacz PT. The neuropathogenesis of delirium: A need to focus our research. Psychosomatics 1994;35:374.

Author: Arthur Sanders

Delivery, Uncomplicated

Clinical Presentation

SIGNS AND SYMPTOMS

- True labor manifests as contractions occurring at least every 5 minutes, and lasting 30–60 seconds. Labor also frequently causes low back pain, and can occasionally present as isolated lower back pain
- Signs of imminent delivery include a fully effaced and dilated cervix (approximately 10 cm in a term infant), palpable fetal parts in the pelvic floor, bulging of the perineum, and widening of the vulvovaginal area
- Labor is not normally associated with significant vaginal bleeding. Symptoms of labor with vaginal bleeding in the third trimester demands immediate assessment for placenta previa or placental abruption

ETIOLOGY

- Delivery in the Emergency Department is relatively rare and is most often associated with one or more of these factors
  —The multiparous patient with a history of prior rapid labor
  —The nulliparous young patient who has not recognized the symptoms of labor
  —Patients with lack of transportation, lack of prenatal care, or premature labor

Pre-Hospital

- Pregnant patients in labor should be placed in the left lateral recumbent position
- EMS personnel should be adequately trained, and have proper equipment available for delivery
- Studies have shown that transport of high risk obstetric patients *before delivery* results in lower neonatal morbidity and mortality, and is faster and less expensive compared to transportation of the neonate after delivery
- The use of air transport for obstetric patients has been shown to be safe and effective
  —If altitude during flight can result in hypoxia for the compromised fetus, pregnant patients should be placed on supplemental oxygen

Diagnosis

ESSENTIAL WORKUP

- The bimanual pelvic exam is the most useful test to assess the presence of labor and the possibility of imminent delivery
  —Dilation and effacement of the cervix and station of the fetus should be noted
  —Bimanual exam should *not* be done in the presence of vaginal bleeding until ultrasound can rule out placenta previa
- Fetal heart tones should be obtained by Doppler

LABORATORY

- If patient is in active labor, CBC, blood typing, and Rh screen should be sent if this information is not already known
- Urinalysis if there is concern for preeclampsia or UTI

IMAGING/SPECIAL TESTS

- Imaging studies are not needed for uncomplicated vaginal deliveries
- Third-trimester vaginal bleeding should have emergent ultrasound to evaluate for placenta previa or placental abruption

DIFFERENTIAL DIAGNOSIS

- "Braxton Hicks" contractions
  —Presents as *irregular* uterine contractions that do not result in dilation or effacement
- Round uterine ligament pain
- Muscular low back pain
- Other causes of abdominal pain including appendicitis, nephrolithiasis, etc

Treatment

INITIAL STABILIZATION

- *Immediate pelvic exam* to assess for cervical dilation, effacement, or presenting parts
- Patients in active labor should be transferred to Labor and Delivery immediately unless delivery is imminent
- If the patient is completely dilated and fetal parts are on the perineal verge, prepare for ED delivery

ED TREATMENT

- The obstetrician should be notified that delivery will be occurring in the Emergency Department
- If the patient is high-risk or less than 36 weeks gestational age, the pediatrician or neonatologist and NICU should be notified
- Begin IV saline and supplemental oxygen, and place patient in lithotomy position
- Assemble bulb syringe, 2 sterile Kelly clamps, sterile Mayo scissors, and an umbilical clamp (usually part of an "OB pack")
  —Neonatal resuscitative equipment should also be available
- If time permits sterilize vaginal area with betadine
- Uncomplicated vaginal delivery should occur as follows
  —As crowning occurs *deliver the head in a controlled fashion,* guiding it through the introitus with each contraction
  —Routine episiotomy is not necessary, however, if the perineum is tearing perform a midline episiotomy by placing two fingers behind the perineum and make a straight incision toward (but not including) the rectum with sterile Mayo scissors
  —After the fetal head is delivered, quickly suction the nasopharynx, then feel around the neck for a nuchal cord. If present, manually reduce over the head. If the nuchal cord is too tight, double clamp, cut the cord, and deliver the infant immediately
  —Apply gentle downward pressure on the fetal head with uterine contractions, and after delivery of the anterior shoulder, the posterior shoulder and remainder of the infant will rapidly deliver
  —After delivery, the infant should be held at the level of the uterus and the oropharynx suctioned again
  —Double clamp the cord with sterile Kelly clamps and cut between them
  —The infant should be stimulated, warmed, and dried. If cyanosis is present, the infant should be given oxygen and resuscitated
  —The placenta will spontaneously deliver in 20–30 minutes and the mother should be observed closely as this is a potentially dangerous time because of postpartum hemorrhage

—Uterine massage can aid in the separation of the placenta from the uterus, and limit uterine atony. *Avoid placing traction on the umbilical cord* as this can lead to inversion of the uterus or rupture of the cord
—If the patient has severe bleeding and the placenta is not passing spontaneously, the patient should be taken to the operating room immediately
—After delivery of the placenta, it should be examined for any irregular or "torn" areas suggestive of retained placental products
—If bleeding persists after delivery of the placenta, continue uterine massage. If necessary, give oxytocin IV and examine for lacerations. If atony appears to be the cause of bleeding, administer methergine IM. If bleeding is still not controlled, IM hemabate can be repeated every 15–60 minutes. The obstetrician and operating room should be notified of continuous bleeding and the need for possible surgical intervention

MEDICATIONS

- Hemabate: 0.25 mg IM (250 µg)
- Methergine: 0.2 mg IM
- Oxytocin: 20 or 40 IU in 1 L of crystalloid; infuse at 200–500 cc/hr

Disposition

ADMISSION CRITERIA

- All women with uncomplicated deliveries and no significant postpartum bleeding should be admitted to Labor and Delivery or the postpartum unit for care and monitoring
- All infants with respiratory distress, gestational age less than 36 weeks, weight less than 5 pounds or low Apgar scores should have immediate pediatric or neonatal consultation and be admitted to neonatal intensive care unit
- Term infants with none of the above complications may be admitted to the nursery or with the mother to a combined maternal-fetal unit

DISCHARGE CRITERIA

- Adequate recovery from delivery

Miscellaneous

ICD9: 650.0

CORE CONTENT CODE: 12.4, 12.6(1–4), 23.4.2.2

SUGGESTED READINGS

Druelinger. L. Postpartum emergencies. Emerg Med Clin North Am 1994;12:219–225.

Gianopoulos JG. Emergency complications of labor and delivery. Emerg Med Clin North Am 1994;12:201–217.

Doan-Wiggins L. Emergency Childbirth. In: Roberts J, Hedges J, eds. Clinical procedures in emergency medicine. Philadelphia: WB Saunders, 1991. 2nd ed. 903-927.

Parer JT. Effects of hypoxia on the mother and fetus with emphasis on maternal air transport. Am J Obstet Gynecol 1982;142:957–961.

Zlatnik FJ. Normal labor and delivery and its conduct. In: Scott J, et al., eds. Danforth's obstetrics and gynecology. 6th ed. 1990.

Authors: S. Brent Barnes; James S. Walker

Dementia

Clinical Presentation

SIGNS AND SYMPTOMS

- Gradual progression of the signs and symptoms
  - —Stage of the underlying dementia frequently deteriorates after an acute illness
- Multiple cognitive deficits including memory impairment; and at least one of the following
  - —Apraxia
  - —Aphasia
  - —Agnosia
  - —Disturbance of executive functioning memory impairment
- Memory disorder
  - —Common initial presentation
  - —Usually for recent events
  - —May appear later in the progression of the disease
- New information encoding impaired
- Remote recall impaired in more progressive disease
- Anomia or poor word list generation
- Paraphasia
- Fluent aphasia
- Poor constructions
- Spatial disorientation
- Irritability
- Indifference
- Apathy
- Aggressive behavior
- Restlessness
- Pacing
- Urinary or fecal incontinence (in later stages)

MECHANISM/DESCRIPTION

- Decline in cognition
  - —Frequently insidious and gradual
- Impairment of independence and daily functioning
- Deficits in memory, speech or language, visuospatial function, higher cognition, and, at times, personality and mood but without impairment of consciousness
- Prevalence of dementia varies according to the criteria used to define the diagnosis
- Range of prevalence is 5–8% in patients over age 65, 15–20% in patients over the age of 75, and 25–50% in patients over 85
- Types of dementias
  - —Alzheimer's disease: 50–75%
  - —Mixed Alzheimer's disease and vascular dementia: 10–15%
  - —Pure vascular: 10–15%

ETIOLOGY

- Secondary to medical illness
- Alzheimer's disease
- Vascular dementia
- Reversible types of dementia
  - —Normal pressure hydrocephalus
  - —Vitamin B_{12} deficiency
  - —Metabolic disturbances

Pre-Hospital

N/A

Diagnosis

ESSENTIAL WORKUP

- All of the testing may be within normal parameters
  - —Must eliminate the possibility of an underlying or superimposed disease process that may resolve or improve the impairment

LABORATORY

- Selected on the basis of history and physical examination that point toward a specific etiology of the patient's cognitive decline
- Full battery of routine blood tests include
  - —CBC
  - —ESR
  - —Electrolytes, BUN/Cr, glucose
  - —Liver function tests
  - —Vitamin B_{12} and folate
  - —Serology tests
    - -Syphilis
    - -HIV
  - —Urinalysis
  - —Thyroid screening
  - —Toxicology screens for drugs either prescribed or illicit
  - —Heavy metals if indicated

IMAGING/SPECIAL TESTS

- CT brain
  - —Not diagnostic
  - —Indicated in patients with rapid decline or unusual presentation
  - —Useful in eliminating confounding presentations (e.g., subdural hematoma, normal pressure hydrocephalus, tumor, or stroke)

DIFFERENTIAL DIAGNOSIS

- Alzheimer's disease
- Vascular dementia
- Binswanger's disease
- AIDS dementia complex
- Frontal lobe dementia
- Parkinson's disease
- Huntington's disease
- Hydrocephalic dementia
- Trauma
- Delirium
- Toxic conditions
- Metabolic disorders
- Tumor
- Depression

Treatment

INITIAL STABILIZATION

- Administer naloxone, dextrose (or Accucheck), and thiamine for altered mental status
- Determine the acute problem that exacerbates the underlying symptoms of dementia

ED TREATMENT

- Differentiate the acute problem from the chronic symptoms and treat the acute illness aggressively
  - —Infections
    - -Urinary tract infection
    - -Pneumonia
    - -Upper respiratory infection
    - -Cellulitis
    - -Meningitis
  - —Cardiac illness
    - -Silent MI
    - -Arrhythmia
  - —CNS event
    - -Stroke
    - -TIA
    - -Delirium
- Treat agitation, irritability and aggressive behavior with
  - —Low-dose antidepressants (trazodone, nefazodone, SSRI)
  - —Anticonvulsants (valproic acid, carbamazepine, neurontin)
  - —Neuroleptics (haloperidol, thiothixene, clozapine)
- Treat psychosis with hallucinations and delusions with
  - —Very low-dose neuroleptics (risperdal, haloperidol, thiothixene, clozapine)
  - —Especially in cases of Parkinson's disease and Lewy body disease
- Anxiety
  - —Use benzodiazepines cautiously
    - -Often disorient the patient (paradoxical reaction in dementia)
- Depression
  - —When superimposed, aggressive treatment often reverses dementia

Medication Guidelines

- Discontinue any noncritical medications
- Avoid and eliminate anticholinergic medications
  - —Can exacerbate symptoms of dementia
- Administer all medications at the lowest possible dose and slowly increase to avoid side effects and overmedicating the patient
  - —Patients with dementia are more sensitive to the effects of medication
- Consider starting donepezil and/or vitamin E as an outpatient

Expected Course and Prognosis

- Dementia is a slow, progressive, deteriorating course of decline in cognitive functioning which leads to eventual physical decline and inability to care for oneself
- 7–10 years after diagnosis is the expected longevity

Disposition

ADMISSION CRITERIA

- Acute deterioration of preexisting dementia
- Unknown diagnosis for change in mental status
- Underlying medical causes resulting in acute deterioration necessitating hospital admission

DISCHARGE CRITERIA

- Stable signs and symptoms of dementia without acute symptoms

Miscellaneous

ICD9: 294.8

CORE CONTENT CODE: 14.8.2

SUGGESTED READINGS

Cassem NH, Bernstein JG. Depressed patients. In: Cassem NH, et al., eds. Handbook of general hospital psychiatry. 4th ed. St. Louis: Mosby-Yearbook, 1997:35–68.

Cassem NH, Murray GB. Delirious patients. In: Cassem NH, et al., eds. Handbook of general hospital psychiatry. 4th ed. St. Louis: Mosby-Yearbook, 1997:101–122.

Devanand DP, Jacobs DM, Tang MX, et al. The course of psychopathologic features in mild to moderate Alzheimer's disease. Arch Gen Psychiatry 1997;54:257–263.

Goff DC, Henderson DC, Manschreck TC. Psychotic patients. In: Cassem NH, et al., eds. Handbook of general hospital psychiatry. 4th ed. St. Louis: Mosby-Yearbook, 1997:149–172.

Martin RL, ed. Geriatric psychiatry: what's new about the old. Psychiatr Clin North Am 1997;20(1):1–268.

Sano M, Ernesto C, Thomas RG, et al. A controlled trial of selegiline, alpha-tocopherol, or both as treatments for Alzheimer's disease. N Engl J Med 1997;336:1216–1222.

Work Group on Alzheimer's Disease and Related Dementias. Practice guideline for the treatment of patients with Alzheimer's disease and other dementias of late life. Am J Psychiatry 1997;154(Suppl):1–39.

Author: M. Cornelia Cremens

Dental Trauma

Clinical Presentation

SIGNS AND SYMPTOMS

- History of facial trauma
- Facial pain
  - —Tooth
  - —Jaw
  - —Ear
  - —Throat
- Exacerbating factors
  - —Chewing
  - —Drinking
  - —Extremes of temperature
- Pain on palpation
- Facial swelling
- Loose or avulsed tooth
- Oral or facial laceration

MECHANISM/DESCRIPTION

- Ellis classification
  - —Class I fracture
    - -Only involves the enamel
    - -Fracture line appears chalky white
    - -Painless to percussion
  - —Class II fracture
    - -Involves the enamel and dentin
    - -Ivory/yellow appearance
    - -Sensitive to cold
  - —Class III fracture
    - -Involves enamel, dentin, and pulp
    - -Exquisitely painful or desensitized
    - -Pinkish blush of blood after wiping the tooth
- Alveolar bone fractures
- Associated with dental fractures, avulsions, or subluxations
- Anterior overbite makes this part of dentition more susceptible to fractures in children
- With avulsed teeth, a 1% chance for successful reimplantation is lost every minute

ETIOLOGY

- Isolated injuries
- Fall
- Athletic
- Event
- Assault
- Laryngoscopy
- Childhood activities
- Child abuse
- Multiple trauma

Pre-Hospital

- Maintain a patent airway
- Account for all teeth
- Immediate reimplantation of tooth if possible
- Otherwise place in a transport solution
  - —Hanks solution (TPS—"tooth preserving system")
  - —Milk
  - —Saline
  - —Saliva (patient or parent's mouth)

Diagnosis

ESSENTIAL WORKUP

- Time of injury
- Mechanism
- Changes in occlusion
- Account for all missing teeth
- Careful inspection of the oral cavity
  - —Soft tissue injuries
  - —Embedded fragments
  - —Associated injuries
    - -Salivary glands
    - -Ducts
    - -Nerves
    - -Blood vessels

LABORATORY

N/A

IMAGING/SPECIAL TESTS

- Plain dental radiograph
  - —Ellis class III fractures
  - —Assess for associated root or alveolar fracture
- Panorex
  - —Indicated if there is a suspicion of associated injuries
    - -Foreign bodies
    - -Displacement of teeth
    - -Alveolar or jaw fractures
- Chest radiograph
  - —Indicated if a tooth or tooth fragment is missing
  - —Bronchoscopic removal is indicated for dental aspiration

DIFFERENTIAL DIAGNOSIS

N/A

Treatment

INITIAL STABILIZATION

- Ensure patent airway as needed
- Control bleeding by having the patient bite on gauze
- Account for all teeth and fragments
- Immediate reimplantation of avulsed tooth

ED TREATMENT

- Ellis class I
  - —Smooth sharp edges with an emory board
  - —Dental referral for cosmetic repair
- Ellis class II
  - —Dressing of calcium hydroxide paste
  - —Cover with dry foil, a metal band, or an enamel-bonded plastic
  - —Dental referral within 24 hours
- Ellis class III
  - —Immediate dental referral when available
    - -Pulpotomy by dentist
  - —If dental consultation is unavailable
    - -Place a piece of moist cotton over the exposed pulp
    - -Cover with dry foil
- Subluxed tooth
  - —Soft diet if minimally mobile
  - —Stabilization for more mobile teeth
- Tooth avulsion
  - —Rinse (do not scrub) in saline
  - —Administer local anesthesia
  - —Reinsert holding the tooth by the crown
  - —Temporary stabilization with a periodontal pack such as a "Coe-Pak"
    - -Mix resin and catalyst in even amounts to a firm consistency
    - -Apply to anterior and posterior surface of the avulsed tooth and adjacent two teeth
  - —Prophylactic antibiotic coverage
  - —Definitive stabilization by a dentist
- Alveolar fracture
  - —Oral surgery consult for stabilization
  - —Prophylactic antibiotic coverage

MEDICATIONS

- Clindamycin: adult: 300 mg po q 8 hrs; peds: 25–30 mg/kg/24hrs po q 8 hrs
- Erythromycin: adult: 500 mg po q 6 hrs; peds: 30–50 mg/kg/24hrs (max 2 g) po q 6 hrs
- Penicillin V: adult: 500 mg po q 6 hrs; peds: 25–50 mg/kg/24hrs (max 3 g) po q 6 hrs
- Tylenol #3: adult: 2 tablets po q 4–6 hrs PRN; peds: codeine: 2.5–5.0 mg/kg/24hrs (max 30 mg) po q 4–6 hrs for children 2–6 years old
- Tylenol and oxycodone: adult: 2 tablets po q 6 hrs PRN; peds: oxycodone: 0.05–0.15 mg/kg/dose (max 10 mg/dose)

Disposition

ADMISSION CRITERIA

- Admission for other associated injuries
- Suspected child abuse and no safe environment available

DISCHARGE CRITERIA

- Isolated dental fractures
- Follow-up with a dentist
- Within 24 hours for avulsions, Ellis class II and Ellis class III fractures

Miscellaneous

ICD9: 525

CORE CONTENT CODE: 18.4.4.6

SUGGESTED READINGS

Amsterdam JT. Dental disorders. In: Rosen P, et al., eds. Emergency medicine: Concepts and clinical practice. 4th ed. St. Louis: CV Mosby, 1998:2680–2697.

Medford HM. Acute care of avulsed teeth. Ann Emerg Med 1982;11:559.

Medford HM, Curtis JW. Acute care of severe tooth fractures. Ann Emerg Med 1983;12:364–365.

Powers MP. Diagnosis and management of dentoalveolar injuries. In: Fonseca RJ, Walker RV, eds. Oral and maxillofacial trauma. Philadelphia: WB Saunders, 1991:323–358.

Author: Marc J. Shapiro

Depression

Clinical Presentation

SIGNS AND SYMPTOMS

- Wide variety of presentations
  - —Dramatically in suicidal crisis
  - —Quietly with somatic complaints, panic attacks, or psychosocial distress
- Vague somatic complaints
  - —Weakness, malaise
  - —Weight loss
  - —Headache
  - —Back pain
- Diminished sense of self-esteem
- Loss of interest in or lack of enjoyment of pleasurable activities
- Loss of energy
- Poor appetite
- Sleep disturbance
- Decreased attention span
- Irritability

MECHANISM/DESCRIPTION

- Major depression
  - —Psychiatric illness with depressed mood and neurovegetative signs and symptoms lasting 2 or more weeks
  - —Significant associated morbidity and mortality
  - —Clinician should try to recognize this disorder in the medically ill

ETIOLOGY

- Major depression with suicidal ideations
  - —Biological illness associated with derangements in several neurotransmitter systems of the brain including serotonin
- Causes of neurobiological derangement include:
  - —Genetic predisposition
  - —Medical illness
  - —Effects of medications
  - —Chronic unremitting stressors in a predisposed individual
- Women are twice as likely to have major depression than men
  - —Men are more likely to successfully complete suicide

PEDIATRIC CONSIDERATIONS

- Depressed children and adolescents are difficult to diagnose because the criteria are not as easily recognized
- Indicators of major depression in children
  - —Irritability
  - —Changes in school, home, and social functioning
  - —Social withdrawal
  - —Substance abuse
- Consultation with a child psychiatrist is crucial in further assessment and disposition

Pre-Hospital

CAUTIONS

- Patients often seek nonpsychiatric medical care shortly before committing suicide
- Search potentially suicidal patients for weapons
- Obtain additional help for potentially suicidal/dangerous patients

Diagnosis

ESSENTIAL WORKUP

- Eliciting the signs and symptoms of major depression is key to making the diagnosis
- DSM-IV diagnostic criteria include
  - —The presence of *depressed mood or loss of interest or pleasure* for 2 weeks or longer accompanied by at least five of the following criteria
    - -Weight loss or gain
    - -Insomnia or hypersomnia
    - -Psychomotor agitation or retardation
    - -Fatigue or loss of energy
    - -Feelings of excessive guilt or worthlessness
    - -Diminished thinking or concentration or indecisiveness
    - -Suicidal ideation or preoccupation with death

LABORATORY

- Focus is on establishing the diagnosis as a psychiatric illness rather than due to a medical condition
- CBC
- Electrolytes, BUN/Cr, glucose
- Liver function tests
- Thyroid screen

DIFFERENTIAL DIAGNOSIS

Depressive-like Psychiatric Illnesses

- Dysthymia
- Adjustment reactions
- Bereavement
- Acute reactions to stress

Medical Causes of Depression

- Drug-induced
  - —Antihypertensives
  - —Oral contraceptives
  - —Steroids
  - —Cimetidine and ranitidine
  - —Sedative-hypnotics
  - —Cocaine and amphetamine
  - —β-Blockers
  - —Metoclopramide
- Endocrine disorders
  - —Thyroid
  - —Adrenal
  - —Diabetes mellitus
  - —Hyperparathyroid
- Tumors
  - —Pancreatic
  - —Lung
  - —Brain
- Neurologic disorders
  - —Dementia (early phase)
  - —Epilepsy
  - —Huntington's disease
  - —Multiple sclerosis
  - —Parkinson's disease
  - —Stroke

—Subdural hematoma
—Syphilis
- Infections
—Hepatitis
—Influenza
—Mononucleosis
- Nutritional disorders
—Folate deficiency
—Pellagra
—Vitamin B_{12} deficiency
- Electrolyte disturbances
- End-stage renal pulmonary and cardiovascular disease
- Chronic pain syndromes

Treatment

INITIAL STABILIZATION

- One-to-one nursing or restrain any potentially suicidal patient for patient safety

ED TREATMENT

Psychological Management

- Empathetic listening to understand the stressors involved in the depression helps focus and encourage patients
- Emphasizing that depression is a treatable condition is reassuring as well as helpful in developing a treatment alliance

Drug Therapy

- For diagnosed neurovegetative, major depression
- Decision to initiate antidepressant medication should be for patients with established follow-up and only with enough medication given until the next appointment
- Low-dose benzodiazepines or neuroleptics maybe used for associated agitation, insomnia, or psychosis
- Usually takes weeks for antidepressant medications to resolve major depression
- Choice of drug for the initiation of antidepressant therapy depends upon
  —Efficacy
  —Side effect profile of the agent
  —Potential lethality if used to overdose
  —Compliance factors
- Tricyclic antidepressants (amitriptyline, imipramine, nortriptyline)
  —Side effects include
    -Anticholinergic effects
    -Postural hypotension
    -Sedation
    -Decreased seizure threshold
    -Overdoses of as little as 1 g of TCA can be fatal
- Monoamine oxidase inhibitors (phenelzine, tranylcypromine)
  —Dietary restrictions to avoid hypertensive crisis
- Selective serotonin reuptake inhibitors (fluoxetine, sertraline, paroxetine)
  —Well-tolerated
  —Side effects include
    -Mild nausea
    -Decreased appetite
    -Agitation
    -Somnolence
    -Sexual dysfunction
    -Minimal overdose potential

Disposition

ADMISSION CRITERIA

- Patient is suicidal or at high risk for suicide
- Minimal or unreliable social supports
- Previous history of suicide or poor treatment response
- Symptoms so severe that continual observation or nursing supportive care is required
- Psychotic features
- *Civil commitment* for psychiatric hospitalization is necessary if the patient is refusing treatment and is suicidal or otherwise judged to be at-risk to harm self or others

DISCHARGE CRITERIA

- Low suicide risk
- Adequate social support
- Close follow up available

Miscellaneous

ICD9: 311

CORE CONTENT CODE: 14.2.2

SUGGESTED READINGS

Hymen SE, et al. Antidepressant drugs. In: Hyman SE, Arana GW, Rosenbaum IF, eds. Handbook of psychiatric drug therapy. 3rd ed. Boston: Little, Brown, and Co., 1995:43–92.

Barreira PL. Depression. In: Hyman SE, Tesar GE, eds. Manual of psychiatric emergencies, 3rd ed. Boston: Little, Brown, and Co., 1994:117–128.

Cassem NH. Depression. In: Cassem NH, ed: Handbook of general hospital psychiatry. 4th ed. St. Louis: Mosby-Yearbook, 1997.

Author: Kathy Sanders

Dermatomyositis/Polymyositis

Clinical Presentation

SIGNS AND SYMPTOMS

- Polymyositis is distinguished from dermatomyositis by the absence of rash. In other respects, the two conditions are considered similar
- Patients with polymyositis (PM) present with muscle weakness and systemic complaints
- Those with dermatomyositis (DM) present with skin rash, and constitutional symptoms including weight loss, fever, anorexia, morning stiffness, myalgias, and arthralgias
- Those with DM/PM often note fatigue doing customary tasks such as brushing hair, climbing stairs, reaching above the head, or rising from a chair. They may also complain of dysphagia, dyspnea, and cough
- Progressive weakness of the proximal limb and girdle muscles is seen early; distal muscle weakness can occur late in the disease
- Skin findings of DM
  —Skin rash occurs with or precedes muscle weakness
  —Heliotrope rash (lilac discoloration) on the upper eyelids associated with edema
  —Gottron's sign: violaceous or erythematous papules over the extensor surfaces of the joints, particularly knuckles, knees, and elbows
  —Shawl sign: a V-shaped erythematous rash occurring on the back and shoulders
  —Periungual telangiectasias: nailbed capillary changes which include thickened irregular and distorted cuticles
  —"Machinist hands": darkened horizontal lines across the lateral and palmar aspects of the fingers

MECHANISM/DESCRIPTION

- DM/PM is a systemic inflammatory myopathy
  —Progression of muscle weakness over weeks to months
  —Respiratory insufficiency from respiratory muscle weakness
  —Aspiration pneumonia due to a weak cough mechanism, pharyngeal muscle dysfunction, and esophageal dysmotility
  —Interstitial lung disease can precede skin and muscle involvement
  —Cardiac manifestations include myocarditis and CHF
  —Arthralgias of the hands, wrists, knees, and shoulders
  —Ocular muscles are not involved and facial muscle weakness may be seen only in advanced cases

ETIOLOGY

- The exact cause of DM/PM is unknown, although an autoimmune etiology is theorized
- The incidence is about 1:100,000 with a female preponderance
- Increased incidence of DM/PM in association with HLA-B8 and HLA-DR3
- There may be an association between PM and viral, bacterial, and parasitic infections
- DM/PM occurs with collagen vascular disease about 20% of the time
- Deposition of complement is the earliest and most specific lesion of DM/PM followed by inflammation, ischemia, microinfarcts, necrosis, and destruction of the muscle fibers

PEDIATRIC CONSIDERATIONS

- While DM is seen in both children and adults, PM is rare in children
- Juvenile form may include vasculitis, ectopic calcifications (calcinosis cutis) and lipodystrophy
- The juvenile form may be associated with Coxsackie virus

Pre-Hospital

N/A

Diagnosis

ESSENTIAL WORKUP

- The most important tests for diagnosis are the serum muscle enzymes: CPK, LDH, aldolase, AST, and SGOT
- Electrocardiogram and urinalysis should also be obtained
- Diagnostic criteria established in 1975 by Bohan and Peter
  —Symmetrical proximal muscle weakness with dysphagia and respiratory muscle weakness
  —Elevation of serum muscle enzymes
  —Electromyographic features of myopathy
  —Muscle biopsy showing features of inflammatory myopathy
- Confidence limits for diagnosis (typical rash must be seen for diagnosis of DM)
  —Definite diagnosis: 3–4 criteria
  —Probable diagnosis: 2 criteria
  —Possible diagnosis: 1 criterion

LABORATORY

- Elevation of CPK is sensitive for muscle injury but not specific for dermatomyositis
- CPK may be normal in juvenile form
- Levels of aldolase, myoglobulin, creatinine, SGPT, SGOT, and LDH may be elevated
- Proteinuria, RBC casts, and sediment may be found on UA
- CBC will generally be normal unless occult bleeding from vasculitis or other cause is present
- EKG may show nonspecific ST-T wave changes in up to 30% of patients

IMAGING/SPECIAL TESTS

- CXR may show interstitial lung disease, evidence of aspiration pneumonia, CHF, or cardiomyopathy
- EMG studies show myopathic potentials that are not specific for DM/PM
- Pulmonary function tests are useful in following the progression of interstitial lung disease
- Renal biopsies of patients may show focal proliferative glomerulonephritis
- *Muscle biopsy is the definitive test*
  —In PM, inflammatory infiltrates are often endomysial, although they may be perivascular
  —In DM, inflammatory infiltrates are mostly perivascular and include a high percentage of B cells

DIFFERENTIAL DIAGNOSIS

- Collagen vascular diseases
- Muscular dystrophies, spinal muscular atrophy, myasthenia gravis, amyotrophic lateral sclerosis, poliomyelitis, Guillain-Barré syndrome
- Hypothyroidism, hyperthyroidism, Cushing syndrome
- Drug-induced: colchicine, AZT, penicillamine, ipecac, ethanol, chloroquine, corticosteroids
- Toxoplasmosis, trichinosis, Coxsackie, HIV, influenza, Epstein-Barr
- Hypokalemia, hypercalcemia, hypomagnesemia, vasculitis, paraneoplastic neuromyopathy, hypereosinophilic myalgia syndrome

Treatment

INITIAL STABILIZATION

- Evaluation and management of respiratory dysfunction is necessary if the swallowing and breathing mechanisms are impaired
- NG suction to prevent aspiration
- Intubation and mechanical ventilation as required
- Pneumothorax has been described as a rare occurrence in childhood DM

ED TREATMENT

- Elevate head of the bed to prevent aspiration
- Begin *high-dose corticosteroids* to suppress inflammation and improve muscle weakness
- Avoid triamcinolone and dexamethasone as there is an associated myopathy
- Efficacy of prednisone determined by objective increase in muscle strength
- Immunosuppressive medications
  —Azathioprine is limited by GI intolerance, and bone marrow suppression
  —Cyclosporine has been used but with limited success
  —Methotrexate
- Do not treat CPK level

OUTCOME

- Mortality rate of patient with DM four times that of the general population
- Death is due to pulmonary, renal, or cardiac complications
- Black females have a poorer prognosis
- 5-year survival rate greater than 75% with steroids

MEDICATIONS

- Azathioprine: 3 mg/kg/day for 4–6 months
- Methotrexate: adults: 15–25 mg per week; peds: 0.5–1 mg/kg per week (not to exceed adult dose)
- Prednisone: adults: 60 mg/day; peds: 1–2 mg/kg/day

Disposition

ADMISSION CRITERIA

- Respiratory insufficiency, aspiration pneumonia, muscle weakness, weakened cough mechanisms, and pharyngeal dysfunction, CHF

DISCHARGE CRITERIA

- Well-appearing patients with no respiratory dysfunction and no risk for aspiration
- Patients who can take oral corticosteroids and immunosuppressive agents as outpatients

Miscellaneous

ICD9: 710.4, 710.3

CORE CONTENT CODE: 8.5.2.2, 8.5.2.1

SUGGESTED READINGS

Bohan A, Peter JB. Polymyositis and dermatomyositis. N Engl J Med 1975;292:344–347.

Bohan A, Peter JB, Bowman RL, et al. A computer-assisted analysis of 153 patients with polymyositis and dermatomyositis. Medicine 1977;56:255–286.

Caro I. Dermatomyositis as a systemic disease. Collagen vascular diseases. Med Clin North Am 1989;73(5):1181–1191.

Dalakas MC. Polymyositis, dermatomyositis and inclusion-body myositis [Review]. N Engl J Med 1991;325:1487–1496.

Norins AL. Juvenile dermatomyositis. Collagen vascular diseases. Med Clin North Am 1989;73(5):1193–1207.

Authors: Lee V. Leak; John Lafleur

Diabetes Mellitus, Juvenile

Clinical Presentation

SIGNS AND SYMPTOMS

- Polydipsia
- Polyuria
- Weight loss
- Fatigue
- 30% present initially as diabetic ketoacidosis
  - —Nausea
  - —Vomiting
  - —Abdominal pain
  - —Altered mental status
  - —Hyperpnea
  - —Ketotic smell on the breath
  - —Marked dehydration
  - —Shock

MECHANISM/DESCRIPTION

- Insulin deficiency
- Elevated counterregulatory hormones
- Decreased peripheral glucose utilization
- Hyperglycemia from increased hepatic gluconeogenesis
- Osmotic diuresis resulting in moderate to severe dehydration
- Ketoacidosis from metabolism of free fatty acids
- Intracellular potassium shifts into the extracellular space due to hydrogen ion exchange
- Potassium is lost from the osmotic diuresis

ETIOLOGY

- Precipitating events leading to DKA
  - —Infection
  - —Emotional stress
  - —Hypoglycemic rebound
  - —Inflammatory reactions

Pre-Hospital

- Monitor the ABCs
- Airway protection if altered mental status
- Establish intravenous access

Diagnosis

ESSENTIAL WORKUP

- Hourly vital signs and neurologic checks
- Frequent blood chemistry

LABORATORY

- Bedside glucose
- Urine analysis
  - —Glycosuria
  - —Ketonuria
- Exclude UTI in patients with polyuria
- Blood chemistries every 2 hours until acidosis has resolved
- Serum glucose
  - —Hyperglycemia
- Electrolytes and venous pH
  - —Anion gap metabolic acidosis
- Serum potassium
  - —High or normal in spite of the total body depletion of potassium
  - —Frequent monitoring during treatment
  - —KCl, KAc, K_2HPO_4 or a combination
  - —No more than half should be given as K_2HPO_4
- Serum sodium
  - —Low or normal
- Serum osmolality
- Urea, creatinine
- CBC
  - —White blood cell count
  - —Often elevated due to stress
  - —Consider underlying infection if elevated
- Calcium
- Phosphate
- Appropriate cultures for underlying infection

DIFFERENTIAL DIAGNOSIS

- Gastroenteritis
- Urinary tract infection
- Sepsis
- Pancreatitis
- Appendicitis

Treatment

INITIAL STABILIZATION

- Oxygen
- Cardiac monitor
- Intravenous access and volume resuscitation

ED TREATMENT

- Fluid replacement
  - —Assume a deficit of at least 10% of the body weight
  - —0.45–0.9% NaCl over the next 24 hours
  - —Initial volume expansion with 10–20 ml/kg of normal saline
  - —Generally give 500 ml/m^2 over the first hour
  - —0.9% NaCl if the sodium <135 mEq
  - —Correct 50% of the volume deficit over the first 8 hours
  - —Replace the deficit of 100 ml/kg in the first 24 hours
- Monitor serum sodium
  - —Risk of cerebral edema if sodium fails to rise as glucose falls
- Intravenous insulin infusion
  - —Drop serum glucose of 50–100 mg/dl per hour
  - —Add dextrose when the blood glucose falls to 250 mg/dl
  - —Decrease after acidosis is corrected and urine ketones are moderate
  - —Change to subcutaneous insulin when pH >7.3
- Replace potassium and phosphate losses
  - —Verify adequate urine output
  - —50/50 mix of KCl and K_3PO_4
  - —20–40 mEq/L of K^+ after the inital fluid bolus
  - —Guide therapy by frequent monitoring of serum potassium
- Sodium bicarbonate
  - —Controversial benefit
  - —Arterial pH <7.1
  - —Amount of bicarbonate = base deficit × body weight × 0.6
    - -Give half over 2 hours and repeat biochemical studies
- Treat cerebral edema as needed
  - —Mortality of 90%
  - —Associated with fluid rate >4 L/m^2/day
  - —Decrease fluid administration
  - —Endotracheal intubation
  - —Hyperventilation to a pCO_2 of 25–30
  - —Administer mannitol

MEDICATIONS

- Insulin drip
  - —Intravenous drip
    - -Start at 0.1 IU/kg/hour
    - -Adjust according to fall in glucose
  - —0.25 IU/kg IM priming dose
  - —0.1 IU/kg IM hourly until serum glucose < 300 mg/dl
- Mannitol: 1 g/kg

Disposition

ADMISSION CRITERIA

- Intensive care unit
  - —Severe or continuing acidosis
  - —Mental status changes
- Wards
  - —New onset diabetics who respond well to treatment
  - —Concern regarding compliance or other social issues

DISCHARGE CRITERIA

- Initial glucose <500 mg/dl
- pH >7.2 or bicarbonate >10 mEq/L
- Known diabetics who respond to therapy
- Able to keep oral fluids down
- Reliable parents
- Reliable follow-up within 24 hours

Miscellaneous

ICD9: 250.1

CORE CONTENT CODE: 13.3.1

SUGGESTED READINGS

Chase HP, Garg SK, Jelley DH. Diabetic ketoacidosis in children and the role of outpatient management. Pediatr Rev 1990;11:297–304.

DeFronzo RA, Matsuda M, Barrett EJ. Diabetic ketoacidosis. Diabetes Rev 1994;2:209–238.

Durr JA, Hoffman WH, et al. Correlates of brain edema in uncontrolled IDDM. Diabetes 1992;41:627–632.

Fleckman AM. Diabetic ketoacidosis. Endocrin Metab Clin North Am 1993;22:2:181–207.

Author: Joan Bothner

Diabetic Ketoacidosis

Clinical Presentation

SIGNS AND SYMPTOMS

- Dehydration
  - —Hypotension
  - —Tachycardia
  - —Sunken eyes
  - —Tenting of skin
  - —Dry mucous membranes
  - —Longitudinally furrowed tongue
- Metabolic acidosis
  - —Tachypnea
  - —Kussmaul respiration (rapid, deep, sighing respiration)
  - —Myocardial depression
  - —Vasodilatation
  - —Fruity odor on breath
- Nausea/vomiting
- Abdominal pain and tenderness

MECHANISM/DESCRIPTION

- Relative insulin deficiency and excess of counter-regulatory hormones (glucagon, growth hormone, catecholamines and cortisol) resulting in a triad of
  - —Ketonemia—primary cause of metabolic acidosis
  - —Hyperglycemia—results in osmotic diuresis
  - —Metabolic acidosis
- Potassium exchanges with hydrogen as an intracellular buffer
- GI symptoms due to acidosis and hypokalemia induced paralytic ileus

ETIOLOGY

- Infectious process
- Noncompliance with insulin/oral hypoglycemic agent
- New onset DM (25%)
- MI
- CVA
- Pregnancy
- GI bleed

PEDIATRIC CONSIDERATIONS

- Overwhelming majority of children with diabetes have type I disease and are ketosis prone
- Diabetic ketoacidosis (DKA) is initial presentation of diabetes in 10% of children

Pre-Hospital

N/A

Diagnosis

ESSENTIAL WORKUP

- Diagnostic criteria
  - —Glucose $>$300 mg/dl
  - —HCO_3^- $<$15 mEq/L
  - —pH $<$7.3 with ketonemia and ketonuria
- Bedside glucose measurement (Accucheck)
- ABG
- Urine dip for ketones
- Search for precipitating factor

LABORATORY

- Serum glucose
  - —Essential to confirm results of reagent strips
- Electrolytes
  - —Increased anion gap metabolic acidosis
  - —Sodium
    - -Measured serum sodium often spuriously lowered by hyperglycemia
    - -Pseudohyponatremia correction factor: 1.6 mEq/L is added to measured value for every 100 mg/dl of blood glucose $>$ 100 mg/dl
    - -Sodium deficit with diabetic ketoacidosis
  - —Potassium
    - -Initial level usually normal to high due to extracellular shift as compensation for acidosis
    - -Level decreases precipitously with fluid and insulin
    - -For every 0.1 increase in pH, potassium decreases by 0.6 mEq/L
    - -Deficit of total body potassium common
- BUN, creatinine
  - —Elevated due to dehydration/renal damage
- Urinalysis
  - —Ketonuria glycosuria, proteinuria
  - —Check for UTI as precipitant
- CBC
  - —WBC often increased to 15–20,000 mm^3 in absence of infection
  - —Suspect infection if left shift of differential present
- Serum HCG
- Ketones
  - —May be spuriously low or absent since only acetone and acetoacetate measured
  - —β hydroxybutyrate not measured by nitroprusside reaction
- Serum osmolality—measured and calculated
  - —Calculated = 2 (Na^+) + glucose/18 + BUN/2.8
  - —Normal range 285–300
  - —Significant hyperosmolarity $>$ 320 mosm/L
- Lab tests of secondary importance
  - —Mg^{++}—decreased (changes follow serum potassium)
  - —Calcium—hypocalcemia may result from phosphate administration
  - —Phosphate—decreased (changes follow serum potassium)
  - —Amylase
  - —Lactate

IMAGING/SPECIAL TESTS

- CXR: for pneumonia
  - —Common precipitant
  - —Aspiration if decreased level of consciousness
- ECG to rule out MI as a precipitant of diabetic ketoacidosis
- CT head—if altered mental status possible, due to primary CNS condition

DIFFERENTIAL DIAGNOSIS

- Nonketotic hyperosmolar coma
- Alcoholic ketoacidosis
- Methanol
- Uremia
- Paraldehyde
- Isoniazid
- Lactic acidosis
- Ethylene glycol
- Sepsis
- Alcohol or drug intoxication
- Starvation ketoacidosis

PEDIATRIC CONSIDERATIONS

- Diabetic ketoacidosis may mimic bacterial sepsis, as well as occur concomitantly with it
  - —If etiology of diabetic ketoacidosis uncertain—consider septic workup (including CBC, blood cultures, U/A, LP) and antibiotics

Treatment

INITIAL STABILIZATION

- ABCs with intubation if comatose
- Narcan, thiamine, Accucheck (or dextrose) for coma of unknown etiology
- Aggressive 0.9%NS fluid resuscitation if hypovolemic

ED TREATMENT

- Rehydration
  - —Average fluid deficit in DKA = 5–10 L
  - —Administer first liter bolus over 30–60 minutes
  - —Initial 2 L use 0.9%NS to replace intravascular deficit then switch to 0.45%NS
  - —Avoid volume overload in patients with CHF
  - —Speed of rehydration may be related to risk of cerebral edema. Many recommend slower rehydration
- Cardiac monitor until electrolyte disorder corrected
- Insulin
  - —Stops ketosis and replenishes cellular glucose
  - —Goal is to decrease glucose by 100 mg/dl/hr
  - —Initiate infusion 5–10 IU/hr (0.1 IU/kg)
  - —Increase insulin drip if glucose fails to respond within one hour
  - —Switch to glucose-containing IV when blood glucose falls to 250 mg/dl
  - —Continue glucose and insulin until pH >7.3
- Potassium
  - —Depletion and imminent hypokalemia may only become apparent as
    - -Rehydration is instituted
    - -Potassium shifts back into cells
    - -Renal excretion returns to normal
  - —Add 20 mEq to each liter of IV fluid once renal function adequate and serum K <5.5 mEq/L
  - —Monitor electrolytes hourly until pH >7.3 and potassium repleted to K >4.0 mEq/L
- Phosphorous
  - —Supplement if phosphorous level <1 mg/dl
  - —Use potassium phosphate 20 mEq/L IV fluid with concomitant potassium depletion
- Sodium bicarbonate
  - —Administer only for pH <7.0
  - —Complications include cerebral edema, alkalosis, paradoxical cerebrospinal fluid acidosis
  - —Administer 44 mEq if pH <7.0 but >6.9
  - —Administer 88 mEq if pH <6.9
- Magnesium repletion if low level
  - —0.35 mEq/kg magnesium in fluids for first 3–4 hours
  - —2.5–3.0 g $MgSO_4$ in 70 kg patient

MEDICATIONS

- D50W: 1 amp (= 25 g) of 50% dextrose (peds: 2–4 ml/kg D25W) IVP
- Insulin (regular, short acting)
- Sodium bicarbonate: (1 amp = 50 CC = 44 mEq) 1–2 mEq/kg IV
- Narcan: 2 mg (peds: 0.1 mg/kg) IVP
- Potassium phosphate: phosphates 3 μmol/ml and potassium 4.4 mEq/ml
- Thiamine: 100 mg (peds: 10–25 mg) IVP

PEDIATRIC CONSIDERATIONS

- Average fluid deficit is 100–150 ml/kg
- Initial volume replacement should be 20 ml/kg NS bolus over 1 hour
  - —Repeat as necessary if in shock
- Replace deficit at 1.5 times maintenance needs over next 24–36 hours
- Switch to D5 0.45%NS when blood glucose <250 mg/dl

Disposition

ADMISSION CRITERIA

- ICU admission for pH <7.0, serious concurrent illness, mental obtundation/coma, age <2 or >60 years
- Telemetry admission if patient has history of CHF or CAD
- Regular admission for moderate diabetic ketoacidosis
- Observation (12–24 hours) admission if bicarbonates >12 mEq/L with no serious precipitating event

DISCHARGE CRITERIA

- Resolution of anion gap acidosis
- Able to tolerate oral fluids
- No evidence of concurrent illness (infection) which may precipitate diabetic ketoacidosis

Miscellaneous

ICD9: 250.1

CORE CONTENT CODE: 4.4.1.1

SUGGESTED READINGS

Fleckman AM. Diabetic ketoacidoses. Endocrinol Metab Clin North Am 1993;22(2):181–207.

Kitabchi AE, Wall BM. Diabetic ketoacidosis. Med Clin North Am 1995;79(1):9–33.

Authors: Steven Friedman; Michelle Ervin

Dialysis Complications

Clinical Presentation

SIGNS AND SYMPTOMS

Vascular Access Related
- Bleeding from puncture sites
- Loss of bruit in the graft
- Local infection/cellulitis/fever
- Decreased sensation, strength distal to access

Nonvascular Access Related
- Hypotension before, during, or after the procedure
- Dysrhythmias
- Chest pain (ischemic/pleuritic)
- Hemorrhage (GI, pleural, retroperitoneal)
- Shortness of breath
- Neurologic (disequilibrium syndrome)
  - —Headache
  - —Malaise
  - —Seizures
  - —Coma

Peritoneal
- Abdominal pain
- Cloudy dialysis effluent
- Vomiting
- Exudates/inflammation at insertion site of Tenckhoff catheter

MECHANISM/DESCRIPTION

Vascular Access Related
- Infections
  - —Due to *Staphylococci aureus*
  - —Bacteremia may be present without local signs of infection

Nonvascular Access Related
- Hypotension
  - —After dialysis: due to acute decrease in circulating blood volume
  - —During dialysis: hypovolemia or onset of cardiac tamponade due to compensated effusion suddenly becoming symptomatic after correction of volume overload
  - —MI, sepsis, dysrhythmias
  - —Hemorrhage secondary to anticoagulation, platelet dysfunction of renal failure
- Shortness of breath
  - —Volume overload
  - —Development of dyspnea *during* dialysis (tamponade, pericardial effusion, hemorrhage, anaphylaxis, pulmonary emboli, or air emboli)
- Chest pain
  - —Ischemic: dialysis creates acute physiologic stressor with transient hypotension and hypoxemia and increased myocardial oxygen demand
  - —Pericarditis if pleuritic
- Neurologic dysfunction: disequilibrium syndrome
  - —Rapid decrease in serum osmolality during dialysis leaving the brain in a comparatively hyperosmolal state

Peritoneal
- Peritonitis
  - —Due to contamination of the peritoneal dialysate or tubing during an exchange
  - —*Staphylococcus aureus* or *Staphylococcus epidermidis* (70%)
- Perforated viscus with severe abdominal pain, fever, brown or fecal material in the effluent, or localized tenderness
- Fibrinous blockage of the catheter resulting from infection or inflammation

Pre-Hospital

CAUTIONS
- Do not perform IVs and BPs in an extremity with a functioning access
- Run IV fluids slowly and keep to a minimum if possible
- Administer furosemide in pulmonary edema (use high doses up to 200 mg in anuric patients)

Diagnosis

ESSENTIAL WORKUP
- Infection
  - —Blood/wound cultures
  - —Cell count, gram stain, and culture of peritoneal fluid
  - —Careful physical exam for occult sources of infection (odontogenic, perirectal abscess)
- Bleeding
  - —CBC to evaluate anemia and platelet count
  - —Coagulation studies
  - —Stool for guiaiac
- Chest pain/shortness of breath
  - —ECG
  - —CXR
  - —ABG
  - —Cardiac enzymes
- Neurologic dysfunction
  - —CT of brain for intracranial hemorrhage

LABORATORY
- Electrolytes, BUN, Cr, glucose
- CBC

SPECIAL TESTS/IMAGING
- Echocardiogram for suspected pericarditis, effusion, or tamponade
- Ultrasonography of access for possible clotted graft/fistula
- Peritoneal catheterogram for catheter blockages

DIFFERENTIAL DIAGNOSIS
- Hypotension
  - —Hypovolemia
  - —Cardiogenic shock, AMI, tamponade, dysrhythmias
  - —Hyper/hypokalemia
  - —Hyper/hypocalcemia
  - —Hypermagnesemia
  - —Embolism: air or pulmonary
  - —Vascular instability: autonomic neuropathy, drug related, dialysate related
- Neurologic Complications
  - —CVA
  - —Intracranial bleed
  - —Meningitis or abscess
  - —Disequilibrium syndrome
  - —Uremia
  - —Hyper/hyponatremia
  - —Hyper/hypoglycemia
  - —Hypoxemia
- Peritoneal
  - —Peritonitis
  - —Hernia incarceration
  - —Perforated viscus
  - —Acute abdominal process: appendicitis, cholecystitis

Treatment

INITIAL STABILIZATION
- ABCs

Vascular Access Related
- Bleeding
  - —Firm pressure to site(s)
    - -Do not totally occlude the graft—may cause clotting
    - -Document presence of thrill postpressure
  - —Apply GelFoam

Nonvascular Access Related
- Hypotension
  - —Search for underlying cause
  - —Vasopressors/fluid/saline
- Shortness of breath
  - —Attempt diuresis if fluid overloaded and arrange dialysis
- Hyperkalemia
  - —Administer IV calcium, bicarbonate, insulin, and glucose
  - —Monitor cardiac rhythm
  - —Administer ion exchange resin (kayexalate)
  - —Arrange for dialysis
- Neurologic complications
  - —Narcan, thiamine, dextrose (or Accucheck) for altered mental status
  - —Control seizures with benzodiazepines

ED TREATMENT

Vascular Access Related Complications
- Infection
  - —Initiate antistaphylococcal IV antibiotics
- Clotted access
  - —Analgesia
  - —Warm compresses
  - —Vascular surgery consult
- Hemorrhage
  - —Control bleeding
  - —Correct coagulopathies
  - —Administer IV fluids/blood products

Nonvascular Access Complications
- Electrolyte imbalances
  - —Treat hypercalcemia or hypermagnesemia with
    - -Saline infusion if tolerated (dilution)
    - -Diuresis with furosemide
    - -Dialysis
- Volume overload
  - —Attempt diuresis
  - —Arrange dialysis
- Pericardial effusion/tamponade
  - —Emergent pericardiocentesis may be necessary
  - —Arrange dialysis
- Acute MI
  - —Consider thrombolytics or angioplasty if candidate
  - —Nitrates to decrease myocardial work load
- Disequilibrium syndrome
  - —Rule out other causes of altered mental status
  - —Resolves over time
  - —May respond to hyperosmolar infusions (mannitol, hypertonic saline)

Peritoneal Complications
- Peritonitis: IV antibiotics/intraperitoneal antibiotics
- Catheter or tunnel infection culture, visible exudates
  - —Oral antibiotics (antistaphylococcal)
  - —If recurrent or tunnel, may need to be unroofed
  - —Meticulous site care
- Perforated viscus
  - —IV antibiotics
  - —Surgical consultation

MEDICATIONS
- Calcium gluconate: 1 g slowly IV (cardioprotective in hyperkalemia)
- Cefazolin: 1 g IV or IM followed by 250 mg/2 L bag × 10 days (peritonitis)
- Dextrose: D50W 1 amp (50 ml or 25 g) (peds: D25W 2–4 ml/kg) IV (hyperkalemia or hypoglycemia)
- Dopamine: 2–20 μg/kg/min IV
- Furosemide: 20–100 mg IV (may require doses of 300 mg or more to effect diuresis in CRF)
- Insulin: 5–10 U regular insulin IV (with D50 for hyperkalemia)
- Kayexalate (sodium polystyrene sulfonate): 1 g/kg up to 15–60 po or 30–50 g retention enema q 6 hr prn hyperkalemia
- Naloxone (Narcan): 2 mg (peds: 0.1 mg/kg) IV or IM initial dose
- Nitroglycerin: 0.4 mg SL; 5–20 μg/min IV
- Sodium bicarbonate: 1 mEq/kg up to 50–100 mEq IV prn
- Thiamine (Vitamin B_1): 100 mg (peds: 50 mg) IV or IM
- Tobramycin: 1.7 mg/kg IV or IM; then 10mg/2 L bag × 10 days (peritonitis)
- Vancomycin: 1g IV or IM; then 50 mg/2 L bag × 10 days (peritonitis)

Disposition

ADMISSION CRITERIA
- ICU admission for severe hyperkalemia, pulmonary edema, volume overload, persistent hypotension, uncontrolled seizures, acute MI, CVA, pericarditis, and sepsis
- Regular admission for fever, vomiting, non-life-threatening electrolyte disturbances or those unable to provide self care for CAPD with antibiotics

DISCHARGE CRITERIA
- Mild infections of the access site or peritonitis without toxic, systemic symptoms
- Same day surgery for some thrombectomy procedures
- Control of hemostasis control at puncture sites

Miscellaneous

ICD9 CODE: N/A

CORE CONTENT CODE: 15.8

SUGGESTED READINGS

Feldman HI, Held PJ, Hutchinson JT, et al. Hemodialysis vascular access morbidity in the United States. Kidney Int 1993;43(Suppl 41):S1091–1096.

Khan IH, Catto GRD. Long-term complications of dialysis: Infection. Kidney Int 1993;43(Suppl 41):S143–S148.

Wolfson AB. Chronic renal failure and dialysis. In: Rosen P, et al, eds. Emergency medicine: Concepts and clinical practice. 4th ed. St. Louis: CV Mosby, 1998.

Author: Mary Stewart

Diaper Rash

Clinical Presentation

SIGNS AND SYMPTOMS

- Shiny glazed appearance of the skin
- Beefy red confluent patches
  - —"Kissing maculopapules"
  - —Candidal rashes
- Pustules
  - —Secondarily infected rash

MECHANISM/DESCRIPTION

- Diaper dermatitis accounts for 20% of skin consultations
- Incidence of perianal dermatitis 7–35% in infants during the first 7 days of life
- Primary irritant dermatitis
  - —Friction in area where the skin contact is the greatest
  - —Trapped moisture causes erythema
  - —Maceration in the intertriginous parts of the diaper area
- Candidiasis
  - —Skin in the diaper area has clusters of erythematous papules and pustules
  - —These coalesce into a beefy red confluent rash with sharp borders
  - —Satellite papules and pustules exist beyond these borders
  - —40% of infants with a diaper dermatitis for more than 72 hours may be presumed to be secondarily infected with candida
- Atopic dermatitis
  - —Similar to primary irritant dermatitis
  - —The rash is more confluent and difficult to treat
  - —Lesions on other body surfaces typical of atopic dermatitis may be found
- Seborrheic dermatitis
  - —Rash with an erythematous base covered with greasy scaling
  - —May find other body areas with similar involvement

ETIOLOGY

- Prolonged presence of urine
  - —Bacterial overgrowth occurs on moist skin over time
  - —Leads to alteration of the epidermal barrier
- Friction
  - —Rubbing of the skin against diaper produces irritation
  - —Less friction is required on wet than dry skin

Pre-Hospital

N/A

Diagnosis

ESSENTIAL WORKUP

- Determine diaper-changing habits and urinary fecal habits of the child
- Examine other body areas to identify other rashes
- Ascertain absence of child abuse and negligence
  - —Burns
  - —Underlying trauma

LABORATORY

- Surface scrapings prepared with potassium hydroxide
  - —Usually the diagnosis of candida is done empirically

IMAGING/SPECIAL TESTS

N/A

DIFFERENTIAL DIAGNOSIS

- Candidiasis
  - —However, this may accompany diaper rash
- Atopic dermatitis
- Psoriasis
- Scabies
- Bullous impetigo
- Bullous pemphigoid
- Papular urticaria
- Herpes simplex
- Varicella
- Burns
- Child abuse
- Trauma
- Congenital syphilis

Treatment

INITIAL STABILIZATION

N/A

ED TREATMENT

- Topical antiyeast agent
  - —Obvious candida impetigo
  - —Spreading rash
  - —Painful rash
  - —Rash greater than 72 hours old
  - —Nystatin, miconazole, clotrimazole

MEDICATIONS

- Clotrimazole: apply to affected area qid or with every other diaper change
- Miconazole: apply to affected area qid or with every other diaper change
- Nystatin: apply to affected area qid or with every other diaper change
- Zinc oxide: apply to area at earliest sign of diaper rash and 2–3 times per day thereafter

Disposition

ADMISSION CRITERIA

- Evidence that the rash may be related to child abuse

DISCHARGE CRITERIA

- Diaper changes every 2 hours
- Dry the area by air exposure after gentle rinsing of the skin with clear water
- Avoid soaps or alcohol (commercial wipes) to prevent further damage to the barrier properties of the skin
- Cornstarch is contraindicated as it serves as a culture medium for *C. albicans*
- Avoid plastic pants or tightly fitting diapers

Miscellaneous

ICD9: 691.0

CORE CONTENT CODE: 13.12.3

SUGGESTED READINGS

Lane AT, Rehder PA, Holm K. Evaluations of diapers containing absorbent gelling material with conventional disposable diapers in newborn infants. Am J Dis Child 1990;144:315–318.

Munz D, Powell KR, Pai CH. Treatment of candidal diaper dermatitis: A double-blinded placebo-controlled comparison of topical nystatin with topical plus oral nystatin. J Pediatr 1982;101:1022–1025.

Sires UL, Mallory SB. Diaper dermatitis. How to treat and prevent. Postgrad Med 1995;98:79–84, 86.

Weston WL, Lane AT, Weston JA. Diaper dermatitis: Current concepts. Pediatrics 1980;66:532–536.

Author: Deepi Goyal

Diaphragmatic Trauma

Clinical Presentation

SIGNS AND SYMPTOMS

- Signs and symptoms vary depending on whether phase is acute, latent, or obstructive
- *Acute phase:* tachypnea, hypotension, absence of breath sounds, abdominal distention, or bowel sounds in the chest
- *Latent phase:* abdominal discomfort caused by intermittent herniation of abdominal contents into thorax
  - —Symptoms are nonspecific such as abdominal pain which is worse postprandially or exacerbated by lying supine
  - —Pain may radiate to the left shoulder, be relieved by sitting or standing, and can be associated with nausea, vomiting, or belching
- *Obstructive phase:* severe abdominal pain, obstipation, nausea, vomiting, and abdominal distention
- Abdominal organs, having become strangulated and necrotic, may perforate and spill abdominal contents into the chest. This rapidly leads to respiratory compromise, sepsis, and death

MECHANISM/DESCRIPTION

- Penetrating injury: direct violation of the diaphragm by the penetrating object (knife and gunshot wounds). Can involve any portion of the diaphragm and defect is usually less than 2 cm in length
- Blunt injury: increased intra-abdominal or intrathoracic pressure is transmitted to the diaphragm, causing rupture
  - —Injuries are typically in a radial orientation, in the posterolateral area of the left side of the diaphragm, corresponding to an embryological point of weakness. Injuries are frequently between 5 and 15 cm in length
- Diaphragmatic defects do not heal spontaneously because of the pleuroperitoneal pressure gradient, which may exceed 100 cm of water during maximal respiratory effort. This gradient promotes herniation of the abdominal contents through the rent in the diaphragm and into the chest

ETIOLOGY

- Incidence is estimated to be 1–6% in all patients sustaining multiple-system trauma
- Lateral torso impact is three times more likely to result in ipsilateral blunt diaphragmatic rupture than frontal impact
- Diaphragmatic injury should be suspected with penetrating trauma to the thoracoabdominal area, or injuries that cross the plane of the diaphragm

Pre-Hospital

CAUTIONS

- Herniation of abdominal contents into the chest wall may mimic hemothorax or tension pneumothorax
  - —Bowel sounds in the chest may help distinguish
  - —Be suspicious of diaphragmatic injury with lateral compression of the chest, and be cautious in placement of needle or tube thoracostomies

Diagnosis

- In the acute phase, there may be no abdominal visceral herniation. This injury may even be missed on initial laparotomy

ESSENTIAL WORKUP

- Chest x-ray is essential and may reveal herniated loops of bowel or other abdominal viscera in the thorax
  - —Pathognomonic finding is the presence of a nasogastric tube above the diaphragm
  - —Findings are often less specific such as a unilaterally elevated diaphragm, mediastinal shift away from the affected side, unilateral pleural thickening, areas of atelectasis or consolidation at the bases, or small hemothorax or pneumothorax
  - —50% of initial chest x-rays may be normal
- Diagnosis may be difficult in the latent phase because of the intermittent nature of herniation. Contrast studies of the gastrointestinal tract can be useful, but the entire tract must be visualized below the diaphragm before the study can be interpreted as normal

LABORATORY

- If diagnostic peritoneal lavage (DPL) is performed, a red blood cell count of 5000 RBC/mm^3 is the recommended level for interpretation as positive
- No laboratory studies confirm or rule out the presence of diaphragmatic injury

IMAGING/SPECIAL TESTS

- Gastrointestinal contrast studies are the most useful in diagnosing chronic herniation of abdominal contents through the diaphragm
- Ultrasound has been successfully used to diagnose traumatic diaphragmatic rupture, particularly on the right side with accompanying hepatic herniation. However, the sensitivity is generally very poor
- Computed tomography (CT) has been used; it is rarely diagnostic and has very poor sensitivity
- Magnetic resonance imaging (MRI) has shown promise and has excellent specificity but experience is limited and sensitivity is unknown
- Diagnostic pneumoperitoneography is a technique where air is injected through a DPL catheter and pneumothorax on subsequent chest x-ray is diagnostic for diaphragmatic injury
  - —Poorly tolerated by unstable patients and may require chest tube placement
- Thoracoscopy and laparoscopy are potentially valuable tools

DIFFERENTIAL DIAGNOSIS

- Atelectasis, hemothorax, pneumothorax
- Gastric dilation, pulmonary contusion, intra-abdominal fluid
- Traumatic pneumatocele, subdiaphragmatic abscess, intrathoracic cyst
- Empyema, congenital eventration of the diaphragm

Treatment

INITIAL STABILIZATION

- Initial stabilization is the same as for all trauma victims and should follow Advanced Trauma Life Support protocols
- If respiratory distress is present, immediate placement of a nasogastric tube may decompress herniated abdominal contents

ED TREATMENT

- Great care must be taken not to injure herniating abdominal viscera or further injure the diaphragm while placing a chest tube in patients with known or suspected diaphragmatic rupture
  —Palpate within the chest wall completely for visceral organs prior to placing tube
- Patients with visceral perforations are septic and need aggressive resuscitation and antibiotic therapy
- Early surgical intervention is paramount
- Empiric broad spectrum antibiotics are indicated in the case of perforated viscera

MEDICATIONS

- Gram-negative aerobes
  —Gentamicin: adult/peds: 2–5 mg/kg IV
- Gram-negative anaerobes
  —Clindamycin: adult: 900 mg IV q 8 hrs; peds: 20–40 mg/kg/day IV div q 8 hrs
  —Metronidazole: adult: 1 g IV load then 500 mg IV q 6 hrs; peds: 15 mg/kg then 7.5 mg/kg IV q 6 hrs
- Both aerobic and anaerobic
  —Ampicillin/sulbactam: adult: 3 g IV q 6 hrs; peds: safety not established
  —Cefotetan: adult: 2 g IV q 12 hrs; peds: dose not established
  —Cefoxitin: adult: 2 g IV q 12 hrs; peds: 80–160 mg/kg/day div q 6 hrs
  —Ticarcillin/clavulanate: adult: 3.1 g IV q 6 hrs; peds: safety not established

Disposition

ADMISSION CRITERIA

- Patients with suspicion for diaphragmatic injury must be admitted to the trauma surgical service
- Patients should be admitted to a monitored or intensive care unit setting

DISCHARGE CRITERIA

- Patients with diaphragmatic injury must not be discharged from the ED

Miscellaneous

ICD9: 862.0

CORE CONTENT CODE: 18.4.11.6

SUGGESTED READINGS

Kanowitz A, Markovchick V. Esophageal and diaphragmatic trauma. In: Rosen P, et al., eds. Emergency medicine: Concepts and clinical practice. 4th ed. St. Louis: CV Mosby, 1998:546–554.

Meyers BF, McCabe CJ. Traumatic diaphragmatic hernia: Occult marker of serious injury. Ann Surg 1993;218(6):783–790.

Pagliarello G, Carter J. Traumatic injury to the diaphragm: Timely diagnosis and treatment. J Trauma 1992;33(2):194–197.

Shah R, Sabanathan S, Mearns AJ, Choudhury AK. Traumatic rupture of the diaphragm. Ann Thorac Surg 1995;60:1444–1449.

Author: Robert S. Hamilton

Diarrhea, Adult

Clinical Presentation

SIGNS AND SYMPTOMS

- Loose, watery bowel movements
- Bloody stools with mucous
- Abdominal pain and cramps, tenesmus, flatulence
- Fever, headache, myalgias
- Nausea, vomiting
- Dehydration, lethargy and stupor
- Perianal inflammation, fissure, fistula

ETIOLOGY

Infectious

Viruses

- 50–70% of all cases

Invasive Bacteria

- Campylobacter
  - —Contaminated food/water, wilderness water, birds and animals
  - —Most common bacterial diarrhea
  - —Gross or occult blood is found in 60–90%
- Salmonella
  - —Contaminated water, eggs, poultry, or dairy products
  - —Typhoid fever (*S. typhi*) characterized by unremitting fever, abdominal pain, rose spots, splenomegaly, and bradycardia
- Shigella
  - —Fecal/oral route
- *Vibrio Parahaemolyticus*
  - —Raw and undercooked seafood
- Yersinia
  - —Contaminated food (pork), water, and milk
  - —May present as mesenteric adenitis or mimic appendicitis

Bacterial Toxin

- *Escherichia coli*
- Major cause of traveler's diarrhea
- Ingestion of food or water contaminated by feces
- *Staphylococcal aureus*
  - —Most common toxin related disease
  - —Symptoms 1–6 hours after ingesting food
- *Bacillus cereus*
  - —Classic source—fried rice left on steam tables
  - —Symptoms within 1–36 hours
- *Clostridium difficile*
  - —Antibiotic associated enteritis linked to pseudomembranous colitis
  - —Incubation period within 10 days of exposure or initiation of antibiotics
- *Aeronomas hydrophilis*
  - —Aquatic sources primarily
  - —Affects children under three years
  - —Fecal leukocytes absent
- Cholera
  - —Caused by an enterotoxin produced by *Vibrio cholerae*
  - —Profuse watery stools with mucous (classic appearance of "rice-water" stools)

Protozoa

- *Giardia lamblia*
  - —Most common cause of parasite gastroenteritis in North America
  - —High risk groups: travelers, children in day care centers, institutionalized people, homosexual men, and campers who drink untreated mountain water
- *Cryptosporidium parvum*
  - —Commonly carried in patients with AIDS
- *Entamoeba histolytica* (entamebiasis)
  - —5–10% extraintestinal manifestations (hepatic amebic abscess)

PEDIATRIC CONSIDERATIONS

- Focus evaluation on state of hydration
  - —Frequency of urination
  - —Weight loss, flat or sunken fontanelle
  - —Tachycardia
  - —Tachypnea (reflecting acidosis)
  - —Dry mucous membranes, lack of tears, decreased skin turgor
- Majority of the cases are of viral origin and self-limited
  - —Rotavirus accounts for up to 50%
- *Shigella:* infections associated with seizures

Pre-Hospital

CAUTIONS

- Difficult IV access with severe dehydration
- Avoid exposure to contaminated clothes or body substances

Diagnosis

ESSENTIAL WORKUP

- Digital rectal examination to determine the presence of gross or occult blood
- Fecal leukocyte determination
  - —Present with invasive bacteria
  - —Absent in protozoal infections, viral, toxin-induced food poisoning

LABORATORY

- CBC—indications
  - —Significant blood loss
  - —Systemic toxicity
- Electrolytes, glucose BUN/Cr—indications
  - —Lethargy, significant dehydration, toxicity, or altered mental status
  - —Diuretic use, persistent diarrhea, chronic liver or renal disease
- Stool culture—indications
  - —Presence of fecal leuckocytes
  - —Historical markers: immunocompromised, travel, homosexual
  - —Public health: food handler, day/health-care worker, institutionalized
- Blood cultures—indications
  - —Suspected bacteremia/systemic infections
  - —Ill patients requiring admission
  - —Immunocompromised
  - —Elderly/infants

IMAGING/SPECIAL TESTS

- Abdominal x-ray films
  - —No value unless an obstruction or a toxic megacolon suspected

DIFFERENTIAL DIAGNOSIS

- Ulcerative colitis
- Crohn's disease
- Mesenteric ischemia
- Diverticulitis, anal fissures, hemorrhoids
- Irritable bowel syndrome
- Milk and food allergies
- Malrotation with midgut volvulus
- Meckel's diverticulum
- Intussusception
- Drugs and toxins: mannitol, sorbital, phenolphthalein, magnesium-containing antacids, quinidine, colchicine, mushrooms, mercury poisoning

PEDIATRIC CONSIDERATIONS

- Laboratory studies not required in most cases
- Rotazyme assay
  - —Detects rotavirus
  - —Rarely indicated in managing outpatients
  - —Helpful to cohort and avoids cross-contamination among inpatients
- Stool cultures—indication
  - —Febrile
  - —Abrupt onset of diarrhea occuring more than four times per day
  - —Blood in the stool

Treatment

INITIAL STABILIZATION

- ABCs
- IV fluid with 0.9%NS resuscitation for severely dehydrated

ED MANAGEMENT

- Oral fluids for mild dehydration (gatorade/pedialyte)
- IV fluids for
  - —Hypotension, nausea/vomiting, obtundation, metabolic acidosis, significant hypernatremia or hyponatremia
  - —0.9%NS bolus (500 ml–1 L adults, 20 ml/kg pediatrics) for resuscitation then 0.9%NS or D5W 0.45%NS (D5W 0.25%NS pediatrics) to maintain an adequate urine output
- Bismuth subsalicylate (pepto-bismol)
  - —Antisecretory agent
  - —Effective clinical relief without adverse effects
- Kaolin-pectin (kaopectate)
  - —Reduces fluidity of stools
  - —Does not influence the course of the disease
- Antimotility drugs: diphenoxylate (lomotil), loperamide (imodium), paregoric, and codeine
  - —Appropriate in noninfectious diarrhea
  - —Initial use of sparse amounts to control symptoms in infectious diarrhea
  - —Avoid prolonged use in infectious diarrhea—may increase the duration of fever, diarrhea, and bacteremia, and may precipitate a toxic megacolon

Antibiotics for Infectious Pathogens

- Campylobacter: quinolone or erythromycin
- Salmonella: quinolone or trimethoprim/sulfamethoxazole (TMP/SMX)
- Ceftriaxone for typhoid fever
- Shigella: quinolone, TMP/SMX, or ampicillin
- *Vibrio parahaemolyticus:* tetracycline or doxycycline
- *Clostridium difficile:* vancomycin
- *Escherichia coli:* quinolone or TMP/SMX
- *Giardia lamblia:* metronidazole or quinacrine
- *Entamoeba histolytica* (entamebiasis): iodoquinol or metronidazole

MEDICATIONS

- Ampicillin: 500 mg (peds: 20 mg/kg/24 hr) po/IV q 6 hr
- Bactrim DS (trimethoprim/sulfamethoxazole): 1 tab (peds: 8–10 mg TMP/40–50 mg SMX/kg/24 hr) po/IV bid
- Ciprofloxacin (quinolone): 500 mg po/IV bid
- Doxycycline: 100 mg po/IV bid
- Erythromycin: 500 mg (peds: 40–50 mg/kg/24 hr) po qid
- Iodoquinol: 650 mg (peds: 30–40 mg/kg/24 hr) po tid
- Metronidazole: 250 mg (peds: 35 mg/kg/24 hr) po tid
- Tetracycline: 500 mg po/IV q 6 hr
- Quinacrine: 100 mg (peds: 6 mg/kg/24 hr) po tid
- Vancomycin: 125–400 mg (peds: 10–50 mg/kg/24 hr) po qid

Disposition

ADMISSION CRITERIA

- Hypotension, unresponsive to IV fluids
- Significant bleeding
- Signs of sepsis/toxicity
- Intractable vomiting or abdominal pain
- Severe electrolyte imbalance/metabolic acidosis
- Altered mental status
- Children with >10–15% dehydration

DISCHARGE CRITERIA

- Mild cases requiring oral hydration
- Dehydration responsive to IV fluids

Miscellaneous

ICD9: 787.91

CORE CONTENT CODE: 22.4.6

SUGGESTED READINGS

Bitterman R. Acute gastroenteritis and constipation. In: Rosen P, Barkin RM, et al, eds. Emergency medicine: Concepts and clinical practice. 4th ed. St. Louis: Mosby-Year Book, 1998: 1917–1958.

Hogan D. The emergency department approach to diarrhea. Emerg Med Clin North Am November 1996;14(4):673–694.

Reisdorff E, Pflug V. Infectious diarrhea: Beyond supportive care. Emerg Med Reports 1996;17(14):141–150.

Author: Isam Nasr

Diarrhea, Pediatric

Clinical Presentation

SIGNS AND SYMPTOMS

- Frequent, loose stools
  - —Watery
  - —Bloody
  - —Mucoid
- Signs of dehydration reflect loss of total body water
- Fever
- Abdominal pain, distention
- Vomiting
- Tenesmus
- Impaired nutritional status or abnormal growth parameters

MECHANISM/DESCRIPTION

- One of the most common pediatric complaints second only to respiratory infections in overall disease frequency
- Acute infectious enteritis (AIE)
  - —Defined as vomiting and diarrhea
  - —2 episodes annually for each child <5 years of age in the United States
  - —responsible for approximately 10% of all pediatric ED visits and hospital admissions
- Acute change in the "normal" bowel pattern that leads to increased stools or volume and lasts less than 7 days
  - —Chronic if the diarrhea persists for more than 2 weeks

ETIOLOGY

Acute enteritis

- Infectious
  - —Viruses: 70–80% of cases
    - -Rotavirus and Norwalk viruses in the winter months
    - -Enteroviruses in the summer and early autumn
  - —Bacteria: 10–20%
    - -E. coli
    - -Campylobacter
    - -Salmonella
    - -Shigella
    - -Yersinia enterocolitica
    - -Clostridium difficile
  - —Parasites 5%
- Postinfection
- Milk allergy
- Associated with other infections
  - —Otitis media
  - —Urinary tract infection

Chronic diarrhea

- Osmotic
  - —Lactose intolerance (increased sorbitol from fruit juices)
- Secretory
  - —Increased secretion due to secretagogues bacterial (toxins, failure reabsorption)
- Altered motility
  - —Increased gut transit (irritable bowel syndrome)
- Exudative diarrhea
  - —Inflammatory conditions where there is disruption of the mucosa of the intestines (Inflammatory Bowel Disease, Henoch Schönlein Purpura, Bacterial colitis)

SIGN	5%	5–10%	>10%
Skin turgor	nl—slight decreased	decreased	very decreased
Color	nl—pale	sallow	ashen
Oral mucosa	tacky	very dry	parched
Tears	± decreased	absent	absent
Fontanelle	normal	depressed	sunken
Heart rate	± increased	increased	extreme tachycardia
Blood pressure	normal	± decreased	decreased
Urine output	mild decrease	oliguria	anuria
Level of consciousness	irritable	lethargic	unresponsive

Pre-Hospital

CAUTIONS

- Severely dehydrated (>10% dehydration) children in shock or near-shock must receive
  - —Immediate IV bolus with 20 cc/kg 0.9%NS
  - —Blood glucose determination
  - —100% O_2 via nonrebreather
  - —Cardiac monitoring

Diagnosis

ESSENTIAL WORKUP

- Gross examination of stool
- Guaiac and Wright stain for fecal leucocytes
  - —Watery diarrhea without blood or mucus associated with viral enteritis or related to bacterial enterotoxins
  - —Diarrhea with blood or mucus suggests an enteroinvasive inflammatory or cytotoxin-mediated process (Salmonella, invasive E. coli)
  - —Microscopic examination of a Wright-stained smear of the mucoid part of stool revealing >5 fecal leucocytes/HPF is suggestive of bacterial infection
    - -Shigella
    - -Salmonella
    - -Campylobacter
    - -Yersinia
    - -Invasive E. coli

LABORATORY

- Serum electrolytes, BUN/Cr assist in the assessment of dehydration
- Urinalysis assists in the assessment of dehydration

IMAGING/SPECIAL TESTS

- Stool culture
  - —Unnecessary in most cases unless there is a high likelihood of identifying bacterial pathogens where the clinical course and period of contagion may be altered by antibiotic therapy

DIFFERENTIAL DIAGNOSIS

- Infectious
  - —Bacterial gastroenteritis
    - -Fever >39°C
    - -Toxic clinical appearance
    - -Crampy abdominal pain
    - -Bloody mucoid stools
  - —Viral gastroenteritis
    - -Seasonal epidemics
    - -Guaiac negative stool
  - —Parasitic
    - -Giardia lamblia
    - -Chronic diarrhea
- Postinfectious
  - —C difficile
- Noninfectious
  - —Milk allergy
    - -Heme-positive stool
    - -Vomiting
  - —Malrotation with midgut volvulus
  - —Inflammatory bowel disease
  - —Intussusception
    - -Currant jelly stool
    - -Abdominal mass

Treatment

INITIAL STABILIZATION

- For severely dehydrated children in shock or near-shock, intravenous or intraosseous access with 20 cc/kg normal saline or Ringers lactate and 1 g/kg dextrose if hypoglycemic
- Pulse oximetry
- Endotracheal intubation may be required for children in shock

ED TREATMENT

- For mild to moderate dehydration, correct dehydration using oral rehydration therapy (ORT) 50 ml/kg and 100 ml/kg respectively over a 4-hour period
  —Replace ongoing losses with 10 ml/kg of ORT for each stool
- If diarrhea is not associated with dehydration, use 10 ml/kg of ORT for each stool alone
- Antibiotics for defined acute enteritis
  —Campylobacter jejuni
    -Erythromycin
  —Salmonella—uncomplicated
    -No antibiotics
  —Salmonella—complicated (infant <6 months, disseminated, bacteremia, immunocompromised host, enteric fever)
    -Ampicillin or TMP/SMX × 10 days
  —Shigella
    -TMP/SMX × 5 days
  —Yersinia
    -None or TMP/SMX × 5 days
  —C. difficile—carrier
    -None
  —C. difficile—severe and or prolonged enteritis
    -Metronidazole or vancomycin × 7 days
  —E. coli—enterotoxigenic, enteropathogenic
    -None
  —E. coli—enteroinvasive
    -TMP/SMX × 5 days
  —E. coli—enteroadherent
    -Neomycin 100 mg/kg/day × 5 days
  —Lamblia
    -Furazolidone or metronidazole × 10 days
- Antidiarrheal agents *not* recommended
  —Alter intestinal motility (loperamide, opiates, opiate-atropine combinations)
  —Alter secretion (bismuth subsalicylate)
  —Adsorb fluid/toxins (kaolin-pectin, fiber, activated charcoal, attapulgite)
  —Alter intestinal microflora (lactobacillus-containing compounds)

Post-ED Diet

- On rehydration, feed children with diarrhea age-appropriate diets
- Well-tolerated foods
  —Rich in complex carbohydrates (rice, potatoes, bread)
  —Lean meats
  —Yogurt
  —Fruits
  —Vegetables
  —Full strength milk and formula unless there is a strong suspicion of lactose intolerance
- Avoid fatty foods and foods high in simple sugars

MEDICATIONS

- Ampicillin: 50–200 mg/kg/24hrs IV/PO divided q 6 hrs
- Erythromycin: 40 mg/kg/24hrs po q 6 hrs; 10–20 mg/kg/24hrs IV divided q 6 hrs
- Furazolidone: 6 mg/kg/24hrs divided q 6 hrs
- Metronidazole: 15–30 mg/kg/24hrs
- Neomycin: 100 mg/kg/24hrs po divided q 4 hrs
- ORT (45–50 mmol/L of sodium): as described above
- TMP (6–12 mg/kg/24hrs) SMX (30–60 mg/kg/24hrs): divided q 12 hrs
- Vancomycin: 20–40 mg/kg/24hrs po divided q 6 hrs

Disposition

ADMISSION CRITERIA

- Surgical abdomen
- Inability to tolerate oral fluids
- ≥10% dehydration
- Suspected salmonella enteritis in immunocompromised
- Toxic-appearing child or in infant <3 months of age

DISCHARGE CRITERIA

- ORT tolerated
- Improvement in the patient's condition
- Child's caretakers can follow through on using appropriate ORT and with feeding an appropriate diet
- Caregivers be able to report signs and symptoms of dehydration

Miscellaneous

ICD9: 009.1, 558

CORE CONTENT CODE: 22.4.6

SUGGESTED READINGS

Bonadio WA. Acute infectious enteritis in children—emergency department diagnosis and management. Emerg Med Clin North Am 1995;13:457–472.

Merrick N, Davidson B, Fox S. Treatment of acute gastroenteritis: too much and too little care. Clin Pediatr 1996;9:429–436.

Provisional Committee on Quality Improvement, Subcommittee on Acute Gastroenteritis. Practice parameter: the management of acute gastroenteritis in young children. Pediatrics 1996;97:424–436.

Author: Richard Lichtenstein

Digoxin, Poisoning

Clinical Presentation

SIGNS AND SYMPTOMS

Cardiovascular

- Dysrhythmias
  - —Paroxysmal atrial tachycardia (PAT) with atrial-ventricular (AV) block
    - -Classic dysrhythmia
    - -Uncommon
  - —Nonparoxysmal accelerated junctional tachycardia
  - —Ventricular tachycardia (VT)
  - —Regularized atrial fibrillation (AFib)
  - —Bigeminy
  - —Premature ventricular contraction (common)
  - —Bradycardia
  - —Nonparoxysmal atrial tachycardia
  - —AV blocks
  - —Sinus arrhythmia
  - —Premature atrial contraction
- CHF exacerbation
- Hypotension
- Shock
- Cardiovascular collapse
- Syncope

CNS

- Mental status changes
  - —Agitation
  - —Lethargy
  - —Seizures
  - —Psychosis
- Visual perception
  - —Blurred
  - —Scotoma
  - —Green/yellow halo
  - —Photophobia
  - —Hallucinations
  - —Color perception changes

GI

- Anorexia
- Nausea/vomiting
- Diarrhea
- Abdominal pain

General

- Headache
- Weakness
- Lightheadedness

MECHANISM/DESCRIPTION

Digitalis Effects

- Inhibit sodium-potassium ATPase in cell membranes
- Allows more calcium ions to enter the cell and cardiac cells to contract more strongly
- Increases K^+ extracellularly
- Increases vagal tone
- Slows AV node conduction
- Increases automaticity and conduction system refractory period

ETIOLOGY

- Onset: 2 hours after PO ingestion and 15 minutes following IV
- Toxicity
  - —Occurs with normal digoxin levels
  - —May be absent with elevated digoxin levels
- Plants containing cardiac glycosides
- Foxglove
- Oleander
- Lily of the valley
- Dogbane
- Red squill

Pre-Hospital

CAUTIONS

- Avoid cardioversion with tachydysrhythmias
  - —May precipitate ventricular fibrillation

Diagnosis

ESSENTIAL WORKUP

- ECG
  - —For dysrhythmia (see above)
- Digoxin level
  - —Normal range: 0.5 to 2.0 ng/ml
  - —Distribution after oral intake not complete until 6 hours
  - —False elevations possible with spironolactone use, pregnancy, hyperbilirubinemia, chronic renal failure
  - —Not useful after digoxin immune Fab antibodies given

LABORATORY

- Electrolytes, BUN/Cr, glucose
  - —Hypokalemia contributes to digitalis toxicity
  - —Hyperkalemia seen in acute toxicity and correlates with acute digitalis toxicity better than digoxin serum levels
  - —Follow K^+ serially
- Calcium/magnesium

DIFFERENTIAL DIAGNOSES

- Overdoses
  - —Calcium channel blockers
  - —β blockers
  - —Quinidine/procainamide
  - —Clonidine
  - —Organophosphates
- Primary cardiac dysrhythmias
- Acute gastroenteritis

Treatment

INITIAL STABILIZATION
- ABCs
- IV, oxygen, monitor
  - —IV fluid bolus if hypovolemic
- Administer naloxone, thiamine, dextrose, (Accucheck) for altered mental status

ED TREATMENT
Cardiac Arrest Resuscitation
- Defibrillate for ventricular fibrillation, pulseless VT
- Standard ACLS protocol
- Administer digoxin specific antibody Fab fragments (digibind) up to 20 vials
- $MgSO_4$ 2 g IV push
- Continue resuscitation for 30 minutes following digoxin immune Fab antibodies

General Measures
- Gastric lavage if <1 to 2 hours postacute ingestion
  - —May cause bradycardia, asystole
  - —Use caution if bradycardia or atrioventricular block present
  - —Consider atropine pretreatment
- Avoid ipecac/induction of emesis
- Activated charcoal if acute ingestion
- Potassium replacement to achieve level above 4.0 mEq/L
  - —Use with caution if bradycardia or AV block
- Replete magnesium
- Treat hyperkalemia with insulin, dextrose, bicarbonate, sodium polystyrene sulfonate
  - —Calcium *contraindicated*

Dysrhythmia Management
- Initiate the following while waiting for digoxin specific immune fragments
  - —Lidocaine for ventricular dysrhythmias without AV block
  - —Phenytoin
    - -Drug of choice for ventricular dysrhythmias
    - -Action at AV node and beneficial response in supraventricular dysrhythmias (atrial tachycardia with AV block)
  - —Atropine, pacing for symptomatic bradydysrhythmia
  - —β blockage (propranolol, esmolol) for supraventricular tachycardia
    - -Avoid with AV block, bradycardia
  - —$MgSO_4$ for ventricular dysrhythmias
  - —Bretylium and catecholamines may exacerbate toxicity
  - —Quinidine, procainamide contraindicated
- Cardioversion contraindicated unless as last resort for severe life threatening dysrhythmia
  - —Start at low energy 10 to 25 joules then increase to high levels if ineffective
  - —Safe if digoxin level <2.0 ng/ml

Digoxin Specific Antibody Fab Fragments (Digibind)
- Indications
  - —Ingestion of >10 mg (adults) or 0.2 mg/kg (children)
  - —Hyperkalemia
  - —Hemodynamically unstable or life threatening dysrhythmias
  - —Ventricular tachycardia, ventricular fibrillation
  - —Atrial tachycardia
  - —Variable AV block
  - —Bradycardia with no response to atropine
  - —Hypotension
- Onset: 20 to 30 minutes
- Digoxin levels increase after therapy due to antibody complexes
- Renal clearance of the drug antibody complexes
- Second dose if rebound toxicity
- Complications
  - —Exacerbation of CHF
  - —Hypokalemia
  - —AFib with rapid ventricular response

MEDICATIONS
- Activated charcoal slurry: 1–2 g/kg up to 90 g PO
- Atropine 0.5 mg (peds: 0.02 mg/kg) IV repeat 0.5–1.0 mg IV (peds: 0.04 mg/kg)
- Dextrose: D50W 1 amp (50 ml or 25 g) (peds: D25W 2–4 ml/kg) IV
- Digoxin specific antibody Fab fragments
  - —40 mg per vial neutralizes 0.6 mg of digoxin
  - —If amount ingested known:
    - -# of vials needed = amount ingested mg/0.6
  - —If steady serum level known:
    - -# of vials needed = serum digoxin level × patient's weight in kg/100
  - —If neither amount ingested or serum level known:
    - -Acute toxicity 10 to 15 vials adults or children
    - -Chronic toxicity 2 to 3 vials adults
  - —Bolus for cardiac arrest
  - —Additional doses as needed
- Esmolol: 50–200 mg/kg/min
- Insulin and glucose: 10 U (peds: 0.25 U/kg) regular insulin + 50 ml 50% (peds: 1g/kg) dextrose IV
- Lidocaine: 1 mg/kg IV then 0.5 mg/kg q 10 min to max 3 mg/kg
- Magnesium sulfate: 2 g (peds: 25–50 mg/kg/dose) IV PB
- Naloxone: 2 mg (peds: 0.1 mg/kg) IV or IM
- Phenytoin: 15–18 mg/kg IV
- Propranolol: 1mg (peds: 0.01–0.1 mg/kg) IV
- Sodium bicarbonate: 1–3 amp (44 mEq) IV over 20–30 min (peds: 1–2 mEq/kg/dose)
- Sodium polystyrene sulfonate (kayexalate)
  - —Oral: 15 g mixed with water or 50 ml of sorbitol
  - —Rectal enema: 50 g in 200ml of sorbitol
  - —peds: 1.0 g/kg po or PR
- Sorbitol: 1–2 g/kg to a max of 100 g (peds: >1 yr old: 1–1.5 g/kg as a 35% solution to a max of 50 g) po
- Thiamine: 100 mg (peds: 50 mg) IV or IM

Disposition

ADMISSION CRITERIA
- ICU
  - —Symptomatic toxicity or digoxin level >2 ng/ml with acute exposure
  - —Post digoxin immune Fab (for 24 hours) administration
  - —Unstable acute or chronic toxicity
- Telemetry
  - —Asymptomatic or mildly symptomatic dysrhythmia especially following large doses
  - —High risk for developing toxicity

DISCHARGE CRITERIA
- Acute ingestion
  - —Digoxin level <2.0 ng/ml
  - —Asymptomatic for 6 hours and no ECG abnormalities
- Chronic exposure
  - —Digoxin level <2.5 ng/ml
  - —Asymptomatic for 6 hours and no ECG abnormalities

Miscellaneous

ICD9: 972.1

CORE CURRICULUM CODE: 17.2.15.3

SUGGESTED READINGS

Bayer MJ. Recognition and management of digitalis intoxication: Implications for emergency medicine. Am J Emerg Med 1991;9(2 Suppl 1):29–31.

Ellenhorn MJ, Schoonwald S, Ordog G, et al. Digitalis. In: Ellenhorn's Medical Toxicology, 2d ed. Baltimore: Williams & Wilkins, 1997:541–546.

Kelly RA, Smith TW. Recognition and management of digitalis toxicity. Am J Cardiol 1992;69(18):108G–119G.

Woolf AD, Wenger TL, Smith TW. Results of multicenter studies of digoxin—specific antibody fragments in managing digitalis intoxication in the pediatric population. Am J Emerg Med 1991;9(2 Suppl 1):16–20.

Author: Leslie Wolf

Disseminated Intravascular Coagulation

Clinical Presentation

SIGNS AND SYMPTOMS

- Excessive bleeding
  —Petechiae
  —Purpura
  —Hemorrhagic bullae
  —Wound bleeding
  —Epistaxis
  —Hemoptysis
  —Gastrointestinal bleeding
- Excessive thrombosis
  —Large vessels
  —Microvascular thrombosis and end organ dysfunction
    -Cardiac, pulmonary, renal, hepatic, CNS
  —Thrombophlebitis
  —Pulmonary embolus
  —Nonbacterial thrombotic endocarditis
  —Gangrene
  —Ischemic infarcts of kidney, liver, CNS, bowel
- Acute DIC
  —Hemorrhagic complications predominate
- Chronic DIC
  —Thrombotic complications predominate

MECHANISM/DESCRIPTION

- Normal coagulation
  —A series of *local* reactions among blood vessels, platelets, and clotting factors
- DIC is *systemic* activation of coagulation and fibrinolysis by some other primary disease process
- Coagulation system activation results in systemic circulation of thrombin and plasmin
  —Role of thrombin in DIC
    -Thrombin circulates and converts fibrinogen to fibrin monomer
    -Fibrin monomer polymerizes into fibrin (clot) in the circulation
    -Clots cause micro- and macrovascular thrombosis with resultant peripheral ischemia and end organ damage
    -Platelets become trapped in clot with resultant thrombocytopenia
  —Role of plasmin in DIC
    -Plasmin circulates systemically converting fibrinogen into fibrin degradation products (FDPs)
    -FDPs combine with fibrin monomers
    -FDP/monomer complexes interfere with normal polymerization and impair hemostasis
    -FDPs also interfere with platelet function
- Acute DIC—uncompensated form
  —Clotting factors used more rapidly than the body can replace them
  —Hemorrhage predominant clinical feature which overshadows ongoing thrombosis
- Chronic DIC—compensated form
  —Body able to keep up with pace of clotting-factor consumption
  —Thrombosis predominant clinical feature

ETIOLOGY

- Precipitated by many disease states
- Complications of pregnancy
  —Retained fetus
  —Amniotic fluid embolism
  —Placental abruption
  —Abortion
  —Eclampsia
- Sepsis
  —Gram-negative (endotoxin mediated meningococcemia)
  —Gram-positive (mucopolysaccharide mediated)
- Trauma
  —Crush injury
  —Severe burns
  —Severe head injury
- Malignancy
  —Metastatic disease
  —Leukemia
- Intravascular hemolysis
  —Transfusion reactions
  —Massive transfusion
- Thrombocytopenia
  —Thrombotic thrombocytopenic purpura
  —Idiopathic thrombocytopenic purpura

Pre-Hospital

N/A

Diagnosis

ESSENTIAL WORKUP

- Depends on precipitating illness
- Diagnosis generally not made in the emergency department
- Platelet count
  —Decreased
  —$<100,000/mm^3$
  —May be normal in chronic DIC
- PT/PTT
  —Increased
  —May be normal in chronic DIC
- Fibrinogen
  —Decreased
  —<150 mg/dl in 70%
  —May be normal in chronic DIC
- FDPs (fibrin degradation products)
  —Increased
  — >40 μg/ml
- D-Dimer
  —Increased

LABORATORY

- CBC/peripheral smear
  —Red cell fragments
  —Low platelets
  —Peripheral smear confirms disease in chronic DIC
- Electrolytes, BUN/Cr, glucose
  —Elevated BUN/Cr due to renal insufficiency
- ABG
  —Oxygen/acid base status

IMAGING/SPECIAL TESTS

- CXR for suspected pneumonia/sepsis
- CT brain for altered mental status

DIFFERENTIAL DIAGNOSIS

- Inherited coagulation disorders
  —Factor deficiencies
- Other acquired coagulation disorders
  —Anti-coagulant therapy
  —Drugs
  —Hepatic disease
- Platelet dysfunction

Treatment

INITIAL STABILIZATION

- ABCs
  - —Control bleeding
  - —Establish IV access
  - —Restore and maintain circulating blood volume
- Initiate therapy of precipitating disease
  - —Antibiotics in sepsis
  - —Evacuate uterus of retained dead fetus
  - —Chemotherapy in malignancy
  - —Debridement of devitalized tissue in trauma

ED TREATMENT

Overview

- Therapy of DIC is controversial and should be individualized based on
  - —Age
  - —Hemodynamic status
  - —Severity of hemorrhage
  - —Severity of thrombosis
- Involve admitting service prior to initiating specific DIC therapy

DIC Therapy

- Replace depleted blood components
  - —FFP
    - -For prolonged PT
    - -Provides clotting factors and volume replacement
    - -Dose: 2 U or 10–15 ml/kg
  - —Platelets
    - -If platelet count <20,000 or platelet count <50,000 with ongoing bleeding
    - -Dose: 1 U/10 kg body weight
  - —Cryoprecipitate
    - -Higher fibrinogen content than whole plasma
    - -For severe hypofibrinogenemia (<50 mg/dl) or for active bleeding with fibrinogen <100 mg/dl
    - -Dose: 8 U
  - —Washed packed cells
  - —Albumin
  - —Nonclotting volume expanders
- Inhibition of intravascular clotting
  - —Heparin (use is controversial)
    - -May be effective in mild to moderate DIC
    - -Efficacy undetermined in severe DIC
    - -Possible indications
      - *Purpura fulminans (gangrene of digits/extremities)
      - *Acute promyelocytic leukemia
      - *"Dead fetus syndrome"—several weeks after intrauterine fetal death
      - *Thromboembolic complications of large vessels
      - *Before surgery with metatstatic carcinoma
    - -Low dose regimen: 5–10 U/kg/hr IV for chronic DIC
    - -High dose regimen: 10,000 U bolus followed by 1000 U/hr; 20–30,000 U every 24 hours via constant infusion
  - —Antithrombin concentrates (controversial)
    - -Used alone or in combination with heparin
- Inhibition of fibrinolysis
  - —Block secondary compensatory fibrinolysis that accompanies DIC
  - —Use complicated by severe thrombosis
  - —Use only when DIC accompanied by primary fibrinolysis
    - -Promyelocytic leukemia
    - -Giant hemangioma
    - -Heat stroke
    - -Amniotic fluid embolism
    - -Metastatic carcinoma of prostate
  - —Initiate in extreme cases only
    - -Profuse bleeding not responding to replacement therapy
    - -Excessive fibrinolysis present (rapid whole blood lysis/short euglobulin lysis time)
  - —ε-amino caproic acid (EACA)

Disposition

ADMISSION CRITERIA

- Severe precipitating illness in combination with DIC requires ICU admission

DISCHARGE CRITERIA

- None

Miscellaneous

ICD9: 286.6

CORE CONTENT CODE: 7.2.2

SUGGESTED READINGS

Bick RL. Disseminated intravascular coagulation: Objective clinical and laboratory diagnosis, treatment and assessment of therapeutic response. Semin Thromb Hemost 1996;22(1):69

Gilbert JA, Scalzi RP. Disseminated intravascular coagulation. Emer Med Clin North Am 1993;11(2):465

Seligsohn U. Disseminated intravascular coagulation. In: Williams W, et al, eds. Williams hematology. 5th ed. New York: McGraw Hill, 1995:1497–1511

Author: Steven Bowman

Disulfiram Reaction

Clinical Presentation

SIGNS AND SYMPTOMS

Disulfiram—Ethanol Reaction

- Facial and truncal erythema and flushing—diaphoresis
- Sensation of "warmth"
- Conjunctival injection
- Nausea, vomiting, abdominal discomfort
- Headache, anxiety, ataxia, dizziness, confusion, lethargy, seizures
- Chest tightness and discomfort, palpitations, dyspnea
- Dysrhythmias and cardiac ischemia
- Hypotension, tachycardia, tachypnea

Disulfiram overdose

- Dysarthria, agitation, hallucinations, acute psychosis, seizures, coma
- Hypotension, tachycardia, fever
- Sulfur odor on breath
- Catatonia; symptoms similar to Parkinsonism may occur late and persist
- Flaccid paresis, symmetric bilateral hypesthesias due to sensory/motor axonopathy

MECHANISM/DESCRIPTION

- Hepatically metabolized to active metabolites which exert their effect on various enzymes
- Disulfiram—ethanol reaction
  - —Disulfiram metabolites covalently bind and inactivate the active site on aldehyde dehydrogenase
  - —Ethanol metabolism blocked at the aldehyde dehydrogenase step leading to accumulation of acetaldehyde
  - —Acetaldehyde results in release of histamine, causing vasodilatation and hypotension
- Disulfiram metabolites inhibit dopamine β-hydroxylase and limit the synthesis of norepinephrine from dopamine
  - —Relative excess of dopamine contributes to mental status changes
  - —Relative depletion of norepinephrine contributes to hypotension
- Disulfiram metabolites inhibit pyridoxal 5-phosphate
  - —Diminishes concentration of pyridoxine available for the formation of γ-aminobutyric acid (GABA) in the CNS
  - —Potentially predisposes to seizures
- Disulfiram metabolites can cause acute toxic hepatitis, often peaking after two months of treatment
- Disulfiram metabolites can cause peripheral neuropathies which are dose and duration dependent

ETIOLOGY

- Used as a deterrent to ethanol consumption in the treatment of chronic ethanol abuse
- Investigated as an inhibitor of HIV replication and as an immune stimulant
- Other agents which can cause a (usually milder) disulfiram-ethanol-like reaction
  - —Antiinfectives: cephalosporins, metronidazole, nitrofurantoin, griseofulvin, monosulfiram (an ascaricide)
  - —CNS drugs: procarbazine, tranylcypromine, pargyline, amitriptyline, chloral hydrate
  - —Sulfonylureas
  - —Industrial: carbon disulfide, carbon tetrachloride, dimethyl formamide, tetraethyl lead, tetrachloroethylene, trichloroethylene

Pre-Hospital

N/A

Diagnosis

ESSENTIAL WORKUP

- Consider disulfiram-ethanol reaction if the above signs and symptoms are present in patients who are being treated for chronic ethanol abuse in conjunction with recent ethanol ingestion, or exposure to ethanol-containing foods or medications

LABORATORY

- Ethanol level
- Electrolytes, BUN, Cr, and glucose
- Liver function tests if hepatitis is suspected
- CPK if seizures or agitation may predispose to rhabdomyolysis

IMAGING/SPECIAL TESTS

- EKG to assess cardiac ischemia
- CT scan
  - —Indicated with altered mental status/seizure
  - —Bilateral, symmetric, low density lesions in the basal ganglia have been seen within days after severe intoxication with disulfiram
- EEG: diffuse slowing without focal abnormalities has been seen in cases of acute toxicity with coma

DIFFERENTIAL DIAGNOSIS

- Sepsis
- Meningitis, encephalitis
- Myocardial ischemia or infarction with cardiogenic shock
- Anaphylactoid/anaphylactic reaction
- Gastroenteritis/pancreatitis with dehydration
- Ethanol withdrawal

Treatment

INITIAL STABILIZATION

- ABCs
  - —Mechanical airway placement: if necessary to protect the airway
  - —Supplemental oxygen
  - —Mechanical ventilation if necessary
  - —0.9%NS IV resuscitation for hypotension
  - —Pressor support with *norepinephrine* for refractory hypotension

ED TREATMENT

- GI decontamination
  - —Activated charcoal in cases of disulfiram overdose
  - —Syrup of ipecac contraindicated (contains ethanol)
- Alleviation of flushing
  - —Histamine antagonists (diphenhydramine)
  - —Prostaglandin inhibitors (indomethacin)
- Antiemetics for intractable vomiting (metoclopramide, prochlorperazine)
- Seizures
  - —Benzodiazepines (diazepam, lorazepam)
  - —Pyridoxine (for disulfiram overdose)
- 4-Methyl pyrazole
  - —Inhibits ethanol metabolism at the alcohol dehydrogenase enzyme, limiting the further production of acetaldehyde
  - —FDA-approved for use in the U.S. for ethylene glycol poisoning only
- Hemodialysis
  - —Used to treat acute disulfiram overdose (reported in case reports)
  - —No studies documenting beneficial effect

MEDICATIONS

- Diazepam: 5–10 mg (peds: 0.2–0.5 mg/kg) IV
- Diphenhydramine: 25-50 mg (peds: 1–2 mg/kg) IV
- Indomethacin: 50 mg po; (peds: 0.6 mg/kg po for age >14 yrs)
- Lorazepam: 2–6 mg (peds: 0.03–0.05 mg/kg) IV
- Metoclopramide: 10 mg (peds: 1–2 mg/kg) IV
- Norepinephrine: 4 cc in 1000 cc of D5W, infused @ 0.1–0.2 μg/kg/min
- Prochlorperazine: 5–10 mg (peds: 0.1–0.15 mg/kg) IV
- Pyridoxine: 1 g IV

Disposition

ADMISSION CRITERIA

- ICU admission for mechanical airway maintenance, or severe agitation, coma, refractory seizures, refractory hypotension requiring pressors, or cardiac ischemia
- Persistent vomiting, abdominal pain, or flushing
- Elderly patients or those who have preexisting cardiac disease

DISCHARGE CRITERIA

- Mild reactions which resolve with supportive care after an observation period of 8–12 hours
  - —Symptoms may recur upon re-challenge with ethanol up to 7–10 days after the last dose of disulfiram or agents which cause disulfiram-like reactions
  - —Abstain from ethanol use until at least two weeks after their last dose of such agents
- Appropriate follow-up needed to assess the development of any hepatic or neurologic sequelae as a result of disulfiram toxicity

Miscellaneous

ICD9: 977.3

CORE CONTENT CODE: N/A

SUGGESTED READINGS

Brewer C. Invited review: Recent developments in disulfiram treatment. Alcohol Alcohol 1993;28(4):383–395

Enghusen Poulsen H, Loft S, Anderson JR, et al. Disulfiram therapy—adverse drug reactions and interactions. Acta Psychiatr Scand 1992;86:59–66

Goldfrank LR. Disulfiram and disulfiram-like reactions. In: Goldfrank LR, ed. Goldfrank's toxicologic emergencies. East Norwalk, CT: Appleton & Lange,1994

Johansson B. A review of the pharmacokinetics and pharmacodynamics of disulfiram and its metabolites. Acta Psychiatr Scand 1992;86:15–26

Petersen EN. The pharmacology and toxicology of disulfiram and its metabolites. Acta Psychiatr Scand 1992;86:7–13

Author: Susan Farrell

Diverticulitis

Clinical Presentation

SIGNS AND SYMPTOMS

General

- Symptoms develop over hours to days
- Anorexia
- Nausea, vomiting
- Low grade fever
- Malaise

GI

- Abdominal pain
  —Persistent
  —Initially vague
  —Becomes localized to left lower abdomen
- Tenderness at left lower quadrant with occasional mass palpated (phlegmon)
  —*Phlegmon*—inflamed bowel loops or abscess
- Abdominal distention
- Bowel sounds normal, increased or decreased
- Rectal tenderness with heme positive stool
  —Massive gross rectal bleeding rare
- Diarrhea (colon irritation) or constipation (inflammatory obstruction)
- Flatulence, heartburn
- Peritoneal signs if
  —Perforation has occurred
- Unremarkable examination if
  —Elderly
  —Immunocompromised
  —On corticosteroids

Other

- Urinary frequency
  —Due to contact of inflamed colon against the bladder
- Resultant complications
  —Bowel obstruction
  —Fistulas after recurrent attacks
    -Colovesicle fistula (most common) presents with dysuria, frequency, urgency, pneumaturia and fecaluria

MECHANISM/DESCRIPTION

- Perforation of a diverticulum

ETIOLOGY

- Fecal material becomes lodged in a diverticulum and hardens forming a fecalith
- Fecalith can either abrade the mucosa or compromise surrounding blood supply causing inflammation
- Inflammation causes microperforation of the bowel wall
  —Peridiverticulitis: inflammation of colonic wall not extending beyond serosa
  —Pericolic abscess: perforation of serosal layer though inflammation remains localized
  —Peritonitis: perforation of serosal layer with generalized spread of inflammation

Pre-Hospital

CAUTION

- Avoid analgesics in abdominal pain when the underlying etiology is uncertain

Diagnosis

ESSENTIAL WORKUP

- CBC
  —Elevated WBC with a "left shift"
  —Iron deficiency anemia suggests underlying carcinoma etiology
- Abdominal (supine and upright) and chest radiographs
  —Perforation indicated by free air
  —Obstruction indicated by air-fluid levels
- CT of abdomen
  —Preferred diagnostic modality
  —Better than contrast studies at diagnosing extraluminal processes (i.e. diverticulitis)
  —Diagnostic criteria include
    -Wall thickening of >5mm
    -Inflammation of pericolic fat
    -Pericolic abscess
  —Nondiagnostic criteria include
    -Stricture
    -Diverticula
    -Fistula
  —Diagnoses nondiverticular causes of abdominal pain
  —CT guided percutaneous needle aspiration of localized abscesses avoids further surgery

LABORATORY

- Urinalysis
  —WBC/RBC common
  —Colovesicle fistula results in WBC, bacteria, or feces
- Blood cultures
  —If hospitalized with peritonitis

IMAGING/SPECIAL TESTS

- Avoid endoscopic procedures and contrast studies in acute cases so as not to cause perforation
  —In select cases, water-soluble contrast may be a safe alternative
- Barium enema
  —Indicated after resolution of acute illness to rule out fistula or other colonic pathology (i.e. carcinoma)
- Endoscopy
  —Not necessary to diagnose acute illness
  —Rigid sigmoidoscopy aids in diagnosing nondiverticular causes of abdominal pain (spasm, stricture, edema, pus, or peridiverticular erythema)
- Ultrasonography
  —For diagnosing colonic wall thickening, inflammation, mass, abscess, or fistula
  —Greatly operator dependent
  —Not reliable in the presence of intestinal gas

DIFFERENTIAL DIAGNOSIS

- Colon carcinoma with perforation
- Ischemic colitis
- Bacterial colitis
- Appendicitis
  - —Left sided pain if peritonitis from ruptured appendix
  - —Right sided diverticular pain with cecal diverticulum (rare) or redundant sigmoid colon
- Inflammatory bowel disease
- Irritable bowel syndrome
- Rupture or torsed ovarian cyst
- Pelvic inflammatory disease
- Peptic ulcer disease
- Renal colic

Treatment

INITIAL STABILIZATION

- Rehydration with 0.9%NS to replace intravascular volume depletion
- Bowel rest
  - —NPO
  - —NG tube if persistent vomiting or bowel obstruction present

ED MANAGEMENT

Analgesia

- Anticholinergics (dicyclomine)
  - —Reduces colonic spasm
  - —Does not mask underlying pathology
- Opiates for more aggressive pain management (IV morphine or demerol)
  - —If hemodynamically stable
  - —When not dependent upon repeat abdominal examinations for diagnostic or therapeutic decisions

Antibiotics

- Mild, uncomplicated cases (without perforation)
  - —Outpatient oral agents include
    - -Trimethoprim-sulfamethoxazole (TMP-SMX) DS
    - -Ciprofloxacin plus metronidazole
    - -Amoxicillin/clavulanate
  - —Duration of therapy is 7 to 10 days or until afebrile for 3 to 5 days
- Complicated cases (with peritonitis from perforation)
  - —Clindamycin or metronidazole plus gentamicin in severe cases
  - —Cefoxitin or ampicillin/sulbactam in moderate disease

Surgery

- Emergent surgery
  - —Indicated for generalized peritonitis from perforation
  - —Two stage procedure with resection of diseased segment of colon and a proximal colostomy followed later with a re-anastomosis
- Elective surgery
  - —Indicated for
    - -Multiple recurrent attacks without generalized peritonitis
    - -Fistula formation
    - -Intractable pain
    - -Unresolved obstruction
    - -Failure of medical therapy
    - -Single serious attack under forty years of age (controversial)
  - —One stage procedure following initial medical therapy allowing resolution of inflammation
- Peridiverticular abscess drainage
  - —Indicated if well circumscribed and easily accessible
  - —Accomplished by CT (or ultrasound) guided percutaneous needle aspiration

Ongoing Therapy

- When acute condition has resolved
- High-fiber, low-fat diet to decrease recurrence of attacks

MEDICATIONS

- Amoxicillin/clavulanate: 875 mg po bid or 500 mg po tid
- Ampicillin/sulbactam: 1.5–3.0 g IV q 6 hrs
- Cefoxitin: 2.0 g IV q 8 hrs
- Ciprofloxacin: 400 mg IV q 12 hrs or 500 mg po bid
- Clindamycin: 450–900 mg IV q 8 hrs
- Dicyclomine: 20 mg po qid (up to 40 mg po qid) or 20 mg IM qid (*not* for IV use)
- Gentamicin: 2 mg/kg load then 1.7 mg/kg IV q 8 hrs or 5.1 mg/kg IV qd (assuming normal renal function)
- Meperidine: 50–100 mg IM q 3–4 hrs PRN or 25–50 mg IV and titrate to clinical response
- Metronidazole: 1.0 g IV loading dose followed by 0.5 g IV q 6 hrs or 1.0 g IV q 12 hrs or 500 mg po q 6 hrs
- Morphine sulfate: 2–10 mg/70 kg body weight IVP slowly
- Trimethoprim-sulfamethoxazole DS: 1 tablet po bid

Disposition

ADMISSION CRITERIA

- Intractable pain
- High fever
- Peritonitis
- Failure to respond to outpatient management
- Immunocompromised or steroid dependent patients
- Extreme of age
- Uncertainty of diagnosis

DISCHARGE CRITERIA

- Mild cases (low grade fever, mild discomfort) of known diverticular disease

Miscellaneous

ICD9 CODE: 562.11

CORE CONTENT CODE: 1.7.2.1

SUGGESTED READINGS

Ambrosetti P, et al. Acute left colonic diverticulitis in young patients. J Am Coll Surg 1994;179:156–160.

Ferzoco LB, Raptopoulos V, Silen W. Acute diverticulitis. NEJM 1998;338:1521–1526.

Freeman SR, McNally PR. Gastrointestinal emergencies: Diverticulitis. Med Clin North Am 1993;77 (5);1149–1165.

Vignati PV, et al. Long-term management of diverticulitis in young patients. Dis Colon Rectum 1995;38:627–629.

Author: Dino Rumero

Diverticulosis

Clinical Presentation

SIGNS AND SYMPTOMS

Subdivisions

- Asymptomatic (90%)
- Symptomatic (painful)
- Hemorrhagic (3%)

GI

- Chronic or intermittent left lower quadrant pain
- Acute, painless bleeding with hematochezia or maroon stools
- Constipation (or diarrhea)
- Flatulence
  —Sometimes relieving the pain
- Dyspepsia
- Abdominal palpation
  —Tenderness in left lower quadrant
  —Firm sigmoid colon in the left lower quadrant
- Rectal exam
  —Predominantly reveals heme negative stool
  —Bleeding typically mild
  —Most common cause of massive gastrointestinal (GI) bleed

Other

- Fever: absent
- Diverticulitis and diverticular bleeding are separate entities and rarely coexist

MECHANISM/DESCRIPTION

- Single (diverticulum) or multiple (diverticula) colonic wall out-pouchings as a result of colonic muscle dysfunction
- Sequence
  —Insufficient amounts of dietary fiber causes diminished stool bulk
  —Increased colonic contractions necessary to propel stool through colon causing an increase in intraluminal pressure
  —Increased pressure forces mucosa and submucosa to herniate through the muscularis propria at its weakest point (site of nutrient artery penetration)

ETIOLOGY

- Occur anywhere in the GI tract though diverticulosis generally refers to colonic disease
  —Sigmoid colon—most common site
- *Pseudodiverticula*
  —Most common form of colonic diverticula
- True diverticula (uncommon) contain all bowel wall layers
- Incidence directly related to increase in age
- Common in Westernized society due to refined diet and low-fiber
- Massive bleeding usually from right colon
  —Fecalith (dry, hard stool) erodes through arterial branch

Pre-Hospital

CAUTION

- Avoid analgesics in abdominal pain when the underlying etiology is uncertain
- Establish 2 large bore IVs with 0.9%NS if significant rectal bleeding/hemodynamic instability
- For hypotension
  —1–2 L (20 cc/kg) bolus 0.9%NS IV
  —Trendelenburg position

Diagnosis

ESSENTIAL WORKUP

- Thorough history and physical examination essential to avoid excessive workup

LABORATORY

- Asymptomatic diverticulosis
  —Requires no testing
- Uncomplicated painful disease (no peritoneal signs) with known history
  —Require no work up
- Uncomplicated painful disease (no peritoneal signs) without previous history
  —Require work up to rule out carcinoma (if weight loss, anorexia, heme-positive stool)
  —CBC for leukocytosis or anemia
  —Urinalysis to exclude hematuria or pyuria
- Hemorrhagic diverticulosis
  —CBC
  —Electrolytes, BUN/Cr, glucose, calcium
  —Type and cross for 4 Units of packed red blood cells (PRBCs)
  —PT, PTT, platelet count
  —ECG

IMAGING /SPECIAL TESTS

- Uncomplicated painful diverticulosis (as an outpatient)
  —Barium enema: search for classic diverticula and exclude carcinoma or polyps
  —Sigmoidoscopy: rule out carcinoma (done before barium studies so as not to have visualization hindered)
- Hemorrhagic diverticulosis
  —Anoscopy: if mild bleeding to rule out hemorrhoids
  —Proctosigmoidoscopy: if no blood in stool above rectum then assume rectal bleed
  —Colonoscopy: requires a clean colon and bleeding cannot be excessive, otherwise difficult to visualize pathology
  —Radionuclide imaging
    -Safe
    -Localizes bleeding site
    -Ideal for detecting intermittent bleeding due to long half-life of radioisotope (24–36 hours)
  —Angiography: identifies site of bleeding (more exact after radionuclide scanning)
  —Barium enema
    -Identify diverticula but not bleeding
    -Can hinder visualization via other imaging techniques therefore rarely indicated

DIFFERENTIAL DIAGNOSIS

- Painful diverticulosis
  - —Irritable bowel syndrome (clinical presentation is almost identical)
  - —Diverticulitis
  - —Colon carcinoma
  - —Crohn's disease
  - —Urologic (renal colic)
  - —Gynecologic (ruptured or torsed ovarian cyst)
- Hemorrhagic diverticulosis
  - —Hemorrhoids
  - —Anal fissure
  - —Proctitis
  - —Colitis
  - —Carcinoma
  - —Polyps
  - —Ischemic enteritis
  - —Angiodysplasia
  - —Amyloidosis
  - —Vascular-enteric fistula
  - —Upper GI source

Treatment

INITIAL STABILIZATION

- Hemorrhagic diverticulosis (massive)
- Airway control (100% oxygen or intubate if unresponsive)
- Intravenous access with at least one large-bore catheter or two if unstable
- 0.9%NS bolus 1–2 L (20 cc/kg) for hypotension
- Central catheter placement if unstable following initial fluid resuscitation for more efficient delivery of fluids and monitoring of central venous pressure
- NG tube to rule out upper GI bleed
- Bladder catheter to monitor urine output
- Transfuse O-negative red blood cells immediately if impending arrest
- Most diverticular bleeding stops spontaneously

ED MANAGEMENT

- Uncomplicated symptomatic diverticulosis
  - —High fiber diet and/or hydrophilic bulk laxative (i.e. psyllium)
  - —Antispasmodic (dicyclomine)
  - —Warm compresses to abdomen
  - —Reassurance
  - —Avoid cathartic laxatives
- Hemorrhagic diverticulitis (massive)
  - —Transfuse IV fluids and PRBCs (monitor electrolytes, calcium)
  - —Monitor fluid status (input/output)
  - —Consult surgeon
  - —Prepare for radionuclide scan followed by angiography if necessary
  - —Surgical intervention for segmental colectomy if bleeding on radionuclide scan
  - —Consider selective angiography with injection of vasopressin to control bleeding
    - -Embolization not recommended for colonic hemorrhage

MEDICATIONS

- Dicyclomine: 20 mg po qid (up to 40 mg po qid) or 20 mg IM qid (*NOT* for IV use)

Disposition

ADMISSION CRITERIA

- ICU admission if unstable with massive hemorrhagic diverticulosis
- Regular admission for mild or intermittent hemorrhagic diverticulosis which is otherwise stable to determine site of bleeding, and to evaluate need for definitive treatment

DISCHARGE CRITERIA

- Uncomplicated, symptomatic diverticulosis
- Stable with trace heme positive stool, negative gastric aspirate, no anemia and without other complaints

Miscellaneous

ICD9 CODE: 562.10

CORE CONTENT CODE: 1.7.2.1

SUGGESTED READINGS

Bono MJ. Gastrointestinal emergencies part I: Lower gastrointestinal tract bleeding. Emerg Med Clin North Am 1996;14(3):547–556.

Kim YI, et al. Injection therapy for colonic diverticular bleeding. J Clin Gastroenterol 1993;17(1):46–48.

McGuire HH. Bleeding colonic diverticula: A reappraisal of natural history and management. Ann Surg 1994;220(5):653–656.

Author: Dino Rumero

Dizziness

Clinical Presentation

SIGNS AND SYMPTOMS

- Dizziness is used to describe a wide range of symptoms
  - —Abnormal sensation of motion
  - —Feeling faint or fainting
  - —Lightheadedness
  - —Unsteadiness
- Classify dizziness into one of four categories by asking the patient to explain the sensation without using the word dizzy
  - —Vertigo
  - —Abnormal sensation of movement and position in space
    - -Nystagmus
  - —Ataxia
    - -Disorder of coordination and rhythm
    - -Loss of equilibrium
  - —Near syncope/syncope
    - -Diaphoresis
    - -Palpitations
    - -Pallor during the episode
  - —Other
    - -Depression
    - -Fatigue
    - -Weakness

MECHANISM/DESCRIPTION

- Most common complaint of patients over age of 75
- Dizziness may be caused by a number of problems
  - —Vestibular dysfunction
  - —Cardiovascular insufficiency
  - —Psychiatric illness
  - —Metabolic derangement
  - —Multiple sensory deficits
  - —Cerebellar disease
- True vertigo suggests vestibular disease
- Faintness that is postural or paroxysmal suggests a cardiovascular disorder
- Constant ill-defined dizziness unrelated to posture suggests a psychogenic etiology
- Disequilibrium suggests a structural central nervous system disorder

ETIOLOGY

Vertigo

- Peripheral
  - —Benign paroxysmal positional
  - —Acute labyrinthitis
  - —Meniere's disease
  - —Vestibule neuritis
  - —Acoustic neuroma
  - —Ototoxic drugs
    - -Aminoglycosides
    - -Antimalarials
    - -Erythromycin
    - -Furosemide
  - —Otitis media and serous otitis with effusion
  - —Foreign body in ear canal
- Central
  - —Cerebellar hemorrhage
  - —Vertebral basilar artery insufficiency
  - —Cerebellar trauma
  - —Temporal lobe epilepsy
  - —Vertebral basilar migraines
  - —Multiple sclerosis
  - —Subclavian steal syndrome
  - —Drugs suppressing the reticular activating system
    - -Sedatives
    - -Anticonvulsants

Ataxia

- Multiple sensory defects
- Frontal lobe disorder
  - —Tumors
    - -Meningioma
    - -Glioma
    - -Metastatic tumor
  - —Anterior cerebral artery syndrome
  - —Hydrocephalus
- Subcortical disorders
  - —Multiple strokes
  - —Ataxic hemiparesis
- Brainstem disorders
  - —Stroke
  - —Multiple sclerosis
- Cerebellar disorders
  - —Cerebellar hemorrhage, infarct, tumor
  - —Spinocerebellar degeneration
  - —Alcoholism
  - —Acute cerebellitis

Cardiac and Vascular Insufficiency

- Hypovolemia
- Anemia
- Cardiac dysrhythmias
  - —Preexcitation
  - —Prolonged QT syndrome
  - —Hypokalemia
  - —Supraventricular tachycardia
  - —Ventricular dysrhythmia
- Pulmonary embolism
- Subarachnoid hemorrhage
- Hypoglycemia
- Hypoxia
- Hypercarbia
- Hyperventilation syndrome
- Vasovagal episode

Other

- Psychogenic
  - —Anxiety
  - —Depression
- Chronic fatigue syndrome
- Familial periodic paralysis
- Hypothyroidism

Pre-Hospital

CAUTIONS

- Acute onset of dizziness may be due to a transischemic attack, stroke, or hemorrhage
  - -Monitor
  - -Supplemental oxygen
- Observe mental status carefully as deterioration may warrant field endotracheal intubation

Diagnosis

ESSENTIAL WORKUP

LABORATORY

- Hematocrit
- Glucose
- Electrolytes
- Toxicological screen

IMAGING/SPECIAL TESTS

- EKG to detect cardiac causes of near syncope and weakness
- CT scan if central vertigo or ataxia are present
- MR angiogram if vertebral basilar insufficiency is suspected

DIFFERENTIAL DIAGNOSIS

See etiology

Treatment

INITIAL STABILIZATION

- Supplemental oxygen
- Stabilization should be determined by more specific classification of dizziness based on the history, physical examination, and ancillary studies

ED TREATMENT

- Treatment should be determined by the underlying cause

MEDICATIONS

- Antivertigo
- Diazepam: 2.5–5 mg IV q 8 hrs *or* 2–10 mg po q 8 hrs
- Diphenhydramine: 25–50 mg IV/IM/PO q 6 hrs
- Meclizine: 25 mg po q 6 hrs PRN
- Promethazine: 12.5 mg IV q 6 hrs *or* 25–50 mg PO/IM/PR q 6 hrs

Disposition

ADMISSION CRITERIA

- Admission of patients with dizziness should be based on the underlying etiology or associated symptoms

DISCHARGE CRITERIA

- Referral for completion of workup as an outpatient to a primary care physician or a neurologist

Miscellaneous

ICD9: 386,780.2

CORE CONTENT CODE: N/A

SUGGESTED READINGS

Baloh RW. Approach to the dizzy patient. In: Baloh RW, ed. Neurotology. Baillieres Clin Neurol 1994;3:453.

Brown JJ. A systematic approach to the dizzy patient. Neurol Clin 1990;8:209–24

Herr RD, Zun L, Mathews JJ. A directed approach to the dizzy patient. Ann Emerg Med 1989;18:664.

Author: Richard Wolfe

Dog Bite

Clinical Presentation

SIGNS AND SYMPTOMS

- Sites (in decreasing order of occurrence)
  - —Upper extremities
  - —Lower extremities
  - —Head and neck
  - —Trunk
- Tissue injury pattern (decreasing order of frequency)
  - —Tearing of tissue
  - —Lacerations
  - —Superficial abrasions
  - —Puncture wounds
- Infection
  - —Cellulitis
  - —Gray malodorous discharge
  - —Regional adenopathy
  - —Fever
  - —Lymphangitis
- Septic arthritis with joint space penetration

MECHANISM/DESCRIPTION

- Large dogs cause the most serious wounds
  - —Pit bulls are responsible for a large share of dog bite related deaths
- Fatal bites more frequent in small children
- Due to exsanguination from a major blood vessel
- Inability to protect self

ETIOLOGY

- Infection risk greatest for crush injuries, puncture wounds, and hand wounds
- Most common aerobic organisms
  - —*Pasteurella multocida*
  - —*Streptococcus sp*
  - —*Staphylococcus aureus*
- Most common anaerobic organisms
  - —*Enterobacter*
  - —*Pseudomonas sp*
  - —*Bacillus subtilis*
- Time of infection post injury
  - —<24 hrs—*P. multocida*
  - —>24 hrs—*Staphylococcus* or *Streptococcus*
- *Capnocytophaga canimorsus*
  - —Very rare
  - —Fastidious, Gram-negative rod
  - —Presents with overwhelming sepsis in immunocompromised hosts
  - —25% fatality rate
  - —PCN G—treatment of choice

Pre-Hospital

N/A

Diagnosis

ESSENTIAL WORKUP

History

- Dog's behavior, provocation, location, ownership
- Time elapsed since attack
- Past medical history: conditions compromising immune function, allergies, and tetanus status

Physical Examination

- Note depth of wound and any crush injury
- Evaluate vascular supply
- Note the status of tendon and nerve function
- Draw a diagram of the location and extent of all injuries
- Document any signs of infection
- Document any joint or bone involvement; include ROM

LABORATORY

- Aerobic and anaerobic cultures from any infected bite wound
- No cultures necessary if wounds not clinically infected

IMAGING/SPECIAL TESTS

- Roentgenography indications
  - —Significant edema and tenderness
  - —If bony penetration or foreign bodies suspected
  - —Subcutaneous emphysema: may represent air introduced during attack or gas from necrotizing infections

DIFFERENTIAL DIAGNOSIS

- Human bite injuries: human teeth cause crush injuries while animal teeth cause more punctures and lacerations
- Cat or other mammalian bite wounds

Treatment

INITIAL STABILIZATION

- ABCs: ensure patent airway and adequate peripheral tissue perfusion

ED TREATMENT

- Wound irrigation
  - —Copious volumes of normal saline pressure irrigation with an 18-gauge plastic catheter tip aimed in the direction of the puncture
  - —Avoid injection of saline through tissue planes due to force of irrigation
- Debridement
  - —Remove any foreign material, necrotic skin tags, or devitalized tissues
  - —Do not débride puncture wounds
  - —Remove any eschar present so that underlying pus may be expressed and irrigated
- Primary closure of wounds
  - —Not recommended on hand due to high morbidity associated with infection
  - —Not recommended on wounds with extensive crush injury or those requiring extensive debridement
  - —Not recommended on puncture wounds—more difficult to clean
  - —Not recommended if wound older than 24 hours or infected at time of presentation
  - —Requires meticulous wound preparation
- Antibiotics (5 days): efficacy has not been conclusively established; agreed to be effective in the following types of wounds
  - —Moderate or severe wounds
  - —Full-thickness puncture of hand, face, or lower extremity
  - —Wounds requiring surgical debridement
  - —Wounds involving joints, tendons, ligaments, or fractures
  - —Immunocompromised patients
  - —Wounds presenting more than 8 hours after the event (controversial)
- Antibiotic choices
  - —Wound prophylaxis
    - -Dicloxacillin
    - -May give one dose of cefazolin in ED prior to discharge
  - —Infections developing <24 hours (*P. Multocida*)—options
    - -Amoxicillin, augmentin, cefazolin, ceftriaxone, cephalexin, penicillin, tetracycline
    - -May give one dose of penicillin G in ED prior to discharge
  - —Infections developing >24 hours (*Staphylococcus* or *Streptococcus*)—options
    - -Dicloxacillin, cephalexin
  - —Initial empiric therapy for inpatient treatment for infections without sepsis—options
    - -Penicillin G, nafcillin
  - —Initial empiric therapy for inpatient treatment of suspected sepsis—options

-Imipenem/cilastatin, ampicillin/sulbactam
- Elevate injured extremity
- Tetanus prophylaxis
- Report to appropriate animal control authority

Rabies Immunoprophylaxis

- In the USA, the main vectors: wild animals (skunks, raccoons, bats, foxes)
- Not required if rabies not known or suspected
- Recommended in following situations
  —Dog unable to be quarantined for 10 days (rabies known area)
  —Previously healthy dog becomes ill during quarantine, and while awaiting results of rabies fluorescent antibody test
  —An ill dog while awaiting rabies test results: immunoprophylaxis to be continued or halted based on results of rabies test
- Active Immunization
  —Human diploid cell vaccine (HDCV): 1 cc IM on days 1, 3, 7, 14, and 28 following exposure
- Passive Immunization
  —Human rabies immune globulin (HRIG): 20 IU/kg
  —Up to one-half in area around wound with the rest IM

MEDICATIONS

- Amoxicillin (amoxil): 500 mg q 8 hrs (peds: 40 mg/kg/24 hrs in three divided doses) po
- Amoxicillin/clavulanic acid (augmentin): 500 mg (40 mg/kg/24 hrs) q 8 hrs po
- Ampicillin/sulbactam (Unasyn): 1.5 to 3.0 g q 6 hrs IV
- Cefazolin (ancef): 1 g (peds: 25 mg/kg) IV
- Ceftriaxone (rocephin): 1 g (peds: 50 mg/kg) IM/IV
- Cephalexin (keflex): 500 mg (peds: 50 mg/kg/24 hrs) po q 6 hrs
- Dicloxacillin (pathocil): 500 mg (peds: 50 mg/kg/24 hrs) po q 6 hrs
- Imipenem/cilastatin (primaxin): 0.5 to 1.0 g (peds: 50 mg/kg/24 hrs) q 6 hrs IV
- Nafcillin (unipen): 1 to 2 g (peds: 50–200 mg/kg/24 hrs) q 4 hours IV
- Penicillin G : 1.2 million U (peds: 25,000 U/kg) IM
- Penicillin VK (pen vee tabs): 500 mg (peds: 50 mg/kg/24 hrs) q 6 hrs po
- Tetracycline: 500 mg q 6 hrs po

Disposition

ADMISSION CRITERIA

- Infected wounds at presentation
- Severe, advancing cellulitis or lymphangitis
- Signs of systemic infection
- Infected wounds that have failed to respond to outpatient (oral) antibiotics

DISCHARGE CRITERIA

- Healthy patient with localized wound infection: discharge on antibiotics with 24 hour follow-up
- 48 hour follow-up for noninfected wounds

Miscellaneous

ICD9 CODE: 879.8

CORE CONTENT CODE: 5.10.2

SUGGESTED READINGS

Brogan TV, et al. Severe dog bites in children. Pediatr 1995;96:947–50.

Dire DJ. Emergency management of dog and cat bite wounds. Emerg Med Clinics North Am 1992;10(4):719–734.

Goldstein EJ. Bite wounds and infection. Clin Infect Dis 1992;14:633–40.

Griego RD, et al. Dog, cat, and human bites: A review. J Am Acad Dermatol. 1995;33:1019–1029.

Wiley JF. Mammalian bites, review of evaluation and management. Clin Pediatr 1990;29(5):283–287.

Author: John Hipskind

Domestic Violence

Clinical Presentation

SIGNS AND SYMPTOMS

- Injuries from domestic violence frequently occur from physical assault and include, but are not limited to: fractures, contusions, lacerations, and penetrating and blunt trauma to the body.
- Patients living with ongoing violence may present with chronic cephalgia, chest pain, chronic abdominal and pelvic pain, multiple somatic complaints, anxiety, depression and suicidal ideation. Domestic violence often contributes to the patient's reason for presenting to the emergency department.
- Traumatic injuries caused by ongoing abuse at home, represent a small subset of clinical presentations in patients seeking medical care.
- Clinical clues of domestic violence victims include the following
  —History not compatible with exam
  —Repeat visits for the same chief complaint
  —Depression or suicidal ideation
  —Delay in seeking care
  —Any injury during pregnancy
  —Interaction between woman and partner that suggests interpersonal problems
  —Evidence of trauma not attributable to a motor vehicle accident
  —Multiple symptoms without obvious physical findings

MECHANISM/DESCRIPTION

- Domestic violence is a subset of family violence which includes child abuse, partner abuse and elder abuse.
- Domestic violence is the infliction or threat of physical harm against an intimate partner. It occurs in dating, married, cohabiting, or separated relationships.
- Domestic violence is a pattern of assaultive and coercive behaviors that includes physical, sexual, and psychological attacks against the victims. These tactics are used to attain compliance and control over their partner.
- All of the following are examples of domestic violence.
  —Pushing, shoving, slapping, punching, kicking, choking
  —Assault with a weapon
  —Holding, tying down, or use of restraints
  —Threats of harm, or intimidation
  —Isolation of a victim physically, or socially
  —Degrading, or humiliating behavior
  —Attempting to perform sexual acts against a persons will
  —Causing physical harm during sex or assaulting genitalia
  —Forcing a victim to have sex without protection against pregnancy

ETIOLOGY

- Most victims are women; most perpetrators are men. However, partners of same sex relationships and men may also be victims. The exact numbers are unknown, but it is estimated that 95% of domestic violence incidents are perpetrated by men against women.

Diagnosis

- Diagnosis and recognition of domestic violence in the emergency department, clinic, or office is difficult and problematic.

ESSENTIAL WORKUP

- Short screening questions of all female patients may be an effective means of identifying victims of domestic violence in the emergency department.
- Asking the patient directly if the seemingly accidental injuries were inflicted by a known past or present partner will aid in detection.
- Patients who have sustained blunt trauma should have a thorough, focused exam of the affected area.

DIFFERENTIAL DIAGNOSIS

- Domestic violence may be the acute precipitant of the patient's reason for presenting to the emergency department, or it may be part of the patient's past or present social history. The spectrum of presentations of domestic violence victims is diverse.

Treatment

INITIAL STABILIZATION

- Provide timely and appropriate medical attention.
- Maintain advocacy by expressing messages of support and validating the victim's dilemma.

ED TREATMENT

- Document the victim's allegations in the chart in his or her own words.
- Diagram or photograph injuries (after consent) and incorporate them into the clinical record.
- Address the patient's safety in returning to the same home environment.
- Important determinants in predicting future danger include violence that is increasing in frequency and severity, threats of homicide or suicide by the partner, or the availability of a lethal weapon.
- With the aid of social services or domestic violence advocates, review the patient's options. This may include outpatient victim services, emergency shelter information, hot lines, restraining order information, and legal services.
- Mandatory reporting requirements vary from state to state.
  —Some states require a health care practitioner to make a report verbally and in writing if they suspect the wound or physical injury is the result of assaultive and abusive conduct.
  —Determine how local authorities respond to reports of domestic violence by health care practitioners.
  —Recognize that mandatory reporting requirements may place the victim in more danger and creates ethical dilemmas for physicians when the victim does not want their case reported to police or social service agencies.

MEDICATIONS

- Acetaminophen: 650–975 mg po
- Ibuprofen: 300–800 mg po
- Meperidine: 1–1.8 mg/kg/dose IV/IM
- Morphine sulfate: 0.1 mg/kg/dose IV/IM

Disposition

ADMISSION CRITERIA

- A victim whose life is in imminent danger and has no place to be safely discharged (home, family, friends, or shelter) may need to be admitted to the hospital.
- Use appropriate admission guidelines depending on the degree of trauma sustained.

DISCHARGE CRITERIA

- A victim whose safety is assured and injuries can be managed as an outpatient may be discharged.

Miscellaneous

ICD9: V15.49, V15.41

CORE CONTENT CODE: 13.8.1, 14.9.2, 14.12.1, 18.1.11.2.1.3, 18.6.1.4

SUGGESTED READINGS

Abbott J. Injuries and illnesses of domestic violence. Ann Emerg Med 1997;29:781–785.

Alpert EJ. Violence in intimate relationships and the practicing internist: New "disease" or new agenda? Ann Intern Med 1995;123:774–781.

Goldberg WG, Tomlanovich MC. Domestic violence victims in the emergency department. JAMA 1984;251:3259–3264.

Hayden SR, Barton ED, Hayden M. Domestic violence in the emergency department: How do women prefer to disclose and discuss the issues? J Emerg Med 1997;15(4):1–5.

Hyman A, Schillinger D, Lo B. Laws mandating reporting of domestic violence: Do they promote well-being? JAMA 1995;273:1781–1787.

Salber PR, Taliaferro E. The physician's guide to domestic violence. Volcano Press, Volcano, CA 1995.

Author: Jim Comes

Duodenal Trauma

Clinical Presentation

SIGNS AND SYMPTOMS

- Complaints are minimal with vague abdominal, flank, and back pain;
- High gastrointestinal obstruction is usually seen with duodenal hematomas

DESCRIPTION/MECHANISM

- The duodenum is 12 inches long, C-shaped, divided into 4 sections (last 3 sections intraperitoneal), and most lie over the first 3 lumbar vertebrae
- The second section is the one most commonly injured
- Types of injury include duodenal wall hematoma, wall perforation, and extensive hemorrhage
- Incidence of duodenal injury is approximately 5% of intra-abdominal injuries
- Penetrating trauma accounts for 85% of duodenal injuries, blunt trauma 15%
- Mortality ranges from 13–28% mostly from exsanguination secondary to delay in diagnosis
- Blunt duodenal injuries have a higher mortality than penetrating, which generally require exploratory laparotomy

DUODENAL INJURY SEVERITY SCALE

GRADE	*INJURY*	*DESCRIPTION*
I	Hematoma	Single portion of duodenum
	Laceration	Partial thickness only
II	Hematoma	Involving more than one portion
	Laceration	Disruption of <50% circumference
III	Laceration	50–75% circumference of D2 50–100% circumference of D1,3,4
IV	Laceration	>75% circumference of D2 Involving ampulla or distal common duct
V	Laceration	Disruption of duodeno-pancreatic complex devascularization of duodenum

- Late mortality is usually from sepsis. If blunt duodenal injury is diagnosed in less than 24 hours the mortality rate is approximately 11%, if more than 24 hours, it then approaches 40%

PEDIATRIC CONSIDERATIONS

- Intramural duodenal hematomas are commonly seen in child abuse, but majority are secondary to recreational injuries (i.e. bicycle injuries)
- In children the hematoma is most commonly seen in the first portion of the duodenum and in adults in the second and third portions.

Pre-Hospital

CAUTIONS

- ABCs: follow trauma protocols
- Important to have pre-hospital personnel provide clear description of the mechanism of injury

Diagnosis

ESSENTIAL WORKUP

Careful physical examination with special attention to tenderness or ecchymosis of upper abdomen or penetrating wounds to right upper quadrant or lower chest

LABORATORY

- Laboratory tests are of little value
  —Only 50% of patients with duodenal injuries have elevated serum amylase

IMAGING/SPECIAL TESTS

Diagnostic Peritoneal Lavage

- Often *positive* for blood, bile, or bowel content; however, a *negative* lavage does not exclude injury

Upright Chest and Abdominal Radiographs

- May show intraperitoneal air, retroperitoneal air, or air in the biliary tree
- Look for scoliosis to the right, loss of psoas shadow, and air around the right kidney
- Injecting air into the nasogastric tube may demonstrate retroperitoneal air more clearly
- Intramural hematomas without leakage may see a coiled spring appearance in plain radiographs of the affected portion

CT With Contrast

- Perhaps the best diagnostic test which will show small amounts of *retroperitoneal gas* and *extravasated contrast material*
- Also used to look for a *sausage-shaped mass* in the duodenal wall, which strongly suggests duodenal hematoma

DIFFERENTIAL DIAGNOSIS

- Injury to hollow organs (stomach, small and large intestines)
- Liver and biliary tree injuries
- Vascular injuries (aortic and mesenteric arteries as well as venous injuries)

Treatment

INITIAL STABILIZATION

- ABCs of multiple trauma care
- Aggressive fluid resuscitation with warmed normal saline or lactated Ringer's
- Central line for unstable patients
- Nasogastric decompression
- Early trauma surgical consultation

ED TREATMENT

- Tetanus prophylaxis for penetrating wounds and antibiotic prophylaxis
- Definitive treatment involves laparotomy in the OR with extensive exploration of the duodenum for injuries
- If unable to maintain perfusion may need to perform open thoracotomy to cross-clamp the aorta in order to survive to the operating room
- Broad-spectrum antibiotics to combat subsequent development of sepsis in patients with known perforation

MEDICATION

- Cefoxitin: 2 g IV in adults; 40 mg/kg IV in peds *plus*
- Gentamicin: 2 mg/kg IV loading dose (adult and peds)

Or

- Cefotetan: 2 g IV in adults; 20 mg/kg IV in peds *plus*
- Gentamicin: 2 mg/kg IV loading dose (adult and peds)

Or

- Clindamycin: 600 mg IV in adults; 20–40 mg/kg/d IV in 3–4 divided doses in peds *plus* Gentamicin: 2 mg/kg IV loading dose (adult and peds)

Or

- Ceftriaxone: 1–2 g IV in adults; 50–75 mg/kg/d in 2 divided doses not to exceed 2 g in peds *plus* Metronidazole: 15 mg/kg IV

PEDIATRIC CONSIDERATIONS

- If child abuse is suspected then prompt referral to appropriate child protective agencies is required along with medical treatment

Disposition

ADMISSION CRITERIA

- Patients with duodenal injuries need admission to a trauma surgical service
- Minor duodenal hematomas that do not require immediate surgery do require nasogastric decompression for obstruction (up to 7 days) and observation for possible expansion or rupture of the hematoma
- Postoperative patients also require nasogastric decompression and need to be observed for possible fistula formation

DISCHARGE CRITERIA

- All patients with duodenal trauma require admission

Miscellaneous

ICD9: 863.21

CORE CONTENT CODE: 18.4.11.4

SUGGESTED READINGS

Carrillo, et al. Evolution in the management of duodenal injuries. J Trauma 1996; 40(6);1037–1046

Ivatury RR, et al. Complex duodenal injuries. Surg Clin North Am 1996; 76(4):797–812

Weigelt JA. Duodenal injuries. Surg Clin North Am 90;70(3);529–539

Author: Hagop Isnar

Dysfunctional Uterine Bleeding

Clinical Presentation

SIGNS AND SYMPTOMS

- Excessive (>80 cc), or prolonged vaginal bleeding
- Vaginal bleeding that is significantly changed from a patients normal pattern
- Pallor, tachycardia, hypotension, orthostasis in severe cases
- Bilateral ovarian enlargement if polycystic ovary disease is the etiology

MECHANISM/DESCRIPTION

- Abnormal uterine bleeding in the absence of systemic or structural disease
  —Includes bleeding between normal menstrual cycles, change in normal pattern of menstrual cycle, increased or decreased amount of menstrual bleeding
- Usually associated with anovulation (75%)
- Diagnosis of exclusion

ETIOLOGY

- Immature hypothalamic-pituitary-ovarian axis
- Perimenopause
- Obesity
- Polycystic ovary syndrome
- Very low calorie diets, intense exercise, rapid weight change, psychological stress

PEDIATRIC CONSIDERATIONS

- Common in adolescence due to immaturity of the hypothalamic-pituitary-ovarian axis

Pre-Hospital

- ABCs

CAUTIONS

- It is rare for women to be hemodynamically unstable simply from dysfunctional uterine bleeding. If such instability is present, concern is for ectopic pregnancy or other cause for perineal hemorrhage

Diagnosis

ESSENTIAL WORKUP

- Exclude causes listed in differential diagnosis
- Thorough history and physical examination will suggest the etiology of bleeding in most cases
- Pregnancy test

LABORATORY

- CBC, PT/PTT, type and screen/crossmatch
- Iron studies, thyroid stimulating hormone, LH, FSH, prolactin level, cervical cultures may be sent for routine follow-up by gynecologist

IMAGING/SPECIAL TESTS

- Endometrial biopsy if over 35
- Pelvic US may be necessary to evaluate for structural uterine/tubal/ovarian abnormality

DIFFERENTIAL DIAGNOSIS

- Pregnancy complication: threatened, incomplete or spontaneous abortion, ectopic or molar pregnancy
- Infectious: vaginitis, cervicitis, pelvic inflammatory disease (PID)
- Coagulopathies: von Willebrand's, idiopathic thrombocytopenic purpura, platelet defects, thalassemia major
- Medications: warfarin, aspirin, oral contraceptives, tricyclic antidepressants, major tranquilizers
- Systemic illness: adrenal, hepatic, renal, thyroid dysfunction, diabetes mellitus or other endocrinopathies
- Anatomic lesions: fibroids, endometriosis, polyps, endometrial hyperplasia, neoplasms
- Intrauterine devices, trauma

Treatment

INITIAL STABILIZATION

- ABCs
  —PRBCs for significant bleeding unresponsive to crystalloids

ED TREATMENT

- Rule out pregnancy
- Gynecology consultation if bleeding is severe and requires crystalloid resuscitation or blood products
- Dilation and curettage may be necessary in the ED for hemodynamic instability
- Hysteroscopy or hysterectomy when symptoms unresponsive to estrogen treatment

MEDICATIONS

- Conjugated estrogen: 20 mg IV over 15 min for hemodynamically unstable patients, repeat every 2–4 hrs until bleeding controlled, then oral estrogen 10 mg po qd
- Multiple hormonal treatments available for outpatient therapy
  —Combination oral contraceptive 4 pills qd for 7 days
  —Medroxyprogesterone: 10 mg qd for 10–12 days q month
  —Depot medroxyprogesterone acetate: 150 mg IM
  —In hemodynamically stable, older patients, defer hormonal therapy until endometrial biopsy can be performed
- NSAIDs, e.g., naproxen sodium 550 mg po then 275 mg q 6 hrs until bleeding stopped

PEDIATRIC CONSIDERATIONS

- Observation may be adequate if no instability
- Oral contraceptives often effective

Disposition

ADMISSION CRITERIA

- Significant blood loss
- Continued bleeding, HCT < 20
- Unresponsive hemodynamic instability for possible D&C or operative treatment

DISCHARGE CRITERIA

- Most patients can be discharged with gynecology referral once bleeding is controlled and hemodynamically stable

Miscellaneous

ICD9: 626.8

CORE CONTENT CODE: 19.1.3.2

SUGGESTED READINGS

Bayer SR, DeCherney AH. Clinical manifestations and treatment of dysfunctional uterine bleeding. JAMA 1993;269(14):1823–1828.

Chuong CJ, Brenner JF. Management of abnormal uterine bleeding. Am J Obstet Gynecol 1996;175(3):787–791.

Mallett V. Gynecology and obstetrics. In: Tintinalli JE, ed. Emergency medicine: A comprehensive study guide. New York: McGraw Hill, 1996:558–559.

Newton E, Hochbaum SR. Vaginal bleeding unrelated to pregnancy. In: Rosen P, et al., eds. Emergency medicine: Concepts and clinical practice. 4th ed. St. Louis: Mosby-Year Book, 1998:2304–2309.

Wathen PI, Henderson MC, Witz CA. Abnormal uterine bleeding. Med Clin North Am 1995;79(2):329–342.

Author: Christy Rosa

Dysphagia

Clinical Presentation

SIGNS AND SYMPTOMS

Oropharyngeal Dysphagia

- Difficulty initiating the swallowing reflex
  - —Immediate, within seconds of swallowing
- Patient aware that the food bolus has not passed below the cervical esophagus
- Swallowing followed by a coughing or a choking fit indicating aspiration of food material into the trachea
- Swallowing followed by a gurgling noise
  - —Suggests the presence of a Zenker's diverticulum
- Difficulty with phonation or hoarseness
  - —Indicates weaknesses in the muscles necessary for a proper swallowing reflex

Esophageal Dysphagia

- "Sticking" sensation with swallowing a food bolus
  - —Often localized between the neck and the xiphoid process
- Nocturnal regurgitation of undigested food
- Cranial nerve weaknesses
- Drooling or regurgitation of undigested food and liquids
  - —Characteristic of esophageal obstruction

MECHANISM/DESCRIPTION

- Dysphagia
  - —Dysfunction in the process of passing food or liquids from the mouth to the stomach following the act of swallowing
- Types of dysphagia
  - —Oropharyngeal
    - -Dysphagia results from problems with *initiating* the voluntary swallowing reflex
    - -Usually occurs as a result of neuromuscular disorders causing weakness or lack of coordination of the muscles involved in swallowing
  - —Esophageal
    - -Sensation of food *sticking* as it passes through the esophagus
    - -Caused by either mechanical obstructions or motility disorders
- Pain pattern
  - —Esophagus is made up of voluntary striated muscle in the upper one-third which transitions to involuntary nonstriated muscle in the lower two-thirds
  - —Somatic nerves, supplied to the upper esophagus, provide for excellent pain localization in this area
  - —Afferents from the vagus nerve and the thoracic and cervical sympathetic ganglia innervate the lower portion of the esophagus resulting in poor discrimination of pain in the distal esophagus
  - —Visceral pain originating in the lower one-third of the esophagus may be quite nebulous and often indistinguishable from that of myocardial ischemia
- Odynophagia
  - —Sensation of *pain* with swallowing
  - —Separate entity from dysphagia

Pre-Hospital

CAUTIONS

- Careful airway precautions with patients complaining of difficulty swallowing
- Place patient in position of comfort with suction immediately available

Diagnosis

ESSENTIAL WORKUP

- ECG
  - —Exclude cardiac etiology for chest discomfort
  - —Heart and esophagus share a common neural pathway
- Four historical questions
  - —What kinds of foods cause the symptoms?
    - -Trouble swallowing *both* solids and liquids suggests a motility disorder
    - -Symptoms occurring only with *solids* or a progression from solids to liquids suggests a mechanical obstruction
  - —Is the current episode the initial presentation or has there been a progressive course?
  - —History of reflux disease?
  - —Is there pain with swallowing?

LABORATORY

- Electrolytes, BUN/Cr, glucose for significant dehydration

IMAGING/SPECIAL TESTS

- CXR for
  - —Food dilating the esophagus
  - —Aspiration pneumonia
  - —Foreign bodies
  - —Compressing masses
- Soft tissue lateral neck radiograph
- Barium swallow
  - —Defines esophageal anatomy
  - —Assesses function
  - —Do not perform if endoscopy anticipated
- Esophagoscopy
  - —Indicated to relieve obstruction and inspect the esophageal anatomy
- CT of the head
  - —Indicated for new onset neuromuscular dysphagia

DIFFERENTIAL DIAGNOSIS

- Neuromuscular
  - —Cerebrovascular accident
  - —Parkinson's disease
  - —ALS
  - —Multiple sclerosis
  - —Brain stem tumors
  - —Myasthenia gravis
  - —Tetanus
- Motility disorders
  - —Scleroderma
  - —Achalasia
  - —Esophageal Spasm
- Mechanical disorders
- Schatzki's ring
- Plummer-Vinson malignancy
- Peptic esophageal stricture
- Zenker's diverticulum
- Foreign body
- Goiter
- Enlarged left atrium

Treatment

INITIAL STABILIZATION

- Secure and maintain an adequate airway
- NPO
  —Due to risk for aspiration
- 0.9%NS 500 cc bolus (peds: 20 cc/kg) IV fluid bolus for dehydration

ED TREATMENT

- Administer glucagon or nitroglycerin (relaxes esophageal smooth muscle) for esophageal spasm or esophageal foreign body
- Treat complications
  —Aspiration
  —Dehydration
  —Poor nutrition
  —Esophageal perforation

MEDICATIONS

- Glucagon: 0.5 mg IV followed by second dose of 1 mg after 5 min if there is no improvement in symptoms
- Nitroglycerin: 0.4 mg SL q 5 min repeated up to 3 times

Disposition

ADMISSION CRITERIA

- Compromised fluid or nutrition status

DISCHARGE CRITERIA

- Well-hydrated patient
- Urgent neurology, otolaryngology, or gastroenterology referral should be made for further evaluation and treatment

Miscellaneous

ICD9: 787.2

CORE CONTENT CODE: 22.1.19

SUGGESTED READINGS

Rothstein RD. A systematic approach to the patient with dysphagia. Hosp Prac 1997;32(3):169–175.

Swann LA, Munter DW. Esophageal emergencies. Emerg Med Clin North Am 1996;14(3):557–570.

Authors: J. Brian Liddy; Timothy J. Mader

Dyspnea

Clinical Presentation

SIGNS AND SYMPTOMS

- Difficult, labored, or uncomfortable breathing
- Upper airway
  - —Stridor
  - —Upper airway obstruction
- Pulmonary
  - —Tachypnea
  - —Accessory muscle use
  - —Wheezing
  - —Rales
  - —Asymmetric breath sounds
  - —Poor air movement
- Cardiovascular
  - —S3 gallop
  - —Murmur
  - —Jugular venous distension
- CNS
  - —Altered levels of consciousness
- General
  - —Diaphoretic/cool vs. hot/dry skin
  - —Pallor
  - —Upright patient position
  - —Clubbing
  - —Cyanosis
  - —Edema
  - —Breath odor
    - -Ketotic

MECHANISM/DESCRIPTION

- Dyspnea comes from the Greek word for "hard breathing"
- Often described as "shortness of breath"
- Usually an unconscious activity, dyspnea is the subjective sensation of breathing, from mild discomfort to feelings of suffocation

ETIOLOGY

- Dyspnea usually reflects an impairment in ventilation, perfusion, metabolic function, or CNS drive
- Mechanisms that control breathing
  - —Control centers
    - -Brain stem and cerebral cortex affect both automatic and voluntary control of breathing
  - —Chemo, stretch, and irritant sensors
    - -CO_2 receptors located centrally and pO_2 receptors located peripherally
    - -Mechanoreceptors lie in respiratory muscles and respond to stretch
    - -Intrapulmonary mechanoreceptors respond to chemical irritation, engorgement, and stretch
  - —Effectors of respiratory center output are in the respiratory muscles and respond to central stimulation to move air in and out of the thoracic cavity
  - —Motorsensory control of the diaphragm and muscles of respiration are controlled by cervical nerves 3–8 and thoracic 1–12
- Derangements of any of these neurosensory pathways produces dyspnea
  - —Many etiologies for the sensation of dyspnea are due to complex nature of mechanisms that control breathing

Pre-Hospital

CAUTIONS

- Place all patients on supplemental oxygen, pulse oximetry, and cardiac monitor
- Initiate therapy for suspected cause of dyspnea when indicated
  - —Asthma
  - —COPD
  - —Congestive heart failure
- Intubate patients in the face of impending respiratory failure

Diagnosis

ESSENTIAL WORKUP

- CXR
  - —For diagnosis of pulmonary conditions
  - —Assess heart size and evidence of congestive heart failure
- Arterial blood gas
  - —Oxygenation
  - —Calculate arterial-alveolar gradient
    - -A-a (at sea level) = $150 - (pO_2 - PCO_2)/0.8$
    - -Normal = 5–20
  - —Assess degree of acidosis
- Pulse oximetry
  - —May be falsely elevated due to increased ventilation or carbon monoxide

LABORATORY

- CBC
  - —Evaluation of anemia
  - —WBC helpful in evaluation of infectious processes
- Electrolyte, BUN/Cr, glucose
  - —For suspected metabolic derangements and renal impairment
- Toxicology screen
- Methemoglobin/carboxyhemoglobin level
- Sputum Gram stain and culture for suspected pneumonia
- Thyroid function tests

IMAGING/SPECIAL TESTS

- ECG for suspected myocardial ischemia/CHF
- Ventilation/perfusion scan for suspected pulmonary embolism
- Soft tissue neck radiograph for suspected upper airway obstruction
- Echocardiography for pericardial effusion/tamponade
- Peak expiratory flow/spirometry to assess for reactive airway disease
- Tensilon test for suspected myasthenia gravis

DIFFERENTIAL DIAGNOSIS

- Upper airway
  - —Epiglottitis
  - —Laryngeal obstruction
  - —Tracheitis or tracheobronchitis
- Pulmonary
  - —Airway mass
  - —Asthma
  - —Bronchitis
  - —Chest wall trauma
  - —Congestive heart failure
  - —Drug-induced conditions (e.g., crack lung, aspirin overdose)
  - —Effusion
  - —Emphysema
  - —Metastatic disease
  - —Pneumonia
  - —Pneumothorax
  - —Pulmonary embolism

—Pulmonary hypertension
—Restrictive lung disease
- Cardiovascular
  —Arrhythmia
  —Coronary artery disease
  —Intracardiac shunt
  —Left ventricular failure
  —Myxoma
  —Pericardial disease
  —Valvular disease
- Neuromuscular
  —CNS disorders
  —Myopathy and neuropathy
  —Phrenic nerve and diaphragmatic disorders
  —Spinal cord disorders
  —Systemic neuromuscular disorders
- Other
  —Acidosis
  —Altitude
  —Anaphylaxis
  —Anemia
  —Thyroid disorders
  —Psychogenic
  —Sepsis

PEDIATRIC CONSIDERATIONS

- Unique conditions in differential diagnosis for age <2 years
  —Croup
  —Congenital anomalies of the airway
  —Congenital heart disease
  —Foreign body aspiration
  —Nasopharyngeal obstruction
  —Shock

Treatment

INITIAL STABILIZATION

- ABCs
- Immediate intubation for impending respiratory distress

ED TREATMENT

- Supplemental oxygen for hypoxia or to increase A-a gradient
- Initiate therapy for underlying condition

Disposition

ADMISSION CRITERIA

- Assisted ventilation
- Hypoxia
- A-a gradient >40
- Medical condition requiring hospital therapy

DISCHARGE CRITERIA

- Adequate oxygenation
- Stable medical illness that can be managed as outpatient

Miscellaneous

ICD9: 786.09

CORE CONTENT CODE: 23.3.3

SUGGESTED READINGS

Schwartzstein RM, Manning HL. Pathophysiology of dyspnea. N Engl J Med 1995;12(3):1547–1552.

Tobin MJ. Dyspnea: pathophysiologic basis, clinical presentation, and management. Arch Intern Med 1990;8:1604–1612.

Weisman IM, Zeballos RJ. Clinical evaluation of unexplained dyspnea. Cardiologia 1996;41(7):621–634.

Author: Elizabeth L. Mitchell

Dystonic Reaction

Clinical Presentation

SIGNS AND SYMPTOMS

General

- Usually occur within 5 hours of ingestion and almost always within the first 3–4 days after exposure to the offending drug
- Age
  - —Twice as often in males
  - —Uncommon in older patients
  - —Children are more susceptible
- Difficulty with vocalization
- Completely alert and able to answer questions

Characteristic Motor Spasms

- Oculogyric crisis
  - —Crisis involves the eye and periorbital muscles
  - —Starts as blepharospasm
  - —Evolves into a painful upward or lateral deviation of the eyes
- Buccolingual crisis
  - —Involves the facial muscles and tongue
  - —Bizarre grimacing
  - —Trismus
  - —Tongue protrusion
  - —Dysarthria
  - —Rarely does it cause spasm of the pharynx and larynx
    - -Can be severe enough to cause choking and respiratory distress
- Torticollic crisis
  - —Twisting of the neck
- Tortipelvic crisis
  - —Abdominal wall muscle spasm
- Opisthotonos
  - —Involves the muscles of the trunk and back
  - —Twisting and arching of the spine

MECHANISM/DESCRIPTION

- Normal pattern of CNS neurotransmission maintained by a balance between dopaminergic and cholinergic receptors
  - —Certain drugs disrupt this balance by blocking dopaminergic receptors
  - —Leads to excess cholinergic stimulation which is manifested as involuntary muscle spasms
- Although the spasms are uncomfortable, they are non-life-threatening

ETIOLOGY

- Usually occur after the patient has taken a neuroleptic drug either for treatment of a psychiatric disorder, as an antiemetic, or for recreational purposes
- Incidence of dystonic reactions in patients taking neuroleptics is 12%
- Neuroleptic agents
  - —Phenothiazine (Thorazine, Mellaril, Prolixin, Compazine)
  - —Thioxanthenes (Navane)
  - —Butyrophenones (Haldol, Droperidol)
  - —Indole (Moban)
  - —Dibenzoxipine (Loxitane)
- Dystonic reactions caused by other agents
  - —Metoclopramide (Reglan)
  - —Trimethobenzamide (Tigan)
    - -Can last for prolonged periods and be difficult to treat
  - —Cyclic antidepressants
  - —Antihistamines
  - —Doxepin
  - —Bromocriptine
  - —Carbamazepine
  - —Cimetidine
  - —Prozac

PEDIATRIC CONSIDERATIONS

- Children are particularly vulnerable to dystonic reactions when dehydrated or febrile

Pre-Hospital

CAUTIONS

- Rarely life-threatening
- Direct attention toward spasm of larynx and tongue to be sure dystonic reaction is not causing respiratory compromise
- Ask family and friends about ingestions of antipsychotic medications, antiemetics, and recreational drugs
- Transport pill bottles

Diagnosis

ESSENTIAL WORKUP

- Clinical diagnosis is based on characteristic signs and symptoms with history of possible drug exposure
- Diagnosis is confirmed by response to treatment

DIFFERENTIAL DIAGNOSIS

- Seizure
  - —History of prior seizures
  - —Not responsive to verbal stimuli
  - —Tonic clonic type motor movements rather than spasm
- Hysteria or pseudoseizure
  - —History of a precipitating emotional event
  - —Tonic clonic motor activity rather than a sustained spasm
- Tetanus
- Strychnine poisoning
- Chronic dystonias
  - —Cerebral palsy, familial choreas
  - —Usually the history of dystonia is associated with a chronic neurologic process
- Scorpion envenomation
  - —Oculogyric crisis and opisthotonos are common manifestations of scorpion envenomation
  - —Patient lacks a history of drug exposure

PEDIATRIC CONSIDERATIONS

- Meningitis and encephalitis may present with atypical seizures that mimic dystonic reaction

Treatment

INITIAL STABILIZATION

- Stabilize airway to prevent spasm of the larynx or tongue from causing respiratory compromise

ED TREATMENT

- Administer diphenhydramine (benadryl) or benztropine mesylate (cogentin)
  —Rapid resolution of the muscular spasm by restoring cholinergic-dopaminergic balance in the CNS
  —IV administration
    -Onset of relief in 2–5 minutes
    -Complete resolution of symptoms in 15 minutes
  —IM administration
    -Begins to work in 15–30 minutes
  —Continue oral administration for 3 days to prevent redevelopment of symptoms
- Diazepam (valium)
  —Administer in cases of dystonia unresponsive to adequate doses of anticholinergic medications
  —A failure to respond to standard treatment should lead the physician to consider other diagnoses

MEDICATIONS

- Benztropine mesylate (Cogentin): 1–2 mg either IV (over 2 min) or IM followed by 1–2 mg po bid for 3 days
  —Not to be used in children under the age of 3 years
  —For children >3 years old: 0.02 mg/kg IV (over 2 min) or IM followed by 0.02 mg/kg po bid for 3 days
- Diazepam: 5–10 mg IV followed by 5 mg po q 4–6 hrs as necessary for 3 days
- Diphenhydramine (Benadryl): 1–2 mg/kg up to 100 mg either IV (over 2 min) or IM followed by 25–50 mg (peds: 1–2 mg/kg) po tid for 3 days

Disposition

ADMISSION CRITERIA

- None

DISCHARGE CRITERIA

- Discharge after resolution of symptoms
- Patient should not drive or perform tasks that require full alertness while taking sedating medications

Miscellaneous

ICD9: N/A

CORE CONTENT CODE: N/A

SUGGESTED READINGS

Black JL, et al. Antipsychotic agents: a clinical update. Mayo Clin Proc 1985;60:777–789.

Ellenhorn MJ, Barceloux DO. Neuroleptic drugs. In: Ellenhorn MJ, ed. Medical toxicology: diagnosis and treatment of human poisoning. New York: Elsevier Science, 1988:478–490.

Krischel S, Jackimczyk K. Cyclic antidepressants, lithium and neuroleptic agents. Emerg Med Clin North Am 1991;9:53–86.

McCormick MA, Manoguerra AS. Dystonic reactions. In: Harwood-Nuss AL, ed. The clinical practice of emergency medicine. New York: Lippincott-Raven, 1996:1319–1321.

Author: Kenneth Jackimczyk

Eating Disorders

Clinical Presentation

SIGNS AND SYMPTOMS

- Prevalence of partial syndrome eating disorders is 5–10% of the population
- A range of disordered eating attitudes and behaviors should be considered

Anorexia Nervosa (AN)

- Refusal to maintain body weight at or above a minimally normal weight for age and height
  —Failure to make expected weight gain during a period of growth
- Intense fear of gaining weight or becoming fat, even though underweight
- Disturbance in the way body weight or shape is experienced
- Undue influence of body weight and shape on self-evaluation
- Denial of seriousness of low body weight
- In postmenarchal females, amenorrhea for 3 consecutive cycles

Bulimia Nervosa (BN)

- Recurrent episodes of binge eating characterized by
  —Eating a larger than usual amount of food in a discrete period of time
  —A sense of loss of control over eating during the episode
- Recurrent inappropriate compensatory behaviors used to prevent weight gain
  —Self-induced vomiting
  —Misuse of laxatives
  —Diuretics
  —Enemas or other medications
  —Fasting
  —Excessive exercise

Binge-Eating Disorder (BED)

- Recurrent episodes of binge eating characterized by
  —Eating a larger than usual amount of food in a discrete period of time
  —A sense of loss of control over eating during the episode
- Binge-eating episodes associated with 3 or more of the following
  —Eating much more rapidly than normal
  —Eating until feeling uncomfortably full
  —Eating large amounts of food when not feeling physically hungry
  —Eating alone because of being embarrassed by how much one is eating
  —Feeling disgusted with oneself, depressed, or very guilty after overeating
  —Marked distress regarding binge eating

Medical Complications

- Endocrine/metabolic
  —Electrolyte imbalances
- Growth retardation
- Nutritionally-based osteoporosis
- Cardiovascular problems
  —Arrhythmias
  —Bradycardia
  —Ipecac cardiomyopathy
- Renal complications
  —Hypokalemia
  —Edema
- Gastrointestinal complications
  —Hematologic changes
  —Anemia
  —Leukopenia
  —Thrombocytopenia
- Potentially irreversible structural brain changes

MECHANISM/DESCRIPTION

- Prevalence
  —AN: 0.5% of the US female population
  —BN: 2%
  —BED: 2%
- Eating disorders tend to be more common among women than among men

ETIOLOGY

- Typical age of onset for AN is bimodal at 13–14 years and 17–18 years
- Typical anorexic is a teenager whose dieting behavior escalates into an obsessive preoccupation with weight and being thin
- BN and BED typically onset in late adolescence or early adulthood
- Typical bulimic
  —Has attempted many diets and failed
  —May have learned purging behaviors from a friend or family member
- BED associated with a history of obesity, weight cycling, and dieting

Pre-Hospital

N/A

Diagnosis

ESSENTIAL WORKUP

- Clinical diagnosis
- Medical evaluation
- Nutritional assessment
- Psychiatric interview
- Family evaluation in cases where the patient lives with her/his family

LABORATORY

- CBC
- Electrolytes, BUN/Cr, glucose
- Liver function tests for serum albumin

DIFFERENTIAL DIAGNOSIS

- Mood disorders
- Anxiety disorders (especially obsessive-compulsive disorder)
- Substance abuse
- Kleptomania
- Variety of personality disorders (especially borderline personality disorder) warrant assessment
- Medical conditions
  —Crohn's disease
  —Diabetes mellitus

Treatment

INITIAL STABILIZATION

- ABCs
- IV 0.9%NS 1 L bolus (peds: 20 cc/kg) for severe dehydration
- Accucheck/correct hypoglycemia with dextrose

ED TREATMENT

- Outpatient treatment
  - —Requires a multimodal, multidisciplinary team approach comprised of
    - -Psychotherapy
    - -Nutritional guidance
    - -Medical monitoring
    - -Pharmacotherapy
    - -Family therapy
    - -Group therapy
  - —Establish modest goals and clear parameters
    - -Expected weight gain for anorexics
  - —Cognitive behavioral therapy and interpersonal psychotherapy
    - -Most effective forms of psychotherapy for eating disorders
- Medical therapy
  - —Pharmacotherapy
    - -Often indicated within the context of psychotherapy
    - -When other psychopathology requires treatment
  - —Antidepressant medications shown to significantly reduce binging and purging behaviors
    - -SSRIs (fluoxetine at doses up to 60 mg/day)
    - -Tricyclic antidepressants
    - -Appetite suppressants in the treatment of BED
    - -No accepted pharmacologic treatment of AN
- Prognosis
  - —Anorexics
    - -20% of anorexics continue on a chronic course
    - -30% improve
    - -50% recover
    - -Mortality rate 5.6% per decade

Disposition

ADMISSION CRITERIA

- Medical risk
  - —Extremely low weight
  - —Rapid weight loss
  - —Serum electrolyte imbalance
- Psychiatric risk
  - —Severe depression
  - —Suicidality
  - —Severe denial
  - —Severe impairment in functioning
  - —Toxic family environment

DISCHARGE CRITERIA

- Safe weight and a decrease in unhealthy eating behaviors in AN patients
- Significant decrease in the frequency, severity, and paralyzing nature of binging and purging behaviors is necessary in BN patients

Miscellaneous

ICD9: 307.50

CORE CONTENT CODE: 13.8.2

SUGGESTED READINGS

American Psychiatric Association. Practice guideline for eating disorders. Am J Psychiatry 1993;2:207–228.

Herzog DB, Becker AE. Eating disorders. In: Nicholi A, ed. The new Harvard guide to psychiatry. Cambridge, MA: Belknap Press (in press).

Herzog DB, Beresin EV. Anorexia nervosa. In: Weiner JM, ed. Textbook of child and adolescent psychiatry. 2nd ed. Washington, DC: American Psychiatric Press, 1997.

Rigotti NA. Approach to eating disorders. In: Goroll AH, May LA, Mulley JB, eds. Primary care medicine: office evaluation and management of the adult patient. 3rd ed. Philadelphia: Lippincott, 1995.

Rigotti NA. Eating disorders. In: Carlson KJ, Eisenstat SA, Frigoletto FD, Schiff IS, eds. Primary care of women. St. Louis: Mosby-Year Book, 1995.

Authors: David Herzog; Ana Richards

Ectopic Pregnancy

Clinical Presentation

SIGNS AND SYMPTOMS

- Amenorrhea (75–95%)
- Abdominal pain (80–100%), frequently unilateral
- Abnormal vaginal bleeding (50–80%)
- Symptoms of Pregnancy (10–25%)
- Orthostatic hypotension, dizziness, and syncope (5–35%)
- Abdominal tenderness (55–95%)
- Adnexal tenderness (75–90%)
- Adnexal mass (35–50%)
- Cervical motion tenderness (43%)
- The classic triad of amenorrhea, vaginal bleeding, and abdominal pain is present in only 15% of women with ectopic pregnancies

MECHANISM/DESCRIPTION

- Implantation of a fertilized ovum outside of the uterus, most commonly the fallopian tube. Incidence is 16.8 cases per 1000 pregnancies
- Risk factors include
  - —Woman >35 yo
  - —African American
  - —Any factor that prevents or delays the fertilized egg from reaching the uterus
    - -Previous fallopian tube damage from infections; e.g., PID
    - -Previous tubal surgery; e.g., history of tubal ligation
    - -History of previous ectopic pregnancy
    - -History of IUD use
    - -DES exposure
  - —43% of women with ectopic pregnancies have no risk factors

Pre-Hospital

CAUTIONS

- Female patients of childbearing age presenting in shock may have an unrecognized ruptured ectopic pregnancy

Diagnosis

ESSENTIAL WORKUP

- Pregnancy testing
  - —Women presenting with vaginal bleeding and abdominal pain *must* have a urine or serum pregnancy test and be ruled out for an ectopic pregnancy

Vital Signs Unstable

- Type and crossmatch
- Culdocentesis or bedside US, if immediately available, simultaneous with resuscitation
- Consult gynecology and prepare for immediate surgical intervention

Vital Signs Stable

- Rapid hemoglobin determination
- Type and Rh
- Ultrasonography

LABORATORY

- Urine ICON can detect β-hCG levels of 50 mIU/L
- β-hCG levels of 25 mIU/L can be detected in serum
- For pregnant patients with no demonstrable intrauterine pregnancy
  - —Quantitative serum β-hCG

ULTRASOUND IN CONJUNCTION WITH QUANTITATIVE β-hcG

- Patients with β-hCG levels of >6500 mIU/L and no gestational sac seen on ultrasound have a 100% chance of having an ectopic pregnancy
- Patients with β-hCG levels of >6500 mIU/L with intrauterine gestational sacs present have a 94% chance of having a normal pregnancy
- Patients with β-hCG of <2000 mIU/L are too early to have a gestational sac seen by abdominal ultrasound and thus cannot be ruled out for an ectopic pregnancy
- Patients with β-hCG of >2000 and <6,500 mIU/L should have an IUP visualized on transvaginal US; suspect ectopic pregnancy if IUP is absent

CULDOCENTESIS

With the wide availability of ultrasound in emergency departments, culdocentesis is performed less frequently. However if ultrasound is not available and the patient is at high risk for an ectopic pregnancy, culdocentesis may be necessary

- Culdocentesis is performed through a speculum by elevating the posterior lip of the cervix with a tenaculum and using an 18-gauge spinal needle on a 10-20-cc syringe and inserting it through the posterior fornix and aspirating the cul-de-sac
- Culdocentesis results
  - —Aspiration of clotted, dark blood: ectopic pregnancy
  - —Aspiration of bright red nonclotting blood: ectopic pregnancy, ruptured corpus luteum, or cyst
  - —Aspiration of clear, straw colored fluid: ruptured follicular cyst infection; e.g., PID

IMAGING

- Sonographic evidence of an intrauterine pregnancy (IUP) makes ectopic pregnancy very unlikely
  - —Positive IUP is indicated by a double-ringed gestational sac and yolk sac, fetal pole, and heart beat seen in the uterus
  - —The use of transvaginal ultrasound allows for the visualization of these structures 1 week earlier
  - —Transvaginal ultrasound; gestational sac at 5 weeks, cardiac activity at 6.5 weeks
  - —Transabdominal ultrasound; gestational sac at 6 weeks, cardiac activity at 8 weeks
  - —Complex adnexal mass and fluid in the cul-de-sac seen in 22% of ectopics and has a 94% positive predictive value when present

DIFFERENTIAL DIAGNOSIS

- Positive pregnancy test with vaginal bleeding
  - —Spontaneous abortion, cervicitis, trauma
  - —Positive pregnancy test with no evidence of an intrauterine pregnancy
  - —Completed spontaneous abortion
  - —Early threatened abortion
- Positive pregnancy test with evidence of an intrauterine pregnancy, abdominal pain, or adnexal tenderness
  - —Septic abortion, threatened abortion, corpus luteal cyst, ovarian torsion, UTI, nephrolithiasis, gastroenteritis, appendicitis

Treatment

INITIAL STABILIZATION

Vital Signs Unstable

- ABCs
- Fluid resuscitation with 2 large-bore IVs
- Consult gynecology and then transport to the OR immediately for surgery

Vital Signs Stable

- IUP present on ultrasound—consider other diagnoses
- IUP absent on ultrasound
  - —Evidence of ectopic pregnancy on ultrasound—OBGyn evaluation for laparoscopy versus outpatient methotrexate treatment
  - —No evidence of ectopic pregnancy (early IUP or early ectopic)
    - *-Desired pregnancy:* β-hCG levels in a normal IUP should double q 2 days. Stable, reliable patients may be followed for serial β-hCGs in conjunction with OBGyn
    - *-Undesired pregnancy:* dilation and curettage (D&C) to evacuate the uterus and confirm the presence of intrauterine products of conception

MEDICATIONS

- RhoGAM in Rh-negative women: 50 μg IM in women <12 weeks pregnant; 300 μg IM in women >12 weeks pregnant
- Methotrexate should be initiated by obstetric consultant

Disposition

ADMISSION CRITERIA

- Any patient that has confirmed ectopic pregnancy or is hemodynamically unstable
- Patients with increased risk factors, no available ultrasound, β-hCG >6500 with no evidence of an IUP, or poor social support should be admitted for observation and serial β-hCGs

DISCHARGE CRITERIA

- Decision for outpatient management should be made in conjunction with OBGyn
- Hemodynamically stable patients with workup that is nondiagnostic
  - —Strict follow-up for serial β-hCG's q 2 days. These patients should be recorded in a log book with phone numbers to ensure follow-up
  - —*Ectopic precautions:* patients should return to the emergency room immediately for increasing abdominal pain, vaginal bleeding, syncope or dizziness. Patients should not be left alone until the diagnosis of ectopic pregnancy can be safely ruled out. Family and friends should also be instructed on the warning signs and symptoms of ruptured/bleeding ectopic pregnancies

Miscellaneous

ICD9: 633.9

CORE CONTENT CODE: 12.3.1

SUGGESTED READINGS

Abbott J. Complications related to pregnancy. In: Rosen P, et al., eds. Emergency medicine: Concepts and clinical practice. 3rd ed., St Louis: CV Mosby, 1992.

Cartwright PS. Diagnosis of ectopic pregnancy. Obstet Gynecol Clin of North Am 1991;18:19.

Hockberger RS. Ectopic pregnancy. Emerg Med Clin North Am 1987;5:481.

Kaplan BC, et al. Ectopic pregnancy: Prospective study with improved diagnostic accuracy. Ann Emerg Med 1996;28:10.

Turner LM. Vaginal bleeding during pregnancy. Emerg Med Clin North Am 1994;12:45.

Author: Aviva Jacoby

Edema

Clinical Presentation

SIGNS AND SYMPTOMS

- Weight gain of several kilograms
- Discomfort in the affected areas
- Swelling
- Tenderness
- Pitting edema
  - —Increased venous hydrostatic pressure or decreased oncotic pressure
- Nonpitting edema
  - —Protein rich extravasated fluid

Generalized Edema (Anasarca)

- Edema is most prominent in dependent areas
  - —Feet
  - —Sacrum
  - —Bilateral lower extremities
- Cardiac
  - —Dyspnea
  - —Orthopnea
  - —Paroxysmal nocturnal dyspnea
  - —Increased JVP
  - —Rales
- Renal
  - —Anorexia
  - —Puffy eyelids
  - —Frothy urine
  - —Oliguria
  - —Dark urine
  - —Hematuria
  - —Hypertension
- Hepatic
  - —Jaundice
  - —Spider angiomas
  - —Palmar erythema
  - —Gynecomastia
  - —Testicular atrophy

Localized

- Ascites
- Hydrothorax
- Associated signs and symptoms by type of disorder
  - —History of trauma
    - -Mechanical, thermal, radiation
  - —Infectious
    - -Chills
    - -Fever
    - -Erythema
    - -Increased warmth
  - —Allergic
    - -Pruritus
    - -Hives
    - -Involvement of the lips and the oral mucosa
  - —Myxedema
    - -Pretibial nonpitting edema
    - -Periorbital edema
    - -Fatigue
    - -Cold intolerance
    - -Weight gain
    - -Constipation
    - -Slowed deep-tendon reflex relaxation
  - —Idiopathic
    - -Diurnal weight gain/loss

MECHANISM/DESCRIPTION

- Clinically apparent accumulation of extravascular fluid due to a derangement in the balance of oncotic and hydrostatic forces
  - —Increase in venous hydrostatic pressure
    - -Systemically as with congestive heart failure
    - -Locally as with deep vein thrombosis
  - —Increase in lymphatic hydrostatic pressure
  - —Decrease in oncotic pressure
    - -Systemically from hypoalbuminemia
    - -Locally from increased capillary permeability
  - —Increased venous hydrostatic pressure or decreased oncotic pressure results in pitting edema
  - —Protein-rich extravasated fluid results in nonpitting edema
    - -Lymphedema
    - -Increased capillary permeability
- In certain disorders, there is no clear relation to Starling forces
  - —Myxedema
  - —Idiopathic (cyclic) edema
    - -Worsened with heat
    - -More common in women
    - -Not necessarily related to menses

ETIOLOGY

Generalized

- Right heart failure
- Constrictive pericarditis
- Acute glomerulonephritis
- Renal failure
- Salt retention
  - —Estrogen therapy
  - —NSAIDs
  - —Vasodilators
  - —Lithium
  - —Acute withdrawal of diuretics
- Idiopathic (cyclic) edema
- Cirrhosis
- Nephrotic syndrome
- Protein-losing enteropathy
- Starvation

Localized

- Thrombophlebitis
- Cellulitis
- Baker's cyst
- Vasculitis
- Angioedema
  - —Allergic
  - —Acquired
- Mechanical trauma
- Thermal injuries
- Radiation injuries
- Chemical burns
- Hemiplegia
- Compressive or invasive tumor
- Postsurgical resection of lymphatics
- Postradiation
- Filariasis

Pre-Hospital

N/A

Diagnosis

ESSENTIAL WORKUP

- Diagnostic studies should be directed by the underlying etiology suggestive by the history and physical examination

LABORATORY

- Renal etiology suspected
  - —Electrolytes
  - —BUN and Creatinine
  - —Urine analysis
  - —Urine electrolytes and protein
- Myxedema suspected
  - —Thyroid function tests

IMAGING/SPECIAL TESTS

- Cardiac etiology suspected
  - —EKG
  - —Chest radiograph
  - —Echocardiography
- Localized edema to an extremity
  - —Ultrasound (duplex scanning) or contrast venography

DIFFERENTIAL DIAGNOSIS

- Cellulitis
- Contact dermatitis
- Diffuse subcutaneous infiltrative process
- Lymphedema
- Obesity

Treatment

INITIAL STABILIZATION

See ED treatment

ED TREATMENT

- Treatment should be directed towards the underlying cause
- Diuretics are indicated in cases of generalized edema but are not required emergently

MEDICATIONS

- Captopril: 25 mg po tid
- Furosemide: 20–40 mg IV; 20–80 mg po qd
- Hydrochlorothiazide: 12.5–50 mg po qd
- Spironolactone: 25–50 mg po qd

Disposition

ADMISSION CRITERIA

- Base the decision to admit the patient on the underlying etiology
- Inability to ambulate without adequate home support
- Hypoxia

DISCHARGE CRITERIA

- Patient should be advised to decrease their salt intake
- Elastic stockings

Miscellaneous

ICD9: 782.3

CORE CONTENT CODE: 4.9.2, 8.8.2

SUGGESTED READINGS

Braunwald E. Edema. In: Fauci AS, et al., eds. Harrison's principles of internal medicine. 14th ed., New York: McGraw Hill, 1998;210–214.

Author: Laura Macnow

Elbow Injuries

Clinical Presentation

SIGNS AND SYMPTOMS

- How patient carries the arm may give clues to diagnosis
  - —Supracondylar fracture
    - –Flexion type: patient supports injured forearm with other arm and elbow in 90° flexion loss of olecranon prominence
    - –Extension type: patient holds arm at side in S-type configuration
  - —Elbow dislocations
    - –Posterior: abnormal prominence of olecranon
    - –Anterior: loss of olecranon prominence
  - —Radial head subluxation
    - –Elbow slightly flexed and forearm pronated, resists moving arm at the elbow

MECHANISM/DESCRIPTION

- Supracondylar fracture
  - —Most common in children
  - —Peak ages 5–10, rarely occurs after age 15
  - —Extension type (98%): FOOSH (*F*all *O*n an *O*ut*S*tretched *H*and) with fully extended or hyperextended arm
    - –Type 1: minimal or no displacement
    - –Type 2: slightly displaced fracture; posterior cortex intact
    - –Type 3: totally displaced fracture; posterior cortex broken
  - —Flexion type: a blow directly to a flexed elbow
    - –Type 1: minimal or no displacement
    - –Type 2: slightly displaced fracture; anterior cortex intact
    - –Type 3: totally displaced fracture; anterior cortex broken
- Radial head fracture
  - —Usually indirect mechanism, i.e., FOOSH
  - —Radial head driven into the capitellum
- Elbow dislocation
  - —Second only to shoulder as most dislocated joint
  - —Most are posterior

ETIOLOGY

- Mechanism aids in determining the expected injury
- Trauma predominates
- Most elbow injuries caused by indirect trauma transmitted through the bones of the forearm (FOOSH)
- Direct blows account for very few fractures or dislocations

PEDIATRIC CONSIDERATIONS

- Subluxed radial head (Nursemaid's elbow)
  - —20% of all upper extremity injuries in children
  - —Peak age 1–4; occurs more frequently in females than males
  - —Sudden longitudinal pull on forearm with forearm pronated

Pre-Hospital

CAUTIONS

- Injuries to the ipsilateral upper limb, particularly fractures to the midshaft humerus and distal forearm are common
- Evaluate for associated neurovascular injuries (up to 20%)

Diagnosis

ESSENTIAL WORKUP

- Radiographs
- Assess wrist and shoulder for associated injury
- Evaluate neurovascular status of limb
- Assess skin integrity
- Examine for compartment syndrome, which is more common in supracondylar fractures

LABORATORY

- None specific for elbow injuries

IMAGING/SPECIAL TESTS

Radiographs

- Routine AP and lateral; add oblique for assessment of subtle injuries to radial head/distal humerus
- Fat pad sign
  - —Seen with intra-articular injuries
  - —Normally the anterior fat pad is a narrow radiolucent strip anterior to humerus, posterior fat pad is normally *not* visible
  - —*Anterior fat pad sign* indicates injury when raised and becomes more perpendicular to the anterior humeral cortex (sail sign)
  - —*Posterior fat pad sign* indicates injury
    - –In adults, posterior fat pad sign implies radial head fracture; in children, it implies supracondylar fracture

DIFFERENTIAL DIAGNOSIS

- Sprain/strain
- Effusion
- Contusion

PEDIATRIC CONSIDERATIONS

- Fractures in children often occur through unossified cartilage making radiographic interpretation confusing
- A line drawn down the anterior surface of the humerus should always bisect the capitellum in lateral view
- If any bony relationships appear questionable on radiographs, obtain a comparison view of the uninvolved elbow
- Suspect child abuse if history does not fit injury

COMPLICATIONS

- Neurovascular injuries to the numerous structures that pass about the elbow, including the anterior interosseus nerve, ulnar and radial nerve, brachial artery
- Volkmann's ischemic contracture is compartment syndrome of the forearm

Treatment

INITIAL STABILIZATION

- Immobilization to prevent further injury before taking radiographs is essential

ED TREATMENT

- Orthopedic consultation is recommended for all but nondisplaced, stable fractures that can generally be splinted with 24–48-hour orthopedic follow-up
- Fractures generally requiring orthopedic consultation
  - —Transcondylar, intercondylar, condylar, epicondylar fractures
  - —Fractures involving articular surfaces such as capitellum or trochlea
- Supracondylar fractures
  - —Type 1 can be handled by ED physician with 24–48-hour orthopedic follow-up
    - -Elbow may be flexed and splinted with posterior splint
  - —Types 2 and 3 require immediate orthopedic consult
    - -Reduce these in ED when fracture is associated with vascular compromise
- Anterior dislocation
  - —Reduce immediately if vascular structures compromised
  - —Then flex to 90° and place posterior splint
- Posterior dislocation
  - —Reduce immediately if vascular structures compromised
  - —Then flex to 90° and place posterior splint
- Radial head fracture
  - —Minimally displaced fractures may be aspirated to remove hemarthrosis, instill Marcaine, and immobilize
  - —Other types should have orthopedic consult
- Radial head subluxation
  - —In one continuous motion, supinate and flex the elbow while placing slight pressure on the radial head
  - —Often will feel a click with reduction
  - —If exam suggests fracture but x-ray is negative, splint and have patient follow-up in 24–48 hours for reevaluation

MEDICATIONS

- Conscious sedation is often required to achieve reduction; see Conscious Sedation Chapter

PEDIATRIC CONSIDERATIONS

- Ossification centers: 1st appears
- Capitellum: 3–6 months
- Radial head: 3–5 years
- Medial epicondyle: 5–7 years
- Trochlea: 9–10 years
- Olecranon: 9–10 years
- Lateral epicondyle: 9–13 years

Disposition

ADMISSION CRITERIA

- Vascular injuries, open fractures
- Fractures requiring operative reduction or internal fixation
- Admit all patients with extensive swelling or ecchymosis for overnight observation and elevation to decrease the risk of compartment syndrome

DISCHARGE CRITERIA

- Stable fractures or reduced dislocations with none of above features
- Splint and arrange orthopedic follow-up in 24–48 hours

Miscellaneous

ICD9: 959.3

CORE CONTENT CODE: 18.4.12.2.2

SUGGESTED READINGS

Minkowitz B, et al. Supracondylar humerus fractures: Current trends and controversies. Orthop Clin North Am 1994;25:4.

Nicholson DA, et al. ABC of emergency radiology: The elbow. BMJ 1993;307:23.

Simon R, Koenigsknecht S. Emergency orthopedics: The extremities. 4th ed. E. Norwalk, CT: Appleton & Lange, 1996.

Author: Christian

Electrical Injury

Clinical Presentation

SIGNS AND SYMPTOMS

General

- Crush-type trauma involving deep tissues which may be extensive relative to small skin burns

Effect of electricity

MILLIAMPERES AT 60 HZ	EFFECT
0.2–2	Tingling sensation
1–4	Pain
6–22	Inability to let go/tetanic contractions
30–50	Diaphragm/intercostal tetany
100	VFib
1000	Ventricular standstill

Cardiac

- Dysrhythmias
  - —PVC
  - —Sinus tachycardia
  - —Atrial fibrillation
- Ventricular fibrillation
  - —Most common cause of death
  - —Induced by alternating current at levels of 50–60 Hz (household current)
- Asystole results from direct current
- Myocardial damage
  - —Occurs rarely
  - —Generally epicardial, not transmural
  - —Patch-like damage does not follow distribution of coronary arteries
  - —ECG will not show standard injury patterns

Respiratory

- Respiratory arrest may occur from
  - —Electrical brain injury causing respiratory center inhibition
  - —Tetanic contraction of chest wall muscles and/or diaphragm
  - —Prolonged paralysis of respiratory muscles
  - —Postcardiac arrest respiratory arrest

Neurologic

- Acute
  - —Respiratory arrest, amnesia, altered mental status, seizures, coma, quadriplegia, localized paresis
- Delayed
  - —Ascending paralysis, transverse myelitis, amyotrophic lateral sclerosis

Vascular

- Venous thrombosis
- Compartment syndromes secondary to edema

Renal

- Renal failure secondary to myoglobinuria

Musculoskeletal

- Forceful muscle contraction from electrostimulation cause
  - —Vertebral column fracture
  - —Posterior shoulder dislocation
- Fractures or dislocations secondary to falls
- Compartment syndrome

Ophthalmologic

- Cataracts (onset 4–6 months postinjury)
- Corneal burns, intraocular hemorrhage, uveitis, retinal injuries, and optic nerve atrophy

Dermatologic

- Thermal burns from current arcing or clothes burning
- Kissing burns from flexor surface arcing as current exits and reenters skin
- Entry/exit wounds

MECHANISM/DESCRIPTION

- Amperage (electron flow) directly proportional to voltage and indirectly proportional to resistance
  - —Decrease in resistance (with moisture) results in worse injury
  - —Increase in voltage leads to worse injury
- Current pathway determines damage
  - —Current through thorax—heart damage
  - —Current through head—brain injury
- High voltage will cause resistant tissues (fat, tendons, bone) to heat and coagulate

PEDIATRIC CONSIDERATIONS

- Fetus much less resistant to electrical shock than mother
  - —All pregnant patients must undergo a period of fetal monitoring
- Oral commissure burn
  - —Results from child biting an electrical cord
  - —Associated with bleeding from the labial artery 3–5 days postinjury
  - —May heal with significant contractures

Pre-Hospital

CAUTIONS

- Care must be exercised in removing patients to ensure that rescuers do not contact live electrical sources
- Spinal precautions for transport
- Standard BLS/ACLS care
- Remove smoldering clothes

Diagnosis

ESSENTIAL WORKUP

- ECG
- Urinalysis for myoglobin
- Cardiac monitor
  - —Controversy abounds on the subject of the need for 24-hour monitoring
  - —Prolonged monitoring is *not* necessary in asymptomatic patients with a normal ECG, no arrhythmias, and an exposure to <240 volts

LABORATORY

- Determined by the nature of the injury
- For most exposures to household current, no testing indicated
- Creatinine kinase (CK) indications
  - —Positive urine myoglobin
  - —High voltage exposures
- CK MB indications
  - —Abnormal ECG
  - —Dysrhythmia
- Electrolytes, BUN, Cr
  - —For high voltage exposures
  - —Provides baseline renal function
  - —Hyperkalemia occurs due to cell death
  - —Metabolic acidosis with significant injury

DIFFERENTIAL DIAGNOSIS

- Thermal burns from electrical arcing flash injuries

Treatment

INITIAL STABILIZATION
- ABCs
- Standard ACLS measures for arrhythmias
- Spine immobilization when indicated

ED TREATMENT
- IV fluid resuscitation
  —Larger fluid volumes required due to extensive third spacing in injured muscle
  —Rapid administration to reach urine output of 1 ml/kg/hr
  —Titrate to urine output and CVP measurement
- Foley catheter
- Prevent renal failure from myoglobinuria
  —Maintain good urine output
  —IV bicarbonate increases solubility of myoglobin in urine
  —Furosemide/mannitol
  —Monitor renal function
- Immobilize/reduce fractures and dislocations
- Local wound care for thermal burns
- Tetanus prophylaxis

MEDICATIONS
- Bicarbonate: 1 amp IV then 2 amps added to 1 L of D5W to maintain urine pH >7.45
- Furosemide: 0.5 mg/kg IV
- Mannitol: 25 g (ped: 0.25–0.5 mg/kg) IV bolus then 12.5 mg/kg/hr IV titrated to urine flow >1 ml/kg/hr

Disposition

ADMISSION CRITERIA
- Documented LOC
- Dysrhythmias observed on monitor
- Abnormal ECG
- Suspicion of deep tissue burns
- Myoglobinuria
- Acidosis
- Significant skin burns/associated injury

DISCHARGE CRITERIA
- Minor, low voltage injury (<240 watts) with no associated injuries

PEDIATRIC CONSIDERATIONS
- Advise parents of children with oral commissure burns of risk of delayed labial artery bleeding and contractures

Miscellaneous

ICD9: 994.8

CORE CONTENT CODE: 5.4

SUGGESTED READINGS

Bailey B, Gaudreault P, Thivierge R, Turgeon J. Cardiac monitoring of children with household electrical injuries. Ann Emerg Med 1995;25(5):612–617.

Fish R. Electric shock, Part II: Nature and mechanisms of injury. J Emerg Med 1993;11:457–462.

Fontanarosa P. Electrical shock and lightning strike. Ann Emerg Med 1993;22(2):378–386.

Garcia C, Smith G, Cohen D, Fernandez K. Electrical injuries in a pediatric emergency department. Ann Emerg Med 1995;26(5):604–608.

Primavesi R. Electrical injuries: Current issues. Can J CME 1996;6:85–96.

Author: Isser Dubinsky

Encephalitis

Clinical Presentation

SIGNS AND SYMPTOMS

- Often begins with a preceding flulike illness over a few days
  —Mild headache, fever, sore throat, reduced appetite, myalgias
- Altered level of consciousness, drowsiness, coma
- Impaired cognitive ability and personality change (sometimes acute psychosis)
- Restlessness, agitation, irritability, delirium
- Seizures
- Fever, headache, vomiting, possibly neck stiffness
- Focal neurologic deficits, tremor, ataxia, cranial nerve palsies
- Papilledema on fundoscopy
- Clinical picture varies from mild headache and mild cognitive/emotional lability to severe agitation, seizures, coma, permanent neurologic sequelae, and death
- Clinical course of symptoms may be slow-moving or rapidly progressive

MECHANISM/DESCRIPTION

- Acute infectious inflammation of the brain
- 20,000 cases per year in United States
- Mortality 10%
- Inflammatory reaction occurs within brain parenchyma with destruction of neurons, parenchymal edema, and petechial hemorrhages
- Infection of the brain usually via hematogenous spread from another site
- Neural migration occurs with rabies, herpes simplex, and varicella zoster encephalitis

ETIOLOGY

- Viral is most common cause
- 50% of cases have no identifiable cause

Specific Viruses

- Herpes simplex
  —15–20% of all encephalitides
  —Primary or reactivation
  —Early treatment improves prognosis
- Arbovirus
  —10–15% of all encephalitides
  —Transmitted by arthropods and mosquitoes in warm months
  —Eastern equine causes a fulminant encephalitis
    -Propensity for the hippocampus
    -Abrupt onset of headache, fever, vomiting
  —Western equine occurs mostly in the western $^2/_3$ of the United States
    -Often preceded by nonspecific upper respiratory/GI tract symptoms
  —Japanese—most prevalent arboviral encephalitis worldwide
    -Indolent course of fever, headache, myalgias, and fatigue followed by confusion, delirium, masklike facies, seizures, brain stem dysfunction, coma, and death
- Enteroviral
  —Occurs mainly in children <10 years old
  —Relatively benign course with little or no long-term consequences
- Measles encephalitis
  —Occurs several days to 2–3 weeks after primary infection and rash
  —Abrupt onset and rapid progression to coma
  —Seizures common (50–60%)
  —Postimmunization incidence of 1 per 1 million vaccinations
- HIV encephalitis
  —Lower CD4 counts correlate with higher incidence of encephalitis
  —Typical features include motor spasticity and dementia
  —Propensity for white matter with extensive neural degeneration
- Rhabdovirus: Rabies

Nonviral

- *Mycoplasma pneumoniae*
- *Toxoplasma gondii*
- *Rickettsia rickettsii*
- *Mycobacterium tuberculosis*
- *Borrelia burgdorferi*
- *Coccidioides immitis*

Immunocompromised/HIV Patients

- *Cryptococcus neoformans*
- *Listeria monocytogenes*
- *Cytomegalovirus*
- *Toxoplasma gondii*

Pre-Hospital

N/A

Diagnosis

ESSENTIAL WORKUP

- Lumbar puncture—CSF analysis for
  - —Cell count/chemistry
    - -Elevated WBC, predominantly lymphocytes
    - -Elevated protein
    - -Glucose usually normal
  - —Viral and bacterial cultures (fungi if indicated by history)
  - —Antigen assays for
    - -Herpes simplex
    - -Cryptococcus
    - -Toxoplasmosis
    - -Other viral antigen and antibody assays if available (enterovirus, adenovirus, cytomegalovirus, mumps, and varicella zoster)

LABORATORY

- CBC
  - —WBC elevated but a normal WBC does not rule out infection
- Electrolytes, glucose, BUN, creatinine
- Bacterial and viral blood cultures
- Liver function tests if hepatic failure suspected
- Carboxyhemoglobin level if CO poisoning suspected
- Toxicology screen if ingestion suspected in differential

IMAGING/SPECIAL TESTS

- CT Scan
  - —To rule out hemorrhagic conditions and mass lesions
  - —Cerebral edema may be the only finding consistent with encephalitis
  - —Parenchymal hemorrhagic areas of the frontal and temporal lobes, along with edema with herpes simplex

DIFFERENTIAL DIAGNOSIS

- Meningitis
- Brain abscess
- Sepsis
- Ischemic stroke
- Head injury
- Subarachnoid hemorrhage
- Encephalopathy (hepatic, uremic)
- Metabolic
  - —Electrolyte abnormalities (Na^+, K^+, Cl^-, Ca^{++}, Mg^{++}, Phosphate)
  - —Hypoglycemia
  - —Hyperglycemic nonketotic coma
- Neoplastic
- Drugs/toxins
- Carbon monoxide inhalation

Treatment

INITIAL STABILIZATION

- ABCs
  - —Intubate obtunded/comatose patients
- Naloxone, thiamine, glucose (or Accucheck) for altered mental status
- For signs of raised intracranial pressure on fundoscopy or CT
  - —Hyperventilate to P_{CO_2} of 25–30 mm Hg
  - —Administer mannitol
- Run IV saline at TKO or half-maintenance to avoid cerebral edema

ED TREATMENT

- Seizure control
  - —Abort with diazepam
  - —Initiate antiseizure medication (dilantin or phenobarbital) if more than 1 seizure has occurred
- No specific treatment for most viral encephalitides
  - —Steroid use controversial
- Treat herpes simplex encephalitis with acyclovir IV
  - —Initiate if considered likely based on clinical grounds, CT, and CSF findings

MEDICATIONS

- Acyclovir: 5–10 mg/kg IV q 8 hrs, maximum 15 mg/kg/day (peds: 250 mg/m^2 IV q 8 hrs, maximum 750 mg/m^2/day)
- Diazepam: 5 mg IV (peds: 0.1–0.2 mg/kg IV or PR) per dose
- Dilantin: loading dose 15 mg/kg IV to a maximum of 1 g
- Mannitol: 0.5–1 g/kg of a 20% solution to run IV over 20–30 min
- Phenobarbital: load 15–20 mg/kg to 300–800 mg IV at 25–50 mg/min

Disposition

ADMISSION CRITERIA

- All patients

DISCHARGE CRITERIA

- None

Miscellaneous

ICD9 CODE: 323.9

CORE CONTENT CODE: 11.4.2

SUGGESTED READINGS

Johnson RT. The pathogenesis of acute viral encephalitis and postinfectious encephalomyelitis. J Infect Dis 1987;155(3):359–364.

Whitley RJ. Viral encephalitis [Review]. N Engl J Med 1990;323(4):242–250.

Whitley RJ, et al. Diseases that mimic herpes simplex encephalitis. JAMA 1989;262(2):234–239.

Author: Murtaza Galamhussein

Endocarditis

Clinical Presentation

SIGNS AND SYMPTOMS

General–HEENT

- Fever
  - —Most common symptom
  - —Often absent in certain settings
    - -Elderly
    - -Congestive heart failure
    - -Severe debility
    - -Chronic renal failure
- "Flu-like illness"
- Chills
- Sweats
- Rigors
- Malaise

Respiratory

- Dyspnea
- Cough

Cardiac

- A new or changing murmur in 80–85% of patients

Abdominal

- Abdominal or back pain
- Splenomegaly (15–50%)

Extremities

- Myalgias
- Arthralgias
- Digital clubbing

Neurologic

- Distant vascular embolization

Skin

- Cutaneous vasculitic lesions
  - —Mucosal and conjunctival petechiae
  - —Splinter hemorrhages
  - —Osler's nodes
    - -Erythematous, painful tender nodules
  - —Janeway lesions
    - -Erythematous or hemorrhagic, macular or nodular lesions, a few millimeters in diameter on the hands and feet
- Retinal hemorrhages or Roth spots

MECHANISM/DESCRIPTION

- A microbial infection of the endothelial surface of the heart
- Characterized by the vegetation (a thrombus with superimposed microorganisms)
- Older population
- Frequently male
- Fewer patients demonstrating the "classic" signs once noted by Osler
- Risk factors
  - —Intravenous drug abuse
    - -Greater risk, than rheumatic heart disease or prosthetic valves
    - -IV drug abuse has a predilection for right-sided heart valves
    - -Risk factor for recurrent endocarditis
  - —Structural heart disease serves as common vegetative sites due to altered intracardiac flow
    - -Mitral valve prolapse
    - -Aortic valve dysfunction
  - —Congenital heart disorders in the pediatric populations
    - -Tetralogy of Fallot
    - -Aortic stenosis
    - -Patent ductus arteriosus
    - -Ventricular septal defects
    - -Aortic coarctation
  - —Prosthetic valves
  - —Indwelling catheters
  - —Any mechanical devices may serve as a portal of entry or attachment for microorganisms

ETIOLOGY

- Major categories
  - —Bacterial endocarditis
  - —Prosthetic valve endocarditis
  - —Nonbacterial thrombotic endocarditis
    - -Malignancy
    - -Uremia
    - -Burns
    - -Systemic lupus erythematosus
- Common organisms
  - —*Streptococcus viridans*—found in oropharynx, common agent in native valve endocarditis
  - —*Streptococcus bovis*—common association with colonic polyps or GI malignancy
  - —*Streptococcus pneumoniae*—causes rapid valvular destruction, abscess, and CHF; risk factor alcoholism
  - —*Staphylococcus epidermidis*—major cause of PVE
  - —*Staphylococcus aureus*—seen in all populations especially IVDA and toxic illness; sometimes metastatic
  - —*Enterococci*—seen in young women and old men following instrumentation or infection
  - —*Candida* and *Aspergillus*—found in IVDA, prosthetic valves, or immunocompromised

Pre-Hospital

N/A

Diagnosis

ESSENTIAL WORKUP

- Identify risk factors for endocarditis in patients with fever of unknown etiology
- Blood cultures
- Echocardiography is needed to confirm the diagnostic

LABORATORY

- CBC
  - —Anemia (sometimes hemolytic)
  - —Leukocytosis (with granulocytosis and bandemia)
- Blood cultures
  - —Multiple sets (minimum of 2–3 sets) should be obtained prior to antibiotic administration
- Elevated sedimentation rate
- Urinalysis
  - —Microscopic hematuria

IMAGING/SPECIAL TESTS

- Chest radiography
  - -CHF
  - -Septic pulmonic emboli which may be seen in right-sided endocarditis
- EKG
  - —Arrhythmia
- Echocardiography
  - —Acute valvular pathology
  - —Abscess
  - —Vegetations
  - —Transesophageal echocardiography provides greater sensitivity

DIFFERENTIAL DIAGNOSIS

- Rheumatic fever
- Atrial myxoma
- Acute pericarditis
- MI
- Aortic dissection with regurgitant valve
- Thrombotic thrombocytopenic purpura
- Systemic lupus erythematosus
- Occult neoplasm with metastasis
- Septicemia

Treatment

INITIAL STABILIZATION

- Monitor for signs of heart failure
- Operative repair
  —Severe valvular dysfunction causing failure
  —Unstable prosthesis
  —Perivalvular extension with intracardiac abscess
  —Antimicrobial therapy failure
  —Large or fungal vegetations
- Antibiotic therapy
  —Intravenous, bactericidal and empiric, pending culture results
  —Native valve or congenital abnormality
    -Penicillin G + nafcillin + gentamycin
    -Vancomycin + gentamycin
  —Prosthetic valve or history of IVDA
    -Vancomycin + gentamycin + rifampin
    -Nafcillin + gentamycin (if MRSA is not suspected)
  —Fungal
    -Amphotericin B

MEDICATIONS

- Penicillin G: 20 million IU IV qd
- Nafcillin: 2 g IV q 4 hrs
- Gentamycin: 1 mg/kg IV q 8 hrs
- Vancomycin: 15 mg/kg IV q 12 hrs
- Rifampin: 600 mg po qd
- Amphotericin B: 0.6 mg/kg IV qd

Disposition

ADMISSION CRITERIA

- Patients with risk factors who exhibit pathologic criteria or clinical findings
- All intravenous drug users with fever
- Admit patients with cardiovascular instability to an ICU/monitored setting

DISCHARGE CRITERIA

None

EXPECTED COURSE

- Most patients will defervesce within 1 week

COMPLICATIONS

- Heart failure
- Right- or left-sided embolic events
- Mycotic aneurysms

Miscellaneous

ICD9: 421

CORE CONTENT CODE: 2.2.4

SUGGESTED READINGS

Berbari E, Cockerill F, et al. Infective endocarditis due to unusual or fastidious microorganisms. Mayo Clin Proc 1997;72:532–542.

Hogevik H, Alestig K. Fungal endocarditis: A report on seven cases and a brief review. Infection 1996;24(1):17–21.

Karchmer A. Infective endocarditis. In: Braunwald E, ed. Heart disease: A textbook of cardiovascular medicine. 5th ed. Philadelphia: WB Saunders, 1997:1077–1104.

Salman L, Prince A, et al. Pediatric infective endocarditis in the modern era. J Pediatr 1993;122:847–853.

Vlessis A, Hovaguimian H, et al. Infective endocarditis: Ten-year review of medical and surgical therapy. Ann Thorac Surg 1996;61:1217–1222.

Author: Michael S. Murphy

Endometriosis

Clinical Presentation

SIGNS AND SYMPTOMS

- Pelvic or back pain, usually cyclic
- Dysmenorrhea, often severe
- Dyspareunia
- Infertility
- Pelvic exam nonspecific, rarely tender, nodular masses are present
- Abdominal exam typically benign unless ruptured endometrioma produces peritoneal signs

ETIOLOGY

- Ectopic endometrial tissue with cyclic hormonal responsiveness
- Invades tissues, spreads locally and hematogenously
- Theories include retrograde menstruation, immunologic factors and metaplastic transformation

PEDIATRIC CONSIDERATIONS

- Not seen prior to menarche

Pre-Hospital

- No specific pre-hospital considerations

Diagnosis

ESSENTIAL WORKUP

- Must rule out other, life-threatening diagnoses, as directed by H&P (e.g., ectopic pregnancy, appendicitis)
- Pregnancy test

IMAGING/SPECIAL TESTS

- Ultrasound, CT, and MRI may show ovarian endometriomas, but rarely reveals implants
- Surgery, usually laparoscopy, required for definitive diagnosis

DIFFERENTIAL DIAGNOSIS

- Appendicitis
- Ovarian cysts
- Ovarian torsion
- Pelvic inflammatory disease
- Menstrual cramps/mittelschmerz
- Inflammatory bowel disease
- Irritable bowel disease
- Diverticulosis
- Gastroenteritis

PEDIATRIC CONSIDERATIONS

- Not seen in premenarchal females

Treatment

INITIAL STABILIZATION

- ABCs
- May require IV crystalloid if pain is severe and unable to tolerate oral fluids/medications

ED TREATMENT

- Once other diagnoses ruled out, adequate analgesia is necessary

MEDICATIONS

- Analgesic of choice
  —Morphine: 2–10 mg IV, repeat as necessary
  —Ketorolac: 15–30 mg IV, IM
  —Oral NSAIDs (ibuprofen): 600 mg po
  —Acetaminophen: 650–1000 mg po
- Oral contraceptives, gonadotropin releasing hormone agonists (e.g., lupron) or other hormonal manipulation may be started in consultation with primary care physician or gynecologist

Disposition

ADMISSION CRITERIA

- Refractory pain
- Unclear diagnosis for exploratory surgery or to follow serial exams
- Ruptured ovarian endometrioma with peritoneal signs

DISCHARGE CRITERIA

- Most patients with a clear exacerbation of endometriosis can be discharged with gynecology follow-up once pain controlled

Miscellaneous

ICD9: 617.9

CORE CONTENT CODE: 19.1.3.1

SUGGESTED READINGS

Cahill D, Wardle P. Treatment options in endometriosis. Practitioner 1996;240:250–254.

Falcone T, Goldberg JM, Miller KF. Endometriosis: Medical and surgical intervention. Curr Opin Obstet Gynecol 1996;8:178–183.

Lu PY, Ory SJ. Endometriosis: Current management. Mayo Clin Proc 1995;70:453–463.

Mallett VT. Endometriosis. In: Tintinalli JE, ed. Emergency medicine: A comprehensive study guide. New York: McGraw Hill, 1996:558.

Author: Christy Rosa

Epididymitis/Orchitis

Clinical Presentation

SIGNS AND SYMPTOMS

- Gradual onset of mild to moderate scrotal pain; may have symptoms in both testes
- Progressive scrotal swelling
  - —Early in course may feel swollen, indurated epididymis
- Dysuria and urethral discharge
  - —Recent urinary tract infection
  - —History of abnormal bladder function
  - —Of patients with gonococcal epididymitis, 30% do not have history of urethral discharge; 50% do not have demonstrable urethral discharge
- Fever (14–28%)
- Recent urinary instrumentation
- Tenderness in groin, lower abdomen, or scrotum
- Scrotal skin commonly erythematous and warm
- Spermatic cord may be edematous
- If pyogenic bacterial orchitis, patients usually are acutely ill with fever, intense discomfort, and swelling of testicle

MECHANISM/DESCRIPTION

Epididymitis

- Definition: inflammation or infection of the epididymis
- Rare in prepubertal boys
- Pathogenesis
  - —Initial stages: cellular inflammation begins in vas deferens and descends to lower pole of epididymis (flank and groin pain)
  - —Acute phase: epididymis is swollen and indurated; spermatic cord thickened
  - —Testis may become edematous due to passive congestion or inflammation
  - —Resolution: may be complete without sequelae; though often peritubular fibrosis develops, occluding ductules
- Complications
  - —Two-thirds of cases will have atrophy due to partial thrombosis of testicular artery
  - —Abscess and infarction are rare (5%)
  - —Incidence of infertility with unilateral epididymitis unknown; 50% incidence of infertility with bilateral epididymitis

Orchitis

- Inflammation or acute infection of the testicle, usually from direct extension of the process within the epididymis
  - —Infection only involving the testicle is rare, but can result from hematogenous spread of bacteria or following a mumps infection
- Categories
  - —Pyogenic bacterial orchitis: secondary to bacterial involvement of epididymis
  - —Viral orchitis: most commonly due to mumps
    - -Rare in prepubertal boys; occurs in 30% of postpubertal boys with mumps
    - -Occurs 4–6 days after parotitis; but can occur without parotitis
    - -Unilateral in 70% of patients
    - -Resolution in 4–5 days
    - ->50% of testes involved have residual atrophy; rarely affects fertility
  - —Granulomatous orchitis: syphilis and mycobacterium and fungal diseases; usually occurs in immunocompromised host

ETIOLOGY

Epididymitis

- Children
  - —Coliform or pseudomonas urinary tract infections
  - —Sexually transmitted diseases rare
  - —Associated with structural, neurological, or functional abnormalities of lower urinary tract
- Young men: age <35 years
  - —Sexually transmitted
  - —*Chlamydia trachomatis* (28–88%)
  - —*Neisseria gonorrhoeae* (3–28%)
  - —Coliform bacteria (7–24%); more common in homosexual males
- Older men: age >35 years
  - —Often associated with underlying urologic pathology
  - —May have acute or chronic bacterial prostatitis
  - —Coliform bacteria most common (23–67%)
  - —*Chlamydia trachomatis* (8–80%)
  - —Pseudomonas species
  - —*Neisseria gonorrhea* (15%)
  - —Gram-positive cocci
- Drug related
  - —Amiodarone has been associated with epididymitis
- Granulomatous: syphilis or mycobacterial and fungal causes; Henoch-Schönlein purpura

Orchitis

- Pyogenic bacterial orchitis
  - —*E. coli*
  - —*Klebsiella pneumoniae*
  - —*Pseudomonas aeruginosa*
  - —Staphylococci
  - —Streptococci
- Viral orchitis
  - —Mumps
  - —Coxsackie A and lymphocytic choriomeningitis virus
- Granulomatous orchitis: syphilis and mycobacterial and fungal diseases
- Posttraumatic orchitis: inflammation

Pre-Hospital

CAUTIONS

- Patients can be toxic in severe cases and may need IV fluid resuscitation

Diagnosis

ESSENTIAL WORKUP

- *Must differentiate from testicular torsion*
- Either color Doppler imaging or testicular scintigraphy should be performed
- Early consultation with urologist for torsion

LABORATORY

- CBC; often leukocytosis in range of 10,000–30,000/mm^3
- Urine analysis and culture
  - —24% of epididymo-orchitis have pyuria
  - —May or may not reveal bacterial source of infection
- Urethral Gram's stain and culture
  - —Especially for postpubertal and sexually active males with a discharge
- Blood culture if systemically ill

IMAGING/SPECIAL TESTS

- Color Doppler ultrasound
  - —82–100% sensitivity, 100% specificity in detecting testicular torsion
    - -Decreased blood flow diagnostic of torsion
  - —Epididymo-orchitis: hyperemia, increased vascularity
  - —Advantages: if torsion not present, can evaluate for epididymitis or other causes of scrotal pain
  - —Disadvantages: highly examiner dependent, difficult in infants or children
- Testicular scintigraphy: radionuclide study to analyze testicular perfusion
  - —Technetium study
  - —90–100% sensitivity, 89–97% specificity in detecting testicular torsion
  - —Inflammatory processes show increased uptake, torsion with decreased uptake
  - —False-positive scans in large fluid collections in scrotum: i.e., abscess, hydrocele, hematocele, bowel herniation
  - —False-negative scans in early torsion, spontaneous detorsion, small children, or infants

DIFFERENTIAL DIAGNOSIS

- *Testicular torsion*
- Testicular tumor
- Torsion of testicular appendages
- Trauma to scrotum
- Acute hernia
- Acute hydrocele

Treatment

INITIAL STABILIZATION

- ABCs
- IV access
- IV fluids, especially if systemically ill

ED TREATMENT

- Antibiotics
  - —Cover for chlamydia and gonococcus if adult or presumed sexually transmitted
  - —Cover for coliforms if child or presumed nonsexually transmitted
  - —Adjust according to culture and sensitivity results
- Bedrest and scrotal support with elevation and ice packs
- Analgesics and anti-inflammatories
- Urologic consultation and follow-up
  - —Children need workup for urologic abnormalities
    - -Voiding cystourethrography and renal ultrasound
  - —Surgical indications
    - -Scrotal abscess
    - -Torsion cannot be excluded
    - -Ischemia caused by severe epididymitis
    - -Scrotal fixation: indicates severe inflammation and potential suppuration

MEDICATIONS

Presumed Sexually Acquired

- Ceftriaxone: 250 mg IM *or*
  - —Ciprofloxacin: 500 mg po bid × 14 d; ofloxacin: 400 mg po bid × 14 d
  - —Followed by
    - -Doxycycline: 100 mg po bid × 14 days *or* tetracycline: 500 mg po qid × 14 d

Presumed Nonsexually Acquired

- TMP-SMX: 1 DS po bid × 14 days *or*
  - —Ciprofloxacin: 500 mg po bid × 14 d *or* ofloxacin: 400 mg po bid × 14 d
- Peds: 8 mg TMP/kg/d div bid; no alternative established

Disposition

ADMISSION CRITERIA

- Surgical indications present
- Older age group and ill appearing as many will have underlying urologic pathology
- Systemically ill: fever, nausea, vomiting
- Scrotal abscess

DISCHARGE CRITERIA

- Fails to meet admission criteria
- Patient with good follow-up
- Able to take oral antibiotics

Miscellaneous

ICD9: 604.90

CORE CONTENT CODE: 19.2.3.1

SUGGESTED READINGS

Berger RE. Acute epididymitis: Etiology and therapy. Semin Urol 1991;9:28–31.

Herberner TE. Ultrasound in the assessment of the acute scrotum. J Clin Ultrasound 1996;24:405–421.

Kass EJ, Lundak B. The acute scrotum. Pediatr Urol 1997;44:1251–1266.

Schul MW, Keating MA. The acute pediatric scrotum. J Emerg Med 1993;11:565–577.

Author: Tami Gash-Kim

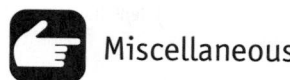

Epidural Abscess

Clinical Presentation

SIGNS AND SYMPTOMS

- *Classic presentation:* severe, progressive back and radicular pain with fever and eventual neurologic deficit (weakness or paralysis, sensory level, sphincter disturbance)
- May present with signs and symptoms of sepsis without prominent back pain
- Occurs at all ages including infants; peak is at ages 60–70 years
- Most patients have predisposing condition (diabetes, malignancy, IV drug abuse, chronic steroids, chronic alcoholism, instrumentation (s/p discogram) or spinal surgery)
- May occur in the absence of identifiable predisposing factors

MECHANISM/DESCRIPTION

- A pyogenic infection of the epidural space
- Most common in the thoracic spine, followed by the lumbar and cervical areas

ETIOLOGY

In most cases, there is a focus of infection followed by either hematogenous spread (~50%) or direct extension. The most common sources are skin structure infections, but any pyogenic infection may be a source. In some cases, no source is identified

- S. aureus accounts for more than 50% of cases with Streptococcus the second most common organism
- H. flu, Gram-negative bacilli, mycobacteria, anaerobic and mixed infections also occur
- May occur after lumbar puncture (usually follows multiple attempts)

PEDIATRIC CONSIDERATIONS

- Children present similar to adults with back pain, fever, and neurologic signs, as well as nonspecific systemic symptoms
- Infants may exhibit only fever, irritability, and associated meningitis
- Sphincter disturbance is frequently seen
- Most cases are secondary to hematogenous spread
- Location and bacteriology similar to adults

Pre-Hospital

N/A

Diagnosis

Fever and severe back pain represent a potentially serious combination. If the pain is radicular or there is a neurologic disturbance, the likelihood of epidural abscess is increased

ESSENTIAL WORKUP

- History should include predisposing conditions when this diagnosis is suspected
- Physical exam for a source of infection, localized spinal tenderness, and neurologic findings, especially decreased sphincter tone, saddle anesthesia, and lower extremity weakness
- MRI is the diagnostic test of choice, however, when this is not available obtain CT myelogram
  —Suspected epidural abscess is a true neurosurgical emergency and requires emergent imaging

LABORATORY

- ESR is almost always elevated (~100%) but is nonspecific
- Blood cultures are often positive (~60%)
- Leukocytosis with a left shift is common (~70%)
- CSF often abnormal but is nondiagnostic; routine lumbar puncture should be avoided when epidural abscess is suspected (may cause meningitis)

IMAGING/SPECIAL TESTS

- MRI is at least 90% sensitive; shows high intensity lesion on T2 imaging
- Myelography and CT myelography are also sensitive but risk dissemination
- Plain films are usually abnormal but nonspecific

DIFFERENTIAL DIAGNOSIS

Diagnosis is difficult due to rarity of the condition and nonspecific symptoms. Multiple physician encounters commonly precede the diagnosis. Most common initial diagnosis is musculoskeletal pathology

- *Early presentation:* muscular or ligamentous pain, degenerative arthritis, compression fracture, discogenic pain
- *Back pain with fever, systemic signs and symptoms:* vertebral osteomyelitis, spinal tumor, meningitis, spinal subdural abscess, discitis, pyelonephritis
- *Back pain with neurologic signs and symptoms:* cord compression, cord ischemia, disc herniation

PEDIATRIC CONSIDERATIONS

- Fever and back pain should be urgently investigated with MRI when epidural abscess is suspected

Treatment

INITIAL STABILIZATION

- Broad spectrum parenteral antibiotics early for signs of sepsis, must include coverage for S. aureus and Streptococcus
- Ceftriaxone and clindamycin are appropriate initial coverage

ED TREATMENT

- Urgent imaging is essential when diagnosis is considered; delay in definitive treatment is associated with a poor outcome
- Urgent neurosurgical consultation or transfer for definitive therapy (surgical decompression) after diagnosis and antibiotic Rx

MEDICATIONS

- Ceftriaxone: 1–2 g IV q 12 hrs
- Clindamycin: 600–900 mg IV q 8 hrs

Disposition

ADMISSION CRITERIA

- Suspected epidural abscess should be admitted; an MRI is needed emergently, transfer the patient if necessary
- Patients with spinal epidural abscess require admission to a facility with neurosurgical capability

DISCHARGE CRITERIA

- Patients with epidural abscess should not be discharged

Miscellaneous

ICD9: 324.9

CORE CONTENT CODE: 11.4.1.2

SUGGESTED READINGS

Martin MJ, Yuan HA. Neurosurgical care of spinal epidural, subdural, and intramedullary abscesses and arachnoiditis. Ortho Clin North Am 1996;27(1):125–136.

Maslin DR, et al. Spinal epidural abscess. Arch Intern Med 1993;153(14):1713–1721.

Redekop GJ, Del Maestro RF. Diagnosis and management of spinal epidural abscess. Can J Neurol Sci 1992;19(2):180–187.

Rubin G, et al. Spinal epidural abscess in the pediatric age group: Case report and review of the literature. Pediatr Infect Dis J 1993;12(12):1007–1011.

Vilke VM, Honingford EA. Cervical spine epidural abscess in a patient with no predisposing risk factors. Ann Emerg Med 1996;27(6):777–780.

Wheeler D, et al. Medical management of spinal epidural abscesses: Case report and review. Clin Infect Dis 1992;15(1):22–27.

Authors: Richard S. Krause; Danielle S. Notebaert

Epidural Hematoma

Clinical Presentation

SIGNS AND SYMPTOMS

- Altered or deteriorating level of consciousness
- Headache, vomiting, lethargy (>90% with at least 1 of these 3 symptoms)
- Unilateral limb weakness
- Pupil asymmetry (30%) is a late finding
  —Hematoma on same side as dilated pupil in >90%
- Posturing is a late finding
- The majority of patients are unconscious when first seen
- Classic description of trauma with unconsciousness, followed by a *lucid interval,* then progressive neurologic deterioration to ipsilateral pupil dilation and contralateral hemiparesis is uncommon (3–12%)

MECHANISM/DESCRIPTION

- Direct trauma over temporoparietal aspect of skull
- Tear of middle meningeal artery (80%), or dural sinus (15%)
- High incidence of associated fracture of the temporal bone

ETIOLOGY

- Accounts for 20% of intracranial hematomas
- Mortality 10–12%
- Male to female ratio is approximately 3:1
- Peak incidence in second to third decade of life
- MVA most common cause in adults
- Assault has the highest association with intracranial injury and need for neurosurgery (excluding GSWs)

PEDIATRIC CONSIDERATIONS

- Falls are most common cause in pediatric group
- In 26% of cases, diagnosis not made until return ED visit
- 38% of children are alert with normal vital signs and neuro exam at time of diagnosis
- If anything about a child's history or presentation makes you consider a CT scan, do the scan

Pre-Hospital

CAUTIONS

- Head-injured patients should be triaged to regional trauma centers and immobilized with backboard and C-collar
- Patients with increased intracranial pressure or signs of impending herniation should be intubated with RSI

Diagnosis

ESSENTIAL WORKUP

- CT of Head
- C-spine series as all head-injured patients are assumed to have cervical spine injury until proven otherwise

LABORATORY

- CBC, ABG, chemistries, PT/PTT as needed
- Blood ETOH/Drug Screen

IMAGING/SPECIAL TESTS

- Characteristic *lenticular/biconvex shaped hemorrhage* visualized on CT
- Fractures seen on plain films are often associated with underlying injury and should always have follow-up CT scan

DIFFERENTIAL DIAGNOSIS

- A history of recent head trauma will usually suggest the diagnosis. Other diagnoses to consider are
  —Cerebral concussion/contusion
  —Subdural hematoma
  —Intracerebral bleed
  —Diffuse axonal injury
  —Subdural hygroma
  —Shaken baby syndrome
  —Toxic, metabolic, or infectious causes

PEDIATRIC CONSIDERATIONS

- In infants with open fontanels, ultrasound can be used to visualize intracerebral structures
- Persistent vomiting, seizure, lethargy, irritability, or a bulging fontanel should suggest hematoma

Treatment

INITIAL STABILIZATION

- ABCs; the presence of hypoxia or shock worsens the prognosis
  —RSI and mild hyperventilation for signs of increased ICP (maintain $PCO_2 = 35$ mmHg)
- Stabilize C-spine
- Elevate head of bed 30°, or gurney in reverse Trendelenburg
- Rapid neurologic assessment
  —Assess brain stem reflexes, pupils, corneal reflex, and gag
- Glasgow Coma Scale
  —GCS of 8 or less = severe head injury
  —GCS of 9–13 = moderate head injury
  —GCS of 14–15 = minor head injury
- Careful secondary survey to uncover coexisting injuries (present in >50%)

ED TREATMENT

- Early surgical intervention (<4 hours) in comatose patients with an acute epidural hematoma significantly reduces mortality and improves outcome
- Factors predictive of poor outcome
  —Best GCS score of 8 or less in first 24 hours
  —Pupillary inequality or nonreactivity
  —Presence of posturing
  —Delayed surgical evacuation of >4 hours
  —Presence of multisystem trauma
  —Prolonged elevated ICP
  —Prolonged hypotension
- Frequent neurologic reassessment
- Avoid narcotics/sedation if possible
- Place A-line and monitor pO_2, pCO_2, mean arterial pressure (MAP)
- Foley catheter to monitor urine output
- IV fluids 0.5%NS at 75% maintenance
  —Adjust fluids to maintain MAP at approximately 110 mm Hg (optimizes cerebral perfusion pressure CPP = MAP − ICP)
  —Induce osmotic diuresis to induce mild hyperosmolar state 295–310 milliosmoles (reduces ICP)
  —Give mannitol followed by Lasix
- Control hypertension
  —Labetalol
  —Hydralazine
- Barbiturate coma only in cases refractory to standard antihypertensive therapy
  —Seizure prophylaxis
  —Dilantin
  —Diazepam
- GI stress ulcer prophylaxis
  —Pepcid
- Prevent hyperglycemia
- Prevent pain/posturing/respiratory effort that fights the ventilator and increases ICP
  —Sedation with versed
  —Neuromuscular blockade with pancuronium
- Steroid therapy is contraindicated
- Antibiotic prophylaxis is unnecessary except with direct contamination of cerebral contents

MEDICATIONS

- Mannitol: adult/peds: 0.5–1.0 g/kg IV q 3–6 hrs
- Lasix: adult/peds: 0.5mg/kg IV
- Labetalol: adult: 15–30 mg/hr IV; peds: safety not established
- Hydralazine: adult: 10 mg/hr IV; peds: safety not established
- Dilantin: adult/peds: load 18 mg/kg at 25–50 mg/min
- Diazepam: adult: 5–10 mg IV; peds: 0.5–1 mg IV to max dose of 5 mg
- Pepcid: adult: 40 mg IV; peds: safety not established
- Versed: 2–4 mg IV/hr PRN; peds: safety not established

PEDIATRIC CONSIDERATIONS

- Serious scalp laceration or hematoma can cause hypotension in an infant

Disposition

ADMISSION CRITERIA

- All severe head injury patients should be admitted to an intensive care unit with neurosurgical consultation
- Moderate head injury patients with persistent mental status changes, alteration of consciousness, or focal neurologic deficit should be admitted to a monitored setting
- Fractures at high risk for complication (overlying meningeal artery, major dural sinus, depressed) should be admitted

DISCHARGE CRITERIA

- Mild head injury patients may be discharged home into the hands of a competent observer with closed head injury instructions. Follow-up should be arranged within the next 48 hours. Tylenol or NSAIDs only for pain
- Intoxicated patients with a negative CT should not be discharged until patient is clinically sober, and neurologic and mental status examinations are normal

Miscellaneous

ICD9: 852.40

CORE CONTENT CODE: 18.4.1.4

SUGGESTED READINGS

Greenberg J. Evaluation and stabilization of head trauma. Surg Rounds 1992;15(6):535–550.

Harad FT, Kerstein MD. Inadequacy of bedside clinical indicators in identifying significant intracranial injury in trauma patients. J Trauma 1992;32(3):359–363.

Miller JD. Head injury. J Neurol Neurosurg Psychiatry 1993;56(5):440–447.

Schutzman SA, Barnes PD, Mantello M, Scott RM. Epidural hematomas in children. Ann Emerg Med 1993;22(3):535–541.

Author: Paul File

Epiglottitis, Adult

Clinical Presentation

SIGNS AND SYMPTOMS

- General
  - —Fever
  - —"Toxic" appearance
  - —Drooling
  - —Stridor
- HEENT
  - —Dysphagia
  - —Sore throat
  - —Voice change
- Respiratory
  - —Respiratory compromise
  - —Sudden loss of airway patency
    - -Often rapid progression from mild symptoms to airway obstruction

MECHANISM/DESCRIPTION

- Inflammation of the supraglottic
  - —Epiglottis
  - —Vallecula
  - —Arytenoids
- Uncommon with an incidence of about 1/100,000
- Twice as common in adults as in children
- Mortality: 4–7%
- Complications
  - —Meningitis
  - —Retropharyngeal abscess
  - —Pneumothorax
  - —Empyema
  - —ARDS
  - —Pulmonary edema

ETIOLOGY

- *Hemophilus influenzae*
- Group A streptococcus
- *Streptococcus pneumonia*
- *Hemophilus parainfluenzae*
- Thermal or caustic injuries

Pre-Hospital

- Transport the patient in most comfortable position, usually sitting up
- Provide supplemental oxygen as necessary
- Intubation may be difficult or impossible and should only be attempted in the patients in extremis
- Racemic epinephrine and β-agonist agents have not been demonstrated to be effective

Diagnosis

ESSENTIAL WORKUP

- Visualization of the epiglottis if no sign of airway compromise
- If airway compromise, no diagnositc studies are needed

LABORATORY

- CBC
  - —WBC >10,000 in 80% of cases
- Cultures of pharynx
- Blood cultures

IMAGING/SPECIAL TESTS

- Nasopharyngoscopy
- Indirect laryngoscopy
- Portable lateral soft-tissue neck x-ray
  - —Epiglottic edema
  - —"Thumb sign"
  - —"Vallecula sign"

DIFFERENTIAL DIAGNOSIS

- Airway obstruction, foreign body
- Anaphylaxis
- Angioedema
- Anxiety
- Laryngitis
- Pharyngitis
- Tracheitis

Treatment

INITIAL STABILIZATION

- Orotracheal intubation in patients with airway obstruction
  —May be required with little warning
  —Airway equipment should be kept at the bedside
  —The neck should be prepped and the equipment ready for a surgical airway
  —When time permits, intubation should be performed in the OR
- Needle-jet insufflation may also be considered to temporarily ventilate a patient

ED TREATMENT

- Administer humidified oxygen
- Intravenous hydration
- Cardiac monitor
- Provide empiric coverage with ceftriaxone or ampicillin/sulbactam
- Chloramphenicol or TMP-SMX if allergic to penicillin/cephalosporins
- Corticosteroids remain controversial

MEDICATIONS

- Ceftriaxone: 1–2 g IV initial dose
- Ampicillin/sulbactam: 3 g IV initial dose
- Chloramphenicol: 1 g IV initial dose
- TMP-SMX: 320 mg (of TMP, 4 amps) IV initial dose
- Rifampin: 20 mg/kg (max 600 mg) qd for 4 d

Disposition

ADMISSION CRITERIA

- All patients with suspected or confirmed diagnosis to an ICU bed

DISCHARGE CRITERIA

- Patients suspected of epiglottitis should not be discharged
- Close contacts should be treated with rifampin prophylaxis

Miscellaneous

ICD9: 464.3, 464.30, 464.31

CORE CONTENT CODE: 6.3.3.2.2

SUGGESTED READINGS

Carey MJ. Epiglottitis in adults. Am J Emerg Med 1996;14:421–424.

Ducic Y, Hebert PC, MacLachlan L, Neugeld K, Lamothe A. Description and evaluation of the vallecula sign: A new radiologic sign in the diagnosis of adult epiglottitis. Ann Emerg Med 1997;30:1–6.

Kornak JM, Freije JE, Campbell BH. Caustic and thermal epiglottitis in the adult. Otolaryngol Head Neck Surg 1996;114:310–312.

Mayo-Smith MF, Hirsch PJ, Wodzinski SF, Schiffman FJ. Acute epiglottitis in adults: An eight-year experience in the state of Rhode Island. N Engl J Med 1986;314:1133–1139.

Wetmore RF, Handler SD. Epiglottitis: Evolution in management during the last decade. Ann Otol Rhinol Laryngol 1979; 88:822.

Author: Jonathan Adler

Epiglottitis, Pediatric

Clinical Presentation

SIGNS AND SYMPTOMS

- Usually fulminant presentation without prodromal illness
- General
  —Irritability
  —Lethargy
  —Toxic appearing
  —High fever is typical (>38.4°C)
- HEENT
  —Sore throat
  —Drooling
  —Dysphagia
  —Muffled voice
- Respiratory
  —Increasing respiratory distress
  —Children usually prefer to sit upright, leaning forward with open mouth ("sniffing position") to maximize air entry
  —Subtle stridor that may progress to severe stridor

MECHANISM/DESCRIPTION

- Inflammation of the epiglottis and surrounding supraglottic region
- Children are at greatest risk of upper airway obstruction because of small caliber airways due to
  —Decreased cross sectional area of the upper airway (R ~1/r4)
  —Cricoid ring is the narrowest part of the airway
  —Loose attachment of mucosal surface and increased vascularity of mucosa allows for edema
  —Dynamic collapse of the airway
- A precipitous decline in the incidence of childhood epiglottitis since the introduction of the *Haemophilus influenza* vaccination
- Typically occurs in children ranging in age from 7 months to 16 years with peak incidence between 2 and 6 years
- Epiglottitis predominates in winter and spring months, but may occur throughout the year

ETIOLOGY

- Infection
  —*Hemophilus influenza*
  —β-hemolytic streptococci
  —Herpes simplex virus (rare)
  —Anaerobes (rare)
  —Klebsiella
  —Aspergillus (usually seen only in patients with underlying disease)
- Caustic
- Thermal
- Traumatic

Pre-Hospital

- Notification to receiving emergency department to prepare OR for visualization and possible airway management in a controlled setting
- Do nothing that agitates any patient, particularly a child with stridor and respiratory distress
- Most children will be most calm when held by or are sitting with a parent
- If the patient allows, administer 100% O_2 by mask or by cannula
- Do not attempt IV access
- Bag valve mask ventilation with 100% O_2 followed by emergency airway procedures if acute obstruction

Diagnosis

ESSENTIAL WORKUP

- Epiglottitis is a clinical diagnosis
- Indirect laryngoscopy or any attempts to directly visualize the epiglottis are not indicated in children with suspected epiglottis unless performed in a controlled environment
- If infection is suspected, obtain cultures of the epiglottis during laryngoscopy

LABORATORY

- Avoid laboratory tests until airway is controlled
- Throat cultures
- Blood cultures
  —Often positive if *Hemophilus influenza* is the pathogen

IMAGING/SPECIAL TESTS

- X-rays of the soft tissue lateral neck
  —Usually not necessary to make the diagnosis
  —Creates additional risk by delaying stabilization of the airway, promoting airway obstruction by agitating the patient and often removing the child from the ED to an uncontrolled environment
  —Variable findings
    -Normal
    -Swelling of the epiglottis and often supraglottic region
    -"Thumbprint" sign from thickened aryepiglottic folds and normal subglottis
    -An EW/C3W (epiglottic width to 3rd cervical vertebral body width) ratio of >0.5
- Laryngoscopy
  —In a controlled environment whenever possible
  —Cultures of the epiglottis during laryngoscopy to clarify pathogens and direct treatment

DIFFERENTIAL DIAGNOSIS

- Other infectious processes
  —Bacterial tracheitis
  —Mononucleosis
  —Diptheria
  —Pertussis
  —Croup (primarily in younger children but there is a significant overlap in the ages of presentation)
  —Ludwig's angina
  —Peritonsillar infection
  —Retropharyngeal abscess
- Allergic reactions
- Angioneurotic edema
- Airway foreign bodies
- Laryngeal trauma
- Laryngospasm
- Inhalation or aspiration of toxins (e.g., hydrocarbons)
- Airway burns (have been related to crack cocaine)

- Systemic diseases: amyloid, sarcoid, pemphigus, pemphigoid, Wegner's granulomatosis
- Hyperventilation
- CNS disorders

Treatment

INITIAL STABILIZATION

- Airway management in patients in extremis
  - —Bag valve mask ventilation with 100% O_2, with cricoid pressure often provides adequate ventilation and provides time to move the patient to the OR
  - —Oral intubation
  - —Use an ETT size 1 mm smaller than indicated by age
  - —Direct compression of the anterior neck in the glottic region may help visualize air bubbles at the opening of the swollen glottis
  - —When oral intubation fails
    - -Emergency cricothyrotomy if age >10–12 years
    - -Needle cricothyrotomy if age <10–12 years

ED TREATMENT

- 100% O_2 as tolerated by patient
- Avoid procedures that agitate the patient
- Empiric invasive airway management may be indicated
  - —Patients with rapidly progressive respiratory difficulty, tachypnea, worsening throat pain, tachycardia, or hypoxemia
  - —Patients at high risk for acute obstruction (e.g., children with immunocompetency disorders)
- Intubate in operating room, or controlled environment by most skilled person
- Inhalational anesthesia is used prior to intubation
- Have appropriate various diameters of ETT available to accommodate the inflamed supraglottic region
- Surgical backup required in case intubation not possible, then emergency tracheotomy or cricothyrotomy can be performed
- Administer IV antibiotics: second- or third-generation cephalosporin is active against β lactamase-producing *H. influenza*
- Equipment for intubation and for a surgical airway or needle cricothyrotomy must be available at the bedside
- Steroids are controversial but frequently given particularly in patients with chemical or thermal epiglottitis

MEDICATIONS

- Ceftriaxone: 50–75 mg/kg/24hrs q 12 hrs IV
- Cefotaxime: 50–150 mg/kg/24hrs q 6 hrs IV
- Ampicillin: 100–200 mg/kg/24hrs q 4 hrs IV
- Chloramphenicol: 75–100 mg/kg/24hrs q 6 hrs IV
- Rifampin: 20 mg/kg (max 600 mg) qd for 4 d

COMPLICATIONS

- Pulmonary edema
- Epiglottic abscesses
- Pulmonary atelectasis

Disposition

ADMISSION CRITERIA

- All patients with suspected epiglottitis

DISCHARGE CRITERIA

- Close contacts should be treated with rifampin prophylaxis

Miscellaneous

ICD9: 464.3, 464.30, 464.31

CORE CONTENT CODE: 13.7.1

SUGGESTED READINGS

Bank D, Krug S. New approaches to upper airway disease. Emerg Med Clin North Am 1995;13(2):473–487.

Brilli R, Benzing G, Cotcamp D. Epiglottitis in infants less than two years of age. Pediatr Emerg Care 1989;5(1):16–22.

Carey M. Epiglottitis in adults. Am J Emerg Med 1996;14(4):421–424.

Frantz T, Ragson B, Quesenberry C. Acute epiglottitis in adults: Analysis of 129 cases. JAMA 1994;272(17):1358–1360.

Gorelick M, Baker M. Epiglottitis in children: 1979 through 1992. Arch Pediatr Adolesc Med 1994;148:47–50.

Kornak J, Freije J, Campbell B. Caustic and thermal epiglottis in the adult. Otolaryngol Head Neck Surg 1996;114(2)310–312.

Rothrock S, Pignatiello G, et al. Radiologic diagnosis of epiglottitis: Objective criteria for all ages. Ann Emerg Med 1990;9:978–982.

Valdepena H, Wald E, Rose E, Ungkanont K, et al. Epiglottitis and *Haemophilus influenza* immunization: The Pittsburgh experience—A five-year review. Pediatrics 1995;96(3):424–427.

Author: Susan J. Duffy

Epiphyseal Injuries

Clinical Presentation

SIGNS AND SYMPTOMS

- Pain
- Inability to use or mobilize affected joint
- Localized tenderness
- Swelling
- Ecchymosis
- Bony deformities

MECHANISM/DESCRIPTION

- More common than sprains in children
  - —Relative weakness of the epiphysis compared to ligaments
- Common mechanisms
  - —Shearing
  - —Bending
  - —Compression
- Salter-Harris classification
  - —Type I
    - -Fracture cleavage is through the physis
    - -Separation of the epiphysis from the metaphysis
    - -No growth disturbance
  - —Type II
    - -Fracture propagates transversely along the physis and out through metaphyseal bone
    - -Periosteum torn on the opposite side of the fracture
    - -Most common epiphyseal fracture
    - -No growth disturbance
  - —Type III
    - -Fracture of the epiphysis extending along and through the physis
    - -Phalanges and distal tibia most commonly affected
    - -Growth disturbance may occur even with anatomic reduction
  - —Type IV
    - -Fracture originates at the articular surface
    - -Extends through the physis and into the metaphysis
    - -Distal humerus and distal tibia most commonly affected
    - -Anatomic reduction essential
  - —Type V
    - -Injury to the focal length of the hypertrophic zone in the physis
    - -Result from significant compressive forces
    - -Usually involve the knee or ankle
    - -Fortunately rare
  - —Type VI
    - -Not described in the original Salter-Harris classification
    - -Involves the pericondylar ring and associated periosteum that surround the physis
    - -May be seen in thermal injuries
- Types I through IV heal without residual deficit with treatment
- Types V and VI require close orthopedic outpatient follow-up for the nearly inevitable focal bone arrest
- Long-term complications
  - —Overreduction
  - —Bone growth disturbances
  - —Reduced joint mobility

ETIOLOGY

N/A

Pre-Hospital

- Immobilize the limb in the position found
- Ice or cold packs over the injured surface
- Neurologic and vascular assessment of the extremity distal to the injury
- Monitor for other signs of injury

Diagnosis

ESSENTIAL WORKUP

- Assess pulses, motor, and sensory function distal to the injury
- Assess integrity of the skin overlying injury
- Assess for other injuries

LABORATORY

N/A

IMAGING/SPECIAL TESTS

- Radiography of the injured bone
  - —Type I fractures
    - -The only abnormality may be a slightly separated physis or an associated joint effusion
    - -May see callous on follow up
  - —Type V and VI
    - -Often no abnormalities on initial film
    - -Subsequent radiographs reveal premature bone arrest at the site of previous injury
  - —Comparison views of the contralateral joint
    - -Needed to detect small slips in type I fractures
- Radionuclide bone scan
  - —Rarely needed
  - —Fractures must be at least 24–48 hours old
  - —Value as an adjunct if child abuse suspected
- CT scan
  - —Helpful in defining the integrity of articular surfaces in Type IV fractures
- MRI
  - —When the diagnosis remains in doubt and a positive finding will alter management

DIFFERENTIAL DIAGNOSIS

- Sprain
- Strain
- Contusion

Treatment

INITIAL STABILIZATION

- Apply sterile dressings to open wounds
- Control hemorrhage
- Reassurance
- Pain control

ED TREATMENT

- Reduction
- Immobilization
  —A splint must immobilize both the joints proximal as well as distal to the injury
  —Administration of analgesics
  —Cold packs applied to the site of injury to reduce the amount of hemorrhage, swelling, and pain
  —Elevation of the injured limb
  —Reduction
    -Circulatory compromise distal to the injury
    -Gross displacement
- Open fractures
  —Intravenous antibiotics
    -Directed towards staphylococcal and streptococcal species
  —Wound must be irrigated with saline
  —Sterile dressing
  —Orthopedic consultation

MEDICATIONS

- Fentanyl: 2–3 mg/kg IV; transmural lollipops 5–15 mg/kg max 400 mg, contraindicated if <10 kg
- Meperidine: 1–1.8 mg/kg IM/po q 3 hrs
- Morphine: 0.1 mg/kg IV/IM
- Cefazolin: 25–50 mg/kg IV/IM divided q 6–8 hrs
- Dicloxacillin: 12–25 mg/kg po divided qid

Disposition

ADMISSION CRITERIA

- Type III and IV fractures
- Orthopedic consultation
- Open surgical reduction required
- Open fractures

DISCHARGE CRITERIA

- Type I, II, V, and VI epiphyseal injuries
- Splint for comfort
- Orthopedic follow-up within 1 week
- Analgesics
- Ice packs
- Elevation of the affected limb

Miscellaneous

ICD9: N/A

CORE CONTENT CODE: 18.6.7.3

SUGGESTED READINGS

England S, Sundberg S. Management of common pediatric fractures. Pediatr Clin North Am 1996;43(5):991.

Olney B. Musculoskeletal injuries. In: Buntain W, ed. Management of pediatric trauma. Philadelphia: WB Saunders, 1995: 394–430.

Rang R. Children's fractures. Philadelphia: JB Lippincott, 1983.

Salter R, Harris W. Injuries involving the epiphyseal plate. J Bone Joint Surg 1963;45A:587.

Thomas M. Musculoskeletal injury. In: Eichelberger M, ed. Pediatric trauma: Prevention, acute care, rehabilitation. St. Louis: CV Mosby, 1992.

Authors: William Sabina; Daniel L. Savitt

Epistaxis

Clinical Presentation

SIGNS AND SYMPTOMS

- Bleeding from one or both nares
- Bleeding into the posterior pharynx
- Massive epistaxis
  - —Tachycardia
  - —Hypotension
  - —Hematemesis
  - —Hemoptysis

MECHANISM/DESCRIPTION

- Bimodal distribution
  - —2–10 years of age
  - —50–80 years of age
- Anterior epistaxis
  - —90% of all cases
  - —Kiesselbach's plexus
    - -Branches of the anterior and posterior ethmoidal arteries
  - —Often self-limited
- Posterior epistaxis
  - —10% of all cases
  - —Posterior branch of the sphenopalatine artery

ETIOLOGY

- Local
  - —Dry nasal mucosa
  - —Drug inhalation
  - —Foreign body
  - —Infection
    - -Rhinitis
    - -Sinusitis
  - —Inflammation
    - -Allergy
    - -Polyps
  - —Neoplasm
  - —Trauma
    - -Nose picking
    - -Facial fractures
- Systemic
  - —Arteriosclerosis
  - —Barotrauma
  - —Coagulopathy (familial)
    - -Hemophilia A or B
    - -Von Willebrand's disease
  - —Coagulopathy (acquired)
    - -Thrombocytopenia
    - -Liver disease
    - -Renal failure/uremia
  - —Drug induced
    - -Salicylates
    - -NSAIDs
    - -Heparin
    - -Coumadin
    - -Heavy metals
  - —Hereditary hemorrhagic telangiectasia (Osler-Weber-Rendu disease)
  - —Hypertension
- Idiopathic

Pre-Hospital

- Stable patients
- Sitting position
- Head down
- Nares pinched closed
- Patients in
  - —Intubation if airway compromise
  - —Intravenous access
  - —Crystalloid resuscitation if signs of hypovolemia

Diagnosis

ESSENTIAL WORKUP

- Assess if anterior or posterior epistaxis
- Assess for a coagulopathy if significant bleeding

LABORATORY

- Needed only if significant bleeding
  - —Type and crossmatch
  - —Hematocrit
  - —PT
  - —PTT
  - —BUN
  - —LFTs

IMAGING/SPECIAL TESTS

- Nasal speculum
  - —Local treatment with a vasoconstricting agent before visualization
  - —Use gloves and protective eyewear
  - —Use headlight with a narrow lightbeam
  - —Optimize visualization of septal mucosa
    - -Have patient blow nose if blood clots obstruct visualization
    - -Advance Frazier suction catheter to clear further bleeding

DIFFERENTIAL DIAGNOSIS

- Hemoptysis
- Hematemesis

Treatment

INITIAL STABILIZATION

- Intubate if airway compromise
  - —Often a difficult airway as oropharyngeal bleeding impairs visualization
- Volume resuscitation if significant bleeding
  - —IV access
  - —Crystalloid
  - —Blood products

ED TREATMENT

- Sedation
  - —Corrects hypertension
  - —Prevents worsening of bleeding
  - —Benzodiazepines
  - —Narcotics

Anterior Epistaxis

- Apply vasoactive and anesthetic agents
- Shape cotton balls into adequate pledgets
  - —Soak pledgets in a vasoactive solution
  - —Insert into both nares with bayonet forceps
  - —Have the patient lean forward with head down
  - —Pinch the nares closed just below the nasal bridge for 10 minutes
  - —Remove pledgets once bleeding has stopped
  - —Posterior epistaxis will often be refractory to vasoactive agents
- Attempt to visualize bleeding site
- Cauterize bleeding site with silver nitrate
  - —Roll silver nitrate stick over the bleeding site for no more than 5–10 seconds
  - —Cautery is impossible if the site is still bleeding significantly
  - —Avoid overzealous application of silver nitrate
    - -Permanent damage to cartilage
    - -Septal perforation
  - —Repeat several times if bleeding persists
- Electric cautery
  - —Little advantage over silver nitrate
  - —Indicated if silver nitrate cautery is unsuccessful
- Nasal packing if medicated pledgets do not arrest the bleeding
  - —Vaseline ribbon gauze (6 feet)
    - -Allow the free end to protrude from the nares
    - -Fold the ribbon upon itself from the inferior aspect of the canal superiorly
    - -The nostril is covered
    - -Both ends of the ribbon should protrude from the nose
  - —Commercially available pressed sponges (Merocel)
    - -Faster and easier than vaseline gauze
    - -Better tolerated by the patient
  - —Intranasal balloon catheter
    - -Single balloon model
    - -Apply water based lubricant to the catheter and balloon
    - -Inflate slowly with saline or sterile water
  - —Antibiotic ointment
    - -Apply to all packing materials before insertion
  - —Complications from anterior nasal packs
    - -Dislodgment
    - -Sinusitis
    - -Toxic shock syndrome
  - —Prophylaxis with systemic antibiotics
    - -Generally used to prevent sinusitis
    - -Cephalexin or amoxicillin/clavulanate
    - -Clindamycin or trimethoprim/sulfamethoxazole are good second-line drugs

Posterior Epistaxis

- Placement of commercially available packing devices (nasostat, epistat)
  - —Device with an anterior and posterior balloon
  - —Coat with antibiotic ointment before insertion
  - —Insert as deep as possible
  - —The posterior balloon should be partially filled (4–8 cc) and pulled forward until the balloon is wedged into the choanae
  - —Maintain gentle traction
  - —Inflate the posterior balloon until the soft palate begins to swell
  - —The anterior balloon is inflated after the posterior balloon
- Placement with a 14- or 16-French Foley catheter with a 5 ml balloon
  - —When the commercial device is not available
  - —The tip of the Foley should be cut off before insertion
  - —Slowly inflate with water until the patient feels discomfort
  - —Anchor the Foley with an umbilical clamp
  - —Pack the anterior canal with vaseline gauze
- Alternatively, tamponade with a gauze buttress
  - —Thread strings through the oral and nasal pharynx
  - —Pull a gauze buttress against the choanae
- More difficult and time consuming than commercial devices
- Prophylaxis with systemic antibiotics
  - —Cephalexin or amoxicillin/clavulanate
  - —Clindamycin or trimethoprim/sulfamethoxazole are good second line drugs
- Complications of posterior packing
  - —Sinusitis
  - —Aspiration
  - —Hypoventilation
  - —Bradycardia
  - —Cardiac arrhythmias
  - —Cerebrovascular accident
  - —Cardiac arrest

MEDICATIONS

- Vasoactive solutions
  - —4% cocaine
  - —1:1 mixture of 2% tetracaine and epinephrine (1:1000)
  - —1:1 mixture of oxymetazoline 0.05% (afrin) and lidocaine solution 4%
  - —Neosynephrine
- Cephalexin: 250 mg po q 6 hrs
- Amoxicillin/clavulanate potassium: 250 mg po q 8 hrs
- Clindamycin: 150 mg po q 6 hrs
- Trimethoprim: 160 mg/sulfamethoxazole 800 mg po q 12 hrs

Disposition

ADMISSION CRITERIA

- Posterior nasal packing
  - —Otolaryngology consult
  - —Hospital admission for observation

DISCHARGE CRITERIA

- Apply a lubricating ointment at home
- Increase home humidity
- Instruct patients not to pick at the nose
- Return if
  - —Recurrent bleeding not controlled with pressure
  - —Fever
  - —Nausea
  - —Vomiting
- With anterior nasal packing follow-up within 2 days for removal

Miscellaneous

ICD9: 784.7

CORE CONTENT CODE: 6.2.1, 6.2.2

SUGGESTED READINGS

Alvi A, Joyner-Triplett N. Acute epistaxis: How to spot the source and stop the flow. Postgrad Med 1996;99(5):83–96.

Pringle MB, Beasley P, Brightwell A. The use of Mecocel nasal packs in the treatment of epistaxis. J Laryngol Otol 1996;110(6):543–546.

Stair TO. Otolaryngologic disorders. In: Rosen P, et al., eds. Emergency medicine: Concepts and clinical practice. 3rd ed. St. Louis: CV Mosby, 1992:2460–2469.

Author: Randel Brown

Erysipelas

Clinical Presentation

SIGNS AND SYMPTOMS

- Most common site of involvement is the face, lower legs, and ears
- Skin has an intense "fiery" red color earning the nickname "St. Anthony's fire"
- The involved skin is an edematous, indurated, well-circumscribed plaque often with a sharp, clearly demarcated edge of induration
- Vesicles and bullae may be present in more serious infection
- Predilection for infants, children, and the elderly
- Systemic symptoms may include malaise, fever, chills, nausea, and vomiting
- Traumatic portal of entry on skin is not always apparent
- Rarely there may be an associated periorbital cellulitis or cavernous sinus involvement

MECHANISM/DESCRIPTION

- Group A β-hemolytic streptococci is the causative organism

PEDIATRIC CONSIDERATIONS

- *Hemophilus influenza* type b causes facial cellulitis in children that appears similar to erysipelas

Pre-Hospital

N/A

Diagnosis

ESSENTIAL WORKUP

- The diagnosis is clinical based on the characteristic skin findings
- Needle-aspirate wound cultures are seldom positive and not indicated

DIFFERENTIAL DIAGNOSIS

- Allergic inflammation
- Cellulitis
- Contact dermatitis
- Herpes zoster
- Impetigo
- Viral exanthem

Treatment

INITIAL STABILIZATION

- Patients with periorbital cellulitis or cavernous sinus thrombosis may be toxic and in need of intravenous fluid resuscitation or pressure support

ED TREATMENT

- Appropriate antibiotic therapy
  - —Patients with extensive involvement may benefit from a parenteral antibiotic dose in the ED
  - —Most patients can be discharged on oral therapy if nontoxic appearing, good compliance, and close follow-up can be assured
  - —Penicillin is the drug of choice when clearly the symptoms are consistent with erysipelas
  - —If there is difficulty in distinguishing from cellulitis, staphylococcal coverage should be added
- Facial cellulitis in children may be caused by *Hemophilus influenza* in patients that have not been vaccinated. Many will be bacteremic and require admission
  - —Cefuroxime or other appropriate. *Hemophilus influenza* coverage is important. *Hemophilus influenza* is less commonly an infectious etiology since the advent of the vaccine

MEDICATIONS

- Penicillin G: adult: 2 million IU every 4 hrs IV; peds: 25,000 IU/kg IV q 6 hrs
- Penicillin VK: adult: 500 mg po q 6 hrs; peds: 25–50 mg/kg/day divided q 6–8 hrs
- Dicloxacillin: adult: 250 mg po q 6 hrs; peds: 30mg/kg/day po divided q 6 hrs
- Cephalexin: adult: 500 mg po q 12 hrs; peds: 40mg/kg/day po divided q 8 hrs
- Cefuroxime: peds: 50–100 mg/kg/d divided q 8 hrs

Disposition

ADMISSION CRITERIA

- Patients with extensive involvement, fever, or toxic appearance will require admission
- Children more often require admission. Intravenous treatment, including coverage for *Hemophilus influenza,* should be initiated for patients that have not been immunized

DISCHARGE CRITERIA

- Minimal facial involvement
- Nontoxic appearing
- Not immunosuppressed
- Able to tolerate and comply with oral therapy
- Adequate follow-up

Miscellaneous

ICD9: 035

CORE CONTENT CODE: 3.2.1.3

SUGGESTED READINGS

Kahn RM, Goldstein EJ. Common bacterial skin infections. Postgrad Med 1993;93(6):175–182.

Ochs MW, Dolwick MF. Facial erysipelas: Report of a case and review of the literature. J Oral Maxillofac Surg 1991;49:1116–1120.

Author: James Larson

Erythema Infectiosum

Clinical Presentation

SIGNS AND SYMPTOMS

- Following the incubation period mild constitutional symptoms
  - —Low grade fever
  - —Headache
  - —During this time the child is contagious

Rash

- Begins 1 week after initial onset of symptoms
- Three stages
  - —First stage
    - -"Slapped cheek" appearance occurs in 75%
    - -Erythematous
    - -Warm
    - -Nontender
  - —Second stage
    - -Occurs 1–4 days following the facial rash
    - -Pink to dull red, lacy macular eruption
    - -Occurs on the extremities and trunk
    - -May be pruritic
    - -Usually spares the palms and soles
  - —Third stage
    - -Rash may recur secondary to cutaneous vasodilation especially during periods of stress, exercise, sun exposure, and bathing
    - -Resolves in 1–3 weeks but can recur over a period of months

Possible Complications

- Arthritis
  - —Common complication in adults
- Transient aplastic crisis in patients with hemolytic anemias
  - —Fever
  - —Pallor
  - —Weakness
  - —Lethargy
  - —Hepatosplenomegaly
  - —Evidence of heart failure

MECHANISM/DESCRIPTION

- Infectious exanthem also known as fifth disease
  - —Derived from the historical numbering of infectious exanthems
    1 Measles
    2 Scarlet fever
    3 Rubella
    4 Filatov-Dukes' disease (this was a variant of scarlet fever that is no longer recognized)
    5 Erythema infectiosum
    6 Roseola

ETIOLOGY

- Caused by human parvovirus B19
- Incubation period typically is 4–14 days
- Seasonal predilection for late winter and spring
- Spreads via respiratory transmission
- School aged children typically infected
- Adults infrequently affected

Pre-Hospital

N/A

Diagnosis

ESSENTIAL WORKUP

- Clinical diagnosis based on typical signs and symptoms

LABORATORY

- No workup necessary unless concerns for an aplastic crisis or arthritis are present
- CBC

IMAGING/SPECIAL TESTS

- IgM-antibody assay
  - —Diagnostic testing is only available at a few sites
  - —Confirms acute infection

DIFFERENTIAL DIAGNOSIS

- Scarlet fever
- Rubella
- Roseola
- Infectious mononucleosis
- Echovirus
- Coxsackie virus
- Drug eruptions

Treatment

INITIAL STABILIZATION

- ABCs for septic or ill-appearing patient

ED TREATMENT

- No specific antiviral treatment or vaccine is available
- Symptomatic treatment with fluids and acetaminophen
- Hospitalization and respiratory isolation for aplastic crisis

Expected Course

- Rash usually resolves in 1–3 weeks but can recur over a period of months; most children do very well
- Exposed pregnant women have an increased incidence of nonimmune hydrops fetalis
- Once the rash is present the patient is no longer contagious
  —May return to school or day care

Disposition

ADMISSION CRITERIA

- Aplastic crisis
- Significant arthritis
- Overall ill appearance

DISCHARGE CRITERIA

- Almost all patients
- Well-appearing with rash and no signs of aplastic crisis or arthritis

Miscellaneous

ICD9: 057.0

CORE CONTENT CODE: 13.12.4.1

SUGGESTED READINGS

Adams DM, Ware RE. Parvovirus B19: how much should you worry? Contemp Pediatr 1996;13(4):85–96.

Anderson MJ, Higgins PG, Davis LR, et al. Experimental parvoviral infection in humans. I. Infect Dis 1985;152:257–265.

Ussery X, Demmler G. Human parvovirus B19. Semin Pediatr Infect Dis 1996;7(2):89–96.

Author: Kathlene Bassett

Erythema Multiforme

Clinical Presentation

SIGNS AND SYMPTOMS

- *Prodrome:* Patients may experience minimal fever and malaise, or systemic symptoms may be completely absent
- *Rash:* The characteristic "target" lesions spread from the extremities toward the trunk and may be mildly pruritic (see description)

MECHANISM/DESCRIPTION

- Erythema Multiforme is sometimes divided into *Major* and *Minor* types
- *E. Multiforme Major* is part of a spectrum of disease that includes the more severe disorders *Toxic Epidermal Necrolysis* (TEN) and *Stevens Johnson Syndrome* (*SJS*), which are described separately
- *E. Multiforme Minor* is characterized by a benign, self-limited rash, which is generally not associated with acute, serious illness. It is simply referred to as *Erythema Multiforme.* It has these features
  —Symmetric dull red macules and papules, evolving into round, well-demarcated "target" lesions with central clearing
  —Distribution involves extremities, dorsal hands and feet, palms and soles, extensor surfaces, especially elbows and knees
  —"Multiforme" refers to the evolution of the rash through various morphologic stages at different times
  —Spreads from extremities toward trunk
  —May involve one mucosal surface (usually mouth)
  —Duration is usually 1–4 weeks, but may become chronic or recurrent
  —Usually affects children and young adults (>50% under age 20), and males are affected more often than females

ETIOLOGY

- Hypersensitivity reaction, probably due to a transient autoimmune defect
- Viral illness often precedes erythema multiforme
- Recurrent herpes simplex is the most common precipitant
- Mycoplasma infections and drug reactions (especially antibiotics, anticonvulsants, and analgesics) are common causes, but are more associated with TEN and SJS. Less common precipitants include other infections and malignancies
- Half of all cases are idiopathic

Pre-Hospital

- There are no relevant pre-hospital care issues, and the rash is not contagious

Diagnosis

ESSENTIAL WORKUP

- Complete history and physical exam, with special attention to the genitourinary system, recent or concomitant infectious symptoms, and medications taken

LABORATORY

- There are no specific laboratory tests needed
- History and physical examination dictate work-up for underlying illnesses

IMAGING/SPECIAL TESTS

- *Skin biopsy* reveals mononuclear cell infiltrate around upper dermal blood vessels, without leukocytoclastic vasculitis. Also, there is necrosis of epidermal keratinocytes

DIFFERENTIAL DIAGNOSIS

- Systemic lupus erythematosus
- Pityriasis rosea
- Secondary syphilis
- Tinea corporis
- Urticaria

Treatment

INITIAL STABILIZATION

- E. multiforme minor is generally a benign, self-limited illness that requires no specific initial stabilization because there are no significant complications

ED TREATMENT

- Attempt to identify, treat or remove any underlying or precipitating cause
- Treat the rash symptomatically with cool compresses

MEDICATIONS

- Diphenhydramine: 25–50 mg po 3–4 times/day; peds: 5 mg/kg/day div q 6 hrs
- If recurrent herpes infection is present
  —Acyclovir: adult: 400 mg po bid (chronic suppressive therapy); peds: 20 mg/kg/dose
- If mycoplasma infection is present
  —Erythromycin: 250 mg po 4 qid for 7–10 days; peds: 40 mg/kg/day div q 6 hrs

Disposition

ADMISSION CRITERIA

- None for uncomplicated cases

DISCHARGE CRITERIA

- E. multiforme is a benign disorder that does not require admission

Miscellaneous

ICD9: 695.1

CORE CONTENT CODE: 3.5.1

SUGGESTED READINGS

Brady WJ, DeBehnke D, Crosby DL. Dermatological emergencies. Am J Emerg Med 1994;12(2):217–237.

Fabbri P, Panconesi E. Erythema multiforme ("minus" and "maius") and drug intake. Clin Dermatol 1993;11(4):479–489.

Stampien TM, Schwartz RA. Erythema multiforme. Am Family Phys 1992;46(4):1171–1176

Weston WL. What is erythema multiforme? Pediatr Ann 1996;25(2):106–109.

Authors: Gregory W. Hendey; Thomas A. Utecht

Erythema Nodosum

Clinical Presentation

SIGNS AND SYMPTOMS

- Acute onset of tender subcutaneous erythematous nodules usually symmetrically distributed on anterior portions of legs
- Lesions can occasionally occur on fingers, hands, arms, calves, and thighs
- In bedridden patients, dependent areas may be involved
- Patients may have fever, malaise, leukocytosis, arthralgias, arthritis, and unilateral or bilateral hilar adenopathy with any form of the disease

MECHANISM/DESCRIPTION

- Erythema nodosum (EN) is characterized by multiple nonulcerative tender nodules on the extensor surface of the lower extremities typically in young adults
  —3:1 female to male predilection
- Nodules are round with poorly demarcated edges and vary in size from 1–10 cm
- Skin lesions are initially red, but become progressively "ecchymotic appearing" as they resolve over a 2–6-week period
- Lesions do not typically ulcerate
- Lesions are caused by inflammation of the septa between subcutaneous fat nodules (septal panniculitis)
- Natural history of idiopathic form or with treatment of underlying disease is spontaneous regression of lesions within 3–6 weeks
- Major disease variants include erythema nodosum migrans (usually mild unilateral disease with little or no systemic symptoms) and chronic erythema nodosum (lesions spread via extension and while associated systemic symptoms occur as with traditional acute form they tend to be milder)

ETIOLOGY

- EN is a common dermatologic disease and is generally considered an immune-mediated response
- EN is often a marker for systemic disease; specific etiologies include
  —Drug reactions (oral contraceptives, sulfonamides, penicillins)
  —Systemic infections including streptococcal, mycobacterium tuberculosis, atypical mycobacteria, and coccidioidomycosis
  —Sarcoidosis (Lofgren's syndrome)
  —Inflammatory bowel disease, particularly ulcerative colitis
  —Miscellaneous infectious agents include viral (hepatitis), spirochetal (syphilis), chlamydial (psittacosis), and rickettsial organisms, as well as enteric pathogens (Campylobacter, yersinia, and salmonella) and parasites (amebiasis and giardiasis)
  —Malignancies such as lymphoma and leukemia
  —HIV infection
  —Leprosy (erythema nodosum leprosum)
  —Rarely can be caused by vaccines for hepatitis and tuberculosis (BCG)
  —Idiopathic (30–50%)
- Incidence of the different etiologies vary according to the time of year as well as the geographic location and ethnicity of the population being studied
- Typically erythema nodosum begins two to three weeks after the onset of pharyngitis in children

Pre-Hospital

N/A

Diagnosis

ESSENTIAL WORKUP

- Careful history and physical examination directed at detecting precipitating etiology

LABORATORY

- CBC, ESR, appropriate chemistry tests. Tuberculosis and coccidioidomycosis skin tests may be useful initial screening tests for lymphoma, leukemia, TB, and cocci

IMAGING/SPECIAL TEST

- Chest radiograph can serve as initial screen for sarcoidosis
- Definitive diagnosis made by deep elliptical biopsy and histopathologic evaluation (punch biopsy inadequate as subcutaneous fat sample must be obtained)

DIFFERENTIAL DIAGNOSIS

- Erythema nodosum migrans and chronic erythema nodosum
- Any type of panniculitis can resemble erythema nodosum
- Differences can be determined histopathologically
- Other disorders include periarteritis nodosum, migratory thrombophlebitis, superficial varicose thrombophlebitis, Scleroderma, systemic lupus erythematosus, α_1-antitrypsin deficiency, Beçhet's syndrome, lipodystrophies, leukemic infiltration of fat, and panniculitis associated with steroid use, cold, and infection

PEDIATRIC CONSIDERATIONS

- In children, streptococcal pharyngitis is the most likely etiology

Treatment

INITIAL STABILIZATION

- ABCs, IV, oxygen, monitoring as appropriate

ED TREATMENT

- Treatment should be directed at the underlying disease
- Typically only supportive therapies, such as analgesics, are necessary for dermatologic lesions
- Treatment of the underlying pathology usually assures disappearance of the lesions within 1–2 months
- Specific therapies such as potassium iodide and systemic corticosteroids are used only when the underlying process is known
- Systemic corticosteroids are contraindicated in presence of certain underlying infections such as tuberculosis or coccidioidomycosis which may disseminate with their use

MEDICATIONS

- Aspirin: 650 mg po q 4–6 hrs PRN; peds: contraindicated
- Nonsteroidal anti-inflammatory agents
  —Ibuprofen: 300–800 mg po q 8 hrs; peds: 5–10 mg/kg po q 6 hrs
  —Indomethacin: 25–50 mg po q 8 hrs
- Potassium iodide/SSKI (used for resistant disease; contraindicated in hyperthyroidism): 900 mg po qd for 3–4 weeks
- Systemic corticosteroids

Disposition

ADMISSION CRITERIA

- Patient admission should be dictated by the severity of symptoms and the etiologic agent

DISCHARGE CRITERIA

- Nontoxic patients, able to take oral fluids without difficulty
- Scheduled follow-up should be arranged

Miscellaneous

ICD9: 695.2

CORE CONTENT CODE: 3.5.2

SUGGESTED READINGS

Fegueux S, Maslo C, de Truncuis P, et al. Erythema nodosum in HIV-infected patients. J Am Acad Dermatol 1991;25(1):113.

Fox MD, Schwartz RA. Erythema nodosum. Am Fam Physician 1992; 46(3): 818–822.

Myerson MS. Erythema nodosum leprosum. Int J Dermatol 1996;35(6):389–392.

Jorizzo JL. Blood vessel-based inflammatory disorders. In: Moschella SL, Hurley HJ, eds. Dermatology. Philadelphia: WB Saunders, 1992:584–586.

Authors: Theresa M. Schwab; Herbert G. Bivins

Esophageal Trauma

Clinical Presentation

SIGNS AND SYMPTOMS

Common to Most

- Dysphagia—difficulty swallowing (gagging, coughing, aspiration risk (liquids > solids)), food "sticks" or "won't go down"
- Odynophagia—painful swallowing, cervical pain, or retrosternal ache
  —May radiate or worsen with swallowing
- Chest pain—anginalike, severe and unrelenting, may radiate to back or neck; colicky
- Hoarseness may be associated

Tears or Perforations

- Bleeding—laceration; Mallory-Weiss tear
- Hematemesis
- Subcutaneous air
- Shock
- Septicemia
- Peritonitis—perforation or Boerhaave's syndrome
- Associated neck, chest, or abdominal injury with trauma (most commonly the trachea)

Ingestions

- Drooling or excessive salivation—corrosive ingestions
- Choking, gagging, vomiting, stridor, wheezing, inability of liquids to pass distally—swallowed foreign bodies or food impactions

ETIOLOGY

External Forces or Agents (30%)

- Penetrating—missile wounds, stab wounds
- Blunt—motor vehicle crash
- Caustic ingestions—acids pH <2, alkalis pH >12
- Swallowed foreign bodies—coins, bones, buttons, marbles, pins, meat bolus, button batteries, cocaine
- Food bolus impaction, tortilla chips, meat

Iatrogenic (55%)

- Perforations secondary to instrumentation

Increased Intrathoracic Pressure (15%)

- Mallory-Weiss
- Boerhaave's Syndrome

MECHANISM/DESCRIPTION

Partial Tears

- Swallowed foreign bodies, sharp objects, or food impactions
  —Common sites of entrapment include upper esophageal sphincter (cricopharyngeus muscle), crossover of aortic arch, and lower esophageal sphincter
- Mallory-Weiss—forceful vomiting; sudden, violent, usually repeated increase in intra-abdominal pressure against a weakened esophageal wall
  —Valsalva or striking the steering wheel or compression during external heart massage can also cause Mallory-Weiss tear

Full-Thickness Tears

- Caustic ingestions
  —Alkali: liquefaction necrosis causing burns, airway edema or compromise, perforation, chronic stricture, and cancer
  —Acid: coagulation necrosis, thermal injury, and dehydration causing perforation, ulceration, and infection
- Injection of sclerosing agents in patients with esophageal varices
- Perforation: penetrating trauma, foreign bodies, instrumentation, can lead to mediastinitis
- Boerhaave's syndrome—full-thickness rupture of distal esophagus, classically associated with ETOH or large meals with violent, repeated vomiting

PEDIATRIC CONSIDERATIONS

- 80% of swallowed foreign bodies occur in children (usually 18–48 months old); location of entrapment is usually the cricopharyngeus muscle

Pre-Hospital

CAUTIONS

- Chest pain patients should be presumed to be cardiac in origin until proven otherwise
- Swallowed foreign bodies may require frequent suctioning
- IV crystalloid if patient is hypotensive or has been vomiting, or if there is any hematemesis

Diagnosis

ESSENTIAL WORKUP

- High level of suspicion and early diagnosis are the keys
  —Mortality <5% if perforation is repaired within 24 hours; if delayed, mortality is 75%
- History of ingestion (type, time, quantity of ingestion)
- Chest x-ray for foreign body or perforation (pneumomediastinum, pneumothorax, or pleural effusion)

LABORATORY

- CBC or hemoglobin testing in cases of upper GI bleeding from esophageal tears as an initial baseline test. Bleeding screen.
- Electrolytes in cases of protracted vomiting or prolonged retained foreign body

IMAGING/SPECIAL TESTS

- Fiberoptic nasopharyngoscopy for foreign bodies
- Esophagram for foreign bodies or water-soluble contrast studies when perforation or thermal injury is suspected
  —May need to be performed in left or right lateral decubitus positions
  —Esophagoscopy only done if perforation is not confirmed with contrast studies or if the patient is unconscious
  —Flexible endoscopy (6–18 hours postingestion)

DIFFERENTIAL DIAGNOSIS

Pulmonary

- Tracheal injury
- Pneumothorax

Cardiovascular

- Myocardial infarction
- Aortic dissection

Other Esophageal Emergencies

- Peptic stricture
- Esophageal neoplasms
- Schatzki's Ring
- Diverticula
- Achalasia
- Diffuse esophageal spasm
- Nutcracker esophagus
- GERD
- Esophagitis

Treatment

INITIAL STABILIZATION

- ABCs, intravenous access, appropriate monitoring
- Early intubation for penetrating neck and chest wounds
- Frequent suction for copious secretions

ED TREATMENT

- Swallowed foreign bodies or food impactions—80% pass, 20% need endoscopy, 1% need surgery
  —Glucagon may be used (see medications)
  —GI consultation and endoscopic extraction
- Ingestions
  —Immediate decontamination—water or milk
  —Emesis/lavage *contraindicated*
  —Charcoal may interfere with endoscopy
  —Consult GI specialist
- Partial thickness tears usually heal spontaneously
- Mallory-Weiss tears usually self-limited venous or arterial bleeding
- Perforation requires surgical consult for thoracotomy and primary repair

MEDICATIONS

- Foreign bodies or food impactions
  —Glucagon: 1–2 mg IV adults or 0.02–0.03 mg/kg in children, may repeat once in 10–20 min
  —Carbonated beverages
- Ingestions: antibiotics if perforated (see below)
- Extensive alkali burn
  —Solumedrol: adults: 125 mg IV; peds: 1–2 mg/kg IV
- Perforation: IV antibiotics
  —Cefoxitin: adults: 1 g IV; peds: 80–160 mg/kg/day in 4–6 divided doses
  —Clindamycin: adults: 300–600 mg IV; peds: 8–12 mg/kg/day in 3–4 divided doses

PEDIATRIC CONSIDERATIONS

- Certain swallowed foreign bodies require GI consultation and possible endoscopic removal
  —Sharp objects—fish bones, straight pins, razor blades
  —Caustic objects—button batteries
- Other objects may pass on their own if below the lower esophageal sphincter and require follow-up only
  —Coins, buttons, marbles, etc.
  —Open safety pins may pass spontaneously if blunt end is forward; consult Pediatric GI specialist

Disposition

ADMISSION CRITERIA

- Caustic ingestion
- Airway compromise
- Penetrating neck or chest trauma
- Evidence of sepsis, mediastinitis, or esophageal perforation
- Significant bleeding
- Inability to tolerate oral fluids

DISCHARGE CRITERIA

- Self-limited bleeding from Mallory-Weiss tear
- Esophageal foreign body or food impaction that has passed distal to the lower esophageal sphincter (objects that are not sharp or caustic as above)

Miscellaneous

ESOPHAGUS INJURY SCALE

Grade	
I	Contusion/hematoma; partial thickness laceration
II	Laceration <50% circumference
III	Laceration >50% circumference
IV	Segmental loss or devascularization <2 cm
V	Segmental loss or devascularization >2 cm

ICD9: 862.22; 862.32

CORE CONTENT CODE: 1.1; 18.4.11.4

SUGGESTED READINGS

Javors B, Panzer D, Goldman I. Acute thermal injury of the esophagus. Dysphagia 1996;11(1):72–74.

Lovejoy F, Woolf A. Corrosive ingestions. Pediatr Rev 1995;16(12):473–474.

Polsky S, Kerstein M. Pharyngo-esophageal perforation due to blunt trauma. Am Surg 1995;61(11):994–996.

Stack L, Munter D., Foreign bodies in the gastrointestinal tract. Emerg Med Clin North Am 1996;14(3):493–521.

Swann L, Munter D. Esophageal emergencies. Emerg Med Clin North Am 1996;14(3):557–570.

Weiman D, et al. Combined tracheal and esophageal trauma from gunshot wounds. South Med J 1996;89(2):208–211.

Authors: James Smith; Susan Dufel

Ethylene Glycol, Poisoning

Clinical Presentation

SIGNS AND SYMPTOMS

Cardiovascular

- Tachycardia/bradycardia/other dysrhythmias
- Hypertension/hypotension

Central Nervous System

- Inebriation/irritability
- Ataxia
- Obtundation
- Coma
- Cerebral edema
- Convulsions

Gastrointestinal

- Nausea/vomiting
- Abdominal pain
- Hematemesis

Pulmonary

- Hyperventilation/tachypnea
- Pulmonary edema

Renal

- Acute renal failure
- Costal-vertebral angle tenderness
- Crystalluria

MECHANISM/DESCRIPTION

- Peak levels in 1–4 hours
- Half-life = 2.5–4.5 hours
- <20% excreted unmetabolized by the kidneys
- *Three stages* (may be overlap)
  —First stage
    -1–12 hours postingestion
    -CNS depression
    -GI symptoms
    -Worsening acidosis
    -Coma, convulsions, cerebral edema
    -Tetany and myoclonus secondary to hypocalcemia
  —Second stage
    -12–24 hours postingestion
    -Cardiopulmonary symptoms
    -Most deaths occur
  —Third stage
    -24–72 hours postingestion
    -Oliguria, flank pain, acute renal failure
    -Bone marrow suppression and pancytopenia

Pathophysiology

- Metabolized by hepatic alcohol dehydrogenase and aldehyde dehydrogenase ultimately to oxalic acid
  —Results in aldehyde and acid metabolites
    -Directly toxic to the CNS, lungs, and kidney
  —Metabolites inhibit metabolic pathways, including oxidative phosphorylation

ETIOLOGY

- Ethylene glycol-containing products
  —Antifreeze
  —Solvents
- Minimum reported lethal dose = 30 ml of 100% ethylene glycol

Pre-Hospital

N/A

Diagnosis

ESSENTIAL WORKUP

- History of all substances ingested
- Drawn *simultaneously*
  —ABG
  —Serum ethylene glycol, methanol, and ethanol levels
  —Electrolytes, BUN/Cr, glucose
  —Measured serum osmolality (by freezing point depression)
  —Serum calcium, phosphorus, magnesium

LABORATORY

- Determine the anion gap
  —Anion gap = $(Na^+) - (Cl^- + HCO_3^-)$
  —Normal anion gap = 8–12
- Determine osmol gap
  —Osmol gap = measured osmolality − calculated osmolarity
    -Calculated osmolarity = $2(Na^+)$ + glucose/18 + BUN/2.8 + ethanol (in mg/dl)/4.6
  —Calculated to screen for ethylene glycol ingestion because toxic alcohol levels are not commonly available in a timely manner from most clinical laboratories
  —Most useful early in the course of ethylene glycol poisoning or with concurrent ethanol ingestion
  —With concurrent ethanol ingestion, osmol gap tends to be larger and acidosis tends to be less severe because relatively less ethylene glycol has been converted to acid-producing metabolites
  —Increased osmol gap: >10
  —Normal osmol gap does not rule out ethylene glycol ingestion
- Ethylene glycol level
- Ethanol level
  —Measured to determine the amount of ethanol bolus necessary to attain a therapeutic level
- Urinalysis
  —Envelope-shaped oxalate crystals—an insensitive but specific finding
  —Ketones may be due to isopropyl alcohol ingestion, starvation, or DKA
- Acetaminophen level with all suicidal ingestions

IMAGING/SPECIAL TESTS

- Wood's lamp inspection of urine or gastric contents
  —Detects the presence of fluorescein, a common antifreeze additive
  —Insensitive but specific marker of antifreeze ingestion

DIFFERENTIAL DIAGNOSIS

- Increased osmol gap: *ME DIE A*
  - —*M*ethanol
  - —*E*thanol
  - —*D*iuretics (mannitol, glycerin, sorbitol)
  - —*I*sopropyl alcohol
  - —*E*thylene glycol
  - —*A*cetone, ammonia
- Elevated anion gap metabolic acidosis: *ACAT MUDPILES*
  - —*A*lcoholic ketoacidosis
  - —*C*yanide, CO, H_2S, others
  - —*A*SA, other salicylates
  - —*T*oluene
  - —*M*ethanol, metformin
  - —*U*remia
  - —*D*iabetic ketoacidosis
  - —*P*araldehyde, phenformin
  - —*I*ron, INH
  - —*L*actic acidosis from other causes
  - —*E*thylene glycol
  - —*S*tarvation ketosis

Treatment

INITIAL STABILIZATION

- ABCs
- Supplemental oxygen, cardiac monitor, secured IV with 0.9%NS
- D50W (or Accucheck), naloxone, and thiamine for altered mental status

ED TREATMENT

Prevent Further Ethylene Glycol Absorption

- Gastric lavage
  - —If <1 hour since ingestion, or if the patient's clinical condition mandates, endotracheal intubation
- Ipecac contraindicated
- Initial dose of activated charcoal for potential co-ingestants
  - —Activated charcoal poorly adsorbs ethylene glycol

Prevent Ethylene Glycol Conversion to Toxic Metabolites

- Ethanol therapy
  - —Initiate before the ethylene glycol level returns if a potentially toxic ingestion suspected
  - —Ethanol—greater affinity than ethylene glycol for alcohol dehydrogenase
    - -Slows conversion to toxic metabolites
  - —Indications
    - -History of accidental ethylene glycol ingestion of greater than a sip or intentional ethylene glycol ingestion
    - -Altered mental status associated with an unexplained osmol gap or elevated anion gap metabolic acidosis
  - —Goal: serum ethanol level of 100–150 mg/dl
  - —Continue ethanol therapy until the ethylene glycol level is zero
- 4-Methylpyrazole (4-MP, Antizol)
  - —Competitive inhibitor of alcohol dehydrogenase
  - —Significantly more expensive than ethanol therapy
  - —Advantages over ethanol
    - -No need for continuous infusion
    - -No inebriation/CNS depression

Enhance Elimination

- Hemodialysis
  - —Decreases the elimination half-life of ethylene glycol and removes toxic metabolites
  - —Indications
    - -Severe acidosis unresponsive to bicarbonate therapy
    - -Persistent electrolyte or fluid disturbance
    - -Renal insufficiency
    - -Pulmonary edema
    - -Cerebral edema
    - -Serum ethylene glycol level >25–50 mg/dl
  - —Continue hemodialysis until ethylene glycol level approaches zero
- Administer thiamine and pyridoxine
  - —Act as cofactors in the degradation of glyoxylic acid into metabolites less toxic than oxalate

Correct Secondary Disorders

- Ensure adequate urine output via IV fluids
- Sodium bicarbonate therapy for acidemia with pH <7.1
- Monitor/replace calcium
  - —Deposition of calcium into tissues can result in hypocalcemia

MEDICATIONS

- Activated charcoal: 1 g/kg po
- Dextrose: D50W 1 amp (50 ml or 25 g) (peds: D25W 2–4 ml/kg) IV
- Ethanol
  - —Oral: 40% ethanol solution (80 proof liquor) via NGT
    - -Loading dose: 2.5 ml/kg
    - -Maintenance dosing
      - *Nonalcoholic patient: 0.3 ml/kg/hr
      - *Alcoholic patient: 0.5 ml/kg/hr
      - *During hemodialysis: 0.75–1 ml/kg/hr
  - —IV: 10% ethanol in D5W
    - -Loading dose: 10 ml/kg over 30–60 min
    - -Maintenance infusion rates
      - *Nonalcoholic patient: 1–1.2 ml/kg/hr
      - *Alcoholic patient: 1.5–2 ml/kg/hr
      - *During hemodialysis: 3–4 ml/kg/hr
- 4-Methylpyrazole
  - —Loading dose: 15 mg/kg slow infusion over 30 min
  - —Maintenance dosing: 10 mg/kg q 12 h for 4 doses, then 15 mg/kg q 12 hrs until ethylen glycol levels reduced below 20 mg/dl
  - —Increase dosing during dialysis
- Naloxone: 2 mg (peds: 0.1 mg/kg) IV or IM initial dose
- Pyridoxine: 50 mg q 6 hrs for 2 days
- Sodium bicarbonate: 1–2 mEq/kg IV
- Thiamine: 100 mg (peds: 50 mg) IV or IM q 6 hrs for 2 days

PEDIATRIC CONSIDERATIONS

- Measure fingerstick glucose hourly to monitor for ethanol-induced hypoglycemia

Disposition

ADMISSION CRITERIA

- All patients with significant ethylene glycol ingestion even if initially asymptomatic
- ICU admission for seriously ill patients
- Transfer to another facility if hemodialysis is indicated but not readily available

DISCHARGE CRITERIA

- Asymptomatic patient with isolated ethylene glycol ingestion if the serum ethylene glycol level is undetectable

Miscellaneous

ICD9: 982.8

CORE CONTENT CODE: 17.2.2.2

SUGGESTED READINGS

Davis D, Bramwell KJ, Hamilton RS, Williams SR. Ethylene glycol poisoning: Case report of a record-high level and a review. J Emerg Med 1997;15(5):653–667.

Jacobsen D, McMartin KE. Antidotes for methanol and ethylene glycol poisonings. J Toxicol Clin Toxicol 1997;35(2):127–143.

Winchester JF. Methanol, isopropyl alcohol, ethylene glycol, cellosolves, acetone, and oxalate. In: Haddad LM, Shannon MW, Winchester JF, eds. Clinical management of poisoning and drug overdose. Philadelphia: WB Saunders, 1998:491–504.

Authors: Saul Melman; Jeffrey Schlab; Theodore Toerne

External Ear Chondritis/Abscess

Clinical Presentation

SIGNS AND SYMPTOMS

- Initially a dull pain that increases in severity
- Pinna
  - —Painful
  - —Exquisite tenderness
  - —Erythematous
  - —Warmth
  - —Loss of contours caused by edema often with sparing of the lobule
- Increase of the auriculocephalic angle
- Fluctuant areas develop with eventual breakdown and suppuration
- Entire ear involvement if untreated
  - —Disfigurement can occur
- Fever
- Chills

MECHANISM/DESCRIPTION

- Inflammation and infection of the pinna
- Cartilage of the external ear is easily damaged due to
  - —Lack of overlying subcutaneous tissue
  - —Relative avascularity
  - —Exposed position
- Chondritis
  - —Most commonly a secondary complication of otic trauma and burns
  - —Onset often insidious and may be delayed until apparent healing has occurred

ETIOLOGY

- Common causes of chondritis include
  - —Chemical or thermal burns
  - —Frostbite
  - —Hematoma formation
  - —Mastoid surgery
  - —Human bites
  - —Deep abrasions
  - —External otitis
  - —High piercing of the ear lobe
- Bacteria involved
  - —*P. aeruginosa*
  - —Staphylococcus
  - —Proteus

Pre-Hospital

N/A

Diagnosis

ESSENTIAL WORKUP

- Clinical diagnosis
  - —Typical physical findings in combination with above causes

LABORATORY

- CBC for systemic symptoms
- Blood culture if systemic signs of infection

Treatment

ED TREATMENT

Antibiotics

- Oral antibiotics for minor cases of early ear lobe inflammation
  - —Ciprofloxacin preferred (>18 years old)
  - —First-generation cephalosporin or dicloxacillin
- IV antibiotics for severe infection
- Apply topical antibiotics when break in skin barrier

ENT Consult

- For chondritis, abscess, and necrosis of the involved cartilage
- Early surgical drainage for chondritis
- Aggressive early management may prevent gross ear deformity

General Postinjury Preventive Measures

- Prevention of chondritis is of the utmost importance
  - —Difficult management and disfiguring potential
- Avoid pressure to the injured ear
- Minimize active débridement of eschars and crusts
- Gentle washing twice daily with antibacterial soap and water followed by complete drying and application of topical antibiotics
- Keep hair away from the ear

Complications

- Disfiguration of the pinna
  - —Occurs without proper treatment
  - —Ranging from being shriveled, cauliflower-like ear to complete loss of the external ear and possible stenosis of the auditory meatus

MEDICATIONS

- Ciprofloxacin: 500 mg po tid (adult)
- Cephalexin: 500 mg (peds: 50 mg/kg/24 hrs) po qid
- Dicloxacillin: 500 mg (peds: 25 mg/kg/24 hrs) po qid

Disposition

ADMISSION CRITERIA

- Parenteral antibiotics and early surgical drainage for patients with chondritis
- Edema, erythema, and significant ear tenderness
- Toxic patient with fever and chills
- Immunocompromised patient
- Unreliable patient or caretaker

DISCHARGE CRITERIA

- Stable patient without systemic signs with close ENT followup

Miscellaneous

ICD9: 733.99

CORE CONTENT CODE: 6.1.1

SUGGESTED READINGS

Bentrem DJ, Bill TJ, Himel HN, et al. Chrondritis of the ear: a late sequela of deep partial thickness burns of the face. J Emerg Med 1996;14:469–471.

Staley R, Fitzgibbon JJ, Anderson C. Auricular infections caused by high ear piercing in adolescents. Pediatrics 1997;99:610–611.

Author: Assaad J. Sayah

Extremity Trauma, Penetrating

Clinical Presentation

SIGNS AND SYMPTOMS

- Entry and exit wound (if present), lacerations
- High muzzle-velocity gunshot wounds produce a shock wave that results in significant tissue injury
- Vascular injury
  - —Arterial injury is indicated by decreased distal pulse, distal ischemic changes, expanding hematoma, bruit, or thrill over the injury
  - —The presence of a pulse does not exclude vascular injury
- Neurological injury
  - —Paresthesias, decreased motor function or sensation distal to the injury
- Musculoskeletal injury
  - —Visible deformity
  - —Ligamentous laxity in joints adjacent to the injury suggests
  - —Tendon injury
  - —An effusion in an adjacent joint indicates fracture or ligamentous injury
- Compartment syndrome
  - —Suggested by severe and constant pain over the involved compartment
  - —Pain on active and passive extension or flexion of the distal extremity
  - —Weakness, pain on palpation of the compartment, and hypesthesia of the nerves in the compartment
  - —Pulselessness is a late finding

Pre-Hospital

CAUTIONS

- Control hemorrhage with direct pressure
  - —Tourniquet, blown-up blood pressure cuff may be necessary
- Elevate extremity
- Evaluate neurovascular status

Diagnosis

ESSENTIAL WORKUP

History

- Mechanism of injury (stab, puncture, gunshot, laceration, bite, high-pressure injection injury)
- Age of wound
- Circumstances of wounding (assault, self-inflicted wound, domestic abuse)
- Comorbid conditions (immunosuppression, diabetes, valvular heart disease, asplenia, peripheral vascular disease)

Physical Examination

- Note location, length, depth and shape of the primary wound and of the exit wound, if present
- Vascular injury
  - —Compare distal pulses by palpation and with Doppler
  - —Ankle-Brachial Index (ABI): A systolic pressure difference of greater than 10 mm Hg suggests vascular injury
  - —Expanding hematoma, bruit, or thrill over the injury also indicates vascular injury
- Neurological injury
  - —Assess distal motor function and sensory function (two-point discrimination, light touch, proprioception)
- Musculoskeletal injury
  - —Note associated crush, tendon, or ligamentous injury and bony deformity
  - —Examine adjacent joints for range of motion
  - —Assess for compartment syndrome
- Explore the wound for *foreign body*

LABORATORY

- Culture of fresh wounds is not indicated
- Wounds with signs of infection may be cultured to guide antibiotic choice

IMAGING/SPECIAL TESTS

- X-ray to evaluate for radiopaque foreign body or underlying fracture
- Radiolucent foreign bodies may be located by fluoroscopy, ultrasound, or CT
- Arteriogram is indicated when vascular injury is suspected, and if emergent vascular surgery is not required

Treatment

INITIAL STABILIZATION

- ABCs of trauma care
- Expose the wound completely and remove constricting clothing or jewelry
- Control hemorrhage with direct pressure
- Blind clamping within the wound is not recommended

ED TREATMENT

- Pain control
- Complete neurological assessment prior to local anesthesia
- Prolonged soaking of wounds, particularly with cytotoxic agents, is *not* recommended
- Remove any visible debris and débride devitalized tissue
- Most important is copious high pressure irrigation with saline
- Tetanus prophylaxis
- Stab wounds and gun shot wounds should receive a single dose of cefazolin in the ED
- Immobilize the extremity if there is suspicion of significant vascular injury, tendon injury, fracture, or joint violation
- Loss of pulse or distal ischemia requires emergent surgery
  - —Do not delay surgical management for arteriogram
- Lacerations may be closed if they have been adequately cleaned, have minimal tissue loss, and are seen within 6–8 hours of injury. Clean face and scalp wounds may generally be closed for up to 24 hours after injury
  - —Delayed primary closure is an alternative for older or contaminated wounds

SPECIAL CONSIDERATIONS

- Plantar puncture wounds
  - —Examine the wound carefully under bright light, remove any foreign material, and clean the wound carefully. Coring the wound is controversial and should be reserved for removal of devitalized tissue or imbedded debris
  - —Probing or high pressure irrigation of a puncture wound will only force particulate matter further into the wound
  - —Prophylactic antibiotics are not recommended (unless the patient is diabetic or immunocompromised)

MEDICATIONS

- Tetanus prophylaxis: TD 0.5 cc IM
- Wounds more than 12 hours old, especially of the hands and lower extremities, crush wounds with devitalized tissue, contaminated wounds
  - —Cefazolin: adults: 1 g IV/IM; peds: 20–40 mg/kg IM/IV single-dose in the ED
  - —Cephalexin: adults: 500 mg po bid; peds: 25–50 mg/kg/day divided bid for 7 days *or*
  - —Amoxicillin clavulanate: adults: 500/125 po tid; peds: 20 mg/kg/day divided tid for 7 days
  - —Erythromycin: adults: 500 mg po qid; peds: 40 mg/kg/day divided q 6 hrs for 7 days
- Contaminated wounds in patients with preexisting valvular heart disease
  - —Cefazolin: 1 g IM/IV then cephalexin 500 mg po bid for 7 days
  - —If penicillin allergic
    - -EES: 800 mg po, then 400 mg po q 6 hrs for 7 days *or*
    - -Clindamycin: 300 mg po, then 150 mg po q 6 hrs for 7 days

Disposition

ADMISSION CRITERIA

- Emergent surgical consultation and admission is required for any penetrating wounds with potential for vascular compromise, with associated compartment syndrome, and with joint penetration
- High muzzle-velocity penetrating gunshot wounds should be admitted
- Diabetic or immunocompromised patients with contaminated wounds should be admitted

DISCHARGE CRITERIA

- Penetrating extremity injuries not requiring surgical intervention may be discharged after appropriate wound care with instructions to elevate the extremity, keep the wound clean, and to return for recheck in 24–48 hours or for any signs of infection

Miscellaneous

ICD9: 959.8

CORE CONTENT CODE: 18.3.2, 18.4.12, 18.4.13

SUGGESTED READINGS

American College of Emergency Physicians. Clinical policy for the initial approach to patients presenting with penetrating extremity trauma. Ann Emerg Med 1994;23:1147–1156.

Nassoura ZE, Ivatury RR, Simon RJ, et al. A reassessment of Doppler pressure indices in the detection of arterial lesions in proximity penetrating injuries of extremities: A prospective study. Am J Emerg Med 1996;14:151–156.

Talan DA. Infectious disease issues in the emergency department. Clin Infect Dis 1996;23:1–14.

Author: Deborah Y. Sanders

Failure to Thrive

Clinical Presentation

SIGNS AND SYMPTOMS

- Child's failure to achieve or maintain a growth rate appropriate for his or her age
  - —Any child growing below the 3rd or 5th percentile
  - —Child whose growth has fallen across two major growth percentiles lines (e.g., from the 75th to the 25th percentiles) in a short time should be evaluated for causes of failure to thrive
- Calorie deprivation initially results in weight loss, followed by impaired linear growth, and a decrease in the enlargement of head circumference
- Wasted thin extremities with loose skin hanging from buttocks
- Temporal wasting
- Thin, sparse hair or alopecia
- Edema

MECHANISM/DESCRIPTION

- Lack of appropriate nourishment
- Poor gastrointestinal function
- Acute or chronic disease
- Psychosocial issues
  - —In the United States, psychosocial causes predominate and may complicate organic causes up to 50% of the time

ETIOLOGY

- Also referred to as "growth deficiency"
- Many causes of growth deficiency, both organic and inorganic

Pre-Hospital

N/A

Diagnosis

ESSENTIAL WORKUP

- Thorough history and physical
  - —Birth history, drug exposures, recent illness, parental development, and family history of inheritable diseases
  - —Examine growth records and gather current height, weight, and head circumference measurements
  - —Evaluate feeding patterns and levels of motor, language, and behavioral development
  - —Observe family interactions within the emergency department
  - —Perform a careful physical exam looking for clues to congenital ailments
  - —Look for signs of poor hygiene or inappropriate behaviors between parent and child may suggest neglect

LABORATORY

- Urinalysis and culture for renal disease and infection
- Electrolytes, BUN/Cr, glucose for
  - —Hydration and acidosis
  - —Metabolic disorders
  - —Diabetes mellitus
- CBC for
  - —Infection
  - —Malignancy
  - —Lead poisoning
  - —Anemia
- ESR for infection

IMAGING/SPECIAL TESTS

- Reducing substances for inborn metabolic errors
- Lead level
- Tuberculin test
- EKG
- Skeletal survey for child abuse
- Bone age radiographs for infection, metabolic and hereditary bone disease

DIFFERENTIAL DIAGNOSIS

Organic Causes

- Congenital
  - —Genetic syndromes (including Turners, Noonan, Williams, and Russell-Silver)
  - —Inborn errors of metabolism (including maple syrup urine disease, methylmalonic aciduria, glycogen storage disease)
  - —Fetal alcohol syndrome
  - —Perinatal infections
  - —Cleft palate, cleft lip, diencephalic syndrome
- Gastrointestinal
  - —Malabsorption syndromes (including cystic fibrosis, celiac disease, lactose intolerance, and milk protein intolerance)
  - —Inflammatory bowel disease, ulcerative colitis

—Hepatobiliary disease (including hepatitis, cirrhosis)
—Obstructive disease (including pyloric stenosis, Hirschsprung disease)
—Gastroesophageal reflux disease
—Pancreatic insufficiency

- Cardiopulmonary
  —Congenital heart disease
  —Cystic fibrosis
  —Chronic lung disease (including bronchopulmonary dysplasia, severe asthma)
  —Anatomic abnormalities of the upper airway
- Renal
  —Anatomic abnormalities with renal failure
  —Renal tubular acidosis
  —Chronic renal insufficiency
- Immunologic
  —Severe combined immunodeficiency
  —DiGeorge Syndrome
  —AIDS
- Endocrinologic
  —Hypopituitarism
  —Thyroid disease
  —Diabetes mellitus
  —Adrenal insufficiency or excess
  —Growth hormone deficiency
- Neurologic
  —Mental retardation
  —Cerebral hemorrhages
  —Degenerative disorders
  —Brain tumors
- Infectious
  —Tuberculosis
  —Parasitic or bacterial infection of the GI tract
  —Recurrent tonsillitis and adenoiditis
  —Chronic urinary tract infection
- Miscellaneous
  —Lead poisoning
  —Malignancy
  —Collagen vascular disease

Nonorganic Causes

- Parent-child dysfunction/psychosocial
  —Maternal-infant bonding problems
  -Feeding problems
  -Breast feeding difficulties
  -Young or inexperienced parent
  —Insufficient family or emotional supports
  —Developmental delay
  —Attention disorders
  —Care requirements for chronic disease
  —Family discord
  —Child abuse or neglect

Treatment

INITIAL STABILIZATION

- Check for hypoglycemia
- Fluid resuscitation when dehydrated
- Correct electrolyte imbalances
- Provide a supportive environment

ED TREATMENT

- Identify a child with failure to thrive
- Rule out organic abnormalities (see Differential Diagnosis)
- Ensure appropriate follow-up
- Contact social services if psychosocial issues suspected
- Children frequently respond well to an appropriate diet in a supportive setting, so they are often admitted to the hospital for further evaluation and family teaching

Disposition

ADMISSION CRITERIA

- Any child who has fallen across two major growth percentiles, unless the underlying etiology has already been identified and is being treated appropriately
- Any child who has suffered abuse or neglect
- Any child under 1 year of age with severe failure to thrive
- Any child with severe dehydration or malnutrition

DISCHARGE CRITERIA

- Outpatient care is preferred when the child has mild growth deficiency, but strong outpatient follow-up with regular physician contact is essential
- Physiologically stable children may be discharged into the care of the family after careful evaluation by a physician and social services personnel
- If child abuse is suspected or neglect is severe, the appropriate child protection agency must be contacted and alternate discharge custody arranged

Miscellaneous

ICD9: N/A

CORE CONTENT CODE: 21.1.21

SUGGESTED READINGS

Bithoney WG, Dubowitz H, Egan H. Failure to thrive/growth deficiency. Pediatr Rev 1992;13:453.

Frank D, Silva M, Needleman R. Failure to thrive: Mystery, myth, and method. Contemp Pediatr 1993;10:114.

Author: Angela Anderson, Delora Snyder

Fatigue

Clinical Presentation

SIGNS AND SYMPTOMS

- Perception of being physically, intellectually, or emotionally exhausted
- Occurs with or without objective findings on physical exam
- Focal or generalized motor weakness may accompany fatigue

MECHANISM/DESCRIPTION

Localized Motor Fatigue

- Deconditioning of nerves or muscle results in loss of function
- Localized muscular fatigue occurs after overuse or trauma to a muscle group

Generalized Motor Fatigue

- Infection and immunologic mechanisms
  —Increase cytokines, inflammation, and immunoglobulin complexes
- Endocrine disorders
  —Alter metabolic status hydration, and electrolyte balance
- Neoplastic disease
  —Alter chemical and cellular mediators
- Drugs
  —Cause electrolyte disturbances
  —Decreased sympathetic tone or energy uncoupling
- Nutritional deficiency
  —Produces catabolism
- Psychiatric disorders
  —Produce imbalances in neurotransmitters
- Chronic fatigue syndrome
  —Associated with abnormalities in the reticular activating system

Pre-Hospital

CAUTIONS

- Apply cardiac monitor
- Insert IV catheter
- Administer oxygen for patient with or suspected to have low oxygen saturation
- Perform accucheck and administer glucose for hypoglycemia

Diagnosis

ESSENTIAL WORKUP

- Chronic fatigue syndrome (CFS) is clinical diagnosis
  —Persistent or relapsing fatigue >6 months
  —Greater than 50% reduction in daily activity
  —Minor symptoms such as
    -Headaches
    -Migratory arthralgia
    -Sleep disturbances
    -Mild fever or chills
    -Myalgia
    -Exercise intolerance
    -Painful lymphadenopathy
  —Exclusion of other diseases or psychiatric illness
- Fatigue may be a symptom of many other disorders

LABORATORY

- Electrolytes, BUN/Cr
  —Hyperkalemia
  —Hypokalemia
  —Renal failure
  —Adrenal insufficiency
- Glucose
  —Hyper- or hypoglycemia
- CBC
  —Leukemia
  —Infection
  —Anemia
- Arterial blood gas or pulse oximetry for oxygen saturation

IMAGING/SPECIAL TESTS

- ECG
  —Silent ischemia
  —Arrhythmias
- Chest x-ray
- Pneumonia
- Congestive heart failure
- Tumors
- Tests for specific diseases include
  —Cosyntropin test
  —Thyroid studies
  —Lyme titers
  —Sedimentation rate

DIFFERENTIAL DIAGNOSIS

- Infection
  —Bacteremia
  —Urosepsis
  —Pneumonia
  —Abscess
  —EBV
  —CMV
  —HIV
  —HHV-6
- Immunologic
  —MS
  —Rheumatologic (RA, SLE, JRA)

—Myasthenia gravis
—Eaton-Lambert
- Neoplastic
  —Solid or hematologic cancers
- Metabolic
  —Electrolyte abnormalities
  —Mitochondrial diseases
  —Bromism
- Hematologic
  —Anemia
  —Hypovolemia
  —Hemoglobinopathy
- Endocrine
  —Hyper- or hypothyroid
  —Adrenal insufficiency
  —Diabetes
- Psychiatric
  —Major depression

Treatment

INITIAL STABILIZATION

- ABCs
- Administer supplemental oxygen for hypoxia
- IV fluid bolus for signs of dehydration

ED TREATMENT

- Exclude serious infection
- Correct metabolic and hematologic disturbances
- Diagnose progressive neurologic disease and acute psychiatric crisis
- Initiate workup for endocrine and neoplastic disease
- Chronic fatigue syndrome treatment options
  —Intravenous IgG
  —Magnesium
  —Monoamine oxidase inhibitors (moclobemide)
  —Cognitive-behavioral therapy
  —Good follow up

Disposition

ADMISSION CRITERIA

- Underlying disease requiring intravenous medication or monitoring
- Failure to thrive as outpatient
- Unable to provide for self

DISCHARGE CRITERIA

- Able to care for self
- Serious disturbances have been excluded
- Adequate followup is arranged

Miscellaneous

ICD9: 780.7

CORE CONTENT CODE: 22.1.22

SUGGESTED READINGS

Buchwald D, Wener MH, Pearlman T, Kith P. Markers of inflammation and immune activation in chronic fatigue and chronic fatigue syndrome. J Rheumatol 1997;24(2):372–376.

Dickinson CJ. Chronic fatigue syndrome—etiological aspects. Eur J Clin Invest 1997;27(4):257–267.

Maul AC. Chronic fatigue syndrome. Immunol Invest 1997;26(1–2):269–273.

Author: Christopher Lipinski

Feeding Problems, Pediatric

Clinical Presentation

SIGNS AND SYMPTOMS

Symptoms

- Define nature of problems
  - —Frequency, duration, and quantity of feeding
  - —Onset, duration, and severity
  - —Findings during feeding
    - -Cough, dyspnea, color change
    - -Vomiting, spitting
- Variability in feeding patterns is typical; parental impression of normal feeding is best guide
  - —Full-term normal infant usually has 2–3 ounces of formula every 2–3 hours
  - —Breast-fed baby eats 10–20 minutes on each breast every 2–3 hours
  - —1-month-old normally eats 4 ounces every 4 hours
- Poor weight gain
- Irritability

Signs

- Vital signs variable
- Hydration variable
- Growth (especially weight) velocity slow; impaired nutritional status
- Cough, tachypnea, color change
- Oropharyngeal inflammation, infection, or anatomic abnormality
- Chest-evidence of aspiration
- Neurologic status: muscle tone, reflexes, mental status

Complication

- Poor nutrition may lead to abnormal brain development, immunocompromise and other long-term adverse outcomes

MECHANISM/DESCRIPTION

- Feeding requires a coordinated series of actions involving several components
- Getting food into the oral cavity: appetite, food seeking behavior, ingestion
- Swallowing good: oral and pharyngeal phases
- Ingestion and absorption: esophageal swallowing, gastrointestinal phase
- Infant requires a minimum of 100–120 calories/kg/day
  - —Formula and human breast milk provide 20 calories/ounce

ETIOLOGY

- Physiologic, developmental, or anatomic disorders may contribute to feeding difficulties
- Family disruption, stress, tension also may contribute to feeding difficulties

Pre-Hospital

- Assess vital signs and hydration, and resuscitate as necessary

Diagnosis

ESSENTIAL WORKUP

- Observation of caretaker feeding child and parental-child interactions

LABORATORY

- Initial assessment if child failing to thrive or dehydrated
  - —CBC, urinalysis, electrolytes, BUN, glucose
- Chest x-ray, oximetry, and ABG if suspected cardiopulmonary concerns
- Cultures of blood, urine, and CSF if evidence of infection

IMAGING/SPECIAL TESTS

- Fluoroscopy, contrast radiographs, endoscopy, and ultrasound may be needed on an individual basis to define nature of swallowing, reflux, and associated conditions

DIFFERENTIAL DIAGNOSIS

- Family dysfunction, stress leading to potential neglect
- Difficulty getting food into the oral cavity
  - —Depression or other behavioral issues
  - —Deprivation
  - —Infection of oropharynx: herpes, aphthous ulcers, etc.
  - —CNS or endocrine disease (thyroid or adrenal dysfunction)
  - —Sensory deficit
  - —Neuromuscular disease
  - —Continued dysphagia and fatigue due to overwhelming infection (sepsis, meningitis, UTI)
  - —Anemia
  - —Cardiopulmonary disease (CHF, congenital heart disease, bronchopulmonary dysplasia, bronchiolitis, pneumonia)
- Difficulty in swallowing
  - —Anatomic abnormalities of oropharynx or esophagus-congenital or acquired
  - —Cardiopulmonary disease
  - —Neuromuscular disorder
  - —Disorder of esophagus-peristalsis, mucosal inflammation, esophagitis, reflux

Treatment

INITIAL STABILIZATION

- Resuscitation as required

ED TREATMENT

- Observe feeding session with primary caretaker; note gagging, coughing, emesis, noisy airway sounds, ability to handle secretions

Disposition

ADMISSION CRITERIA

- Suspected system infection
- Moderate to severe dehydration
- Significant failure to thrive
- Decompensated cardiopulmonary disease
- Severe esophagitis or reflux
- Symptomatic anemia or endocrine dysfunction
- Negligent caretaker

DISCHARGE CRITERIA

- Demonstrated ability to tolerate oral feedings
- Reliable caretaker and followup
- Behavioral therapy may be needed

Miscellaneous

ICD9: 783.3

CORE CONTENT CODE: 13.1.3

SUGGESTED READINGS

Rudolph CD. Feeding disorders in infants and children. J Pediatr 1994;125:S116–S124.

Author: Niels Ratlev

Feeding Tube Complications

Clinical Presentation

SIGNS AND SYMPTOMS

Extubation
- Tube removed from source

Occlusion
- Unable to pass liquid through tube

Tube Migration
- Distal displacement of PEG tube
- Obstruction at or distal to the pylorus
- Dumping syndrome
- Ischemia
- Intussusception
- Evidence of distal prolapse on external tube (if marked)

Peristomal Wound Infections
- Cellulitis
- Necrotizing fasciitis
- Abscess formation

Stoma Leak
- Leakage of feedings/GI contents around stoma
- Usually mild and short-lived

Aspiration Pneumonia
- Cough
- Dyspnea
- Hypoxia
- Food coloring in pulmonary secretions
- Fever
- Misplacement of nasoenteric tube (NET) in the pulmonary tree
  —Pneumothorax
  —Pleural effusion
  —Bronchopleural fistula

Diarrhea
- Frequent loose stools
- Dehydration

MECHANISM/DESCRIPTION

Extubation
- Accidental or intentional
- More common with NET compared with percutaneous endoscopic gastrostomy (PEG) tubes, gastrostomy (G-tube), or jejunostomy (J-tube) tubes

Occlusion
- Due to small diameter
  —Most common with NET
  —Polyurethane tubes and solution with high pH less likely to occlude
- Due to pill fragments (especially if enteric coated, or sustained release)
- Physical incompatibilities between formula and medications
  —Adherence of formula residue to the inner wall
- Essential to R/O malposition, fracture, and dislodgment

Peristomal Wound Infections
- Risk factors
  —Malnutrition
  —Poor wound healing
  —Stomal leak
  —Local irritation
  —Poor wound care
  —Immunosuppression
  —Diabetes mellitus
  —Obesity
  —Excessive traction on the tube
- Leads to delayed maturation of gastrocutaneous tract

Stoma Leak
- Problematic with distal obstruction (mechanical or dysmotility); more common with high gastric residual

Aspiration Pneumonia
- At risk
  —Impaired cough/gag reflex
  —Delayed gastric emptying due to ileus
  —Obstruction
  —Gastroparesis (in DM or head trauma)
  —Gastroesophageal reflux (frequent with large NET)

Diarrhea
- Medication-induced
  —Antibiotics
  —Sorbitol or magnesium-containing medications
  —Overgrowth of *C. difficile,* other bacteria, or candida
- Formula intolerance
  —Too rapid delivery
  —High osmolarity
  —Lactose or fat intolerance
  —Low serum albumin

Pre-Hospital

CAUTIONS
- If extubation of tube has occurred, transport tube with patient to facilitate easier replacement

Diagnosis

ESSENTIAL WORKUP
- Careful examination of feeding tube site and position of feeding tube within wound

LABORATORY

Peristomal Wound Infections
- CBC for significant infections

Aspiration Pneumonia
- ABG or pulse oximeter
- CBC
- Electrolytes, BUN/Cr, glucose
- U/A
- Blood and sputum culture

Diarrhea
- Stool for WBC/culture/*C. difficile* toxin

IMAGING/SPECIAL TESTS
- CXR
  —For NET tube position
  —Aspiration pneumonia

Tube Migration
- Endoscopy or upper GI barium study to confirm migration of tube into GI tract

Treatment

INITIAL STABILIZATION

- ABCs
- IV fluid resuscitation for dehydration/sepsis

ED TREATMENT

Extubation

- Nasoenteric tube (NET)
  —Replaced in the ED
  —Confirm position by x-ray before use
- Percutaneous endoscopic gastrostomy (PEG) tube
  —Takes up to 6 weeks for the gastrocutaneous tract/fistula to mature
    -Improper or aggressive attempt at tube replacement could lead to disruption of the gastrocutaneous tract and subsequent peritonitis
  —PEG tube in place >1 week prior to extubation
    -Replace in ED
    -May use a Foley catheter
    -Confirm by gastrografin study if there is doubt about placement
    -Secure the catheter to the abdominal wall to prevent distal migration
  —PEG tube in place <1 week prior to extubation
    -Fistula may not close promptly
    -Do not replace the tube in the ED
    -Watch for signs of peritonitis due to intraperitoneal leak of gastric contents
    -May need hospital admission and endoscopic tube replacement
- Surgical gastrostomy (G-tube) or jejunostomy (J-tube)
  —Management similar to PEG tube
  —Early dislodgment within first 3 days requires emergency surgical consult and antibiotic coverage for peritonitis

Occlusion

- Attempt gentle irrigation with normal saline, water, or carbonated soda
- If irrigation fails, replace the tube
- Do not use meat tenderizer or pancreatic enzymes

Tube Migration

- If retraction of the tube is possible and well tolerated
  —Secure the tube externally
  —Discharge home after brief trial of tube feeding
- If the feeding is not tolerated, or if there are signs of persistent obstruction, or peritonitis
  —Admit with consult to the appropriate service (surgical/GI)
- If the external tube is cut (accidental or intentional)
  —The inner bumper usually passes through the GI tract
  —Cases of obstruction, subsequent perforation, and peritonitis have been reported, especially in children

Peristomal Wound Infections

- Local wound care with hydrogen peroxide
- Antibiotics
  —First generation cephalosporin (cefazolin or cephalexin)
  —Ampicillin/sulbactam
  —Amoxicillin/clavulanic acid
- Outpatient management for milder cases
- More severe cases require surgical consult for possible drainage/debridement and inpatient care
- Prophylactic use of antibiotic (cefazolin) before tube placement does decrease wound infection

Stoma Leak

- Change from intermittent to continuous delivery
- Decrease the rate of infusion
- Administer prokinetic agents (e.g., metoclopramide, cisapride, or erythromycin)
- Local care
  —Keep the site clean and dry
  —Use sucralfate powder or stoma adhesive powder

Aspiration Pneumonia

- Stop enteral feeding
- Administer oxygen and broad spectrum antibiotics
- Endotracheal intubation with mechanical ventilation for respiratory failure and airway protection when indicated
- Prevent by
  —Elevation of head of bed
  —Monitoring gastric residual
  —Use of continuous infusion at graduated rate
  —Use of prokinetic agent

Diarrhea

- Manage etiology
- Correct fluid and electrolyte imbalance
- Try isotonic, hypotonic, or fat- or lactose-free formulas
- High-fiber formula if above measures fail
- Antimotility agents
  —Loperamide
  —Kaopectate
  —Cholestyramine

MEDICATIONS

- Amoxicillin/clavulanic acid (augmentin): 250–500 mg (peds: 40 mg/kg/24hrs) po tid
- Ampicillin/sulbactam: 1.5–3 g IV q 6 hrs
- Cefazolin (ancef, kefzol): 500 mg–1 g (peds: 25–100 mg/kg/24hrs) IV q 6 hrs
- Cephalexin (keflex): 250–500 mg (peds: 25–50 mg/kg/24hrs) po qid
- Cholestyramine: 4 g po 1–6 times/day
- Kaopectate: 30 ml (peds: 7.5 mg 3–6 years old; 15 ml 6–12 years old) po after each loose BM up to 7 times per day
- Loperamide (imodium): 4 mg initially then 2 mg (peds: 1 mg tid if 13–20 kg; 2 mg bid if 20–30 kg; 2 mg tid if >30 kg) po up to 16 mg/day

Disposition

ADMISSION CRITERIA

- PEG tube extubation within 1 week of placement
- Surgical gastrostomy (G-tube) or jejunostomy (J-tube) extubation within 3 days of placement
- Significant peristomal wound infection with fever/leukocytosis
- Aspiration pneumonia
- Diarrhea associated with dehydration
- Peritonitis

DISCHARGE CRITERIA

- Successful replacement of extubated feeding tube

Miscellaneous

ICD9: N/A

CORE CONTENT CODE: N/A

SUGGESTED READINGS

Fleming CR. Enteral nutrition. Gastrointest Dis Today 1996;5(2):1–9.

Kirby DF, Delegg MH, Fleming CR. American Gastroenterological Association technical review on tube feeding for enteral nutrition. Gastroenterol 1995;108:1282–1301.

Schapira GD, Edmundowicz SA. Complications of percutaneous endoscopic gastrostomy. Gastrointest Endosc Clin North Am 1996;6:409–422.

Author: Abbas Zagnoon

Felon

Clinical Presentation

SIGNS AND SYMPTOMS

- Swelling and tension of distal finger tip
- Throbbing pain
- Patients often elevate the finger to avoid increased pain in the dependant position
- Kanavel's signs of pyogenic flexor tenosynovitis
  —Flexed resting position of involved digit
  —Tenderness over flexor sheath
  —Fusiform swelling
  —Severe pain in passive extension

MECHANISM/DESCRIPTION

- A felon is a palmer closed-space infection of the distal pulp of the finger
- Felons can develop into serious infections resulting in significant patient disability. Neglect or incomplete incision and drainage may result in soft tissue and bony tuft necrosis, osteomyelitis, septic arthritis, lymphangitis, and flexor tenosynovitis. Improper surgical interventions can also result in an insensate, unstable palmer pad

ETIOLOGY

- The distal finger is anatomically a closed compartment, separate from the rest of the finger
- Multiple fibrous septa connect the volar skin fat pad to the periosteum
- Septa form compartments causing infections to be closed-space
- Worsening infection increases compartmental pressure resulting in ischemia and necrosis
- Spread of the infection can result in osteomyelitis
- Inoculating site rarely identified; wooden or glass splinters, minor cuts, or repeated trauma from fingerstick blood testing are common etiologies
- *S. aureus* is the most common organism; Streptococcus and Gram-negatives are also reported

Pre-Hospital

N/A

Diagnosis

ESSENTIAL WORKUP

- Thorough neurologic and vascular examination of finger pulp and digit function
- Cessation of pain indicates extensive tissue necrosis and nerve damage
  —Orthopedic consult should be obtained

LABORATORY

- Culture from I & D should be routinely performed because of the increased risk of osteomyelitis and prolonged infections

IMAGING/SPECIAL TESTS

- Finger radiographs should be obtained if there is suspicion of retained foreign body or osteomyelitis

DIFFERENTIAL DIAGNOSIS

- Herpetic whitlow—examine for vesicles
- Osteomyelitis
- Flexor tenosynovitis

Treatment

INITIAL STABILIZATION

No specific measures indicated

ED TREATMENT

- Digit block utilizing a long-acting agent (bupivacaine)
- Apply a tourniquet for the procedure to provide a bloodless field during incision
- Establish a sterile field
- Unilateral incision along side of the finger from 0.5 cm distal to the DIP crease to the free edge of the nail
  - —Incision must be dorsal to neurovascular bundle of the fingertip
- Bluntly dissect subcutaneous tissue to break up loculations in the septa
- Débride necrotic tissue
- Frank pus may not be evident
- The incision and dissection must not cross the DIP flexor crease; increased risk of inoculating the flexor tendon sheath
- Pack wound with sterile gauze or packing strip
- Splint finger to immobilize both digit and wrist
- Previously advocated fishmouth and lateral through-and-through incisions are associated with severe iatrogenic complications (i.e., unstable finger pad, permanent anesthesia) and should not be part of initial management

MEDICATIONS

- Antibiotics for 5–7 days
  - —Dicloxacillin: adult: 250–500 mg q 6 hrs po; peds: 25–100 mg/kg/d (qid) po
  - —Nafcillin: adult: 1–2 g q 4–6 hrs IV; peds: 50 mg/kg q 6 hrs IV
  - —Clindamycin: adult: 150–300 mg q 6 hrs po; peds: 10–25 mg/kg/d (qid) po
- Alternative antibiotics
  - —Cephalexin: adult: 250–500 mg q 6 hrs po; peds: 25–50 mg/kg/d (qid) po
  - —Cefazolin: adult: 1 g q 8 hrs IV; peds: 100 mg/kg/d (q 8 hrs) IV
  - —Erythromycin: adult: 250–500 mg q 6 hrs po; peds: 20–50 mg/kg/d (qid) po
- While wound culture results are pending, coverage for *S. aureus* is mandatory

Disposition

ADMISSION CRITERIA

- Flexor tenosynovitis, frank necrosis or other reasons for debridement in the OR

DISCHARGE CRITERIA

- Provided that reliable follow-up can be ensured and no indications of extension of infection from pulp, felons can be managed as an outpatient
- Wound check in 48 hours to include packing removal and wound irrigation
- Replace packing if continued drainage and follow up in 24 hours
- Otherwise, warm soaks and dressing changes
- Adjust antimicrobial coverage as indicated by cultures
- Symptoms usually resolve quickly; healing process can take up to 2 weeks
- Early consultation recommended for resistant infections

Miscellaneous

ICD9: 681.01

CORE CONTENT CODE: 10.6.4

SUGGESTED READINGS

Abrams RA, Botte MJ. Hand infections: Treatment recommendations for specific types. J Am Acad Orthop Surg 1996;4(4):219–230.

Canales FL, Newmeyer WI, Kilgore ES. The treatment of felons and paronychias. Hand Clin 1989;5(4):515–523.

Lammers RL, Freemyer BC. Hand. In: Rosen P, et al. Emergency medicine: Concepts and clinical practice. 3rd ed. St. Louis: CV Mosby, 1992:580–581.

Warden TM, Fourré MW. Incision and drainage of cutaneous abscesses and soft tissue infections. In: Roberts H, ed. Clinical procedures in emergency medicine. 2d ed. Philadelphia: WB Saunders, 1991:605–608.

Author: Allen Marino

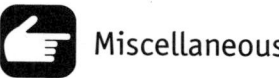

Femur Fracture

Clinical Presentation

SIGNS AND SYMPTOMS

- Usually obvious with pain, deformity, swelling, and thigh shortening
- Patient unable to move hip or knee
- Commonly presents with associated injuries: chest or abdominal trauma, hip or knee injury, including dislocation
- Rarely open fracture unless injury is due to penetrating trauma
- Patient may be hypotensive due to hemorrhagic into the thigh
- Patient may have impaired circulation in the foot due to vascular compromise

MECHANISM/DESCRIPTION

- Fractures classified according to
  —Location
    -Proximal third (subtrochanteric region)
    -For fractures of the femoral head, neck, and intertrochanteric regions, see chapter: Hip Injury
    -Middle third
    -Distal third (distal metaphyseal-diaphyseal junction)
  —Geometry of major fracture line
    -Transverse, oblique, spiral, longitudinal, or segmental
  —Degree of comminution—Winquist and Hansen classification
    -Grade I: small fragment of bone has been broken off; stable lengthwise and rotationally
    -Grade II: >50% contact between abutting cortices; stable lengthwise; may or may not have rotational stability
    -Grade III: <50% contact between abutting cortices; unstable lengthwise and rotationally
    -Grade IV: circumferential loss of cortex; unstable lengthwise and rotationally
- Usually requires major trauma
- Patients are mostly young adults with high-energy injuries (MVAs, GSWs, falls)
- Occasionally seen as a pathologic fracture
- Rarely seen as a stress fracture

PEDIATRIC CONSIDERATIONS

- 70% of femoral fractures in children <3 years old are the result of nonaccidental trauma
- Spiral fractures of the femur strongly suggest child abuse

Pre-Hospital

- Immobilization of the extremity and application of a traction splint is important as it can tamponade further blood loss into the thigh
- Contraindications to traction
  —Fractures close to the knee
  —Fracture or dislocation of the ipsilateral hip
  —Fractures of the pelvis
  —Fractures of the lower leg

CAUTIONS

- Do not attempt to reduce open fractures in the field; cover open wounds with sterile dressings

Diagnosis

ESSENTIAL WORKUP

- Radiographs (see below)
- Assess distal pulses, palpate compartments, evaluate sensation and motor function
- If pulses are not equal or palpable, bedside Doppler may be necessary
- Search for associated injuries
- In suspected child abuse, obtain skeletal survey or bone scan

LABORATORY

- CBC, type, and crossmatch

IMAGING/SPECIAL TESTS

- AP pelvis; true lateral of the hip; AP and lateral views of the femur; and complete knee series
- Baseline CXR, other films as indicated by trauma protocols

DIFFERENTIAL DIAGNOSIS

- Hip fracture or dislocation
- Knee fracture or dislocation
- Thigh contusion or hematoma

PEDIATRIC CONSIDERATIONS

- Cartilaginous components of the proximal and distal ends of the developing femur alter the fracture patterns seen in hip and knee injuries in children

Treatment

INITIAL STABILIZATION

- ABCs of trauma care
- Monitor blood pressure continuously; the thigh can contain 4–6 units of blood

ED TREATMENT

- Pain control is essential; parenteral analgesia acceptable in isolated femur injuries
  —A femoral nerve block can be performed in multiple trauma patients or pediatric patients
- Orthopedic consultation is necessary for all femoral fractures and is emergent in cases of fracture with neurovascular compromise
- Femur fractures with diminished or absent distal pulses, an expanding hematoma, or a palpable pulsatile mass require immediate angiography or femoral artery exploration
- Skeletal traction should be applied if the patient will not go to the OR immediately
- For closed fractures that require internal fixation, give cefazolin within 24 hours prior to operation
- Open fractures must go directly to the OR for irrigation and débridement
  —For open fractures with a laceration of >1 cm, extensive soft-tissue injury, or obvious contamination, give cefazolin and gentamicin or tobramycin in the ED, as well as tetanus booster if indicated
  —For injuries with highly contaminated wounds add penicillin G to cover Clostridial species
  —For gunshot wounds to the femur, culture the missile track and cover with an iodine dressing

MEDICATIONS

- Cefazolin: adult: 2 g IM/IV; peds: 20 mg/kg IM/IV
- Gentamicin/tobramycin: 1.5 mg/kg IV
- Penicillin G: adults: 2 million IU IV; peds: 25,000 IU/kg/day IV divided q 8 hrs

PEDIATRIC CONSIDERATIONS

- Assess markers for nonaccidental trauma
  —Delay in presentation; history of mechanism inconsistent with the injury
  —Isolated trauma to the thigh, associated burns, bruises, or linear abrasions
- Assess for dislocation of the femoral capital epiphysis
- Depending on the age of the patient and the fracture type, pediatric femoral fractures may not require operative treatment

Disposition

ADMISSION CRITERIA

- All femur fractures must be admitted except as noted below in discharge criteria
- Any suspicion of nonaccidental trauma in children

DISCHARGE CRITERIA

- In certain rare circumstances of pathologic fracture, or femur fractures in patients that are not ambulatory and would not undergo operative fixation, discharge can be considered in consultation with orthopedics if adequate pain control can be achieved and proper follow-up assured

Miscellaneous

ICD9: 821.00

CORE CONTENT CODE: 18.4.13.1.7

SUGGESTED READINGS

Brien W, et al. Management of gunshot wounds to the femur. Orthop Clin North Am 1995;26(1):133–138.

Buckley S. Current trends in the treatment of femoral shaft fractures in children and adolescents. Clin Orthop 1997;338:60–73.

Rockwood C, et al. Fractures of the femoral shaft. Chap. 19. In: Rockwood and Green's Fractures in adults and children. Philadelphia: Lippincott-Raven, 1991.

Author: Chris Ho

Fever, Adult

Clinical Presentation

SIGNS AND SYMPTOMS

- Anorexia
- Chills and sweating
  - —Occur during variation of body temperature
- Fatigue
- Headache
- Malaise
- Myalgias
- Night sweats
  - —Suggestive of chronic inflammatory conditions
- Elevated core temperature
  - —Oral temperature >37.5°C or 99.5°F
  - —Rectal temperature >38.0°C or 100.4°F
  - —Temperature >106°F suggests failure of thermoregulation
- Fever every other day or every third day
  - -Malaria
- Relapsing fever
  - -Fever daily for 3–6 days followed by a fever-free interval for about 1 week
  - -Borrelia infections
  - -Rat-bite fever
- Undulating fever
  - -Brucellosis
  - -Typhoid
- Periodic pyrexia
  - -Hodgkin's disease
- Heart rate is increased
  - —Dissociation of the heart rate and temperature suggests certain types of infection
    - -Typhoid fever
    - -Legionnaire's disease
    - -Psittacosis
    - -Brucellosis
    - -Factitious fever
- Increased respiratory rate
  - —Absent with factitious fever

MECHANISM/DESCRIPTION

- Fever is defined as an elevation of the thermoregulatory set point resulting in an abnormal elevation of core body temperature
  - —Core body temperature is tightly regulated at a set point of about 37°C
  - —A normal circadian rhythm allows for variations up to 2°C
  - —Core body temperature elevation also occurs when the body is unable to adequately dissipate heat or failure of thermoregulation
- Cells of the immune system release pyrogenic cytokines that bind to receptors on vascular endothelial cells within the hypothalamus
- Thermoregulatory mechanisms are controlled by the preoptic area of the anterior hypothalamus
  - —A local sensing mechanism links blood temperature to sympathetic autonomic discharge
    - -Shivering thermogenesis
    - -Dermal vasoconstriction
  - —Cooling mechanisms involve a mixture of sympathetic and parasympathetic pathways
  - —Sweating
  - —Dermal vasodilation

ETIOLOGY

- *All infectious etiologies may cause fever*
- Common infections in the United States
  - —Upper respiratory illnesses
  - —Urinary tract infections
  - —Cellulitis
  - —Abscesses (superficial and deep)
  - —Pneumonia
  - —Sepsis
- Common regional infections
  - —Southeastern United States
    - -Rocky Mountain Spotted Fever
  - —New England
    - -Tularemia
    - -Babesiosis
  - —Asia, Africa, Central and South America
    - -Malaria
    - -Dengue fever
- Pharmacologic
  - —Almost all medication may cause drug fevers
    - -Sulfonamides
    - -Penicillins
    - -Thiouracils
    - -Barbiturates
    - -Quinidine
    - -Laxatives especially with phenolphthalein
- Endocrine
  - —Thyrotoxicosis
- Inflammatory
  - —Collagen vascular disease
    - -Rheumatic fever
    - -Systemic lupus erythematosus
    - -Rheumatoid arthritis
    - -Vasculitis
  - —Granulomatous
    - -Sarcoidosis
    - -Granulomatous hepatitis
    - -Crohn's disease
  - —Tissue injury
    - -Pulmonary emboli
    - -Sickle cell disease
    - -Hemolytic anemia
  - —Neoplastic diseases
    - -Lymphoma/leukemia
    - -Hodgkin's and non-Hodgkin's lymphoma
    - -Acute leukemias
    - -Carcinoma especially when metastatic
    - -Atrial myxomas
- Factitious illnesses
  - —Injections of toxic materials
- Other causes
  - —Familial Mediterranean fever
  - —Fabry's disease
  - —Cyclic neutropenia

Pre-Hospital

CAUTIONS

- Fever does not require specific field interventions
- Pre-hospital interventions such as intravenous access and monitoring should be determined by patient stability or altered mental status

Diagnosis

ESSENTIAL WORKUP

- Rectal temperatures are the only reliable ED method to accurately measure a patient's temperature
- A careful physical examination including a rectal examination to assess for occult blood should guide the ordering of ancillary studies

LABORATORY

- Urinalysis
  - —Indicated if the cause of fever is not clearly identified by the physical examination
  - —Culture specifically for mycobacterium if tuberculosis is suspected
- CBC
  - —The white blood cell count is rarely helpful in managing febrile patients in the ED
  - —Critical to use to determine if neutropenia is present in patients receiving chemotherapy
  - —The differential may provide some indication as to the type of infection
    - -Neutrophilia suggests bacterial infections
    - -Monocytosis suggests tuberculosis, brucellosis, chronic inflammation
    - -Lymphopenia suggests immunodeficiency or a malignancy
    - -The total lymphocyte count is a reliable means of predicting the T cell count in HIV patients
  - —Platelet count below 150,000 is a weak predictor of sepsis
- Sedimentation rate (ESR)
  - —Rarely indicated in the ED evaluation as nonspecific and time-consuming
  - —When very elevated, suggestive of temporal arteritis, polymyalgia rheumatica, Still's disease, or bacterial endocarditis
  - —A normal ESR does not rule out life-threatening infections
- Blood cultures
  - —Indicated when sepsis is suspected
  - —Obtain before initiating antibiotic therapy whenever possible
  - —When ordering blood cultures in adults, patients should generally be admitted for observation

IMAGING/SPECIAL TESTS

- Chest radiograph
  - —Indicated if the cause of fever can not be ascertained by the physical examination
- Lumbar puncture
  - —Antibiotics should never be delayed to perform this procedure
  - —Indicated when fever is associated with altered mental status or a severe headache
  - —CT may be considered before procedure.

DIFFERENTIAL DIAGNOSIS

- Failure of thermoregulation
  - —Adrenergic syndrome
  - —Anticholinergic syndrome
  - —Neuroleptic malignant syndrome
  - —Malignant hyperthermia
- Hyperthermia from impaired heat loss
  - —Climatic temperatures exceeding body heat
    - -Heat stroke
  - —Congenital absence of sweat glands during hot weather
- Factitious elevations in temperature
  - —Manipulation or exchange of thermometers

Treatment

INITIAL STABILIZATION

- Immediate treatment of fever is rarely warranted
- Initiate antibiotics rapidly in the ED in patients with unstable vital signs, altered mental status, or immunosuppression

ED TREATMENT

- Certain patients require early treatment to reduce fever
  - —Myocardial ischemia
  - —History of seizures
  - —Pregnancy
  - —Temperature >106°F
- Acetaminophen
- Salicylates
- Nonsteroidal anti-inflammatory drugs
  - —Blocking the synthesis of prostaglandins within the endothelium of the hypothalamic vasculature
  - —Do not lower body temperature beneath its normal set point
- Glucocorticoid hormones
  - —Impede the production of endogenous pyrogens
  - —May be used to treat fever from chronic inflammatory conditions
  - —Never indicated to reduce fever in patients with infectious etiologies

MEDICATIONS

- Acetaminophen: 10–15 mg/kg po q 4–6 hrs
- Aspirin: 650 mg po q 4 hrs (avoid in children)
- Ibuprofen: 10 mg/kg po q 6 hrs

Disposition

ADMISSION CRITERIA

- Intensive care unit in patients with unstable vital signs
- All intravenous drug abusers with fever require admission to rule out endocarditis

DISCHARGE CRITERIA

- Outpatient etiology of fever determined during the ED evaluation
- Stable vital signs at discharge

Miscellaneous

ICD9: 780.6

CORE CONTENT CODE: N/A

SUGGESTED READING

Beutler B, Beutler SM. The pathogenesis of fever. In: Bennett JC, ed. Cecil's textbook of medicine. 20th ed. Philadelphia: WB Saunders, 1996:1533–535.

Author: Richard Wolfe

Fever, Pediatric

Clinical Presentation

SIGNS AND SYMPTOMS

- Clinical appearance must be evaluated
- Toxicity associated with lethargy, poor perfusion, hypo/hyperventilation, weak cry; purpuric or petechial rash
- Altered mental status
  - —Lethargy presenting with decreased level of consciousness
  - —Irritability
  - —Impaired interaction with environment, parents, physician, toys
- Physical examination to search for underlying condition
- Febrile seizures
- 10% of children <2 years old with temperature >41.1°C have bacterial meningitis
- 53% of children with temperature >41.1°C have serious illness
- Temperatures >42°C often have a noninfectious etiology
- Serious infection may occur in the absence of fever
- Antipyretics may change findings without impacting underlying disease

MECHANISM/DESCRIPTION

- Fever is defined as a temperature of 38.0°C rectally
  - —Oral and tympanic temperatures are generally 0.6–1.0°C lower
- Tympanic temperatures are not accurate in children <6 months
- Axillary temperatures are generally unreliable

ETIOLOGY

- General: bacteremia, septicemia, viral exanthem (varicella, roseola, rubella), coxsackie (hand-foot-mouth disease), abscess
- CNS: meningitis, encephalitis
- HEENT: otitis media, facial cellulitis, orbital/periorbital cellulitis, pharyngitis (group A β-hemolytic streptococcus, herpangina, adenovirus pharyngoconjunctival fever), viral gingivostomatitis (herpes and coxsackie), cervical adenitis, retropharyngeal abscess, peritonsillar abscess, sinusitis, mastoiditis, conjunctivitis
- Respiratory: croup (paramyxovirus), epiglottitis, bronchiolitis (RSV), pneumonia, empyema
- Cardiovascular: purulent pericarditis, endocarditis, myocarditis
- GU: cystitis, pyelonephritis
- GI: bacterial diarrhea, intussusception, appendicitis, hepatitis
- Extremity: osteomyelitis, septic arthritis, cellulitis
- Miscellaneous: Kawasaki syndrome, vaccine (DPT) reaction, heat exhaustion/stroke, factitious, familial dysautonomia, thyrotoxicosis, collagen vascular disease, vasculitis, rheumatic fever, malignancy, drug-induced, overbundling (recheck 15 minutes after unbundling)

Pre-Hospital

- Resuscitate as appropriate
- Begin cooling either with antipyretics or tepid towels

Diagnosis

ESSENTIAL WORKUP

- Resuscitate as appropriate
- Determine duration of illness, degree and height of fever, use of antipyretics, past medical history, drug allergies, immune status, recent medications/antibiotics, birth history if <6 months of age, exposures, feeding, activity, urine/bowel habits, travel history and relevant review of systems
- Physical examination searching for underlying condition
- Initiate antipyretic therapy

LABORATORY

- CBC with differential
- Sedimentation rate
- Urinalysis and culture in all male children <6 months and females <2 years of age
- Cultures: blood, CSF, stool
- Stool for WBCs

IMAGING/SPECIAL TESTS

- Chest x-ray to exclude pneumonia
- Lumbar puncture as indicated
- Other studies as indicated to evaluate for underlying infection

DIFFERENTIAL DIAGNOSIS

See etiology

Treatment

INITIAL STABILIZATION

- Treat any life-threatening conditions
- Antipyretic therapy
- Evaporative cooling techniques such as sponge bath

ED TREATMENT

- Focal infections require evaluation and treatment
- Empiric antibiotics if cultures done and awaiting results or child toxic
- Toxic children require prompt septic workup and appropriate antibiotics
- All potential life-threatening conditions must be excluded before treating a minor acute illness which is more common
- Infants 0–30 days need a full septic workup: CBC, UA, cultures (blood, urine, CSF), lumbar puncture, chest x-ray
  —Antibiotics: cefotaxime and ampicillin
  —Admit
- Infants 30–90 days need septic workup; selective admission and antibiotics (ceftriaxone)
- Children 3 months to 3 years are evaluated selectively. Antibiotic use is individualized for specific identifiable infections and pending appropriate cultures
  —Children with WBC >15-20,000/mm³ and temperature over 39.4°C are at increased risk of bacteremia and may benefit from empirical antibiotics pending culture results
- Immunocompromised children need aggressive evaluation as do children with fever and petechiae/purpura

MEDICATIONS

- Acetaminophen: 15 mg/kg/dose PO/PR q 6 hrs
- Ibuprofen: 10 mg/kg/dose po q 6 hrs
- Amoxicillin: 50 mg/kg/day po tid
- Penicillin V: 25–50 mg/kg/day po BID-QID
- Ceftriaxone: 50–100 mg/kg/day IM/IV q 12 hrs
- Cefotaxime: 100 mg/kg/day IV q 6–8 hrs
- Ampicillin: 150 mg/kg/day IV q 4–6 hrs

Disposition

ADMISSION CRITERIA

- All toxic patients
- Infants 0–30 days of age with fever > 38°C
- Infants 30–90 days of age with fever >38°C if any aspect of clinical or laboratory evaluation abnormal
- Poor compliance or followup

DISCHARGE CRITERIA

- Infants 30–90 days meeting low risk criteria
  —No prior hospitalizations, chronic illness, antibiotic therapy, prematurity
  —Reliable, mature parents with home phone, available care, thermometer, and living in relative proximity to ED
  —No evidence of focal infection (except otitis media), nontoxic appearing, normal activity, perfusion and hydration with age-appropriate vital signs
  —WBC count between 5,000 and 15,000/mm³, normal urinalysis (<5 WBC/hpf), and when stool examination warranted <5 WBC/hfp
- Infants 91 days to 36 months who are nontoxic and previously healthy with good followup
  —Antipyretics
  —Consider ceftriaxone and close followup
- Followup by phone in 12–24 hours and reevaluation in 24–48 hours with parental instructions to return if concerns develop or patient worsens

Miscellaneous

ICD9: 780.6

CORE CONTENT CODE: 13.0

SUGGESTED READINGS

Baraff LJ, Bass JW, Fleischer GR, et al. Practice guidelines for the management of infants and children 0 to 36 months of age with fever without a source. Pediatrics 1993;92:1–12.

Bulloch B, Craig WR, Klassen TP. The use of antibiotics to prevent serious sequelae in children at risk for occult bacteremia: a meta-analysis. Acad Emerg Med 1997;4:679–683.

Jones RG, Bass JW. Febrile children with no focus of infection: a survey of their management by primary care physicians. Pediatr Infect Dis J 1993;12:179–183.

Kramer MS, Shapiro ED. Management of the young febrile child: a commentary on recent practice guidelines. Pediatrics 1997;100:128–134.

Authors: David A. Peak; Andrew S. Ulrich; Paul Ishimine

Fibrocystic Breast Disease

Clinical Presentation

SIGNS AND SYMPTOMS

- Pain (mastodynia) and tenderness
  - —Usually bilateral, can be unilateral
  - —Especially premenstrual phase of normal menstrual cycle
- Lumpiness, nodularity—may be localized or generalized, unilateral or bilateral
- Excessive nodularity
- Increased engorgement and breast density; breasts described as being dull and heavy with fluctuations in the size of the cystic areas
- Occasional spontaneous nipple discharge

MECHANISM/DESCRIPTION

- Synonyms: fibrocystic breast, cystic mastitis, symptomatic chronic cystic mastopathy, Schimmelbusch's disease, Reclus's disease, mammary dysplasia
- Defined as palpable lumps in the breast, associated with pain and tenderness, that fluctuates with the menstrual cycle. Often become progressively worse until menopause
- Fibrocystic changes (FCC) are found histologically in 50% of women
- *Three clinical stages of fibrocystic changes*
  - —*Mazoplasia:* intense proliferation of the breast stroma. Pain usually in upper outer breast quadrant with most tender area in axillary tail. Generally affects women in their 20s
  - —*Adenosis:* marked proliferation and hyperplasia of ducts, ductules, and alveolar cells. Multiple breast nodules (2–10 mm) in size. Premenstrual pain and tenderness. Generally affects women in their 20s and 30s
  - —*Cystic:* solitary (Cooper's disease) or multiple (Reclus' disease). Lumps are cystic when palpated and tender, slightly mobile, and well delineated. Vary in size from microscopic to 5 cm in diameter. Deeply imbedded or clustered. Usually not painful, unless rapid increases in cyst size and lump appears. Fluid aspirated is straw colored or dark brown to green

ETIOLOGY

- Enhanced or exaggerated reaction by breast tissue to cyclic levels of ovarian hormones; therefore, most common in reproductive, premenopausal years
- Risk factors: nulliparity, late age of natural menopause, high social status. Age, genetic makeup, and lactational history may affect the development of FCC as well

Pre-Hospital

N/A

Diagnosis

ESSENTIAL WORKUP

- Clinical examination: ideally 7–9 days after onset of menstrual flow when breasts are least congested
- Ultrasonography: can differentiate cystic from solid breast masses. Useful in palpable masses as well as nonpalpable masses that appear on screening mammography. Benign cystic masses typically have uniform outer margin without asymmetry or irregular thickness of the cyst wall. There are no echoes centrally and posterior wall enhancement is noted. Can assist in aspiration of deep cysts or those not palpated. Alternatively, can conservatively follow size of cysts

IMAGING/SPECIAL TESTS

- Mammography: sensitivity of approximately 85% in detecting malignancies. However, mammographic findings of benign processes of the breast can appear as malignant and vice versa. Should be done either before aspiration or 7–10 days after aspiration (to avoid artifacts after aspiration)
- Needle aspiration: should completely evacuate cyst. Can be done for symptomatic or large masses
- Excisional biopsy: Gold Standard diagnostic test for patients with abnormal results of mammogram, a breast mass, or normal results of mammogram and a palpable mass that has not been proved cystic

DIFFERENTIAL DIAGNOSIS

- Benign breast masses
- Malignant breast masses

Treatment

INITIAL STABILIZATION

Not applicable

ED TREATMENT

- Referral to primary care physician
- Reassurance if only minimal symptoms
- *Conservative therapy*
  - —Support bra: reduces tension on supporting ligaments of breast and can reduce inflammatory response and edema
  - —Mild diuretic for 2–3 days before onset of menses
  - —Dietary changes: reduction in dietary methylxanthines reduces level of cAMP and cGMP and has been found by some authors to reduce symptoms and changes of fibrocystic changes
  - —NSAIDs
- *Hormonal therapy*
  - —Oral contraceptives: can decrease the symptoms of fibrocystic changes, particularly after 1 year of treatment. Mechanism is thought to be reduction in ovarian estradiol production with alteration of breast estrogen receptors by the progestin component of the pill. Most studies are with the older oral contraceptive pills with higher progesterone content
- *Sex hormone inhibitors* (should be prescribed by primary care physician to enable follow-up during course of treatment)
  - —Danazol: a synthetic androgen with greater anabolic than androgenic activity. Reduces breast nodularity in 47–75% of cases. Mechanism is related to its inhibitory effect on sex steroid synthesis by competitively inhibiting the binding of sex steroids to receptors. Contraindicated in pregnancy and in patients with abnormal uterine bleeding or with abnormal hepatic, renal, or cardiac function. Many side effects
  - —Tamoxifen: a partial estrogen antagonist. Response rate of 65–75%. Fewer side effects than Danazol
  - —Bromocriptine: inhibits prolactin production. Most patients (75%) have relief from mastalgia and reduced nodularity. However, significant side effects of nausea, vomiting, alopecia, dizziness, edema, and headache occur in 50–60% of those treated. Should be prescribed by primary care physician and only used in very selected patients with very careful assessment and close follow-up
- *Surgical intervention:* If a nodule in a breast remains, excision is recommended regardless of mammographic or ultrasonic findings. If a large cyst recurs after aspiration on two occasions, it should be excised and studied histologically. Referral to general surgeon

MEDICATIONS

- Danazol: 100–400 mg/day in 2 divided doses for 6 months
- Oral contraceptives: for example, combination with 0.02 mg of ethinyl estradiol and 1 mg norethindrone acetate—1 tablet/day
- Tamoxifen: 10 mg/day

Disposition

ADMISSION CRITERIA

None

DISCHARGE CRITERIA

- All patients may be discharged if the diagnosis is fibrocystic changes
- It is important for patient satisfaction, as well as patient health and disease prevention, to ensure follow-up for all patients with breast masses. Referral to a primary care physician or even a general surgeon should be provided

Miscellaneous

ICD9: 610.1

CORE CONTENT CODE: 16.2.1

SUGGESTED READINGS

Drukker BH. Fibrocystic change of the breast. Clin Obstet Gynecol 1994;37:903.

Fiorica JV. Fibrocystic changes. Obstet Gynecol Clin North Am 1994;21:445.

Hutter RVP. Consensus meetings. Is "fibrocystic disease" of the breast precancerous? Arch Pathol Lab Med 1986;110:171.

Scanlon EF. The early diagnosis of breast cancer. Cancer 1981;48:523.

Author: Tami Gash-Kim

Fibromyalgia

Clinical Presentation

SIGNS AND SYMPTOMS

- Generalized musculoskeletal pain and stiffness
- Weakness and fatigue
- Sleep disturbance
- Tension headaches
- Gastrointestinal complaints (e.g., irritable bowel syndrome)
- Paresthesias
- Sensation of swollen hands
- Skin fold tenderness
- Postexertional pain
- Cold intolerance
- Dermatographism

MECHANISM/DESCRIPTION

- Fibromyalgia is a nonarticular form of rheumatism with limited physical findings
- Predominantly affects women between the ages of 20 and 50
- It is not an inflammatory process so the term *fibrositis* is no longer used

ETIOLOGY

- The etiology is unknown
- Sleep studies have suggested that disturbance of normal stage 3–4 sleep (non-REM) may play a role in the development of fibromyalgia
  - —Normal stage 3–4 sleep is characterized by low frequency *delta* waves. In fibromyalgia patients, sleep studies show that this stage of sleep is interrupted by high frequency alpha waves termed *alpha wave intrusion*
- Muscle biopsies from tender points have shown no reproducible abnormalities
- Immunologic and endocrinologic dysfunction have also been proposed in the etiology of fibromyalgia

Pre-Hospital

N/A

Diagnosis

ESSENTIAL WORKUP

- History is the key to making the diagnosis
  - —Characteristic *widespread* axial pain distribution on both the left and right sides of the body and pain above and below the waist
  - —11 or more of 18 specific tender points on digital palpation with a force of 4 kg (the amount of pressure required to blanch a thumbnail.) The *9 paired* tender points are
    - -Occiput: suboccipital muscle insertions
    - -Trapezius: midpoint of the upper border
    - -Supraspinatus: above the medial border of the scapular spine
    - -Low cervical: anterior aspects of the C5, C7 intertransverse spaces
    - -Second rib: second costochondral junction about 3 cm lateral to the sternal border
    - -Lateral epicondyle: about 2 cm below the bony prominence
    - -Gluteal: upper outer-quadrant of the buttocks
    - -Greater trochanter: posterior to the trochanteric prominence
    - -Knee: medial fat pad proximal to the joint line

LABORATORY

- Complete blood count, blood chemistries, erythrocyte sedimentation rate (ESR), and thyroid function tests may help rule out alternate diagnoses
- No specific laboratory abnormalities are present with fibromyalgia

IMAGING/SPECIAL TESTS

- No specific radiographic abnormalities present

DIFFERENTIAL DIAGNOSIS

- Myofascial pain syndrome (*trigger points present* not *tender points*)
- Polymyalgia rheumatica
- Axial arthritis
- Hypothyroidism
- Electrolyte imbalance
- Metabolic myopathies
- Early collagen disease
- Osteomalacia
- Psychogenic rheumatism
- Chronic fatigue syndrome
- Eosinophilia-myalgia syndrome

Treatment

INITIAL STABILIZATION

- None required

ED TREATMENT

- *Patient education and reassurance:* emphasize that fibromyalgia is not life-threatening and does not reduce life expectancy. The disorder is chronic but not crippling or deforming. Effective treatment is available to manage pain and make patients more functional
- *Psyche:* emphasize that fibromyalgia is not a psychiatric disease
  —Patients with poor coping skills will require psychologic intervention
  —Specific problems such as depression, alcoholism, anxiety, and childhood abuse once diagnosed should be referred early for appropriate treatment

Pharmacologic Therapy

- Amitriptyline, cyclobenzaprine, and alprazolam given at bedtime have been shown in blind, randomized placebo-controlled trials to be effective. These medications are beneficial in improving sleep quality
- Nonsteroidal anti-inflammatory drugs (NSAIDs) and corticosteroids have *not* been shown to be effective. However, they may be required for the treatment of coexistent disease
- Injecting tender points with steroids or local anesthetics is controversial. No studies available to prove efficacy
- Narcotics should be avoided

MEDICATIONS

- Amitriptyline: 10–25 mg at bedtime
- Cyclobenzaprine: 10–20 mg at bedtime
- Alprazolam: 0.5–1 mg at bedtime

Lifestyle Modifications

- Physical exercise should be encouraged. Exercise program should be gradual to avoid overexertion and discouragement. Aerobic exercise may be more beneficial than simple stretching
- Good sleep *hygiene* should also be discussed; e.g., establishing a nightly ritual in preparation for sleep, avoiding caffeine-containing beverages or foods in the afternoons or evenings, and removing distractions from the bedroom such as radios, televisions, books, exercise equipment, pets, or a snoring restless sleeper
- Patients should also be encouraged to learn stress management and coping strategies

Disposition

ADMISSION CRITERIA

- Patients with serious underlying disease or immunocompromised
- Patients with suicidal ideation

DISCHARGE CRITERIA

- Patients with uncomplicated fibromyalgia can be managed as outpatients

Miscellaneous

ICD9: 729.1

CORE CONTENT CODE: 10.4.3

SUGGESTED READINGS

Wolfe F, Smythe HA, Yunus MB, et al. The American College of Rheumatology 1990 criteria for the classification of fibromyalgia. Arthritis Rheum 1990;33:160.

Author: Karlene Chin

Flail Chest

Clinical Presentation

SIGNS AND SYMPTOMS

- *Flail chest* paradoxically moves inward during inspiration and outward during expiration
  - —Initially this may not be seen because of muscle splinting
- Localized chest wall pain increases with deep inspiration or coughing
- Ecchymosis, bony crepitus, and tenderness associated with multiple rib fractures
- Splinting respirations
- Intercostal muscle spasm
- Dyspnea, tachypnea; onset may be insidious, increasing over time
- Hemoptysis
- Cyanosis, tachycardia, hypotension
- Auscultation: initially normal breath sounds progressing to wet rales or absent breath sounds
- Flail chest is most commonly associated with *pulmonary contusion*

MECHANISM/DESCRIPTION

- Direct chest wall trauma, fall from height, motor vehicle accident
- Flail chest is a free-floating segment of chest wall resulting when three or more adjacent ribs are fractured in two or more places or from rib fractures in conjunction with sternal fractures or costochondral separations
- Ribs usually break at the point of impact or the posterior angle, which is the structurally weakest region
- Direct injury from the transfer of kinetic energy to the lung parenchyma causes disruption of the alveolocapillary membrane and development of pulmonary contusion
- Arteriovenous shunting, ventilation-perfusion mismatch, hypoxemia, and potential respiratory failure result
- *The main problem with flail chest is the resultant pulmonary contusion, not alteration in ventilatory mechanics due to the free-floating segment*

PEDIATRIC CONSIDERATIONS

- Relatively elastic chest wall make rib fractures less common in children

Pre-Hospital

CAUTIONS

- In the field, positioning the patient injured side down can stabilize the flail segment and improve ventilation in the noninjured hemithorax
- Patients with thoracic trauma associated with a motor vehicle accident, significant fall, or preexisting lung disease should be routed to the nearest available trauma facility

Diagnosis

ESSENTIAL WORKUP

- Diagnosis is based on clinical examination
  - —Inspection under tangential light may magnify the paradoxical motion of the chest wall segment
  - —The thorax should be palpated in search of tenderness and crepitus
- Chest radiography aids diagnosis, revealing multiple rib fractures
  - —Associated intrathoracic pathology such as pneumothorax, hemothorax, and widened mediastinum
  - —*Pulmonary contusion* appears within 6–12 hours postinjury and ranges from patchy alveolar infiltrates to frank consolidation

LABORATORY

- Arterial blood gas may reveal hypoxemia and an elevated A-a gradient

IMAGING/SPECIAL TESTS

- Thoracic computed tomography (CT) may be a useful adjunct in defining associated thoracic injuries not identified on chest x-ray

DIFFERENTIAL DIAGNOSIS

- Rib contusion or intercostal muscle strain
- Costochondral separation
- Sternal fracture and dislocation
- Radiographic differential diagnosis includes
  - —Adult respiratory distress syndrome (ARDS)
  - —Pulmonary laceration
  - —Congestive heart failure
  - —Pneumonia or other infectious process
  - —Noncardiogenic causes of pulmonary edema

Treatment

INITIAL STABILIZATION

- ABCs, IV, O_2, continuous cardiac and pulse ox monitoring
- Control airway
  - —Endotracheal intubation is indicated for patients with severe hypoxemia ($PaO_2 < 60$ mm Hg on room air, < 80 mm Hg on 100% O_2), significant underlying lung disease or impending respiratory failure

ED TREATMENT

- Maintain adequate oxygenation, monitor O_2 saturation and respiratory rate
- In the conscious and alert patient, O_2 administration via facemask is first-line therapy
  - —If the patient cannot maintain a $PaO_2 >$ 80 mmHg on high flow oxygen then continuous positive airway pressure (CPAP) via mask or nasal BiPAP can be attempted
- If adequate oxygenation cannot be maintained with mask/CPAP/BiPAP, early endotracheal intubation and mechanical ventilation should be instituted with positive end expiratory pressure (PEEP)
  - —This results in a physiologic internal fixation of the flail segment
- External fixation or stabilization of the flail segment is not indicated
- Adequate pain control is the key to maintaining adequate pulmonary function, avoiding splinting, atelectasis, and subsequent pneumonia
- Search for associated injuries, treat exacerbation of underlying lung disease
- *Intercostal nerve blocks with 0.5% bupivacaine are safe and effective when performed properly, providing 6–12 hours of pain relief*
  - —The intercostal nerve can be blocked posteriorly 2-3 fingerbreadths from the midline
  - —The neurovascular bundle runs just along the undersurface of the rib; aspirate first to be sure the intercostal vessels have not been punctured
- *Avoid overhydration:* in the setting of pulmonary contusion the need for intravenous crystalloid resuscitation must be weighed against the risk of increasing interstitial pulmonary edema. Frequent reexaminations and serial chest radiographs are required to monitor alveolar fluid accumulation
- Prophylactic antibiotics are not indicated

MEDICATIONS

- Acetaminophen: 325 mg/oxycodone 5 mg (percocet) 1–2 tabs po q 6 hrs
- Morphine sulfate: adult: 2–10 mg; peds: 0.05–0.1 mg/kg IV/IM/SC q 4–6 hrs
- Hydromorphone (dilaudid): 1–2 mg IV/IM/SC q 4–6 hrs
- Meperidine (demerol): adult: 50–150 mg; peds: 0.75–2.0 mg/kg IV/IM q 3–4 hrs
- Bupivacaine 0.5% for intercostal nerve blocks
- For the admitted patient epidural or patient-controlled analgesia (PCA) is an effective alternative to traditional parenteral narcotics. Consider these for patients with refractory pain, oversedation, or hypoventilation secondary to narcotic analgesics

Disposition

ADMISSION CRITERIA

- All patients with flail chest are admitted to a critical care setting for close monitoring and pain control

DISCHARGE CRITERIA

- Patients found to have flail chest, with or without pulmonary contusion, should not be discharged

Miscellaneous

ICD9: 807.4

CORE CONTENT CODE: 18.4.10.4

SUGGESTED READINGS

Committee on Trauma, American College of Surgeons. Advanced trauma life support instructor manual. 5th ed. Chicago: American College of Surgeons, 1993.

Vukich D, Markovchick V. Thoracic trauma. In: Rosen P, et al., eds. Emergency medicine: Concepts and clinical practice. 4th ed. St. Louis: CV Mosby, 1998:514.

Wilson R. Thoracic trauma. In: Tintinalli J, et al., eds. Emergency medicine: A comprehensive study guide. 4th ed. New York: McGraw Hill, 1996:1156.

Author: Greg Lampe

Forearm Fractures, Shaft/Distal

Clinical Presentation

SIGNS AND SYMPTOMS

- Forearm pain, crepitus, tenderness to palpation, deformity, shortening of the forearm
- Forearm edema, ecchymosis, elbow or wrist joint effusions
- Abnormal mobility or loss of function at elbow/wrist/hand
- Neurological deficits, vascular compromise

MECHANISM/DESCRIPTION

- Direct blow to forearm
- Longitudinal compression load, fall on outstretched hand (FOOSH)
- Excessive pronation, supination, hyperextension, or hyperflexion
- Forearm fractures are classified by the bone(s) involved, anatomic location, alignment, angulation, rotation, comminution, whether open or closed, and concurrent dislocations
- Shaft fractures (single and paired) are often displaced by contraction of the muscles of the arm, and are sometimes associated with dislocations
  —*Galeazzi* fracture is a distal radius fracture, associated with distal radioulnar dislocation
  —*Monteggia* fracture is a proximal ulnar fracture, associated with dislocation of the radial head
- Distal fractures include extension, flexion, and intra-articular classifications
  —*Colles'* fracture is a hyperextension fracture of the distal radius (distal fragment displaced dorsally with radial deviation) that may also involve the ulnar styloid and the distal radioulnar joint
  —*Smith's* fracture is a hyperflexion fracture of the distal radius (distal fragment displaced volarly)
  —*Barton's* fracture is an intra-articular fracture of the dorsal or volar rim of the distal radius, often associated with dislocation of the carpal bones
  —*Hutchinson's* fracture is an intra-articular fracture of the radial styloid

PEDIATRIC CONSIDERATIONS

- Shaft fractures
  —*Torus* fracture involves compression (buckling) of the cortex on one or both sides
  —*Greenstick* fracture involves distraction of one side of the cortex with the opposite side intact
  —*Plastic deformity* results in bowing of the radius or ulna without apparent disruption of the cortex (multiple microfractures)
- Distal fractures
  —*Salter-Harris*-type fractures (see chapter on Salter-Harris classification)

Pre-Hospital

CAUTIONS

- All suspected forearm fractures should be splinted and immobilized, including the elbow and wrist joints
- All open fractures should be wrapped with a sterile dressing before splinting/immobilization
  —Do not reduce open fractures back under the skin in the field

Diagnosis

ESSENTIAL WORKUP

- Physical examination with special attention to skin integrity, deformity, and neurovascular status
- All suspected forearm fractures require AP and lateral x-rays, including wrist and elbow

IMAGING/SPECIAL TESTS

- Compartment pressures should be measured for suspected compartment syndrome
- Some intra-articular fractures may require CT imaging

DIFFERENTIAL DIAGNOSIS

- Upper extremity muscle, ligamentous injury
- Elbow or wrist dislocations, including the Pediatric Nursemaid's elbow
- Forearm contusions, hematomas, cellulitis, abscesses, soft-tissue masses
- Forearm osteogenic tumors, osteomyelitis
- Upper extremity vascular or neurologic injuries
- Elbow or wrist arthritis, joint effusions
- Pediatric growth plates, nutrient vessels may be mistaken for fractures

Treatment

INITIAL STABILIZATION

- All suspected forearm fractures should be immobilized, elevated, and have a cold compress applied
- Appropriate pain medication
- Open fractures need early systemic antibiotics

ED TREATMENT

- Shaft fractures, nondisplaced
  —Long-arm splint
  —Orthopedic referral
- Shaft fractures, displaced
  —Orthopedic consultation (often require open reduction, internal fixation)
- Distal fractures, nondisplaced
  —Forearm sugar-tong or anterior-posterior splint; orthopedic referral
- Distal fractures—*Colles'/Smith's*
  —Simple, noncomminuted, extra-articular Colles' and Smith's fractures may be reduced, splinted (long-arm sugar-tong splint), placed in a sling, and referred to orthopedics
  —Complicated Colles' and Smith's fractures require orthopedic consultation
- Distal fractures—*Barton's/Hutchinson's*
  —Uncomplicated Barton's and Hutchinson's fractures can be splinted (anterior-posterior or sugar-tong splint), placed in a sling, and referred to orthopedics
  —Complicated fractures require orthopedic consultation
- Open fractures
  —Open fractures should be covered with sterile dressings, given IM/IV antibiotics, tetanus immunization (if indicated), and splinted, and require immediate orthopedic consultation
  —Forearm fractures associated with compartment syndrome or neurovascular compromise require immediate orthopedic consultation
- Special pediatric considerations
  —*Torus* and *Greeenstick* fractures with less than 10° of angulation may be treated with a long-arm splint, sling, and orthopedic referral
  —*Plastic deformities* require orthopedic consultation. Some minimally displaced plastic deformities may be placed in a long-arm splint and sling
  —*Salter-Harris*-type fractures require orthopedic consultation

MEDICATIONS

- Antibiotics
  —Open fractures require IM/IV antibiotics
  —Cefazolin 1 g or equivalent first generation cephalosporin. If contaminated, add an aminoglycoside
- Acetaminophen: peds: 10–15 mg/kg q 4 hrs po; adult: 325–1000 mg po q 4 hrs
- Codeine: peds: >2 yrs 0.5–1.0 mg/kg q 4 hrs po/IM; adult: 15–60 mg po/IM q 4 hrs
- Hydrocodone: adult: 5–10 mg po q 4 hrs
- Ibuprofen: peds: >6 mos 5–10 mg/kg/dose q 6 h; adult: 200–800 mg q 4–8 hrs
- Meperidine: peds: 1–1.5 mg/kg q 3 hrs po/IM/IV; adult: 50–100 mg po/IM/IV q 3 hrs
- Morphine sulfate: peds: 0.01 mg/kg/dose IV/IM; adult: 2–10 mg IV/IM titrate to pain
- Tetanus (Td): 0.5 ml IM q 10 yrs

Disposition

ADMISSION CRITERIA

- Open fractures
- Fractures with compartment syndrome or neurovascular compromise
- Fractures needing immediate operative management or general anesthesia for reduction

DISCHARGE CRITERIA

- Appropriate immobilization
- Arranged orthopedic follow-up
- Adequate pain control measures
- Cast/splint care discharge instructions provided and understood by patient
- Documentation of intact neurovascular function following ED treatment

Miscellaneous

ICD9: 813.20; 813.40

CORE CONTENT CODE: 18.4.12.1.4; 18.4.12.2.3

SUGGESTED READINGS

Dicke TE, Nunley JA. Distal forearm fractures in children: Complications and surgical indications. Orthop Clin North Am 1993;24(2):333.

Patzakis MJ, Wilkens J. Factors influencing infection rate in open fracture wounds. Clin Orthop 1988;243:36.

Price CT. Injuries to the shafts of the radius and ulna. In: Rockwood CA, Wilkins KE, Beaty JH, eds. Fractures in children. Vol 3. 4th ed. Philadelphia: JB Lippincott, 1996:449–586.

Richards RR, Corley FG. Fractures of the shafts of the radius and ulna. in Rockwood CA, Green DP, Bucholz RW, Heckman JD, eds. Fractures in adults. Vol 1. 4th ed. Philadelphia: JB Lippincott, 1996:869–929.

Szabo RM. Extra-articular fractures of the distal radius. Orthop Clin North Am 1993;24(2):229.

Wilkins KE, O'Brien E. Fractures of the distal radius and ulna. In: Rockwood CA, Wilkins KE, Beaty JH, eds. Fractures in children. Vol 3. 4th ed. Philadelphia: JB Lippincott, 1996:586–653.

Authors: Trevor J. Mills; Peter M. C. DeBlieux

Foreign Body, Esophageal

Clinical Presentation

SIGNS AND SYMPTOMS

Acute Ingestion

- Dysphagia
- Odynophagia
- Drooling
- Vomiting
- Choking
- Gagging
- Blood-stained saliva

Chronically Retained

- Respiratory symptoms predominate (due to paraesophageal tissue swelling compromising airflow through trachea)
  - —Cough
  - —Stridor
  - —Hoarseness

General

- Anxiety
- Weight loss
- Irritability
- Anorexia
- Substernal chest pain
- Fever
- Foreign body (FB) sensation site usually corresponds to the level in the esophagus where the foreign body lodges
- Esophageal perforation
  - —Redness
  - —Swelling
  - —Crepitus in the neck
- Asymptomatic (<20%)

MECHANISM/DESCRIPTION

- Typically lodge at one of three sites of physiologic constriction
  - —Cricopharyngeal muscle (C6) (most common)
  - —Aortic arch (T4)
  - —Gastroesophageal junction (T11)
- Less commonly at tracheal bifurcation (T6) and thoracic inlet (T1)
- 90% of ingested FB pass spontaneously

ETIOLOGY

- Most common FBs in adolescents and adults are food boluses and bones
  - —Esophageal pathology almost always underlies food impactions
- Increased risk for
  - —Edentulous adults
  - —Intoxicated patients
  - —Predisposing esophageal disease

PEDIATRIC CONSIDERATIONS

- Infants
  - —Refusal to eat, stridor, upper respiratory infection, neck/throat pain
  - —*Uncommon:* esophageal-aortic fistula, tracheoesophageal fistula
  - —80% of FB ingestions occur in the pediatric age group, particularly <2 years
- Coins—80% of esophageal FB
- Predisposing factor—esophageal strictures

Pre-Hospital

CAUTIONS

- Airway maintenance and prevention of aspiration paramount
- Oxygen for all patients in distress
- Place patients in whatever position gives them the most comfort
- Ipecac and cathartics contraindicated

Diagnosis

ESSENTIAL WORKUP

- History regarding the object ingested
- Focus physical examination on degree of distress
  - —Search for complications: esophageal obstruction, perforation, hemorrhage
  - —Careful oropharynx examination for erythema, irritated throat, or palatal abrasions
  - —Direct or indirect laryngoscopy
  - —Lung—evidence of stridor and wheezing
  - —Abdomen—evidence of peritonitis or bowel obstruction

LABORATORY

N/A

IMAGING/SPECIAL TESTS

- CXR including the neck
  - —For all patients with suspected FB ingestions for localization whether symptomatic or not
  - —Esophageal FB align in the coronal plane
  - —Tracheal FB align in sagittal plane
  - —Esophageal perforation—air in the retropharyngeal space, in the soft tissues of the neck, or by pneumomediastinum
- Esophageal contrast studies for nonradiopaque foreign bodies
  - —Changes in the contour of the barium column
  - —Check for passage of the contrast solution into the stomach—partial versus complete obstruction
  - —*Caution*
    - -Oral contrast in high grade esophageal obstructions can increase the risk of aspiration
    - -Barium may coat the mucosa limiting subsequent endoscopy
    - -Traditional water soluble contrast can cause severe tissue reaction in perforations due to its hyperosmolarity
- Metal detectors have been used in localizing ingested metal, particularly coins
- Endoscopy
  - —Method of choice for localizing and managing esophageal FB
  - —Ability to inspect the surrounding esophageal mucosa for pathology
- CT detects FB not identified by other means

DIFFERENTIAL DIAGNOSIS

- Globus phenomenon
- Esophagitis
- Croup
- Epiglottitis
- Upper respiratory infection
- Retropharyngeal abscess

Treatment

INITIAL STABILIZATION

- ABCs
- Prevent aspiration

ED TREATMENT

- Foreign bodies lodged in the upper or mid-esophagus
  - —Extraction required
- Asymptomatic patients with coins or smooth objects in the distal esophagus
  - —Observe up to 24 hours to see if it will pass into the stomach
- Impacted food bolus completely obstructing the esophagus
  - —Emergent removal indicated
  - —Digestion with proteolytic enzymes (papain) not advocated due to associated serious morbidity including esophageal perforation and aspiration
- Extricate sharp or pointed esophageal FB regardless of their location
- Button batteries
  - —Emergent extraction indicated wherever they lodge in the esophagus
  - —Frequently leak potassium hydroxide and mercury
  - —Mucosal burns can occur within 4–6 hours

Removal Techniques

- Fluoroscopically guided Foley catheter extraction
  - —Successful and safe in experienced hands
  - —Foley catheter (10–16F) placed nasally and passed into the esophagus with the tip and balloon pushed beyond the FB under fluoroscopic control
  - —Foley balloon inflated with barium contrast material and the catheter slowly withdrawn
  - —Contraindicated in chronic ingestions, uncooperative patients, sharp pointed objects
- Push a distal foreign body into the stomach with a Foley catheter
- Endoscopy
  - —Preferred method to remove acute or chronic foreign bodies
  - —Always be used with impactions of long duration >2–4 days because of associated esophageal irritation/edema
  - —General endotracheal anesthesia needed in difficult cases (infants, psychiatric patients, difficult FB)
- IV glucagon
  - —Decreases LES tone without interfering with esophageal contractions
  - —Often permits distal food boluses to pass into the stomach
  - —Recommended for impactions <24 hours duration
- Gas-forming agents
  - —Useful in patients with esophageal food impactions of <24 hours
  - —May combine with glucagon followed by oral gas-forming agents
- Surgical intervention
  - —Reserved for patients in which the FB cannot be removed by other methods
  - —Approximately 2% of all patients
  - —Toothpicks and bones common objects

MEDICATIONS

- E-Z Gas: 30 ml solution ($NaHCO_3$, citric acid, and simethicone) po
- Glucagon: 1–2 mg IV push after test dose to determine hypersensitivity

Disposition

ADMISSION CRITERIA

- Seriously ill patients and those with complications such as esophageal perforation, migration of foreign body through the wall of the esophagus, significant bleeding
- Airway compromise
- Symptomatic patients with unsuccessful attempts to remove the foreign body

DISCHARGE CRITERIA

- Asymptomatic patients in whom the foreign body has been removed or passed distal to the esophagus
- Asymptomatic patients with distal esophageal smooth foreign bodies need reexamination within 12–24 hours to ascertain if spontaneous passage into the stomach has occurred

Miscellaneous

ICD9: 935.1

CORE CONTENT CODE: 1.1.2.6

SUGGESTED READINGS

Conners GP, Chamberling JM, Ochsenschlager DW. Symptoms and spontaneous passage of esophageal coins. Arch Pediatr Adolesc Med 1995;149:36–39.

Gingsberg GG. Management of ingested foreign objects and food bolus impactions. Gastrointest Endosc 1995;41:33–38.

MacPherson RI, Hill JG, Othersen HB, et. al. Esophageal foreign bodies in children: Diagnosis, treatment and complications. AJR 1996;166:911–924.

Schunk JE, Harrison AM, Corneli HM, et al. Fluoroscopic Foley catheter removal of esophageal foreign bodies in children: Experience with 415 episodes. Pediatrics 1994;94:709–714.

Webb WA. Management of foreign bodies of the upper gastrointestinal tract: Update. Gastrointest Endosc 1995;41:39–51.

Author: Thomas Lukens

Foreign Body, Ear

Clinical Presentation

SIGNS AND SYMPTOMS

- Decreased hearing
- Unilateral ear pain
- Fullness
- Loud noises
  - —Live insects
    - -Buzzing sound
    - -Severe pain
    - -Nausea
    - -Dizziness
    - -Ipsilateral tearing
- Purulent discharge from the external ear

MECHANISM/DESCRIPTION

- Foreign bodies lodged in the external auditory canal (EAC)
- Types of foreign bodies
  - —Children
    - -Stones
    - -Small beads
    - -Paper
    - -Toys
    - -Seeds
    - -Beans
  - —Competent adults
    - -Cotton-swab tips
    - -Earplugs
  - —Insects at any age
- Inanimate objects often have delayed presentations
- Most objects tend to become trapped in the outer two-thirds of the canal
- Children and psychiatric patients may place anything sufficiently small to enter the EAC
- Ear foreign bodies are most common under 8 years of age
- Nasal foreign bodies are the most common under 3 years of age
- Complications
  - —Perforation of the tympanic membrane
    - -Usually as a result of the removal
  - —Otitis externa
  - —Symptoms usually resolve within a few days after foreign body removal

ETIOLOGY

N/A

Pre-Hospital

CAUTIONS

- If severe ear pain and a loud buzzing sound
  - —Clear signs of a live insect in the external auditory canal
  - —Instill warm lidocaine or mineral oil in the affected ear to kill the insect

CONTROVERSIES

- Attempts at removal in the field are not indicated
  - —Lack of appropriate equipment
  - —Prior failed attempts may make future attempts more difficult

Diagnosis

ESSENTIAL WORKUP

- Always seek to identify the nature of the foreign body before trying to remove it
  - —Live insect
  - —Vegetable
  - —Inanimate object
- Careful otoscopic examination
  - —Minimize pain
  - —Gain the patient's trust
  - —Optimal visualization is achieved by having an assistant exert gentle, steady traction on the patient's lobule
  - —Perform a bilateral examination
    - -Especially in children and psychiatric patients
    - -Avoids missing a quiescent foreign body in the contralateral ear
    - -After removal, examination for evidence of perforation of the tympanic membrane

LABORATORY

N/A

IMAGING/SPECIAL TESTS

- Operating microscope
  - —Indicated if ED removal fails
  - —Radiographs are not needed

DIFFERENTIAL DIAGNOSIS

- Cerumen impaction
- Granuloma
- Hematoma
- Injury
- Otitis externa
- Perforated tympanic membrane
- Residual otitis externa after self-extraction of the foreign body

Treatment

INITIAL STABILIZATION

- Patients in distress because of live insects
  - —The insect should be killed before trying to remove it
  - —Instill solution into the EAC
    - -Mineral oil
    - -Viscous lidocaine
    - -Ether
    - -2% lidocaine
  - —Cold fluids should not be used so as to avoid a caloric response

ED TREATMENT

- Appropriate instruments
  - —Alligator forceps
  - —Cupped forceps
  - —Number 3, 5, and 7 suction tips, preferably with Frazier suction cups
  - —A wire loop
  - —Ear curettes
  - —A right-angle blunt hook
- Vegetable matter
  - —Visualize
    - -Attempt removal with forceps
    - -Be certain to delineate clearly between foreign body and inflamed EAC tissue
  - —The EAC should not be irrigated if the foreign body is of such a nature that it might swell
  - —Attempt visualization and removal
- Nonvegetable inanimate foreign bodies
  - —Visualize
  - —If easily grasped, attempt removal with forceps
  - —If this is not the case, attempt to remove the foreign body with irrigation
    - -Under careful visualization
    - -An angiocath catheter can be placed adjacent to—or preferably, distal to—the foreign body
    - -Warm water or sterile saline is injected through it via a syringe
  - —Backwash the foreign body out
  - —Polished or smooth objects
    - -Direct suction
    - -Blunt right angle probe: pass beyond the foreign body; rotate 90°; remove it with the foreign body
    - -Fogarty catheter: carefully pass beyond the foreign body; inflate and withdraw; this approach puts the tympanic membrane at particular risk for inadvertent injury
    - -Cyanoacrylate glue (Super-Glue): place on the tip of a blunt probe; place on the foreign body; quick bonding may allow foreign body removal with the probe
- Anesthesia or analgesia
  - —None needed in adults for simple foreign body removal
  - —Four-quadrant local anesthetic block
    - -1% or 2% lidocaine, with or without epinephrine
    - -Infiltrate around the EAC
  - —Conscious sedation
    - -Children and uncooperative adults
    - -Place before attempts as unsuccessful efforts may produce bleeding, edema or injury to the tympanic membrane
    - -Ketamine for children
    - -Benzodiazepines for older patients

MEDICATIONS

- Ketamine: 1–2 mg/kg IV or 4 mg/kg IM
- Midazolam: 1 mg IV slowly q 2–3 min up to 5 mg; 6 mo–5 yrs: 0.05–0.1 mg/kg, titrate to maximum of 0.6 mg/kg; 6–12 years: 0.025–0.05 mg/kg, titrate to maximum of 0.4 mg/kg
- Fentanyl: 2–3 μg/kg IV

Disposition

ADMISSION CRITERIA

- Hospital admission is usually not necessary

DISCHARGE CRITERIA

- The patient should be instructed not to place any objects in the ear
- A short course of analgesics after traumatic foreign body removal
- Otitis externa
  - —Topical antimicrobial such as cortisporin suspension
- Immunocompromised patients may require oral antibiotics
- Perforated tympanic membrane
  - —Prophylaxis with antibiotics
  - —ENT follow-up

Miscellaneous

ICD9: 931

CORE CONTENT CODE: 6.1.2

SUGGESTED READINGS

Bressler K, Shelton C. Ear foreign body removal: A review of 98 consecutive cases. Laryngoscope 1993;103:367–370.

Hanson RM, Stephens M. Cyanoacrylate-assisted foreign body removal from the ear and nose in children. J Paediatr Child Health 1994;30:77–78.

Author: Charles V. Pollack, Jr.

Foreign Body, Nasal

Clinical Presentation

SIGNS AND SYMPTOMS

- Most nasal foreign bodies are asymptomatic
- Someone witnesses the child putting an object into their nose
- Foreign body is noticed by the parent or caretaker
- Nasal discharge
  - —Acute or chronic
  - —Unilateral
  - —Foul smelling
  - —Halitosis
- Sinus discomfort
- Epistaxis
- Local inflammation
- Septal perforation
- Ingestion or aspiration of the foreign body

MECHANISM/DESCRIPTION

- Types of foreign bodies
  - —Limited only by nostril size and the imagination and activity of the child
  - —Most are innocuous with sinusitis being the principal risk
    - -Food
    - -Paper
    - -Pieces of toys
    - -Beads
    - -Rocks
    - -Button batteries: high risk of complications as compared with other foreign bodies; tissue necrosis; septal perforation; require rapid removal
- Average age is 2–4 years
- Age is not associated with a particular type of foreign body

ETIOLOGY

N/A

Pre-Hospital

CAUTIONS

- Transport in the sitting position
  - —Avoid posterior displacement and possible aspiration of the foreign body
- Avoid interventions that will upset the child

Diagnosis

ESSENTIAL WORKUP

- Visualization of the foreign body in the nostril

LABORATORY

N/A

IMAGING/SPECIAL TESTS

- Fiberoptic visualization of the foreign body if it cannot be visualized on rhinoscopy
- Sinus films if present for an extended period
  - —Clinical signs of sinusitis
  - —Persistence of symptoms despite removal of the foreign body and antibiotics

DIFFERENTIAL DIAGNOSIS

- Sinusitis
- Epistaxis
- Intranasal mass

Treatment

INITIAL STABILIZATION

N/A

ED TREATMENT

- Topical vasoconstrictors
  - —When mucosal edema is present or when bleeding has occurred secondary to removal attempts
    - -Nebulized epinephrine
    - -Cocaine 4%
    - -Lidocaine 4%
- Positive pressure
  - —Occlude the contralateral nostril
  - —Positive pressure is applied to the mouth only
  - —Deliver a brisk puff as the child begins to inhale using mouth-to-mouth
    - -The parent may tell the child that they will be given a "big kiss"
    - -The foreign body dislodges onto the cheek of the provider or into the room
    - -Placement of 4×4 gauze pads on the caregiver's cheek
    - -May be repeated as necessary
  - —Alternatively deliver the puff with a bag-mask over the mouth and O_2 at 10–15 L/min
- Hooked probe, alligator forceps
  - —Best with very anterior foreign bodies that are easily grasped
  - —Headlamp and nasal speculum facilitate use
  - —The risk is further posterior displacement
- Balloon catheters
  - —Used primarily when instrumentation fails
  - —A 5F or 6F Foley or Fogarty balloon catheter is lubricated with 2% lidocaine jelly
  - —Advance catheter past the object
  - —Following inflation with 2–3 ml of air, the catheter is gently withdrawn
- Suction catheter
  - —Optimal retrieval may be with the Schunkt-neck suction catheter
    - -Metal with plastic umbrella at the tip
  - —The tip is place against the object
  - —Suction is turned to 100–140 mm Hg
  - —The catheter and object are removed
  - —Best for round, smooth objects
- Cyanoacrylate tissue glue
  - —A fine film of cyanoacrylate glue is applied to the cut end of a hollow plastic swab stick
  - —Apply against the object for 60 seconds, then withdraw
  - —Cyanoacrylate tissue glue is presently being approved by the FDA
  - —Caution with other cyanoacrylate glues because tissue irritation may occur
- Referral for ambulatory surgical removal
  - —The foreign body cannot be recovered
  - —Removal under general anesthesia is required

MEDICATIONS

- Cocaine: 4% solution, 2 drops in the affected nares
- Lidocaine: 4% solution, 2 drops in the affected nares
- Phenylephrine 2–3 sprays per nostril q3–4h 0.125–0.5%

Disposition

ADMISSION CRITERIA

N/A

DISCHARGE CRITERIA

- Ensuring all foreign bodies have been removed, patients may be discharged home
- Return if bleeding or evidence of infection (nasal discharge)
- If a button battery was removed
  - —Mandatory follow-up with an ENT specialist
  - —Monitor for any delayed sequelae
    - -Ischemic mucosa
    - -Turbinate or septal damage
    - -Saddle-nose deformity

Miscellaneous

ICD9: 933.0

CORE CONTENT CODE: 6.2.3, 13.7.2

SUGGESTED READINGS

Backlin SA. Positive-pressure technique for nasal foreign body removal in children. Ann Emerg Med 1995;25(4):554–555.

Browne CRS. Intranasal button battery causing septal perforation: A case report. J Laryngol Otol 1994;108:589–590.

Douglas AR. Use of nebulized adrenaline to aid expulsion of intranasal foreign bodies in children. J Laryngol Otol 1996;110:559–560.

Hanson RM, Stephens M. Cyanoacrylate-assisted foreign body removal from the ear and nose in children. J Paediatr Child Health 1994;30:77–78.

Kadish HA, Corneli HM. Removal of nasal foreign bodies in the pediatric population. Am J Emerg Med 1997;15(1):54–56.

Palmer O, Natarajan B, Johnstone A, Sheikh S. Button battery in the nose—An unusual foreign body. J Laryngol Otol 1994;108:871–872.

Tong MC, Ying SY, van Hasselt CA. Nasal foreign bodies in children. Int J Pediatr Otorhinolaryngol 1996;35(3):207–211.

Author: Paul Blackburn

Foreign Body, Rectal

Clinical Presentation

SIGNS AND SYMPTOMS

- Complaint of rectal foreign body
- Rectal fullness
- Rectal pain
- Perirectal abscess (with imbedded bones/toothpick)
- Foreign body on rectal examination

MECHANISM/DESCRIPTION

- Self-insertion (autoeroticism)
  —Phallic substitutes inserted by patient or partner
  —Foreign bodies used to aid in removal of feces
- Ingested
  —Chicken bones
  —Fish bones
  —Toothpick
- Iatrogenic
  —Thermometer
  —Enema tips
- Assault
  —Knife or pipe forcibly inserted
  —Incidence of perforation is very high

Pre-Hospital

CAUTIONS

- Patient has usually tried to remove the foreign body and failed
- Further attempts at extraction will not work and could cause a perforation

Diagnosis

ESSENTIAL WORKUP

- Identify the number, type, and duration of foreign body(s) and mechanism of insertion
- Physical exam with emphasis on abdominal and rectal examinations
- Biplane x-ray films to confirm number and size of foreign body(s)
- For assaulted patients, workup as for blunt trauma to abdomen

LABORATORY

- CBC
  —For bleeding or peritonitis
- Urinalysis
  —For urethral/bladder injuries

DIFFERENTIAL DIAGNOSIS

- Pseudoforeign body
  —Patients insist there is a foreign body when x-ray, rectal examinations, and proctoscopy are normal
- Perirectal abscess
- Hemorrhoid

Treatment

INITIAL STABILIZATION

- Perforation with peritonitis and sepsis
  - —0.9%NS IV fluid 500 cc bolus
  - —Broad spectrum antibiotics
  - —Gentamicin, clindamycin, ampicillin
  - —Urgent surgical consult
- ATLS with multiple trauma victims

ED TREATMENT

Foreign Body Removal

- Small objects that are not fragile or sharp
  - —Can be removed if the object can be firmly held
  - —Remove with gentle but firm continuous traction to overcome the anal sphincter
  - —Colonic mucosa tightly adherent to distal end of foreign body creates vacuum and impedes withdrawl of object
  - —Passage of a Foley catheter beyond the object with insufflation of air breaks vacuum and permits retrieval
- Removal with some direct visualization and a large operating anoscope (following blockage of sphincter and pudendal nerve with local anesthesia) for
  - —Larger objects
  - —Objects that have remained >24 hours with resulting edema
  - —Objects with sharp edges
- Proctoscopy/sigmoidoscopy post extraction to examine the colonic mucosa

MEDICATIONS

- Ampicillin: 1–2 g (peds: 50–200 mg/kg/24hrs) IV q 4–6 hrs
- Clindamycin: 600–900 mg (peds: 20–40 mg/kg/24hrs) IV q 8 hrs
- Gentamicin: 1 mg/kg (peds: 2–2.5 mg/kg) IV q 8 hrs

PEDIATRIC CONSIDERATIONS

- Removal under general anesthesia for children who are too young to cooperate
- It is probably child abuse if a foreign body other than enema tips or thermometer is present

Disposition

ADMISSION CRITERIA

- Failed extraction in ED requires surgical removal in operating room
- Evidence of mucosal tear on proctoscopy should be observed for 24 hours (no antibiotic indicated)
- Symptoms of rectal pain associated with removal of a sharp foreign body indicates the possibility of a small perforation with developing abscess and requires examination under anesthesia

DISCHARGE CRITERIA

- Reliable patient with an atraumatic insertion and removal of a rectal foreign body.
  - —Instruct to return for rectal pain, abdominal pain, fever or massive rectal bleeding

Miscellaneous

ICD9: 937

CORE CONTENT CODE: 1.8.1.5

SUGGESTED READINGS

Abcarian H. Colorectal foreign bodies. In: Mazier PW, et al., eds. Surgery of the colon, rectum, and anus. Philadelphia: WB Saunders, 1995.

Eftaiha M, Hambrick E, Abcarian H. Principles of management of colorectal foreign bodies. Dis Colon Rectum 1977;112:691–695.

Janicke DM, Pundt MR. Anorectal disorders. Emerg Med Clinic North Am 1996;14:757–788.

Nehme-Kingsley A, Abcarian H. Colorectal foreign bodies management update. Dis Colon Rectum 1985;28:941–944.

Author: Charles Orsay

Fournier's Gangrene

Clinical Presentation

SIGNS AND SYMPTOMS

- A *rapidly progressive* necrotizing subcutaneous and fascial infection of the *perineum;* usually seen in diabetics or immunocompromised patients
- Patients are often *toxic* in appearance with nausea, vomiting, fever, and chills
- Sources of infection may be *genitourinary, rectal,* or *penile/scrotal*
- Skin findings include bronze or violaceous discoloration of the skin, a thin brown watery discharge, ulceration, bullous vesicles, subcutaneous gas, frank necrosis, and eschar formation
- Early on pain is out of proportion to the examination, but eventually the dead tissue becomes *insensate*
- Lethargy and an *inappropriate indifference to the illness* are common

MECHANISM/DESCRIPTION

- Hygiene problems lead to *skin maceration* and *excoriation* providing bacteria access to the subcutaneous tissue
- Once the skin barrier is broken, polymicrobial flora spread along the *fascial planes* of the perineum
- Colles' fascia fuses with the urogenital diaphragm slowing propagation posteriorly and laterally
- Anteriorly, Buck's and Scarpa's fascia are continuous allowing rapid extension to anterior abdominal wall, as well as laterally along the fascia lata
- *The testes are usually spared*
- Three anatomic origins account for the majority of cases
  —40% lower urinary tract: urethral strictures, indwelling catheters
  —30% penile or scrotal: condom catheters, hydradenitis, and balanitis
  —30% anorectal: fistulae, perirectal infections, and hemorrhoids
- Rarely, intra-abdominal sources such as perforating appendicitis, diverticulitis or pancreatitis has produced Fournier's gangrene by dependent contiguous spread

ETIOLOGY

- An infection by *polymicrobial flora* (mixed aerobic and anaerobic organisms)
- The mixed bacteria exert a synergistic tissue destructive effect
- End arterial thrombosis in the subcutaneous tissues produces an anaerobic environment promoting extension of the infection
- Bacterial toxins and tissue necrosis factors may contribute to the clinical presentation

Risk factors

IMMUNOCOMPROMISED	*HYGIENE PROBLEMS*	*POSTSURGICAL*
Diabetes mellitus	Homeless	Circumcision
Alcoholism	Paraplegic	Anal biopsy
HIV, cancer	Indwelling catheters	Vasectomy
	Hydradenitis suppurativa	Orchiectomy
	Tinea cruris	Hemorrhoidectomy
	Nursing home resident	Herniorrhaphy
	Abscess I & D	

- The original description was by the French specifically identified a penile and scrotal source

PEDIATRIC CONSIDERATIONS

- Though unusual in children, over 50 cases in children have been described
- Circumcision, balanitis, strictures, and severe diaper rash may precede the disease
- Organisms are more frequently *Staphylococcus* or *Streptococcus*
- Pediatric patients have more local disease and are less toxic

Pre-Hospital

CAUTIONS

- Patients may be hypotensive from septic shock

Diagnosis

ESSENTIAL WORKUP

- Fournier's gangrene is a clinical diagnosis
- History and physical exam with special attention to the perineum, and evaluating for signs of sepsis
- *Early surgical consultation* for emergent debridement is essential
- Other workup directed toward the relevant comorbid factors such as diabetes, alcoholism (alcohol withdrawal), and cardiovascular disease

LABORATORY

- Other than Gram stain of tissue and the associated drainage, there are *no specific laboratory tests* that are diagnostic of Fournier's gangrene
- Urinalysis should be performed in all cases
- Leukocytosis, anemia, electrolyte imbalances, acidosis, and renal failure are common
- Disseminated intravascular coagulation may be present. PT, PTT, fibrin-split products, and fibrinogen levels help identify
- If patient is suspected or known diabetic, glucose, electrolytes, and serum ketones to evaluate for diabetes and DKA
- Culture of blood, urine, and tissue (when available)

IMAGING/SPECIAL TESTS

- Plain films of the pelvis may reveal *subcutaneous emphysema* and an ileus
- CT scanning helps if an intra-abdominal or ischiorectal source is suspected
- Ultrasound has been used to demonstrate scrotal gas with a normal underlying testicle
- Chest radiographs may reveal ARDS (and associated comorbid factors)
- Retrograde urethrography, anoscopy, proctosigmoidoscopy, and barium enemas may be helpful to localize anatomic sources of infection

DIFFERENTIAL DIAGNOSIS

- Testicular torsion
- Scrotal cellulitis
- Epididymitis/orchitis
- Tinea cruris
- Scrotal abscess/inguinal abscess
- Perirectal infections
- Insect and human bites

PEDIATRIC CONSIDERATIONS

- Pediatric consultation to assist with medical management and guide a *more conservative* surgical approach

Treatment

INITIAL STABILIZATION

- ABCs
- Central venous access, fluid resuscitation, and pressure support as indicated
- Avoid femoral access, femoral venipuncture, and lower extremity venous access

ED TREATMENT

- Empiric *broad spectrum antibiotics*
- Early *emergent aggressive surgical debridement*
- *Hyperbaric oxygen therapy* coordinated with surgical care (preoperatively if available)
  - —Early transfer to a facility with appropriate surgical and hyperbaric capability may be lifesaving
- Electrolyte correction (dehydration, hypokalemia, or hyperkalemia)
- Metabolic control directed at diabetes if present
- Prophylaxis for the complications of alcoholism and alcohol withdrawal
- Blood products as needed for DIC or anemia. As with other causes of life-threatening sepsis, oxygen debt can be minimized by keeping the hematocrit >30%
- Tetanus prophylaxis

MEDICATIONS

- Antibiotic regimens
  - —Multidrug regimen
    - -Ampicillin: 2 g IV q 6 hrs (peds: 50 mg/kg) *and*
    - -Clindamycin: 900 mg IV q 8 hrs (peds: 10 mg/kg) *and*
    - -Gentamicin: 5 mg/kg daily load IV div q 8 hrs
  - —Single drug regimens (peds: safety not established)
    - -Ticarcillin/clavulanate: 3.1 g IV initial ED dose *or*
    - -Ampicillin/sulbactam: 3 g IV initial ED dose
- Blood products as indicated
- Dopamine or dobutamine IV drips starting at 5 μg/kg/min titrating to effect if hypotensive
- Insulin adjusted to control glucose and acidosis

PEDIATRIC CONSIDERATIONS

- More conservative surgical approach
- Adequate *Staphylococcal* coverage

Disposition

ADMISSION CRITERIA

- *All* patients with Fournier's gangrene require admission and surgical *intensive care unit* admission
- Mortality estimates of 10% to 50% emphasize the need for early aggressive care

DISCHARGE CRITERIA

- No patients with Fournier's gangrene should be discharged

Miscellaneous

ICD9: 608.83

CORE CONTENT CODE: 19.2.3.3

SUGGESTED READINGS

Adams JR, Mata JA, Venable DD, et al. Fournier's gangrene in children. Urology 1990;35(5):439–441.

Clayton MD, Fowler JE, Sharifi R, et al. Causes, presentation and survival of fifty-seven patients with necrotizing fasciitis of the male genitalia. Surg Gynecol Obstet 1990;170:49–55.

Eltorai IM, Hart GB, Strauss MB, et al. The role of hyperbaric oxygen in the management of Fournier's gangrene. Int Surg 1986;71:53–58.

Grant RW, Mitchell-Heggs P. Radiologic features of Fournier gangrene. Radiology 1981;140:641–643.

Spirnak JP, Resnick MI, Hampel N, et al. Fournier's gangrene: Report of 20 patients J Urol 1984;131:289–291.

Authors: Lance Brown; William Mallon

Fracture, Open

Clinical Presentation

SIGNS AND SYMPTOMS

- Deformity with nearby violation in skin integrity
- Neurovascular compromise may be present

MECHANISM/DESCRIPTION

- Continuity between skin violation and fracture site
- Type I: puncture wound with minimal soft tissue injury
- Type II: larger wound with larger soft tissue damage
- Type III: larger wound with massive soft tissue damage and severe contamination
- Predisposition to complications
  —Massive soft tissue damage
  —Severe wound contamination
  —Compromised vascularity
  —Fracture instability
  —Compromised host (diabetes, vascular disease, etc.)

Pre-Hospital

- Sterile dressings over open wound
- Immobilize the joints above and below the fracture
- Do not reduce long bone fractures unless severely angulated or neurovascularly compromised
- Military antishock trousers (MAST) can be used to immobilize the hip in femur fractures if a traction device is not available

Diagnosis

ESSENTIAL WORKUP

- Complete neurologic and vascular examination
- Plain radiographs including joints above and below the affected area
- Perform saline arthrogram by intra-articular injection of saline or methylene blue if joint involvement suspected

LABORATORY

- CBC, coagulation studies for large bone (femur, pelvis) fractures
- Type and screen or type and crossmatch for significant blood loss

IMAGING/SPECIAL TESTS

- Angiography to assess vascular damage with the following indications
  —Ischemic extremity
  —Knee dislocation
  —High energy fracture patterns
  —Massive soft tissue injury in high risk areas
- Measurement of compartment pressures if compartment syndrome suspected

DIFFERENTIAL DIAGNOSIS

- Laceration
- Abrasion

Treatment

INITIAL STABILIZATION

- ABCs of trauma care
  —30% of patients with open lower extremity fractures are multiple trauma victims
- Reduction of fracture with steady, longitudinal traction
- Immobilization with nonradiopaque device

ED TREATMENT

- Intravenous access
- Administer tetanus if needed, and parenteral antibiotics (cefazolin)
- Early orthopedic consultation for formal irrigation, débridement, and operative fixation, if needed, within 6 hours to reduce likelihood of infection
- Minimize the number of times dressing is removed to avoid secondary contamination
- Examine regularly for compartment syndrome and neurovascular status

MEDICATIONS

- Cefazolin: adult: 1–2 g; peds: 20 mg/kg IM/IV within 3 hrs of injury
- Gentamicin: 2–5 mg/kg IM/IV, or other aminoglycoside, for type II or III open fractures
- Morphine sulfate: adult: 2–10 mg; peds: 0.1 mg/kg/dose IV or equivalent analgesic
- Tetanus booster: 0.5 cc IM
- Tetanus immunoglobulin (TIG): 250 IU IM if not previously immunized against tetanus

PEDIATRIC CONSIDERATIONS

- Diphtheria-pertussis-tetanus booster for children under 7

Disposition

ADMISSION CRITERIA

- The vast majority of patients will be admitted for washout and possibly débridement or operative fixation as well as IV antibiotics

DISCHARGE CRITERIA

- Simple type I open fractures may be washed out and immobilized in the Emergency Department and discharged with oral antibiotics and very close follow-up in 24 hours

Miscellaneous

ICD9: 829.1

CORE CONTENT CODE: 18.4.12.1, 18.4.13.1

SUGGESTED READINGS

Alonso JE, Lee J, Burgess AR, Browner BD. The management of complex orthopedic injuries. Surg Clin North Am 1996;76(4):879–901.

Geiderman JM. Orthopedic injuries: Management principles. In: Rosen P, et al., eds. Emergency medicine: Concepts and clinical practice. 4th ed.St. Louis: Mosby-Year Book, 1998:602–624.

Kefer MP. Fractures and dislocations. In: Tintinalli JE, ed. Emergency medicine: A comprehensive study guide. New York: McGraw Hill, 1996:1206–1208.

O'Meara PM. Management of open fractures. Orthop Rev 1992;21(10):1177–1185.

Author: Christy Rosa

Fractures, Pediatric

Clinical Presentation

SIGNS AND SYMPTOMS

- Decreased limb movement, "pseudoparalysis"
- Swelling
- Tenderness
- Deformity
- Ecchymoses
- Crepitus
- Limp
- Abnormal neurovascular status of extremity
  - —Absence of pulse does not always indicate compromise
  - —Presence of pulse does not assure adequate circulation
  - —Severe pain in forearm or calf, pain with passive stretching of fingers or toes or sensory deficit in the distal extremity are more sensitive indicators of ischemia
- Open fracture may be obvious or subtle (collection of blood with fat globules under skin)
- Complications (long-term)
  - —Nonunion of capitulum fracture
  - —Avascular necrosis of femoral head after femoral neck fracture
  - —Neurovascular compromise
  - —Posttraumatic ossification of elbow after displaced fracture or dislocation
  - —Growth arrest if growth plate crushed
  - —Angulation or rotational deformity from initial injury or subsequent differential growth

MECHANISM/DESCRIPTION

- Bones are highly resilient, elastic, and "springy"
- Cartilaginous growth plates are potential areas of injury
- Ligaments are more resistant to injury than are growth plates
  - —Fractures often accompany dislocations
- Nonaccidental trauma if history not consistent with findings
- Salter-Harris classification
  - —Risk of growth disturbance increases from Type I to Type V
  - —Type I
    - -Separation of epiphysis from metaphysis without displacement or injury to the growth plate
    - -Tenderness and pain at point of growth plate without other findings
    - -X-ray normal initially but when repeated in 7–10 days may show calcification and new bone formation
    - -Growth disturbance is rare
  - —Type II
    - -Epiphyseal plate slip with fracture through the metaphysis, producing a triangular metaphyseal fragment
    - -Most common
    - -Growth disturbance is rare
  - —Type III
    - -Epiphyseal plate slip with an intra-articular fracture involving the epiphysis
    - -Most common site is distal tibial epiphysis
  - —Type IV
    - -Intra-articular fracture extending through the epiphysis, epiphyseal plate, and metaphysis. Lateral condyle of humerus is most common site
  - —Type V
    - -Crush injury to epiphyseal plate, producing growth arrest
    - -Usually occurs in joints such as knee

ETIOLOGY

- Mechanism is useful in defining the potential and type of injury
  - —Falls, motor vehicle accidents, blunt trauma, nonaccidental trauma
- Obesity and rapid growth spurts are risk factors
- Commonly fractures involve lower forearm, clavicle, tibia or fibula, supracondylar fracture of humerus
- Nonaccidental trauma—consider if specific fractures
  - —Fractures of the radius/ulna, tibia/fibula, or femur in children <1 year
  - —Midshaft or metaphyseal fractures of the humerus in children <3 years
  - —Epiphyseal lesions (especially chip fractures)
  - —Rib fractures
  - —Skull fractures, especially in children <1 year
  - —Unexplained, inconsistent, or multiple fractures (especially at different stages of healing)
  - —Subperiosteal ossification without previous known fracture
  - —Unusual behavior in child or parent

Pre-Hospital

CAUTIONS

- Immobilize/splint involved extremity
- Assess for neurovascular status

Diagnosis

ESSENTIAL WORKUP

- Assess neurovascular status
- Exclude concurrent injuries
- Assure that history consistent with injury
- AP, lateral, and oblique radiographs as necessary, including the joint above and below the fracture
  - —Comparison views may be useful if growth plates involved

LABORATORY

- Required only if concomitant injuries, surgery anticipated, or multiple/major bone involvement
- CBC and sedimentation rate to evaluate for infection

IMAGING/SPECIAL TESTS

- Followup radiographs may be required to exclude Salter I fracture
- Bone scans may be useful to exclude fractures if plain radiographs are unhelpful or to evaluate for infection

DIFFERENTIAL DIAGNOSIS

- Infection
- Tumor
- Neurologic deficits
- Subtle dislocations such as radial head subluxation (Nursemaid's elbow)
- Nonaccidental trauma

Treatment

INITIAL STABILIZATION

- Resuscitation for concurrent injuries

ED TREATMENT

- Management of life-threatening concurrent injuries
- Dislocations require immediate assessment and attention to neurovascular compromise
- Mechanism may help in understanding the direction of the force required to relocate
- Alignment is essential, particularly when it involves a joint surface
- Angulation of metaphyseal fractures is tolerated; remodeling often dealing with up to 30°
- Open fractures require attention to convert an open wound to a clean closed wound
- Appropriate reporting of nonaccidental trauma

Salter-Harris Fractures

- Type I and Type II require 3 weeks immobilization for upper extremity and 6 weeks for lower extremities
- Type II distal femur fractures, Type III and Type IV require referral for anatomic reduction
- Type V requires immobilization and consultation

Clavicle Fracture

- Figure-of-eight splint and sling as tolerated for comfort
- Distal third clavicle fractures may be referred with initial sling and swathe or shoulder immobilizer

Supracondylar Humerus Fracture

- Orthopedic consultation because of potential complications
  - —Brachial artery injury
  - —Volar-compartment syndrome of forearm
  - —Epiphyseal injury with long-term growth abnormalities

Distal Radius and Ulnar Fractures

- Rotational deformities must be eliminated
- Reduce angulated fractures >15°
- Immobilize for 4–6 weeks
- Torus fracture (buckling or angulation of cortex)
  - —Immobilize in long arm splint for 4–6 weeks
- Greenstick fracture (diaphysis of long bone with fracture on one side of cortex)
  - —Immobilize in long-arm splint for 4–6 weeks
- Colles fracture
  - —Reduce by traction in the line of deformity to disimpact the fragments, followed by pressure on the dorsal aspect of the distal fragment and volar aspect of the proximal fragment
  - —Correct radial deviation
  - —Immobilize the hand in ulnar deviation, wrist in neutral, and forearm in full pronation
  - —Orthopedic consultation

Tibial or Fibular Fracture

- Isolated fibular fractures: short-leg walking cast
- Undisplaced tibial fracture: long-leg posterior splint, nonweight-bearing
- Displaced tibial fracture and complex fractures require consultation

MEDICATIONS

- For sedation/analgesia during reduction
  - —Fentanyl (Sublimaze): 1–5 μg/kg IV slowly (20-min half-life)
  - —Midazolam (Versed): 0.05–0.10 mg/kg/dose IV over 1–2 min (max: 4 mg/dose)
    - -Often used with fentanyl
  - —Ketamine: 1–5 mg/kg IM (max: 50 mg/dose) with atropine 0.01 mg/kg
    - -Most useful in children 3 months to 7 years because of side effects

Disposition

ADMISSION CRITERIA

- Nonaccidental trauma (or per social services)
- Potential neurovascular compromise
  - —Condylar or supracondylar humerus fracture
  - —Femoral shaft
  - —Complete patella

DISCHARGE CRITERIA

- Uncomplicated fracture: no concurrent injury or neurovascular/compartment compromise
- Followup arranged and parents understand injury and management

Miscellaneous

ICD9: 829.0

CORE CONTENT CODE: 18.6.7

SUGGESTED READINGS

Adams J, Hamblen D. Outline of fractures. 10th ed. New York: Churchill Livingstone, 1992.

Leventhal J, et al. Fractures in young children. Distinguishing child abuse from unintentional injuries. Am J Dis Child 1993;147:87–92.

Authors: Leslie Milne; Adam Barkin

Frontal Sinus Fracture

Clinical Presentation

SIGNS AND SYMPTOMS

- Contusion, bruise, or laceration on the forehead overlying the frontal sinus
- Depression or swelling over the frontal sinus area
- Crepitus over the frontal sinus
- Loss of consciousness or altered mental status secondary to associated brain injury or posterior table fracture
- Associated facial trauma with supraorbital, orbital, nasal, frontonasoethmoid, or maxillary fractures
- Associated ocular trauma may be present
- Bloody discharge from the nose, without visible nasal source
- Clear rhinorrhea indicative of cerebrospinal fluid leak
- Absent tearing which may be indicative of nasofrontal duct injury

MECHANISM/DESCRIPTION

- Typically due to high-velocity blunt trauma localized to the frontal sinus area
- Because the anterior table is thick it requires 800–2200 pounds of force to cause frontal sinus fracture (twice the force required to fracture other facial bones)
- Most frontal sinus fractures are from motor vehicle accidents, although altercations or assaults, usually with a weapon such as a cue stick or baseball bat, can also create enough localized force to cause the injury

PEDIATRIC CONSIDERATIONS

- The frontal sinuses are not fully formed in children and this is a rare injury. The force required to create this injury is usually transmitted to the frontal bones and brain

Pre-Hospital

CAUTIONS

- Airway control takes precedence
  —Associated facial injuries may preclude the use of oral intubation
  —Nasotracheal intubation is contraindicated in massive facial or nasal trauma
  —Cricothyrotomy is the airway of choice if intubation using RSI cannot be performed
- Most patients with frontal sinus fractures have serious associated injuries due to amount of force needed to create the injury
  —If associated injuries are present, protect the cervical spine
- 75% of patients with frontal sinus fractures lose consciousness
- The frontal sinus fracture is not the immediate concern in a multiple trauma victim

Diagnosis

ESSENTIAL WORKUP

- The physical examination is the most important aspect of the evaluation. Failure to diagnose a frontal sinus fracture can lead to abscess formation, meningitis, mucocele formation, osteomyelitis of the calvarium, or permanent cosmetic deformity
- Look for more serious injuries first, and treat life-threats
- Carefully palpate the frontal area for crepitus or depression
- Lacerations over the frontal sinus area mandate digital palpation for a fracture line and a careful visual exploration for underlying fractures
- Perform a nasal speculum examination looking for blood, septal hematoma, or CSF high in the nasal cavity
- Perform a careful neurologic examination to look for CNS injury
- Perform a careful ophthalmologic exam

IMAGING/SPECIAL TESTS

- Caldwell and lateral views are good for preliminary evaluation but frontal sinus fractures can be subtle on these films
- *CT scanning is the imaging modality of choice.* Altered mental status or history of loss of consciousness, or discovery of an anterior table fracture by exam or on plain films should be further investigated by CT to rule out associated posterior table fracture or intracranial injury
  —Associated intracranial injuries on CT may include subdural hemorrhage or pneumocephalus

ASSOCIATED CONDITIONS

- Frontal sinus fractures may disrupt the frontonasal duct
- Intracranial injuries are present in 12–17% of patients with frontal sinus fractures
- About 15% of patients with frontal sinus fractures have an associated CSF leak
- Ocular injuries are present in up to 59%

DIFFERENTIAL DIAGNOSIS

- Nasofrontoethmoid fractures, cribriform plate fractures, and facial fractures including the orbits, maxilla, nasal, and zygomatic bones
- Frontal fractures not involving the frontal sinus may have a similar presentation

Treatment

INITIAL STABILIZATION

- ABCs of trauma care, attend to the airway as the first priority
  - —RSI is the initial airway management of choice
  - —Massive facial injuries may require a surgical airway if RSI is unsuccessful
- If associated injuries are present, protect the cervical spine until cleared
- Other major injuries and life-threats take precedence over the frontal sinus fracture

ED TREATMENT

- If while irrigating a laceration overlying the frontal sinus the patient can taste the irrigating solution or notes the irrigating fluid in the nose, the frontal sinus is disrupted
- If a simple anterior table fracture is noted, and posterior table fracture and intracranial injuries are ruled out, the presence of a frontonasal duct injury should be evaluated by instilling fluorescein into the frontal sinus. Lack of visualization of the fluorescein in the nose is indicative of disruption of the duct
- Antibiotics are indicated in all patients with frontal sinus fractures. Intravenous antibiotics are indicated in patients with posterior table fractures or CSF leaks
- Lacerations overlying frontal sinus fractures involving only the anterior table may be sutured in the ED. ENT or plastic surgery should evaluate lacerations associated with more complex sinus injuries

MEDICATIONS

- Cefotaxime: adult: 2 g IV; peds: 50 mg/kg IV single dose
- Cephalexin: adult: 250–500 mg po qid; peds: 25–50 mg/kg/day div qid

Disposition

ADMISSION CRITERIA

- Patients with other significant associated trauma
- Patients with posterior table fractures (to neurosurgery or ENT)
- Patients with associated intracranial injuries (neurosurgery)
- Patients with CSF leak

DISCHARGE CRITERIA

- Patients with frontal sinus fractures who may be discharged are those with isolated injuries only who have no involvement of the posterior table or evidence of an intracranial injury on CT. Oral antibiotics are indicated in these patients. Referral to ENT in 24–36 hours is appropriate

Miscellaneous

ICD9: 801.00

CORE CONTENT CODE: 18.4.4.1

SUGGESTED READINGS

Keefe SD, et al. Frontal sinus fractures. In: English GM, ed. Otolaryngology. Vol 4. Rev ed. Philadelphia: JB Lippincott, 1994: 342–364.

Manson PN. Maxillofacial injuries. Emerg Med Clin North Am 1984;2(4):761–82.

Rohrich RJ, et al. Management of frontal sinus fractures: Changing concepts. Clin Plast Surg 1992;19(1):219–32.

Authors: Mark L. Madenwald; David W. Munter MD, MBA, FACEP

Frostbite

Clinical Presentation

SIGNS AND SYMPTOMS

- Penis, fingers, toes, ears, and nose most commonly affected
- Initial appearance of an injury often fails to predict eventual depth or outcome

Superficial Frostbite

- Skin structures only involved
- Appearance
  - —Initially white/waxy/mottled
  - —Becomes hyperemic and edematous as warming progresses
- Loss of sensation to touch, pain, or temperature with frozen skin
- Stinging, numbness, burning
- No tissue loss ultimately

Deep Frostbite

- Subcutaneous, muscle, nerve, or bone involved
- Tissue feels hard like a wood log
- Initially no sensation with severe pain/burning with rewarming
- Reduced mobility even after rewarming if deep structures damaged
- Tissue loss inevitable

Postrewarming Appearance

- Postrewarming edema begins within 3 hours and lasts 5 days
- Large clear blebs form within 6–24 hours
- Small, hemorrhagic blebs form after 24 hours
  - —Associated with deeper injury
- Eschar forms in 9–15 days
- Mummification in 3–6 weeks
- Persistent mottling and anesthesia despite edema after rewarming are unfavorable prognostic indicators

MECHANISM/DESCRIPTION

- Tissue damage results from
  - —*Direct cell damage*—due to intracellular ice crystal formation
  - —*Indirect cell damage*—extracellular ice crystal formation leads to intracellular dehydration through osmosis
  - —*Microvascular stasis and thrombosis*—erythrocyte sludging leads to hypoxia then vasospasm, ischemia, tissue necrosis
  - —*Progressive dermal ischemia*—mediated by thromboxane and prostaglandins in blisters
  - —*Reperfusion injury*—after thawing, caused by edema then thrombosis, inflammatory leukocyte infiltration, and necrosis
  - —*Thermal shock*—direct cell death due to the extreme cold
- Devitalized tissue demarcates as the injury evolves over weeks to months

PEDIATRIC CONSIDERATIONS

- Children are more vulnerable to cold stress and frostbite

Pre-Hospital

CAUTIONS

- Protect and immobilize frostbitten area during transport
- Remove restrictive or wet garments
- Avoid dry rewarming of the frostbitten limb if there is a likelihood of refreezing of the injury
  - —If evacuation will be delayed and suitable facilities are available, field rewarming in warm (40–42° C) water can be attempted
- Rubbing, manipulating the limb or applying snow while it is still frozen is contraindicated
- Hypothermia
  - —Common in frostbite victims
  - —Avoid rough handling to minimize possibility of cardiac dysrhythmias in the seriously hypothermic patient
- Look for evidence of intoxication, head injury, trauma, hypoglycemia, cardiac, or neurologic problems as underlying etiologies and treat them appropriately

Diagnosis

ESSENTIAL WORKUP

- Diagnosis is based on the clinical presentation

LABORATORY

- None indicated in most cases
- Baseline studies for severe frostbite
  - —CBC
  - —Electrolytes, BUN/Cr, glucose
- Urinalysis for evidence for myoglobinuria in severe frostbite
- Cultures and Gram stains from open areas when infection suspected

DIFFERENTIAL DIAGNOSIS

- Frostnip
  - —Superficial, reversible ice crystal formation without tissue destruction
  - —Transient numbness and paraesthesia resolve after rewarming
- Trench foot
  - —Exposure to wet cold for prolonged periods
  - —Neurovascular damage without ice crystal formation
  - —Pallor, mottling, paraesthesiae, pulselessness, paralysis, and numbness
  - —Hyperemia with rewarming lasting up to 6 weeks
- Chilblains
  - —Chronic repeated exposure to dry cold
  - —Localized erythema, cyanosis, plaques, and vesicles

Treatment

INITIAL STABILIZATION

- ABCs
- Identify and correct hypothermia
- IV fluid volume expansion with 0.9%NS for severe frostbite
- Protect frostbitten areas from excessive handling or dry warming during resuscitation

ED TREATMENT

- If the injury is less than 24 hours old and has not yet been rewarmed
  - —Initiate rapid thawing of the injured extremity for 10–30 minutes in 40–42° C water
  - —Stop treatment when the limb is warm, red, and pliable
  - —Monitor water temperature closely to prevent thermal injury
- Analgesia
- NSAID (ibuprofen)
  - —Combat the effects of prostaglandins on skin necrosis
- Aloe vera topical cream
  - —Combats the arachidonic cascade
  - —Recommended for all intact blisters
- Blister débridement or aspiration
  - —Indicated for clear blebs (removes thromboxane and prostaglandins)
  - —Contraindicated for hemorrhagic blebs (exposes deeper structures to dehydration and infection)
- Tetanus prophylaxis
- Antibacterial prophylaxis
  - —Consider during the hyperemic recovery phase (at least 2-3 days) in severely frostbitten areas
  - —Against streptococci, staphylococci, and pseudomonas species (cephelosporin, penicillinase-resistant penicillin, quinolone)
  - —Topical antibacterial agents interfere with the use of aloe vera cream and should be considered a second line approach
- Elevation and splinting of frostbitten area
- Change dressing 2–4 times daily
- Avoid vasoconstrictive agents (including tobacco)

MEDICATIONS

- Aloe vera: topical cream 70% concentration q 6 hrs. Avoid preparations containing alcohol, scent, salicylates, which interfere with its effectiveness
- Cephalexin (cephalosporin): 500 mg (ped: 25–50 mg/kg/24hrs q 6 hrs) po qid
- Ciprofloxacin (quinolone): 500 mg po bid
- Dicloxacillin (penicillinase-resistant penicillin): 500 mg (ped: 25–100 mg/kg/24hrs q 6 hrs) po qid
- Ibuprofen (NSAID): 800 mg (ped: 40 mg/kg/24hrs q 6–8 hrs) po tid

Disposition

ADMISSION CRITERIA

- All but the most superficial and painless cases should be admitted for at least 24–48 hours after rewarming
- Lower admission threshold where risk of refreezing exists

DISCHARGE CRITERIA

- Rewarmed injury with evidence of only superficial injury with close follow-up

Miscellaneous

ICD9: 991.3

CORE CONTENT CODE: 5.8.2.2

SUGGESTED READINGS

Danzl DF. Frostbite. In: Rosen P, Barkin R, et al. eds. Emergency medicine: Concepts and clinical practice. 4th ed. St. Louis: CV Mosby, 1998:953–962.

McCauley RL, et al. Frostbite and other cold-induced injuries. In: Auerbach PS, ed. Wilderness medicine. St. Louis: CV Mosby, 1995:129–145.

McCauley RL, et al. Frostbite: Methods to minimize tissue loss. Postgrad Med 1990;88(8):67–77.

Skolnick AA. Early data suggest clot-dissolving drug may help save frostbitten limbs from amputation. JAMA 1992;267(15):2008–2009.

Author: Paul Arnold

Gallstone Ileus

Clinical Presentation

SIGNS AND SYMPTOMS

- Abdominal cramping
  - —Pain episodic
- Nausea
- Vomiting
  - —Can be feculent
- Obstipation
- Abdominal distention
- Abdominal tenderness
  - —Peritoneal findings late
- Abnormal bowel sounds
- Jaundice in 10%
- Initial pain may be suggestive of biliary colic

MECHANISM/DESCRIPTION

- Mechanical intestinal obstruction secondary to the impaction of a gallstone in the bowel lumen
- Gallstone ileus is responsible for
  - —1–4% of all intestinal obstructions
  - —Approximately 25% of those found in patients over age 65

ETIOLOGY

- Chronic stone inflammation in the gallbladder leads to the development of adhesions between the gallbladder and adjacent bowel wall
- A cholecystenteric fistula develops permitting stone passage into the intestine
- Majority of fistulas occur between the gall bladder and duodenum
- Stones usually lodge in the terminal ileum (narrowest portion of the small intestine) causing complete or partial obstruction of the bowel
  - —Gallstone obstruction of large bowel is rare
- Cholecystocolic fistulas occur in 15%
- Stones spilled during cholecystectomy—open or laparoscopic—intraperitoneally may also lead to bowel obstruction
- Recurrent obstruction in 2–10% because of additional stones present in the bowel or migration of common duct stones

PEDIATRIC CONSIDERATIONS

- Very uncommon in children but reported in a 13-year-old

Pre-Hospital

CAUTIONS

- IV hydration for dehydration/hypotension

Diagnosis

ESSENTIAL WORKUP

- Evaluation for intestinal obstruction

LABORATORY

- Electrolytes, BUN, Cr, glucose
  - —Vomiting leads to hypochloremia, hypokalemia, hyponatremia, alkalosis
- Amylase—elevated in late obstructions
- CBC/hematocrit
  - —Hemoconcentration secondary to dehydration

IMAGING/SPECIAL TESTS

- Flat and upright abdominal radiographs
  - —Multiple air fluid levels and distended bowel consistent with bowel obstruction
  - —Direct visualization of the stone uncommon on plain films
- Chest x-ray
  - —Evaluate for pneumoperitoneum
- Criteria for radiographic diagnosis of gallstone ileus (2 of 3 needed)
  - —Air in the biliary tree (pneumobilia)
  - —Partial or complete bowel obstruction
  - —Aberrant gallstone visualized or indirect visualization via contrast medium in the bowel
- Abdominal CT scan
  - —Effective in delineating causes of bowel obstruction including gallstone ileus
- Abdominal ultrasound
  - —Can make diagnosis with visualization of gallstone

DIFFERENTIAL DIAGNOSIS

- Paralytic ileus
- Extrinsic bowel obstruction—adhesions, volvulus, hernia, intussusception
- GI malignancy
- Diverticulitis
- Bezoar
- Inflammatory bowel disease
- Pseudo-obstruction

Treatment

INITIAL STABILIZATION

- IV fluid resuscitation

ED TREATMENT

- Nasogastric suction to decompress the stomach and intestine
- NPO
- Electrolyte replacement
- Monitor urine output
- Analgesics
- Surgical consultation

Disposition

ADMISSION CRITERIA

- Admit all patients with bowel obstruction

DISCHARGE CRITERIA

- None

Miscellaneous

ICD9: 575.10

CORE CONTENT CODE: 1.3.4

SUGGESTED READINGS

Davies JB, Sedman PC, Benson EA. Gallstone ileus—beware of the silent second stone. Postgrad Med 1996;72:300–301.

Huynh T, Mercer CD. Early post-operative small bowel obstruction caused by spilled gallstones during laparoscopic cholecystectomy. Surgery 1996;119:352–353.

Resiner RM, Cohen JR. Gallstone ileus: A review of 1,001 reported cases. Am Surg 1994;60:441–446.

Tadurel PH, Fabre JM, Pradel JA, et al. Value of CT in the diagnosis and management of patients with suspected acute small-bowel obstruction. AJR 1995;165:1187–1192.

Author: Thomas Lukens

Gangrene

Clinical Presentation

SIGNS AND SYMPTOMS

- Sudden severe pain of extremity or involved area
- Low-grade fever
- Tachycardia out of proportion to fever
- Bronzing of the skin over involved area
- Crepitus
- Formation of blebs and bullae
- Thin, serosanguinous exudate with a sweet odor
- Rapid local extension
- Obtunded sensorium
- Systemic toxicity

MECHANISM/DESCRIPTION

- Gas gangrene or clostridial myonecrosis is an acute, rapidly progressive, gas-forming necrotizing infection of muscle and subcutaneous tissue that can be seen in posttraumatic or postoperative situations

ETIOLOGY

- Clostridial organisms, a facultative anaerobic, spore forming, Gram-positive bacillus produces a number of toxins, the most prevalent and lethal is α-toxin
- *Clostridial perfringens* is the most common bacteria; found in 80–90% of wounds
- Other clostridial bacteria isolated include *C. novyi, C. septicum, C. histolyticum, C. bifermentans* and *C. fallux*
- Two distinct mechanisms for introduction of clostridial organisms
  - —Traumatic and postoperative
  - —Nontraumatic (associated with diabetes mellitus, peripheral vascular disease, alcoholism, IVDA, and malignancies)

PEDIATRIC CONSIDERATIONS

- Similar presentation as adults

Pre-Hospital

N/A

Diagnosis

ESSENTIAL WORKUP

- History and physical examination with special attention to clinical evidence of crepitus in soft tissue
- Soft tissue x-rays of involved area to detect gas dissecting along fascial planes (however, the absence of gas does not rule out significant disease)
- Stat Gram stain of wound exudate for Gram-positive bacillus with paucity of leukocytes

LABORATORY

- CBC with differential, electrolytes, BUN, and creatinine
- Coagulation studies to evaluate for hemolysis
- Anaerobic cultures of wound or tissue biopsy

IMAGING/SPECIAL TESTS

- X-rays may reveal soft tissue gas
- CT if area involves abdomen or flank

DIFFERENTIAL DIAGNOSIS

- Cellulitis
- Necrotizing fasciitis
- Nonclostridial myositis and myonecrosis
- Other causes of gas in tissues, as from dissection from respiratory or gastrointestinal tracts

Treatment

INITIAL STABILIZATION

- ABCs
  - —Control airway as needed
  - —Supplemental oxygen; cardiac and oxygen saturation monitors should be placed
  - —Intravenous access; consider central venous pressure monitoring
  - —Aggressive volume expansion including crystalloid, plasma, packed red blood cells, and albumin

ED TREATMENT

- Parental antibiotic therapy
  - —Primary: penicillin G plus clindamycin
  - —Alternative: ceftriaxone or erythromycin
  - —If mixed infection: penicillin plus clindamycin, metronidazole, or vancomycin and Gram-negative coverage with gentamicin
- Surgical consultation
  - —Débridement, amputation, or fasciotomy are required
- Hyperbaric oxygen as adjunctive therapy
  - —Early transfer to hyperbaric facility may be life saving
- Tetanus prophylaxis
- Observe for major complication including ARDS, renal failure, myocardial irritability, and DIC
- Polyvalent antitoxin is not made in the U.S. and studies have not demonstrated efficacy. Due to the unacceptable hypersensitivity reactions it is not routinely recommended

MEDICATIONS

- Ceftriaxone: adult: 2.0 g q 12 hrs IV; peds: 100 mg/kg/dose
- Clindamycin: adult: 900 mg q 8 hrs IV; peds: 40 mg/kg/d divided q 6 hrs
- Gentamicin: adult and peds: 2.0 mg/kg IV q 8 hrs
- Metronidazole: adult: 500 mg IV q 8 hrs; peds: safety not established
- Penicillin G: adult: 24 million IU/day divided q 4–6 hrs IV; peds: 250,000 IU/kg/day IV divided q 4 hrs
- Tetanus immune globulin: 500 IU IM
- Tetanus toxoid: 0.5 mg IM

Disposition

ADMISSION CRITERIA

- All patients with gas gangrene and evidence of myonecrosis *must be admitted* for surgical debridement and IV antibiotics
- Adjunctive use of hyperbaric oxygen therapy is an important adjunct

Miscellaneous

ICD9: 040.0

CORE CONTENT CODE: 10.6.2

SUGGESTED READINGS

Corey EC. Nontraumatic gas gangrene: Case report and review of emergency therapeutics. J Emerg Med 1991;9(6):431–436.

Hart GB, Lamb RC, Strauss MB. Gas gangrene. A collective review. II. A 15-year experience with hyperbaric oxygen. J Trauma 1983;23:991.

Heimbach RD. Gas gangrene. In: Kindwall EP, ed. Hyperbaric medicine practice. Best Publishing, 1995:373–394.

Author: Karen Van Hoesen

Gastric Outlet Obstruction

Clinical Presentation

SIGNS AND SYMPTOMS

- Postprandial fullness
- Epigastric discomfort relieved with emesis
- Vomiting
  - —Occurs approximately 20–30 minutes after eating
  - —With blood if bleeding ulcer/Mallory-Weiss tear
- Vital signs
  - —Usually normal
  - —Tachycardia, hypotension with significant volume depletion
- Abdominal examination
  - —Minimal epigastric distention
  - —Tympany

MECHANISM/DESCRIPTION

- Scarring, stricture, or hyperplasia at pylorus or duodenum
- Intrinsic or extrinsic mass causing compression at pylorus or proximal duodenum

ETIOLOGY

- Peptic ulcer disease
- Pyloric stenosis
- Neoplasms
- Caustic ingestions
- Tuberculosis

PEDIATRIC CONSIDERATIONS

- Pyloric stenosis
  - —Most common cause in pediatric population
  - —May present as early as 1st week after birth and up to age 3 months
  - —Presentation
    - -Initially occasional nonprojectile postprandial vomiting
    - -Progress to nonbilious projectile vomiting
  - —Midepigastric peristaltic wave may be seen prior to vomiting
  - —Epigastric rounded mass "olive" palpable in 80–90% of patients

Pre-Hospital

N/A

Diagnosis

ESSENTIAL WORKUP

- Careful history and physical exam reveals diagnosis
- Abdominal ultrasound in pediatric patients
  - —Reveals if elongated hypertrophic pyloric sphincter

LABORATORY

- CBC
  - —Anemia if blood loss from ulcer
  - —High hematocrit indicates hemoconcentration
- Electrolytes, BUN/Cr, glucose
  - —Hypokalemia
  - —Hypochloremic metabolic alkalosis
  - —Hypoglycemia
  - —Prerenal azotemia
- Urinalysis
- Amylase/lipase

IMAGING/SPECIAL TESTS

- Plain abdominal radiographs
  - —Dilated stomach
  - —Absence of air distally in bowel
- Abdominal CT for detecting neoplastic cause of obstruction
- ECG in elderly/at risk for coronary artery disease
- Upper GI/endoscopy to define and diagnose etiology

DIFFERENTIAL DIAGNOSIS

- Proximal bowel obstruction
- Exacerbation of peptic ulcer disease
- Gastroenteritis
- Psychogenic vomiting
- Cholelithiasis
- Cholecystitis

Treatment

INITIAL STABILIZATION

- 0.9%NS IV fluid resuscitation for prolonged obstruction and significant volume depletion
  —1 L bolus in adult
  —20 cc/kg bolus in children
- Correct electrolyte abnormalities, especially hypokalemia

ED TREATMENT

- Nasogastric tube
- Foley to monitor urine output
- Surgical consultation

Disposition

ADMISSION CRITERIA

- All patients with gastric outlet obstruction will require admission for fluid resuscitation and possible surgical intervention

DISCHARGE CRITERIA

- None

Miscellaneous

ICD9: 537.0

CORE CONTENT CODE: 1.5.1.4

SUGGESTED READINGS

Holder W. Intestinal Obstruction. Gastroenterol Clin North Am 1988;17(2):317.

Shaffer H. Perforation and obstruction of the gastrointestinal tract. Radiol Clin North Am 1992;30(2):405.

Sivit C. Gastrointestinal emergencies in older infants and children. Radiol Clin North Am 1997;35(4):865.

Author: Julio Silva

Gastritis

Clinical Presentation

SIGNS AND SYMPTOMS

- Dyspepsia
- Epigastric pain or discomfort (episodic and chronic)
- Bloating, indigestion, eructation, flatulence, and heartburn
- Anorexia, nausea/vomiting
- Dehydration, tachycardia, and electrolyte disturbances (with vomiting)
- Hematemesis, melena, pallor, and signs of volume depletion (hemorrhagic gastritis)

MECHANISM/DESCRIPTION

- Inflammatory response of the gastric mucosa to injury
- Three lines of defense of the gastric mucosa
  —Mucus layer that forms a protective pH gradient
  —Surface epithelial cells that can repair small defects
  —Postepithelial barrier that neutralizes the acid that has traversed the first two layers
- No definite link between histologic gastritis and dyspeptic symptoms

ETIOLOGY

Acute Gastritis

- Caused by
  —Aspirin
  —Steroids
  —Alcohol
  —NSAIDs
  —Burns
  —Sepsis
  —Trauma
- Stress (sepsis, burns, trauma)
  —Decrease in splanchnic blood flow leading to decreased mucus production, bicarbonate secretion, and prostaglandin synthesis
  —Results in mucosal erosions and hemorrhage
- Alcohol
  —Induces production of leukotrienes that cause microvascular stasis, engorgement, and increased vascular permeability
  —Leads to hemorrhage
- NSAIDs
  —Interfere with prostaglandin synthesis leading to a similar cascade as induced by alcohol
  —Results in mucosal erosions

Chronic Gastritis

- Produced by *Helicobacter pylori*
- Mechanism of *H. pylori* unclear
  —Gram-negative spiral bacteria found in the gastric mucus layer
  —Contains an enzyme urease that allows it to change the pH (alkaline) of its microenvironment

Pre-Hospital

CAUTIONS

- ABCs with significant blood loss producing tachycardia and hypotension
  —2 large-bore IV's infusing LR or 0.9%NS for fluid resuscitation
- Do not underestimate the degree of blood loss in a patient with a history of hypertension with a normal blood pressure

Diagnosis

ESSENTIAL WORKUP

- Careful physical examination including stool hemoccult testing and vital signs with orthostatics
- NG tube when history of hematemesis or unstable vital signs
- Hct determination

LABORATORY

- Normal lab values in uncomplicated gastritis
- CBC
  —Anemia with acute hemorrhagic gastritis
  —Leukocytosis—infection
- Amylase/lipase for pancreatitis in differential
- Urinalysis
  —Assess dehydration/ketosis (starvation)
  —Bilirubin present with hepatitis

IMAGING/SPECIAL TESTS

- EKG
  —For elderly patients
  —Myocardial ischemia in differential
- Endoscopy
  —Outpatient unless significant hemorrhage
  —Allows for visualization of the bleeding sites, histologic confirmation of mucosal inflammation, and detection of *H. pylori*
- Noninvasive *H. pylori* testing
  —Urea breath test
  —Serology to detect antibodies to *H. pylori*

DIFFERENTIAL DIAGNOSIS

- Peptic ulcer disease (PUD)
- "Nonulcer dyspepsia" (symptoms and no ulcer on endoscopy)
- Gastroesophageal reflux
- Biliary colic
- Cholecystitis
- Pancreatitis
- Hepatitis
- Abdominal aortic aneurysm
- Aortic dissection
- Myocardial infarction

Treatment

INITIAL STABILIZATION

- ABCs with acute erosive or hemorrhagic gastritis that presents with hemodynamic instability
- IV fluid resuscitation with LR or 0.9%NS via 2 large-bore catheters
- NG tube for gastric decompression and lavage
- Foley catheterization to assess volume replacement

ED TREATMENT

- Pain control with
  - —Antacids
  - —GI cocktail—30 cc antacids plus 10–20 cc viscous lidocaine
  - —H_2 antagonists
  - —Sucralfate
  - —Avoid narcotics as may mask serious illness

Acute Hemorrhagic Gastritis

- IV fluid resuscitation
- Blood transfusion if low Hct
- Reverse causes (alcohol, sepsis, NSAIDs, or trauma)
- Prevent *acute* or *erosive gastritis* in critically ill
  - —Antacids hourly or IV H_2 antagonists
  - —Goal is to keep pH >4

Chronic Gastritis

- Treatment of *H. pylori* infection
  - —Invasive or noninvasive testing to confirm infection
  - —Oral (po) eradication antibiotic therapy options
    - -Proton pump inhibitor (omeprazole 20 mg bid) and two antibiotics (clarithromycin 250 mg bid plus metronidazole 500 mg bid) for 7 days
    - -H_2 blocker, bismuth subsalicylate (Pepto Bismol) plus either amoxicillin 500 mg qid or tetracycline 500 mg qid (>8 years old) in combination with either metronidazole 250 mg tid or clarithromycin 500 mg tid for 14 days
  - —Treatment controversial for asymptomatic or nonulcer dyspepsia gastritis
- Vitamin B_{12} supplementation for *atrophic gastritis*

MEDICATIONS

- Bismuth subsalicylate: 262 mg tabs 2 po qid
- Cimetidine (H_2 blocker): 800 mg po qhs for 6–8 weeks
- Famotidine (H_2 blocker): 40 mg po qhs for 6–8 weeks
- Misoprostol: 100–200 μg po qid
- Maalox plus: 2–4 tablets po qid
- Mylanta II: 2–4 tablets po qid
- Nizatidine (H_2 blocker): 300 mg po qhs for 6–8 weeks
- Omeprazole: 20 mg po QD for 4 weeks
- Ranitidine (H_2 blocker): 300 mg po qhs for 6–8 weeks
- Sucralfate: 1 g po qid for 6–8 weeks

Disposition

ADMISSION CRITERIA

- Acute hemorrhagic or erosive gastritis that presents with UGI bleeding, tachycardia and hypotension
- Uncontrolled pain or vomiting
- Coagulopathy from medication or liver disease

DISCHARGE CRITERIA

- Unremarkable physical examination with normal CBC and heme-negative stools
- If heme-positive stools, discharge if stable vital signs, normal Hct, and negative NG tube aspiration for upper GI hemorrhage
- Outpatient evaluation for endoscopy

Miscellaneous

ICD9: 535.5

CORE CONTENT CODE: 1.5.2.1

SUGGESTED READINGS

Heatley RV, et al. Gastritis and duodenitis. In: Bockus, ed. Gastroenterology. Vol 1. 5th ed. 1995:635–643.

McGuirk TD, et al. Upper gastrointestinal tract bleeding. Emerg Med Clin North Am 1996;14(3):530–533.

Soll AH, Isenberg JI, Graham DY. Gastritis, peptic ulcer disease, medical therapy. In: Bennett JC, Plum F, eds. Cecil's textbook of medicine. Philadelphia: WB Saunders, 1996:659–669.

Sung JJ, Chung SC, et al. Antibacterial treatment of gastric ulcers associated with *Helicobacter pylori*. N Eng J Med 1995;332:139–142.

Author: Marco Cordero

Gastroenteritis

Clinical Presentation

SIGNS AND SYMPTOMS

- Nausea, vomiting, diarrhea
- Bloody/mucous diarrhea
- Abdominal cramps or pain
- Fever
- Malaise, myalgias, headache, anorexia
- Tachycardia, hypotension, lethargy, and dehydration (severe cases)

ETIOLOGY

Infections

Viruses

- 50–70% of all cases

Invasive Bacteria

- Campylobacter: contaminated food/water, wilderness water, birds, and other animals
  —Most common cause
  —Gross or occult blood is found in 60–90%
- Salmonella: contaminated water, eggs, poultry or dairy products
  —*Typhoid fever* (*S. typhi*) characterized by unremitting fever, abdominal pain, rose spots, splenomegaly, and bradycardia
  —Immunocompromised susceptible
- Shigella: fecal-oral route
- Vibrio parahaemolyticus: raw and undercooked seafood
- Yersinia: contaminated food (pork), water, and milk
  —May present as mesenteric adenitis or mimic appendicitis

Specific Food-Borne Disease (Food Poisoning)

- *Staphylococcal aureus*
  —Most common toxin-related disease
  —Symptoms 1–6 hours after ingesting food
- *Bacillus cereus*
  —Classic source is fried rice left on steam tables
  —Symptoms within 1–36 hours
- Cholera: profuse watery stools with mucous ("rice-water" stools)
- Ciguatera
  —Fish intoxication
  —Onset 5 minutes to 30 hours (average 6 hours) after ingestion
  —Paresthesias, hypotension, peripheral muscle weakness
  —Amitriptyline may be therapeutic
- Scombroid
  —Caused by "blood fish": tuna, albacore, mackerel and mahi-mahi
  —Flushing, headache, erythema, dizziness, blurred vision, and generalized burning sensation
  —Symptoms last <6 hours
  —Treatment includes antihistamines

Protozoa

- *Giardia lamblia*
  —High-risk groups: travelers, day care children, homosexual men, and campers who drink untreated mountain water

Noninfectious Causes

- Toxins
  —Zinc, copper, cadmium
  —Organic chemicals: polyvinylchlorides
  —Pesticides—organophosphates
  —Radioactive substances
  —Alkyl mercury
- Altered-host response to a food substance (tyramine, monosodium glutamate, tryptamine)

PEDIATRIC CONSIDERATIONS

- Focus evaluation on state of hydration
- Majority of viral origin and self-limited
- Rotavirus accounts for up to 50%
- *Shigella* infections associated with seizures

Pre-Hospital

CAUTIONS

- Difficult IV access in severe dehydration
- Avoid exposure to contaminated clothes or body substances

Diagnosis

ESSENTIAL WORKUP

- Digital rectal examination to determine the presence of gross or occult blood
- Fecal leukocyte determination
  —Present with invasive bacteria
  —Absent in protozoal infections, viral, toxin-induced food poisoning

LABORATORY

- CBC—indications
  —Significant blood loss
  —Systemic toxicity
- Electrolytes, glucose, BUN/Cr—indications
  —Lethargy, significantly dehydration, toxicity, or altered mental status
  —Duiretic use, persistent diarrhea, chronic liver or renal disease
- Stool culture—indications
  —Presence of fecal leukocytes
  —Historical markers (immunocompromised, travel, homosexual)
  —Public health (food handler, day/health care worker)
- Blood cultures—indications
  —Suspected bacteremia/systemic infections
  —Ill patients requiring admission

IMAGING/SPECIAL TESTS

- Abdominal x-ray films have no value unless an obstruction or a toxic megacolon suspected

DIFFERENTIAL DIAGNOSIS

- Gastritis/peptic ulcer disease
- Milk and food allergies
- Appendicitis
- Irritable bowel syndrome
- Ulcerative colitis/Crohn's disease
- Malrotation with midget volvulus
- Meckel's diverticulum
- Drugs and toxins: mannitol, sorbitol, phenolphthalein, magnesium-containing antacids, quinidine, colchicine, mushrooms, mercury poisoning

PEDIATRIC CONSIDERATIONS

- Laboratory studies not required in most cases
- Rotazyme assay detects rotavirus
  —Rarely indicated in managing outpatients
  —Helpful to cohort and avoid cross-contamination among inpatients
- Stool cultures—indication
  —Fecal leukocytes
  —Toxic
  —Infants
  —Immunocompromised

Treatment

INITIAL STABILIZATION

- IV fluid with 0.9%NS resuscitation for severely dehydrated

ED TREATMENT

- Oral fluids for mild dehydration (Gatorade/Pedialyte)
- IV fluids for
  - —Hypotension, nausea/vomiting, obtundation, metabolic acidosis, significant hypernatremia or hyponatremia
  - —0.9%NS 500 ml–1 L bolus (peds: 20 ml/kg) for resuscitation then 0.9%NS or D5.45%NS (peds: D5.25%NS) to maintain an adequate urine output
- Bismuth subsalicylate (Pepto-Bismol)
  - —Antisecretory agent
  - —Effective clinical relief without adverse effects
- Kaolin-pectin (Kaopectate)
  - —Reduces fluidity of stools
  - —Does not influence the course of the disease
- Antimotility drugs (diphenoxylate (lomotil), loperamide (imodium), paregoric, and codeine)
  - —Appropriate in noninfectious diarrhea
  - —Initial use of sparse amounts to control symptoms in infectious diarrhea
  - —Avoid prolonged use in infectious diarrhea—may increase the duration of fever, diarrhea, and bacteremia, and may precipitate a toxic megacolon
- Antiemetics: prochlorperazine (compazine) and promethazine (phenergan) for nausea/vomiting

Antibiotics for Infectious Pathogens

- Campylobacter: quinolone or erythromycin
- Salmonella: quinolone or trimethoprin/sulfamethaxozole (tmp/smx)
- Ceftriaxone for typhoid fever
- Shigella: quinolone, tmp/smx, or ampicillin
- *Vibrio parahaemolyticus:* tetracycline or doxycycline
- *Clostridium difficile:* vancomycin
- *Escherichia coli:* quinolone or tmp/smx
- *Giardia lamblia:* metronidazole or quinacrine

MEDICATIONS

- Ampicillin: 500 mg (peds: 20 mg/kg/24hrs) PO/IV q 6 hrs
- Bactrim DS (trimethoprin/sulfamethaxozole): 1 tab (peds: 8–10 mg tmp/40–50 mg smx/kg/24hrs) PO/IV bid
- Ciprofloxacin (quinolone): 500 mg PO/IV bid (>18 years old)
- Doxycycline: 100 mg PO/IV bid
- Erythromycin: 500 mg (peds: 40–50 mg/kg/24hrs) po qid
- Metronidazole: 250 mg (peds: 35 mg/kg/24hrs) po tid (>8 years old)
- Tetracycline: 500 mg PO/IV q 6 hrs
- Prochlorperazine (compazine): 5–10 mg IVP q 3–4 hrs; 10 mg po q 8 hrs; 25 mg PR; q 12 hrs PRN (peds: >2 yrs: 0.06 mg/lb IM 1 dose only)
- Promethazine (phenergan): 25 mg IM/IVP q 4 hrs, 25mg PO/PR q 12 hrs PRN (peds: >2 yrs: 6.25–12.5 mg IM/IV q 4 hrs; 12.5–25 mg po PR q 12 hrs)
- Quinacrine: 100 mg (6 mg/kg/24hrs) po tid

Disposition

ADMISSION CRITERIA

- Hypotension unresponsive to IV fluids
- Significant bleeding
- Signs of sepsis/toxicity
- Intractable vomiting or abdominal pain
- Severe electrolyte imbalance
- Metabolic acidosis
- Altered mental status
- Children with >10–15% dehydration

DISCHARGE CRITERIA

- Mild cases requiring oral hydration
- Dehydration responsive to IV fluids

Miscellaneous

ICD9: 558.9

CORE CONTENT CODE: N/A

SUGGESTED READINGS

Bitterman R. Acute gastroenteritis and constipation. In: Rosen P, Barkin RM, et al., eds. Emergency medicine: Concepts and clinical practice. 4th ed. St. Louis: Mosby-Year Book, 1998:1917–1958.

Blacklow NR, Greenberg HB. Viral gastroenteritis. N Engl J Med 1991;325:252.

DuPont H, Miranda A. Small intestine: Infections with common bacterial and viral pathogens. In: Yamada T, et al., eds. Textbook of gastroenterology. 2d ed. Philadelphia: JB Lippincott, 1995:1605–1629.

Fleisher GR. Gastrointestinal infections. In: Fleisher G, Ludwig S, eds. Pediatric emergency medicine. 3rd ed. Baltimore: Williams & Wilkins, 1993:628–633.

Author: Isam Nasr

Gastroesophageal Reflux

Clinical Presentation

SIGNS AND SYMPTOMS

- Heartburn (pyrosis)
  - —Retrosternal burning pain
  - —May radiate from the epigastrium through the chest to the neck and throat
- Dysphagia
  - —Suggests esophageal spasm or stricture
- Odynophagia
  - —Suggests ulcerative esophagitis
- Regurgitation
- Water brash
- Belching
- Early satiety, nausea, anorexia, weight loss
- Symptoms worse with recumbency or bending over
- Symptoms usually temporarily relieved with antacids
- GI bleeding
- Barrett esophagus (metaplastic mucosa)
- Esophageal strictures

Atypical Signs

- Noncardiac chest pain
- Asthma
- Persistent cough, hiccups
- Hoarseness
- Globus sensation
- Pharyngeal/laryngeal ulcers and carcinoma
- Frequent throat clearing
- Recurrent pneumonitis
- Nocturnal choking
- Upper GI bleeding

MECHANISM/DESCRIPTION

- Spectrum of pathology in which gastric reflux causes symptoms and damage to the esophageal mucosa
- 40% of the general population experiences symptoms monthly

ETIOLOGY

- Incompetent reflux barrier allowing an increase in the frequency and duration of gastric contents into the esophagus
  - —Exposed esophageal mucosa becomes acidified and with time necrosed
- Main antireflux barriers
  - —Lower esophageal sphincter (LES) and the crural diaphragm attachment (diaphragmatic sphincter)
  - —Both contribute to the pressure barrier at the gastroesophageal junction
  - —Peristalsis clears esophageal acid
  - —Esophageal mucosal resistance
- Brief episodes of postprandial reflux occur in the great majority of healthy individuals without causing symptoms
- Decreased LES tone due to
  - —Smoking
  - —Certain foods and drugs (calcium channel blockers, morphine, meperidine, barbiturates, theophylline, anticholinergics, alcohol, chocolate, onion)
- Delayed gastric emptying and gastric distention contribute to reflux
- Hiatal hernias associated with GERD, but their significance varies in any given individual
  - —Most persons with hiatal hernia do not have clinically evident reflux disease
- Acid secretion is the same in those with or without GERD

PEDIATRIC CONSIDERATIONS

- Regurgitation common in infants
  - —Incidence decreases from twice daily in 50% of those age 2 months to 1% of 1-year-old infants
- Frequent vomiting, irritability, cough, crying, and malaise can be signs of GERD in infants
- Arching the body (hyperextension) at feeding and refusals of feedings are signs for esophagitis

Pre-Hospital

CAUTIONS

- Esophageal pain may mimic angina
  - —Direct treatment toward the more serious condition
  - —Maintain airway—vomiting can lead to aspiration

Diagnosis

ESSENTIAL WORKUP

- Differentiate GERD symptoms from more emergent conditions such as ischemic heart pain or esophageal perforation
- History typically reveals the diagnosis
- Physical examination nonspecific
- Diagnostic trial of antacid

LABORATORY

- CBC
  - —Chronic anemia from esophagitis

IMAGING/SPECIAL TESTS

- Chest radiograph for
  - —Esophageal perforation
  - —Hiatal hernia
- ECG for chest pain in at-risk individuals
- Endoscopy
  - —Outpatient referral for all patients with persistent reflux symptoms
- Barium esophagram
  - —Outpatient referral if dysphagia prominent
- Esophageal manometry and pH monitoring
  - —Consider in referral
  - —Esophageal pH monitoring—best test for evaluation of suspected acid-related chest pain

DIFFERENTIAL DIAGNOSIS

- Ischemic heart disease
  - —Asthma
  - —Peptic ulcer disease
  - —Gastritis
  - —Esophageal perforation
  - —Esophageal foreign body
  - —Esophageal infection
  - —Cholecystitis

PEDIATRIC CONSIDERATIONS

- Differential diagnosis
  - —Failure to thrive
  - —Formula intolerance
  - —Sepsis
  - —Gastroenteritis

Treatment

INITIAL STABILIZATION

- ABCs need to be evaluated
- IV fluid resuscitation for blood loss or shock

ED TREATMENT

- Symptomatic relief
  —Antacids
  —Antacids with viscous lidocaine
  —Sublingual nitroglycerine relieves esophageal spasm
  —Analgesics
- Lifestyle modifications
  —Avoid late night meals
  —Minimize time in the supine position after eating
  —Elevation of the head of the bed on blocks
  —Avoid direct esophageal irritants such as citric juices and coffee
  —Avoid foods that decrease LES pressures (fatty foods, chocolate, coffee)
  —Avoid drugs that lower LES tone
- Antacids
  —Useful for treating mild and infrequent reflux symptoms
  —Not effective for healing esophagitis
  —Alginic acid forms a viscous slurry that floats on the surface of the gastric contents providing a mechanical barrier
  —Sucralfate slurry binds pepsin, bile salts and exposed submucosa, thereby limiting inflammation
- H_2 blockers
  —Effective for mild to moderate disease
  —Severe disease requires greater medication dosage than used for peptic ulcer disease
- Proton pump inhibitors
  —Potent long-acting inhibitors of gastric acid secretion
  —Result in faster healing than other drug therapies
  —More efficacious in severe GERD and frank esophagitis
- Prokinetic medications—cisapride
  —Effective in improving peristalsis, accelerating gastric emptying, and increasing LES pressure
  —Other similar drugs—metoclopramide and bethanechol
  —Considerable incidence of side effects
  —Of questionable value
- Antireflux surgery for
  —Chronic reflux
  —Younger patients
  —Nonhealing ulceration
  —Severe bleeding
  —Fundoplication can be more effective than medical therapy in selected cases

MEDICATIONS

- Antacids: 30 cc + viscous lidocaine 10cc po
- Bethanechol (urecholine): 10–50 mg po BID/QID
- Cimetidine: 400–800 mg bid
- Cisapride: 10 mg 30 min before meals and qhs
- Famotidine: 20–40 mg bid
- Lansoprazole: 15–30 mg qd
- Metoclopramide (reglan): 10 mg IV/IM; 10–30 mg po qid 30 min prior to meals and qhs
- Nizatidine: 150–300 mg bid
- Omeprazole: 20–40 mg qd
- Ranitidine: 150–300 mg bid
- Sucralfate: 1 g qid

Disposition

ADMISSION CRITERIA

- Seriously ill patients
- Significant esophageal bleeding
- Uncontrolled reactive asthma
- Dehydration
- Starvation and failure to thrive

DISCHARGE CRITERIA

- Discharge uncomplicated GERD with referral to their primary care physician or a gastroenterologist for further evaluation

Miscellaneous

ICD9: 530.11

CORE CONTENT CODE: 1.1.3.1

SUGGESTED READINGS

Fennerty MB, Castell D, Fendrick AM, et al. The diagnosis and treatment of gastroesophageal disease in a managed care environment. Arch Intern Med 1996;156:477–484.

Hyman PE. Gastroesophageal reflux: One reason why baby won't eat. J Pediatr 1994;125:103–109.

Kahrilas PJ. Gastroesophageal reflux disease. JAMA 1996;276:983–988.

Mittal RK, Balaban DH. The esophagogastric junction. N Engl J Med 1997;336:924–932.

Richter JE. Typical and atypical presentations of gastroesophageal reflux disease. Gastroenterol Clin North Am 1996;25:75–103.

Author: Thomas Lukens

Gastrointestinal Bleeding

Clinical Presentation

SIGNS AND SYMPTOMS

- Fatigue
- Weakness
- Dyspnea on exertion
- Anxiety
- Altered level of consciousness
- Tachycardia
- Orthostasis
- Pale appearance
- Pale conjunctiva
- Mucous membranes
- Pale nail beds

Upper Gastrointestinal Bleeding

- Hematemesis
- Abdominal pain
  - —Sharp, burning
  - —Epigastric
- Coffee ground emesis
- Black stools

Lower Gastrointestinal Bleeding

- Bright red blood per rectum
- Melena
- Black stools
- Blood in toilet bowl

MECHANISM/DESCRIPTION

- Black melanotic stool requires rapid loss of at least 100 ml of blood
- Mortality rate for gastrointestinal bleeding
  - —Increases as age increases
  - —Ranges from <5% in children to as high as 25% in adults >70 years of age
- Two categories
  - —Upper—proximal to the ligament of Treitz
  - —Lower—distal to the ligament of Treitz
- Range
  - —Occult—a heme-positive stool or new anemia
  - —Massive

ETIOLOGY

- Most common causes of upper gastrointestinal bleeding include
  - —Peptic ulcer disease
  - —Gastritis
  - —Esophageal varices
  - —Mallory-Weiss tear
  - —Caustic ingestions
- Most common causes of lower gastrointestinal bleeding include
  - —Diverticular disease
  - —Angiodysplasia
  - —Gastrointestinal polyps
  - —Hemorrhoids
  - —Anal fissures

PEDIATRIC CONSIDERATIONS

- Common causes of lower gastrointestinal bleeding
  - —Meckel's diverticulum
  - —Intussusception

Pre-Hospital

CAUTIONS

- Stabilize the airway
  - —Place the patient on 100% oxygen via mask
  - —Intubation for massive upper gastrointestinal (GI) bleeding
- Insert at least one large-bore IV line (14g–16g) and administer crystalloids to attempt to maintain a blood pressure greater than 90 mm Hg systolic
  - —Attempt second IV while transport is undertaken
  - —Do not remain at the scene for a second IV line

Diagnosis

ESSENTIAL WORKUP

- Hematocrit
- Nasogastric aspiration for suspected upper GI bleeding
  - —Most useful test for determining current upper GI bleeding
  - —Follow by room-temperature saline lavage to demonstrate any active bleeding
  - —25% falsely negative if bleeding source duodenal
    - -Lower false-negative rate if aspirate contains bile
  - —Iced lavage is not useful
    - -Causes hypothermia and does not stop bleeding
- Rectal examination with stool for melena and hemoccult testing
  - —False-positive hemoccult
    - -Raw meat
    - -Some iron preparations
  - —Agents causing black stools aside from GI bleeding
    - -Iron
    - -Charcoal
    - -Bismuth
    - -Food dyes
    - -Beets

LABORATORY

- CBC
  - —For anemia
  - —Low MCV associated with chronic blood loss
  - —For thrombocytopenia
- Electrolytes, BUN/Cr, glucose
- PT/PTT/INR
- Type and cross for active bleeding or unstable patient

IMAGING/SPECIAL TESTS

- Panendoscopy
  - —Reveals the location of gastrointestinal bleeding in up to 90% of cases
  - —May be therapeutic
- Upright CXR/abdominal series
  - —If signs of acute peritonitis
  - —For perforation or obstruction
- Angiography
  - —Diagnostic and therapeutic
- Radionuclide scans for slow bleeding in attempt to locate source
- ECG for cardiac ischemia

DIFFERENTIAL DIAGNOSIS

- Acute abdomen
- Aortoenteric fistula
- Visceral trauma

Treatment

INITIAL STABILIZATION

- Control airway in massive GI bleed with unstable vital signs and altered mental status
- Administer oxygen
- Place cardiac, pulse oximetry, and noninvasive blood pressure monitors
- Initiate 2 large-bore IV access with 0.9%NS
  - —Administer 1-L bolus (peds: 20 cc/kg)
  - —Administer blood if no response to initial 2-L bolus
- Place central line for CVP/Swan Ganz measurements if unsure of volume status in hypotensive patient

ED TREATMENT

- Consult gastroenterology service for emergent endoscopy if significant ongoing bleeding
- Follow serial hematocrit
  - —May take several hours for level to reflect blood loss
- Place Foley to follow urine output
  - —Good indicator of response to volume resuscitation
- Blood transfusion
  - —For patients with ongoing chest pain or ischemic changes on ECG
  - —For continued hypotension unresponsive to crystalloid infusion with ongoing bleeding regardless of hematocrit

Upper GI Bleeding

- Place nasogastric tube
  - —Aspirate for blood
  - —Place on suction
  - —Lavage with water to determine if continued bleeding
  - —May not detect duodenal bleed with competent pyloric sphincter
- Initiate H_2 blockers (cimetidine, famotidine, ranitidine)
  - —Helps to prevent rebleeding in gastritis
- Emergent endoscopy
  - —Indications
    - -Active bleeding that does not clear with lavage
    - -Hemodynamic instability in setting of liver disease
  - —Therapeutic options
    - -Cauterization of bleeding ulcers or vessels
    - -Injection sclerosis of visible vessels
- Variceal bleeding treatment
  - —Endoscopic sclerotherapy
    - -Most effective
  - —Vasopressin
    - -Potent vasoconstrictor
    - -May be used concurrently with sclerotherapy
    - -Administered concurrently with IV nitroglycerin to prevent tissue necrosis/myocardial ischemia
  - —Balloon tamponade
    - -Sengstaken-Blakemore tube
    - -For confirmed variceal bleeding unresponsive to above measures
- Spontaneous resolution
  - —60% from variceal bleeding
  - —80% from other upper gastrointestinal sources

Lower GI Bleeding

- Anoscopy for suspected hemorrhoidal bleeding
- Flexible fiberoptic colonoscopy
  - —Best if done electively after adequate bowel preparation
- Angiography for massive or continuous bleeding
  - —Diagnostic and therapeutic
- Spontaneous resolution
  - —80% of the time
  - —25% rate of rebleeding

MEDICATIONS

- Cimetidine: 300 mg IV q 6 hrs; 400 mg po bid
- Famotidine: 20 mg IV q 12 hrs; 40 mg po q HS
- Nitroglycerin: 5–20 μg/min IV
- Ranitidine: 50 mg IV q 8 hrs; 300 mg po q HS
- Vasopressin: 0.2–0.4 IU/min (peds: 0.1–0.3 IU/min) initial dose then titrate up IV

Disposition

ADMISSION CRITERIA

- Unstable vital signs at any time
- Decreased hematocrit with recent GI bleed
- Coagulopathy
- Advanced age/comorbid conditions
- Active upper GI bleeding
- Lower GI bleeding
  - —Significant initial blood loss
  - —Continued bleeding

DISCHARGE CRITERIA

- Resolution of upper GI bleeding with negative NG tube aspirate
- Minor, resolved lower GI bleed
- Stable vital signs
- Stable hematocrit >30%
- Normal coagulation function

Miscellaneous

ICD9: 578.9

CORE CONTENT CODE: 22.4.16, 22.4.27, 22.4.20,

SUGGESTED READINGS

Bono MJ. Lower gastrointestinal tract bleeding. Emerg Med Clin North Am 1996;14(3):547–555.

McGuirck TD, Coyle WJ. Upper gastrointestinal tract bleeding. Emerg Med Clin North Am 1996;14(3):523–539.

Author: Dean E. Johnson

Glaucoma

Clinical Presentation

SIGNS AND SYMPTOMS

Acute Closed-Angle

- Severe eye or forehead pain
- Blurred vision
- Halos around lights
- Injected sclera
- Hazy cornea
- Shallow anterior chamber angle
- Mid-dilated pupils
- Decreased visual acuity
- Firm eyes with digital ballottement
- Nausea and vomiting
- Abdominal pain (nonspecific)

Open-Angle

- Painless, gradual loss of vision
- Disc pallor and cupping
- Visual field defects

MECHANISM/DESCRIPTION

- Increased intraocular pressure due to overproduction of aqueous humor or decreased aqueous humor outflow leads to
  —Corneal edema
  —Pupillary sphincter paralysis
  —Optic nerve degeneration
  —Eventual blindness

ETIOLOGY

- Glaucoma classifications
  —*Primary* (unknown cause)—open-angle, closed-angle, or congenital
  —*Developmental*—developmental abnormality in the aqueous outflow tract
  —*Secondary*—a condition that leads to a secondary rise in intraocular pressure
    -Inflammation (uveitis, scleritis, keratitis)
    -Trauma (blunt or penetrating)
    -Intraocular blood
    -Systemic diseases (amyloidosis, diabetes mellitus, thyroid disease)

Closed-Angle

- Most common type presenting to ED because of the rapid onset and painful nature
- Abnormally narrow anterior chamber angles allow for occlusion of aqueous humor outflow
- Inciting agents
  —Trauma
  —Stress
  —Entering a darkened room
  —Sneezing
  —Pharmacological dilation of the eye
    -Intentional with an ophthalmological examination
    -Unintentional as with inhaled β-agonists or atropine, or intranasal use of cocaine that accidentally enters the eye
- Both eyes are at risk—abnormality usually bilateral

Open-Angle

- Normal anterior chamber angle
- Risk factors
  —Age >35 years old
  —Diabetics (three times more likely)

PEDIATRIC CONSIDERATIONS

- Tearing, photophobia, blepharospasm, and irritability
  —Often the first signs
  —Secondary to corneal irritation from corneal edema
- Cornea appearance
  —Hazy due to edema
  —Haab's striae (breaks in Descemet's membrane, which causes linear ridging)
  —Enlarged due to the elasticity of a child's eye
- Entire eye may be enlarged (buphthalmos, "ox eye")
- Older children have progressive myopia due to the eye's change in shape from continued intraocular pressure

Pre-Hospital

N/A

Diagnosis

ESSENTIAL WORKUP

- Detailed history and ocular examination
- Visual acuity
- Tonometry (normal intraocular pressure = 10–21 mm Hg)
  —Pressures >21 mm Hg suspicious
  —Pressures >24 mm Hg abnormal

DIFFERENTIAL DIAGNOSIS

- Broad differential depending on whether the chief symptom is a painful red eye, headache, gastrointestinal complaint, or chronic loss of vision
  —Diagnosis of glaucoma made with increased intraocular pressure
- Headache
  —Migraine
  —Cluster
  —Tension
- Red eye
  —Conjunctivitis
  —Iritis
  —Allergic/toxic
  —Corneal abrasion
  —Trauma

PEDIATRIC CONSIDERATIONS

- Consider developmental glaucoma (relatively rare: 1:10,000 live births) in an irritable photophobic child or when "big eyes" noted
- Children (<5 years) may need general anesthesia for a good ophthalmological examination

Treatment

INITIAL STABILIZATION

- Initiate steps to lower intraocular pressure in acute closed-angle glaucoma

ED TREATMENT

Acute Closed-Angle

- Goals of treatment
  - —Decreasing intraocular pressure in the affected eye
  - —Preventing an episode in the other eye
- Decrease aqueous humor production
  - —*Carbonic anhydrase inhibitors* (acetazolamide)
    - -Inhibits the generation of carbonic acid needed in the production of aqueous humor
    - -Results in less aqueous humor formation
    - -Do not administer acetazolamide in sickle cell patients secondary to a hyphema—may induce sickling and worsen the prognosis
  - —β-Blockers (timolol, betaxolol) decrease aqueous production and increase outflow
- Decrease intraocular volume
  - —Hyperosmotic drugs (mannitol, glycerol) raise blood osmolality rapidly thereby inducing an osmotic gradient between the blood and ocular fluids
    - -Water moves to the plasma from the eye decreasing the intraocular volume
- Decrease pupil size
  - —Cholinergic drugs (pilocarpine)—miotics that cause pupillary constriction
    - -Allows for angle widening and increased aqueous outflow
    - -Cholinergic drugs may worsen the condition in cases of pupillary ischemia due to pupillary block as the pupil will not constrict but the lens will move forward
- Move lens posteriorly
  - —Supine position uses gravity to allow the lens to move posteriorly
  - —May relieve some degree of pupillary block

Open-Angle

- Not generally treated in the emergency department
- Symptoms occur gradually and the patients do not come to ED for this complaint
- If increased intraocular pressure found, refer to an ophthalmologist

PEDIATRIC CONSIDERATIONS

- Complications of β-adrenergic antagonist (asthma, bradycardia, drowsiness, and hyperactivity) more common in children

MEDICATIONS

- Acetazolamide
  - —IV: 500 mg (peds: 20–40 mg/kg/24hrs q 6 hrs) initially followed by 250 mg every 4 hrs
  - —po: 500 mg sustained-release (peds: 8–30 mg/kg/24hrs q 6–8 hrs) po bid
- Betaxolol: 0.5% 1 drop bid
- Glycerol: 1–1.5 ml/kg po
- Mannitol: 1.5–2 g/kg IV
- Timolol: 0.25–0.5% 1 drop bid
- Pilocarpine 2%
  - —Affected eye: 1 drop q 15 min for 5 times then 1 drop q 2–3 hrs
  - —Unaffected eye: 1 drop q 6 hrs

Disposition

ADMISSION CRITERIA

- Acute closed-angle glaucoma with immediate ophthalmological consultation

DISCHARGE CRITERIA

- Primary open-angle glaucoma with ophthalmological follow-up as this is a chronic progressive disease

Miscellaneous

ICD9: 365.9

CORE CONTENT CODE: 6.4.2.2

SUGGESTED READINGS

Bertolini J, Pelucio M. The red eye. Emerg Med Clin North Am 1995;13:561–580.

Patel KH, Javitt JC, et al. Incidence of acute angle-closure glaucoma after pharmacologic mydriasis. Am J Opthtalmol 1995:120(6):709–717.

Author: Loice Swisher

Globe Rupture

Clinical Presentation

SIGNS AND SYMPTOMS

- Markedly decreased visual acuity
- Severe subconjunctival hemorrhage and edema
- Abnormally deep anterior chamber
- Hyphema (sometimes with clotted blood)
- Limited extraocular motion
- Extrusion of intraocular contents
- Full thickness scleral or corneal laceration (indicates penetrating injury)
- Low intraocular pressure (occasionally can be normal or high)
- Irregular pupil
- Iridodialysis/cyclodialysis
- Subluxed lens
- Commotio retinae
  - —Gray-white discoloration of the retina
- Choroidal rupture
- Traumatic optic neuropathy

MECHANISM/DESCRIPTION

- Blunt trauma to the eye
  - —Causes an abrupt rise in intraocular pressure
  - —Subsequent rupture of the eye at the weakest points
    - -At an extraocular muscle insertion
    - -At the corneoscleral junction
- Penetrating injuries
  - —Occur with sharp or pointed objects or projectiles injuring the scleral or anterior eye directly
  - —Most common anteriorly, because the orbital bone protects posteriorly
  - —Posterior injury can occur with fracture of the surrounding orbit or with penetrating injuries of the eyelid or eyebrow
- Hemorrhage within the eye portends a poor prognosis
  - —Blood is both a source of fibrosis and an aggravating influence on fibrosis in the posterior portion of the eye

ETIOLOGY

- Falls, impact injuries
- Sport-related injuries (e.g., elbow impacts, ball impacts, etc.)
- Indirect concussive injuries (explosions)
- Sharp instrument/stabbing injuries, accidental or intentional
- Projectile injuries (industrial, firearms, etc.)

Pre-Hospital

CAUTIONS

- Do not manipulate the eye if possible ruptured globe
- Place a shield (not patch) over eye with no pressure on the globe

Diagnosis

ESSENTIAL WORKUP

- Penlight or slitlamp examination observing for signs of globe rupture
- Defer complete ocular examination until the time of surgical repair in the operating room once the diagnosis of ruptured globe is made
  - —Prevents placing any undue pressure onto the eye and risking extrusion of the intraocular contents
- If no evidence of globe rupture on initial survey proceed with thorough ophthalmologic examination
  - —Visual acuity
  - —Slitlamp
    - -Corneal
    - -Anterior chamber
    - -Iris
    - -Sclera
    - -Posterior chamber
  - —Fluorescein
    - -Observe if fluorescein moves away as contents leak out of globe (Seidel test: positive indicates rupture)
  - —Visualize fundus/retina
  - —Measure intraocular pressure

LABORATORY

- Preoperative labs as indicated
  - —CBC
  - —Electrolytes, BUN/Cr, glucose

IMAGING/SPECIAL TESTS

- Orbital radiograph (AP/lat) for metallic intraocular foreign body with penetrating injuries
- CT scan of the orbits and brain, axial, and coronal views
- B-scan ultrasound of the eye

DIFFERENTIAL DIAGNOSIS

- Intraocular foreign body
- Hypemia
- Severe subconjunctival hemorrhage and chemosis
- Partial corneal laceration
- Partial scleral laceration

PEDIATRIC CONSIDERATIONS

- Childhood injuries are generally much more devastating secondary to more marked and more rapid fibrosis
- Early aggressive therapy indicated to establish best visual stimulus as quickly as possible to prevent amblyopia

Treatment

INITIAL STABILIZATION

- Protect eye with shield

ED TREATMENT

- Urgent ophthalmological consultation
- Bedrest
- No food or drink (NPO)
- Administer antiemetic for nausea/vomiting
  - —Compazine
  - —Droperidol
- Administer tetanus prophylaxis
- Administer prophylactic antibiotics
  - —First-generation cephalosporin with an aminoglycoside
- Avoid succinylcholine if rapid sequence intubation required (increase intraocular pressure)

MEDICATIONS

- Cefazolin (ancef): 1 g (peds: 25–50 mg/kg/24hrs) IV q 6–8 hrs
- Gentamicin: 1 mg/kg (peds: 2–2.5 mg/kg) IV q 8 hrs
- Prochlorperazine (compazine): 5–10 mg IV/IM (peds: 0.13 mg/kg/dose IM)
- Droperidol: 2.5 mg (peds: 0.05–0.06 mg/kg/dose) IV/IM q 6–8 hrs

Disposition

ADMISSION CRITERIA

- All patients with globe-rupture/penetrating eye injuries
- Early enucleation for devastating eye injury in which there is no hope of salvageable vision

DISCHARGE CRITERIA

- Globe penetration excluded

Miscellaneous

ICD9: 871.0

CORE CONTENT CODE: 18.4.6.8

SUGGESTED READINGS

Coles WH. Indirect global ruptures and sharp scleral injuries. In: Current Ocular Therapy. 3rd ed. Philadelphia: WB Saunders, 1990.

DeJuan E Jr, Sternberg P Jr, Michels RG. Penetrating ocular injury: Types of injuries and visual results. Ophthalmology 1983;90(11):1313–1322.

Klystra JA, Lamkin JC, Runyan DR. Clinical predictors of scleral rupture after blunt ocular trauma. Am J Ophthalmol 1993;115(4):530–535.

Author: Evan Liu

Glomerulonephritis

Clinical Presentation

SIGNS AND SYMPTOMS

- Cardinal signs
  - —Proteinuria
  - —Hematuria
- Edema
  - —Periorbital
  - —Ascites
  - —Pleural effusion
  - —Due to renal salt and water retention
- Hypertension (diastolic)
  - —Mild in 50%
  - —+/− Oliguria
- Azotemia—commonly in older patients
- Congestive heart failure—older patients with associated hypertension
- Renal failure
- Autoimmune disorders
  - —Arthralgias
  - —Arthritis
  - —Rash
  - —Fever
- Nonspecific manifestations: fatigue, weight loss, abdominal pain, nausea, and vomiting

MECHANISM/DESCRIPTION

- Group of conditions affecting the glomerulus resulting in
  - —Proteinuria
  - —Edema
  - —Hypertension
  - —Azotemia
  - —Abnormal urine sediment (excretion of red blood cells, casts, leukocytes, etc.)
- Immunologic mechanism
  - —Due to individual host response to specific antigen, reticuloendothelial system function, and genetic makeup of host, resulting in diffuse inflammatory changes in renal glomeruli

ETIOLOGY

- Grouping according to presentation
  - —Acute nephritic syndrome (see Nephritic chapter)
  - —Rapidly progressive glomerulonephritis (RPGN)
  - —Idiopathic renal hematuric syndrome
  - —Nephrotic syndrome (see Nephrotic chapter)
  - —Chronic nephritic syndrome
- Causes
  - —Infectious: poststreptococcal GN (PSGN) most common
  - —Systemic diseases: vasculitis, Henoch-Schonlein purpura, Goodpasture's disease, SLE
  - —Primary glomerular diseases: membranoproliferative GN (MPGN), IgA nephropathy (Berger's disease)
  - —Drugs (penicillamine, hydralazine, rifampin)
  - —Rarer causes: hemolytic uremic syndrome, acute hypersensitivity interstitial nephritis, serum sickness

Rapidly Progressive Glomerulonephritis (RPGN)

- Development of *acute renal failure* within weeks to months after episode of acute GN
- Onset insidious with fatigue, fever, weakness, anorexia, and abdominal pain
- *Edema* in 50%
- Hypertension uncommon
- >50% require dialysis within 6 months of onset

Idiopathic Renal Hematuric Syndrome

- Asymptomatic, persistent, minimal urinary abnormalities
  - —Mild proteinuria
  - —+/− Hematuria
  - —*Without* edema, azotemia, and hypertension
- *Proteinuria alone (nonnephrotic)*—most common: "orthostatic" proteinuria, focal and segmental glomerulosclerosis, MPGN, diabetes, amyloidosis
- Occurs 1–2 days after URI; onset of hematuria *coincides* with illness (differing from PSGN)

Chronic Glomerulonephritis

- *Persistent abnormal proteinuria* (*nonnephrotic*) with associated hypertension, reduced GFR, and abnormal urinary sediment
- Irreversible end-stage renal failure occurs over a number of years

Pre-Hospital

N/A

Diagnosis

ESSENTIAL WORKUP

- Urinalysis for
  - —Hematuria, red blood cell casts, and proteinuria

LABORATORY

- Electrolytes, BUN, Cr, glucose
  - —Baseline renal function
  - —Hyperkalemia
  - —For diabetes
- Albumin, total protein
  - —Varying degrees of hypoalbuminemia depending on clinical process
- CBC
  - —Anemia secondary to chronic renal disease or neoplasm
  - —Leukocytosis or normal WBC in infections
- PT, PTT, platelets (abnormal in neoplasms)
- ABG if renal failure

IMAGING/SPECIAL TESTS

- KUB film /renal ultrasound
  - —Evaluate kidney size
  - —CXR: normal or slightly enlarged heart +/− edema
  - —Ultrasound for neoplasm, trauma, cystic malformation, stone, obstruction, reflux
  - —Renal biopsy: discern primary glomerulopathies versus other causes

Diagnostic Tests

- Cultures—throat, skin, blood (if infection suspected)
- Calcium—hypocalcemia (nephrotic patients)
- 24-hour urine collection—protein, urine electrolytes
- Streptozyme or antistreptolysin O titer
- Complement levels (C3, C4, CH_{50})—decreased in PSGN, MPGN, SLE
- ANA, rheumatoid factor—connective tissue diseases
- Serum and urine protein electrophoresis—multiple myeloma, amyloidosis
- Viral studies—hepatitis serology, IgM and IgG titers (CMV and Ebstein-Barr virus), CMV
- Cryoglobulins and immune complexes—vasculitis, various acute GN
- Endocrine—glucose tolerance test, thyroid function test (hypothyroidism; nephrotic syndrome)

DIFFERENTIAL DIAGNOSIS

- *Hematologic*—Sickle cell disease, coagulopathy
- *Renal*—infectious, malformation, neoplasm, ischemic, trauma, vasculitis
- *Postrenal*
  —Mechanical (stones, reflux, obstruction, catheterization)
  —Inflammatory (cystitis, prostatitis, epididymitis, endometriosis, periurethritis)
  —Neoplasm
- *Factitious*—food, drugs, pigmenturia (myoglobin, porphyria, hemoglobinemia), vaginal bleeding

Treatment

INITIAL STABILIZATION

- ABCs

ED TREATMENT

- Treatment is mainly supportive care
- Fluid and sodium restriction (withhold oral intake for first 24 hours)
- Loop diuretics
  —Furosemide
  —May precipitate acute renal failure with intrinsic renal disease
- Lower blood pressure for hypertensive emergency
  —Nitroprusside
  —Diazoxide
- Dialysis for
  —Severe hyperkalemia
  —Fluid overload
  —Uremia

Specific Medical Treatments

- Antibiotics
  —If infectious cause suspected
  —Penicillin for PSGN
- Dopamine
  —Controversial
  —Low dose in early renal failure to increase renal perfusion
- Albumin, plasmapheresis—not recommended
- Erythropoietin—anemia due to chronic renal disease; still in experimental stages

RPGN Treatment

- Steroid pulse therapy—methylprednisolone, followed by daily prednisone
- Cytotoxic agents—azathioprine, cyclosporine
- Anticoagulants, antithrombotics (heparin)—due to coagulation involvement in crescent formation
  —Anticoagulants may be harmful in advanced renal failure or pulmonary hemorrhage
- Plasma exchange—controversial
  —Combined with steroids and cytotoxic agent to accelerate disappearance of circulating anti-GBM antibody
- Dialysis

MEDICATIONS

- Azathioprine: 2 mg/kg/day
- Cyclophosphamide: 2 mg/kg/day
- Diazoxide: 1–3 mg/kg IV, max 150 mg, repeat q 15 min
- Dopamine: 1–3 mg/min IV
- Erythromycin: 250 mg (peds: 30–50 mg/kg/24hrs) po q 6 hrs for 7–10 days
- Furosemide: 20–100 mg (peds: 1 mg/kg/dose max 6 mg/kg) IV; max 2 mg/kg day
- Heparin: 80 IU/kg bolus followed by 18 IU/kg drip IV
- Methylprednisolone: 30 mg/kg IV over at least 30 min; max 3 g
- Morphine sulfate: 2–4 mg (peds: 0.1 mg/kg/dose; max 15 mg/dose) IV q 5 min
- Nitroprusside: 0.5–10 mg/kg/min IV
- Penicillin
  —Benzathine penicillin: 1.2 million units (peds: 0.6 million units for <30 kg) IM
  —Penicillin: 2 million units po q 6 hrs for 7–10 days
- Prednisone: 0.5–1 mg/kg/day

Disposition

ADMISSION CRITERIA

- Unstable vital signs
- Oliguria, anuria
- Uremia
- Acute renal failure
- Electrolyte abnormality
- Malignant hypertension
- Congestive heart failure
- Infectious cause of GN

DISCHARGE CRITERIA

- Healthy patients with no comorbid illness who present with mild proteinuria and hematuria with
  —Stable vital signs
  —No signs of infection
  —Otherwise normal lab work
  —Close follow-up

Miscellaneous

ICD9: 583.9

CORE CONTENT CODE: 15.3.1

SUGGESTED READINGS

Glassock R. The primary glomerulopathies. Dis Mon 1996;42(6):340–348.

Glassock RJ, Cohen AH, Adler SG. Primary glomerular diseases. In: Brenner , Rector, eds. The kidney. Vol. 3. Chap. 30. 5th ed. Philadelphia: WB Saunders, 1996:1392–1423.

Mason PD, Pusey CD. Glomerulonephritis: Diagnosis and treatment. Br Med J 1994;309:1557–1563.

Author: Shirley Lee

Gonococcal Disease

Clinical Presentation

SIGNS AND SYMPTOMS

Female

- Cervicitis
  —Yellow or white thick mucopurulent endocervical discharge
  —Cervical edema, congestion, and friability
  —Abnormal vaginal bleeding
- Pelvic inflammatory disease
  —Abdominal pain/tenderness
  —Fever
  —Cervical motion tenderness
  —Bilateral adnexal tenderness
  —Nausea/vomiting
  —Fitz-Hugh-Curtis syndrome
    -Right upper-quadrant pain/tenderness
- Vaginal itching
- Dysuria
- 30–40% asymptomatic carriers

Male

- Urethritis with yellow-white thick discharge
- Urinary tract infection symptoms
  —Dysuria
- Prostatitis
- Epididymitis
- Proctitis

Disseminated

- Fever
- Chills
- Migratory tenosynovitis
  —Involve flexor tendon sheaths of wrist/Achilles tendon
- Rash
- Two-thirds accompanies tenosynovitis
- Hemorrhagic, necrotic pustules on erythematous base
- Begin distally
- Resembles meningococcus
- Healing crust in 4 days
- Arthralgia
- Arthritis
  —Especially of knees, ankle, and wrist
  —Swollen, warm joint with effusion
- Endocarditis

Other

- Pharyngitis
- Conjunctivitis
  —Severe purulent discharge
  —Conjunctival injection/irritation

MECHANISM/DESCRIPTION

- Common sexually transmitted disease
- Often seen with Chlamydia
- Humans only known host for *Neisseria gonorrhea*
- 60–80% of females in contact with males with urethral gonorrhea develop infection
- 20–30% of males in contact with females with gonorrhea develop infection

ETIOLOGY

- *Neisseria gonorrhea*
  —Gram-negative aerobic, diplococcus bacteria
  —Die rapidly when outside normal environment

PEDIATRIC CONSIDERATIONS

- Ophthalmia neonatorum
  —Bilateral conjunctivitis 2–5 days postbirth

Pre-Hospital

N/A

Diagnosis

ESSENTAL WORKUP

- Clinical diagnosis in male gonorrhea
  —Gram's stain of urethral exudate with 95% sensitivity and 97% specificity
- Cervical culture in female gonorrhea
  —Gram's stain cervical discharge with 50% sensitivity and 90% specificity

LABORATORY

- Monoclonal antibodies and DNA probes
  —From simple cervical or urethral swabs
  —Accurate
- Blood cultures for disseminated GC
- Joint arthrocentesis/analysis
  —Neutrophilic leukocytosis (usually >50,000 leukocytes/mm^3)
  —Positive culture when >80,000 leukocytes/mm^3
- Pharyngeal/rectal cultures for local symptoms in high-risk individuals
- CBC for suspected PID
- Urinalysis for suspected PID/lower abdominal pain in females
- Pregnancy test for lower abdominal pain

DIFFERENTIAL DIAGNOSIS

- Urethritis
  —Chlamydia
  —Trichomonas
  —Urinary tract infection
  —Syphilis
- Disseminated GC
  —Meningococcus (rash)
  —Reiter's syndrome
  —Rheumatic fever
  —Systemic lupus
  —Hepatitis

Treatment

INITIAL STABILIZATION

- 0.9%NS 500 cc IV fluid bolus for dehydration due to nausea/vomiting

ED TREATMENT

Genital Infection

- Uncomplicated male genital or female/male pharyngeal/rectal infection
  - —1 dose of the following plus 7-day course of doxycyline or 1 dose of azithromycin
    - -Ceftriaxone 250 mg IM
    - -Cefixime 400 mg po
    - -Ofloxacin 400 mg po
    - -Ciprofloxin 500 mg po
- Salpingitis/pelvic inflammatory disease
  - —Outpatient options
    - -1 dose cefixime/ceftriaxone/spectinomycin plus 14-day course of doxycycline
    - -Ofloxacin 400 mg bid plus clindamycin 450 mg tid or metronidazole 500 mg bid for 14 days
  - —Inpatient options
    - -Cefoxitin IV plus doxycycline IV
- Gonorrhea in pregnancy
  - —1 dose ceftriaxone or spectinomycin plus 7-day course of erythromycin
- Treat sexual partners
- Recommend syphilis (RPR)/HIV testing

Nongenital Infections

- Disseminated GC
  - —Open drainage of septic joints rarely indicated
  - —Inpatient antibiotics for moderate to severe infection
    - -Oral outpatient antibiotics to conclude 7-day course once improvement
  - —Outpatient antibiotics for mild infection not involving weight-bearing joints
  - —Antibiotic options
    - -Ceftriaxone 1 g IM q 24 hrs
    - -Ceftizoxime 1 g IV q 8
    - -Cefotaxime 1 g IV q 8
    - -Spectinomycin 2 mg IM q 12 hrs
    - -Cefixime 400 mg po bid
    - -Ciprofloxacin 500 mg po bid
- Conjunctivitis
  - —Ophthalmia neonatorum options
    - -Penicillin G 100,000 IU/kg/24hrs q 6 hrs
    - -Ceftriaxone 25–50 mg/kg/24hrs q day
    - -Ceftriaxone 125 mg IM/IV

MEDICATIONS

- Azithromycin: 1 g po
- Cefixime: 400 mg po
- Cefotaxime: 1 g IV 8 hrs
- Cefoxitin: 2 g IV q 6 hrs
- Ceftizoxime: 1 g IV q 8 hrs
- Ceftriaxone: 125–250 mg IM; 1 g (peds: 25–50 mg/kg/24hrs) IV q 24 hrs
- Ciprofloxin: 500 mg po
- Clindamycin: 450 mg po tid
- Doxycycline: 100 mg IV/PO q 12 hrs
- Erythromycin: 500 mg po q 6 hrs
- Metronidazole: 500 mg po bid
- Ofloxacin: 400 mg po
- Penicillin G: 100,000 IU/kg/24hrs q 6 hrs
- Spectinomycin: 2 g IM q 12 hrs

Disposition

ADMISSION CRITERIA

- Moderate to severe disseminated GC with arthritis involving weight-bearing joints
- PID with
  - —Peritoneal signs
  - —WBC >15,000/mm^3
  - —Vomiting
  - —Conjunctivitis requiring IV antibiotics

DISCHARGE CRITERIA

- Uncomplicated genital, pharyngeal, or conjunctival infection
- Mild disseminated GC in nontoxic patient without arthritis in weight-bearing joints
- Encourage treatment of sexual partners

Miscellaneous

ICD9: 98.0

CORE CONTENT CODE: 9.1.2

SUGGESTED READINGS

Adimora AA, Hamilton H, Holmes KK, Sparling PF. Sexually transmitted diseases—companion handbook. New York: McGraw Hill, 1994.

Berger RE. Sexually transmitted diseases. Adv Urol 1997;2:97.

Centers for Disease Control and Prevention. 1993 Sexually transmitted disease treatment guidelines. MMWR 1993;42:1–102.

Author: David Levine

Gout/Pseudogout

Clinical Presentation

SIGNS AND SYMPTOMS

- *Gout and pseudogout* both present abruptly as monoarticular arthritis
- Increased warmth, erythema, swelling of the joint
- Early attacks subside spontaneously within 3–10 days, even without treatment
- Later attacks may last longer, cluster, and be more severe
- Crystalline deposition presents as a subacute, acute, or chronic arthritis
  - —Primarily affects articular cartilage, synovium, and nearby tendons or ligaments

Gout

- Symptoms present maximally within 12–24 hours
- Gout also affects bone and subcutaneous tissues (tophi and joint desquamation)
- In women, there is polyarticular predominance (up to 70%)
- Less dramatic presentations in the immunosuppressed and the elderly
- Most common: 1st metatarsophalangeal joint (75%) > ankle; tarsal area; knee > hand; wrist

Pseudogout

- Typically involves larger joints than gout
- Most common: knee > wrist > metacarpals; shoulder; elbow; ankle > hip; tarsal joints
- Monoarticular (25%)
- Asymptomatic (25%)
- Pseudo-osteoarthritis (45%): progressive degeneration, often symmetric
- Pseudorheumatoid arthritis (in the elderly): a polyarticular variant with fever and confusion

MECHANISM/DESCRIPTION

- Gout is the most common of the crystalline diseases
- Renal dysfunction due to urologic deposition of uric acid calculi
- It affects mainly middle-aged men and postmenopausal women
- Risk factors
  - —Male:Female ratio = 9:1
  - —Age >40
  - —Obesity; hypertension; diabetes; hyperlipidemia; vascular disease

Four Phases

- Asymptomatic hyperuricemia (up to 20 years)
- Acute gout
- Intercritical gout: initially no signs or symptoms
- Tophaceous gout (up to 45% of cases)
  - —Attributed to inadequate treatment, and frequent or persistent attacks
  - —Evident usually 10 years after first attack
  - —A deforming arthritis
  - —Associated with avascular necrosis
  - —Tophi
    - -Early in postmenopausal women
    - -Most frequent in previously damaged joints; synovium; subchondral bone, bursae (olecranon; infrapatellar; prepatellar); Achilles tendon; extensor surface of the forearms; toes; fingers; ear; rarely CNS or cardiac (valves)
    - -May coalesce later

Pseudogout (Chondrocalcinosis)

- The most common cause of acute monarthritis after age 60
- Risk factors
  - —Hypercalcemia (e.g., hyperparathyroidism, familial); hemochromatosis; hemosiderosis;
  - —Hypo- and hyperthyroidism, hypophosphatemia, hypomagnesemia, amyloidosis, or gout

ETIOLOGY

- Gout is caused by deposition of *monosodium urate crystals* in tissues from supersaturated extracellular fluid, due to
  - —Underexcretion of uric acid
  - —Any rapid change in uric acid levels (e.g., the initiation or cessation of diuretics, alcohol, salicylates, cyclosporine, lead acetate poisoning, and uricosurics or allopurinol)
- Pseudogout occurs secondary to excess synovial accumulation of *calcium pyrophosphate* crystals
- Precipitants for both gout and pseudogout include minor trauma and acute illnesses (e.g., surgery, ischemic heart disease)

Pre-Hospital

N/A

Diagnosis

ESSENTIAL WORKUP

- Arthrocentesis and aspiration of tophi
  - —Examine aspirant for crystals, Gram's stain, cultures, leukocyte count, and differential
  - —Fluid is typically thick pasty white
  - —*Gout:* 20,000–100,000 WBC/mm^3; poor string and mucin clot; no bacteria
  - —*Pseudogout:* up to 50,000 WBC/mm^3; no bacteria
- Microscopic examination of crystals under polarized light
  - —*Gout:* needle-shaped; strong birefringence; negative elongation
  - —*Pseudogout:* rhomboid; weak birefringence; positive elongation

LABORATORY

- CBC often shows a leukocytosis that does not differentiate infectious from crystalline etiology
- Chemistry panel to assess for renal impairment
- Magnesium and calcium, TSH, and serum iron
- Uric acid level has limited value
  - —It is normal in 30% of acute gouty attacks
  - —In screening general populations, hyperuricemia is mostly asymptomatic (90% of cases)
- If infectious arthritis is suspected
  - —Blood and urine cultures
  - —Urethral, cervical, rectal, or pharyngeal gonococcal cultures

IMAGING/SPECIAL TESTS

- Plain radiographs to assess the presence of
  - —Effusion
  - —Joint space narrowing
  - —The baseline status of the joint
  - —Contiguous osteomyelitis
  - —Fractures or foreign body
    - -*Acute Gout:* soft tissue swelling; normal mineralization; joint space preservation
    - -*Chronic Gout:* calcified tophi; asymmetric bony erosions; overhanging edges; bony shaft tapering
    - -*Pseudogout:* chondrocalcinosis; subchondral sclerosis or cysts (wrist); radiopaque calcification of cartilage, tendons, and ligaments; radiopaque osteophytes
- 24-hour urine uric acid may detect uric acid underexcretion

DIFFERENTIAL DIAGNOSIS

- Infectious arthritis
- Trauma
- Osteoarthritis
- Reactive arthritis
- Miscellaneous crystalline arthritis
- Aseptic necrosis
- Rheumatoid arthritis
- Systemic lupus erythematosus
- Sickle Cell
- Osteomyelitis

Treatment

INITIAL STABILIZATION

- Relieve pain
- Rule out an infectious etiology

ED TREATMENT

- NSAIDs are the first line treatment
- If ineffective or contraindicated
  - —Oral prednisone
  - —Colchicine (limited by toxicity)
- Joint aspiration with or without intra-articular steroid injection
- Avoid aspirin
- The reduction of hyperuricemia and the long-term management of gout and pseudogout are not within the usual scope of ED care. Strategies include
  - —The careful withdrawal of gout-producing agent
  - —In gout, uricosurics or allopurinol can be used to reduce uric acid
  - —Uricosurics (e.g., probenecid, sulfinpyrazone) increase uric acid excretion
  - —Increased fluid intake and urine alkalization to prevent renal stones
  - —Allopurinol is the most effective agent. It is recommended for overproducers, renal disease, those undergoing cytotoxic therapy, uricosuric failure, frequent attacks, and tophaceous disease
  - —Long-term colchicine or NSAIDs may be effective prophylactically against pseudogout and gout

MEDICATIONS

- NSAIDs in maximal doses initially × 3 d, then taper over 4 d
  - —Indomethacin: 50 mg po tid qid
  - —Ketorolac: 15–30 mg IM/IV in ED, may repeat × 1 dose
  - —Naproxen: 500 mg po tid
  - —Sulindac: 200 mg po tid
- Corticosteroids
  - —Prednisone: 40 mg po qd × 3–4 d; taper over 7–14 d
  - —Methylprednisolone: 40 mg IM or IV qd × 3–4 d
  - —Triamcinolone: 10–40 mg plus dexamethasone 2–10 mg intra-articular
- Colchicine: 0.5mg/hr po up to pain relief, 8 mg total, or GI toxicity
- Probenecid: 250–500 mg po bid 1st dose
- Allopurinol: 100–300 mg po qd 1st dose

Disposition

ADMISSION CRITERIA

- Suspected infectious arthritis
- Acute renal failure
- Intractable pain

DISCHARGE CRITERIA

- No evidence of infection
- Adequate pain relief

Miscellaneous

ICD9: 274.9, 275.49

CORE CONTENT CODE: 10.2.1.2

SUGGESTED READINGS

Buckley TJ. Radiologic features of gout. Am Fam Physician 1996;54(4):1232–1238.

Joseph J, McGrath H. Gout or "pseudogout": How to differentiate crystal-induced arthropathies. Geriatrics 1995;50(4):33–39.

McGill NW. Gout and other crystal arthropathies. Med J Aust 1997;166:33–38.

Schumacher HR. Crystal-induced arthritis: An overview. Am J Med 1996;100(Suppl 2A):46S–51S.

Authors: Delaram Ghadishah; A. Antoine Kazzi

Granulocytopenia

Clinical Presentation

SIGNS AND SYMPTOMS

- Fever (may be only sign of infection)
- Localized erythema or fluctuances (indicates abscess)
- Signs of lung consolidation
  - —Rales
  - —Rhonchi
  - —Dullness
- Dysuria
- Urinary retention, urgency, or frequency
- Change in bowel habits
- Mucosal lesions

MECHANISM/DESCRIPTION

- Less than normal number of polymorphonuclear leukocytes
- Number of PMN + bands $<500/mm^3$
  - —Patients with a count below 1,000 that has recently or rapidly fallen are at greater risk for infection than those with a count below 500 but rising
  - —Patients with myelodysplastic syndromes should be considered granulocytopenic with higher counts because of defective neutrophils

ETIOLOGY

- Most commonly seen in patients undergoing myelosuppressive drug therapy or radiation treatment for neoplasms
- Chemicals
  - —NO
  - —Benzene
  - —Arsenic
  - —Bismuth
- Immune-related
  - —Bone marrow infiltration
- Infection
  - —Bacterial
    - -Primarily staphylococcal and Gram-negative
  - —Fungal
- Vitamin deficiency (B_{12}/folate)

Pre-Hospital

N/A

Diagnosis

ESSENTIAL WORKUP

- Complete physical examination
- Detailed examination of oral mucosa and perianal area
- Palpation of skin, searching for fluctuances or tenderness
- Careful lung examination may reveal pneumonia
- Rectal examination

LABORATORY

- CBC with differential
- Blood culture from two different sites, with one from IV catheter site if present
- Urinalysis and urine culture
  - —Urinalysis may be normal

IMAGING/SPECIAL TESTS

- Chest radiography even in absence of lung findings
- CSF analysis for altered mental status/signs of meningitis

DIFFERENTIAL DIAGNOSIS

- Infection
  - —Bacterial
  - —Fungal
  - —Viral
  - —Protozoal/parasitic
- Immune suppression
  - —Cell-mediated
  - —Antineoplastic agents

Treatment

INITIAL STABILIZATION

- ABCs
- Initiate IV, O_2 , monitor
- For hypotension
  —Administer 1 L 0.9%NS IV fluid bolus (peds: 20 cc/kg)
  —Initiate pressors as needed to stabilize blood pressure if no response to IV fluids

ED TREATMENT

- Strict isolation
- Administer broad-spectrum combination antibiotics after cultures for suspected or documented infection
  —Imipenem-cilastatin
  —Ceftazidime alone or with aminoglycoside (amikacin, tobramycin, gentamycin)
  —Aminoglycoside plus antipseudomonal β-lactam (mezlocillin, piperacillin, or ticarcillin)
  —Vancomycin
    -Add if patient is at risk to be carrier of *Staphylococcus aureus* or has a history of previous staphylococcal infections

MEDICATIONS

- Amikacin: 15 mg/kg/24hrs (peds: 15–30 mg/kg/24hrs) divided q 8–24 hrs IV
- Ceftazidime: 1–2 g (peds: 100–150 mg/kg/24hrs) q 8–12 hrs IV
- Gentamycin: 1 mg/kg (peds 2–2.5 mg/kg) q 8 hrs or 5 mg/kg q 24 hrs
- Imipenem-cilastatin: 250 mg–1000 mg q 6–8 hrs
- Mezlocillin: 3 g q 4 hrs over 30 min
- Piperacillin: 3 g q 4 hrs over 30 min
- Ticarcillin: 3 g (peds: 200–300 mg/kg/24hrs) q 4 hrs over 30 min
- Tobramycin: 3–5mg/kg/24hrs (peds: 6–8 mg/kg/24hrs) divided q 8 hrs IV
- Vancomycin: 1–2 mg/kg q 8–12 hrs IV

Disposition

ADMISSION CRITERIA

- Signs of infection
- Unreliable patient
- Close followup unavailable

DISCHARGE CRITERIA

- Previously diagnosed granulocytopenia
- Completely asymptomatic
- Close followup assured
- Reliable patient

Miscellaneous

ICD9: 288.0

CORE CONTENT CODE: 7.7.3

SUGGESTED READINGS

Bagby GC. Disorders of neutrophil production. In: Bennett JC, et al. Cecil's textbook of medicine. Philadelphia: WB Saunders, 1996:908–915.

Calandra T. Spectrum and treatment of bacterial infections in cancer patients with granulocytopenia. Rec Res Can Res 1991;121:329–336.

Schimpff SC. Infections in the cancer patient—diagnosis, prevention, and treatment. In: Mandel G, et al., eds. Mandel, Douglas and Bennet's principles and practice of infectious disease. New York: Churchill Livingstone, 1995:2666–2684.

Vogelzang NJ, Flaherty JP. Fever and granulocytopenia: a viewpoint from an academic setting. Rec Res Can Res 1993;132:79–88.

Authors: Andrzej Dmowki; Elicia Sinor Kennedy

Greenstick Fracture

Clinical Presentation

SIGNS AND SYMPTOMS

- Pain
- Inability to use or mobilize the affected extremity
- Localized tenderness
- Swelling
- Ecchymosis
- Palpation of bony deformities
- Crepitus
- Pseudoparalysis
- Ecchymosis

MECHANISM/DESCRIPTION

- An incomplete fracture of the diaphysis of a long bone
  - —A break in the cortex and periosteum of one side
  - —An intact periosteum on the other side of the fracture
- Compared with adults, children's bones are more
  - —Porous
  - —Compliant
  - —Resilient
  - —Soft
- Stresses and forces applied result often in incomplete fractures
  - —These fractures are more stable
  - —Somewhat less painful than complete fractures
  - —May have some degree of angulation and rotation
- Most common type of pediatric fracture
  - —50% of all fractures prior to the age of 12
  - —May occur into the teenage years
- Complete healing is the most common outcome
- Complications
  - —Plastic/bowing deformities
  - —Reduction of limb mobility
  - —Rarely growth plate disturbances

ETIOLOGY

N/A

Pre-Hospital

- Cold packs to affected area
- Splint the injured extremity in the position found
  - —Air cushions
  - —Boards
  - —Plain tape
  - —Rolled towels

Diagnosis

ESSENTIAL WORKUP

- Assessment of the extremity distal to the injury
  - —Circulation
  - —Motor function
  - —Sensation
- Assess for associated injuries
- Obtain appropriate radiographs

LABORATORY

N/A

IMAGING/SPECIAL TESTS

- AP and lateral radiograph of the involved limb
  - —Cortical disruption
  - —Periosteal tearing on the convex side of the bone
  - —Intact periosteum on the concave side
  - —Greenstick fractures are never compound
- Oblique views are sometimes helpful
- Repeat radiograph after reduction

DIFFERENTIAL DIAGNOSIS

- Contusions
- Sprains
- Bowing deformities
- Other fractures
- Infection
- Tumor

Treatment

INITIAL STABILIZATION

- Immobilization of the injured extremity
- Pain control
- Reduction of angulation or rotation using conscious sedation

ED TREATMENT

- Splint or cast the injured limb
  —Immobilize the joints proximal and distal to the injury

MEDICATIONS

Conscious Sedation

- Fentanyl: 1–2 μg/kg IV
- Ketamine: 0.5–1 mg/kg IV
- Meperidine: 1–1.5 mg/kg IV
- Midazolam: 0.05–0.1 mg/kg (max 2.5 mg) IV
- Morphine sulfate: 0.1 mg/kg (max 15 mg) IV

Pain Control

- Acetaminophen with codeine: 0.5–1.0 mg/kg (max 60 mg) q 4 hrs po
- Ibuprofen: 4–10 mg/kg (max 3200 mg/24hrs) po

Disposition

ADMISSION CRITERIA

- Suspicion of nonaccidental trauma

DISCHARGE CRITERIA

- Pain is well controlled
- Immobilization does not severely impede the child
- Orthopedic referral within 1 week
- Splint or cast instructions
  —Ice/cold pack application
  —Elevation of the injured limb
  —Analgesic medication

Miscellaneous

ICD9: N/A

CORE CONTENT CODE: N/A

SUGGESTED READINGS

Davis D, Green D. Forearm fractures in children: Pitfalls and complications. Clin Orthop 1976;120:172.

England S, Sundberg S. Management of common pediatric fractures. Pediatr Clin North Am 1996;43:991.

Olney B. Musculoskeletal injuries. In: Buntain W, ed. Management of pediatric trauma. Philadelphia: WB Saunders, 1995.

Rang R. Children's fractures. Philadelphia: JB Lippincott, 1983.

Authors: William Sabina; Daniel L. Savitt

Guillain-Barré Syndrome

Clinical Presentation

SIGNS AND SYMPTOMS

- Guillain-Barré Syndrome (GBS) presents in the classic pattern in approximately 90–95% patients
- Two features required for diagnosis according to standards of National Institute of Neurological and Communicative Disorders (NINCDS);
  —Progressive motor weakness/paralysis of more than one limb
    -Weakness classically begins in the lower extremities and *ascends* to the upper extremities
    -Weakness is most often *proximal* in distribution
    -Motor weakness is most commonly the initial presenting complaint
    -Weakness progresses rapidly reaching symptomatic peak in 1–4 weeks
  —Loss of tendon reflexes
    -Initial hyporeflexia followed by complete areflexia in affected limbs
    -75% areflexic on initial presentation
- NINCDS features strongly suggestive of diagnosis;
  —Symptoms progress rapidly, reaching a peak at 2 weeks in 50% of patients and at 4 weeks in 90% of patients
  —Sensory symptoms
    -Paresthesias of the fingertips or toes are common and can precede weakness by 7–10 days
    -Pain (33%) commonly in the shoulders, thighs, or muscles of the lumbar or pelvic region
  —Cranial nerve (CN) involvement
    -Facial weakness (50%) (CN VII), most commonly bilateral
    -Bulbar weakness (25–50%) (CN IX, X); dysphasia, dysarthria, drooling
    -Extraocular (15%) (CN III, IV); ophthalmoplegia, ptosis
    -Pupillary abnormalities not seen in GBS
  —Respiratory weakness; 25–33% will require mechanical ventilation
  —Respiratory failure occurs due to
    -Bulbar weakness and inability to protect upper airway
    -Inadequate ventilation from respiratory muscle weakness
    -Atelectasis (42%), pneumonia (25–40%), pulmonary embolus (2%)
  —Some degree of autonomic dysfunction occurs in 70%
    -Most common is sinus tachycardia
    -Labile hypertension, orthostatic hypotension, dysrhythmias
  —No fever on initial presentation
  —Bowel and bladder function is commonly preserved
- Features which should suggest an alternative diagnosis
  —Fever
  —Marked asymmetry of weakness
  —Normal reflexes
  —Sharply demarcated sensory level
  —Bowel/bladder dysfunction, decreased rectal tone
- GBS Variants
  —Miller-Fisher syndrome presents with triad of ophthalmoplegia, ataxia, and areflexia
    -Weakness may not be significant
    -Accounts for approximately 5% of GBS patients
  —Many rare variants

MECHANISM/DESCRIPTION

- GBS is an acute inflammatory, symmetrically progressive, demyelinating neuropathy
- Involves peripheral nervous system only, central nervous system spared
- It is the most common cause of acute generalized paralysis
- Incidence of 0.6–2.0 per 100,000 population
- All ages affected with slight bimodal distribution in young adults and the elderly
- No sexual predilection
- Mortality 3–12%
- Aberrant autoimmune response directed against myelin or axonal antigens in peripheral nerve
- Recovery usually begins 2–4 weeks after symptom progression stops
  —15% patients will recover with no residual deficit
  —66% will have minor residual neurologic deficits
  —5–10% will be permanently disabled due to weakness or paralysis

ETIOLOGY

- Postinfectious
  —66% patients have mild illness involving the respiratory or GI tract 1–4 weeks prior
    -Campylobacter jejuni
    -Hepatitis virus
    -Mycoplasma pneumoniae
    -Human immunodeficiency virus
    -Cytomegalovirus, Epstein-Barr virus
    -Varicella
- Post vaccination; influenza, rabies
- Hodgkin's disease
- Surgery
- Drugs: heroin, streptokinase, captopril, danazol, penicillamine, vincristine

PEDIATRIC CONSIDERATIONS

- GBS highly variable in children
- Pain and irritability will be initial symptoms in 20% of younger children

Pre-Hospital

CAUTIONS

- Patients may need ventilatory support

Diagnosis

ESSENTIAL WORKUP

- Initial diagnosis suspected based on clinical presentation
- Definitive diagnosis based on clinical, laboratory, and electrodiagnostic criteria
- Assess cardiorespiratory status; ECG, CXR, arterial blood gas
- Vital capacity (VC)
  —Respiratory therapist should formally perform, <15 ml/kg may require ventilatory support
  —Ability to count from 1–25 in a single breath reflects a VC of approximately 20 ml/kg
- Electrolytes
  —Serum Na and K^+; SIADH associated with GBS
- Lumbar puncture
  —CSF protein will be elevated between 55 and 250
  —CSF cell count should be <10 mononuclear leukocytes/mm^3

IMAGING/SPECIAL TESTS

- MRI, CT myelogram to evaluate for suspected cord compression
- Electromyography for evaluation of peripheral nerve function

DIFFERENTIAL DIAGNOSIS

- The most acute condition to rule out is acute cord compression
  —Cord compression is suggested by more acute onset, bowel and bladder dysfunction, decreased rectal tone, and sharply demarcated sensory loss
- Transverse myelitis
- Trauma, recent invasive procedure of spine
- Myasthenia gravis, Lyme disease, tick paralysis
- Lambert-Eaton syndrome
- Acute intermittent porphyria, poliomyelitis
- Systemic lupus erythematosus
- Botulism, diphtheria, viral syndrome
- Acute alcoholic myopathy
- Heavy metals (lead, arsenic)
- Psychogenic/hysteria, malingering
- Drugs

Treatment

INITIAL STABILIZATION

Airway

- The progression to respiratory failure can occur rapidly
- Intubate patients with the following
  —Severe hypoxia (PO_2 <50)
  —Tachypnea (RR >30)
  —Poor patient appearance/fatigue
  —Respiratory acidosis and hypercarbia (pH <7.25, PCO_2 >50)
  —Rapid progression of symptoms
  —*Vital capacity measurement of <15 ml/kg* is an indication for elective intubation
- *Administration of succinylcholine in GBS patients is contraindicated* because of the potential for lethal hyperkalemia. Use nondepolarizing paralytic

ED TREATMENT

- Mode of ventilation
  —Weak/paralyzed patient; SIMV with a tidal volume of 10–15 ml/kg, PEEP of 5
- Plasmapheresis is first-line therapy
- Intravenous immunoglobulin (IVIG) should be considered second-line therapy
- There is no role for the use of corticosteroids in the treatment of GBS
- Neurology should be consulted

MEDICATIONS

- Plasmapheresis: 50 ml/kg albumin equals 1 plasma volume
- Immunoglobulin: 0.4 g/kg/day IV

Disposition

ADMISSION CRITERIA

- Patients with GBS should be admitted for observation
- Admission to the ICU is recommended for any patient with respiratory compromise, inability to walk, autonomic or bulbar symptoms

DISCHARGE CRITERIA

- Patients with suspected GBS should not be discharged

Miscellaneous

ICD9: 357.0

CORE CONTENT CODE: 11.5.1

SUGGESTED READINGS

Brody AJ, Sternbach G, Varon J. Octave Landry: Guillain-Barré syndrome. J Emerg Med 1994;12(6):833–7.

Jones HR. Childhood Guillain-Barré syndrome: Clinical presentation, diagnosis, and therapy. J Child Neurol 1996;11(1):4–12.

Kissel JT. Treatment and prognosis of Guillain-Barré syndrome and variants. Annual Meeting of American Academy of Neurology 1996:336-1–336-14.

Ng KK, Howard RS, Fish DR, et al. Management and outcome of severe Guillain-Barré syndrome. QJM 1995;88(4):243–50.

Rees J. Guillain-Barré syndrome. Clinical manifestations and directions for treatment. Drugs 1995;49(6):912–920.

Teitelbaum JS, Borel CO. Respiratory dysfunction in Guillain-Barré syndrome. Clin Chest Med 1994;15(4):705–714.

Author: Paul File

Hallucinogen, Poisoning

Clinical Presentation

SIGNS AND SYMPTOMS

- Considerable individual variation
- Usually oriented and able to give a history of exposure, even while having illusions
- Initial symptoms
  - —Nausea
  - —Flushing
  - —Chills
  - —Tachycardia
  - —Hypertension
  - —Piloerection
  - —Tremor

NEUROLOGIC SYMPTOMS

- Restlessness and dizziness within 20 to 30 minutes of ingestion
- Affective lability
- Desire to laugh (especially with *Psilocybe* mushrooms)
- Anxiety, despair, helplessness, incipient dread
- Exaggeration of preexisting mood (medical personnel are more likely to see patients with exaggeration of anxious moods, or "bad trips")
- Intensified perceptions
- Visual distortions
- Auditory distortions (less than visual distortions)
- Tactile distortions (especially with mescaline)
- Distortions of reality
- Synesthesia: blending of sensory modalities (e.g., seeing sounds)
- Time-space distortions
- Sensation of rapid aging
- Loss of ego boundaries and feeling of unity with the universe
- Religious or mystical experiences
- Sleep disruption

NEUROLOGICAL SIGNS

- Unusual behavior
- Speech disruption
- Markedly dilated pupils (especially with LSD)
- Piloerection
- Hyperreflexia
- Coma, with massive exposures
- Convulsions, with massive exposures and in children who become hyperpyrexic after *Psilocybe* mushroom ingestion

PULMONARY

- Mild tachypnea
- Respiratory arrest, with massive exposures

CARDIOVASCULAR

- Tachycardia
- Hypertension
- Dysrhythmias (with methamphetamine and amphetamine use)

GASTROINTESTINAL

- Nausea/ vomiting (especially with mescaline)

METABOLIC

- Hyperpyrexia (especially with MDMA use at "Rave" clubs)

HEMOPOIETIC

- Coagulopathies and hemorrhage due to disruption of platelet serotonin function, has been reported at high doses

MECHANISM/DESCRIPTION

- Characteristics
  - —Predominantly alters perception, cognition, and mood
  - —Minimal memory loss, intellectual deficits, stupor, autonomic nervous system dysfunction
- Symptoms characterized by sympathetic arousal
- Structurally similar to neurotransmitters
  - —Serotonin (5-HT)
  - —Involved in the production of hallucinations
  - —Norepinephrine (NE)
  - —Epinephrine (EPI)
  - —Dopamine (DA)
- Hallucinogens act as agonists at some 5-HT receptor subtypes and as antagonists at other 5-HT receptor subtypes resulting in intracellular changes that ultimately produce hallucinations

ETIOLOGY

- Most exposures are intentional
- Common hallucinogens include (see Table 1)
  - —Lysergic acid diethylamide (LSD)
  - —Mescaline (Peyote cactus)
  - —Hallucinogenic amphetamines
    - -Methylenedioxyamphetamine (MDA)
    - -Methylenedioxyethamphetamine (MDEA)
    - -Methylenedioxymethamphetamine (MDMA)
    - -Dimethoxyamphetamine (DOM or STP)
  - —Psilocybin (*Psilocybe* mushrooms)
- LSD
  - —Prototypical hallucinogen
  - —Street-marketed Peyote cactus "buttons" and *Psilocybe* mushrooms are often adulterated with LSD
  - —Focus for the signs and symptoms described above
  - —Other hallucinogens present similarly

Pre-Hospital

CONTROVERSIES

- Sedation with benzodiazepines versus haloperidol versus physical restraints
  - —Sedation masks the symptoms and may limit the history
- Recommend benzodiazepines over haloperidol, especially for amphetamines

CAUTIONS

- Sedate or restrain patient to insure safe transport
- For the hyperthermic patient: employ sedation rather than physical restraint to limit progressive hyperthermia

Table 1

HALLUCINOGEN	CHEMICAL CLASS	SOURCE	DURATION OF EFFECT
LSD	Indolyl alkylamine	Synthetic derivatives of fungus in rye	6–12 hrs
Mescaline	Phenyl alkylamine	Peyote cactus	6–12 hrs
MDA	Phenyl alkylamine	Synthetic	8–12 hrs
MDMA (Ecstasy)	Phenyl alkylamine	Synthetic	4–6 hrs
Psilocybin	Indolyl alkylamine	Mushrooms	

Diagnosis

ESSENTIAL WORKUP

- Measure core temperature
- Determine risk of rhabdomyolysis
  - —Urine dip for myoglobin
  - —CPK level

LABORATORY

- Electrolytes, BUN/Cr, glucose
- Urine toxicology screen
  - —Rarely indicated
    - -Distinguishing between hallucinogens is of little value
    - -The clinical syndromes and treatments are similar
  - —Most do not detect LSD

IMAGING/SPECIAL TESTS

- Gas chromatography mass spectrometry
  - —Yields true positives for LSD 53% of the time
- Radioimmunoassays for LSD and its major metabolite
  - —May detect LSD for up to 24 hours
- *Psilocybe* mushrooms
  - —Stain blue when bruised or when painted with the photographic developer Metol

DIFFERENTIAL DIAGNOSIS

- Meningitis
- Intracranial bleeds or lesions
- Psychiatric illnesses
  - —LSD associated with prolonged psychoses, resembling schizo-affective disorders
  - —Patients with true psychosis are usually not oriented or able to give their own history
- Other hallucinogenic substances
  - —Anticholinergic drugs (e.g., diphenhydramine)
  - —Plants (e.g., jimsonweed and marijuana)
  - —Phencyclidine (PCP)
  - —Chronic amphetamine abuse
  - —Chronic cocaine abuse
  - —Steroids
- Infectious/febrile seizures in the hyperpyretic child

PEDIATRIC CONSIDERATIONS

Assess parent/child relationships for possibility of neglect or abuse

Treatment

INITIAL STABILIZATION

- ABCs
- IV access/rehydration with 0.9%NS if significant fluid loss
- Aggressive cooling if hyperthermic
- Narcan, Accucheck, and dextrose, and thiamine if altered mental status

ED TREATMENT

- Cooling measures
  - —Cool mist and fans
  - —Benzodiazepines if agitated
  - —Paralytics if needed (*not* succinylcholine)
- Sedate if agitated
  - —Benzodiazepines
  - —Rarely neuroleptics
    - -May intensify hallucinogenic experience
    - -May lower seizure threshold
    - -Haloperidol neuroleptic of choice, if given
- Activated charcoal if oral ingestion
- Place in a quiet, calm environment
- Urine alkalinization for treatment of rhabdomyolysis

MEDICATIONS

- Dextrose: D50W 1 amp (25 g /50 ml) (peds D25W 0.5–1 g/kg or 2–4 ml/kg) IV
- Diazepam (benzodiazepine): 5–10 mg (peds 0.2–0.5 mg/kg) IV
- Haloperidol (haldol): 2.5–10 mg IV/IM
- Mannitol: 1 g/kg IV over 30 min
- Naloxone (narcan): 2 mg (peds 0.01–0.1 mg/kg) IV or IM initial dose
- Sodium bicarbonate drip: 2 amp in 1 L of D5W to run at 1.5–2 times maintenance rates and to keep urine alkalinized
- Thiamine (Vitamin B_1): 100 mg (peds 25 mg) IV or IM

PEDIATRIC CONSIDERATIONS

Avoid haloperidol in children

Disposition

ADMISSION CRITERIA

- Severely intoxicated
- Atypical presentations or prolonged symptoms
- Prolonged periods of agitation and hyperthermia
  - —Risk of rhabdomyolysis

DISCHARGE CRITERIA

Most patients, after receiving supportive therapy and observation can be discharged once asymptomatic

PEDIATRIC CONSIDERATIONS

Suspected cases of child abuse or neglect require referral to child protection agencies

Miscellaneous

ICD9: 969.6

CORE CONTENT CODE: 17.2.19

SUGGESTED READINGS

Abraham HD, Aldridge AM, Gogia P. The psychopharmacology of hallucinogens. Neuropsychopharmacology 1996;14:285–298.

Glennon RA. Classical hallucinogens: An introductory overview. NIDA Res Monogr 1994;146:4–32.

Kulig K. LSD. Emerg Med Clin North Am 1990;8(3):551–558.

McKenna DJ. Plant hallucinogens: Springboards for psychotherapeutic drug discovery. Behav Brain Res 1996;73:109–115.

Spoerke DG, Hall AH. Plants and mushrooms of abuse. Emerg Med Clin North Am 1990;8(3):579–593.

Author: Kimberlie Graeme

Hand Infection

Clinical Presentation

SIGNS AND SYMPTOMS

Paronychia

- Localized edema, erythema, and pain in proximal portion of lateral nail fold
- Fluctuance may be present and may extend beneath the nail margin to the nail bed
- Systemic signs and symptoms are usually not present

Felon

- Erythema and tense swelling of the distal pulp space that does *not* extend proximal to the PIP
- Aching pain early, severe throbbing pain late
- Systemic signs and symptoms are usually not present

Herpetic Whitlow

- Distal pulp space is swollen, but remains soft
- Lateral nail folds may be affected
- Throbbing pain of the distal pulp space
- Vesicles containing nonpurulent fluid are present and may form bullae
- Systemic symptoms may be present, as fever, lymphadenopathy, and constitutional symptoms

Flexor Tenosynovitis

- Severe pain and symmetric edema of the digit, usually the thumb, index finger, or middle finger
- Severe tenderness over the course of the tendon sheath
- Flexed position of the finger at rest
- Pain on passive extension of the finger—may be the only finding in early infection

Clenched Fist Injury

- Laceration over the MCP from striking an object with a clenched fist
- Any laceration over the MCP must be assumed to be a human bite wound until proven otherwise

Web Space Abscess

- Pain and edema of the affected web space and adjacent palm
- Fingers are held abducted

Palmar Space Infections

- Thenar space infection
  - —Pain, tenderness, tense edema of thenar eminence
  - —Dorsal edema without tenderness
  - —Thumb is held abducted and flexed, and passive adduction is painful
- Midpalmar space infection
  - —Pain, edema, and tenderness of the midpalmar space
  - —Dorsal edema without tenderness
  - —Motion of middle and ring fingers is painful
- Hypothenar space infection
  - —Pain and fullness over hypothenar eminence
  - —No limitation of finger movement

ETIOLOGY

- Bacterial infection of the hand is associated with skin pathogens, *Staphylococcus* or *Streptococcus* species, and history of a puncture wound
- Anaerobes are identified in 75% of paronychia in children due to thumb sucking and nail biting
- Chronic paronychia may be caused by *Candida albicans*
- Herpetic whitlow is caused by type 1 or 2 herpes simplex virus
- Clenched fist injuries involve a variety of pathogens, including anaerobic *Streptococcus* and *Eikenella*

Pre-Hospital

- No specific considerations

Diagnosis

ESSENTIAL WORKUP

- Most hand infections are diagnosed by history and physical examination with special attention to neurovascular status

LABORATORY

- Although usually not necessary, herpetic whitlow may be confirmed by Tzank test
- Gram stain and culture may guide antibiotic choice in felons
- Blood cultures are not routinely indicated

IMAGING/SPECIAL TESTS

- Radiographs are usually not helpful in paronychia unless there has been trauma or a suspected foreign body
- With felon, flexor tenosynovitis, and palmar space infection, radiograph may identify osteomyelitis or foreign body
- Radiographs in clenched fist injury may reveal a fracture

DIFFERENTIAL DIAGNOSIS

- Paronychia should be differentiated from herpetic whitlow and felon
- The differential for palmar space infection includes flexor tenosynovitis, cellulitis, and web space infection

Treatment

INITIAL STABILIZATION

- ABCs if patient is toxic or above conditions occur in the setting of sepsis or other injury

ED TREATMENT

Paronychia

- Early paronychia without purulence present may be managed with oral antibiotics and rest
  —Cephalexin, dicloxacillin
  —Clindamycin or erythromycin if associated with nail biting or oral contact
- Superficial infections are drained by inserting an 11-blade between nail and eponychium and lifting the eponychium from the nail
- If necessary, the lateral nail fold may be incised tangential to the curvature of the nail
- When pus is present under the adjacent nail, one-fourth of the nail should be removed
- When pus is present under the dorsal roof of the proximal nail, remove one-third of the proximal nail

Felon

- Felons are drained through a unilateral longitudinal incision which does not cross the DIP flexor crease
  —A lateral incision is preferred to drain distal pulp infection
  —Make sure the incision avoids the neurovascular bundle
- Disruption of fibrous septa is no longer recommended because it results in an unstable fingertip
- Give oral antibiotics to cover skin pathogens, place a drain, and recheck in 48 hours
  —Cephalexin, dicloxacillin

Herpetic Whitlow

- Usually self-limited; do not incise and drain
- Oral acyclovir may be given to patients with systemic infection

Flexor Tenosynovitis, Web Space Abscess, Palmar Space Infection

- Elevation, IV antibiotics, and pain control in the ED
  —Ampicillin/sulbactam, cefoxitin, ticarcillin/clavulanate
- All of these infections require consultation with a hand surgeon for admission and drainage

Clenched Fist Injury

- Elevation, IV antibiotics, tetanus prophylaxis, and pain control in the ED
  —Ampicillin/sulbactam, cefoxitin, ticarcillin/clavulanate
- All bite wounds with evidence of infection or joint involvement require emergent consultation with a hand surgeon
- If there are no signs of infection and no joint penetration, patients may be considered for outpatient treatment with oral antibiotics after appropriate irrigation and wound care
  —Ampicillin/clavulanate or penicillin V plus cephalexin or dicloxacillin
  —Do not primarily close lacerations associated with a human bite; delayed primary closure or healing by secondary intention is appropriate

MEDICATIONS

- Acyclovir: adult: 400 mg po tid for 10 d; peds: not recommended for herpetic whitlow
- Ampicillin/clavulanate: adult: 875/125 mg po bid; peds: 40 mg/kg/d po div q 6 hrs
- Ampicillin/sulbactam: adult: 2 g IV q 6 hrs; peds: safety not established
- Cefoxitin: adult: 2 g IV q 8 hrs; peds: 80–160 mg/kg/d IV or IM div q 6 hrs
- Cephalexin: adult: 500 g po qid for 7 d; peds: 40 mg/kg/d po div q 6 hrs
- Clindamycin: adult: 300 mg po qid for 7 d; peds: 20–40 mg/kg/d div q 6 hrs po, IV, IM
- Dicloxacillin: adult: 500 mg po qid for 7 d; peds: 12.5–50 mg/kg/d po div q 6 hrs
- Erythromycin: adult: 500 mg po qid for 7d; peds: 40 mg/kg/d div q 6 hrs po
- Penicillin V: adult: 250 mg po qid; peds: 40 mg/kg/d po div q 6 hrs
- Ticarcillin/clavulanate: adult: 3.1 g IV q 6 hrs; peds: safety not established

Disposition

ADMISSION CRITERIA

Flexor Tenosynovitis, Web Space Abscess, Palmar Space Infections

- All these infections require admission for IV antibiotics and drainage

Clenched Fist Injury with Signs of Infection

- Requires admission for surgical debridement and IV antimicrobials

DISCHARGE CRITERIA

Paronychia and Felons

- Patients with uncomplicated paronychia or felon may be discharged from the ED with a recheck and drain removal in 48 hours

Herpetic Whitlow

- Patients with herpetic whitlow may be discharged from the ED with appropriate follow-up

Clenched Fist Injury Without Infection

- May be discharged on oral antibiotics with follow-up in 24 hours

Miscellaneous

ICD9: 136.9

CORE CONTENT CODE: 3.2

SUGGESTED READINGS

Brown DM, Young VL. Hand infections. South Med J 1993;86(1):56–66.

Hausman MR, Lisser SP. Hand infections. Orthop Clin North Am 1992;23(1):171–185.

Antosia RE, Lyn E. The hand. In: Rosen P, et al., eds. Emergency medicine: Concepts and clinical practice. 4th ed. St. Louis: CV Mosby, 1998:625–668.

Authors: Deborah Sanders; Robert Galli

Head Trauma, Blunt

Clinical Presentation

SIGNS AND SYMPTOMS

- Evidence of trauma to head includes
  - —Scalp laceration, cephalohematoma, or ecchymosis
  - —Raccoon's eyes: bilateral ecchymosis of orbits associated with basilar skull fractures
  - —Battle's sign: ecchymosis behind the ear at mastoid process associated with basilar skull fracture
  - —Hemotympanum
  - —Cerebral spinal fluid rhinorrhea or otorrhea
- Evidence of increasing intracranial pressure (ICP) includes
  - —Decreasing level of consciousness, falling Glasgow Coma Score (GCS)
  - —Cushing's response; bradycardia, hypertension, and diminished respiratory rate
  - —Dilated pupils associated with decorticate or decerebrate posturing

ETIOLOGY

- Blunt trauma to head may cause several types of closed head injuries
  - —*Concussion:* head trauma associated with transient loss of consciousness or amnesia with no evidence of intracranial pathology on computed tomography
  - —*Subdural hematoma:* mass intracranial lesion arising from tearing of subdural bridging veins and bleeding into the subdural space
  - —*Epidural hematoma:* mass intracranial lesion usually associated with a skull fracture and dural arterial injury, especially the middle meningeal artery
    - -Classically, transient loss of consciousness followed by a *lucid interval,* then rapid demise
  - —*Subarachnoid hemorrhage:* bleeding into the subarachnoid space following trauma. This is not a mass lesion
  - —*Cerebral contusion:* focal injuries to the brain characterized as coup (beneath area of impact) or contrecoup (area remote from impact)
  - —*Intracerebral hemorrhage:* mass intracranial lesion with bleeding into the brain parenchyma
  - —*Diffuse axonal injury:* microscopic injuries scattered throughout the brain, without a mass lesion, in a patient in deep coma

Pre-Hospital

- Blunt head trauma patients with risk for intracranial lesion must go to a trauma center. *High-risk* patients include depressed consciousness, focal neurologic signs, multiple trauma, or palpable depressed skull fractures
- Blunt head trauma patients with *moderate risk* for intracranial lesion should go to a hospital with the ability to obtain prompt neurosurgical consultation. Moderate risk patients include those with progressive headache, alcohol or drug intoxication, unreliable history, posttraumatic seizure, repeated vomiting, posttraumatic amnesia, signs of basilar skull fracture, possible skull penetration, or depressed skull fracture
- If patient is showing evidence of increased intracranial pressure (obtundation with Cushing's reflex, GCS <8), initiate measures to decrease pressure, including
  - —Rapid sequence induction (RSI) intubation with mild hyperventilation
  - —Elevating head of bed 20–30°
- C-spine precautions must be maintained in all patients

CAUTIONS

- Hypotension (systolic blood pressure (SBP) <90 mm Hg) should be avoided
- Hypoxia should be avoided; administer 100% O_2

Diagnosis

ESSENTIAL WORKUP

- *Head computed tomography (CT)* should be performed in patients with any of the following
  - —Loss of consciousness or amnesia
  - —Progressive headache, alcohol or drug intoxication, unreliable history, posttraumatic seizure, repeated vomiting, signs of basilar skull fracture, possible skull penetration or depressed skull fracture, GCS <15, or focal neurological findings
  - —Patients on coumadin, heparin, or with history of bleeding dyscrasias (i.e., hemophilia) must be imaged even only with a trivial history of head trauma
  - —Elderly patients and alcoholics are at higher risk for intracranial hemorrhage and have low threshold to scan

LABORATORY

- Rapid check of blood glucose
- CBC, platelet count, coagulation perimeters
- Type and crossmatch for surgical candidates
- Baseline electrolytes, BUN, and creatinine levels
- Alcohol levels if indicated

IMAGING/SPECIAL TESTS

- Head CT as above
- Cervical spine x-ray, including AP, lateral, and odontoid, should be obtained when indicated

DIFFERENTIAL DIAGNOSIS

- Penetrating head trauma
- Any condition that alters mental status that may have produced a fall and caused external evidence of head trauma (e.g., hypoglycemic episode, seizure)

Treatment

INITIAL STABILIZATION

- ABCs of trauma care
  - —Control airway as needed. RSI intubation if GCS <8, unable to protect airway, or evidence of hypoxia
  - —Pretreatment with lidocaine, etomidate, or fentanyl as induction agent, rocuronium or vecuronium as the paralytic
  - —IV catheter placement, normal saline, and bolus as needed to avoid hypotension (SBP >90 mm Hg)
  - —Cervical spine precautions
  - —Elevate head of bed 20–30°

ED TREATMENT

- Early neurosurgical consultation
- If patient has evidence of increased ICP, initiate measures to decrease ICP, including
  - —Mild hyperventilation, keep $PaCO_2$ ~35
  - —Morphine sulfate for ongoing sedation
  - —Mannitol boluses if evidence of increased ICP, provided SBP >100 mm Hg
  - —Foley catheter will be needed in these patients
- Phenytoin to prevent *early* posttraumatic seizures
- The use of glucocorticoids is *not* recommended to lower ICP in head trauma patients
- If definitive neurosurgical care is not immediately available, a single burr hole may preserve life until neurosurgical intervention can be obtained
  - —This should only be done in comatose patients with decerebrate or decorticate posturing on the side of a known mass lesion who have not responded to hyperventilation and mannitol
  - —If computed tomography is not available to localize a lesion, the burr may be placed on the side of the dilated pupil

MEDICATIONS

- Chlorpromazine: adult: 50 mg IM; peds: 0.5–1.0 mg/kg
- Etomidate: 0.2–0.3 mg/kg IV
- Fentanyl: 3–5 μg/kg IV if SBP >100 mm Hg
- Lidocaine: 1.0 mg/kg IV
- Mannitol: 1.0 g/kg IV
- Morphine sulfate: adult: 2–10 mg IV; peds: 0.1 mg/kg up to adult doses
- Phenytoin: 15–20 mg/kg IV up to 1000 g
- Rocuronium: 0.6 mg/kg IV
- Vecuronium bromide: 0.1 mg/kg IV

Disposition

ADMISSION CRITERIA

- All patients with any mass lesion associated with head trauma must be admitted to the ICU or OR
- Patients with subarachnoid hemorrhage and diffuse axonal injury should be initially admitted to the ICU
- Patients with ongoing symptoms including repetitive questioning, anterograde amnesia, or disorientation should be admitted to a monitored unit for neurological evaluation

DISCHARGE CRITERIA

- Patients with resolved symptoms, negative head CT, and no other comorbid factors (e.g., intoxication, additional trauma needing treatment) may be discharged home with a friend or family member
- Patients with minor head trauma, no loss of consciousness or amnesia, and normal neurological exam can be discharged home with a friend or family member with head injury instructions

Miscellaneous

ICD9: 959.01

CORE CONTENT CODE: 18.4.1, 18.3.1

SUGGESTED READINGS

Committee on Trauma. Head trauma. In: Advanced trauma life support. American College of Surgeons: Chicago , IL 1993;3:159–183.

Brain Trauma Foundation. Guidelines for the management of severe head injury. July 1995.

Chestnut RM, Marshall LF, Klauber MR, et al. The role of secondary brain injury in determining outcome from severe head injury. J Trauma 1993;34:216–222.

Cold GE. Cerebral blood flow in acute head injury. Acta Neurochir 1990;(Suppl 49):3–64.

Gennarelli TA. Emergency department management of head injuries. Emerg Med Clin North Am 1984;2:749–760.

Author: Gary M. Vilke

Head Trauma, Penetrating

Clinical Presentation

SIGNS AND SYMPTOMS

- Alteration in level of consciousness and neurological exam varies based on object and location
- Evidence of increasing intracranial pressure (ICP) include
  —Decreasing level of consciousness, falling Glasgow Coma Score (GCS)
  —Cushing's response: bradycardia, hypertension, and diminished respiratory rate
  —Blown pupil associated with decorticate or decerebrate posturing
- Evidence of penetrating injury to head or basilar skull fracture, or object still remaining in head
  —Raccoon's eyes: bilateral ecchymosis of orbits associated with basilar skull fractures
  —Battle's sign: ecchymosis behind the ear at mastoid process associated with basilar skull fracture
  —Hemotympanum
  —Cerebral spinal fluid rhinorrhea or otorrhea

MECHANISM/DESCRIPTION

- Penetrating injury to the intracranial contents
  —*High velocity penetration: usually* bullets, which cause trauma directly to brain tissue, but also have a "shock wave" injury to local surrounding brain tissue along the bullet's path
  —*Low velocity penetration: usually* knives, picks or other sharp objects, with direct local trauma to brain issue

ETIOLOGY

- Direct penetration of the skull into the intracranial cavity by foreign objects
- The object itself may cause direct or local damage to brain tissue
- The trauma can cause intracranial hemorrhage, including subdural, epidural, and intraparenchymal bleeds
- A bullet that hits the skull, ricochets off, and does not fracture the skull can still cause significant trauma to the underlying brain tissue

Pre-Hospital

CAUTIONS

- If the foreign object is still in the patient's head (e.g., a knife), stabilize it, but *do not* remove
- Determine the weapon type or caliber of weapon at scene
- If there is evidence of increased ICP (obtundation with Cushing's reflex, GCS <8), initiate measures to decrease ICP including
  —Rapid sequence induction (RSI) intubation with *mild* hyperventilation
  —Elevating head of bed 20–30°
- Maintain C-spine precautions
- Patient must go to a trauma center
- Hypotension (systolic blood pressure (SBP) <90 mm Hg), and hypoxia should be avoided as worse neurologic outcome can result

Diagnosis

ESSENTIAL WORKUP

- *Head computed tomography:* location of the lesion and extent of damage can be best evaluated with this study. Side-to-side injuries and those lower in the brain tend to be more ominous

LABORATORY

- CBC, platelet count, coagulation perimeters
- Type and crossmatch
- Electrolytes, BUN, and creatinine baseline levels

IMAGING/SPECIAL TESTS

- Head computed tomography as listed above
- Occasionally, skull radiographs can assess depth of impalement, location of bone fragments, and whether multiple fragments are within the cranium
- Cervical spine evaluation, including AP, lateral, and odontoid, should be obtained when indicated

DIFFERENTIAL DIAGNOSIS

- Blunt head trauma
- Basilar skull fracture
- Any condition that alters mental status that may have induced a fall and caused secondary penetrating trauma

Treatment

INITIAL STABILIZATION

- ABCs
  - —Control airway as needed. RSI intubation if GCS <8, unable to protect airway, or evidence of hypoxia or increased ICP
  - —Medications for RSI should include lidocaine pretreatment, etomidate, or fentanyl as induction agent, rocuronium or vecuronium as the paralytic. Morphine sulfate for ongoing sedation
  - —Intravenous catheter placement, normal saline, and bolus as needed to keep SBP >90 mm Hg
  - —Address other sources of associated trauma
  - —Cervical spine precautions should be maintained

ED TREATMENT

- Early neurosurgical consultation is necessary
- If patient demonstrates evidence of increased ICP (obtundation with Cushing's reflex, GCS <8), initiate measures to decrease ICP including
  - —Mild hyperventilation to keep $PaCO_2$ ~35, which correlates to an end-tidal CO_2 of 32–35
  - —Mannitol boluses IV if evidence of increased ICP
    - -Do not administer mannitol unless SBP >100 mm Hg
    - -Foley catheter will be needed in these patients
  - —Elevate head of bed 20–30°
- Phenytoin IV to prevent *early* posttraumatic seizures
- The use of glucocorticoids is *not* recommended to lower ICP in head trauma patients
- Barbiturates are *not* recommended in the initial ED treatment of penetrating head-injured patients until all other medical and surgical techniques have been utilized
- Transfuse as needed to keep hematocrit above 30%
- If definitive neurosurgical care is not immediately available, a single burr hole may preserve life until neurosurgical intervention can be attained. This should only be done in comatose patients with decerebrate or decorticate posturing on the side of a known mass lesion/hematoma who have not responded to hyperventilation and mannitol
- Avoid hyperthermia, as this increases the rate of brain metabolism and levels of carbon dioxide
  - —Treat with a cooling blankets
  - —Shivering should be controlled with chlorpromazine
- Avoid hypothermia, as this will increase risks of coagulopathy during surgery

MEDICATIONS

- Chlorpromazine: adult: 50 mg IM; peds: 0.5–1.0 mg/kg
- Etomidate: 0.2–0.3 mg/kg IV
- Fentanyl: 3–5 μg/kg IV if SBP >100 mm Hg
- Lidocaine: 1 mg/kg IV
- Mannitol: 1 g/kg IV
- Morphine sulfate: adult: 2–10 mg IV; peds: 0.1 mg/kg up to adult doses
- Phenytoin: 15–20 mg/kg IV up to 1000 mg
- Rocuronium: 0.6 mg/kg IV
- Vecuronium bromide: 0.1 mg/kg IV

Disposition

ADMISSION CRITERIA

- All patients with penetrating head trauma must be admitted to the ICU, if not directly to the operating room

DISCHARGE CRITERIA

- Patients with penetrating head injury should not be discharged

Miscellaneous

ICD9: 959.01

CORE CONTENT CODE: 18.4.1.6

SUGGESTED READINGS

Committee on Trauma. Head trauma. In: Advanced Trauma Life Support. American College of Surgeons, Chicago, IL, 1993: 159–183.

Brain Trauma Foundation. Guidelines for the management of severe head injury. July 1995.

Chestnut RM, Marshall LF, Klauber MR, et al. The role of secondary brain injury in determining outcome from severe head injury. J Trauma 1993;34:216–222.

Cold GE. Cerebral blood flow in acute head injury. Acta Neuorochir 1990;(Suppl 49):3–64.

Author: Gary M. Vilke

Headache

Clinical Presentation

SIGNS AND SYMPTOMS

- Migraine
  - —Aura (usually visual)
  - —Recurring
  - —Unilateral
  - —Pulsating
  - —Moderate to severe intensity
  - —4–72-hr duration
  - —Nausea and vomiting
  - —Photophobia
  - —Phonophobia
- Tension
  - —Recurring
  - —Bilateral
  - —Nonpulsatile
  - —Bandlike
  - —Mild to moderate intensity
  - —30 min to 7 days duration
  - —Anorexia
  - —Photophobia
  - —Phonophobia
- Cluster
  - —Recurring
  - —Unilateral
  - —Penetrating
  - —Severe intensity
  - —Sudden onset
  - —45–60-min duration
  - —Lacrimation
  - —Conjunctival injection
  - —Rhinorrhea
  - —Ptosis
  - —No aura
- Potentially life-threatening headaches
- Less common
- New onset severe headache or "worst headache of my life"
  - —New onset in elderly
  - —Abnormal vital signs, particularly diastolic BP >130 mm Hg or fever
  - —Altered level of consciousness
  - —Altered mental status
  - —Abnormal neurologic findings or meningismus

MECHANISM/DESCRIPTION

- Vascular
  - —Severe, throbbing headache
  - —Divided into migraine (the majority) and vascular nonmigrainous
  - —Triggered by stress, hormone fluctuations, lack of sleep, certain foods
- Tension (muscle contraction headache)
  - —Most common type of chronic recurring headache
  - —Secondary to sustained contraction of head and neck muscles
  - —Triggered by poor posture, stress, anxiety, depression, cervical osteoarthritis
- Cluster headaches
  - —Triggered by alcohol, certain foods, altered sleep habits, strong emotions
- Intracranial (traction)
  - —Mass lesions inside the calvarium stretching arteries and other pain sensitive structures
- Extracranial (nontension)
  - —Pathology from an extracranial site causing pain in a peripheral nerve of the head and neck

ETIOLOGY

- Vascular
  - —Intra/extracranial vasodilatation and constriction of pain-sensitive blood vessels
- Tension
  - —Unknown (possibly serotonin imbalance, decreased endorphins)
- Other headaches
  - —Multiple etiologies depending on cause (see differential diagnosis)
  - —Generally through traction, tension or inflammation of the pain-sensitive structures; the vasculature, meninges, and cranial nerves V, IX, and X

PEDIATRIC CONSIDERATIONS

- Migraine
  - —Most common headache in children
  - —70–90% have positive family history
  - —May only manifest as cyclic vomiting or vertigo

Pre-Hospital

N/A

Diagnosis

ESSENTIAL WORKUP

- Detailed history and CNS examination
- Workup is strongly dependent on the clinical differential diagnosis

LABORATORY

- ESR
  - —If temporal arteritis or other inflammatory disorders suspected
- Tests appropriate for patient's underlying medical condition (e.g., ABG, glucose)
- Tests appropriate for physical examination abnormalities

IMAGING/SPECIAL TESTS

- Head CT scan
  - —Indications
    - -Unclear diagnosis based on H&P
    - -Signs of increased ICP
    - -Worst or first headache
    - -Acute onset
    - -Focal neurologic abnormalities
    - -Papilledema
    - -Recurrent morning headache
    - -Persistent vomiting
    - -Headache associated with fever, rash, and nausea without systemic illness
    - -Head trauma with LOC, focal neurologic findings, or lethargy
    - -Altered mental status, meningismus
  - —90% Sensitive for subarachnoid hemorrhage (SAH)
    - -Must do LP if SAH suspected and CT is negative
- Lumbar puncture indications
  - —Intracranial infections
  - —Detect blood not evident on CT scan
- Sinus imaging
  - —Suspect sinusitis
- Vascular assessment with angiogram or MR angiography
  - —May be indicated if nonmigrainous vascular cause suspected
- MRI
  - —Suspected posterior fossa lesion

DIFFERENTIAL DIAGNOSIS

- Vascular
  - —Migraine: classic (with aura), common (without aura), cluster, ophthalmoplegic, hemiplegic, migraine equivalents
  - —Hypertensive headache: throbbing, occipital, SBP >130 mm Hg
  - —Anoxic: carbon monoxide toxicity, sleep apnea, anemia
- Tension
  - —Muscular contraction
  - —Conversion reaction
  - —Chronic anxiety states
- Intracranial (traction)

—Subarachnoid hemorrhage: "first or worst," sudden onset, vomiting, meningismus
—Aneurysm/AVM: sudden onset, unilateral, severe, decreased vision
—Meningitis/encephalitis: fever, nonfocal, meningismus
—Acute subdural hematoma: mental status, depression, or focal findings
—Chronic subdural hematoma: hemiparesis, focal seizures
—Epidural hematoma: trauma, brief LOC, rapid progression of neurologic symptoms
—Brain tumor: pain on awakening, progressively worsens, worse with Valsalva, ataxia
—Brain abscess: fever, nausea/vomiting, seizures
—Pseudotumor cerebri: young obese female, irregular menses, papilledema

- Extracranial
  —Trigeminal neuralgia: transient, shocklike facial pain
  —Temporal arteritis: elderly, severe, scalp artery tenderness/swelling
  —Sinusitis: stabbing/aching, worse with bending or coughing
  —Metabolic: fever, hypoglycemia, high altitude, acute anemia
  —Acute glaucoma: nausea/vomiting, eye pain, conjunctival injection, increased IOP
  —Cervical: spondylosis, trauma, arthritis
  —Temporomandibular joint syndrome

Treatment

INITIAL STABILIZATION

- ABCs
- IV fluids, oxygen, and monitoring if necessary

ED TREATMENT

- Migraine
  —Abortive therapy
    -Ergotamine
    -Phenothiazine
    -Serotonin agonists
    -NSAID
  —Analgesia/comfort
    -Narcotics (most common but suboptimal)
    -Dark quiet room
  —Prophylactic measures
    -Not recommended for ED use
- Tension
  —Aspirin
  —Acetaminophen
  —NSAID
- Cluster
  —Oxygen
  —Intranasal lidocaine
  —Migraine medications excluding β-blockers
- Temporal arteritis
  —Steroids
- Intracranial infection: see meningitis chapter
- Intracranial hemorrhage: see subarachnoid hemorrhage chapter

MEDICATIONS

- Chlorpromazine: 25–50 mg IM/IV (peds: 0.5–1 mg/kg/dose IM/IV/PO) q 4–6 hrs
- Dihydroergotamine: 0.5–1.5 mg IM/IV, repeat hourly; max dose 3 mg
- Ergotamine: 2 mg PO/SL at onset, then 1 mg po q 30 min; max dose 10 mg/wk
- Ketorolac: 30–60 mg IM; 15–30 mg IV once, then 15–30 mg q 6 hrs
- Lidocaine 4%: 1 ml intranasal on same side as symptoms
- Meperidine: 50–150 mg (peds: 1–1.5 mg/kg/dose) PO/IV/IM/SC q 3–4 hrs
- Metoclopramide: 1–2 mg/kg IV q 2–4 hrs
- Morphine: 2.5–20 mg (peds: 0.1–0.2 mg/kg/dose) IM/IV/SC q 2–6 hrs
- Prochlorperazine (compazine): 10 mg IV
- Sumatriptan: 6 mg SQ, repeat in 1 hr, up to 12 mg/24hrs

Disposition

ADMISSION CRITERIA

- Headache secondary to suspected organic disease
- Chronic daily headache, pain refractory to outpatient management
- Persistent migraine with intractable vomiting and dehydration
- Headache complicated by significant surgical or medical history
- Intracranial infection
- Intracranial hemorrhage
- Consider ICU admission
  —Suspected aneurysm
  —Acute subdural hematoma
  —Subarachnoid hemorrhage
  —Stroke
  —Increased ICP
  —Severe headache following trauma
  —Intracranial infection

DISCHARGE CRITERIA

- Most migraine, cluster, and tension headaches after pain relief
- Local or minor systemic infections

Miscellaneous

ICD9: 784.0

CORE CONTENT CODE: 22.2.12

SUGGESTED READINGS

Goadsby PJ, Olesen J. Diagnosis and treatment of migraine. Br Med J 1996;312:1279–1283.

Henry GL. Headache. In: Rosen P, et al., eds. Emergency medicine: concepts and clinical practice. 4th ed. St. Louis: CV Mosby, 1997;2119–2130.

Perkins AT, Ondo W. When to worry about headache: head pain as a clue to intracranial disease. Postgrad Med 1995;98(2):197–208.

Thomas SH, Stone CK. Emergency department treatment of migraine, tension, and mixed-type headache. J Emerg Med 1994;12(5):657–664.

Authors: Matthew R. Harmody; Robert J. Vissers

HELLP Syndrome

*H*emolysis, *E*levated *L*iver Enzymes, and *L*ow *P*latelets)

Clinical Presentation

SIGNS AND SYMPTOMS

- Classically white, multiparous woman presenting before 37 weeks gestation
  - —Nearly one-third occur after delivery
  - —May develop HELLP syndrome during second trimester
- Most cases with epigastric, upper abdominal, or right upper-quadrant pain and tenderness
  - —Nausea and vomiting in half of patients
- Many with nonspecific viral, flulike symptoms such as fatigue or malaise
- Often vague clinical features; delay in diagnosis of several days is common due to the nonspecific nature of symptoms
- Majority of patients have moderate or severe hypertension
  - —HELLP syndrome can occur with normal or only mildly elevated blood pressures
- Other features include convulsions, jaundice, GI bleeding, hypovolemic shock, hematuria, bleeding from mucosal surfaces, chest or shoulder pain, and peripheral edema

MECHANISM/DESCRIPTION

- HELLP syndrome is a rare complication of eclampsia or preeclampsia, complicating 0.3% of all pregnancies and up to 20% of women with severe preeclampsia or eclampsia
- First described as a syndrome of hemolysis, coagulopathy, and liver abnormalities, later termed HELLP
- Often involves organ systems other than liver and hematologic systems, especially the kidney and the brain
- Complications of syndrome include DIC, abruptio placenta, acute renal failure, pulmonary edema, subcapsular liver hematoma, retinal detachment, GI bleeding, pleural effusions, ARDS, and cerebral edema
- Syndrome is associated with poor maternal and fetal outcomes with maternal mortality of up to 24% and perinatal mortality of up to 33%

ETIOLOGY

- Many theories proposed, but the etiology and pathogenesis of the syndrome remains unclear
- Endothelial cell injury with resulting vasospasm, platelet activation, abnormal platelet prostacyclin-thromboxane ratio, and decreased release of endothelium-derived relaxing factor play a central role in pathogenesis of syndrome

Pre-Hospital

CAUTIONS

- The same precautions apply to patients with HELLP as those with preeclampsia or eclampsia, mainly that of seizure management and protection of patient
- *Main concern is for rapid transport to facility capable of caring for complicated OB patients*

Diagnosis

ESSENTIAL WORKUP

- Diagnosis is based mainly on these lab findings
  - —Hemolysis defined by abnormal smear (burrs and schistocytes)
  - —LDH >600 IU/L and bilirubin >1.2 mg/dl
  - —Elevated liver enzymes defined by SGOT >72 IU/L
  - —Thrombocytopenia defined as platelet count <100,000/ml

LABORATORY

- CBC will reveal anemia and thrombocytopenia
- Peripheral smear will show findings of microangiopathic hemolytic anemia (burr cells or schistocytes)
- Other hemolysis markers include elevated reticulocyte counts, decreased haptoglobin, elevated LDH, bilirubin, free hemoglobin, and urobilinogen levels
- Liver transaminases (SGOT/SGPT) will be elevated, as may alkaline phosphatase
- PT/PTT or entire DIC panel if DIC suspected
- BUN/Cr to evaluate renal function
- Urinalysis for proteinuria

IMAGING/SPECIAL TESTS

- CXR if pulmonary edema is suspected
- Emergent CT of head if cerebral edema is suspected (altered mental status)
- Abdominal ultrasound may be helpful to rule out other etiologies
- Ultrasound imaging of placenta and fetus is mandatory

DIFFERENTIAL DIAGNOSIS

- Gastritis, biliary colic, cholecystitis, hepatitis, pancreatitis, hiatal hernia, PUD, acute fatty liver of pregnancy, Budd-Chiari syndrome
- ITP, "gestational" thrombocytopenia, preeclampsia-associated thrombocytopenia, TTP, HUS

Treatment

INITIAL STABILIZATION

- ABCs
  - —Airway control as indicated (e.g., patients with cerebral edema, pulmonary edema, or status epilepticus)
  - —IV access; 2 large-bore peripheral IVs recommended in hemodynamically unstable patient, e.g., GI bleed
  - —Supplemental O_2, 100% via face mask to increase O_2 content to both mother and fetus
  - —Cardiac and pulse oximetry monitoring as well as fetal monitoring
  - —Place patient on left lateral decubitus position to prevent IVC syndrome

ED TREATMENT

- Control hypertension with hydralazine (see chapter on preeclampsia/eclampsia)
- Treat preeclampsia or eclampsia if present with IV $MgSO_4$
- Type, cross, and administer blood products as indicated (see below)
- Obtain emergent OB or perinatology consult
- Consider antenatal corticosteroids to promote fetal lung maturity in consultation with perinatologist if delivery is not immediately indicated
- The definitive treatment of HELLP syndrome is delivery
- Monitor urine output with Foley catheter: maintain at >25 ml/hr
- Limit IV fluid administration unless resuscitation indicated
- Monitor for and treat hypoglycemia if present

Blood Products

- Correct thrombocytopenia by platelet transfusion in women with PLT platelet counts of less than 20,000/μL, even without active bleeding, as risk of postpartum bleeding is significantly increased
  - —Platelet counts above 40,000/μL are generally considered safe for vaginal delivery
- Correct thrombocytopenia to platelet counts >50,000/μL if delivery by Cesarean section is planned
- If coagulation dysfunction is present, transfusion with FFP, PRBC, and antithrombin III is indicated
- Transfusion with fresh whole blood or PRBC is recommended for hemoglobin less than 10g/dl

MEDICATIONS

- Hydralazine: 5–10 mg every 15–20 min to keep diastolic BP <110
- Magnesium sulfate: 4–6 g in 100 ml IV over 15–20 min loading dose, then maintenance drip starting at 2 g/hr and titrate to clinical effect and toxicity (antidote is calcium gluconate 10%, 10 ml IV over 3 min)

Disposition

ADMISSION CRITERIA

- All women with HELLP should be admitted
- If woman is remote from term, arrange for transfer to tertiary referral center once maternal condition stabilized in ED
- Patients with pulmonary edema/respiratory failure, cerebral edema, or heavy GI bleeding with hemodynamic instability should be admitted to an ICU setting
- Noncritically ill patients with HELLP syndrome should be admitted to the OB ward for close continuous monitoring of both mother and fetus

Miscellaneous

ICD9: 642.50

CORE CONTENT CODE: 7.0

SUGGESTED READINGS

Abbott J. Complications related to pregnancy. In: Rosen P, et al., eds. Emergency medicine: Concepts and clinical practice. 3rd ed. St. Louis: CV Mosby, 1998:2342–2364.

Geary M. The HELLP syndrome. Br J Obstet Gynaecol 1997;104(8):887–891.

Jean T. Abbott. Hypertensive disorders in pregnancy. In: Cunningham FG, et al., eds. Williams' obstetrics. 20th ed. Stamford, CT: Appleton and Lange, 1997:2342–2364.

Mushambi MC, Halligan AW, Williamson K. Recent developments in the pathophysiology and management of pre-eclampsia. Br J Anaesth 1996;76(1):133–148.

Author: Sam Torbati

Hemophilia

Clinical Presentation

SIGNS AND SYMPTOMS

- Bleeding
  - —Hemarthrosis (most common)
    - -Knee (most common) > elbow > ankle > shoulder > wrist (least common)
  - —Muscle hemorrhage
  - —Postextraction or oral mucosal bleeding
  - —Hematuria
  - —Sustained, from minor trauma
  - —Intracranial hemorrhage
  - —Gastrointestinal bleeding
  - —Epistaxis (only in severe disease)

MECHANISM/DESCRIPTION

- Caused by deficiency of Factor VIII or Factor IX
- Absence of factors causes partial inactivation of coagulation cascade and impaired hemostasis
- Two types
  - —Hemophilia A: Factor VIII deficiency
  - —Hemophilia B (Christmas disease): Factor IX deficiency
- Severity varies among different individuals reflecting available natural factor activity
  - —70% of type A hemophiliacs are severe

	AVAILABLE FACTOR ACTIVITY	*CLINICAL PRESENTATION*
Mild	5–30%	Bleeding almost exclusively with trauma
Moderate	1–5%	Occasional spontaneous hemorrhages
Severe	<1%	Frequent spontaneous hemorrhages

ETIOLOGY

- Genetic transmission; sex-linked recessive occurring in males
- Rare disease
  - —Hemophilia A occurs in approximately 1 in 5000 males
  - —Hemophilia B occurs in approximately 1 in 30,000 males

Pre-Hospital

CAUTIONS

- Control bleeding with direct pressure

Diagnosis

- Generally not made in emergency department
- Consider in undiagnosed patients if
  - —Positive family history
  - —Recurrent prior episodes of bleeding

ESSENTIAL WORKUP

- Thorough physical examination
- Factor specific assays (see below)

LABORATORY

- CBC
- Platelet count: normal
- PT/PTT
  - —PT: normal
  - —PTT: increased
- Bleeding time: normal
- Consider if indicated
  - —Urinalysis—asymptomatic hematuria is a common finding

IMAGING/SPECIAL TESTS

- Specific factor assays
  - —Factor VIII:Ag (measures Factor VIII quantity): decreased
  - —Factor VIII:c (measures Factor VIII activity): decreased
  - —VWF (measures von Willebrand factor activity): normal
  - —VWF:Ag (measures von Willebrand factor quantity): normal
- Radiographic studies may be required in certain circumstances. Consider
  - —Head CT to evaluate or exclude intracranial bleed
  - —Renal US/IVP to evaluate excessive hematuria or renal trauma
  - —Abdominal CT to evaluate or exclude retroperitoneal bleeding

DIFFERENTIAL DIAGNOSIS

- Von Willebrand's disease
- Anticoagulant drugs
- Antiplatelet agents
- Thrombocytopenia
- Hepatic dysfunction

Treatment

INITIAL STABILIZATION

- ABCs
  - —Control bleeding
  - —Establish IV access

ED TREATMENT

General

- Goals of emergency department therapy
  - —Abort current bleeding episode by raising factor level
  - —Prevent additional morbidity
  - —Coordinate ED care with primary provider (hematologist)
- Approach to therapy
  - —Patients generally have excellent understanding of their disease
  - —Determine desired factor level based on risk of bleeding and location/system
  - —Factor VIII required (in units) = wt (kg) × 0.5 × (% factor activity desired)
    - -1 IU Factor VIII/kg raises activity approximately 2%
  - —Factor IX required (in units) = wt (kg) × 1.0 × (% factor activity desired)
    - -1 IU Factor IX/kg raises activity approximately 1%
  - —May need to increase dose if inhibitors (antibodies to factor) are present or use special factor replacement
    - -Patient/primary care provider usually has this information
  - —Avoid all IM injections
  - —Avoid the following medications
    - -Aspirin
    - -Aspirin containing products
    - -Antihistamines (chlorpheniramine)
    - -Cough syrup (Robitussin)

Factor Replacement Options

- Cryoprecipitates
  - —Obtained from FFP after thawing at 4° C
  - —Contains multiple proteins but high in VIII, vWF, and fibrinogen
  - —Only use if purified factor not available
  - —Not useful in hemophilia B; does not contain factor IX
- Factor VIII concentrates
  - —Mainstay of modern hemophilia therapy
  - —Choice based on patient's profile, prior agents, cost
  - —Intermediate purity products
    - -Low factor VIII specific activity
    - -Contain fibronectin, fibrinogen, other proteins
    - -Viruses killed by solvent detergent extraction, or pasteurization
    - -Indicated for older hemophiliacs, patients with prior exposure to blood products
    - -Examples: Humate-P, Profilate
  - —High purity products
    - -High factor VIII specific activity

–Contain fewer plasma proteins
–Examples: Alphanate
—Very high purity products
–Highest Factor VIII specific activity
–Contains no plasma proteins
–Either plasma derived and monoclonal antibody purified or produced using recombinant DNA technology
–Indications: pediatric patients; those with limited prior exposure to blood products
–Very expensive
–Examples: Monoclate-P
- Factor IX concentrates
—Fewer options
—Low purity products also known as prothrombin complex concentrates (PCCs)
—Plasma derived; contain Factors VII, X, and prothrombin
—May be activated, i.e., able to initiate coagulation cascade (APCCs)
—If administered at frequent or prolonged intervals, may cause DIC or thrombosis
—Examples: Profilnine (PCC); Autoplex (APCC)
—High purity concentrates
–Plasma derived; purified either using chromatography or immunoaffinity
–Expensive
–Example: Alphanine
- Adjuncts
—DDAVP
–Synthetic analogue of the antidiuretic hormone L-arginine vasopressin
–Raises factor VIII level 2–4 times in patients with activity >5%
–Not useful in patients with Hemophilia B
–Maximal effect occurs 15–30 minutes after infusion
–Side effects: mild flushing, headache, tachycardia, hypotension, hyponatremia
–Dose 0.3 μg/kg of DDAVP diluted in 50 ml 0.9%NS given over 15–30 minutes
—Amicar
–Only for mucosal bleeding
–Do not use in children
–Do not use in hemarthrosis or hematuria

Specific Management Considerations

- Hemarthrosis
—Replace factor promptly
—Splint
—Ace, ice
—Avoid aspirin
—Arthrocentesis rarely indicated
- Muscle hemorrhage
—Replace factor promptly
—Forearm/calf—consider compartment syndrome
—Avoid cylindrical casts
—Psoas hematoma—groin pain, femoral nerve paresthesias
- Postextraction or oral mucosal bleeding
—Treat locally with avitene or microfibrillar collagen
—Replace factor if severe
—Amicar may be useful
- Hematuria
—Generally mild
—Replace factor if symptoms >2 days (50–100%)
—Hydrate
—Avoid Amicar and cryoprecipitate
- Intracranial hemorrhage
—All head injuries should be considered significant, especially in children
—Don't delay therapy for diagnostic testing
—Replace factor to 100%
—CT scan aggressively
—Gastrointestinal bleeding
—Secondary to ulcers, polyps, hemorrhoids
—Replace factor promptly (50–100%)
—Replace factor prior to endoscopy

SITE/MECHANISM	RISK	DESIRED HEMOSTATIC FACTOR LEVEL	EMPIRICAL THERAPY (FACTOR VIII)
Soft tissue injury Joint or muscle bleeding	Low to moderate	30–50%	25–50 IU/kg
GI/GU bleeding	Moderate to severe	50–100%	25–50 IU/kg
CNS injury Major trauma Presurgery	Severe	100%	50 IU/kg

Disposition

ADMISSION CRITERIA

- Low threshold for admission
- Generally observe 23 hours for resolution of bleeding
- Bleeding episodes may require multiple infusions
- Severe complications
- Head trauma

DISCHARGE CRITERIA

- Minor bleeding with resolution
- If subjective symptoms only

Miscellaneous

ICD9: 286.0

CORE CONTENT CODE: 7.2.1.1

SUGGESTED READINGS

Cohen AJ, Kessler CM. Treatment of inherited coagulation disorders. Am J Med 1995;99:675.

DiMichele D. Hemophilia 1996: New approach to an old disease. Pediatr Clin North Am 1996;43:709.

Furie B, Limentani SA, Rosenfield C. A practical guide to the evaluation and treatment of hemophilia. Blood 1994;84:3.

Pfaff JA, Geninatti M. Hemophilia. Emerg Med Clin North Am 1993;11:337.

Author: Steven Bowman

Hemoptysis

Clinical Presentation

SIGNS AND SYMPTOMS

- Expectoration of blood
- Presence of blood in sputum
- *Essential to differentiate between hemoptysis and hematemesis*
  - —Blood originating in the airway
    - -Bright red and frothy
    - -Alkaline
    - -Often mixed with sputum
    - -Accompanied by coughing or preceded by a gurgling noise
  - —Gastrointestinal blood
    - -Usually has a dark red, brown, or "coffee grounds" color
    - -Acidic
    - -May contain food particles
    - -Usually accompanied by nausea, wretching, or emesis
  - —Gastric lavage and stool testing for occult blood may be necessary to distinguish the source

General

- Acute infectious symptoms
  - —Cough
  - —Fever
  - —Chest pain
  - —Upper respiratory congestion/rhinorrhea
  - —General malaise
  - —Chronic constitutional symptoms (malignancy or tuberculosis)
    - -Weight loss
    - -Night sweats
    - -Development of adenopathy
    - -Pulmonary embolism
- Chest pain
  - —Dyspnea
  - —Coagulopathy
- Hematuria
- Gingival bleeding
- Epistaxis
- Petechiae
- Spontaneous bruising
- Goodpasture's syndrome or Legionella pneumonia
- URI or sinusitis
- Nasal and sinus pain or bleeding

MECHANISM/DESCRIPTION

- Hemoptysis
  - —Expectoration of blood or the presence of blood in sputum
  - —May be the manifestation of a wide variety of disease processes or entities in patients of any age
  - —More common in adults (children under age 6 usually swallow their sputum and rarely present with hemoptysis unless they have substantial bleeding)
- Massive hemoptysis
  - —100–600 ml over 24 hours (>8 ml/kg per 24 hours in child) or 1000 ml over several days
  - —Rare (<5%)

ETIOLOGY

Infection

- URI most common
  - —Sinusitis
  - —Tracheobronchitis, pneumonia (especially Staphylococcus, Klebsiella, Legionella, Pneumococcus)
  - —Lung abscess
  - —Tuberculosis
  - —Mycetoma
- Fungal
- Viral
- Parasitic

Neoplastic

- Lung cancer (squamous cell, small cell, carcinoid) second most common
- Bronchial adenoma
- Metastasis

Cardiac

- Mitral stenosis
- CHF
- Any left-sided obstructive lesion

Pulmonary

- Bronchiectasis
- Cystic fibrosis
- Pulmonary embolism/infarction
- Bullous emphysema

Systemic Disease

- Goodpasture's syndrome
- Systemic lupus erythematosus
- Vasculitis (e.g., Wegener's granulomatosis, Henoch-Schönlein purpura)

Hematologic

- Coagulopathy
- Thrombocytopenia
- Platelet dysfunction
- DIC

Vascular

- Pulmonary hypertension
- Arteriovenous malformation
- Aortic aneurysm
- Aortobronchial fistula
- Aortic aneurysm

Drugs/Toxins

- Aspirin
- Anticoagulants
- Penicillamine
- Solvents

Trauma

- Fat embolism
- Tracheobronchial rupture

Iatrogenic

- Bronchoscopy
- Lung biopsy
- Transtracheal aspirate

Miscellaneous

- Foreign body
- Endometriosis
- Amyloidosis
- Bronchopleural fistula
- Factitious or Munchausen's syndrome
- Idiopathic

Pre-Hospital

- Airway management
  - —Oxygen
  - —Endotracheal intubation for respiratory difficulty
- IV access
- Cardiac monitoring

Diagnosis

ESSENTIAL WORKUP

- Careful history
- Smoking or chronic lung disease
- Chronic alcohol abuse (increased risk of lung abscess or tuberculosis)
- New onset orthopnea, pedal edema, and dyspnea (possible CHF)
- Recent travel abroad (parasitic disease or tuberculosis)

PEDIATRIC CONSIDERATIONS

- Chronic productive cough or wheezing
- Congenital or rheumatic heart disease
- Foreign body aspiration (majority of cases in children <4 years old)
- Physical examination
- Thoroughly inspect oropharynx and nose to exclude an oral lesion or epistaxis
- Poor dentition may predispose to lung abscess
- Wheezing over one lung segment may suggest a focal obstruction or foreign body
- Crackles may point to pneumonia, CHF, or alveolar hemorrhage
- Digital clubbing suggests chronic lung disease, cancer, or congenital heart disease
- Diffuse petechiae or purpura points to a possible coagulopathy
- Telangiectasias or hemangiomas may indicate the presence of arteriovenous malformations

LABORATORY

- CBC with platelet count and differential
- PT, PTT
- Blood type and cross
  —With massive hemoptysis
  —Sputum Gram's and acid-fast stains with cultures and cytology
  —Arterial blood gases
- If massive bleeding or signs of respiratory failure
  —Urinalysis for hematuria
  —Electrolytes, BUN/Cr, Glucose
- Pregnancy testing in women of child-bearing potential

IMAGING/SPECIAL TESTS

- Chest radiography
  —If foreign body aspiration is suspected
  —Inspiratory and expiratory films to check for unilateral hyperinflation
- Ventilation-perfusion scan and/or pulmonary arteriography for pulmonary embolism
- Bronchoscopy
  —Initial invasive procedure of choice for significant hemoptysis
- CT, nuclear medicine studies, and bronchial/pulmonary arteriography for patients with massive hemoptysis after initial bronchoscopy by a pulmonologist or surgeon

PEDIATRIC CONSIDERATIONS

- Sweat chloride test if cystic fibrosis suspected
- CT of chest more useful in children, as part of the initial evaluation of stable patients, particularly if the CXR reveals a mass, foreign body, or other abnormality

Treatment

INITIAL STABILIZATION

- Massive hemoptysis
  —IV access
  —Supplemental oxygen
  —Place patient in upright position
  —Cardiac monitor
  —Pulse oximetry
- Asphyxia
  —Most immediate threat to life
  —Control airway
  —Oral endotracheal intubation for impending respiratory failure
  —Large-diameter tube (8Fr or larger)
  —Careful suctioning once intubated to prevent further airway trauma

ED TREATMENT

- Volume resuscitation as needed with IV fluid and blood
- Correct coagulation abnormalities with
  —Fresh frozen plasma
  —Platelets
  —Specific factor/cryoprecipitate
  —Vitamin K
  —Heparin reversal (e.g., protamine) as indicated by coagulation studies
  —Consult with pulmonologist *and* thoracic surgeon
- Place patient in lateral decubitus position with involved side down
- If bleeding can be localized to one lung and airway is adequately controlled, minimizes soiling of nonbleeding lung
- Treat underlying pathology
- Ensure respiratory isolation measures until proven that the patient does not have *active pulmonary tuberculosis*

Disposition

ADMISSION CRITERIA

- ICU
  —Massive hemoptysis
  —Hypovolemic shock
  —Severe hypoxemia
  —Threatened airway
  —Intubation/mechanical ventilation
  —Suspected pulmonary embolism
  —Cavitary lung disease
  —Lung abscess
  —Suspected active pulmonary tuberculosis
  —Foreign bodies for bronchoscopy or surgical removal

DISCHARGE CRITERIA

- Minor hemoptysis due to tracheobronchitis
- Pneumonia amenable to outpatient treatment
- Bronchogenic carcinoma
- Discharge with cough suppressants (codeine, etc.) and an appropriate oral antibiotic for coverage of possible pathogens
- Close followup

Miscellaneous

ICD9: 786.3

CORE CONTENT CODE: 22.3.4

SUGGESTED READINGS

Cahill B, Ingbar D. Massive hemoptysis: assessment and management. Clin Chest Med 1994;15(1):147–67.

Goldman J. Hemoptysis: emergency assessment and management. Emerg Med Clin North Am 1989;7(2):325–38.

Pianosi P, Al-Sadoon H. Hemoptysis in children. Pediatr Rev 1996;17(10):344–8.

Author: Gregory S. Hall

Hemorrhagic Shock

Clinical Presentation

SIGNS AND SYMPTOMS

- *Class I hemorrhage:* loss of up to 15% of blood volume
  - —Minimal tachycardia, possible increase in pulse pressure, slightly anxious
- *Class II hemorrhage:* loss of 15–30% of blood volume
  - —Tachycardia, tachypnea, decreased pulse pressure, elevated diastolic BP
  - —Mild anxiety
  - —Small decrease in urine output
- *Class III hemorrhage:* loss of 30–40% of blood volume
  - —Marked tachycardia, tachypnea, decreased pulse pressure, falls in systolic BP
  - —Significant change in mental status (anxious and confused)
  - —Marked decrease in urine output
- *Class IV hemorrhage:* loss of greater than 40% of blood volume
  - —Marked tachycardia, very narrow pulse pressure, significant fall in systolic BP
  - —Depressed mental status with confusion, lethargy, possible LOC
  - —Negligible urine output
  - —Skin is cold and pale

ETIOLOGY

- The most common cause of hemorrhagic shock is blunt or penetrating trauma
- Other causes of hemorrhagic shock include acute GI or gynecologic bleeding and massive hemoptysis

MECHANISM/DESCRIPTION

- Shock occurs when loss of effective circulating blood volume results in inadequate tissue perfusion
- At the tissue level, inadequate perfusion leads to hypoxia
- Compensated shock occurs when the patient's physiologic reserve prevents significant alteration in vital signs until there is loss of a large amount of circulating volume
- Blood loss can be estimated by multiplying 70 ml/kg (adult blood volume) by body weight in kg and the class of hemorrhage in decimal

PEDIATRIC CONSIDERATIONS

- Children often have greater physiologic reserve and can preserve normal vital signs longer
- Systemic responses to blood loss in the pediatric patient include
  - —<25% volume loss: weak, thready pulse and tachycardia; lethargy, irritability, confusion; cool, clammy skin; decreased urine output (UO) with increased urine specific gravity
  - —25–40% volume loss: tachycardia; marked change in consciousness, dulled response to pain; cyanotic, cold extremities with decreased capillary refill; minimal UO
  - —>45% volume loss: hypotension, tachycardia, or bradycardia; comatose; pale, cold skin; no UO

Pre-Hospital

CONTROVERSIES

- The current standard of care calls for IV crystalloid resuscitation in trauma patients; follow local protocols

Diagnosis

ESSENTIAL WORKUP

- Blood type and crossmatch
- Hemoglobin/hematocrit

LABORATORY

- Coagulation studies (PT/PTT and platelet count) may be useful
- Other measures of shock and tissue hypoperfusion include arterial blood gas, base deficit, and serum lactate level
- Serum electrolytes to assess renal function and intravascular volume status

IMAGING/SPECIAL TESTS

- Chest x-ray is useful in assessing for hemothorax in blunt chest injuries
- Pelvic x-ray is useful in assessing for pelvic fracture that may be associated with significant hemorrhage in trauma victims
- DPL, abdominal and pelvic CT scan, and ultrasound are necessary to detect intra-abdominal bleeding. See chapters: Abdominal Trauma, Blunt and Abdominal Trauma, Imaging
- Endoscopy is useful in the setting of upper and lower gastrointestinal bleeding
- Angiography is useful in the settings of pelvic fracture, retroperitoneal hemorrhage, lower gastrointestinal bleeding, and neck trauma with suspected vascular injuries
- Embolization therapy for bleeding from arterial sources can be performed

DIFFERENTIAL DIAGNOSIS

- Other etiologies of shock
  - —Hypovolemic shock (burn, abnormal intake/output, etc.)
  - —Cardiogenic shock
  - —Neurogenic shock
  - —Septic shock
  - —Anaphylactic shock
- Cardiac tamponade; tension pneumothorax
- Gastric dilation in the trauma patient may cause unexplained hypotension
- Hypothermia

Treatment

INITIAL STABILIZATION

- Airway and breathing
  - —Intubation as indicated by patient's respiratory and mental status
  - —100% oxygen via face mask should be administered
- Circulation
  - —Two large-bore peripheral IV lines should be established (16-gauge or larger)
  - —Venous cutdown (saphenous) may be necessary
  - —Aggressive crystalloid resuscitation should be initiated in the ED
  - —3:1 rule: for 1 unit volume of blood loss, give 3 volumes of crystalloid
- With evidence of Class III or IV hemorrhage initiate blood transfusion early
  - —Type and crossmatch blood is preferred when time permits, often 1 hour
  - —Type-specific blood is usually available within 10–15 minutes
  - —Type O-negative blood can be used in life-threatening situations

ED TREATMENT

- Place patient on continuous monitor; insert Foley catheter to monitor urine output
- Central venous access may be indicated for CVP monitoring, but placement of such lines should not interfere with resuscitation measures
- Continually reassess patient for clinical response or deterioration
  - —Monitor vital signs, mental status, urine output
  - —Follow serial blood gas, lactate level, hemoglobin/hematocrit measurements
  - —Maintain urine output at 50 cc/hr
- The response to initial fluid resuscitation is the key to determining subsequent therapy
  - —Rapid response to fluid administration indicates minimal (<20%) blood loss
  - —Transient response to volume resuscitation indicates ongoing hemorrhage or inadequate resuscitation; continue fluid and blood administration and rapidly obtain necessary studies and consultations
  - —Minimal or no response to volume resuscitation indicates ongoing severe blood loss; immediate angiography or surgical intervention is warranted
- Use fluids warmed (approximately 39°C) by means of microwave ovens, warm water baths, or blood warmers
- Transfuse platelets and coagulation factors as indicated by laboratory testing

MEDICATIONS

- Crystalloids: normal saline or lactated ringers IV: adults: 1–2 L bolus, reassess for perfusion; peds: 20 ml/kg bolus
- Blood products: crossmatched, type-specific, or O-negative: adult: initiate with 4–6 units PRBC; peds: 10 ml/kg of PRBC

PEDIATRIC CONSIDERATIONS

- In children less than 6 years old, access may be obtained by intraosseous route after one or two unsuccessful attempts at peripheral access
- Maintain urine output at 1 cc/kg/hr for children and 2 cc/kg/hr for infants

Disposition

ADMISSION CRITERIA

- All patients with hemorrhage should be admitted to the appropriate service

DISCHARGE CRITERIA

- No patients with acute hemorrhagic shock in the ED should be discharged home

Miscellaneous

ICD9: 958.4, 785.59

CORE CONTENT CODE: 18.1.3.1

SUGGESTED READINGS

American College of Surgeons, Committee on Trauma. Advanced trauma life support course. Student manual. Chicago: American College of Surgeons, 1993.

Baron BJ, Scalea TM. Acute blood loss. Emerg Med Clin North Am 1996;14(1):35.

Bickell WH, Wall MJ Jr, Pepe PE, et al. Immediate versus delayed fluid resuscitation for hypotensive patients with penetrating torso injuries. N Engl J Med 1994;331:1105.

Author: Theodore C. Chan

Hemorrhoid

Clinical Presentation

SIGNS AND SYMPTOMS

- Painless, rectal bleeding with defection
- Bleeding is usually limited
- Blood usually found
  - —On the stool
  - —Toilet tissue paper
  - —Dripping into the toilet bowl
- Prolapse of hemorrhoidal tissue
- Pain
  - —Uncommon with uncomplicated hemorrhoids
  - —Associated with thrombosed external hemorrhoids and strangulated thrombosed internal hemorrhoids
  - —May be associated with coexistent fissure
- Thrombosed external hemorrhoids appear as enlarged, painful, bluish mass at anal verge
- Pruritus ani

MECHANISM/DESCRIPTION

- Dilated arteriovenous vascular cushions
- Dentate line
  - —Separates the columnar epithelium of the GI tract from the squamous epithelium of the anal canal
  - —Differentiates internal and external hemorrhoids
- *Internal hemorrhoids*
  - —Occur proximal to the dentate line and drain into the portal system
  - —Not usually visible but may protrude externally
  - —Occur in the right posterolateral, right anterolateral, and left lateral positions with the patient prone (2, 5, and 9 o'clock)
- *External hemorrhoids*
  - —Originate below the dentate line
  - —Drain into the iliac system
  - —Covered with skin
  - —Clearly visible

Classification of Internal Hemorrhoids

GRADE	*SYMPTOMS*
1	Bleeding
2	Prolapse with defecation, reduce spontaneously, + bleeding
3	Prolapse with defecation, manual reduction, + bleeding
4	Prolapsed, not reducible

ETIOLOGY

- Increased hydrostatic pressure in the erect position
- Intrinsic weakness of vessel walls
- Increased intra-abdominal pressures (straining at stool)
- Obstruction to outflow (pregnancy)
- Portal hypertension

PEDIATRIC CONSIDERATIONS

- Internal hemorrhoids rare in children even with portal hypertension

Pre-Hospital

N/A

Diagnosis

ESSENTIAL WORKUP

- History important
- Visual inspection of the anal area and digital examination mandatory
- External hemorrhoids
  - —Skin covered and visible externally
  - —If thrombosed, appear dark blue with a palpable clot
- Internal hemorrhoids, unless thrombosed, are not palpable

LABORATORY

- Hct if history of significant blood loss

IMAGING/SPECIAL TESTS

- Anoscopic exam allows excellent exposure of the anoderm and allows hemorrhoidal tissue to protrude into the scope for identification

DIFFERENTIAL DIAGNOSIS

- Rectal prolapse
- Perirectal abscess
- Anal fissure

Treatment

INITIAL STABILIZATION

- Control bleeding with manual pressure

ED TREATMENT

- Conservative therapy
  - —Hot sitz baths for 15 minutes 3 times per day and after each bowel movement
  - —Increased roughage and generous oral fluids to provide soft, formed, regular movements
  - —Stool softener
  - —Bulk-forming laxative
  - —Topical antibiotics, anesthetics, and steroid creams are of limited value and may cause delayed healing
- Conservative therapy for
  - —External hemorrhoids if pain tolerable and the swelling not tense
  - —Grades 1 and 2 internal hemorrhoids
- Clot excision for thrombosed external hemorrhoids with severe pain and recent clot; follow with conservative therapy
  - —Infiltrate the overlying skin using a 30-gauge needle with lidocaine containing epinephrine
  - —Provide gentle traction to the overlying skin
  - —Make an elliptical incision to expose and evacuate the thrombosed vein
  - —Place a small piece of gauze into the wound and place a pressure dressing externally
  - —Remove pressure dressing at the time of the first sitz bath 6–12 hours later
- Manually reduce nonthrombosed prolapsed internal hemorrhoids and follow with conservative therapy
- Nonreducible hemorrhoids
  - —Surgical referral
- Analgesia
  - —NSAIDs/acetaminophin
  - —Nitroglycerin ointment to external anal canal to reduce pain by decreasing internal sphincter spasm
  - —Use narcotics sparingly due to worsening constipation
- Surgical therapy
  - —Rubber band ligation
  - —Sclerosing injections
  - —Cryotherapy
  - —Laser therapy
  - —Hemorrhoidectomy

MEDICATIONS

- Acetaminophen: 325–650 mg (peds: 15 mg/kg) with codeine 15–30mg (peds: codeine 0.5 mg/kg) po q 4 hrs PRN
- Docusate (colace): 60–360 mg/24hrs (peds: 3-5 mg/kg/24hrs) po tid
- Bran/fiber: 10 g/day po (0.5–1 tsp/day)
- Ibuprofen: 400–600 mg (40 mg/kg/24hrs) po q 6hrs
- Psyllium seeds: 30 g/day (0.5–1 tsp/day) po

Disposition

ADMISSION CRITERIA

- Surgical consult for painful, edematous, incarcerated grade 4 hemorroids

DISCHARGE CRITERIA

- Nearly all patients will be discharged
- Discharge with surgical referral for
  - —Grades 3 and 4 internal hemorrhoids
  - —Incarcerated/strangulated hemorrhoids
  - —Patients with inflammatory bowel disease, coagulopathy, pregnancy, immunocompromised, or with suspected anorectal or colonic tumors

Miscellaneous

ICD9: 455.6

CORE CONTENT CODE: 1.8.1.3.1, 1.8.1.3.2

SUGGESTED READINGS

Gorfine SR. Treatment of benign anal disease with topical nitroglycerin. Dis Colon Rectum 1995;38:453–457.

Hancock BD. Hemorrhoids. Br Med J 1992;304:1042–1044.

Janicke DM, Pundt MR. Anorectal disorders. Emerg Med Clin North Am 1996;14(4):757–788.

Mazier WP. Hemorrhoids, fissures, and pruritus ani. Surg Clin North Am 1994;74(6):1277–1291.

Pfenninger JL, Surrell J. Nonsurgical treatment options for internal hemorrhoids. Am Fam Physician 1995;52:821–834.

Smith LE. Hemorrhoids—a review of current techniques and management. Gastroenterol Clin North Am 1987;16(1):79–90.

Author: Anthony Best

Hemothorax

Clinical Presentation

SIGNS AND SYMPTOMS

- Small amount of blood in thorax (less than 400 cc): little or no change in patient's appearance, vital signs, or physical findings
- Large amount of blood (more than 1000 cc): restlessness, anxiety, pallor, pleuritic pain, hemoptysis, dyspnea, or air hunger
- Tachycardia, tachypnea, hypotension
- Chest inspection: asymmetric expansion, paradoxical wall movement, abrasion, contusion
- Chest wall palpation: tenderness or crepitus over ribs, clavicles, scapulae, or the sternum; subcutaneous emphysema, dullness to percussion
- Auscultation: ipsilateral decreased breath sounds

MECHANISM/DESCRIPTION

- Accumulation of blood in the intrapleural space causing lung compression. This results in decreased vital capacity, hypoxia, and respiratory compromise
- Hemothorax can cause increased intrathoracic pressure resulting in compromised venous return and decreased cardiac output
- Loss of large intravascular volume results in hemodynamic instability
- Large hemothoraces cause the release of substances that can act as anticoagulants and contribute to continued intrathoracic bleeding

ETIOLOGY

- Traumatic injuries to major vessels: laceration of major blood vessels, including pulmonary artery, pulmonary vein, intercostal artery, internal mammary artery, aorta, vena cava, and heart are associated with hemorrhage into the thoracic cavity
- Traumatic lung parenchymal injuries: often stops spontaneously by nature of the low pulmonary pressures and high concentrations of tissue thromboplastin in the lung
- Nontraumatic spontaneous hemothoraces: very rare. Coagulation disorder, malignancy, primary vascular event (such as aortic dissection), infection, and complication of spontaneous pneumothoraces

Pre-Hospital

CAUTIONS

- It is difficult to differentiate hemothoraces from pneumothoraces or hemopneumothoraces by clinical presentation and examination. All may present with dyspnea, pleuritic chest pain, decreased breath sounds, and hemodynamic instability
- Certain clues aid in making the diagnosis such as subcutaneous emphysema for pneumothorax, and dullness to percussion for hemothorax
- If the patient shows signs of significant hemodynamic instability, it is necessary to perform needle thoracostomy to treat a potential tension pneumothorax

Diagnosis

ESSENTIAL WORKUP

- Chest radiography is the single best diagnostic tool. Fluid collections >200–300 cc can usually be seen on good upright to decubitus radiograph of the chest
  - —In the supine position, which is often the initial view available, up to 1000 cc of blood may not be readily apparent. Hemothorax appears as a slight haziness over the involved hemithorax on the AP radiograph
  - —In the hemodynamically stable patient, the optimal technique is an upright PA projection at full inspiration. A lateral chest film should be added when practical, and an end-expiratory film may be helpful in confirming a small pneumothorax
- Pulse-oximetry, arterial blood gas

LABORATORY

- Hematocrit may be helpful if it shows a drop or changes on serial evaluations
- Type and crossmatch

IMAGING/SPECIAL TESTS

- Ultrasound diagnostic imaging is a valuable tool in the evaluation of intrapleural fluid collection. It has the advantage of being a rapid, sensitive, and specific diagnostic modality in the trauma patient
- Computerized tomography (CT) is useful in detecting small amounts of intrapleural fluid not visible on the chest radiograph

DIFFERENTIAL DIAGNOSIS

- Hemopneumothorax
- Pneumothorax
- Pulmonary contusion

Treatment

INITIAL STABILIZATION

- ABCs
  - —Control airway as needed. Endotracheal intubation for patients with impending respiratory failure
  - —Supplemental oxygen: 100% non-rebreather mask
  - —Intravenous access: Two large-bore intravenous catheters to restore circulating blood volume
  - —Needle thoracostomy should be performed in patients with hemodynamic instability. This will aid in differentiating pneumothorax from hemothorax

ED TREATMENT

- Hemothorax is treated by evacuating accumulated blood in the intrapleural space
- Tube thoracostomy evacuates blood; allows for reexpansion of the lung as well as constant monitoring of blood loss
- Tube thoracostomy: use a large-bore chest tube (36–40 French) inserted in the fourth or fifth intercostal space at the midaxillary line aiming posteriorly and superiorly. The tube is then connected to underwater-seal drainage and suction (20–30 ml H_2O)
- Autotransfusion should be used if available to replace blood loss
- Indications for thoracotomy
  - —Initial tube drainage greater than 20 cc/kg of blood
  - —Persistent bleeding at a rate greater than 7 cc/kg/hr
  - —Increasing hemothorax seen on chest radiography
  - —Patient remains hypotensive despite adequate blood replacement and other sites of blood loss have been ruled out
  - —Patient decompensates after initial response to resuscitation

MEDICATIONS

- Local anesthetics for cutaneous anesthesia prior to tube thoracostomy in awake, conscious patients
- Conscious sedation (midazolam) and analgesia (fentanyl) should be used for stable, awake patients prior to tube thoracostomy
  - —Fentanyl: adult/peds: 2–5 μg/kg/dose
  - —Midazolam: adult/peds: 0.02–0.04 mg/kg/dose

Disposition

ADMISSION CRITERIA

- Hemothoraces large enough to require tube thoracostomies should be admitted for monitoring and thoracostomy tube management

DISCHARGE CRITERIA

- Isolated small hemothoraces (detected incidentally on ultrasound or CT imaging) may be considered for discharge after 4–6 hours of observation if there is no evidence of continued bleeding and the patient is not hypoxic

Miscellaneous

ICD9: 511.8

CORE CONTENT CODE: 18.4.10.13

SUGGESTED READINGS

Eddy CA, Carrico CJ, Rusch VW. Injury to the lung and pleura. In: Moore EE, Mattox KL, Feliciano DV, eds. Trauma. 2d ed. East Norwalk, CT: Appleton & Lange, 1991.

Meredith JW. Chest wall injury. In: Trunkey D, Lewis FR Jr, eds. Current therapy of trauma. 3rd ed. Philadelphia: BC Decker, 1991:216–219.

Parry GW, Morgan WE, Salama FD. Management of haemothorax. Ann R Coll Surg Engl 1996;78(4):325–326.

Vukich DJ, Markovchick V. Thoracic trauma. In: Rosen P, et al., eds. Emergency medicine: Concept and clinical practice. 4th ed. St. Louis: CV Mosby, 1998:514–526.

Author: Thomas C. Lee

Henoch Schönlein Purpura

Clinical Presentation

SIGNS AND SYMPTOMS

General

- History of an upper respiratory tract infection
- Malaise
- Low grade fever
- Hypertension
  - —Uncommon finding associated with renal failure

Abdominal

- Abdominal findings may precede the rash by 4 weeks
- Abdominal pain
  - —70–80% of cases
  - —Colicky to severe
- Gastrointestinal bleeding
  - —75% of cases
  - —Occult to severe blood loss
  - —Intussusception

Extremities

- Arthritis
  - —70–80% of cases
  - —Migratory periarticular pain
  - —Most frequent in knees and ankles
  - —Angioedema

Skin

- Purpura
  - —Only present 50% at the time of onset
  - —Ultimately 100% of patients develop purpura
  - —First appears as pink rounded papules that blanch
  - —Progresses to 2–3 cm circular palpable purpura within 24 hours
  - —Specific anatomic distribution
    - -Symmetric
    - -Extensor surface of the extremities
    - -Buttocks
    - -Lower back
    - -Rarely the face
- Erythema multiforme
- Erythema nodosum
- Children <3 months commonly only have skin manifestations
- Rash begins on dependent areas of legs and buttocks
- May reoccur in 40% of patients within 6 weeks

Renal-Genitourinary

- Asymptomatic hematuria
  - —Occurs in 80% of cases
- Scrotal pain
- Testicular swelling
- Renal failure

Neurologic

- Headache
- Seizure
- Focal deficits

MECHANISM/DESCRIPTION

- Vasculitis
- Peak incidence school-aged children and young adults
- More common in Caucasians
- Males > females
- Occurs more often in winter months
- Multisystem involvement can lead to life-threatening or long-term complications
  - —Intussusception
  - —Proliferative glomerulonephritis
  - —Chronic renal failure
  - —Intracranial hemorrhage

ETIOLOGY

- Increased serum IgA
  - —Circulating IgA complexes
  - —Glomerular mesangial deposition of IgA
- Associated with
  - —Infections
    - -Group A strep
    - -Mycoplasma
    - -Varicella
    - -Epstein-Barr virus
  - —Drugs
  - —Allergens

Pre-Hospital

N/A

Diagnosis

ESSENTIAL WORKUP

- Essentially a clinical diagnosis
- Ancillary studies are used to rule out other etiologies and assess for complications

LABORATORY

- CBC
  - —Platelet count normal
  - —WBC often elevated
- PT, PTT, Bleeding time
- Serum complement level C3
- Electrolytes
- BUN, Creatinine
  - —May be elevated in cases with serious renal complications
- Urinalysis
  - —Hematuria is common
  - —Proteinuria is suggestive of glomerulonephritis

IMAGING/SPECIAL TESTS

- Abdominal imaging studies
  - —Indicated if abdominal pain or gastrointestinal bleeding
  - —Upright and abdominal flat plate
  - —Abdominal ultrasound
  - —Barium enema to rule out intussusception
- Testicular ultrasound
  - —Indicated in patients with testicular pain and swelling

DIFFERENTIAL DIAGNOSIS

- Abdominal pain
  - —Appendicitis
  - —Inflammatory bowel disease
  - —Meckel's diverticulum
- Arthralgias
  - —Acute rheumatic fever
  - —Polyarthritis nodosa
  - —Juvenile rheumatoid arthritis
  - —Systemic lupus erythematosus
- Purpura
  - —Thrombocytopenia
  - —Functional platelet disorders
  - —Trauma/child abuse
  - —Meningococcemia
  - —Viral exanthema
  - —Infectious mononucleosis
  - —Bacterial endocarditis
  - —Rocky Mountain Spotted Fever
  - —Streptococcal infection
  - —Drugs/toxins
    - -Sulfonamides
    - -Iodides
    - -Belladonna
    - -Bismuth
    - -Penicillins
    - -Chloral hydrate
    - -Mercurial compounds

- Renal disease
  - —Acute glomerulonephritis
- Testicular swelling
  - —Incarcerated hernia
  - —Orchitis
  - —Testicular torsion

Treatment

INITIAL STABILIZATION

- Parenteral fluids and blood in massive GI hemorrhage

ED TREATMENT

- Nonsteroidal anti-inflammatory drugs
  - —Arthralgias
- Prednisone
  - —Painful subcutaneous edema
  - —Renal disease
  - —Central nervous system involvement

MEDICATIONS

- Ibuprofen: 5–10 mg/kg po q 6 hrs
- Prednisone: 1–2 mg/kg for 5–7 days po qd

Disposition

ADMISSION CRITERIA

- Severe abdominal pain
- Gastrointestinal bleeding
- Intussusception
- Evidence of renal failure

DISCHARGE CRITERIA

- Normal platelet count
- Minimal abdominal pain
- Follow-up for routine urinalysis and kidney function test
- If steroids started, follow up within 24 hours

Miscellaneous

ICD9: 287.0

CORE CONTENT CODE: 13.11.3

SUGGESTED READINGS

Causey AL, Woodall BN, Wahl NG, et al. Henoch-Schönlein purpura: four cases and a review. J Emerg Med 994;12(3):331–341.

Fleisher GR, Ludwig S. Textbook of pediatric emergency medicine. 3rd ed. Baltimore: Williams & Wilkins, 1993:710–711.

Hurwitz S. Clinical pediatric dermatology. 2d ed. Philadelphia: WB Saunders, 1993:539–541.

Szer IS. Henoch-Schönlein purpura: When and how to treat. J Rheumatol 1996;23(9):1661–1665.

Authors: David Nelson; Lydia Ciarallo

Hepatic Encephalopathy

Clinical Presentation

SIGNS AND SYMPTOMS

- Wide range of mental status changes affecting the behavioral, intellectual, neuromuscular function and the level of consciousness
- Rate of progression variable
- Constructional apraxia
  —Inability to draw a clock or a star
  —In early stages of hepatic encephalopathy (HE)
- *Fetor hepaticus*—peculiar sweet odor
- Symptoms and signs of chronic liver disease, portal hypertension, or fulminant hepatic failure

Grading

- Grade 0
  —No apparent clinical changes
  —Abnormal psychometric tests
- Grade I
  —Euphoria or depression
  —Reversal of normal sleep pattern
  —Irritability and impairment of writing and drawing
- Grade II
  —Lethargy/slow responses
  —Inappropriate behavior
  —Asterixis
  —Slurred speech
  —Ataxia
- Grade III
  —Disorientation to time and place
  —Amnesia
  —Paranoia
  —Nystagmus
  —Hyperactive reflexes
  —Positive Babinski reflex
  —Marked drowsiness
- Grade IV
  —Dilated pupils
  —Opisthion
  —Stupor or unconscious

MECHANISM/DESCRIPTION

- Multifactorial leading to disturbances of blood brain barrier as well as
  —Neurotoxins, including ammonia (produced by protein degradation by colonic bacteria), short-chain fatty acids, phenols, mercaptans, and elevated ratio of aromatic to branched-chain amino acids (BCAA)
  —Increased inhibitory neurotransmitters including endogenous benzodiazepines, GABA, and serotonin
  —Decreased excitatory neurotransmitters including glutamate, dopamine, aspartate, and catecholamine
  —Decreased cerebral blood flow and oxygen, and glucose consumption
  —Zinc deficiency
- Although HE is thought to be a reversible metabolic condition of episodic nature, there is a suggestion that it is a progressive neurodegenerative disorder

ETIOLOGY

- Advanced cirrhosis often in association with portal hypertension
- Postsurgical or transjugular intrahepatic portosystemic stent/shunt (TIPS)
- Fulminant hepatic failure (FHF)
- Precipitating causes
  —GI bleeding (more common in elderly)
  —Sepsis (e.g., spontaneous bacterial peritonitis)
  —Constipation
  —Noncompliance with lactulose
  —High-protein diet
  —Hypokalemia
  —Alkalosis
  —Hypoglycemia
  —Hypovolemia (e.g., postlarge-volume paracentesis)
  —Azotemia (e.g., diuretic-induced)
  —Use of narcotics or sedatives, including alcohol
  —Zinc deficiency—zinc important for normal nitrogen metabolism
  —Hepatocellular injury including viral- or drug-induced hepatitis

Pre-Hospital

CAUTIONS

- With advanced grades HE or associated active GI bleeding, attention to
  —Maintaining the airway
  —Providing adequate ventilation
  —Prompt treatment of hypoglycemia

Diagnosis

ESSENTIAL WORKUP

- Clinical diagnosis: altered mental status with evidence of liver failure or portal hypertension
- Search for precipitating cause (particularly GI bleeding and sepsis)
- Paracentesis to detect spontaneous bacterial peritonitis

LABORATORY

- Arterial ammonia level
  —Increased in the majority of patients with HE
  —Level correlates poorly with the degree of HE
  —Helpful in detecting HE in cases of altered mental status of unknown cause
  —Normal ammonia level with suspected HE warrants search for other causes of altered mental status
  —Serial measurements helpful in monitoring individual patients
  —Level affected by azotemia, infusion of amino acid solution, or massive tissue breakdown
- CBC
  —Anemia
  —Leukocytosis points to infection
- Electrolytes, BUN, Cr, glucose
- PT, PTT
- Liver profile
- Liver enzymes
- ABG
- Toxicology screen including acetaminophen and alcohol level
- TSH
- Urinalysis
- Magnesium
- Zinc level
- Viral serology
- Blood and urine cultures

IMAGING/SPECIAL TESTS

- CXR for pneumonia and signs of CHF
- ECG for arrhythmia and electrolyte imbalance
- Head CT scan in new-onset altered mental status, focal neurological deficit, or suspected trauma
- CSF examination
  —For new onset or unexplained worsening of HE
  —CSF glutamine level correlates with the severity of HE

DIFFERENTIAL DIAGNOSIS

- *Alcohol withdrawal syndromes including delirium tremens (DTs)*
  —Signs of sympathetic hyperactivity, hallucinations, anxiety, seizures
- *Asterixis* is seen in other metabolic encephalopathies including
  —Uremia

—CO_2 narcosis
—CHF
—Sedative overdose
- Uremia
- Hypoglycemia
- Sedatives including alcohol intoxication
- Medications or drug-induced toxic confusional states
- Head injury
- Cerebrovascular accident and neuropsychiatric disorders
- Meningitis or encephalitis

PEDIATRIC CONSIDERATIONS

- Consider Reye's syndrome early (most common cause of FHF in children) even if PT is only mildly prolonged
- Consider fatty acid β-oxidation disorder
  —Freeze serum and urine sample for subsequent testing

Treatment

INITIAL STABILIZATION

- In advanced grades of HE
  —Oxygen and airway protection due to loss of gag reflex and risk of aspiration
  —Cardiac monitor
  —Fluid resuscitation
- Narcan, D50W (or Accucheck) and thiamine for altered mental status

ED TREATMENT

- Aggressive treatment of complicating conditions:
  —Acute GI bleeding
  —Sepsis
  —Coagulopathy
  —Renal and electrolytes disturbances: hypokalemia, hypoglycemia, and alkalosis
- Avoid sedative/narcotics
  —For agitation use agents not metabolized by the liver
  -Oxazepam 10–30 mg carefully titrated
- Increase nitrogen elimination with
  —Lactulose
  —Lactitol
- Decrease ammonia producing intestinal flora (in combination with lactulose)
  —Metronidazole
  —Neomycin (nephrotoxic and ototoxic)
- Clean bowel with Fleet's, sorbitol, or lactulose enema
- Correct zinc deficiency with zinc acetate or sulfate
- Restrict protein intake in diet
- If not contraindicated, a trial of flumazenil could provide moderate but not sustained improvement in patients who have received benzodiazepines
- *Liver transplantation provides cure* for severe, spontaneous, or recurrent HE

MEDICATIONS:

- Flumazenil (romazicon)
  —Initial: 0.2 mg IV over 30 sec
  —If no response: 0.3 mg IV after 30 sec
  —If still no response: 0.5 mg IV and repeat q 30–60 sec if needed up to maximum dose of 3–5 mg
- Dextrose: D50W 1 amp (50 ml or 25 g) (peds: D25W 2–4 ml/kg) IV
- Lactulose: 30 ml (peds: 0.3 ml/kg) po or via NG tube qid titrated to produce 2–3 soft stools per day and stool pH <5
- Metronidazole: 250 mg (peds: 10–30 mg/kg/day) tid for 2 weeks
- Naloxone (narcan): 2 mg (peds: 0.1 mg/kg) IV or IM initial dose
- Neomycin: 1–2 g (peds: 50–100 mg/kg/24hrs) po q 4 hrs
- Thiamine (vitamin B_1): 100 mg (peds: 50 mg) IV or IM
- Zinc acetate or sulfate: 200 mg po tid

Disposition

ADMISSION CRITERIA

- HE Grade II, III, or IV, or inadequate social support
- Advanced stages of HE to ICU with urgent GI consult
- Associated complicating condition (GI bleeding and sepsis)
- Uncertainty about the cause of altered mental status

DISCHARGE CRITERIA

- Known chronic or intermittent HE, in grades 0 or I, with remediable cause, adequate supervision at home, and close follow-up

Miscellaneous

ICD9: 572.2

CORE CONTENT CODE: 1.2.3

SUGGESTED READINGS

Bosch J, Bruix J, Mas A, et al. The treatment of major complications of cirrhosis. Aliment Pharmacol Ther 1994;8:639.

Jalan R, Seery JP, Taylor-Robinson SD. Pathogenesis and treatment of chronic hepatic encephalopathy. Aliment Pharmacol Ther 1996;10:681.

Marsano L, McClain C. How to manage both acute and chronic hepatic encephalopathy. J Crit Illness 1993;8:579.

Riordan SM, Williams R. Treatment of hepatic encephalopathy. N Engl J Med 1997;337:473–479.

Author: Abbas Zagnoon

Hepatic Injury

Clinical Presentation

SIGNS AND SYMPTOMS

- Systemic signs due to acute blood loss
  - —May present with dizziness and weakness
  - —Profound hypotension, or clinical shock
- Local signs include right upper-quadrant tenderness, guarding, abdominal distention, rigidity, or rebound
- Contusions, abrasions, or penetrating wounds to the right chest, flank, or abdomen may be indicative of underlying hepatic injury
- Fractures of lower right ribs are commonly seen in association with hepatic injuries
- Physical exam is neither sensitive nor specific for hepatic injury

MECHANISM/DESCRIPTION

- The size of the liver alone, occupying most of the right upper-quadrant places it at significant risk for any penetrating injury
- The position of the liver, under the lower rib cage, makes it highly susceptible to blunt injuries, either by direct blow or deceleration forces
- Mechanism of injury and kinematic forces are important factors in evaluating patients for possible hepatic injury
  - —For blunt trauma obtain information about the forces and direction (horizontal or vertical) of any deceleration or compressive forces
  - —In penetrating trauma the type and caliber of the weapon, distance from the weapon, variety and length of knife or impaling object are important to discern
- Hepatic injuries are graded by severity, ranging from subcapsular hematoma and lacerations to severe hepatic fragmentation

PEDIATRIC CONSIDERATIONS

- Poorly developed musculature and relatively smaller anterior-posterior diameter increase the vulnerability of abdominal contents to compressive forces in children

Pre-Hospital

CAUTIONS

- Obtain details of mechanism of injury from the pre-hospital providers
- Initiate IV access as hemorrhage is major threat to life
- Penetrating wounds or evisceration should be covered with moist saline dressings

Diagnosis

ESSENTIAL WORKUP

- Physical exam is neither specific nor sensitive for hepatic injury
- Objective evaluation for intraperitoneal bleeding and liver injury is mandatory for significant abdominal injuries

LABORATORY

- No hematologic laboratory studies are specific for diagnosis of injury to the liver
- Obtain baseline hemoglobin
- Liver function tests are not helpful in the acute setting

IMAGING/SPECIAL TESTS

- Plain abdominal x-rays are of little value
- Bedside ultrasound is rapidly becoming the initial procedure of choice as it detects intra-abdominal fluid and other findings that may be suggestive of hepatic injury
- Diagnostic peritoneal lavage is extremely sensitive for the presence of hemoperitoneum although nonspecific for source of bleeding
- CT scan best depicts the presence and extent of hepatic injury as well as injuries to adjacent organs
  - —Patient must be stable enough to go to the CT scanner

DIFFERENTIAL DIAGNOSIS

- Other causes of intraperitoneal injury
- Retroperitoneal injury
- Thoracic injury

Treatment

INITIAL STABILIZATION

- ABCs (including C-spine immobilization)
  - —Control airway as needed; may have associated injuries including closed head injury
  - —Supplemental oxygen, cardiac monitor, pulse oximetry
  - —Adequate IV access, including central lines and cutdowns as dictated by the patient's hemodynamic status
  - —Fluid resuscitation, initially with 2 L of crystalloid (NS or LR), followed by blood products as needed

ED TREATMENT

- Immediate laparotomy may be appropriate in the acutely injured patient who is hemodynamically unstable with presumed hemoperitoneum and hepatic injury
- Bedside US or DPL may be helpful in confirming clinically suspected intra-abdominal hemorrhage in the patient with blunt multiple trauma
- Adjunctive diagnostic procedures should be performed early in the evaluation followed by laparotomy when indicated by positive diagnostic findings
- Gun shot wounds to the anterior abdomen are routinely explored in the OR
- Stab wounds can be managed by local wound exploration followed by US or DPL when intraperitoneal penetration is demonstrated or equivocal
- Operative versus nonoperative management
  - —Patients with frank signs of intraperitoneal hemorrhage, those with indications based on diagnostic procedures and those who fail nonoperative management should undergo laparotomy
  - —Nonoperative management may be considered for those that are hemodynamically stable, no evidence of other intra-abdominal injury, and isolated hepatic injury confirmed by imaging study, most commonly CT scan
  - —Patients over 55 should not routinely be considered for nonoperative management because of decreased tolerance to insult and reduced physiologic reserve

Disposition

ADMISSION CRITERIA

- All patients with hepatic injury require hospitalization for definitive laparotomy or observation with serial exams and hematocrit determinations

DISCHARGE CRITERIA

- Patients with hepatic injuries should not be discharged

Miscellaneous

ICD9: 864.00

CORE CONTENT CODE: 18.4.11.3

SUGGESTED READINGS

Croce MA, et al. Nonoperative management of blunt hepatic trauma is the treatment of choice for hemodynamically stable patients. Ann Surg 1995;221(6):744–755.

Marx J. Abdominal trauma. In: Rosen P, et al., eds. Emergency medicine: Concepts and clinical practice. 4th ed. St. Louis: CV Mosby, 1998:555–581.

Ochsner MG, Jaffin JH, Golocovsky M, Jones RC. Major hepatic trauma. Surg Clin North Am 1993;73(2):337–352.

Pachter HL, Liang HG, Hofstetter SR. Liver and biliary tract trauma. In: Felicano D, et al., eds. Trauma. 3rd ed. Stamford, CT: Appleton and Lange, 1996:487–524.

Author: Tom Moats

Hepatitis

Clinical Presentation

SIGNS AND SYMPTOMS

- Often asymptomatic and subclinical
- Preicteric phase
  —Flulike illness with fever, chills, malaise
  —Nausea/vomiting/anorexia
  —Aversion to smoking or certain foods
  —60% remain anicteric
- Icteric phase
  —Tender hepatomegaly
  —Jaundice
  —Itching
  —Dark urine
- May present in fulminant hepatic failure (FHF), with ascites or hepatic encephalopathy (HE)
- FHF in
  —2% of hepatitis B (HBV)
  —3% of hepatitis D (HDV) coinfection with HBV
  —30% of HDV superinfection or chronic HBV
  —0.2% of hepatitis A (HAV)
  —1% of hepatitis E (HEV)
  —Up to 20% of pregnant women with HEV
- Chronic viral hepatitis
  —Often asymptomatic or nonspecific symptom
  —Abnormal liver tests
  —With hepatitis C/C-GB and B (with or without HDV)
  —May first present as cirrhosis or hepatocellular carcinoma
- Extrahepatic manifestation of HCV or HBV
  —Urticaria/angioedema
  —Porphyria
  —Polyarteritis nodosa
  —Synovitis
  —Glomerulonephritis

ETIOLOGY

- Hepatitis C/C-GB
  —Unknown mode of transmission in one-fourth of patients
- Secondary hepatitis viruses
  —Epstein-Barr, cytomegalovirus, herpes viruses, HIV, adenovirus, coxsackie
  —Seen mostly in immune-compromised host

MECHANISM/DESCRIPTION

- Primary hepatitis viruses (A, B, C/C-GB, D, and E)
  —Account for 95% of cases
  —Attack primarily the liver
- Secondary hepatitis viruses
  —Involve the liver in the course of infection of other organs
- In acute hepatitis, liver biopsy shows hepatocellular necrosis and mononuclear infiltrate

PEDIATRIC CONSIDERATIONS

- Majority of cases are hepatitis A
- Usually subclinical
- Up to 90% of newborns of HB_sAg-positive mothers (especially if HB_eAg is positive) develop chronic HBV

Pre-Hospital

N/A

HEPATITIS:	*INCUBATION (WEEKS)*	*BLOOD PRODUCT*	*TRANSMISSION ENTERIC*	*SEXUAL*	*BODY FLUID*
A (HAV)	2–6	Rarely	Yes	No	Very Rare
B (HBV)	12–26	Yes	Yes	Yes	Yes
C (HCV/C-GB)	6–7	Yes	No	Rarely	No
E (HEV)	2–6	Rarely	Yes	No	No
D (HDV)	4–7	Occurs as coinfection/ superinfection with hepatitis B			

Diagnosis

ESSENTIAL WORKUP

- Detailed history for *risk factors* for hepatitis
- Clinical picture consistent with hepatitis

LABORATORY

- Electrolytes, BUN, Cr, glucose
  —Azotemia with hepatorenal syndrome
  —Hypoglycemia with severe liver damage
- Urinalysis
  —Dark-tea colored
  —+ Bilirubin
- CBC for
  —Leukopenia
  —Thrombocytopenia
  —Aplastic anemia is a rare complication of HBV and HCV

Liver Function Tests

- Liver enzymes
  —Elevation reflects injury
  —AST and ALT increased 10–1000 times
  —Degree of elevation does not correlate with severity
  —Lower enzyme elevation in chronic hepatitis
- Alkaline phosphatase
  —Mild to moderate elevation except in the less common cholestatic form (seen with HAV)
- Conjugated bilirubin
  —Mild to moderate elevation
- Prolongation of PT reflects more severe diseases
- Serum albumin, globulin

Viral Serology

- Hepatitis A
  —IgM anti-HAV—excellent marker for acute infection
  —IgG anti-HAV—previous exposure and immunity
- Hepatitis B
  —Acute hepatitis B
    -HB_sAg may or may not be positive
    -IgM anti-HB_C—almost always positive
  —Chronic hepatitis
    -HB_sAg-positive
    -Positive HB_eAg indicates active viral replication and high infectivity
    -Negative HB_eAg indicates low viral replication or a carrier state if liver enzymes and histology are normal
  —HB_s antibody (titer of >10 mIU/ml)—reflects immunity
  —Isolated presence of IgG anti-HB_c (with all other serologic markers negative) reflects remote infection with hepatitis B or rarely false-positive test
- Hepatitis C
  —ELISA II is negative in the acute stage but viral RNA (by PCR) is usually positive

—ELISA III, RIBA II, or viral RNA (tested by PCR) may be used to confirm the diagnosis
—Only few laboratories can test for HC-GB viral RNA

- Hepatitis D
  —Hepatitis D antibody (IgM or IgG) or viral RNA
- Hepatitis E
  —Hepatitis E antibody (IgM or IgG) or viral RNA

Additional Testing

- α-fetoprotein—every 12 months for surveillance for hepatocellular carcinoma in long-standing hepatitis B or C/C-GB
- Monospot—for Epstein Barr Virus

IMAGING/SPECIAL TESTS

- Head CT scan in cases of hepatic encephalopathy
- RUQ US for biliary obstruction

DIFFERENTIAL DIAGNOSIS

- Drug- or toxin-induced hepatitis: isoniazid, acetaminophen, α-methyldopa, amiodarone, valproate, phenytoin, halothane, cocaine
- Ischemic or hypoxic hepatitis: hypotension, hypoxemia, or CHF
- Alcoholic hepatitis
  —Elevation of AST is 2–3 times more than ALT
  —Elevation is usually less than 300 units
  —Encephalopathy, high bilirubin, and prolonged PT indicate poor prognosis
- Autoimmune hepatitis
- Wilson's disease (adolescents)
- Pregnancy-associated hepatitis
  —HELLP syndrome
  —Acute fatty liver of pregnancy
- Reye's syndrome
- Infectious mononucleosis

Treatment

INITIAL STABILIZATION

- ABCs for fulminant hepatic failure
- Narcan, thiamine, glucose (or Accucheck) for altered mental status

ED TREATMENT

- Treat hypovolemia with IV 0.9%NS
- Correct electrolytes imbalance
- Control vomiting with metoclopramide or trimethobenzamide
- Avoid hepatotoxic agents, or those metabolized in the liver (phenothiazines, alcohol, and acetaminophen)
- Vitamin K 10 mg SQ (give daily for 3 days) if PT is prolonged
- Ursodeoxycholic acid or cholestyramine for cholestasis-induced itching

Contact Immunoprophylaxis

- Hepatitis A
  —Immune globulin 0.02 ml/kg IM (within 2 weeks of exposure)
  -For household, day care, or institutional contacts
  —HAV vaccine 1 ml (peds: 2–17 yrs: 0.5 ml) IM, repeated in 6 months
  -Complete 2 weeks before expected exposure (e.g., travel)
- Hepatitis B
  —Hepatitis B immune globulin 0.06 ml/kg IM
  -Within 10 days of HBV exposure
  -Sexual contact, percutaneous, transmucosal exposure
  —HBV vaccine 1 ml (peds: 0.5 ml) IM given at 0, 1, and 6 months
  -For infants and children; particularly newborns of HB_sAg-positive mothers
  -Post-HBV exposure
- Hepatitis C: no vaccine or effective immune prophylaxis
- Hepatitis D: prevent HBV
- Hepatitis E: no vaccine or effective immune prophylaxis
  —Interferon SQ 3 times a week
  -For chronic hepatitis B: 10 million units (6 million units/m^2) for 4–6 months;
  -For chronic hepatitis C: 3 million units (3 million units/m^2) for 12 months

MEDICATIONS

- Cholestyramine: 4 g po 1–6 times/day
- Dextrose: D50W 1 amp (50 ml or 25 g) (peds: D25W 2–4 ml/kg) IV
- Meteclopromide (reglan): 10 mg IV/IM q 6–8 hrs PRN; 10–30 mg po qid
- Naloxone (narcan): 2 mg (peds: 0.1 mg/kg) IV or IM initial dose
- Thiamine (vitamin B_1): 100 mg (peds: 50 mg) IV or IM
- Trimethobenzamide (tigan): 250 mg po TID/QID; 200 mg IM/PR q 6–8 hrs (peds: 100–200 mg/dose if >15 kg)
- Ursodeoxycholic acid: 8–10 mg/kg/24hrs tid

Disposition

ADMISSION CRITERIA

- Intractable vomiting, dehydration, or electrolyte imbalance not responding to ED treatment
- Acute hepatitis with evidence of liver dysfunction
  —PT >3 seconds above control
  —Bilirubin >20 mg/dl
  —Hypoglycemia
  —Albumin <2.5 g/dl
- ICU admission for fulminant hepatic failure
- Hepatic encephalopathy
- Pregnancy, immunocompromised host, or possible toxic hepatitis

DISCHARGE CRITERIA

- Outpatient management usual
- Food handlers with enteric pathogens should not return to work as long as they are infectious

Miscellaneous

ICD9: 573.3

CORE CONTENT CODE: 1.2.1

SUGGESTED READINGS

Bondesson JD, Saperston AR. Hepatitis. Emerg Med Clin North Am 1996;14:695–718.

Lemon SM, Thomas DL. Vaccines to prevents viral hepatitis. N Engl J Med 1997;336:196.

Sjogren M. Serologic diagnosis of viral hepatitis. Med Clin North Am 1996;80:929.

Wolf JL. Liver disease in pregnancy. Med Clin North Am 1996;80:1167.

Author: Abbas Zagnoon

Hepatorenal Syndrome

Clinical Presentation

SIGNS AND SYMPTOMS

- Progressive oliguria
- Ascites, often tense
- Jaundice or hepatic encephalopathy
- Signs of acute or chronic liver disease
- Signs of portal hypertension
- Hypotension
- Tachycardia
- Warm extremities

MECHANISMS/DESCRIPTION

- Functional defect
  - —Kidneys have normal histology and structure
  - —Worsening of tubular function with worsening of hepatic function and hyperaldosteronism
- Renal hypoperfusion because of intense renal cortical vasoconstriction due to hepatorenal reflex secondary to portal hypertension
- Low effective blood volume due to peripheral and splanchnic vasodilatation and impaired cardiac function
- Contributing factors include
  - —Activated sympathetic and renin-angiotensin systems
  - —ADH
  - —Decreased atrial natriuretic factor
  - —Altered production of renal prostaglandins
  - —Nitric oxide
  - —Adenosine
  - —Kinin

ETIOLOGY

- Chronic liver disease, especially alcoholic
- Fulminant hepatic failure
- Obstructive jaundice
- Precipitating factors
  - —Decreased effective blood volume due to GI bleeding, vigorous diuresis, or paracentesis; hypotensive event
  - —Use of nephrotoxic agent (NSAIDs and aminoglycoside)
  - —Sepsis
  - —Worsening jaundice

Pre-Hospital

CAUTIONS

- Attention to hypotension, active GI bleeding, respiratory distress

Diagnosis

ESSENTIAL WORKUP

- Azotemia in setting of cirrhosis
- Search for precipitating causes including paracentesis (for peritonitis)

LABORATORY

- CBC
  - —Anemia due to GI bleed
- Electrolytes
  - —Hyperkalemia
  - —Acidosis
- Glucose
- Elevated BUN, Cr
  - —Normal Cr found with low GFR in association with muscle wasting, poor nutrition, and ascites
  - —Cr increased by some medications: cimetidine, trimethoprim, and spironolactone due to inhibition of tubular secretion of creatinine
  - —Hyperbilirubinemia
    - -Can artifactually lower serum creatinine (as tested by automated analyzers)
- PT, PTT
- Urinalysis
  - —Absence of ATN casts
  - —Check for UTI
- Spot urine sodium and creatinine, and serum and urine osmolality
  - —Spot urine Na+ <10 mEq/L
  - —Fractional excretion of Na+ <1%
  - —Urine/plasma creatinine >30:1
  - —Hyperosmolar urine
- Blood, ascitic fluid, and urine culture as indicated
- Urinary excretion of β_2-microglobulin—useful marker of acute tubular damage

IMAGING/SPECIAL TESTS

- CXR: for signs of CHF or fluid overload
- ECG: for dysrhythmia or signs of hyperkalemia
- Renal ultrasound: for obstruction as etiology
- Central venous pressure (CVP) measurements
  - —Differentiates prerenal (low) from hepatorenal (elevated)

DIFFERENTIAL DIAGNOSIS

- Acute tubular necrosis
  - —Urine sodium >30 mEq/L
  - —Urine osmolality equals plasma osmolality
  - —Urine casts and cellular debris
- Prerenal azotemia
  - —Urine output improves following correction of hypovolemia
- Obstruction
- Interstitial nephritis
- Postliver transplant renal dysfunction due to
  - —HRS: due to failure of transplanted liver
  - —Medications, e.g., cyclosporin
  - —Preexisting renal disease
  - —Perioperative hypovolemia

Treatment

INITIAL STABILIZATION

- ABCs
- Aggressive correction of hypovolemia with
  - —0.9%NS IV fluid
  - —Colloid volume expanders: 100 g albumin in 500 ml of normal saline
  - —Closely monitor clinical status including use of CVP
  - —Urine output should improve with prerenal azotemia
- Manage life-threatening emergencies of renal failure
  - —Hyperkalemia
  - —Severe acidosis

ED MANAGEMENT

- Supportive care
- *Do no harm*—discontinue potentially nephrotoxic agents
  - —NSAIDs
  - —Aminoglycosides
  - —Demeclocycline
- Search for and treat coexisting renal disease
- Correct electrolyte imbalances
- Treat any associated cardiopulmonary disorder and hypoxia
- Initiate broad spectrum antibiotics if sepsis suspected
- Correct liver associated complications
  - —Obstructive jaundice
  - —Hepatic encephalopathy
  - —Hypoglycemia
- Large volume paracentesis with IV albumin replacement (to relieve tense acites)
  - —Increases renal blood flow, and may briefly improve HRS
- Dialysis
  - —Useful in correcting fluid, electrolytes, acid-base imbalances, and pulmonary edema
  - —Indicated in patients awaiting liver transplant, fulminant liver failure, coexisting renal disease, azotemia-induced hepatic encephalopathy, and acute renal failure of unknown etiology
- Renal dose dopamine: 2 μg/kg/min
  - —May improve renal function
  - —Not curative
- Liver transplant
  - —Only available cure

Disposition

ADMISSION CRITERIA

- All suspected hepatic renal syndrome with gastroenterology and nephrology consult
- ICU admission for associated cardiopulmonary disease, hepatic encephalopathy, marked electrolyte imbalances

DISCHARGE CRITERIA

- None

Miscellaneous

ICD9: N/A

CORE CONTENT CODE: 1.2.3

SUGGESTED READINGS

Badalamenti S, Graziani G, Salerno F, et al. Hepatorenal syndrome. Arch Intern Med 1993;153:1957

Forrest EH, Jalan R, Hayes PC. Renal and circulatory changes in cirrhosis—pathogenesis and therapeutic perspective. Aliment Pharmacol Ther 1996;10:219

Roberts LR, Kamath PS. Ascites and hepatorenal syndrome: Pathophysiology and management. Mayo Clin Proc 1996;71:874

Author: Abbas Zagnoon

Hernia

Clinical Presentation

SIGNS AND SYMPTOMS

General

- Pain/swelling
  - —Localized to region of hernia
- Constant pain, vomiting, fever may indicate
  - —Incarceration
  - —Strangulation
  - —Obstruction

Inguinal Hernia

- Pain
  - —Localized to inguinal region
  - —Exacerbated by straining/positional changes
  - —Relieved by rest
- Swelling
  - —Males: intermittent bulge in scrotum
  - —Females: bulge immediately inferior to inguinal ligament or in labia
- Swelling of spermatic cord, scrotum, or testes
- Valsalva maneuver done while finger directed toward internal ring—may allow hernia sac to descend against finger

Femoral Hernia

- Pain/swelling
  - —Localized to femoral orifice inferior to inguinal ligament

Incisional Hernia

- Pain/swelling
  - —Localized to previous incision/scar

Obturator Hernia

- Nonspecific abdominal pain
- Intermittent intestinal obstruction
- Weight loss
- Pain
  - —Due to pressure on obturator nerve from hernia (Howship-Romberg sign)
  - —Along medial thigh
  - —Radiating to hip
  - —Relieved with thigh flexion
  - —Exacerbated by hip extension, adduction, or external rotation

Spigelian Hernia

- Abdominal pain/mass along anterior abdominal wall
- Increased pain with maneuvers increasing intra-abdominal pressure
- Intermittent bowel obstruction
- Palpable mass along Spigelian line
  - —Convex line extending from costal arch to pubic tubercle along lateral edge of rectus muscle

MECHANISM/DESCRIPTION

- Abnormal protrusion of peritoneal contents through a defect in the abdominal wall
- Incarceration
  - —When contents in hernia sac cannot be manipulated back into abdomen
- Strangulation
  - —Compromise of vascular supply to bowel contained in hernia leading to ischemia and gangrene
  - —Tender irreducible hernia with nausea/vomiting, fever, leukocytosis

ETIOLOGY

- Indirect inguinal hernia
  - —Results from persistent process vaginalis
  - —Herniation of peritoneal contents through internal ring
  - —Right side more common than left
- Direct inguinal hernia
  - —Due to defect or weakness in transversalis area in Hesselbach's triangle
    - -Inguinal ligament inferiorly
    - -Inferior epigastric vessels laterally
    - -Lateral border of rectus abdominus medially
  - —Herniation through Hesselbach's triangle
- Incisonal hernia
  - —Resultant breakdown of surgical fascial closure
  - —Herniation through surgical fascia
- Femoral hernia
  - —Peritoneum herniates into the femoral canal beneath the inguinal ligament
- Obturator hernia
  - —Passes through obturator membrane and exits beneath pectineal muscle
- Umbilical hernia
  - —Failure of umbilical ring closure
  - —Herniation through umbilical ring/umbilicus

PEDIATRIC CONSIDERATIONS

- Diagnosis difficult
  - —Parents complain of a bulge in inguinal area often no longer present at time of exam
  - —Incarcerated hernias may present with irritability, abdominal pain, or intermittent vomiting
- Incidence of incarceration/strangulation is 10–20%
  - —Greater than 50% occurring in patients less than 6 months of age
- Incidence of incarceration higher in girls than boys
- Umbilical hernias
  - —Strangulation and incarceration rare
  - —Majority close spontaneously
  - —Most surgeons will delay closure until age 4

Pre-Hospital

N/A

Diagnosis

ESSENTIAL WORKUP

- Diagnosis based on history and careful clinical exam
  - —Palpate inguinal/femoral area for tenderness/masses
  - —Repeat examination while standing/straining

LABORATORY

- CBC
  - —Leukocytosis with strangulation
- Electrolytes, BUN/Cr, glucose
  - —If vomiting/dehydration
- Urinalysis
  - —For identifying GU causes of groin pain

IMAGING/SPECIAL TESTS

- Plain abdominal radiographs
  - —Bowel obstructive pattern with incarceration or strangulation
- Ultrasound
  - —For identifying testicular source of scrotal swelling

DIFFERENTIAL DIAGNOSIS

- Hydrocele
- Varicocele
- Lymphadenitis
- Testicular torsion
- Testicular tumor
- Undescended testis
- Lymphogranuloma venereum

Treatment

INITIAL STABILIZATION

- 0.9%NS IV fluid resuscitation when bowel strangulation, obstruction, or sepsis
  —Adults: 1 L bolus
  —Children: 20 cc/kg

ED TREATMENT

Incarceration Irreducible/Strangulation

- IVF
- Nasogastric tube
- Immediate surgical consultation
- Preoperative antibiotics for strangulated hernia

Hernia Reduction Method

- Intravenous sedation (benzodiazepine) and analgesia (opiate)
- Place in Trendelenburg position
- Allow 20–30 minutes for spontaneous reduction of hernia
- Manual reduction
  —Place constant, gentle pressure on hernia
  —For inguinal hernias, achieve reduction by putting fingers of one hand on internal ring while gently pulling then pressing on hernia distal to external ring
- Obtain surgical consultation if reduction is unsuccessful after one or two attempts
- Contraindications to reduction include
  —Fever
  —Leukocytosis
- Complications
  —Reduction of strangulated bowel into abdomen
    -Further ischemia/necrosis occurs with no clinical improvement

MEDICATIONS

- Cefoxitin: 1–2 g q 6–8 hrs (peds: 0–7 d 40 mg/kg/24hrs q 12 hrs; >7 d 80–160 mg/kg/24hrs q 6 hrs) IV PB
- Fentanyl: 1–4 μg/kg IVP
- Meperidine (demerol): 25 mg increments (peds: 1mg/kg) IV PRN
- Midazolam (versed): 2.5–5 mg (peds: 0.07 mg/kg) IV
- Morphine sulfate: 2–4 mg increments (peds: 0.1 mg/kg) IV PRN

PEDIATRIC CONSIDERATIONS

- Reduction in girls is harder since ovary may be wrapped in hernia

Disposition

ADMISSION CRITERIA

- Strangulated hernias require immediate surgical intervention
- Incarcerated hernias require admission for urgent surgical intervention
- Intestinal obstruction
- Peritonitis
- Vomiting
- Severe pain

DISCHARGE CRITERIA

- After successful reduction has been achieved
- Scheduled reevaluation in 24 hours and referral to surgery

Miscellaneous

ICD9: 553.9

CORE CONTENT CODE: 1.9.1, 13.1.9

SUGGESTED READINGS

Mensching JJ, Musielewicz AJ. Abdominal wall hernias. Emerg Med Clin North Am 1996;14(4):739–756.

Miller PA, Mezwa DG, Feczko PJ, Jafri ZH, Madrazo BL. Imaging of abdominal hernias. Radiographics 1995;15(2):333–347.

Author: Julio Silva

Herpes Simplex

Clinical Presentation

SIGNS AND SYMPTOMS

- HSV commonly causes 6 syndromes
  - —All may present with the classic grouped 1–3 mm vesicles on an erythematous base
  - —Vesicles may be filled with clear or cloudy fluid, or may appear as frank pustules

Orofacial Infection

- Primary infection
  - —Gingivostomatitis or pharyngitis
  - —Fever, malaise, irritability, cervical adenopathy, and myalgia
  - —Inability to eat due to pain
- Recurrent infection
  - —Commonly incited by sunlight, heat, stress, trauma, or immunosuppression
  - —Prodrome of itching, tingling, throbbing, or burning
  - —Involves the vermilion border

Genital infection

- See chapter on genital herpes

Encephalitis

- Acute onset of fever, altered mental status, and focal neurologic deficits
- Ages 5–30 and age >50 most commonly affected
- Can complicate either primary or recurrent disease

Neonatal Infection—Three Syndromes

- Skin, eye, mouth disease (SEM)
  - —Vesicular lesions on presenting birth part (usually face, eyes, mouth), or areas such as scalp monitor sites
- CNS disease
  - —Cranial nerve abnormalities; focal and generalized seizures
  - —Apnea and bradycardia
  - —May develop skin lesions
  - —Presents in 2nd–3rd week of life
- Disseminated disease
  - —Any organ system may be involved
  - —Presents in first week of life

Skin Other than Orofacial—Herpetic Whitlow and Herpes Gladiatorum

- History of exposure to infected secretions
- Abrupt onset fever, edema, erythema, and localized tenderness
- Epitrochlear and axillary lymphadenopathy

Eye

- Caused by extension of facial lesions or direct inoculation
- Acute onset of pain and photophobia, blurring of vision, chemosis, and conjunctivitis
- Dendritic lesions of cornea noted on fluorescein exam

MECHANISM/DESCRIPTION

- Disease of viral origin which classically produces recurrent painful vesicular lesions of mucocutaneous areas
- Lips, genitalia, rectum, hands, and eyes most commonly involved

ETIOLOGY

- Disease is caused by DNA virus's herpes simplex type 1 or type 2
- Viruses belong to the *Herpesviridae* family
  - —Characterized by latency and reactivation
- Virus transmission occurs through mucosa or abraded skin
- Both viruses infect oral or genital mucosa

PEDIATRIC CONSIDERATIONS

- See neonatal disease above
- Primary maternal HSV infection will result in CNS or disseminated disease in 70% of exposed neonates
- Vesicular skin lesions may or may not be present on initial exam
- Orofacial disease is most likely to present as gingivostomatitis in children less than 5 years
- Whitlow may be caused by thumb-sucking children with oral herpes

Pre-Hospital

CAUTIONS

- Maintain universal precautions

Diagnosis

ESSENTIAL WORKUP

- Orofacial
  - —Presumptive diagnosis made by history and exam
  - —If definitive diagnosis is necessary (e.g., invasive disease, child abuse)
    - -Viral culture of vesicles
    - -Fluorescent antibody detection of antigen; serum antibody studies
    - -Scrapings for Tzanck smear or Papanicolaou stain
- Encephalitis
  - —CT or MRI
  - —EEG diagnostic if spike and slow waves in temporal region
  - —Lumbar puncture with CSF pleocytosis and negative bacterial antigens
- Neonatal
  - —CT or MRI, EEG, and lumbar puncture
  - —Liver function studies and chest x-ray
- Eye
  - —Dendritic corneal lesions by fluorescein exam
  - —Swab of affected area for viral culture or fluorescent antibody detection

LABORATORY

- Lesion scrapings
  - —Virus isolation by tissue culture or fluorescent antibody
  - —Tzanck smear demonstrating multinucleated giant cells, atypical keratinocytes, and large nuclei
  - —Brain biopsy is Gold Standard for encephalitis
- Serum
  - —ELISA testing may demonstrate HSV antibodies, but it has many limitations
    - -Cannot distinguish HSV-1 from HSV-2
- CSF
  - —Ratio of CSF antibody to serum antibody of >20:1 indicates encephalitis
    - -Not usually elevated until 7–10 days into disease
  - —Polymerase Chain Reaction (PCR): newer test which may have high specificity and sensitivity

DIFFERENTIAL DIAGNOSIS

- Orofacial and skin
  - —Bacterial pharyngitis and mycoplasma pneumoniae pharyngitis
  - —Stevens-Johnson syndrome
  - —Herpes zoster
  - —Varicella
  - —Pemphigus
  - —Contact or chemical dermatitis
  - —Impetigo
- Encephalitis/meningitis
  - —Bacterial, viral, fungal, tuberculous, parasitic, or vasculitic
  - —Cerebrovascular accident
  - —Brain tumor
- Neonatal
  - —Sepsis of any etiology
- Eye
  - —Conjunctivitis: viral, bacterial, or allergic
  - —Herpes zoster ophthalmicus
  - —Scleritis/episcleritis
  - —Angle closure glaucoma

PEDIATRIC CONSIDERATIONS

- *All* neonatal disease mandates complete work up because progression to systemic disease is likely

Treatment

INITIAL STABILIZATION

- Protect airway in comatose or obtunded patients with suspected CNS disease
- Parenteral antiviral is indicated for neonatal HSV, encephalitis, and infections in immunocompromised patients

ED TREATMENT

- Orofacial
  - —Primary disease
    - -Supportive: hydration and topical anesthetics (viscous lidocaine, diphenhydramine elixir)
    - -Acyclovir for severe disease or immunocompromised patients
  - —Recurrent disease
    - -Supportive care with analgesics and hydration
    - -Antiviral therapy in immunocompromised patients or patients with eczema
- Encephalitis
  - —Acyclovir IV is the drug of choice for adults
    - -No benefit of acyclovir over vidarabine has been demonstrated in neonates
- Neonatal
  - —All types treated with an intravenous antiviral drug
  - —Acyclovir and vidarabine appear to have equal efficacy
- Skin (other than orofacial or genital)
  - —May be treated with oral acyclovir
  - —Antibiotics if secondary bacterial infection
  - —*Do not incise and drain,* may lead to spread of infection
- Eye
  - —Topical antiviral therapy with trifluridine, alternatives include idoxuridine and vidarabine
  - —*Do not treat with steroids,* may cause increased viral replication
  - —Consult with ophthalmology

MEDICATIONS

- Acyclovir
  - —Orofacial: adults: 400 mg po tid for 10 days or 5 mg/kg IV q 8 hrs for 7–10 days; peds: not recommended
  - —Encephalitis: adults: 10 mg/kg IV q 8 hrs; peds: 10 mg/kg IV q 8 hrs for 14–21 days; neonatal: 10 mg/kg IV q 8 hrs
  - —Skin (not orofacial or genital): adults: 400 mg po tid for 10 days; peds: 20 mg/kg po tid for 10 days
- Idoxuridine: adults: 1 drop 0.1% solution to eye qh; peds: 1 drop 0.1% solution to eye qh
- Trifluridine: adults and peds: 1 drop of 1% ophthalmic solution to eye q 2 hrs while awake (max. 9 drops per day)
- Vidarabine: adults: 10 mg/kg IV q 8 hrs; peds: 10 mg/kg IV q 8 hrs; adults or peds: topical 0.5-inch ribbon of 3% ophthalmic ointment to eye 5 times per day

PEDIATRIC CONSIDERATIONS

- Children may refuse liquids and food and dehydration may require admission

Disposition

ADMISSION CRITERIA

- Encephalitis, disseminated disease, dehydration, need for continued IV hydration
- Severe local disease or immunocompromised host
- Neonatal HSV
  - —ICU vs ward based on toxicity and need for airway support

DISCHARGE CRITERIA

- Uncomplicated local disease

Miscellaneous

ICD9: 054.9

CORE CONTENT CODE: 3.2.4.2

SUGGESTED READINGS

Annunziato PW, Gershon A. Herpes simplex virus infections. Pediatr Rev 1996;17:415–423.

Miller CS, Redding SW. Diagnosis and management of orofacial herpes simplex virus infections. Dent Clin North Am 1992; 36:879–895.

Whitley RJ, Lakeman FL. Herpes simplex virus infections of the central nervous system: therapeutic and diagnostic considerations. Clin Infect Dis 1995;20:414–420.

Authors: Mark G. Richmond; Steven M. Green

Herpes Zoster

Clinical Presentation

SIGNS AND SYMPTOMS

- Prodrome of pain and paresthesias in a dermatomal distribution
  —Character of pain may be sharp, dull, tingling, burning, or intense pruritus
  —Pain precedes rash by 1–10 days
  —Young patients are less likely to have a prodrome
- Classical rash is grouped vesicles on an erythematous base
  —The lesions begin as patches of erythema
  —Vesicles rapidly follow erythema
  —Initially appear clear, become cloudy, then progress to scab and crust formation over 10–12 days,
  —Crusts fall off in 2–3 weeks
  —Lesions evolve synchronously as opposed to primary varicella in which lesions of varying stages of development is pathognomonic
  —One dermatome typically affected, rarely crosses midline
  —Second thoracic to second lumbar nerve distributions are most commonly involved, followed by trigeminal and cervical
- Ocular involvement occurs in half of cases involving the ophthalmic division of the trigeminal nerve
  —Closely associated with disease occurring at the tip of the nose or the eyelid
  —Corneal involvement is most common, beginning as a punctate keratitis, which may coalesce to form a pseudodendritic or stellate pattern
- Disseminated disease may cause signs and symptoms of meningoencephalitis, myelitis, peripheral neuropathy, and hepatic disease
- Immunosuppressed patients generally have similar signs and symptoms, but of greater severity

MECHANISM/DESCRIPTION

- Commonly known as "shingles," may be referred to as "dermatomal zoster" or "zona"
- Most common in 50–80-year-old patients
- Disease disseminates in 1–2% of normal hosts and frequently in immunocompromised hosts
- *Ramsay-Hunt syndrome* is characterized by zoster oticus, peripheral facial palsy, regional adenopathy, vertigo, and anesthesia of the anterior two-thirds of the hemitongue
  —This is secondary to seventh and eighth cranial nerve involvement
- Postherpetic neuralgia is pain that is either spontaneous, provoked by minimal stimuli, or persists at the site of zoster lesions for more than 1 month after the cutaneous disease has healed
  —10–70% of patients will have pain after resolution of lesions
  —Incidence increases with age
- A syndrome of identical signs and symptoms as herpes zoster occurring without rash is known as zoster sine herpete

ETIOLOGY

- Caused by varicella zoster virus (VZV), which is a DNA virus in the Herpesviridae family
- Occurs exclusively in individuals with a prior history of chickenpox
- Herpes zoster is reactivation disease from virus that lays dormant in the dorsal root ganglia

PEDIATRIC CONSIDERATIONS

- Herpes zoster during pregnancy is associated with an extremely low rate of fetal complications, there is no need to consider termination
- Childhood zoster is most common when varicella occurred in utero or within the first 6 months of life

Pre-Hospital

CAUTIONS

- Zoster is potentially contagious and may cause varicella in nonimmune health care workers
- Maintain universal precautions

Diagnosis

ESSENTIAL WORKUP

- Clinical presentation is sufficient for diagnosis in most patients
- If definitive diagnosis is necessary, tissue culture is the Gold Standard
- The patient should be isolated and considered contagious until there is crust on every vesicle
- Herpes zoster ophthalmicus (HZO) is diagnosed by slitlamp exam
  —The pseudodendrites of HZO are broader, more opaque, and stain less brightly with fluorescein than the lesions of herpes simplex

LABORATORY

- Cell yields are highest if the base of vesicular lesions are scraped into collection device
- Numerous rapid immunofluorescence assays exist to detect VZV in vesicular fluid
- Tzanck smear demonstrating giant cells and intranuclear inclusions
- IgM and IgG is most commonly measured by ELISA; antibody titers rise 2 weeks after acute infection

DIFFERENTIAL DIAGNOSIS

- Zosteriform herpes simplex
- Varicella
- Herpes simplex
- Nonherpetic conjunctivitis
- Enteroviral infections such as hand, foot, and mouth disease
- Insect bites
- Bullous impetigo
- *Molluscum contagiosum*

PEDIATRIC CONSIDERATIONS

- Zoster may be the first manifestation of VZV infection because primary infection may have occurred in utero

Treatment

INITIAL STABILIZATION

- Rarely necessary
- Disseminated disease to CNS or lungs may require intubation to control airway
- IV access to administer fluids and antiviral therapy

ED TREATMENT

- Burrow's solution compresses
- Ocular involvement
  —Necessitates ophthalmologic consultation
  —Acyclovir oral or intravenous is best if started within 72 hours but is beneficial up to 1 week after symptom onset
- Acyclovir, valacyclovir, or famciclovir is recommended for immunocompromised patients and the elderly
  —Should be instituted within 72 hours of rash formation
- Foscarnet for acyclovir-resistant VZV in immunocompromised patients
- Analgesia with NSAIDs, narcotics, or nerve blocks
- Postherpetic neuralgia is difficult to manage; famciclovir may prevent it
  —Topical lidocaine or lidocaine and prilocaine cream provides short-term relief
  —Topical capsaicin is the only FDA-approved medication for this disorder but its use is controversial and should not be initiated in the ED
  —Tricyclic antidepressants, anticonvulsants, and NMDA-receptor antagonists have some efficacy
  —A list of pain clinics can be obtained from the American Pain Society (708) 966-5595

MEDICATIONS

- Acyclovir: adults: 800 mg po 5 times/d for 7–10 days; immunocompromised with severe disease 10–12 mg/kg IV over 1 hr q 8 hrs; peds: 20 mg/kg po qid × 5 days
- Famciclovir: adults: 500 mg po tid × 7 days; peds: not approved
- Valacyclovir: 1000 mg po tid × 7 days; peds: not approved

PEDIATRIC CONSIDERATIONS

- Aspirin should be avoided as in varicella because of the potential risk of Reye's syndrome

Disposition

ADMISSION CRITERIA

- Disseminated disease or disease involving more than two dermatomes in the immunocompromised patient requires admission for IV acyclovir
- Herpes zoster ophthalmicus in the immunocompromised patient requires admission for IV acyclovir
- Ramsay-Hunt syndrome requires admission and IV acyclovir
- Intractable pain
- ICU versus ward depends on severity of disease

DISCHARGE CRITERIA

- Most patients are managed as outpatients with referral to primary care or specialist as needed
- Postherpetic neuralgia may require long-term follow-up and management, these patients may need to be referred to a pain specialist
- Patients should be instructed that lesions may heal with scarring or may leave depigmented areas

PEDIATRIC CONSIDERATIONS

- Zoster in the neonate requires admission and treatment with IV acyclovir; ward versus ICU depends on severity of disease

Miscellaneous

ICD9: 053.9

CORE CONTENT CODE: 3.2.4.3

SUGGESTED READINGS

Karlin JD. Herpes zoster ophthalmicus: The virus strikes back. Ann Ophthalmol 1993;25:208–215.

Kost RG, Straus SE, Wood AJ. Postherpetic neuralgia—pathogenesis, treatment, and prevention. N Engl J Med 1996;335:32–42.

Nikkels AF, Pierard GE. Recognition and treatment of shingles. Drugs 1994;48:528–548.

Wood MJ. Current experience with antiviral therapy for acute Herpes zoster. Ann Neurol 1994;35:S65–S68.

Authors: Mark G. Richmond; Steven M. Green

Herpes, Genital

Clinical Presentation

SIGNS AND SYMPTOMS

- Local pain and itching
- Grouped vesicles on an erythematous base
- Lesions ulcerate, crust over, then heal
- Lesions on vulva, vagina, cervix, perineum, buttocks; penile shaft or glans
- Vesicles may not be apparent on moist mucosal surfaces, ulcers may predominate
- Herpetic cervicitis, vaginitis, or urethritis may present with dysuria, urinary hesitancy, or retention, vaginal discharge, or pelvic pain
- Systemic symptoms like fever, headache, malaise, photophobia, anorexia, myalgias, and lymphadenopathy are more common with primary infection

MECHANISM/DISEASE

Primary HSV Infection

- More prominent clinical syndrome
- 2–12 day incubation; symptoms peak 8–10 days after onset; lesions heal in 3 weeks
- More likely to have systemic symptoms or complications (e.g., encephalitis, meningitis)

Recurrent HSV Infection

- 50% of patients have 3–4 recurrences per year
- Virus reactivated from dorsal root ganglia
- Triggered by local trauma, emotional stress, fever, sunlight, etc.
- 1–2 day prodrome of local tingling, burning, itching, or pain prior to eruption (can mimic sciatica)
- Milder clinical syndrome; fewer lesions that usually heal within 10 days
- Associated with cervical cancer
- No cure for chronic recurrences

Asymptomatic HSV Infection

- Positive cultures without lesions or symptoms can occur

ETIOLOGY

- 70–90% of cases caused by Herpes simplex virus, type 2 (HSV-2), a DNA virus that may also cause aseptic meningitis
- 10–30% of cases caused by Herpes simplex virus, type 1 (HSV-1), which usually causes herpes labialis (cold sores) and can be associated with herpes encephalitis

PEDIATRIC CONSIDERATIONS

- Neonatal infections are often disseminated or involve the CNS
- Congenital HSV in the neonate without vesicles may mimic rubella, CMV, or toxoplasmosis

Pre-Hospital

CAUTIONS

- Contact isolation should be maintained in the form of gloves to protect health care workers

Diagnosis

ESSENTIAL WORKUP

- Diagnosis usually based on typical history and physical examination

LABORATORY

- Tzanck prep (Wright's or Giemsa stain of vesicle fluid or ulcer base) positive in half of cases
- Viral culture of vesicle fluid or ulcer base positive in 85–95% of cases

DIFFERENTIAL DIAGNOSIS

- Chancroid
- Syphilis
- Lymphogranuloma venereum (LGV)
- Granuloma inguinale
- Candidiasis
- Beçhet's syndrome

Treatment

INITIAL STABILIZATION

- Culture suspected lesions in pregnant patients

ED TREATMENT

- Acyclovir (zovirax) interferes with viral DNA polymerase. Oral or intravenous therapy is almost always preferable to topical therapy. Alternative medications with less frequent dosing regimens are famciclovir and valacyclovir
  - —Primary infection: acyclovir 200 mg po, 5 times/day for 10 days (or until clinical resolution) decreases the duration and severity of symptoms
  - —Recurrent infection: acyclovir is not routinely recommended because it offers marginal clinical benefit
  - —Immunocompromised patients or patients with systemic symptoms: acyclovir 5 mg/kg IV q 8 hrs times 7 days (or until clinical resolution)
  - —Frequent painful recurrences: treat as primary infection during prodrome or at first sign of infection. Consider suppressive therapy with acyclovir 200 mg 3–5 times daily or 400 mg bid for 6 months
- Analgesics and antipruritics as needed
- Urinary retention may be relieved with sitz baths or voiding in a warm bathtub
- Avoid any sexual contact from prodrome until healing
- Practice safe sex techniques even if there are no lesions
- Consider testing for concomitant STDs

MEDICATIONS

Acyclovir (zovirax)

- Acute therapy
  - —Adult: 200 mg po, 5 times/day × 10 days *or* 5 mg/kg IV q 8 hrs × 7 days
  - —Peds: 20 mg/kg po q 8 hrs × 5 days *or* 5 mg/kg IV q 8 hrs over 1 hr
- Suppressive Therapy
  - —Adults: 400 mg po tid; peds: 5 mg/kg q 8 hrs

Famciclovir

- Acute Therapy
  - —Adults: 250–500 mg po bid for 5 days; peds: not approved
- Suppressive Therapy
  - —Adults: 125 mg po bid for 5 days; peds: not approved

Valacyclovir

- Acute Therapy
  - —Adults: 1000 mg po bid for 5 days; peds: not approved
- Suppressive Therapy
  - —Adults: 500 mg po bid for 5 days; peds: not approved

PEDIATRIC CONSIDERATIONS

- Consider sexual abuse in children with genital HSV. Culture lesions and test for other STDs in all suspected cases

Disposition

ADMISSION CRITERIA

- Systemic involvement (encephalitis, meningitis), significant dissemination
- Severe local symptoms (pain, urinary retention)
- Severely immunocompromised patient

DISCHARGE CRITERIA

- Immunocompetent patient without systemic involvement

Miscellaneous

ICD9: 054.10

CORE CONTENT CODE: 19.4, 3.2.4.2

SUGGESTED READINGS

Polis M. Viral infections. In: Rosen P, et al., eds. Emergency medicine: Concepts and clinical practice. 3rd ed. St. Louis: CV Mosby, 1998:2532–2552.

Crumpacker C. Herpes simplex. In: Fitzpatrick T, et al., eds. Dermatology in general medicine. 3rd ed. New York: McGraw Hill, 1987.

Kuhn G. Vulvovaginitis. In: Tintinalli J, et al., eds. Emergency medicine: A comprehensive study guide. 3rd ed. New York: McGraw-Hill, 1992.

Authors: Mark Richmond; Steven Green

Hiccups

Clinical Presentation

SIGNS AND SYMPTOMS

- Characteristic sound abruptly ending an inspiratory effort
- Attacks usually occur at brief intervals and last only a few seconds or minutes
- Attacks lasting more than 48 hours suggest an underlying disorder

MECHANISM/DESCRIPTION

- Sudden, involuntary, contraction of the diaphragm and other inspiratory muscles terminated by abrupt closure of the glottis
- Usually occur with a frequency of 4–60 per minute
- Results from stimulation of one or more limbs of the hiccup reflex arc
  - —Requires involvement of the vagus and phrenic nerves
  - —"Hiccup center" is located in the upper spinal cord
- Diaphragmatic flutter
  - —Rare disorder in which rhythmic contractions of the diaphragm occur at a rate of 1–8 per second
- Male > Female 4:1
  - —In men, greater than 90% have an organic basis
  - —In women, a psychogenic cause is more likely

ETIOLOGY

- In most cases a cause is not found
- Gastrointestinal
  - —Gastric distention
  - —Esophageal lesions
    - -Reflux esophagitis
    - -Achalasia
    - -Candida esophagitis
    - -Carcinoma
    - -Obstruction
  - —Gastric lesions
    - -Ulcer
    - -Cancer
  - —Hepatic lesions
    - -Hepatitis
    - -Hepatoma
  - —Pancreatic lesions
    - -Pancreatitis
    - -Pseudocysts
    - -Cancer
  - —Inflammatory bowel disease
  - —Cholelithiasis
  - —Cholecystitis
  - —Appendicitis
  - —Postoperative, abdominal procedures
- Diaphragmatic irritation
  - —Tumors
  - —Pericarditis
  - —Eventration
  - —Splenomegaly
  - —Hepatomegaly
  - —Peritonitis
- CNS lesions
  - —Encephalitis
  - —Stroke
  - —Brainstem tumors
  - —Parkinson's disease
- Mediastinal and other thoracic lesions
  - —Pneumonia
  - —Aortic aneurysm
  - —Tuberculosis
  - —Myocardial infarction
  - —Lung cancer
- Toxic metabolic causes
  - —Uremia
  - —Alcoholism
  - —Hyponatremia
  - —Gout
  - —Diabetes
- Drug induced
  - —α-Methyldopa
  - —Benzodiazepines
  - —Steroids
- Psychogenic causes
  - —Hysterical neurosis
  - —Grief
  - —Malingering
- Other
  - —Herpes zoster
  - —Otic foreign body irritating the tympanic membrane
  - —Pharyngitis
  - —Laryngitis
  - —Prostatic disorders
  - —Idiopathic

Pre-Hospital

N/A

Diagnosis

ESSENTIAL WORKUP

- Careful physical examination in search of an underlying cause
  - —Examine mouth and throat for candida esophagitis
  - —Otoscopic examination to rule out a foreign body
- In the vast majority of cases, laboratory and imaging studies are not indicated in the ED

LABORATORY

- Indicated if uremia is suspected
  - —Intractable hiccups
  - —Peripheral edema
  - —Anuria
  - —Order electrolytes, BUN, creatinine

IMAGING/SPECIAL TESTS

- Fluoroscopy
  - —Not indicated in the ED
  - —Rarely useful in the outpatient setting to determine if one hemidiaphragm is dominant

DIFFERENTIAL DIAGNOSIS

- Eructation

Treatment

INITIAL STABILIZATION

N/A

ED TREATMENT

- Rarely required as hiccups generally subside spontaneously or as the initiating disease improves
- Treat specific causes when these are identified
  —Remove foreign bodies from the ear
  —Antifungal treatment of candida esophagitis
  —Relieve gastric distention with a nasogastric tube
- Catheter stimulation of the posterior pharynx through the nares will often ablate most cases in the ED
- Pharmacologic treatment
  —Chlorpromazine
  —Haldol
- Rarely indicated, counterirritation of the vagus nerve can ablate the attack
  —Supraorbital pressure
  —Carotid sinus massage
  —Digital rectal massage

MEDICATIONS

- Baclofen: 10 mg tid
- Chlorpromazine: 25–50 mg IV
- Haloperidol: 2–12 mg IM

Disposition

ADMISSION CRITERIA

- Admission is not indicated

DISCHARGE CRITERIA

- Remedies that can be tried at home in case of reoccurrence
  —Swallowing a spoonful of sugar
  —Sucking on a hard candy or swallowing peanut butter
  —Holding breath and increasing pressure on diaphragm (Valsalva maneuver)
  —Tongue traction
  —Lifting the uvula with a cold spoon
  —Drinking from the far side of a glass
  —Inducing fright
  —Smelling salts
  —Rebreathing into a paper bag
  —Sipping ice water
- Referral in cases of intractable hiccups for investigation into an underlying cause and more definitive therapeutic measures
  —Phrenic nerve block of dominant hemidiaphragm
  —Phrenic nerve crush or transection
  —Psychiatric interventions
    -Hypnosis
    -Behavioral modification

Miscellaneous

ICD9: 786.8

CORE CONTENT CODE: N/A

SUGGESTED READINGS

Lewis JH. Hiccups: Reasons and remedies. In: Lewis JH, ed. A pharmacologic approach to gastrointestinal disorders. Baltimore: Williams & Wilkins, 1994;11–16.

Rousseau P. Hiccups. South Med J 1995;88(2):175–81.

Author: Richard Wolfe

High Altitude Illness

Clinical Presentation

SIGNS AND SYMPTOMS

Acute Mountain Sickness (AMS)

- Generally benign and self-limited
- Symptoms may become debilitating
- Onset 4–12 hours after ascent
- Headache
- Anorexia/nausea/vomiting
- Fatigue
- Weakness
- Dizziness
- Lightheadedness
- Difficulty sleeping

High Altitude Pulmonary Edema (HAPE)

- Occurs 2–4 days after ascent
- Dyspnea at rest (early)
- Cough (dry at first then productive)
- Tachypnea
- Rales
- Cyanosis
- Severe respiratory distress and death may occur

High Altitude Cerebral Edema (HACE)

- Life-threatening
- Occurs in presence of HAPE
  —Seen rarely as an isolated entity
- Onset
- May occur 12 hours after the onset of AMS
- Usually requires 2–4 days for development
- Ataxia
- Severe headache
- Altered mental status
- Nausea/vomiting
- Seizure
- Focal neurologic deficit
- Coma

MECHANISM/DESCRIPTION

- Incidence dependent on
  —Rate of ascent
  —Final altitude
  —Sleeping altitude
  —Duration at altitude
- AMS incidence
  —Up to 67% incidence with rapid ascent (1–2 days) >14,000 ft
  —20% incidence for skiers visiting resorts and sleeping <9000 ft
- HAPE incidence
  —<1–2%
  —Varies with rate of ascent
- HACE incidence <1%

PEDIATRIC CONSIDERATIONS

- AMS in infants and young children manifested by
  —Increased fussiness
  —Decreased playfulness
  —Decreased appetite
  —Vomiting
  —Sleep disturbances
- Incidence of HAPE greater in younger individuals (<20 years) than adults
- No cases of HAPE or HACE reported in children <4 years old

Pre-Hospital

CAUTIONS

- Severe cases require immediate evacuation to a lower altitude
- Do not proceed to higher altitude in the presence of symptoms
- Oxygen delivery or simulated descent in a portable hyperbaric chamber (Gamow bag) can be a life-saving temporary measure making self-rescue possible

Diagnosis

ESSENTIAL WORKUP

- Clinical diagnosis in setting of recent altitude gain

AMS

- Diagnosis made with a history of a headache plus at least one of the following
  —Decreased appetite
  —Nausea/vomiting
  —Weakness/fatigue
  —Dizziness
  —Difficulty sleeping
- No diagnostic laboratory or imaging studies

HAPE

- Dyspnea on exertion—universal finding at altitude
- Dyspnea at rest—early symptom of HAPE
- Rales, cyanosis or cough support the diagnosis

HACE

- Cerebellar ataxia with or without other symptoms of AMS

LABORATORY

- ABG for HAPE

IMAGING AND SPECIAL TESTS

- CXR in HAPE
  —Reveal fluffy (alveolar) infiltrates which are patchy in distribution, with areas of clearing between the patches
  —Unilateral or bilateral infiltrates (right midlung field being most common)
  —Cardiomegaly, "batwing" distribution of infiltrates, and Kerley B lines (typical of cardiogenic pulmonary edema)—absent in HAPE
- Swan Ganz monitoring in HAPE
  —Increased pulmonary vascular resistance
  —Elevated pulmonary artery
  —Normal pulmonary wedge pressures
- ECG in HAPE
  —Tachycardia
  —Evidence of right-heart strain
- CT and MRI scans in HACE
  —Vasogenic edema of the white matter

DIFFERENTIAL DIAGNOSIS

AMS

- Viral syndrome
- Exhaustion
- Alcohol hangover
- Carbon monoxide poisoning

HAPE

- Pneumonia
- High altitude bronchitis and pharyngitis
- Pulmonary embolism
  —More rapid onset
  —Pleuritic chest pain

HACE

- Cerebrovascular accidents/transient ischemic attacks
  —Focal neurologic signs suggest a vascular lesion

Treatment

INITIAL STABILIZATION

HAPE and HACE

- ABCs
  - —Endotracheal intubation for impending respiratory failure, hyperventilation, or airway protection
- Establish IV access
- Supplemental oxygen and monitoring
- Continuous positive airway pressure (CPAP) for HAPE

ED MANAGEMENT

AMS

- Mild cases usually self-limited
  - —Symptomatic treatment
  - —Halt ascent until symptoms resolve
- Acetazolamide for moderate to severe symptoms
- Aspirin or acetaminophen for headache
- Prochlorperazine for nausea
- Supplemental oxygen in severe cases
- Descent for severe or persistent symptoms

HAPE

- Descent
  - —Immediate descent for moderate/severe symptoms
  - —Mild cases may be managed without descent if
    - -Adequate oxygen supplies available
    - -Serial medical examinations possible
    - -Immediate descent for any deterioration in clinical status
- Bed rest (to avoid exercise induced pulmonary hypertension)
- Supplemental oxygen
  - —High flow rates (6–8 L/min) of oxygen until improvement then continue with lower flow rates
- Nifedipine when other interventions are unavailable

HACE

- *Immediate evacuation to lower altitude*
- Oxygen
- Dexamethasone
- Bed rest with elevation of head at 30° and in severe cases the aggressive management of elevated intracranial pressure

MEDICATIONS

- Acetazolamide: 250 mg (peds: 5 mg/kg) po bid
- Prochlorperazine: 5–10 mg (peds: 0.13 mg/kg/dose) IM/po tid; 25 mg PR bid
- Nifedipine: 10 mg po then 30 mg SR po bid
- Dexamethasone: 8 mg IV then 4 mg po/IV qid

Disposition

ADMISSION CRITERIA

- Descent to a lower facility mandatory in severe cases
- Persistent symptoms after observation in the lower altitude ED require admission

DISCHARGE CRITERIA

- Once clinical improvement seen and oxygen saturation >95% on room air
- Offer prophylactic therapy for future ascents in patients with recurrent AMS (acetazolamide) or HAPE (nifedipine)

Miscellaneous

ICD9: 993.2

CORE CONTENT CODE: 5.5

SUGGESTED READINGS

Bärtsch P, Maggiorini M, Ritter M, Noti C, Vock P, Oelz O. Prevention of high altitude pulmonary edema by nifedipine. N Engl J Med 1991;325:1284–1289.

Grissom CK, Roach RC, Sarnquist FH, Hackett PH. Acetazolamide in the treatment of acute mountain sickness: Clinical efficacy and effect on gas exchange. Ann Intern Med 1992;116:6:461–465.

Honigman B, Theis MK, McLain J, Roach RC, Yip R, Houston C, et al. Acute mountain sickness in a general tourist population at moderate altitudes. Ann Intern Med 1993;118(8):587–592.

Author: Michael Yaron

Hip Injury

Clinical Presentation

SIGNS AND SYMPTOMS

- Groin pain, medial knee pain, pain with ambulation/weight-bearing
- History of chronic bone loss or high-impact trauma
- Obvious signs of trauma
  - —Deformity or angulation, swelling, open fracture, or missile entrance wound
- Lower extremity held in position of comfort
  - —Hip fracture: flexion, abduction, external rotation of hip
  - —Posterior hip dislocation: flexion, *adduction, internal rotation* of hip, flexion of knee, hip totally immobile
  - —Anterior hip dislocation: flexion, *abduction, external rotation* of hip, thigh shortening due to spasm, hip totally immobile

MECHANISM/DESCRIPTION

- Hip fracture = fracture of proximal femur; classified by
  - —Location
  - —Displacement and angulation
  - —Open or closed, and degree of comminution
  - —Arrangement of fracture lines and fragments
- Hip dislocation = disarticulation of femoral head from acetabulum
  - —Often coexists with fracture
- Femoral head/neck fracture (intracapsular)
  - —Usually elderly patients with bone loss
  - —Trauma often minor
  - —Patient may or may not be ambulatory
- Intertrochanteric fracture (extracapsular)
  - —Usually elderly patients with bone loss
  - —Nonambulatory with significant pain
  - —Often due to fall
  - —Extremity often shortened
- Subtrochanteric fracture
  - —Usually due to direct trauma
  - —Common site for pathologic fracture
  - —Occasional site of stress fracture in runners and military recruits
  - —Extremity may be shortened with noticeable displacement of the proximal fragment
- Posterior dislocation
  - —Often due to MVA in which the knees strike the dashboard
  - —Much more common than anterior
- Anterior dislocation
  - —Often due to fall or trauma resulting in sudden abduction of thigh

PEDIATRIC CONSIDERATIONS

- Fracture usually requires high-impact trauma
- Must suspect nonaccidental trauma
- Must consider pathologic fracture if trauma is minor

Pre-Hospital

- Neurovascular exam is essential

CAUTIONS

- DO NOT apply traction
- Monitor closely for development of hemorrhagic shock

Diagnosis

ESSENTIAL WORKUP

- Radiographs as outlined below
  - —Remove splints and clothing prior to taking films
  - —A patient with a worrisome exam and negative standard films has a hip fracture until proven otherwise
- Assess distal pulses, palpate compartments, evaluate sensation and motor function
- If pulses are not equal or palpable, bedside Doppler may be necessary
- Search for associated injuries
- In suspected child abuse, obtain skeletal survey or bone scan

LABORATORY

- CBC, type, and screen

IMAGING/SPECIAL TESTS

- Standard films—AP pelvis and true lateral of hip
- AP pelvis with hip internally rotated 15–20° will optimally image the femoral neck
- Pelvic inlet and outlet views may identify associated or symptomatic pubic ramus or acetabular fractures
- Judet views (oblique films of the hip) aid in the evaluation of the acetabulum
- CT, MRI, or bone scan if fracture not identified; MRI is preferred
- Joint aspiration +/− arthrogram under fluoroscope if suspect a septic joint, foreign body, or hemarthrosis, especially in GSW to hip

DIFFERENTIAL DIAGNOSIS

- Pubic ramus fracture
- Acetabular fracture
- Septic joint
- Isolated fractures of the greater or lesser trochanters
- Thigh, knee, ankle, or foot injury
- Trochanteric bursitis
- Ileotibial band tendinitis
- Hip contusion

PEDIATRIC CONSIDERATIONS

- Pediatric fracture patterns are different because of the developing cartilaginous components; fracture classification and management are also different
- Suspect nonaccidental trauma in the absence of an obvious mechanism
- Be concerned about hip pain that may be due to a separate process (limb-length discrepancy, neuromuscular disorders, neoplastic invasion of bone)

Treatment

INITIAL STABILIZATION

- ABCs of trauma care
- Monitor blood pressure continuously; the thigh can contain 4–6 units of blood

ED TREATMENT

- Remove splint and clothing; maintain pelvis and hip stability
- Pain control is essential; parenteral analgesia acceptable in isolated hip injuries
  —A femoral nerve block can be performed in multiple trauma patients or pediatric patients
- Orthopedic consultation is necessary for all hip fractures and is emergent in cases of fracture with neurovascular compromise
- For closed fractures that require internal fixation, give cefazolin within 24 hours prior to operation
- Open fractures must go directly to the OR for irrigation and débridement
  —For open fractures with a laceration of >1 cm, extensive soft-tissue injury, or obvious contamination, give cefazolin and gentamicin or tobramycin in the ED, as well as tetanus booster if indicated
- For injuries with highly contaminated wounds add penicillin G to cover Clostridial species
- For gunshot wounds to the femur, culture the missile track and cover with an iodine dressing

Hip Dislocation

- A true orthopedic emergency, incidence of posttraumatic arthritis increases linearly with time
- Perform reduction in ED
- Often requires deep sedation or neuromuscular blockade to reduce
- Patients with prior hip arthroplasty may be reduced in the ED with conscious sedation

MEDICATIONS

- Cefazolin: adult: 2 g IM/IV; peds: 20 mg/kg IM/IV
- Gentamicin/tobramycin: 1.5 mg/kg IV
- Penicillin G: adults: 2 million IU IV; peds: 25,000 IU/kg/day IV divided q 8 hrs

PEDIATRIC CONSIDERATIONS

- Assess markers for nonaccidental trauma
  —Delay in presentation; history of mechanism inconsistent with the injury
  —Isolated trauma to the thigh, associated burns, bruises, or linear abrasions
  —Assess for dislocation of the femoral capital epiphysis

Disposition

ADMISSION CRITERIA

- All hip fractures or dislocations
- Septic joint
- Suspicion of occult fracture
- Suspicion of nonaccidental trauma in children

DISCHARGE CRITERIA

- Hip pain attributable to other cause
- Fracture ruled out (negative radiographs *plus* negative clinical exam)
- Patient with successful reduction of dislocated hip arthroplasty may be considered for discharge in consultation with orthopedics and with appropriate follow-up arranged

Miscellaneous

ICD9: 959.6

CORE CONTENT CODE: 18.4.13.1.8

SUGGESTED READINGS

Hughes L, Beaty J. Fractures of the head and neck of the femur in children. J Bone Joint Surg 1994;76A(2): 283–292.

Long W, et al. Management of civilian gunshot injuries to the hip. Orthop Clin North Am 1995;26(1):123–131.

Lyons R. Clinical outcomes and treatment of hip fractures. Am J Med 1997;103(2A):51S–64S.

Zuckerman J. Hip fracture. N Engl J Med 1996;334(23):1519–1525.

Author: Chris Ho

HIV/AIDS

Clinical Presentation

SIGNS AND SYMPTOMS

- Primary HIV infection
  - —fever, malaise, rash on face and trunk
  - —Headache, photophobia, meningismus
  - —Flulike syndrome with lymphadenopathy and hepatosplenomegaly
  - —Asymptomatic period averaging 8 or more years after initial infection
- Advanced disease (CD4 <200)
  - —Weight loss, fatigue, fevers, night sweats
  - —Chronic diarrhea with severe dehydration and electrolyte abnormalities
  - —Respiratory distress
  - —Chronic low-grade headache, altered mental status, seizures, neurologic deficits
  - —Skin lesions (Kaposi's Sarcoma (KS)), painless visual loss

ETIOLOGY

- The HIV retrovirus impedes the immune system by destroying CD4 lymphocytes
- Risk factors include prostitution, intravenous drug abuse, homosexuality, blood transfusions prior to 1985, and unprotected sex with partners at-risk, and children of women who engage in high-risk behavior

MECHANISM/DESCRIPTION

- As the CD4 cell population decreases, the patient becomes susceptible to a variety of opportunistic diseases
  - —CD4 <200 cells/mm^3: *Pneumocystis carinii* pneumonia (PCP)
  - —CD4 <100 cells/mm^3: cryptococcal infection, toxoplasmosis
  - —CD4 <50 cells/mm^3: CNS lymphoma, mycobacterium avium complex
- Pulmonary
  - —PCP pneumonia
    - -Subacute, progressive shortness of breath, fever, dry cough
  - —Mycobacterial pneumonia, tuberculosis
    - -Hemoptysis, weight loss, dyspnea
  - —Bacterial pneumonia
    - -High fever, productive cough
- Neurologic
  - —Cryptococcal meningitis
    - -Chronic headache, fever, vomiting, blurred vision
  - —Toxoplasmosis
    - -Necrotizing encephalitis, focal signs, chorea
  - —CNS lymphoma
  - —AIDS dementia
  - —Progressive multifocal leukoencephalopathy
    - -Progressive demyelinating disorder, seizures, focal deficits, visual field deficits
    - -Peripheral neruopathy
- Gastrointestinal
  - —Diarrhea caused by routine bacteria, uncommon parasites, and viruses
  - —Dysphagia caused by candida esophagitis, herpes, or cytomegalovirus
  - —Mycobacterium avium-intracellulare complex (MAC) can cause severe weight loss and diarrhea
- Medication complications
  - —Zidovudine (AZT) has serious hematologic and cardiovascular side effects
  - —Both dideoxyinosine (DDI) and dideoxycytidine (DDC) can cause pancreatitis
  - —DDC and stavudine (D4T) can cause peripheral neuropathy

PEDIATRIC CONSIDERATIONS

- Infants infected with HIV may present with failure to thrive, recurrent bacterial infections, unexplained organomegaly or lymphadenopathy, and unexplained developmental delay

Pre-Hospital

CAUTIONS

- Universal precautions are essential

Diagnosis

ESSENTIAL WORKUP

- HIV serologic tests as noted below
  - —There is a "window" of 6 months between primary infection and seroconversion, during which tests may be negative
- Respiratory symptoms
  - —Chest x-ray, ABG, and induced sputum for Gram stain, silver stain, AFB, and culture
- Neurologic symptoms
  - —Head CT and lumbar puncture
  - —CSF for glucose, protein, Gram stain and culture, cell count with differential, AFB smear, India ink stain, cryptococcus titer, and VDRL
- GI symptoms
  - —Stool for O&P, Gram stain, culture, *C. difficile* toxin, acid fast, and viral culture
- Fever workup must include aerobic/anaerobic, fungal, AFB, and MAC blood cultures

LABORATORY

- HIV infection
  - —The ELISA, enzyme immunoassay, detects IgG antibody against HIV. The sensitivity and specificity are approximately 99%
    - -Test can be negative during window period
  - —Western blot detects IgG antibody against HIV proteins p24, gp120, gp41
    - -This test is more specific than the ELISA and is used to confirm a positive ELISA
  - —The p24 antigen assay and PCR and viral cultures for HIV are able to detect HIV during the window period
- Opportunistic infections
  - —PCP pneumonia: increased A-a gradient on blood gas analysis, an elevated serum LDH, and pneumocystis on sputum silver stain
  - —Cryptococcal meningitis: positive CSF India ink

IMAGING/SPECIAL TESTS

- CXR
  - —Bilateral interstitial infiltrates or pneumothorax = PCP
  - —Reticulonodular infiltrates = TB, KS, fungal pneumonia
  - —Consolidation = bacterial
  - —Cavitation = TB, necrotizing bacterial pneumonia, coccidioidomycosis
- Head CT (with IV contrast)
  - —Toxoplasmosis—multiple ring-enhancing lesions with edema in basal ganglia or cortex
  - —CNS lymphoma—weakly enhancing periventricular lesions with edema
  - —Progressive multifocal leukoencephalopathy—multiple subcortical nonenhancing lesions

DIFFERENTIAL DIAGNOSIS

- Mononucleosis, hepatitis, syphilis, rubella, disseminated gonococcal infection
- Pulmonary emboli, tuberculosis, bacterial, viral, or fungal pneumonia, pulmonary malignancies, and lymphocytic interstitial pneumonitis
- Neurosyphilis, CMV encephalitis, CNS lymphoma, coccidioidal meningitis, subarachnoid hemorrhage, cerebral infarction, or edema

Treatment

INITIAL STABILIZATION

- ABCs
  —Supplemental oxygen or intubate as necessary
  —Prior to intubation identify code status

ED TREATMENT

- Patients should receive their first dose of specific antibiotics in the emergency department

MEDICATIONS

Primary HIV Infection and Maintenance

- HIV treatment strategies use three antiretroviral medications: two nucleoside analogs and a protease inhibitor
- Antiretroviral nucleoside analogs
  —Zidovudine (AZT): 100 mg po 5 times a day
  —Dideoxyinosine (DDI): 125–300 mg po twice a day
  —Dideoxycytidine (DDC): 0.75 mg po 3 times a day
  —Stavudine (D4T): 40 mg po twice a day
  —Lamivudine (3TC): 150 mg po twice a day
- Protease inhibitors
  —Saquinavir: 600 mg po 3 times a day
  —Indinavir: 800 mg po 3 times a day
- Specific AIDS-related diseases
  —Candidiasis, esophageal: ketoconazole 400 mg/day po *or* fluconazole 100–200 mg/day po
  —Cryptococcal meningitis: amphotericin B 0.3–0.6 mg/kg/day IV with or without flucytosine 25–37.5 mg/kg po q 6 hrs
  —MAC: rifabutin 300 mg po qd
  —PCP pneumonia: trimethoprim (TMP)/sulfamethoxazole 20 mg/kg/day as IV/PO divided qid; pentamidine 4 mg/kg IV for sulfa-allergic patients; if $PaO_2 < 70$ mm Hg or A-a gradient is >35 mm Hg, add prednisone 80 mg po for 5 days, then taper
  —PCP prophylaxis (CD4<200): septra DS 1 tab po bid or pentamidine 300 mg inhaled every month

PEDIATRIC CONSIDERATIONS

- The oral polio vaccine is contraindicated in HIV positive patients
- Immunization with the pneumococcal vaccine and tetanus booster is recommended

Disposition

ADMISSION CRITERIA

- The following should be admitted to the hospital
  —Unexplained fever with CNS involvement
  —Severe hypoxemia ($PaO_2 < 70$ mm Hg), suspected bacterial pneumonia or tuberculosis
  —A change in neurologic status, new onset seizures
  —Inability to ambulate or to tolerate oral intake
  —Intractable diarrhea with dehydration

DISCHARGE CRITERIA

- The patient can maintain adequate oral intake, provide self-care, and ambulate
- Communication with the patient's primary care doctor is essential

Miscellaneous

ICD9: 042

CORE CONTENT CODE: 8.6.1, 9.5.1

SUGGESTED READINGS

Fein JA, Friedland LR, Rutstein R, Bell LM. Children with unrecognized human immunodeficiency virus infection. An emergency department perspective. Am J Dis Child 1993;147(10):1104–1108.

Guss DA. The acquired immune deficiency syndrome: An overview for the emergency physician, Part 1. J Emerg Med 1994;12(3):375–384.

Guss DA. The acquired immune deficiency syndrome: An overview for the Emergency physician, Part 2. J Emerg Med 1994;12(4):491–497.

Author: Lori Shore

Hordeolum

Clinical Presentation

SIGNS AND SYMPTOMS

- Red tender painful swollen mass on the eyelid
- Typically solitary lesion but may be multiple
- Develops acutely
- Nontoxic appearing patient
- Internal versus external depending on the gland affected
  - —External hordeolum
    - -Tender mass at the base of the lash or between the lashes pointing anteriorly
  - —Internal hordeolum
    - -Tender mass originating on the inner aspect of the lid margin
    - -May discharge through the conjunctiva or through the skin
    - -Typically more inflamed, larger, and more painful
- Palpable preauricular lymph node
- May be associated with preseptal cellulitis

MECHANISM/DESCRIPTION

- Tarsal plate contains secreting glands
  - —Superficial sebaceous glands of Zeis—external
  - —Superficial sweat glands of Moll—external
  - —Deeper modified sebaceous Meibomian glands—internal
- Develops due to obstruction of one of the glands and subsequent abscess formation

ETIOLOGY

- Caused by *Staphylococcus aureus*
  - —More commonly seen with chronic staphylococcal blepharitis

Pre-Hospital

N/A

Diagnosis

ESSENTIAL WORKUP

- Identify the origin of the abscess
- Determine extent of surrounding cellulitis

IMAGING/SPECIAL TESTS

- Not indicated in nontoxic patient with localized swelling
- Orbital CT
  - —If deep tissue involvement suspected (rare)

DIFFERENTIAL DIAGNOSIS

- Chalazion
- Dacryoadenitis
- Sebaceous cell carcinoma
- Pyogenic granuloma
- Preseptal cellulitis

Treatment

INITIAL STABILIZATION

- Initial approach and immediate concerns
  - —Clinically determine likelihood of deep tissue involvement

ED TREATMENT

- Warm compresses for 15 minutes 4–6 times a day
- Gentle massage of the nodule to open the duct and express purulent material
- Topical antistaphylococcal antibiotic ointment
- Incision and drainage in severe cases of internal hordeolum
  - —Typically done by an ophthalmologist
  - —If pointed toward the skin, perform a horizontal incision for good cosmetic effect
  - —If pointed toward the conjunctiva, perform a vertical incision to avoid injury to the Meibomian glands

MEDICATIONS

- Erythromycin ophthalmic ointment
  - —Place in cul de sac and massage along lid margins every 4 hours

Disposition

ADMISSION CRITERIA

- Severe associated preseptal cellulitis

DISCHARGE CRITERIA

- All uncomplicated cases
- If incision and drainage is done follow-up within 1 week is appropriate
- Symptoms should resolve within 3–4 weeks
- If mass persists, chalazion may develop and incision and curettage may ultimately be necessary

Miscellaneous

ICD9: 373.11

CORE CONTENT CODE: 6.4.1.7

SUGGESTED READINGS

Cullom R. The Will's eye manual: Office and emergency room diagnosis and treatment of eye disease. Philadelphia: Lippincott-Raven, 1994:133–134.

Kanski JJ. Clinical ophthalmology. London:Butterworth-Heinemann, 1994:2–4.

Lavrich JB, Nelson LB. Disorders of the lacrimal system apparatus. Pediatr Clin North Am 1993;40:767–804.

Rubin S, Hallagan L. Lids, lacrimals and lashes. Emerg Med Clin North Am 1995;13(3):631–647.

Author: Shari Schabowski

Horner's Syndrome

Clinical Presentation

SIGNS AND SYMPTOMS

- Horner's syndrome is characterized by
  - —*Ptosis:* drooping of the eyelid on the affected side, usually slight
  - —*Miosis:* a decrease in pupillary size on the involved side (pupillary asymmetry ≥1 mm)
  - —*Anhidrosis:* lack of sweating on the involved side of the face
- The importance of Horner's syndrome is its association with certain disease states

MECHANISM/DESCRIPTION

- Unilateral sympathetic denervation produces the signs of Horner's syndrome
  - —Relaxation of the retracting muscles in the upper and lower lids—ptosis
  - —Loss of pupillary dilator innervation—miosis (unopposed pupillary constriction)
  - —Loss of sympathetic stimulation of the sweat glands—anhidrosis

ETIOLOGY

- Malignant tumors: tumors of the lung or metastases to the cervical nodes can interrupt the preganglionic sympathetic fibers (between the thoracic sympathetic trunk and superior cervical ganglion)
- Trauma: penetrating neck wounds
- Pneumothorax: tension pneumothorax may cause traction on the sympathetic fibers due to shift of mediastinal structures
- Infiltration or infection of cervical nodes: sarcoidosis, tuberculosis
- Vascular disorders: migraine or cluster headaches, carotid artery dissection

PEDIATRIC CONSIDERATIONS

- Hereditary Horner's syndrome: associated with a blue iris (or irregular coloration) on the affected side and brown on the unaffected side (heterochromia iridis)
- Birth trauma: may cause damage to the sympathetic chain

Pre-Hospital

CAUTIONS

- The importance of Horner's syndrome is its association with more serious underlying conditions. Patients with increased ICP or tension pneumothorax must be recognized immediately

Diagnosis

ESSENTIAL WORKUP

- History and physical exam focused on neurologic findings
- Chest x-ray to screen for tumor or pneumothorax

IMAGING/SPECIAL TESTS

- Pharmacologic (cocaine) testing confirms the diagnosis of a sympathetic ocular lesion. One drop of 5% ocular cocaine solution is instilled into each eye. Failure of pupil on the involved side to dilate as much as the other pupil (an increase in the amount of anisocoria) in 1 hour is confirmatory (positive test)
- CT or MRI of the head, neck, or chest may be indicated depending on the signs and symptoms
- Ocular tonometry for suspected glaucoma
- Carotid Doppler US may be indicated to evaluate for carotid dissection

DIFFERENTIAL DIAGNOSIS

- Increased ICP: almost always associated with altered LOC
- *Simple anisocoria (pseudo-Horner's syndrome):* 15–20% of the population has anisocoria and 3–4% also have miosis and ptosis. The cocaine test is negative (both pupils dilate equally). Inspect photo ID for preexisting anisocoria
- Topical medications or exposures
- Migraine or cluster headache
- Glaucoma, inflammatory ocular diseases, or ocular trauma

PEDIATRIC CONSIDERATIONS

- Birth trauma in newborns
- Hereditary Horner's syndrome

Treatment

INITIAL STABILIZATION

- If increased ICP is suspected, measures to control ICP (intubation and hyperventilation, osmotic diuretics, steroids) are used as indicated
- Tension pneumothorax: needle thoracostomy followed by chest tube

ED TREATMENT

- Horner's syndrome per se requires no ED treatment

MEDICATIONS

- Cocaine; 5% (adult), 2.5% (pediatric) ophthalmic solution: 1 drop in each eye is diagnostic

Disposition

ADMISSION CRITERIA

- Admission for isolated Horner's syndrome is not needed. Admission may be needed for the underlying condition

DISCHARGE CRITERIA

- Patients with Horner's syndrome may be discharged with appropriate follow-up arranged for continued workup as an outpatient

Miscellaneous

ICD9: 337.9

CORE CONTENT CODE: 11.6

SUGGESTED READINGS

Cook T, Kietzman L, Leibold R. "Pneumoptosis" in the emergency department. Am J Emerg Med 1992;10:431–434.

Corbett J, Thompson H. Pupillary function and dysfunction. In: Asbury A, McKhann G, MacDonald W, eds. Diseases of the nervous system: Clinical neurobiology. Philadelphia: WB Saunders, 1992:495–500.

Fields C, Barker F. Review of Horner's syndrome and a case report. Optom Vis Sci 1992;69(6):481–485.

Wilheim H, et al. Horner's syndrome: A retrospective analysis of 90 cases and recommendations for clinical handling. Ger J Ophthalmol 1992;1(2):96–102.

Authors: Andrew Jenis; Richard S. Krause

Human Bite

Clinical Presentation

SIGNS AND SYMPTOMS

- Paronychia (from biting fingernails)
  - —Collection of pus at edges of nail beds
- Occlusal bites
  - —Laceration or crush injury to affected body part

Clenched Fist Injuries (Most Serious Type)

- Wound/laceration in hand
  - —Location
    - -Metacarpophalangeal joint most common
    - -Proximal interphalangeal joint
    - -Distal interphalangeal joint
  - —Most commonly injured digits in decreasing order of frequency
    - -Long finger
    - -Index finger
    - -Ring finger
    - -Small finger
    - -Thumb
- Frequent complications
  - —Cellulitis
    - -Serious deep-space infections (septic arthritis and osteomyelitis)
- Limited ROM due to edema restricting the ability of tendons to glide in their sheaths

MECHANISM/DESCRIPTION

Paronychia

- Occurs among children who suck their fingers or individuals who bite their nails

Occlusal Bites

- Human teeth bite into the skin
- Same risk of infection as other wounds

Clenched Fist Injuries (CFI)

- Sustained from a clenched fist striking the mouth and teeth of another person
- With joint relaxation from the clenched position
  - —Puncture site sealed
  - —Oral bacteria inoculated in the anaerobic setting within the joint
- Bacterial inoculation carried by the tendons deeper into the potential spaces of the hand
  - —Increases chances for a more extensive infection

ETIOLOGY

- Aerobic and anaerobic organisms
  - —*Streptococcus, Staphylococcus aureus,* and *Haemophilus influenzae*
  - —*Enterobacter, Proteus, Serratia,* and *Eikenella corrodens*
- *E. corrodens* exhibits synergism with *Streptococcus, S. aureus, Bacteroides,* and Gram-negative organisms

PEDIATRIC CONSIDERATIONS

- Human bite marks rarely occur accidentally—good indicators of inflicted injury

Pre-Hospital

N/A

Diagnosis

ESSENTIAL WORKUP

Physical Examination

- Record the location and extent of all injuries
- Document any swelling, crush injuries, or devitalized tissue
- Note the range of motion of affected areas
- Note the status of tendon and nerve function
- Document any signs of infection, including regional adenopathy
- Document any joint or bone involvement

LABORATORY

- Aerobic and anaerobic cultures from any infected bite wound
- Cultures not indicated if wounds not clinically infected

IMAGING/SPECIAL TESTS

- Plain radiographs indications
  - —Fracture
  - —Foreign body, e.g., tooth, is considered possible
  - —Baseline film if a bone or joint space has been violated in evaluating for osteomyelitis
  - —For infection in proximity to a bone or joint space

DIFFERENTIAL DIAGNOSIS

- Bite injuries from animals
  - —Sharper teeth cause more punctures and lacerations than human teeth, which usually cause more crush type injuries

PEDIATRIC CONSIDERATIONS

- In suspected sexual abuse
  - —Check for a central area of bruising or "hickey" from suction
- Linear abrasions or bruises on both the dorsal and palmar/plantar surfaces of the hand or foot
  - —Highly suggestive of bite marks
  - —Lesions on one extremity should prompt a search for lesions on the other extremities
- An intercanine distance of >3 cm indicates permanent dentition (present only if the attacker is >8 years old)
- If abuse suspected
  - —Rub a saline-moistened swab in the wound to collect any saliva and then place in a paper envelope (no plastic components) to be sent for ABO blood antigen determination
  - —Obtain photographs

Treatment

INITIAL STABILIZATION

- ABCs: ensure patent airway and adequate peripheral tissue perfusion

ED TREATMENT

- Wound irrigation
  —Copious volumes of normal saline with an 18-gauge plastic catheter tip aimed in the direction of the puncture
- Debridement
  —Remove any foreign material, necrotic skin tags, or devitalized tissues
  —Do not débride puncture wounds
  —Remove any eschar present so that underlying pus may be expressed and irrigated
- Closed fist injuries
  —Immobilization
    -Splint in a position of function that maintains the maximal length of ligaments and intrinsic muscles
    -Use a bulky hand-dressing
  —Consultation with hand surgeon regarding operative irrigation/exploration of wound/wound closure
  —Elevation for several days until any edema resolved
    -Sling for outpatients
    -Place the hand in a tubular stockinette attached to an IV pole for inpatients
- Do not perform primary repair of avulsion wounds
- Repair guidelines
  —Do not suture infected wounds or wounds >24 hours postinjury
  —Repair of wounds >8 hours—controversial
    -Close facial wounds (warn patient of high risk of infection)
    -May approximate the wound edges with steri-strips and perform a delayed primary closure
  —Do not suture closed fist injuries
- Antibiotics (augmentin or combination penicillin/dicloxacillin) (5 days) for outpatients with
  —Moderate to severe injuries with crush injury or edema
  —Involve the bones or a joint
  —Hand bites
  —Wounds near a prosthetic joint
  —Underlying disease (diabetes, prior splenectomy, or immunosuppression) that increases their risk of developing a more serious infection
- Tetanus prophylaxis
- Refer for possible testing/surveillance for HIV infection

MEDICATIONS

- Amoxicillin/clavulanic acid (augmentin): 500 mg (peds: 40 mg/kg/24hrs) q 8 hrs po
- Cefoxitin (mefoxin): 1–2 g (peds: 80–160 mg/kg/24hrs) q 6 hrs IV
- Ciprofloxacin (cipro): 500–750 mg q 12 hrs po or 400 mg q 12 hrs IV
  —Poor anaerobic coverage
- Clindamycin (cleocin): 150–450 mg (peds: 8–20 mg/kg/24hrs) po q 6 hrs or 600–900 mg (peds: 20–40 mg/kg/24hrs) IV q 8 hrs
  —No coverage against *E. corrodens*
- Dicloxacillin (pathocil): 500 mg (peds: 50 mg/kg/24hrs) po q 6 hrs
- Penicillin (penicillin VK): 500 mg (peds: 50 mg/kg/24hrs) po q 6 hrs
- Ticarcillin/clavulanic acid (timentin): 3.1 g q 4–6 hrs
- Trimethoprim-sulfamethoxazole (septra DS): 1 tab q 12 hrs (peds: 8 mg/kg trimethoprim and 40 mg/kg sulfamethoxazole per day divided into 2 daily doses) po
  —Poor anaerobic coverage

Disposition

ADMISSION CRITERIA

- Infected wounds at presentation
- Severe/advancing cellulitis/lymphangitis
- Signs of systemic infection
- Infected wounds that have failed to respond to outpatient (oral) antibiotics

DISCHARGE CRITERIA

- Healthy patient with localized wound infection: discharge on antibiotics with 24-hour follow-up
- 48-hour follow-up for noninfected wounds

Miscellaneous

ICD9 CODE: 879.8

CORE CONTENT CODE: 5.10.2

SUGGESTED READINGS

Fischer H, et al. Picture of the month. Arch Pediatr Adolesc Med 1996;150:429–430.

Goldstein EJ. Bite wounds and infection. Clin Infect Dis 1992;14:633–640.

Griego RD, et al. Dog, cat, and human bites: A review. J Am Acad Dermatol 1995;33:1019–1029.

Stucker FJ, et al. Management of animal and human bites in the head and neck. Arch Otolaryngol Head Neck Surg 1990;116:789–793.

Author: John Hipskind

Humeral Head Fracture

Clinical Presentation

SIGNS AND SYMPTOMS

- Pain, swelling, and tenderness about the shoulder, especially around the greater tuberosity
- Difficulty in initiating active motion
- Position of patient is often with arm closely held against the chest
- Crepitus may be present
- Ecchymoses within 24–48 hours at area of fracture and may spread to chest wall, flank, and distal extremity
- Diminished peripheral pulses, or decreased sensation especially over the deltoid muscle (axillary nerve)

MECHANISM/DESCRIPTION

- Proximal humeral fractures involve fractures of the humeral head, lesser tuberosity, greater tuberosity, bicipital groove, and proximal humeral shaft
- Mechanisms of injury
  - —Fall onto an outstretched hand
  - —High energy direct trauma
  - —Excessive rotation of the arm in the abducted position
  - —Electrical shock or seizure
  - —Pathologic fracture from metastatic disease
- Typically seen in adults over the age of 45 years and the elderly
- Proximal humeral fractures account for 5% of all fractures

Pre-Hospital

CAUTIONS

- Excessive movement of the arm may produce further neurovascular injury

CONTROVERSIES

- Pre-hospital reduction is not recommended as manipulation may induce neurovascular injury or displace a fracture

Diagnosis

ESSENTIAL WORKUP

- Careful history and physical examination to localize the injury and to rule out any other significant injuries
- Assessment of neurovascular status
  - —Assess function of radial, median, ulnar, axillary (sensation to the lateral aspect of the shoulder), and musculocutaneous nerve (sensation to the extensor aspect of the forearm)
  - —Presence of radial, ulnar, and brachial pulses, and good capillary refill in all digits
- Shoulder radiographs

IMAGING/SPECIAL TESTS

- Anteroposterior, lateral and axillary views or Transthoracic or 'y' view
  - —The axillary view is necessary to assess tuberosity displacement, the glenoid articular surface, and the relationship of the humeral head to the glenoid
  - —CT scan can be useful in evaluating articular surfaces of glenoid and humeral head

DIFFERENTIAL DIAGNOSIS

- Acute hemorrhagic bursitis
- Traumatic rotator cuff tear
- Dislocation
- Acromioclavicular separation
- Calcific tendinitis
- Pathologic fracture

PEDIATRIC CONSIDERATIONS

- In children, proximal humeral fractures consist of metaphyseal fractures and physeal separations. Three fracture patterns tend to be displayed depending on the age group
- Children <5 years: Salter-Harris I fractures are seen
  - —Neonatal fractures occur from obstetric trauma and pseudoparalysis are often seen
  - —Physeal separation in the infant may also be the result of physical abuse
- Children 5–10 years: metaphyseal fractures tend to occur in this age group because rapid growth causes thinning of the metaphyseal cortex. Most fractures are transverse or short oblique
- Children >11 years: Salter-Harris II fractures tend to be seen in the adolescent

Treatment

INITIAL STABILIZATION

- ABCs and secondary survey for associated injuries
- Immediate immobilization is important to prevent further fracture displacement or neurovascular injury
  —Sling with arm supported at the side or in the Velpeau position
  —Axillary pad may also be used for comfort
  —After immobilization perform another neurovascular exam

ED TREATMENT

- Emergency Department treatment consists of proper immobilization, orthopedic consultation, and providing pain management
- *Operative versus nonoperative treatment* is decided in conjunction with orthopedics
- *Neer classification:* this system identifies the number of fragments and their location
  —The fractures consist of 2-part to 4-part fractures, and the locations include the anatomical neck, the surgical neck, the greater tuberosity, and the lesser tuberosity
  —Fracture-dislocation and humeral head splitting are also part of the Neer classification
  —In general, the higher the number of fragments in the fracture and the greater the degree of displacement, the more difficult it is to manage the patient with a closed reduction
- *Nonoperative treatment*
  —Initial immobilization and early motion: succeeds in many cases as most proximal humeral fractures are minimally displaced
  —Use a sling, swathe, and axillary pad to immobilize
  —Closed reduction should be performed with consultation of an orthopedic surgeon
  —Conscious sedation should be used for all closed reductions
  —Following reduction, the stability of the fracture can be tested in different positions to ascertain that significant displacement requiring surgical intervention will not occur
  —1-part and 2-part fractures are often successfully treated with closed reduction, but 3-part and 4-part fractures are unstable and may need ORIF

MEDICATIONS

- Pain medications are indicated for comfort
- Conscious sedation should be used if attempting a closed reduction. (See chapter on conscious sedation)

PEDIATRIC CONSIDERATIONS

- In children nearing skeletal maturity, determining the degree of displacement or separation of the proximal humeral epiphysis is essential as exact reduction is important to prevent later growth disturbance

Disposition

ADMISSION CRITERIA

- Open fractures for operative management and parenteral antibiotic therapy
- Displaced fracture which cannot be treated through closed reduction and therefore requires operation
- Significant associated injuries which require admission and observation

DISCHARGE CRITERIA

- Patients with either a nondisplaced fracture or a fracture that is successfully treated through closed reduction and who has no associated injuries

PEDIATRIC CONSIDERATIONS

- Pediatric patients are often less compliant with immobilization and less able to verbalize complaints and may benefit from admission to the hospital for observation and neurovascular checks

Miscellaneous

ICD9: 812.09

CORE CONTENT CODE: 18.4.12.1.6

SUGGESTED READINGS

Hawkins RJ, Angelo RL. Displaced proximal humeral fractures: Selecting treatment, avoiding pitfalls. Orthop Clin North Am 1987;18(3):421–431.

Morrissy RT, Weinstein SL. Lovell and Winter's pediatric orthopaedics. Vol. II. 4th ed. Philadelphia: Lippincott-Raven, 1996.

Neer CS. Displaced proximal humeral fractures: I. Classification and evaluation. J Bone Joint Surg 1970;52A:1077–1089.

Rasmussen S, Hvass I, Dalsgaard J, Christensen S, Holstad E. Displaced proximal humeral fractures: Results of conservative treatment. Injury 1992;23(1):41–42.

Rockwood CA, Green DP, Bucholz RW, Heckman JD. Rockwood and Green's fractures in adults. 4th ed. Philadelphia: Lippincott-Raven, 1996.

Authors: Nancy Kwon; Wallace Carter

Humeral Shaft Fracture

Clinical Presentation

SIGNS AND SYMPTOMS

- Pain and swelling over the area of the humeral shaft
- Shortening, deformity, or decreased mobility
- Crepitus on gentle motion
- Possible weakness or numbness
  - —Associated nerve injury is the radial nerve

MECHANISM

- Most commonly direct trauma from a fall or direct blow to the upper arm
- Fall on elbow or outstretched arm
- Ball throwing

MECHANISM/DESCRIPTION

- 3 types
  - —Nondisplaced
  - —Displaced or angulated
  - —Severely displaced or associated with neurovascular damage
- 3% of all fractures

PEDIATRIC CONSIDERATIONS

- Always consider child abuse especially with spiral fractures of the humerus which implies a rotational component to the injury

Pre-Hospital

CAUTIONS

- Immobilization with sling and swath and transport
- Rapid transport in presence of neurologic or vascular deficits

Diagnosis

ESSENTIAL WORKUP

- History and examination with special attention to a thorough neurovascular exam and skin integrity
- Consider associated injuries
- Diagnosis is confirmed by x-ray

IMAGING/SPECIAL TESTS

- AP and lateral views of the entire humerus are mandatory
  - —Include shoulder and elbow views to exclude associated joint involvement

DIFFERENTIAL DIAGNOSIS

- Contusion
- Tendon rupture
- Neuropraxia

Treatment

INITIAL STABILIZATION

- Pain control with NSAIDs or narcotic analgesics
- Immobilization with sling and swath or shoulder immobilizer pending definitive diagnosis
- Application of ice to limit swelling
- Open humerus fractures require covering with a sterile dressing, tetanus prophylaxis, and parenteral prophylactic antibiotics

ED MANAGEMENT

- These fractures usually don't require elaborate reduction or immobilization
- Nondisplaced fractures can be treated with a sugar-tong splint of the upper extremity
- Grossly displaced or comminuted fractures require immobilization with a light hanging cast
- Open fractures or fractures associated with neurovascular compromise require immediate orthopedic consultation

Disposition

ADMISSION CRITERIA

- Open fractures or fractures associated with neurovascular compromise

DISCHARGE CRITERIA

- Uncomplicated humeral shaft fractures should be referred to an orthopedic surgeon for follow-up
- Orthopedic consultation in the ED is required for patients with grossly displaced or comminuted fractures

Miscellaneous

- Always repeat the neurological examination after splint or cast application
- Consider pathologic fractures with any humerus fracture produced by low energy mechanism as the humerus can be a common site of metastatic disease

ICD9: 812.21

CORE CONTENT CODE: 18.4.12.1.6

SUGGESTED READINGS

Magnusson AR. Humerus and elbow. In: Rosen P, et al., eds. Emergency medicine: Concepts and clinical practice. 4th ed. St. Louis: CV Mosby, 1998.

Simon R, Koenigskhecht S. Emergency orthopedics, the extremities. 3rd ed. Norwalk, CT: Appleton & Lange, 1993.

Zuckerman J, Koval K. Fractures of the shaft of the humerus. In: Rockwood and Green, Fractures in adults. 4th ed. Philadelphia: Lippincott-Raven, 1996.

Authors: William Goldberg; Wallace Carter

Hydatidiform Mole

Clinical Presentation

SIGNS AND SYMPTOMS

- Findings consistent with pregnancy, usually exaggerated subjective symptoms
- Vaginal bleeding is most common symptom (97%)
  —Usually late first trimester or early second trimester
  —Usually painless bleeding
  —May have passage of tissue; edematous trophoblasts passed through dilated cervical os
- Discrepancy between size of uterus on palpation and size expected by date of LMP (50–66%)
  —Usually larger than dates; due to marked trophoblastic growth
  —Can be smaller than dates, especially partial mole
- Adnexal masses
  —Prominent ovarian theca lutein cysts, due to high levels of circulating human chorionic gonadotrophin (hCG)

Complete Mole

- Toxemia (27%): visual changes, hypertension, proteinuria, hyperreflexia, rarely convulsions
- Hyperthyroidism (7%): marked tachycardia, tremor
- Acute respiratory distress (2%): tachypnea, tachycardia, mental status changes (agitation, confusion)
  —Cause is multifactorial: trophoblastic pulmonary embolism or cardiopulmonary changes from toxemia, hyperthyroidism, vigorous fluid replacement
  —Diffuse rales
- Absent fetal heart tones

Partial Mole

- Usually do not exhibit the dramatic clinical features of complete mole
- Often presents at more advanced gestational age
- Typically uterine growth is less than expected for gestational age
- May have fetal heart tones

DISEASE DESCRIPTION

CHARACTERISTIC	*COMPLETE HYDATIDIFORM MOLE*	*PARTIAL HYDATIDIFORM MOLE*
Chorionic villi swelling	Diffuse	Focal
Trophoblastic hyperplasia	Diffuse	Focal
Fetal or embryonic tissue	Absent	Present
Karyotype	46,XY (90%) 46,XY (10%)	Triploid (90%) Diploid (10%)
Nuclear DNA	Paternal	Paternal and maternal
Mechanism	1 or 2 sperm "fertilize" empty egg	2 sperm fertilize normal egg
Risk of persistent GTT	20%	2–4%

- Risk factors for gestational trophoblastic tumor (GTT): marked trophoblastic proliferation (elevated hCG, excessive uterine enlargement, prominent theca lutein ovarian cysts), older patients, and repetitive molar pregnancies

ETIOLOGY

- Largely unknown
- Frequency more common in Asian countries, 1 per 125 live births, and less common in Western Europe and United States, 1 per 1500 live births
- Socioeconomic and nutritional factors; vitamin A deficiency
- Advanced maternal age; women older than 40 have a 5- to 10-fold greater risk

Pre-Hospital

CAUTIONS

- As with any pregnant patient, ensure patent airway, provide oxygen, and establish IV access
- If convulsions are present, treat with diazepam
- Save any passed tissue for histological evaluation

Diagnosis

ESSENTIAL WORKUP

- Ultrasonography
  —Complete molar pregnancy produces characteristic vesicular sonographic pattern from swelling of chorionic villi ("snowstorm" appearance)
  —Partial molar pregnancy may have cystic changes in placenta and changes in the shape of gestational sac (transverse to anteroposterior dimension ratio of 1:5)
  —Theca lutein ovarian cysts, associated with high hCG levels
- hCG and free subunits
  —Complete mole: mean ratio of β-hCG to α-hCG is 20.9. Higher serum level of percent free β-hCG
  —Partial mole: mean ratio of β-hCG to α-hCG is 2.4. Higher serum level of percent free α-hCG
  —Prognostic indicator: pretreatment hCG $>$40,000 mIU/ml is poor prognosis
  —Can be followed as indication of persistent disease

LABORATORY

- Hemoglobin and hematocrit
- Blood type and Rh (RhoGAM should be given as in normal pregnancy when indicated)
- CBC, electrolytes, liver function tests, urinalysis if toxemia suspected
- TSH, thyroxine (free T_4) if hyperthyroidism suspected

IMAGING

- Chest x-ray if suspect acute respiratory distress or for baseline to check for metastatic disease

DIFFERENTIAL DIAGNOSIS

- Threatened abortion
- Missed abortion
- Incomplete abortion
- Ectopic pregnancy

Treatment

INITIAL STABILIZATION

- ABCs
- IV access
- Type and cross for blood, especially if patient needs uterine extraction

ED MANAGEMENT

Acute Respiratory Distress

- CXR: may show bilateral pulmonary infiltrates
- Intubation and mechanical ventilation

Hyperthyroidism

- β-Adrenergic blockers. Administer before molar evacuation. Stress of anesthesia or surgery may precipitate thyroid storm with tachydysrhythmia, high-output failure, hyperthermia, and convulsions

Preeclampsia

- Benzodiazepine if convulsions
- Magnesium

Suction Curettage

- Done by obstetrician, possibly in emergency department
- Method of choice in women wishing to preserve fertility
- Oxytocin infusion after anesthesia started to induce myometrial tone
- Cervix carefully dilated
- 12-mm cannula to permit rapid evacuation and involution of the uterus to control bleeding
- Sharp curettage to remove residual chorionic tissue
- Submit suction and curettage specimen separately

Chemoprophylaxis

- Should be prescribed by obstetrician for patients with follow-up
- Use of chemoprophylaxis at time of evacuation remains controversial
- Kim et al. showed chemoprophylaxis reduced the incidence of postmolar tumor from 47% to 14% in patients with high-risk complete mole
- Berkowitz et al. showed that actinomycin D reduces risk of persistent gestational trophoblastic tumors (GTT) in patients with high-risk complete mole
- Chemoprophylaxis may be useful in high-risk complete mole or if hormonal follow-up is unavailable or unreliable

MEDICATIONS

- Actinomycin D: 12 μg/kg/d IV for 5 days q 2 wk *or* 1.5 mg IV q 14 days
- Methotrexate: 0.4 μg/kg/d for 5 days IM q 2 wk
- Oxytocin: postpartum bleeding: 10 IU IM or 10–40 IU in 1000 ml NS IV
- Propranolol: 1 mg IV increments q 2 min
- RhoGAM: 1 vial within 72 hrs if mother Rh^-
- Diazepam: 0.2–0.4 mg/kg up to 5–10 mg IV *or* 0.3–0.5 mg/kg PR

Disposition

ADMISSION CRITERIA

- Enlargement of uterus beyond 16 weeks gestational size; the larger the uterus, the greater the risk for uterine perforation during suction curettage, hemorrhage, and pulmonary complications
- Clinical evidence of preeclampsia, hyperthyroidism, respiratory distress
- Indications for hysterectomy
  —Patient in older age group or patient who does not want to preserve fertility
  —Should be considered in patient with high-risk disease
  —Hysterectomy ensures removal of entire primary neoplasm but does not prevent metastases
  —Partial molar pregnancies: often need larger grasping instruments to remove abnormal fetus
  —Hemodynamic instability

DISCHARGE CRITERIA

- Uncomplicated dilation and curettage of low-risk and small size mole (less than 16 weeks) in reliable patient with good OBGyn follow-up

Miscellaneous

ICD9: 630

CORE CONTENT CODE: 12.3.8

SUGGESTED READINGS

Berkowitz RS, Goldstein DP. Management of molar pregnancy and gestational trophoblastic tumors. In: Knapp RC, Berkowitz RS, eds. Gynecologic oncology. 2d ed. New York: McGraw Hill, 1993:328–338.

Goldstein DP, Berkowitz RS. Current management of complete and partial molar pregnancy. J Reprod Med 1994;39:139–146.

Homesley HD. Development of single-agent chemotherapy regimens for gestational trophoblastic disease. J Reprod Med 1994;39:185–192.

Kim DS, et al. Effects of prophylactic chemotherapy on persistent trophoblastic disease in patients with complete hydatidiform mole. Obstet Gynecol 1986;67:690–694.

Soper JT. Surgical therapy for gestational trophoblastic disease. J Reprod Med 1994;39:168–174.

Author: Tami Gash-Kim

Hydrocarbon, Poisoning

Clinical Presentation

SIGNS AND SYMPTOMS

- Often asymptomatic at presentation
- Odor of hydrocarbons on breath
- Pulmonary
  - —Mild to severe respiratory distress
  - —Cyanosis
  - —Aspiration (primary complication)
- CNS
  - —Intoxication
  - —Euphoria
  - —Slurred speech
  - —Lethargy
  - —Coma
- GI
  - —Local mucosal irritation
  - —Gastritis
  - —Diarrhea
- Cardiac
  - —Tachycardia
  - —Dysrhythmias (volatile substance abuse)
- Dermal
  - —Local erythema
  - —Maculopapular or vesicular eruptions
  - —Chronic exposure leads to a defatting dermatitis
  - —Huffer's rash of the face seen in chronic abusers

ETIOLOGY

- Accidental exposures—typical in young children
- Abuse of volatile hydrocarbons and suicidal gestures are seen in adolescents and adults

Major Classes of Hydrocarbons

- Aliphatics, or straight-chain compounds
  - —Include kerosene, mineral oil, seal oil, gasoline, solvents, and paint thinners
  - —Pulmonary toxicity via aspiration
  - —Asphyxiation with the gaseous methane and butane by displacement of alveolar oxygen
- Halogenated hydrocarbons
  - —Carbon tetrachloride, and trichloroethane
  - —Found in industrial settings as solvents
  - —Well absorbed by the lungs and the gut—high toxicity
  - —Liver and renal failure are associated with ingestion
- Cyclics, or aromatic compounds
  - —Toluene and xylene highly volatile and well absorbed from the gut
  - —Death from benzene reported with 15 ml ingestion
- Terpenes, or wood distillates (turpentine and pine oil)
  - —Significant GI absorption
  - —Great degree of CNS depression

MECHANISM/DESCRIPTION

- Physical properties that determine the type and extent of toxicity
  - —Viscosity (resistance to flow): aspiration risk
  - —Volatility (ability of a substance to vaporize): aromatic hydrocarbons capable of giving off gas and displacing alveolar air leading to hypoxia
  - —Surface tension (the ability to adhere to itself at the liquid's surface): low surface tension allows easy spread from the oropharynx to the trachea, promoting aspiration, e.g., mineral oil, seal oil
- Volatile substance abuse
  - —Common solvents abused: typewriter correction fluid, adhesive, or other halogenated hydrocarbons such as gasoline or cigarette-lighter fluid
  - —*Huffing:* product inhaled through a soaked rag held to face
  - —*Bagging:* product poured into a bag and multiple inhalations take place
  - —Symptoms
    - -Initial: euphoria and disinhibition
    - -Later: dysphoria, ataxia, confusion, and hallucination
    - -Sudden sniffing death: cardiac arrest in volatile substance abusers secondary to hypersensitization of the myocardium leading to malignant dysrhythmias upon adrenergic stimulation

Pre-Hospital

CAUTIONS

- Keep volatile-substance abusers calm and avoid interventions that cause anxiety or distress

CONTROVERSIES

- Management of accidental hydrocarbon exposures at home
  - —<1% required physician intervention
  - —For asymptomatic or quickly asymptomatic after ingestion with reliable observer available
  - —Only applies when the exact product and its components are known and there is no indication for gastric decontamination or possibility for delayed organ toxicity
  - —Ipecac contraindicated due to increased risk of aspiration

Diagnosis

ESSENTIAL WORKUP

- Obtain
  - —Product: exact name on label, manufacturer, and ingredients
  - —Nature of ingestion or exposure: accidental or intentional
  - —Estimated amount ingested
  - —In industrial settings, the manufacturer safety data sheets (MSDS)

LABORATORY

- Pulse oximetry
  - —If abnormal follow with ABG
- Electrolytes, BUN, Cr, glucose, liver function tests
  - —For halogenated and aromatic hydrocarbon exposure
  - —Metabolic acidosis
  - —Hypokalemia
- Carboxyhemoglobin levels for methylene chloride exposure
  - —Methylene chloride metabolized to carbon monoxide in vivo

IMAGING/SPECIAL TESTS

- ECG for volatile substance abusers who are intoxicated
- CXR
  - —Abnormalities occur as early as 20 minutes or as late as 24 hours
  - —Increased bronchovascular marking and bibasilar and perihilar infiltrates (typical)
  - —Lobar consolidation (uncommon)
  - —Pneumothorax, pneumomediastinum and pleural effusion (rare)
  - —Pneumatocoeles—resolve over weeks
- Abdominal radiograph
  - —Radiopaque halogenated hydrocarbons visible

DIFFERENTIAL DIAGNOSIS

- Caustic, pesticide, or toxic alcohol ingestions
- Accidental vs. intentional: psychiatric evaluation for all intentional ingestions
- Child neglect—poor supervision or unsafe home environment

Treatment

INITIAL STABILIZATION

- ABCs
- Naloxone, thiamine, glucose (or Accucheck) for altered mental status
- IV access and fluid resuscitation if hypotensive or ongoing fluid losses
- Cardiac monitoring for halogenated hydrocarbons (*baggers* and *huffers*)

ED TREATMENT

- Supportive care
- Respiratory symptoms
  - —Oxygen
  - —Nebulized β_2-agonist for bronchospasm (albuterol)
  - —Endotracheal intubation and mechanical ventilation possibly with CPAP or PEEP for respiratory failure
  - —Steroids not indicated for bronchospasm
- Gastric evacuation generally not indicated
  - —Risk of aspiration is higher than the risk of systemic absorption for aliphatic hydrocarbon mixtures which account for most ingestions
  - —Contraindicated if spontaneous emesis has occurred
  - —Evacuation indicated for CHAMP containing hydrocarbon ingestions
    - -CHAMP: mnemonic for camphor, halogenated hydrocarbons, aromatic hydrocarbons, metals (e.g., lead, mercury), pesticides
    - -Use small-bore lavage tube (petroleum distillates are liquids)
    - -Endotracheal intubation with a cuffed tube for airway protection during lavage if no gag reflex or altered mental status
- Activated charcoal not indicated except for significant coingestants
- Cathartics not indicated—diarrhea from the hydrocarbon common

MEDICATIONS

- Dextrose: D50W 1 amp (50 ml or 25 g) (peds: D25W 2–4 ml/kg) IV
- Naloxone (narcan): 2 mg (peds: 0.1 mg/kg) IV or IM initial dose
- Thiamine (vitamin B_1): 100 mg (peds: 50 mg) IV or IM

Disposition

ADMISSION CRITERIA

- All symptomatic patients
- Potential delayed organ toxicity (carbon tetrachloride or other toxic additives)

DISCHARGE CRITERIA

- Observe for 6 hours, then discharge
  - —Asymptomatic patients with a normal chest x-ray and pulse oximetry
  - —Asymptomatic patients with abnormal chest x-ray and normal oxygenation and respiratory rate may be discharged if reliable follow-up ensured
  - —Symptomatic patients on presentation who quickly become asymptomatic may be evaluated as above
- Observe volatile substance abusers until mental status clears

Miscellaneous

ICD9: 987.1

CORE CONTENT CODE: 17.2.24

SUGGESTED READINGS

Anas N, Namasonthi V, Ginsburg C. Criteria for hospitalizing children who have ingested products containing hydrocarbons. JAMA 1981;246:840–843.

Ellenhorn MJ, Schoonwald S, Ordog G, Wasserberger J. The hydrocarbon products. In: Ellenhorn's medical toxicology. 2d ed. Baltimore: Williams & Wilkins, 1997:1158–1563.

King GS, Smialek JE, Troutman WG. Sudden death in adolescents resulting from the inhalation of typewriter correction fluid. JAMA 1985;253:1604–1606.

Machado B, Cross K, Snodgrass WR. Accidental hydrocarbon ingestion cases telephoned to a regional poison center. Ann Emerg Med 1988;17:804–807.

Author: Bonnie McManus

Hydrocele

Clinical Presentation

SIGNS AND SYMPTOMS

- Progressive painless swelling on the involved side of the scrotum
- May be unilateral or bilateral
- Symptoms may include sensation of heaviness

MECHANISM/DESCRIPTION

- *Communicating hydrocele* occurs in those patients with patent processus vaginalis and the scrotum fills and empties with peritoneal fluid depending on body position
- *Noncommunicating hydrocele* is due to the production of serous fluid by a disease process

ETIOLOGY

- Hydrocele results from an imbalance between the production and resorption of fluid within the space between the tunica vaginalis and the tunica albuginea
- Disease processes causing adult noncommunicating hydrocele include
  - —Epididymitis
  - —Hypoalbuminemia
  - —Tuberculosis
  - —Trauma
  - —Mumps
  - —Spermatic vein ligation
  - —In the Third World, hydrocele is primarily caused by infections such as *Wucheria bancrofti* or *Loa Loa*
  - —Rarely malignancy (1° testicular neoplasm or lymphoma)
- Rare etiology is the "abdominoscrotal hydrocele" that may cause hydroureter or unilateral limb edema due to compression
  - —Ultrasound reveals single sac extending from scrotum into the abdominal cavity via the deep inguinal ring

PEDIATRIC CONSIDERATIONS

- Congenital in 6% of newborn males
- Usually diagnosed in the newborn nursery
- Caused by a patent processus vaginalis, a structure that remains patent in 85% of newborns
- As it communicates with the abdominal cavity, it may vary in size due to position or crying. Patients may present with a history of a scrotal mass that has resolved

Pre-Hospital

N/A

Diagnosis

ESSENTIAL WORKUP

- History and examination with special attention to identifying torsion of the testicle
- Initial diagnostic test is transillumination of the affected side
- Due to the possibility in adults that a hydrocele may be due to a primary neoplasm, the testicle must be palpated in its entirety
- In cases of massive hydrocele, or if the testicle can not be palpated, direct visualization with ultrasound is indicated

LABORATORY

- No specific laboratory tests are indicated unless underlying etiology demands it

IMAGING/SPECIAL TESTS

- Ultrasound is diagnostic and allows visualization of testicular anatomy
  - —Appears as a large fluid filled space surrounding the testicle

Treatment

INITIAL STABILIZATION

- Stabilization should focus on the underlying cause (e.g., trauma)

ED MANAGEMENT

- Appropriate examination of testicle to exclude primary neoplasm and referral

MEDICATIONS

- Treat underlying etiology

Pediatric Considerations

- See Disposition below

Disposition

ADMISSION CRITERIA

- Patients with secondary hydrocele may need admission for further evaluation of underlying pathology (e.g., neoplasm, trauma)

DISCHARGE CRITERIA

- Otherwise healthy patients without comorbid illness may be referred for further evaluation to a urologist
- Hydrocele is usually repaired if cosmesis is a factor or in cases where it causes discomfort
- Repair may be
  —Surgical
  —Medical—with aspiration of hydrocele contents and sclerotherapy to prevent recurrence

PEDIATRIC CONSIDERATIONS

- Most hydroceles in the infant population will spontaneously resolve by 12 months of age; referral and observation are appropriate once the diagnosis is made
- After the age of 12–18 months refer for surgical repair as communicating hydroceles usually have a hernia that needs repair.

Miscellaneous

ICD9: 603.9

CORE CONTENT CODE: 19.2.1.1

SUGGESTED READINGS

Schul MW, Keating MA. The acute pediatric scrotum. J Emerg Med 1993;11:565–577.

Rabinowitz R, Hulbert WC. Acute scrotal swelling. Urol Clin North Am 1995;22:101–105.

Sivam NS, Ananthakrishnan N, Kate V, Daniala C. Abdominal hydrocele: Diagnosis by sonography. J Clin Ultrasound 1995;25:210–211.

Gomella LG. Paratesticular tumors and masses. In: Seidman EJ, Hanno PM, eds. Current urologic therapy. 3rd ed. Philadelphia: WB Saunders, 1994:500–501.

Authors: Sean O. Henderson

Hydrocephalus

Clinical Presentation

SIGNS AND SYMPTOMS

Obstructive (Noncommunicating) Hydrocephalus

- *Headache,* with nausea and vomiting, decreased level of consciousness (LOC), urinary incontinence
- Ocular palsies, papilledema, decreased vision
- Pupillary dilation and the Cushing's response (raised systolic pressure and bradycardia)
- *Pediatric patients:* full fontanelle, irritability, and lethargy
- May present like nonobstructive hydrocephalus if obstruction develops slowly

Nonobstructing (Communicating) Hydrocephalus

- Progressive dementia, somnolence
- Gait disturbance, urinary incontinence, impaired upward gaze, generalized weakness, and lethargy
- Dementia is often insidious with subacute onset of progressive intellectual deterioration
- No headache or papilledema
- Pediatric patients increase CSF volume slowly resulting in craniomegaly, retardation, prominent scalp veins, and impaired upward gaze ("setting sun" sign)

MECHANISM/DESCRIPTION

- The signs and symptoms of hydrocephalus result from increased fluid in the cranium
- *Obstructive hydrocephalus* is the most common form
  - —The obstruction is within the ventricular system or in the subarachnoid space
- Acute obstructive hydrocephalus may cause acute rises in ICP, rapidly leading to death or permanent cerebral damage
- *Nonobstructive hydrocephalus* causes subacute symptoms and is a potentially treatable form of dementia

ETIOLOGY

- *Obstructive hydrocephalus*
  - —Obstruction of the foramen of Monro, third ventricle, fourth ventricle, aqueduct of Sylvius, or foramina of Luschka and Magendie (tumor or other masses) or the subarachnoid space around the brainstem (postinfectious or post-SAH)
  - —Acute presentations usually secondary to CSF shunt blockage, SAH, or severe head trauma
- *Nonobstructive hydrocephalus*
  - —Normal pressure hydrocephalus: increased intracranial volume without intracranial hypertension
  - —Increased ventricular size on CT
- *Pediatric hydrocephalus*
  - —Congenital hydrocephalus due to neonatal hemorrhages, congenital malformations, or acquired postmeningitis secondary to subarachnoid scarring around the brain stem

Pre-Hospital

CAUTIONS

- Elevated ICP cannot be definitively diagnosed in the field
- When it is suspected, supplemental O_2 and aggressive airway management are indicated
- If not contraindicated, patients should be transported with head elevated at 30°

Diagnosis

ESSENTIAL WORKUP

- CT scan of the head will allow assessment of ventricular size and symmetry and aid in the diagnosis of cerebral edema, mass lesions, and hemorrhage

LABORATORY

- Lumbar puncture is typically performed after head CT
  - —The opening pressure on LP will reflect increased ICP in nonobstructive hydrocephalus
  - —CSF should be sent for routine tests (Gram stain, culture, protein, and glucose) if an infectious or inflammatory process is suspected

IMAGING/SPECIAL TESTS

- MRI of brain reveals ventricular size and symmetry and may allow for better visualization of masses than CT

DIFFERENTIAL DIAGNOSIS

- Acute cerebral infarction or hemorrhage
- Intracranial infection
- Mass effect from fast-growing tumor or hematoma
- Dementia or delirium of other cause
- Toxic or metabolic encephalopathies

PEDIATRIC CONSIDERATIONS

- Suspect hydrocephalus in an infant whose head circumference is increasing excessively
- Congenital anomalies, e.g., constitutional macrocrania, megalencephaly, Dandy-Walker malformation, Arnold-Chiari malformation, meningomyelocele, choroid plexus papilloma, hypoplasia/dysfunction of arachnoid villi
- Infections, e.g., rubella, CMV, toxoplasmosis, syphilis, bacterial meningitis, Reye's syndrome
- Tumors, especially posterior fossa tumors, e.g., medulloblastoma, astrocytoma, ependymoma
- Hemorrhage, e.g., intraventricular bleed and fibrosis, subarachnoid bleed

Treatment

INITIAL STABILIZATION

- Signs of impending herniation
  - —RSI with lidocaine pretreatment; thiopental or etomidate for induction. Paralytic choice is controversial
    - -Depolarizing agents (succinylcholine) may increase ICP though this effect may not be clinically significant
    - -Nondepolarizing agents (rocuronium, vecuronium) may be preferable
  - —Ventilation to maintain $PaCO_2$ ~35 mm Hg
  - —Maintain systolic bp >100 mm Hg (adult) with fluids or pressors
  - —Mannitol
- If a CSF shunt is present and there are signs of impending herniation
  - —Forced pumping of shunt chamber: flush the device with 1 cc saline to remove distal obstruction; slow drainage of CSF from the reservoir to achieve pressure <20 cm H_2O; IV mannitol to lower ICP

ED TREATMENT

- Signs of impending herniation or acute shunt malfunction are absent—hydrocephalus does not require ED treatment
- Ultimate treatment of hydrocephalus involves either placement (or revision) of a shunting device or treatment of the underlying cause (e.g., tumor)
- Increased ICP refractory to other treatments may respond to controlled lumbar drainage
- Neurologic symptoms (gait disturbance) or severe headache associated with normal pressure hydrocephalus may respond to removal of 25–30 cc of CSF

MEDICATIONS

- Atropine: 0.02 mg/kg IV (max 0.1 mg)
- Etomidate: 0.2–0.3 mg/kg
- Lidocaine: 1 mg/kg IV
- Mannitol: 0.5–1 mg/kg
- Rocuronium: 0.6 mg/kg IV
- Vecuronium: 0.1 mg/kg
- Succinylcholine: 1–1.5 mg/kg IV

Disposition

ADMISSION CRITERIA

- Evidence of increased ICP or shunt malfunction requires admission

DISCHARGE CRITERIA

- Patients with presumed normal pressure hydrocephalus may be discharged for follow-up with a neurosurgeon or neurologist

Miscellaneous

ICD9: 331.4

CORE CONTENT CODE: 11.8, 13.5.4

SUGGESTED READINGS

Adams RD, Victor M, Ropper AH. Principles of neurology. 6th ed. New York: McGraw Hill, 1997:539–553.

Del Bigio MR. Neuropathological changes caused by hydrocephalus. Acta Neuropathol 1993;85(6):573–585.

Ledin T, Bynke O, Odkvist LM. Influence of cerebrospinal fluid tapping on dynamic equilibrium in suspected hydrocephalus. Acta Otolaryngol 1995;520(Part 2 Suppl):317–319.

Marmarou A, Foda M, Bandoh K, et al. Posttraumatic ventriculomegaly: hydrocephalus or atrophy? A new approach for diagnosis using CSF dynamics. J Neurosurg 1996;85:1026–1035.

Mori K. Current concept of hydrocephalus: evolution of new classifications. Childs Nerv Syst 1995;11(9):523–531.

Rowland LP. Merritt's textbook of neurology. 9th ed. Baltimore: Williams & Wilkins, 1995:294–309.

Vanaclocha V, Saiz-Sapena N, Leiva J. Shunt malfunction as related to shunt infection. Acta Neurochir 1996;138(7):829–834.

Authors: Sucharita Paul; Richard S. Krause

Hymenoptera Envenomation

Clinical Presentation

SIGNS AND SYMPTOMS

Local Reaction

- Initial "stabbing" pain at site of injection
- Later "burning, throbbing" pain
- Wheal and flare reactions
- Severe local reactions can cause edema and erythema of an entire extremity without causing systemic effects

Systemic reaction

Symptoms

- Anxiety
- Sensation of throat "closing"
- Pruritus
- Abdominal pain
- Nausea
- Diarrhea
- Lightheadedness
- Shortness of breath
- Chest pain

Signs

- Skin
  —Urticaria
  —Flushing
  —Vasodilatation
- Cardiovascular
  —Tachycardia
  —Hypotension
  —Shock
- Pulmonary
- Dyspnea
- Hoarseness
- Wheezing/bronchospasm
- Laryngeal edema
- Pulmonary edema
- GI
  —Abdominal tenderness
  —Vomiting
  —Diarrhea
- CNS: loss of consciousness

MECHANISM/DESCRIPTION

- Injection of hymenoptera venom causes
  —Release of biologic amines
  —Local or systemic allergic reactions
- Reactions are
  —Usually IgE mediated type I hypersensitivity reaction
  —Type III (Arthrus) hypersensitivity reactions rare

ETIOLOGY

- Hymenoptera—order of the phylum arthropoda
- Includes bees, wasps, and fire ants

Pre-Hospital

CAUTIONS

- Majority of deaths occur within the first hour due to either respiratory obstruction or anaphylaxis causing cardiovascular and respiratory collapse
- When signs of systemic reactions
  —Assess for a patent airway
  —Establish IV access

Diagnosis

ESSENTIAL WORKUP

- History and physical—keys to diagnosis
- *No* radiologic or laboratory test will confirm hymenoptera envenomation or anaphylaxis

LABORATORY

- CBC, electrolytes, BUN, Cr, glucose, ABG
  —Consider when significant systemic effects present

SPECIAL TEST/IMAGING

- ECG
  —When significant systemic effects in patients at risk for cardiovascular disease

DIFFERENTIAL DIAGNOSIS

- Difficult to differentiate a persistent severe local reaction with that of a cellulitis
  —Infections of hymenoptera envenomations are rare and usually caused by wasp envenomations
  —Severe local symptoms usually peak between the 2nd and 3rd day and do not cause lymphangitis
  —Local reaction resembles periorbital cellulitis
- Local reaction
  —Cellulitis
  —Gout
  —Soft tissue trauma
- Systemic reaction
  —Pulmonary embolus
  —Anaphylaxis from a different agent
  —Hyperventilatory syndrome/anxiety

Treatment

INITIAL STABILIZATION

Acute Severe Systemic Reaction/ Anaphylaxis

- ABCs
  - —Intubation /ventilation with rapidly increasing signs of laryngeal compromise
  - —Oxygen
  - —0.9%NS IV access
- Epinephrine SQ/IV
- Antihistamines IV

ED MANAGEMENT

Systemic Reactions

- Epinephrine for respiratory symptoms/hypotension
- Antihistamines—H_1(diphenhydramine) and H_2 (cimetidine) blockers
- Steroids (prednisone, methylprednisolone)
- Inhaled β-agonist for wheezing/shortness of breath
- For persistent hypotension
  - —0.9%NS IV fluid resuscitation
  - —Vasopressor (epinephrine/α-adrenergic) for hypotension resistant to IV fluids
  - —Removal of remnants of stinger at site of envenomation (bees may leave stingers) by scraping not squeezing

Local reactions

- Cool compress
- Elevation
- Remove constrictive clothing or jewelry
- Topical antihistamine/topical steroidal cream as needed
- Oral antihistamine or steroids as needed

MEDICATIONS

- Albuterol, β-agonist (inhaled): 3 mg in 5 ml solvent (ped: 0.03 ml/kg of 5 mg/ml concentration) via nebulization
- Cimetidine: 300 mg (5 mg/kg) IV
- Diphenhydramine:
  - —50–100 mg (peds: 0.5–1.0 mg/kg) IV for severe reactions
  - —25–50 mg (peds 1 mg/kg) po qid for severe local reactions
- Epinephrine
  - —0.1 mg (10 ml of 1:100,000 dilution) (peds: 0.01 mg/kg = 1 ml/kg of 1:100,000 dilution up to 10 ml) IV over 5 min for shock
  - —0.1 ml/kg up to 0.3 ml of 1:1,000 dilution SQ for severe reactions but not in shock
- Prednisone: 60 mg (peds: 1–2 mg/kg) po
- Methylprednisolone: 125 mg (peds: 1–2 mg/kg) IV
- Norepinephrine: 4–12 μg/min (peds: 0.1 μg/kg/min) titrated continuous infusion

Disposition

ADMISSION CRITERIA

- Persistent unstable vital signs require ICU admission
- Life-threatening reaction requires 24-hour observation
- Systemic reaction require a minimum of 6 hours of observation

DISCHARGE CRITERIA

- Minimal isolated local reaction
- Systemic reactions that resolve and do not recur during 6-hour observation period
- Follow-up
  - —Provide patients with life threatening reactions emergency anaphylaxis kits (EpiPen) and medical identification bracelets (Medi-Alert)
  - —Systemic reaction requires follow-up for possible immunotherapy

Miscellaneous

ICD9: 989.5

CORE CONTENT CODE: 5.10.1

SUGGEST READINGS

Ellenhorn MJ. Envenomations—bites and stings. In: Ellenhorn MJ, et al., eds. Ellenhorn's medical toxicology. 2d ed. Baltimore: Williams & Wilkins, 1997; 1733–1799.

McDougle L, Klein G, Hoehler FK. Management of hymenoptera sting anaphylaxis: A preventive medicine survey. J Emerg Med 1995;13:9–13.

Author: David Lee

Hyperbaric Oxygen Therapy

Clinical Presentation

INDICATIONS FOR HYPERBARIC OXYGEN (HBO)

- Arterial gas embolism
- Decompression sickness
- Toxic inhalations
  - —Carbon monoxide
  - —Cyanide
  - —Hydrogen sulfide
- Wound care (requires multiple treatments)
  - —Gas gangrene
  - —Osteomyelitis
  - —Postradiation tissue injury
  - —Burns
  - —Crush injuries and acute peripheral extremity ischemic injuries
- Indications continuously evolving

MECHANISM/DESCRIPTION

- Definition: administration of 100% oxygen at pressure greater than sea level (1 ATM)
- Two effects of HBO
  - —Mechanical effect—compression of any gas bubbles
  - —Increase in the amount of oxygen available at the cellular level due to increased oxygen dissolved in plasma
    - -At 3 ATM pressure and breathing 100% oxygen—enough oxygen is dissolved in plasma to supply baseline tissue requirements and hemoglobin is not necessary for oxygen transport
- Types of HBO chambers
  - —Monoplace
    - -Accommodates a single supine patient monitored by a technician outside the clear tube
    - -Compressed with 100% oxygen
  - —Multiplace
    - -Holds multiple patients as well as tenders who "dive" with the patients
    - -Air locks allow for transfer of medication and equipment in and out of the chamber
    - -Compressed with air: patients breathe oxygen by mask, face tent, or endotracheal tube
- Due to the risk of oxygen toxicity and seizures, most hyperbaric protocols limit depth to 2–2.8 ATM (60 feet) for no more that 90–120 minutes

Pre-Hospital

CAUTIONS

- Administer 100% oxygen for all patients being transported to HBO facility
- Establish IV access

Diagnosis

ESSENTIAL WORKUP

- Determine need for HBO treatment by above diagnosis

LABORATORY

- ABG
  - —Baseline measure useful for hypoxic patients
  - —Serial measurements of the suspected inhaled toxin (CO, CN, HS) may be necessary

IMAGING

- CXR to rule out any untreated pneumothorax

Treatment

INITIAL STABILIZATION

- Only absolute contraindication to HBO therapy
  - —Untreated pneumothorax
    - -Increased pressure converts a simple pneumothorax into a tension pneumothorax
- Cardiovascular stability required for treatment in monoplace chambers
- Multiplace chambers allow for nursing and other personnel to provide ongoing care

ED TREATMENT

- Patient equipment/devices with balloons (i.e., Foley catheters, endotracheal tubes) must be filled with fluid to avoid rupture
- Pretreatment with decongestants if sinus congestion present
- Tympanostomy tubes for patients who experience middle ear discomfort (squeeze) during compression and who cannot equalize the ear pressures
- Multiplace chambers can accommodate IVs, ventilators, and most medical therapies
- No smoking or any potentially flammable devices
- Divers Alert Network (DAN)
  - —Based at Duke University Medical Center in North Carolina
  - —Provides a 24-hour emergency hotline for medical consultation on the treatment of dive-related injuries and for referrals to hyperbaric chambers
  - —Telephone: (919) 684-8111

MEDICATIONS

- Pseudoephedrine (sudafed): 60 mg (peds: 6–12 years old, 30 mg; 2–5 years old, 15 mg/dose) po q 4–6 hrs

Disposition

ADMISSION CRITERIA

- Arterial gas embolism/decompression sickness should be admitted for repeat neurologic exam
- Severe inhalational injury with CO or CN

DISCHARGE CRITERIA

- Mild toxic inhalations may be discharged post-HBO therapy if their oxygenation status is acceptable and there are no other injuries

Miscellaneous

ICD9: N/A

CORE CONTENT CODE: N/A

SUGGESTED READINGS

Kindwall, EP. Hyperbaric medicine practice. Best Publishing, 1995.

Tibbles PM, Edelsberg JS. Hyperbaric oxygen therapy. N Engl J Med 1996;334(25):1642–1648

Author: Jeffrey Gordon

Hypercalcemia

Clinical Presentation

SIGNS AND SYMPTOMS

General

- Severity depends on level of serum calcium and rate of its rise
- Hypercalcemic crisis, usually above 14 mg/dl, associated with serious signs and symptoms

Neurologic

- Headache
- Fatigue
- Weakness
- Difficulty concentrating
- Confusion
- Irritable
- Lethargy
- Stupor
- Coma
- Hyporeflexia

Cardiovascular

- Hypotension, if severely volume depleted or hypertension
- ECG
  —Shortening of QT interval
  —Prolongation of PR interval
  —QRS widening
- Accentuates side effects of digoxin
- Sinus bradycardia, bundle branch block, AV block, cardiac arrest with severe hypercalcemia (rare)

Renal

- Dehydration
- Polyuria, polydipsia
- Oliguric renal failure
- Chronically: renal calculi, nephrocalcinosis, interstitial nephritis

Gastrointestinal

- Anorexia
- Nausea
- Vomiting
- Abdominal pain
- Constipation
- Intestinal ileus
- Chronically: increased risk of peptic ulcer disease and pancreatitis

Dermatologic

- Pruritus
- Band keratopathy
- Ectopic calcification

MECHANISM/DESCRIPTION

- 0.1–10% of patients on routine laboratory screening
- Most cases mild (<12 mg/dl) and asymptomatic
- Calcium in bloodstream in three forms
  —Ionized: 45%
  —Bound to protein (primarily albumin): 40%
  —Bound to other anions: 15%
- Ionized calcium—only physiologically active form

PEDIATRIC CONSIDERATIONS

Infantile Hypercalcemia

- Characteristic facies: pug nose, fat nasal bridge, "cupid's bow" upper lip
- Failure to thrive
- Slow development
- Hypotonia
- Associated with pulmonic and supravalvular aortic stenosis
- Mental retardation may ensue

Pre-Hospital

N/A

Diagnosis

ESSENTIAL WORKUP

- Ionized and total serum calcium levels, albumin levels
  —Normal total calcium level is <10.5 mg/dl
  —Must correct for calcium that is protein-bound, primarily to albumin
  —Corrected total calcium (mg/dl) = measured total calcium (mg/dl) + 0.8 × {4.0-albumin concentration (g/dl)}
- Electrolytes, BUN/Cr, glucose
- ECG

LABORATORY

- Phosphate
- Protein
- Urinalysis
- Parathyroid hormone level
- Vitamin D level, if suspected
- Digoxin level, if taking
- Thyroid function tests

IMAGING/SPECIAL TESTS

- CT head, if altered mental status
- Work-up for occult malignancy, if no other cause

DIFFERENTIAL DIAGNOSIS

Primary Hyperparathyroidism

- Most common cause in outpatients
- Usually mild, less than 11.2 mg/dl
- Increased bone resorption, relative decrease in calcium excretion, increased intestinal calcium absorption

Malignancy

- Most common cause in hospitalized patients
- Most common paraneoplastic complication of cancer
- Most commonly from production of parathyroid hormone-related protein with similar actions
- May result from production of other bone-resorbing substances by tumor
- May result from local effects of osteolytic skeletal metastasis

MISCELLANEOUS

- Thiazide diuretics increase renal reabsorption
- Granulomatous disorders may lead to activation of vitamin D
- Acute vitamin A intoxication
- Increased exogenous vitamin D intake
- Milk-alkali syndrome from excessive ingestion of calcium and nonabsorbable antacids such as milk or calcium carbonate
- Long-term lithium therapy
- Renal transplantation
- Acute tubular necrosis

PEDIATRIC CONSIDERATIONS

- Differential diagnosis: differences from adults
  - —Primary hyperparathyroidism
    - -Less common than in adults
  - —Infantile hypercalcemia
    - -Uncertain etiology
    - -Possibly, hypersensitivity and in utero excessive exposure to vitamin D
  - —Immobilization hypercalcemia
    - -Typically adolescent who is growing rapidly
    - -Prolonged immobilization, especially in traction, leads to hypercalciuria and then hypercalcemia
    - -Presumably from increased bone resorption with decreased or arrested bone mineralization

Treatment

INITIAL STABILIZATION

- ABCs, intravenous access, oxygen, cardiac monitor
- 0.9%NS 1 L bolus (20 ml/kg) for hypotension or severe dehydration
- Naloxone, thiamine, D50W (or Accucheck) for altered mental status

ED TREATMENT

General

- Immediate therapy for severe hypercalcemia (corrected total >14mg/dl) regardless of symptoms, and for symptomatic hypercalcemia
- Asymptomatic, mild hypercalcemia does not require emergency treatment

Fluid Administration

- Isotonic saline for restoration of intravascular volume
- Often need 2–5 L per day
- Correct other electrolyte abnormalities
- Cardiovascular status of patient may necessitate central venous pressure monitoring to adjust fluid administration rates

Renal Elimination

- After volume expansion and if needed to avoid overload, administer loop diuretics like furosemide
- Avoid thiazide diuretics
- May need peritoneal or hemodialysis against a low calcium diasylate in renal failure

Inhibition of Osteoclastic Activity

- Reduce mobilization of calcium from bone
- Administer drug therapy when corrected calcium level >14 mg/dl or signs or symptoms
- First-line drug therapy
  - —Biphosphonates
    - -Pamidronate more potent and possibly less toxic
    - -Etidronate
  - —Calcitonin
    - -Rapid onset but modest decrease in levels
- Other potential drug therapy
  - —Plicamycin
    - -Efficacious but numerous side effects
  - —Hydrocortisone
    - -Especially useful with malignancies, granulomatous disorders, or vitamin D intoxication
- Encourage ambulation in appropriate patients

Underlying Disorder

- Prepare to treat underlying cause
- Parathyroidectomy for primary hyperparathyroidism resulting in symptomatic or severe hypercalcemia
- Treat tumor for malignancy
- Discontinue medication if cause

MEDICATIONS

- Calcitonin: 4 IU/kg q 12 hrs IV
- Etidronate: 7.5 mg/kg over 4 hrs daily for 3–7 days IV
- Furosemide: 10–40 mg q 6–8 hrs (peds: 1–2 mg/kg) IV
- Gallium nitrate: continuous infusion of 200 $mg/m^2/d$ for 5 days IV
- Hydrocortisone: 200–300 mg/day IV (peds: consult pediatrician)
- Pamidronate: single 24-hr infusion of 60–90 mg IV (peds: consult pediatrician)
- Plicamycin: 25 μg/kg over 4 hrs IV

PEDIATRIC CONSIDERATIONS

- Fluid at 2–3 times daily maintenance in otherwise normal patients

Disposition

ADMISSION CRITERIA

- Corrected total calcium level above 13.0 mg/dl
- Signs or symptoms attributed to hypercalcemia
- Monitored bed or ICU for corrected level >14 or serious signs and symptoms

DISCHARGE CRITERIA

- Corrected calcium level below 13.0 mg/dl and no signs or symptoms of hypercalcemia
- Rapid follow-up arranged to determine cause and long-term therapy

Miscellaneous

ICD9: 275.4

CORE CONTENT CODE: 4.3.1

SUGGESTED READINGS

Bilezikian JP. Clinical review 51: Management of hypercalcemia. J Clin Endocrinol Metab 1993;77(6):1445–1449.

Cronan KM, Norman ME. Renal and electrolyte emergencies. In: Fleisher GR, Ludwig S, et al., eds. Textbook of pediatric emergency medicine. 3rd ed. Baltimore: Williams & Wilkins, 1993:670–717.

Edelson GW, Kleerekoper M. Hypercalcemic crisis. Med Clin North Am 1995;79(1):79–92.

Gibbs MA, Wolfson AB, Tayal VS. Electrolyte disturbances. In: Rosen P, et al., eds. Emergency medicine: Concepts and clinical practice. 4th ed. St. Louis: CV Mosby, 1998:2432–2455.

Kaye TB. Hypercalcemia. How to pinpoint the cause and customize treatment. Postgrad Med 1995;97(1):153–155, 159–160.

Author: Jeff King

Hyperemesis Gravidarum

Clinical Presentation

SIGNS AND SYMPTOMS

- Nausea and vomiting normally occurs in most pregnancies
- Onset of symptoms by the 4th–8th week of pregnancy and resolution by the 20th
- Hyperemesis gravidarum is defined by the following
  —Persistent, severe nausea and vomiting
  —Dehydration
  —Weight loss, often up to 5% of total body weight
  —Laboratory findings: *ketonuria, increased urine specific gravity*

MECHANISM/DESCRIPTION

- Hyperemesis is at the severe end of the continuum of symptoms found in pregnancy

Pre-Hospital

N/A

Diagnosis

ESSENTIAL WORKUP

- History and physical examination with special attention to state of hydration and abdominal exam for other diagnoses associated with vomiting (appendicitis, etc.)
- The *only mandated test is an uncontaminated urinalysis*
- Other lab testing is indicated by the presence of fever, abdominal pain, jaundice, or failure of the patient to resolve her symptoms with hydration and antiemetics (see below)

LABORATORY

- Urinalysis
  —Increased specific gravity and ketonuria
  —Presence of glucose mandates checking serum glucose to rule out diabetes
  —Presence of bilirubin mandates a search to rule out hepatobiliary cause for the vomiting
- The following labs are *not* routinely necessary unless there is no response to initial treatment
- CBC
  —May have an elevated hematocrit
  —White blood cell count is usually normal
- Electrolytes
  —Elevated blood urea nitrogen indicating volume depletion
  —Hyponatremia, hypokalemia, hypochloremia, and metabolic alkalosis from loss of HcT in emesis
- Liver function tests
  —Mild increases in bilirubin may occur but should be below 4 mg/dl
  —AST and ALT may also be mildly elevated, but not over 100 IU/L
- Amylase/lipase should be normal

DIFFERENTIAL DIAGNOSIS

- Pyelonephritis; most commonly missed
- Gastroenteritis
- Hepatobiliary disease; hepatitis, cholecystitis
- Pancreatitis
- Appendicitis
- Diabetic ketoacidosis
- Hyperthyroidism
- Uremia; persistent nausea and vomiting are seen with severe renal dysfunction

Treatment

INITIAL STABILIZATION

- IV hydration using a crystalloid with dextrose (D5LR or D5NS)

ED TREATMENT

- IV hydration using up to 3 L of D5LR or D5NS
- The dextrose is added to help break the cycle of the ketosis
- Treat until the patient is no longer symptomatic from hypovolemia
- Antiemetics administered IV are given to break the vomiting cycle
- The most commonly used medications are the phenothiazines (promethazine, chlorpromazine, droperidol), which are FDA Category C, or metoclopramide, which is FDA Category B
    - —These medications have been used extensively in pregnancy and there is little or no evidence that these antiemetics are associated with increased risk of congenital anomalies
    - —Parenteral antiemetics are clearly preferable to the risk of prolonged ketosis and the associated hypovolemia
- Oral rehydration in the ED after the initial fluid resuscitation and the antiemetics are given

MEDICATIONS

- Metoclopramide: 10–20 mg IV
- Prochlorperazine: 5–10 mg IV not to exceed 40 mg/day
- Promethazine: 12.5–25 mg IV
- Droperidol: 0.625–1.25 mg IV

DISCHARGE MEDICATIONS

- Consider the first-line medications and elevate to the second-line for repeated visits
- Meclizine: 25 mg po q 6 hrs PRN, FDA Category B first line
- Prochlorperazine: 5–10 mg po q 6 hrs or 25 mg PR bid PRN, FDA Category C second line
- Promethazine: 12.5–25 mg po or PR q 4–6 hrs PRN, FDA Category C second line
- Pyridoxine (vitamin B_6): 25 mg po tid first line (over-the-counter)

Disposition

ADMISSION CRITERIA

- Inability to tolerate oral intake after treatment
- Inability to control the emesis despite treatment
- Severe electrolyte or metabolic disturbances

DISCHARGE CRITERIA

- The majority of patients can be discharged to home as long as they are able to tolerate oral intake and have adequate follow-up
- Correction of the dehydration and associate symptoms
- Patients should be counseled to eat small, frequent meals, stopping short of satiety. They should avoid all irritant or spicy foods. Their meals should contain simple carbohydrates as opposed to complex fats
- Decreased ketonuria

Miscellaneous

ICD9: 643.00

CORE CONTENT CODE: 12.3.2

SUGGESTED READINGS

Abell TL, Riely CA. Hyperemesis gravidarum. Gastroenterol Clin North Am 1992;21(4)835–849.

Abbott J. Acute complications related to pregnancy. In: Rosen P, et al., eds. Emergency medicine: Concepts and clinical practice. 4th ed. St. Louis: CV Mosby, 1998:2342–2364.

Hod M, et al. Hyperemesis gravidarum. J Reprod Med 1994;39:605–612.

Author: David Della-Giustina, Marco Coppola

Hyperkalemia

Clinical Presentation

SIGNS AND SYMPTOMS

- Muscular weakness (rare except in severe cases)
  - —Generalized weakness—may progress to flaccid paralysis
  - —Dyspnea due to respiratory muscle weakness
- Cardiac dysrhythmias—initial manifestation
  - —See ECG below

MECHANISM/DESCRIPTION

- Potassium distribution
  - —Extracellular space: 2%
  - —Intracellular space: 98%
- Renal and extrarenal mechanisms maintain plasma concentration between 3.8–5.5 mmol/L
- Renal excretion of potassium affected by
  - —Dietary intake
  - —Distal renal tubular function
  - —Acid-base balance
  - —Mineralocorticoids
- Regulation between intracellular and extracellular potassium balance, affected by
  - —Acid-base balance
  - —Insulin
  - —Mineralocorticoids
  - —Sympathetic activity

ETIOLOGY

Decreased Potassium Excretion

- Most common cause: renal failure (acute or chronic)
- Distal tubular diseases
  - —Acute interstitial nephritis
  - —Renal transplant rejection
  - —Sickle cell nephropathy
- Mineralocorticoid deficiency
  - —Addison's disease
  - —Hypoaldosteronism
- Drugs
  - —ACE inhibitors
  - —Potassium sparing diuretics
  - —NSAIDs
  - —Cyclosporine
  - —High dose trimethoprim
  - —Lithium toxicity

Intracellular to Extracellular Potassium Shifts

- Metabolic acidosis
  - —Serum K^+ rises 0.5–1.3 mmol/L for each 0.1 unit fall in arterial pH
- Hyperosmolar states
- Insulin deficiency
- Cell necrosis
- Rhabdomyolysis
- Hemolysis
- Chemotherapy
- Drugs
  - —Digitalis toxicity
  - —Depolarizing muscle relaxants (e.g., succinylcholine)
  - —β-Adrenergic blockers
  - —α-Adrenergic agonists
- Hyperkalemic periodic paralysis

Excess Exogenous Potassium Load

- Salt substitutes
- Oral potassium
- Potassium penicillin G
- Rapidly infused massive transfusions of banked blood

Pseudohyperkalemia

- Traumatic venipuncture with hemolysis
- Post venipuncture release of potassium can occur in the setting of
  - —Thrombocytosis (platelets >800,000/mm^3)
  - —Extreme leukocytosis (WBCs >100,000/mm^3)

Pre-Hospital

CAUTIONS

- Treatment of hyperkalemic induced dysrhythmias/cardiac arrest involves different drugs from usual ACLS measures (see Treatment below)
- Diagnosis suggested by the pre-hospital rhythm strip or in at-risk populations (renal failure)

Diagnosis

ESSENTIAL WORKUP

- Serum potassium >5.5 mmol/L
- Collect in heparinized tube if pseudohyperkalemia suspected

LABORATORY

- Electrolytes, BUN, Cr, glucose
  - —Elevated BUN, Cr in renal failure
  - —Hyponatremia with mineralocorticoid deficiency
  - —Mild metabolic acidosis with type IV renal tubular acidosis
- Arterial blood gases
  - —Assesses acid-base status
- Creatinine kinase
- Ca^{++}
- For hyperkalemia in the face of normal renal function, calculate transtubular potassium gradient (TTKG)
  - —TTKG = Urine K × Posm/Plasma K × Uosm
    - -Posm = plasma osmolality; Uosm= urine osmolality
  - —TTKG >8 suggests an extrarenal cause; TTKG <6 indicates a renal excretory defect

IMAGING/SPECIAL TESTS

- ECG: Changes correlate with the degree of hyperkalemia
  - —>6.0: peaking of T waves; shortening of QT_c interval
  - —>7.5–8.0: loss of P waves; widening of QRS complexes
  - —>10–12: sine wave complex

DIFFERENTIAL DIAGNOSIS

- Pseudohyperkalemia

Treatment

INITIAL STABILIZATION

- ABCs
- IV access
- Cardiac monitor

ED TREATMENT

Marked ECG Changes (Widened QRS Complexes/Dysrhythmia): Antagonize Potassium-Mediated Cardiotoxicity

- Administer calcium gluconate or calcium chloride
  - —Immediate onset
  - —30-minute duration
  - —No effect on serum potassium levels

Severe (>7.0) or Moderate (6.0–7.0) with ECG Changes: Shift Potassium Intracellularly

- Administer combination of insulin and glucose
  - —Onset over 20–30 minutes
  - —2-hour duration
- IV sodium bicarbonate
  - —Onset over 20 minutes
  - —2-hour duration
  - —Caution in patients at risk for volume overload
  - —Worsens concomitant hypocalcemia
- Inhaled albuterol
  - —Onset within 30 minutes
  - —4–6-hour duration

Enhanced Excretion for K^+ >6.0

- Administer cation exchange resin
  - —Calcium or sodium polystyrene sulfonate po or PR

All Patients

- Limit exogenous potassium and potassium-sparing drugs
- Treat the underlying cause

Special situations

- Renal failure
  - —Arrange for dialysis
  - —Hemodialysis extremely effective at removing potassium
- Furosemide
  - —Effective in the absence of oliguric renal failure
  - —Causes a potassium-losing diuresis
- Cardiac arrest
  - —Administer $CaCl_2$ and $NaHCO_3$ with known or suspected hyperkalemia
- Digoxin toxicity
  - —Avoid calcium
    - -When necessary, administer small doses extremely slowly
  - —Consider digibind administration
- Mineralocorticoid deficiency
  - —Hydrocortisone

MEDICATIONS

- —Albuterol: 10–20 mg (peds: 2.5 mg if <25 kg; 5.0 mg if >25 kg) nebulized over 10 min
- —Calcium chloride 10%: 10-ml amp (peds: 0.2–0.3 ml/kg/dose) IV over 2–5 min
- —Calcium gluconate 10%: 20-ml amp (peds: 0.1 ml/kg) IV over 2–5 min
- —Hydrocortisone: 100 mg (peds: 1–2 mg/kg) IV
- —Furosemide: 40–80 mg (peds: 1.0 mg/kg) IV—modify dose to achieve appropriate diuresis
- —Insulin and glucose: 10 IU (peds: 0.1 IU/kg) regular insulin plus 50 ml 50% (peds: 0.5–1 g/kg) dextrose IV
- —Sodium bicarbonate: 1–3 amp (44 mEq per amp) IV over 20–30 min (peds: 1.0–2.0 mEq/kg/dose)
- —Sodium polystyrene sulfonate (kayexalate) or calcium polystyrene sulfonate (preferred with volume overload)
  - -Oral: 15 g mixed with water or 50 ml of sorbitol q 2 hrs to a total of 5 doses
  - -Rectal enema: 50 g in 200 ml of sorbitol q 4–6 hrs
  - -Peds: 1.0 g/kg orally or rectally

Disposition

ADMISSION CRITERIA

- Admit most cases
  - —Process of potassium removal relatively slow
  - —Levels may continue to rise

DISCHARGE CRITERIA

- Mild hyperkalemia (<6.0 mmol/L) provided that
  - —Response to treatment has been demonstrated
  - —Known correctable cause
  - —Further rises in serum potassium not anticipated
  - —Early follow-up possible

Miscellaneous

ICD9: 276.7

CORE CONTENT CODE: 4.3.5

SUGGESTED READINGS

Clark BA, Brown RS. Potassium homeostasis and hyperkalemic syndromes. Endocrinol Metab Clin North Am 1995;24(3):573–591.

Allon M. Hyperkalemia in end-stage renal disease: Mechanisms and management. J Am Soc Nephrol 1995;6(4):1134–1142.

Rodríguez-Soriano J. Potassium homeostasis and its disturbances in children. Pediatr Nephrol 1995;9(3):364–74.

Author: Joel Yaphe

Hypernatremia

Clinical Presentation

SIGNS AND SYMPTOMS

General

- Most symptoms attributed to the underlying cause (dehydration)
- More marked with acute changes
- May see the following, usually at levels ≥160 mEq/L
- Death likely to occur with sodium of ≥185 mEq/L

Neurologic

- Tremulous
- Irritability
- Ataxia
- Mental confusion
- Delirium
- Seizures
- Coma
- Subarachnoid, intracerebral, and subdural hemorrhages

Musculoskeletal

- Spasticity
- Muscle weakness

Other

- Venous sinus thrombosis

Hypovolemic Hypernatremia

- Tachycardia
- Orthostasis
- Dry mucous membranes
- Oliguria
- Azotemia

Hypervolemic Hypernatremia

- Pulmonary edema
- Peripheral edema

MECHANISM/DESCRIPTION

- Hypernatremia definition: sodium >146 mEq/L
  —Mild hypernatremia serum sodium 146–155 mEq/L
  —Severe hypernatremia serum sodium >155 mEq/L

ETIOLOGY

- Divided into 3 categories

Hypovolemic hypernatremia

- Most common
- Loss or deficiency of water and sodium with water losses being greater than sodium losses
- Examples
  —Diuretics
  —Glucosuria
  —Mannitol
  —Renal failure
  —High protein feedings
  —Lactulose
  —Excess sweating
  —Respiratory loss
  —Defective thirst mechanism
  —Lack of access to water
  —Diarrhea/vomiting

Isovolemic Hypernatremia

- Water deficiency without sodium loss
- Examples
  —Polycystic kidney disease
  —Sickle cell nephropathy
  —Diabetes
  —Diabetes insipidus
  —Lithium
  —Fever
  —Tachypnea

Hypervolemic Hypernatremia

- Gain of water and sodium with sodium gain greater than water gain
- Examples
  —Iatrogenic—most common cause
    -Sodium bicarbonate administration
    -NaCl tablets
    -Hypertonic IVF
    -Hypertonic dialysis
  —Cushing's disease
  —Adrenal hyperplasia
  —Primary aldosteronism

PEDIATRIC CONSIDERATIONS

- More prone to iatrogenic causes
- More likely to die or to have permanent neurologic sequella
- Morbidity anywhere from 25–50%
- May present with high pitched cry, lethargy, irritable

Pre-Hospital

N/A

Diagnosis

ESSENTIAL WORKUP
- Serum Na^+ level

LABORATORY
- Electrolytes, BUN/Cr, glucose
- CBC
- Urinalysis
  - —Specific gravity

IMAGING/SPECIAL TESTS
- CXR
  - —For infection/aspiration
  - —Pulmonary edema with hypervolemia hypernatremia
- CT brain
  - —For altered mental status
  - —Urine/serum osmolality
  - —Urine Na^+

DIFFERENTIAL DIAGNOSIS
- Diabetic ketoacidosis
- Hyperosmolar coma
- Primary CNS lesions

Treatment

INITIAL STABILIZATION
- ABCs
- 0.9%NS IV bolus for severe hypotension
- Narcan, thiamine, D50W (or Accucheck) for altered mental status

ED TREATMENT

General
- Do not rapidly correct hypertonicity to a normal serum osmolality
  - —Rapid correction may cause seizures
  - —Reduce serum sodium level by <0.5–0.7 mEq/L/hr

Hypovolemic Hypernatremia
- Replace volume contraction with 0.9%NS IV bolus
- Change to D5W or hypotonic saline once volume repleted and hemodynamically stable

Isovolemic Hypernatremia
- Calculate water deficit
  - —Water deficit = 0.6 (weight in kg) × (actual Na^+ − desired Na^+)/(actual Na^+)
- Correct water deficit with D5W or hypotonic saline
  - —Replace half of deficit in first 24 hours then remainder over 1–2 days

Hypervolemic Hypernatremia
- Remove excess water with diuretics or dialysis
- When euvolemic replace water deficit with D5W
- Avoid hypotonic saline solutions because already have an excess of total body sodium

Diabetes Insipidus (DI) Hypernatremia
- Sodium restriction
- Desmopressin
  - —Vasopressin agonist
  - —Best therapeutic agent
- Chlorpropamide enhances effect of vasopressin at renal tubule
- Carbamazepine causes release of vasopressin
- Hydrochlorothiazide enhances sodium excretion
- Discontinue DI-inducing drugs

MEDICATIONS
- Chlorpropamide (diabinese): 100–500 mg/day
- Desmopressin: 0.05 mg po bid; 0.1–0.4 mg/d intranasal divided BID/TID; 1–2 μg IV/SC q 12 hrs
- Dextrose: D50W 1 amp (50 ml or 25 g) (peds: D25W 2–4 ml/kg) IV
- Hydrochlorothiazide: 25 mg po
- Naloxone (narcan): 2 mg (peds: 0.1 mg/kg) IV or IM initial dose
- Thiamine (vitamin B_1): 100 mg (peds: 50 mg) IV or IM

Disposition

ADMISSION CRITERIA
- Newly diagnosed sodium >150 mEq/L for monitoring and treatment
- Admit sodium >160 mEq/L or symptomatic patients to ICU

DISCHARGE CRITERIA
- Sodium <150 mEq/L in asymptomatic patient
- Sodium >150 mEq/L in patients with history of chronically elevated sodium who are at their baseline and asymptomatic

Miscellaneous

ICD9: 276.0

CORE CONTENT CODE: 4.3.6

SUGGESTED READINGS

Barton I, Mansell M. Fluid and electrolyte disorders-sodium. Brit J Hosp Med 1984;32(1):15–18.

Gibbs MA, Wolfson AB, Tayal VS. Electrolyte disturbances. In: Rosen P, et al., eds. Emergency medicine concepts and clinical practice. 4th ed. St. Louis: CV Mosby, 1998;2432–2455.

Author: Linda Mueller

Hyperosmolar Syndrome

Clinical Presentation

SIGNS AND SYMPTOMS

- Polyuria/polydipsia/weight loss
- Dizziness/weakness
- Marked dehydration
- Decreased sweating, dry mucous membranes
- Orthostasis
- Hypotension
- Tachycardia
- Collapsed neck veins
- Decreased skin turgor
- Urinary output maintained until late
- Lethargy/drowsiness
- Seizures/focal neurological deficits/coma

MECHANISM/DESCRIPTION

- Results from a relative insulin deficiency in the undiagnosed or undertreated diabetic
  —Sufficient insulin to prevent ketogenesis but not control hyperglycemia
- Sustained hyperglycemia creates an osmotic diuresis and dehydration
  —Extracellular space maintained by the osmotic gradient at the expense of the intracellular space
  —Eventually profound intracellular dehydration occurs
- Total body deficits of H_2O, Na^+, K^+, PO_4^- and Mg^+
- Most commonly occurs in mild Type 2 elderly diabetic with renal insufficiency who experiences some stressful illness that precipitates worsening hyperglycemia and reduced renal function
- Less common than DKA but with a greater mortality

ETIOLOGY

- Factors that may contribute to the hyperosmolar state include
  —Increase in endogenous glucose: in the under-treated diabetic
  —Increase in exogenous glucose: with dietary indiscretion or improperly managed parenteral hyperalimentation
  —Decreased insulin: caused by excess catecholamines during periods of physiological stress, such as serious infections, burns, trauma, pancreatitis, myocardial ischemia, pulmonary emboli, CVA, GI bleeding, or as side effect of common medications such as β-blockers, dilantin, and diazoxide
  —Impaired peripheral action of insulin as with Type 2 diabetes, exogenous steroids
  —Decrease in patient's ability to keep up with fluid loss: particularly in older debilitated patients, altered mental status, and those with impaired thirst
  —Increased renal glucose threshold with renal insufficiency
  —Impaired renal elimination of glucose—use of thiazide diuretics

PEDIATRIC CONSIDERATIONS

- Rare in childhood

Pre-Hospital

CAUTIONS

- Avoid routine use of D50W in all cases of altered mental state without first performing a fingerstick glucose check
  —Exacerbates the hyperosmolar state

Diagnosis

ESSENTIAL WORKUP

- Diagnostic criteria
  —Serum glucose ≥600 mg/dl (usually >1000 mg/dl)
  —Absence of ketosis—acetest ≤2+, pH ≥7.3
  —Increased serum osmolarity
    ->350 Osm/L or
    -≥320 Osm/L with at least mild disturbance in mentation

LABORATORY

- Electrolytes
  —Initially elevated levels of K^+ found even in presence of total body deficit due to shift from intracellular space to extracellular space
  —Mild anion gap metabolic acidosis due to lactic acid, β-hydroxybutyric acid or renal insufficiency
  —Increased sodium—must correct for hyperglycemia (raise Na1 by 1.6 for each 100 mg/dl of glucose over 100)
- BUN, Cr
  —Azotemia with elevated BUN/Cr ratio due to prerenal and renal causes
- ABG to rapidly determine pH
- Serum osmolarity = 2 ×Na^+ glucose/18 + BUN/2.8
- CBC
  —Leukocytosis
  —Increased Hct due to hemoconcentration
- Amylase
  —Pancreatitis common
- Urinalysis
  —Check for ketones/glucose
  —Assess renal function
  —Investigate for UTI
- Magnesium, phosphate
- Blood cultures if febrile

IMAGING/SPECIAL TESTS

- EKG for ischemia or infarction
- CXR to check for pneumonia, the most common precipitant
- Head CT (noncontrast-enhanced) indicated if comatose or with a focal neuro deficit

DIFFERENTIAL DIAGNOSIS

- Differentiate from DKA
  —If acidosis present: determine if from ketosis (DKA) or from lactate (hypoperfusion, sepsis, or postictal)

Treatment

INITIAL STABILIZATION

- ABCs
  - —Secure airway in comatose patients
  - —Place on cardiac monitor
  - —Naloxane, thiamine, and Accucheck glucose for coma of unknown etiology
- Restore hemodynamic stability with IV fluids
  - —0.9%NS 1–2 L over the first hour
  - —Larger volumes of fluid may be needed to normalize the vital signs and establish urine output

ED TREATMENT

General Strategy

- Frequent reassessment of volume status and mental status
- Electrolyte assessment difficult
  - —Serum levels of Na^+, K^+, PO_4^- do not accurately reflect the total body solute deficits, nor the intracellular environment
  - —Repeat $Na^+$and K^+ levels to determine replacement therapy
- Search for a precipitating illness

Fluids

- Once hemodynamic stability is restored, the fluid should be switched to 0.45%NS
- Replace 50% of the predicted volume deficit within the first 12 hours
  - —Average deficit is = 9 L
- Lower the serum glucose no faster than 100–200 mg/dl each hour

Potassium

- Anticipate hypokalemia
  - —Total body deficit of approximately 5–10 mEq/kg body weight (replace over 3 days)
- Begin potassium repletion as soon as urine output is established
  - —If the initial K^+ is normal (3.5–5.5 mEq/l) give 20–30 mEq KCl in the first liter of fluids, then give 20 mEq/hr
  - —If the initial K^+ is low ($\leq$3.5 mEq/l), begin 40 mEq KCl/hr and avoid insulin
- Follow repeat serum K^+ levels every 1–2 hours and adjust treatment accordingly

Insulin

- Begin insulin only after restoring hemodynamic stability and after instituting K^+ replacement
- Earlier use of insulin may cause rapid correction of hyperglycemia with collapse of the intravascular space, hypotension, and shock. Overzealous use of insulin can contribute to unnecessary morbidity

Other Electrolyte Replacement

- Phosphate
  - —Supplement if phosphorous level <1 mg/dl
  - —Potassium phosphate 20 mEq/L IV fluid with concomitant potassium depletion
- Magnesium
  - —0.35 mEq/kg magnesium in fluids for first 3–4 hours (= 2.5–3.0 g $MgSO_4$ in 70-kg patient)

Pitfalls to Avoid

- Too rapid correction of glucose—may lead to hypotension
- Continuing isotonic fluids after volume resuscitation—may lead to hypernatremia
- Continuing hypotonic fluids without frequent electrolytes—may lead to cellular edema, cerebral edema
- Failure to prevent hypokalemia: respiratory depression, dysrhythmias
- Avoid dilantin in the event of seizure activity
  - —Inhibits the endogenous release of insulin

MEDICATIONS

- D50W: 1 amp
- Insulin: begin with 0.05–0.1 IU/kg/hr, modify after assessing clinical response
- $MgSO_4$ (magnesium sulfate): 50% (5 g/10 ml; dilute to at least 20% before IV use)
- Narcan: 2 mg (peds: 0.1 mg/kg) IVP
- Potassium phosphate: phosphates 3 mmol/ml and potassium 4.4 mEq/ml
- Thiamine: 100 mg (peds: 10–25 mg) IVP

Disposition

ADMISSION CRITERIA

- All but the mildest cases should be admitted to ICU
  - —Frequent serial labs for the first 24 hours
  - —Rapid shifts in fluids and electrolytes and the potential for deterioration in mental status and arrhythmias mandate close monitoring
- Mild cases may be managed in an observation unit over 12–24 hours

DISCHARGE CRITERIA

- Patients meeting the diagnostic criteria for hyperosmolar syndrome should not be discharged
- Mild hyperglycemia with mild volume deficits and normal serum osmolarity can be discharged after hydration and correction of hyperglycemia

Miscellaneous

ICD9: 276.0

CORE CONTENT CODE: 4.4.1.2

SUGGESTED READINGS

Levine SN, Sanson TH. Treatment of hyperglycemic hyperosmolar non-latotic syndrome.Drugs 1989;38(3):462–472.

Lorber D. Nonketotic hypertonicity in diabetes mellitus. Med Clin North Am 1995;79(1):39–52.

Pope DW, Dansky D. Hyperosmolar hyperglycemic nonketotic coma. Emerg Med Clin North Am 1989;7(4):849–857.

Umpierrez GE, et al. Review: Diabetic ketoacidosis and hyperglycemia hyperosmolar nonketotic syndrome. Am J Med Sci 1996;311(5):225–33.

Author: Karen Cosby

Hyperparathyroidism

Clinical Presentation

SIGNS AND SYMPTOMS

- Dehydration
- Depend upon the severity and rapidity of hypercalcemia
- Cardiac
  - —Hypertension (even in the face of dehydration)
  - —Cardiac conduction abnormalities (*not* proportional to degree of hypercalcemia)
    - -Bradyrhythmia
    - -Bundle branch blocks
    - -Complete heart block
    - -Asystole
    - -Short QT interval
    - -Potentiation of digitalis effects
- Neurologic
  - —Headaches
  - —Decreased reflexes
  - —Proximal muscle weakness
  - —Dementia
  - —Lethargy
  - —Coma
- Psychiatric
  - —Personality changes
  - —Depression
  - —Inability to concentrate
  - —Anxiety
  - —Psychosis
- GI
  - —Anorexia, nausea, vomiting
  - —Constipation
  - —Peptic ulcer disease
  - —Pancreatitis
- General
  - —Fatigue
  - —Weight loss
  - —Polyuria and polydipsia
- Musculoskeletal
  - —Gout/pseudogout
  - —Bone pain, bone cysts (osteitis cystica)
  - —Arthralgias
  - —Chondrocalcinosis
- Renal
  - —Kidney stones
  - —Nephrocalcinosis
  - —Decreased renal concentrating ability

Hypercalcemic Crisis

- Anorexia
- Nausea, vomiting
- Mental obtundation

MECHANISM/DESCRIPTION

- Parathyroid hormone (PTH) actions
  - —Decreases urinary Ca^{++} loss
  - —Increases urinary PO_4^{-2} loss
  - —Stimulates vitamin D conversion from 25 (OH)-D to 1,25 $(OH)_2$-D in kidney
  - —Liberates Ca^{++} and PO_4^{-2} from bone
- Magnesium
  - —Cofactor in production of PTH
  - —Essential for action of PTH in target tissues
  - —Hypercalcuria produces increased magnesium losses in urine

ETIOLOGY

- Excess secretion of PTH due to
  - —Primary hyperparathyroidism
    - -Adenoma 85%
    - -Hyperplasia 14%
    - -Carcinoma <1%
  - —Secondary hyperparathyroidism
    - -Response to decreased formation of 1,25 dihydroxycholecalciferol by kidney and decreased renal phosphate excretion
  - —Tertiary hyperparathyroidism
    - -Onset of autonomous parathyroid function following prolonged secondary hyperparathyroidism

PEDIATRIC CONSIDERATIONS

- Hypotonia, weakness, and listlessness
- May present as critically ill infant with calcium as high as 25 mg/dl
- Mid-teens presentation with nonspecific symptoms of hypercalcemia
- Associated with Multiple Endocrine Neoplasia Syndromes I and II
- Newborns following delivery to hypoparathyroid mothers
- Hypercalcemic infants present with
  - —Broad forehead
  - —Epicanthal folds
  - —Underdeveloped nasal bridge
  - —Prominent upper lip
  - —Mental retardation

Pre-Hospital

CAUTIONS

- May present as a primarily psychiatric disorder

Diagnosis

ESSENTIAL WORKUP

- Calcium level
  - —Elevated albumin—falsely elevated calcium level
  - —Low albumin—falsely lowered calcium level
- Evaluate for symptoms of hypercalcemia especially impending parathyroid storm
- Review history for medication ingestion. (See differential diagnosis)
- No further workup except follow-up if
  - —Asymptomatic
  - —Normal EKG
  - —Calcium level <13 g/dl
- If symptomatic or calcium level >13 mg/dl check
  - —CXR
  - —Phosphorus
  - —Albumin
  - —Electrolytes, BUN, creatinine
  - —Sed rate
  - —Alkaline phosphatase
  - —Magnesium
  - —TSH
  - —CBC

LABORATORY

- Calcium correction for albumin
  - —Corrected Ca^{++} (mg/dl) = measured Ca^{++} (mg/dl) + .8 (4.0 − albumin (g/dl))
  - —Acidosis
    - -Shifts binding to albumin—increases ionized (metabolically active) Ca^{++}
    - -Decrease of 0.1 pH Unit increases the ionized Ca^{++} by 3–8%
- Phosphorus
  - —Low in primary hyperparathyroidism
  - —Variable in secondary hyperparathyroidism
  - —Normal or high in malignancy related hypercalcemia
- Chloride /PO_4^{-2} ratio
  - —>33 hyperparathyroidism
  - —<30 malignancy
- Alkaline phosphatase
  - —Increased in 50% of patients with hyperparathyroidism
  - —Normal with vitamin D excess
- ESR
  - —Normal in hyperparathyroidism
  - —Elevated in malignancy or granulomatous diseases
- Anemia
  - —Present with malignancy or granulomatous disease
  - —Absent in hyperparathyroidism
- Magnesium
  - —Low or low normal
- Parathyroid hormone (PTH)
  - —Elevated in primary and secondary hyperparathyroidism

- Parathyroid hormone related peptide
  - —Secreted by squamous cell carcinomas of lung, head, neck; renal carcinomas, bladder carcinomas, adenocarcinomas, and lymphomas

IMAGING/SPECIAL TESTS

- CXR—granulomatous disease or malignancy
- Hand radiograph
  - —Subperiosteal bone resorption in hyperparathyroidism

DIFFERENTIAL DIAGNOSIS

Causes of Hypercalcemia

- Parathyroid hormone related
  - —Primary or secondary hyperparathyroidism
  - —Familial hypocalciuric hypercalcemia
  - —Tumor secreting parathyroid hormone
- Malignancy related
  - —Parathyroid hormone-related peptide or Ca^{++} release from osteolytic tumor
- Vitamin D related
  - —Excess vitamin D intake or vitamin D production by granulomas
- Immobilization—associated with Paget's disease
- Drug induced
  - —Thiazide diuretics
  - —Lithium
  - —Vitamin D
  - —Aluminum-containing antacids
  - —Tamoxifen
  - —Estrogens
  - —Androgens
  - —Vitamin A

Treatment

INITIAL STABILIZATION

- Cardiac monitor for
  - —Symptoms of hypercalcemia
  - —Ca^{++} level >14 mg/dl
- Hydration with IV 0.9%NS

ED TREATMENT

- Treat hypercalcemia
  - —Vigorous hydration with 0.9%NS at minimum of 250 ml/hr
    - -Lowers calcium 1.5–2.0 mg/dl in 24 hours
    - -Achieve urine output 100 ml/hr
  - —Administer furosemide or other loop diuretic (calciuric) after adequate volume replacement or in presence of CHF
    - -Common error: administration of furosemide before adequate hydration. If urinary sodium losses exceed replacement sodium, then renal conservation measures retard calcium excretion
  - —Avoid thiazide diuretics (retard calcium excretion)
  - —Consider steroid administration (prednisone/hydrocortisone)
    - -Decreases gut absorption and increases renal excretion of Ca^{++}
    - -Most effective with vitamin D intoxication or granulomatous diseases
  - —Administer calcitonin if poor response to saline diuresis
  - —Poor response to mithramycin with hyperparathyroid induced hypercalcemia
  - —Start biphosphonates (etidronate) in conjunction with primary physician
    - -Inhibits calcium mobilization from bone
- Treatment of cardiac dysrhythmias
- Determine the etiology of the hypercalcemia
- Stop all medications that may contribute to hypercalcemia
- Extreme caution in use of digoxin
- Anticipate CHF and electrolyte imbalance with frequent reassessment of patient and monitoring of serum electrolytes and magnesium levels
- Emergent dialysis with renal failure

MEDICATIONS

- Calcitonin: 4–8 IU/kg SQ q 6 hr
- Etidronate (didronel): 7.5 mg/kg in 250 ml 0.9%NS over 2 hrs
- Furosemide: 20–80 mg IV after assurance of adequate hydration
- Hydrocortisone: 100 mg (peds: 1–2 mg/kg) IV
- Prednisone: 40–80 mg po

Dispostion

ADMISSION CRITERIA

- Calcium >14 mg/dl
- Symptomatic hypercalcemia
- Evidence of abnormal cardiac rhythm or conduction

DISCHARGE CRITERIA

- Able to maintain adequate hydration

Miscellaneous

ICD9: 252.0, 259.3, 588.8

CORE CONTENT CODE: 4.6

SUGGESTED READINGS

Andreoli T, et al. Cecil's essentials of medicine. 4th ed. Philadelphia: WB Saunders, 1997.

Edelson GW, Kleerekoper M. Hypercalcemic crisis. Med Clin North Am 1995;79:79–92.

Fleisher G, Ludwig S. Textbook of pediatric emergency medicine. 3rd ed. Baltimore: Williams & Wilkins, 1993.

Fromm RE Jr. Hypercalcemia complicating an industrial near drowning. Ann Emerg Med 1991;20:669–671.

Minisola S, et al. Parathyroid storm: Immediate recognition and pathophysiological considerations. Bone 1993;14:703–706.

Noble J, ed. Textbook of primary care medicine. 2d ed. St. Louis: CV Mosby, 1996.

Olinger ML. Disorders of calcium and magnesium. Emerg Med Clin North Am 1989;7:795–822.

Author: Hugh Schuckman

Hypertension

Clinical Presentation

SIGNS AND SYMPTOMS

- Mild to moderate hypertension are asymptomatic until end-organ damage occurs

Neurologic

- Headache
- Nausea
- Vomiting
- Visual disturbances
- Confusion
- Seizures
- Physical findings
  —Focal neurologic deficits
  —Papilledema

Cardiovascular

- Chest pain
- Dyspnea
- Acute aortic dissection
  —Severe tearing chest pain
  —Pulse deficit
  —New murmur of aortic insufficiency
  —Pericardial friction rub
- Left ventricular dysfunction
  —Rales
  —Third heart sound
  —Jugular venous distension
  —Tachycardia
- Renal involvement suggested by nonspecific symptoms
  —Weakness
  —Pedal edema
  —Oliguria
  —Hematuria

MECHANISM/DESCRIPTION

- More than 15% of the adult population in the United States has an elevated blood pressure
- Higher percentage among African-Americans and in older age groups

Definitions

- Hypertension definition
  —Systolic BP >140 mm Hg or diastolic pressure >90 mm Hg
- Hypertensive emergency
  —Systolic BP higher than 200 mm Hg or diastolic BP higher than 120 mm Hg, with new or progressive end-organ damage of the neurologic, cardiovascular, or renal system
- Hypertensive urgency
  —Severe hypertension without evidence of end-organ damage

ETIOLOGY

- Predisposing factors to hypertensive emergencies and urgencies
  —Central nervous system abnormalities
    -Subarachnoid hemorrhage
    -Intracranial hemorrhage
    -Thrombotic infarction
    -Encephalopathy
    -Head trauma
    -Transient ischemic attacks
  —Cardiovascular abnormalities
    -Acute coronary insufficiency
    -Acute aortic dissection
    -Accelerated hypertension
    -Acute heart failure
    -Myocardial infarction
    -Unstable angina
  —Renal system abnormalities
    -Acute renal insufficiency
    -Acute glomerulonephritis
  —Excessive catecholamine states
    -Pheochromocytoma crisis
    -Monoamine oxidase inhibitor interactions
    -Antihypertensive medication withdrawal
  —Pregnancy—preeclampsia
  —Drugs
    -Cocaine
    -Amphetamines
    -Oral contraceptives
    -Corticosteroids
  —Toxin
    -Heavy metal (lead)

Pre-Hospital

CAUTIONS

- ABCs
- IV access
- O_2 therapy
- Cardiac monitoring
- Pulse oximetry
- Patients with respiratory compromise require intubation

Diagnosis

ESSENTIAL WORKUP

- Determine blood pressure in both arms and legs
- Take repeated measurements to ensure accuracy and sustained hypertension
- ECG for myocardial ischemia/infarction or hyperkalemia

LABORATORY

- CBC for microangiopathic hemolytic anemia seen in malignant hypertension
- Electrolytes, BUN/Cr, glucose for renal failure
- Urinalysis for microscopic hematuria or large proteinuria—evidence of acute compromise
- Red cell casts suggest glomerulonephritis

IMAGING/SPECIAL TESTS

- CXR for
  —Cardiomegaly
  —Pulmonary edema
  —Wide mediastinum suggesting aortic aneurysm
- CT scan of head for
  —intracranial hemorrhage
  —Stroke
  —Encephalopathy
- Echocardiography, CT scan, or angiography to detect aortic dissection

DIFFERENTIAL DIAGNOSIS

- Pseudohypertensive emergencies can be caused by
  —Hypoxia
  —Hypercarbia
  —Hypoglycemia

Treatment

INITIAL STABILIZATION

- Scrupulously monitor BP with noninvasive blood pressure monitor or arterial line
- Intubation for intracranial abnormalities that alter respiratory status

ED TREATMENT

Hypertensive Emergency

- Goals
  - —Decrease BP while maintaining organ perfusion
  - —Lower mean arterial pressure by approximately 20%, depending on patients underlying condition and previous BP measurements

Medications

- Sodium nitroprusside (NTP)
  - —"Gold standard" for treatment of most hypertensive emergencies
  - —Easily titratable
  - —Requires meticulous BP monitoring
- Labetalol
  - —α- and β-adrenoreceptor blocker
  - —Contraindicated in patients with bronchospasm, severe sinus bradycardia, heart block, or congestive heart failure
- Nicardipine hydrochloride
  - —Calcium channel blocking agent
- Esmolol
  - —May be combined with nitroprusside to abrogate reflex tachycardia
  - —Short half-life advantageous
  - —Contraindicated in patients with bronchospasm, severe sinus bradycardia, heart block, or congestive heart failure

Hypertensive Urgency

- No need to lower BP in ED acutely
- Initiate oral antihypertensive medications in ED or as outpatient with close followup

MEDICATIONS

- Nitroprusside IV infusion: initiate at 0.5 μg/kg/min; titrate to response
- Labetalol IV bolus: 20 mg or 1–2 mg/kg (whichever is lower) over 2 min; if no response after 10 min, additional doses in increments of 20, 40, or 80 mg to total of 300 mg
- Nicardipine IV load: 5–15 mg/hr (safety not known in pediatrics)
- Esmolol IV load: 500 μg/kg over 1 min; infusion at 50–100 μg/kg/min

Disposition

ADMISSION CRITERIA

- New signs of end-organ damage
- ICU admission for
  - —Hepatic encephalopathy
  - —Myocardial ischemia
  - —Pulmonary edema
  - —Patients requiring closely monitored BP (i.e., on nitroprusside)

DISCHARGE CRITERIA

- No signs of end-organ damage
- Close followup

Miscellaneous

ICD9: 401.9

CORE CONTENT CODE: 2.8.2

SUGGESTED READINGS

Murphy C. Hypertensive emergencies. Emerg Med Clin North Am 1995;13(4):973–1007.

Thach AM, Schultz PJ. Nonemergent hypertension: New perspectives for the emergency medicine physician. Emerg Med Clin North Am 1995;13(4):1009–1035.

Author: Kenneth H. Butler

Hypertensive Emergencies

Clinical Presentation

SIGNS AND SYMPTOMS

- Malignant hypertension
  - —Headache
  - —Visual changes
  - —Nocturia
  - —Weakness
  - —Chest pain
  - —Dyspnea
  - —Funduscopic abnormalities
  - —Papilledema (most common finding)
  - —Retinal flame hemorrhages
  - —Soft exudates
- Hypertensive encephalopathy
  - —Headaches
  - —Nausea
  - —Vomiting
  - —Visual changes
  - —Confusion
  - —Weakness
  - —Disorientation
  - —Altered mental status
  - —Papilledema
  - —Focal weakness
  - —Seizures

MECHANISM/DESCRIPTION

- A severe elevation in blood pressure
  - —Diastolic pressure of greater than 140 mm Hg
    - -Acute progressive end-organ damage
- Abrupt increase in systemic vascular resistance
  - —Increase in circulating vasoconstrictors
    - -Norepinephrine
    - -Angiotensin II
  - —Arteriolar fibrinoid necrosis
  - —Endothelial damage
  - —Platelet and fibrin deposition
  - —Loss of autoregulation of blood flow
  - —End-organ ischemia
    - -Prompts the renewed release of vasoconstrictors
    - -Triggers a vicious cycle
  - —2% of hypertensive patients will have a hypertensive emergency
  - —Malignant hypertension
    - -Young black men
    - -Underlying renal disease

ETIOLOGY

- Central nervous system abnormalities
  - —Subarachnoid hemorrhage
  - —Intracranial hemorrhage
  - —Thrombotic infarction
  - —Encephalopathy
  - —Head trauma
  - —Transient ischemic attacks
- Cardiovascular abnormalities
  - —Acute coronary insufficiency
  - —Acute aortic dissection
  - —Accelerated hypertension
  - —Acute heart failure
  - —Myocardial infarction
  - —Unstable angina
- Renal system abnormalities
  - —Acute renal insufficiency
  - —Acute glomerulonephritis
- Excessive catecholamine states
  - —Pheochromocytoma
  - —Adrenocortice tumors
  - —Monoamine oxidase inhibitor interactions
- Antihypertensive medication withdrawal
- Pregnancy-induced hypertension
- Preeclampsia
- Drugs
  - —Cocaine
  - —Amphetamines
  - —Oral contraceptives
  - —Corticosteroids
  - —Toxins
  - —Heavy metals

Pre-Hospital

CAUTIONS

- Intravenous access
- Cardiac monitoring
- Pulse oximetry
- Oxygen administration
- Twelve lead electrocardiography (ECG) when available
- Follow standard pre-hospital protocols
  - —Chest pain
  - —Congestive heart failure

Diagnosis

ESSENTIAL WORKUP

- Exclusion of other causes of severe symptomatic hypertension

LABORATORY

- BUN, creatinine
  - —Acute elevation if renal damage
- Serum electrolytes
- Urinalysis
  - —Proteinuria and casts

IMAGING/SPECIAL TESTS

- EKG
  - —Assess for myocardial ischemia
- Intra-arterial line
  - —Continuous blood pressure monitoring during initial treatment
- Head CT
  - —Exclude subarachnoid and intracerebral hemorrhage
- Lumbar puncture
  - —Exclude subarachnoid hemorrhage
  - —When CT is negative

DIFFERENTIAL DIAGNOSIS

- Subarachnoid hemorrhage
- Intracerebral hemorrhage
- Cerebral infarction
- Acute myocardial ischemia
- Acute myocardial infarction
- Acute pulmonary edema
- Aortic dissection
- Preeclampsia/eclampsia
- Withdrawal syndromes
  - —β-Blockers
  - —Central acting antihypertensive agents (e.g., clonidine)
- States of catecholamine excess
  - —Pheochromocytoma
  - —Cocaine/sympathomimetic drug intoxication
  - —Tyramine ingestion in patients on monoamine oxidase inhibitors

Treatment

INITIAL STABILIZATION

- Cardiac monitoring
- Pulse oximetry
- Oxygen administration
- Intravenous access
- Anti-ischemic therapy
  - —With signs of acute myocardial ischemia or infarction

ED TREATMENT

Goals of Parenteral Antihypertensive Therapy

- Reduce the mean arterial pressure by 25%
- Decrease the diastolic blood pressure to 100–110 mm Hg
  - —The reduction should occur over several minutes to hours
  - —More gradual reduction in certain settings
    - -Long history of poorly controlled hypertension
    - -Acute ongoing injury to the central nervous system
    - -Cardiac involvement
  - —Further blood pressure reduction should be avoided in the ED

Nitroprusside

- Potent vasodilator
- Immediate onset
- Brief (2–3 minutes) duration of action
- Indications
  - —First-line agent
  - —Malignant hypertension
  - —Hypertensive encephalopathy
  - —Aortic dissection
    - -Administer concomitantly with β-blockers to reduce aortic wall stress and eliminate reflex tachycardia caused by nitroprusside
- Complications
  - —Hypotension
  - —Nausea and vomiting
  - —Reflex tachycardia
- Contraindications
  - —Pregnancy

Labetalol

- A combined α- and β-blocker
- Onset of action of 5–10 minutes
- 3-6-hour duration of action
- Does not cause reflex tachycardia
- Easily converted to oral therapy
- Indications
  - —Acceptable alternative to nitroprusside
  - —All hypertensive emergencies
- Contraindications
  - —To β blockers

Diazoxide

- A smooth-muscle relaxant
- Indications
  - —Hypertensive encephalopathy
  - —Malignant hypertension
  - —Pregnancy induced hypertension
  - —Preeclampsia/eclampsia
- Complications
  - —Reflex sympathetic stimulation
- Contraindications
  - —Aortic dissection
  - —Acute myocardial ischemia

Phentolamine

- α-Blocker
- Agent of choice in states of catecholamine excess
- Indications
  - —Pheochromocytoma
  - —MAO inhibitor reactions
  - —Stimulant abuse
  - —Antihypertensive drug withdrawal states
- Caution
  - —β Blockers should be avoided in states of catecholamine excess
  - —Only after α blockade
  - —Only for tachydysrhythmias

Second-Line Agents

- Trimethaphan camsylate
  - —A ganglionic blocker
  - —Lowers aortic wall stress
  - —Indicated in aortic dissection
- Nicardipine
  - —Intravenous calcium channel blocker
- Enalapril
  - —An intravenous angiotensin-converting enzyme inhibitor
  - —Useful in patients with high renin states
  - —Congestive heart failure
- Hydralazine
  - —Eclampsia
- Nitroglycerin
  - —Myocardial ischemia
  - —Heart failure

MEDICATIONS

- Diazoxide: 50–100 mg IV q 5–10 min or 10–30 mg/min IV infusion
- Enalapril: 1.25–5 mg q 6 hrs
- Hydralazine: 5–10 mg IV or IM q 20 min up to 20 mg
- Labetalol: 20–80 mg IV q 5–10 min or 0.5–2.0 mg/kg IV infusion
- Nicardipine: 5–15 mg/hr IV infusion
- Nitroglycerin: 5–200 μg/min IV infusion
- Nitroprusside: 0.2–0.5 μg/kg/min initial IV; infusion up to 8–10 μg/kg/min
- Phentolamine: 5–10 mg IV q 5–15 min
- Trimethaphan: 1–15 mg/min IV infusion

Disposition

ADMISSION CRITERIA

- All patients hypertensive emergencies
  - —Signs of end organ damage
  - —Intensive care unit for cardiac and blood pressure monitoring

DISCHARGE CRITERIA: N/A

- Hypertensive urgencies
  - —Absence of ocular, cardiac, or renal damage
- Instruct to return with chest pain or headache

Miscellaneous

ICD9: 401.0, 401.1, 401.9

CORE CONTENT CODE: 2.8.1

SUGGESTED READINGS

Abdelwahab W, Frishman W, Landau A. Management of hypertensive urgencies and emergencies. J Clin Pharmacol 1995;35:747–762.

Calhoun DA, Oparil S. Treatment of hypertensive crisis. N Engl J Med 1990;323:1177–1183.

Houston M. Hypertensive emergencies and urgencies: Pathophysiology and clinical aspects. Am Heart J 1986;111:205–210.

Rubenstein EB, Escalante C. Hypertensive crisis. Crit Care Clin 1989;5:477–495.

Author: David M. Brown

Hyperthermia

Clinical Presentation

SIGNS AND SYMPTOMS

Heat Stroke

- Core temp: >105°F
- CNS: severe confusion/lethargy, coma, seizure, ataxia, or focal deficits
- CV: tachycardia, hypotension
- Pulmonary: tachypnea
- GI: nausea, vomiting, diarrhea
- Skin: in most cases dry and hot
- Acute oliguric renal failure due to rhabdomyolysis/dehydration
- Hepatic failure

Heat Exhaustion

- Core temp: <104°F
- CNS: headache, fatigue, malaise, confusion, agitation
- CV: mild tachycardia, dehydration
- Pulmonary: tachypnea
- GI: nausea, vomiting

Heat Cramps

- Cramps in heavily exercised muscles
- During or after exercise
- Primarily in lower extremities

Heat Tetany

- Carpal-pedal spasm—secondary to hyperventilation

Heat Edema

- Swelling of dependent areas of body
- Resolves after acclimatization

MECHANISM/DESCRIPTION

- Continuum of increasingly severe illnesses secondary to overwhelming heat stress
- Begins with dehydration and electrolyte abnormalities and progresses to thermoregulatory dysfunction and multisystem organ failure

Heat Stroke

- Loss of thermoregulatory function, severe CNS dysfunction, and multisystem organ failure
- Classic heat stroke
  - —Occurs in those with compromised homeostatic mechanisms (elderly, debilitated)
  - —Develops over days to weeks
  - —Severe dehydration
- Exertional heat stroke
  - —Occurs in younger, athletic individuals with a combined environmental and exertional heat stress
  - —Develops over hours
  - —Internal heat production overwhelms dissipating mechanisms
  - —May be sweating

Heat Exhaustion

- Fluid and electrolyte depletion
- Thermoregulatory function is maintained

Heat Cramps

- Secondary to excessive sweating and sodium loss

ETIOLOGY

- Circulatory insufficiency
  - —Age extremes
  - —Dehydration
  - —CHF
  - —Obesity
  - —Diuretics
  - —Laxatives
- Pharmacologic causes
  - —Sympathomimetics
  - —LSD
  - —MAO inhibitors
  - —PCP
  - —Anticholinergics
  - —Antihistamines
  - —Drug or alcohol withdrawal
- Excessive heat load
  - —Environmental
  - —Fever
  - —Exertional
  - —Lack of acclimatization
- Decreased cardiovascular function
  - —β-Blockers
  - —Sympatholytics

PEDIATRIC CONSIDERATIONS

- Children are at increased risk of heat illness due to increased body surface area to mass ratio

Pre-Hospital

CAUTIONS

- Institute cooling measures for severe heat illness
  - —Remove from heat stress
  - —Disrobe patient
  - —Ice packs to axilla, groin, and neck
  - —Cover body with wet sheet
- IV 0.9%NS 500 cc fluid bolus if hypotensive
- If altered mental status: glucose (or Accucheck), thiamine, naloxone

Diagnosis

ESSENTIAL WORKUP

- Accurate core temperature
- Obtain history of heat exposure
- Heat exhaustion—diagnosis by exclusion of other causes

LABORATORY

For Heat Stroke and Heat Exhaustion

- CBC
  —Leukocytosis might point toward infection
- Electrolytes, BUN, Cr, glucose
  —Hypernatremia with severe dehydration
  —Acute renal failure
- UA
  —Myoglobin present in rhabdomyolysis
  —Bacteria/WBC

For Heat Stroke

- Liver function tests
  —Hepatic necrosis
- PT/PTT/DIC panel
  —Clotting abnormalities

IMAGING/SPECIAL TESTS

- EKG indicated in elderly or at cardiac risk
- CT head for altered mental status
- CXR for ARDS, aspiration pneumonia

DIFFERENTIAL DIAGNOSIS

Febrile illness/sepsis

- Thyroid storm
- Pheochromocytoma
- Malignant hyperthermia
- Cocaine
- PCP
- Anticholinergics
- MAO inhibitors
- Meningitis
- Encephalitis
- Cerebral falciparum malaria
- Delirium tremens

Treatment

INITIAL STABILIZATION

- ABCs
- Immediate/rapid cooling if temperature >40°C

ED MANAGEMENT

Cooling Measures

- Initiate for body temperature >40°C
- Evaporative
  —Extremely effective (0.05–0.3°C/min)
  —Spray disrobed patient with fine mist of warm water (prevents shivering)
  —Airflow with fans blow over patient
- Conductive
  —Ice packs to groin/axilla—combine with evaporative adjunctive treatment above
  —Iced or cold water immersion—very effective but impractical
- Iced peritoneal lavage and cardiopulmonary bypass for refractory cases
- To avoid hypothermia stop cooling therapy at 39°C

Supportive Measures

- Rehydration for heat stroke/heat exhaustion
  —Initial rehydration with 0.5–1.0 L 0.9%NS
  —Avoid overhydration may contribute to development of ARDS
  —Peds: 20 cc/kg bolus
- Glucose/naloxone/thiamine for altered mental status
- Chlorpromazine to stop shivering
- Benzodiazepine for seizure
- Analgesics and oral or IV hydration with electrolyte containing fluid for heat cramps
- Reassurance/calming measures/rebreathing in closed system (bag or nonrebreather without oxygen) for hyperventilation heat tetany
- Lower extremity elevation/removal from heat stress for heat edema

MEDICATIONS

- Chlorpromazine: 25–50 mg IV push (pediatric use not documented)
- Dextrose: 50–100 cc D50 (peds: 2 cc/kg of D25W over 1 min) IV
- Diazepam (benzodiazepine): 5–10 mg (peds: 0.2–0.4 mg/kg) IV push
- Nalaxone (narcan): 2 mg (peds: 0.1 mg/kg) IV

Disposition

ADMISSION CRITERIA

- Heat stroke to the ICU
- Heat exhaustion
  —Severe electrolyte abnormalities
  —Renal failure/evidence of rhabdomyolysis
  —Elderly

DISCHARGE CRITERIA

- All patients except those with heat stroke or severe heat stroke may be discharged

Miscellaneous

ICD9: 780.6

CORE CONTENT CODE: 5.9.1

SUGGESTED READINGS

Lee-Chiong TL, Stitt JT. Heat stroke and other heat-related illnesses. Postgrad Med 1995;98(1):26–36.

Simon HB. Hyperthermia. New Engl J Med 1993;329(7):483–487.

Tek D, Olshaker J. Heat illness. Emerg Med Clin North Am 1992;10(2):299–310.

Author: Charles Everly

Hyperthyroidism

Clinical Presentation

SIGNS AND SYMPTOMS

- Reflect end organ responsiveness to thyroid hormone

Symptoms

- Weight loss
- Palpitations
- Dyspnea
- Chest pain
- Weakness
- Diarrhea
- Abdominal pain
- Myalgia
- Nervousness
- Heat intolerance

Signs

- Fever
- Tachycardia disproportional to fever
- CHF
- Wide pulse pressure
- Thyromegaly
- Shock
- Jaundice
- Tremor
- Disorientation
- Psychosis
- Coma
- Tender liver
- Thyrotoxic stare

Apathetic hyperthyroidism

- Seen in the elderly
- Due to multinodular goiter
- Subtle clinical findings
  - —Often reflecting single organ dysfunction (CHF)
  - —Weight loss
  - —Depressed mentation
  - —Tremor
  - —Hyperactivity

MECHANISM/DESCRIPTION

- Excessive thyroid function results in continuum of disease
  - —Mild hyperthyroidism
  - —Thyrotoxicosis
  - —Thyroid storm or thyrotoxic crisis with life-threatening manifestations
- 1–2% of patients with hyperthyroidism progress to thyroid storm

ETIOLOGY

- Toxic diffuse goiter (Graves' disease)
- Toxic multinodular or uninodular goiter
- Factitious thyrotoxicosis
- T_3 toxicosis
- Hashimoto's thyroiditis
- Malignancy
- Hypothalamic hyperthyroidism
- TSH-producing pituitary tumor

Pre-Hospital

N/A

Diagnosis

- Laboratory confirmation of the diagnosis usually not possible in the ED
  - —Strong clinical picture should prompt initiation of therapy
- Thyroid storm–exaggerated signs and symptoms of thyrotoxicosis
  - —Goiter
  - —Extreme tachycardia
  - —Hyperpyrexia
- Disorientation and mental status changes common

ESSENTIAL WORKUP

- Thyroid function tests for
  - —Elderly patient with new onset CHF
  - —New AFib/SVT
- Free T_4
  - —If free T_4 is unavailable, total T_4 and resin T_3 uptake
- TSH
- ECG
  - —Tachydysrhythmias
  - —Atrial fibrillation
- CBC
  - —Anemia
- Electrolytes, BUN, Cr, glucose
  - —BUN, creatinine 2° dehydration
  - —Hypokalemia
- Calcium
- Liver function tests
- Arterial blood gases for hypoxemia
- Search for the underlying etiology

DIFFERENTIAL DIAGNOSIS

- Pheochromocytoma
- Sepsis
- Sympathomimetic ingestion
- Psychosis

Treatment

INITIAL STABILIZATION

- ABCs
- Cardiac monitor
- Supplemental oxygen to meet metabolic needs
- Initiate cooling measures
  —Avoid aspirin

ED TREATMENT

- Inhibit hormone synthesis using thioamides
  —Propylthiouracil (PTU)
- Block hormone release
  —Potassium iodide or
  —Oral Lugol's solutions or
  —Sodium iodide
  —Administer iodine therapy at least 1 hour after thionamides to prevent organification of the iodine
- Prevent peripheral conversion of T_4 to T_3
  —PTU or
  —Dexamethasone
- Block the peripheral effects of thyroid hormone
  —β Blockade
    -Propranolol
    -Esmolol
    -Contraindicated with CHF, diabetes mellitus, and reactive airway disease
  —When β-blockers contraindicated use
    -Reserpine
    -Guanethidine
- Treatment of thyrotoxicosis 2° thyroiditis consists of
  —β Blockade
  —Anti-inflammatory medications
- General support
  —Acetaminophen for hyperpyrexia (aspirin contraindicated; displaces thyroid hormone from thyroglobulin)
  —Control congestive heart failure
  —Manage dehydration
- Identify and treat the precipitating event

MEDICATIONS

- Dexamethasone: 2 mg (peds: 0.15 mg/kg) IV q 6 hrs
- Esmolol: 500 µg/kg IV over 1 min followed by maintenance dose of 50 µg/kg min IV titrate to effect
- Guanethidine: 10 mg/day initially, then increased to 25–50 mg/day in 3 divided doses
- Lugol's solutions: 30 drops q 12 hrs
- Potassium iodide: 5–10 drops SSKI
- Propranolol: 1–2 mg IV repeated every 10–15 min
- Propylthiouracil (PTU): 300 mg (peds: 5–7 mg/kg/24hrs) q 6 hrs po or per NGT
- Reserpine: 1–5 mg IM every 4–6 hrs up to 15 mg/24hrs
- Sodium iodide: 1 g q 8–12 hrs

Disposition

ADMISSION CRITERIA

- Thyroid storm
- Requiring IV medications to control HR
- Symptomatic patients(tachycardia, fever)

DISCHARGE CRITERIA

- Minimally symptomatic individuals that respond well to oral therapy

Miscellaneous

ICD9: 242.9

CORE CONTENT CODE: 4.9.1

SUGGESTED READINGS

Burch HB, Wartofsky L. Life-threatening thyrotoxicosis. Thyroid storm. Endincrinol Metab Clin North Am 1993;22:263–277.

Holmes L, Lakshmanan M. The patient with chronic endocrine disease. In: Herr RD, Cydulka RK, eds. Emergency care of the compromised patient. Philadelphia: JB Lippincott, 1994:123–133.

Tietgens ST, Leinung MC. Thyroid storm. Med Clin North Am 1995;79;169–184

Toft AD. Thyroxine therapy. N Engl J Med 1994;331:174–180.

Wogan JM. Endocrine disorders. In: Rosen P, et al., eds. Emergency medicine: Concepts and clinical practice. 4th ed. St. Louis: CV Mosby, 1998:2488–2503.

Author: Rita Cydulka

Hypertrophic Cardiomyopathy

Clinical Presentation

SIGNS AND SYMPTOMS

General

- Symptoms correlate with exertion, Valsalva, or suddenly assuming upright position
- Severity depends on the location and degree of ventricular wall thickening

Symptoms

- Shortness of breath
- Dyspnea on exertion
- Exertional or postprandial angina
- Presyncope
- Syncope
- Congestive heart failure (CHF)
- Cardiovascular collapse
- Dysrhythmias
  —Paroxysmal atrial fibrillation (Afib)
    -Often leads to significant, rapid clinical deterioration when present with CHF
  —Supraventricular tachycardia
  —Nonsustained ventricular tachycardia (VT) occurs in young adults
  —Bradydysrhythmias less common
  —Ventricular tachycardia/ventricular fibrillation may lead to sudden death

Signs

- No or subtle physical findings
- Double apical cardiac impulse at the mid to upper sternum
- Loud, left-sided S_4
- Murmur
  —Crescendo-decrescendo midsystolic murmur at the apex
    -Increasing in intensity with Valsalva maneuver or standing up
    -Quieter with recumbency, swatting, or handgrips
  —With more severe obstruction, a more apparent murmur with radiation to the left sternal border
  —Radiation to the axilla if there is associated mitral insufficiency

MECHANISM/DESCRIPTION

- Hypertrophic cardiomyopathy (HCM)
  —Hypertrophied, nondilated left ventricle in the absence of another cause of left ventricular hypertrophy
  —Predominant abnormality identified (one-third of the cases) in young (<35 years old) athletes suffering sudden atraumatic death
  —Occurs in all ages from neonate to elderly
    -Average age of diagnosis is 30–40 years old
- Structural abnormality
  —Irregular marked ventricular wall thickening with disarray of myofibrils in the thickened regions and fibrin deposition
  —Thickening usually asymmetric involving the septum to a greater extent than the free ventricular wall
  —Atrial dilatation

Four Clinical Patterns

- Diastolic dysfunction
  —Due to impaired relaxation, with normal to supranormal systolic function until end-stage disease
    -Accounts for a loud S_4
  —Ultimately leads to atrial overload and dilatation, with associated atrial fibrillation
  —Frequently provokes CHF because of the diastolic filling dependence on atrial contribution
- Ischemia
  —Usually due to phenomena affecting small intramural vessels with normal coronary arteries
- Subaortic obstruction
- Systolic dysfunction

ETIOLOGY

- Autosomal dominant inherited disorder of cardiac muscle with variable phenotypic expression
- Hypertrophied, nondilated left ventricle in the absence of clinical settings can lead to ventricular hypertrophy (systemic hypertension (HTN), aortic stenosis (AS) or "athlete's heart")

PEDIATRIC CONSIDERATIONS

- Prepubescent manifestation is generally much more severe
- Infants present with severe, progressive congestive heart failure
- Marked progression often occurs during the rapid growth years of 12 to 18

Pre-Hospital

CAUTIONS

- Consider HCM in patients who decompensate during standard treatments for CHF, ischemia, or supraventricular tachycardia, and in young athletes who collapse during or just after exertion

Diagnosis

ESSENTIAL WORKUP

- Transthoracic cardiac echo/Doppler establishes the diagnosis of HCM
- Electrocardiogram (ECG) findings
  —Normal in 15% of patients
  —LV hypertrophy with strain
  —Large Q waves or deep inverted T waves, particularly with apical hypertrophy
  —Apical infarction
- Chest radiography findings
  —Normal
  —Bulge along left heart border representing hypertrophy of free wall of left ventricle
  —Right or left atrial enlargement
  —Pulmonary vascular redistribution

IMAGING/SPECIAL TESTS

- Nuclear angiography assesses systolic and diastolic function
- Stress thallium and positron emission tomography evaluates ischemia
- Nuclear magnetic resonance imaging supplements indeterminate echocardiography

DIFFERENTIAL DIAGNOSIS

- Aortic stenosis
- Pulmonic stenosis
- Ventricular septal defect
- Mitral regurgitation
- Mitral valve prolapse
- Arteriosclerotic coronary vascular disease
- Differentiate in patients presenting with CHF or angina
- Conventional therapy for these diagnoses may have catastrophic consequences
- Syncopal or presyncopal episodes
- More ominous in the setting of HCM

Treatment

INITIAL STABILIZATION

- ABCs
- Intravenous catheterization
- Supplemental oxygen
- Cardiac monitor
- Pulse oximetry

ED TREATMENT

- Do *not* place in seated or Fowler's position
  —Patient may need to remain supine
- Control heart rate and improve diastolic filling
  —Underlying principles in treating HCM associated CHF and angina
  —β Blockers
    -Mainstay of therapy
    -Decrease dysrhythmias and lower elevation of pressure gradient across the left ventricular outflow tract
  —Calcium channel blockers
    -Verapamil reduces obstruction by decreasing contractility and improving diastolic relaxation and filling
    -Nifedipine relatively contraindicated
  —Standard CHF or anginal vasodilator therapy may lead to cardiovascular collapse
- Administer anticoagulants for recurrent paroxysmal atrial fibrillation
- Dysrhythmia management
  —Amiodarone
    -Drug of choice for ventricular dysrhythmias
    -Used when β blockers and calcium channel blockers fail
  —Disopyramide
    -Effective for supraventricular and ventricular dysrhythmias
  —Electrical cardioversion
    -Used early in HCM with atrial fibrillation, and CHF
- Surgical therapy
  —Septal myomectomy for patients with large systolic gradients that do not respond to drug therapy
  —Relatively high operative mortality

MEDICATIONS

- Amiodarone: 150 mg over 10 min, then 360 mg over 6 hrs, then 540 mg over next 18 hrs (peds: 5 mg/kg IV over 1 hr, with a starting-maintenance dose of 5 μg/kg/min)
- Diltiazem: 0.25 mg/kg IV over 2 min; may repeat in 15 min at 0.35 mg/kg
- Disopyramide: 100 mg IV over 10 min (10 mg every 3 min)—dysrhythmias and CHF
- Esmolol: 500 μg/kg/min load over 1 min, then 50 μg/kg/min for 4 min titrate up to 200 μg/kg/min depending on response
- Propranolol: 1–3 mg slow IV bolus
- Verapamil: 2.5 mg IV bolus over 1–2 min, may repeat as 5.0 mg in 15–30 min

Disposition

ADMISSION CRITERIA

- Telemetry admission for dysrhythmia
- ICU admission
  —Syncopal episodes
  —CHF
  —Angina
  —Hemodynamically significant tachydysrhythmias

DISCHARGE CRITERIA

- When HCM is an incidental finding during the ED evaluation for another presentation
  —Need urgent followup with a cardiologist
  —Counsel against any activities that may decrease diastolic filling pending followup

Miscellaneous

ICD9: 425.4

CORE CONTENT CODE: 2.2.2

SUGGESTED READINGS

Maron BJ, Pelliccia A, Spirito P. Cardiac disease in young trained athletes. Insights into methods for distinguishing athlete's heart from structural heart disease, with particular emphasis on hypertrophic cardiomyopathy. Circulation 1995;91(5):1596–601.

McKenna WJ, Sadoul N, Slade AK, Saumarez RC. The prognostic significance of nonsustained ventricular tachycardia in hypertrophic cardiomyopathy. Circulation 1994;90(6):3115–117.

Spirito P, Rapezzi C, Autore C, et al. Prognosis of asymptomatic patients with hypertrophic cardiomyopathy and nonsustained ventricular tachycardia. Circulation 1994;90:2743–747.

Spirito P, Seidman CE, McKenna WJ, Maron BJ. The management of hypertrophic cardiomyopathy. N Engl J Med 1997;336(11):775–85.

Wigle ED, Rakowski H, Kimball BP, Williams WG. Hypertrophic cardiomyopathy. Clinical spectrum and treatment. Circulation 1995;92(7):1680–692.

Author: L. Kristian Arnold

Hyperventilation

Clinical Presentation

SIGNS AND SYMPTOMS

- Cardiac
  - —Chest pain
  - —Dyspnea
  - —"Air hunger"
  - —Palpitations
- Neurological
  - —Dizziness
  - —Lightheadedness
  - —Syncope
  - —Paresthesias
  - —Carpopedal spasm
  - —Tetany
- Psychiatric
  - —Intense fear, anxiety
  - —Giddiness
  - —Feeling of unreality
- General
  - —Fatigue
  - —Weakness
  - —Malaise
- Clinical signs are rare and varied
  - —Tachypnea may not be present
    - -Patient may increase tidal volume rather than respiratory rate
- Carpopedal spasm
  - —May be dramatic
  - —Chovstek's sign may be present

MECHANISM/DESCRIPTION

- Constellation of symptoms produced by a *nonphysiologic* increase in minute ventilation
- More common in females
- Incidence is approximately 10–15% in the general population

ETIOLOGY

- Usually a response to psychological stressors
- Therapy directed at alleviating those stressors

Pre-Hospital

CAUTIONS

- IV access and pulse oximetry with abnormal vital signs
- Supplemental oxygen if hypoxic

Diagnosis

ESSENTIAL WORKUP

- Diagnosis of exclusion
  - —Physiologic causes must be investigated and excluded
- Clinical diagnosis based on the history and physical exam
- All patients with abnormal vital signs at presentation need further investigation
- Pulse oximetry

LABORATORY

- Arterial blood gas in any hypoxic patient
- Electrolytes, BUN/ Cr, glucose for suspected acidosis/diabetic ketoacidosis

IMAGING/SPECIAL TESTS

- Chest x-ray study in any hypoxic patient
- Electrocardiogram if chest pain present

DIFFERENTIAL DIAGNOSIS

- Organic
  - —Hypoxia (secondary to asthma, CHF, pulmonary embolus, pneumonia)
  - —Severe pain (including myocardial infarction, ischemia)
  - —CNS lesions (e.g., thalamic infarct, postictal)
  - —Hypoglycemia
- Physiologic
  - —Response to acidosis
  - —Pregnancy
  - —Pyrexia
  - —Altitude
- Drugs
  - —Aspirin intoxication
  - —Withdrawal syndrome (e.g., alcohol, benzodiazepines)

Treatment

INITIAL STABILIZATION

- IV access and pulse oximetry for patients with abnormal vital signs
- Initiate therapy for cause of hyperventilation (i.e., asthma, congestive heart failure, fever, alcohol or benzodiazepine withdrawal)

ED TREATMENT

- Initiate the treatment below if
  - —Initial work up does not support a physiologic cause and
  - —The history and physical suggests the diagnosis of hyperventilation syndrome
- Reassurance, calming, and explanation of the voluntary component of the patient's symptoms often have immediate dramatic results
- Benzodiazepine if symptoms persist
  - —used to break the cycle of anxiety and hyperventilation.
- Clarification of the psychological stressors help the patient avoid further attacks
  - —Assess for need of psychiatric evaluation (i.e., suicidal ideation)
- Anxiolytics
  - —Short course of anxiolytics may benefit certain patients with definable temporary stressors

MEDICATIONS

- Buspirone: 5 mg po tid for outpatient treatment
- Lorazepam: 1–2 mg po or IV for ED treatment
- Valium: 2–5 mg po or IV for ED or outpatient treatment

Disposition

ADMISSION CRITERIA

- Hyperventilation syndrome does not require admission

DISCHARGE CRITERIA

- Exclusion or treatment of physiologic causes of hyperventilation
- No acute psychiatric issues (i.e., suicidal ideation)
- Adequate follow up with a primary care physician

Miscellaneous

ICD9: 306.1

CORE CONTENT CODE: 16.4

SUGGESTED READINGS

Block M, Szidon P. Hyperventilation syndromes. Compr Ther 1994;20(5):306–311.

Gardner WN, Bass C. Hyperventilation in clinical practice. Br J Hosp Med 1989;41(1):73–81.

Hanashiro PK. Hyperventilation. Benign symptom or harbinger of catastrophe? Postgrad Med 1990;88(1):191–193.

Jozefowicz RF. Neurological manifestations of pulmonary disease. Neurol Clin 1989;7(3):605–616.

Tobin MJ. Dyspnea. Pathologic basis, clinical presentation, and management. Arch Intern Med 1990;150(8):1604–1613.

Author: Robert F. McCormack

Hyperviscosity Syndrome

Clinical Presentation

SIGNS AND SYMPTOMS

- May be a combination of hematologic, ocular, neurologic, and cardiovascular findings
  - —Bleeding—most common manifestation
  - —Visual and neurologic symptoms—second most common manifestation
  - —Cardiovascular complications—less frequent manifestation
- Hematologic
  - —Epistaxis
  - —Gingival, rectal, uterine bleeding
  - —Hematuria
  - —Prolonged postprocedural bleeding
  - —Anemia (normocytic, normochromic)
- Ocular
  - —Change in visual acuity (blurring, diplopia, visual loss)
  - —Retinal vein distention
  - —Retinal hemorrhage, detachment,
  - —Exudate, microaneurysm formation
  - —Papilledema
- Neurologic
  - —Dizziness, vertigo, nystagmus
  - —Tinnitus, hearing loss
  - —Ataxia
  - —Paresthesia, peripheral neuropathy
  - —Headache
  - —Mental status changes/coma
  - —Seizure
- Cardiovascular
  - —Angina
  - —Dysrhythmias
  - —Myocardial infarction
  - —Congestive heart failure

MECHANISM/DESCRIPTION

- Hyperviscosity syndrome (HVS) includes the disorders of blood viscosity such as
  - —Polycythemia
  - —Leukemia
  - —Sickle cell disease
  - —Dysproteinemias
- Primary HVS
  - —Conditions in which a primary blood abnormality causes impairment in blood flow such as in polycythemia or leukemia
- Secondary HVS
  - —Conditions in which vascular obstruction or stenosis causes a reduction of blood flow provoking tissue ischemia such as in myocardial infarction or stroke
- Syndromes *associated* with blood hyperviscosity include
  - —Diabetes
  - —Shock
  - —Surgery
  - —Rheumatologic diseases

ETIOLOGY

- Increased concentration of circulating cells and blood volume
- Decreased deformability of erythrocytes or increased amounts of rigid leukemic cells
- Waldenström's macroglobulinemia
  - —Most common cause of HVS accounting for 85–90% of cases
  - —HVS is the presenting feature in 10–30% of cases
- Multiple myeloma
  - —Second most common cause of HVS
- Blastic phase of leukemias
  - —WBC >100,000
- Polycythemia vera

Pre-Hospital

CAUTIONS

- IV fluid resuscitation with hemorrhage

Diagnosis

ESSENTIAL WORKUP

- Classic clinical presentation
- Direct measurement of the serum or whole blood viscosity
- Suspect diagnosis if the laboratory evaluation is hampered by serum stasis and increased viscosity causing analyzer blockage

LABORATORY

- CBC with WBC differential
  - —Anemia is a frequent finding in HVS
    - -Usually normocytic and normochromic
  - —Rouleaux of erythrocytes on the peripheral smear—important diagnostic clue
  - —WBC for leukemia
- Electrolyte, BUN/Cr, glucose
  - —Renal dysfunction is commonly noted in HVS
  - —Hypercalcemia and pseudohyponatremia in multiple myeloma
- Coagulation profile
- Serum and urine protein electrophoresis
- Measurement of serum viscosity
  - —By an Ostwald viscosimeter
  - —Normal range for the serum viscosity relative to water is 1.4 to 1.8
  - —Minimal viscosity at which symptoms develop is 4.0 centipoise (cp)

DIFFERENTIAL DIAGNOSIS

- Bleeding and clotting disorders
  - —Platelet disorders (qualitative and quantitative)
  - —Hereditary factor deficiencies
  - —Acquired disorders (vitamin K deficiency, liver disease)
  - —Disseminated intravascular coagulation

Treatment

INITIAL STABILIZATION

- Rehydrate with 0.9%NS IV fluid
- Bleeding may not be controlled by any treatment except plasmapheresis
- In patients with anemia and a leukemic picture, avoid blood transfusion until pheresis is performed as an exacerbation of HVS may occur

ED TREATMENT

- Plasmapheresis/leukapheresis
  - —Recommended exchange
    - -40 ml/kg of body weight in stable patients
    - -60 ml/kg of body weight in critical patients
  - —Many patients require more than one plasmapheresis
  - —Side effects
    - -Hypocalcemia with use of a citrate-containing anticoagulant
    - -Dysrhythmias (rare)
- Phlebotomy
  - —Useful in acute severe cases if plasmapheresis not readily available
  - —100–200 ml of blood

Disposition

ADMISSION CRITERIA

- ICU admission for
  - —Hemorrhage
  - —Altered mental status
  - —Acute myocardial infarction
- Regular admission for less severe presentations

DISCHARGE CRITERIA

- Definitive treatment of the underlying disorder

Miscellaneous

ICD9: 273.3

CORE CONTENT CODE: 7.7

SUGGESTED READINGS

Forconi S, Pieragalli D, Guerrini M, Galigani C, Cappelli R. Primary and secondary blood hyperviscosity syndromes and syndromes associated with blood hyperviscosity. Drug 1987;33(Suppl 2):19–26.

Geraci JM, Hansen RM, Kueck BD. Plasma cell leukemia and hyperviscosity syndrome. South Med J 1990;83(7):800–805.

Pimentel L. Medical complications of oncologic disease. Emerg Med Clin North Am 1993;22(2):407–419.

Somer T, Meiselman HJ. Disorders of blood viscosity. Ann Med 1993;25:31–39.

Stolz JF, Donner M, Larcan A. Introduction to hemorheology: theoretical aspects and hyperviscosity syndromes. Int Angiol 1987;6:119–132.

Author: Verena T. Valley

Hyphema

Clinical Presentation

SIGNS AND SYMPTOMS

- Photophobia
- Blurring of vision/decreased visual acuity
- Ocular pain
- Blood in the anterior chamber
  —Noted on slitlamp examination
  —Red-pigmented substance settling to the bottom of the anterior chamber in an individual whose head is elevated
- Evidence of blunt periorbital or orbital eye trauma including ecchymosis, corneal abrasion or subconjunctival hemorrhage
- Penetrating corneal injuries

MECHANISM/DESCRIPTION

- Defined as blood in the anterior chamber of the eye
- Four grades (classifications) depending on the percentage of the anterior chamber occluded by blood
  —Grade I: <1/3 of the anterior chamber
  —Grade II: 1/3 to 1/2 of the anterior chamber
  —Grade III: >1/2 of the anterior chamber
  —Grade IV: total (also called "eight-ball hyphema")
- Higher grade hyphemas are
  —More likely to rebleed (25% of grade I rebleed compared to 67% of grade III)
  —More likely to experience glaucoma
  —More likely to experience corneal staining
  —Less likely to recover visual acuity
- Blunt trauma
  —An orbital blow deforms the cornea inward causing an acute elevation of intraocular pressure and an anterior chamber fluid wave
  —Limbal tissue stretches and blood vessels tear at the angle
- Penetrating trauma—stromal vessels directly injured or ruptured by sudden decrease in intraocular pressure
- Spontaneous—any vessel in the anterior chamber begins to bleed without trauma

ETIOLOGY

- Traumatic (blunt or penetrating), surgical, or spontaneous
- Most traumatic hyphemas result from blunt ocular trauma (71–94%)
- Spontaneous causes include
  —Tumors: melanoma, retinoblastoma, metastatic tumors, xanthogranulomas
  —Blood dyscrasias: hemophilia, leukemia, and coagulopathies
  —Drugs: aspirin, alcohol, anticoagulants
  —Vascular anomalies: neovascularization
  —Sudden lowering of an inflamed eyes intraocular pressure

Pre-Hospital

CAUTIONS

- Place an eye shield in case of corneal perforation
- Keep head upright to allow the blood to settle to bottom of anterior chamber

Diagnosis

ESSENTIAL WORKUP

- Thorough history including previous visual acuity, prior eye surgery, medications, sickle cell disease, other injuries, and concurrent medical problems
- Visual acuity (mandatory)
- Inspection of the cornea and anterior chamber for perforation
- Slitlamp examination
- Fluorescein evaluation
- Tonometry

LABORATORY TEST

- Laboratory tests should be individualized depending on etiology
- Sickle cell screen
- PT/PTT/bleeding time if bleeding disorder suspected
- Platelet count for those at risk for thrombocytopenia
- BUN and Cr if aminocaproic acid to be used

IMAGING/SPECIAL TESTS

- Orbital radiographs, CT, ultrasound, or MRI if the retina and vitreous chamber cannot be visualized or an intraocular foreign body is suspected

Treatment

INITIAL STABILIZATION

- Hard metal shield

ED TREATMENT

- Restrict activity that increases eye movements (e.g., reading)
- Avoid bending, straining, or exertion
- Elevate the head of the bed to 45°
- Antiemetics for nausea/vomiting (increases IOP)
- Analgesics
  —Avoid NSAID- or aspirin-containing products
- Treat elevated intraocular pressure if present (>21–24 mm Hg) as in glaucoma
  —Carbonic anhydrase inhibitors (acetazolamide)
  —β-Blockers (timolol, betaxolol)
  —Hyperosmotic drugs (mannitol, glycerol)
  —Cholinergic drugs (pilocarpine)
  —In sickle cell patients, avoid acetazolamide, pilocarpine, epinephrine, or hyperosmotics, which can increase sickling and lead to increased intraocular pressure
- Stop anticoagulants and aspirin if possible
- Topical steroids may decrease inflammation from iritis but do not decrease rebleeds
- Cycloplegics may help decrease the pain from iritis
- Oral steroids and antifibrinolytics (aminocaproic acid)
  —Extremely controversial
  —Best left to the discretion of the consulting ophthalmologist

MEDICATIONS

- Aminocaproic acid: 50 mg/kg every 4 hrs for 5 days orally (30 g/day max)
- Acetazolamide
  —IV: 500 mg (peds: 20–40 mg/kg/24hrs q 6 hrs) initially, followed by 250 mg every 4 hrs
  —po: 500 mg sustained-release (peds: 8–30 mg/kg/24hrs q 6–8 hrs) po bid
- Betaxolol 0.5%: 1 drop bid
- Glycerol: 1–1.5 ml/kg po
- Mannitol: 1.5–2 g/kg IV
- Timolol 0.25–0.5%: 1 drop bid
- Pilocarpine 2%: affected eye—1 drop q 15 min for 5 times then q 2–3 hrs

Disposition

ADMISSION CRITERIA

- Unreliable patient
- Disease that increases the risk of rebleeding or increases the risk of increased intraocular pressure (Sickle Cell disease)
- Ongoing bleeding
- Ruptured globe
- Visibility of the vitreous chamber is obscured by blood

DISCHARGE CRITERIA

- No patient should be discharged before consultation with an ophthalmologist
- Treat small hyphemas on an outpatient basis with daily follow-up to assess the complications of corneal staining, rebleeding, increased intraocular pressure, and synechiae

Miscellaneous

ICD9: 364.41

CORE CONTENT CODE: 6.4.2.3

SUGGESTED READINGS

Berrios RR, Dreyer EB. Traumatic hyphema. Int Ophthalmol Clin 1995;35:93–103.

Endo EG, Mead MD. The management of traumatic hyphema. Int Ophthalmol Clin 1994;34:1–7.

Hemphill RR, Doe EA. Right eye pain and redness. Acad Emerg Med 1997;4(2)142–143, 147–149.

Linder JA, Renner GS. Trauma to the globe. Emerg Med Clinic North Am 1995;13:581–601.

Author: Loice Swisher

Hypocalcemia

Clinical Presentation

SIGNS AND SYMPTOMS

- Occur when ionized calcium falls below 3.2 mg/dl
- Reflect both the absolute and the rate of fall in calcium concentration

Neuromuscular

- Paresthesias
- Hyperreflexia
- Muscle spasm
- Latent tetany (Chvostek's and Trousseau's sign)
- Tetany
- Laryngeal stridor
- Seizures

Cardiovascular

- Arrhythmias
- Hypotension
- Impaired contractility (CHF)
- QT and ST prolongation
- T-wave abnormalities

Psychiatric

- Irritability
- Mental status changes
- Psychosis
- Depression
- Confusion
- Delusions

Ocular

- Papilledema
- Cataracts

MECHANISM/DESCRIPTION

- Intravascular calcium circulates in three forms
  —Bound to proteins (mainly albumin): 45–50%
  —Bound to complexing ions (citrate, phosphate, carbonate): 5–10%
  —Ionized (free) calcium (physiologically active form): 45–50%
- Normal total serum calcium concentrations = 8.7–10.5 mg/dl
  —Under normal conditions the ionized calcium level = approximately half of the total calcium level
  —In critically ill patients, the total calcium level is a poor indicator of ionized calcium levels
- Hypocalcemia = total plasma calcium levels below 8.7mg/dl
  —Ionized calcium may be normal and therefore have no clinical manifestations occurring
- Incidence in the general population = 0.6%

ETIOLOGY

- Serum levels of calcium controlled primarily by the activity of three hormones
  —Parathyroid hormone (PTH)
    -Decrease in calcium levels leads to an increase in PTH secretion (increasing: bone resorption, renal absorption, intestinal absorption, and urinary phosphate excretion)
  —Vitamin D (1.25 dihydroxyvitamin D)
    -Decrease in calcium levels activates vitamin D (increasing bone resorption and intestinal absorption)
  —Calcitonin
    -Causes a direct inhibition of bone resorption with increased calcium levels
- Hypoalbuminemia is most common cause of hypocalcemia
  —Each g/dl decrease in serum albumin decreases protein-bound serum calcium by 0.8 mg/dl
    -Will not change ionized (free) calcium

PEDIATRIC CONSIDERATIONS

- Children have higher values of normal calcium (9.2–11 mg/dl)
- Neonatal hypocalcemia = total serum calcium concentrations <7.0 mg/dl or serum-ionized calcium levels <4.4 mg/dl
- Frequent symptoms of hypocalcemia in infancy
  —Hyperactivity, jitteriness
  —Tachypnea
  —Apneic spells with cyanosis
  —Vomiting

Pre-Hospital

N/A

Diagnosis

ESSENTIAL WORKUP

- Serum-ionized calcium level confirms the diagnosis

LABORATORY

- Arterial blood gas
  —Change from normal pH of 0.1 units equals a reciprocal change in ionized calcium of approximately 1.7 mg/dl
- Serum albumin
  —Total serum calcium reduced by approximately 0.8 mg/dl for every g/dl by which the albumin is below the normal value
- Electrolytes, BUN/Cr, glucose
- Magnesium
  —Hypomagnesemia can cause hypocalcemia
- Phosphate
  —Differentiates hypoparathyroidism from vitamin D deficiency
  —Increase in phosphate associated with hypoparathyroidism
  —Decrease in phosphate associated with vitamin D deficiency
- PTH
  —Very high levels of PTH associated with pseudohypoparathyroidism
  —High levels of PTH associated with vitamin D deficiency
  —Low levels of PTH associated with hypoparathyroidism

DIFFERENTIAL DIAGNOSIS

- Impaired PTH action or secretion
  —Autoimmune congenital neck surgery or irradiation
  —Neonatal secondary to maternal hyperparathyroidism
  —Magnesium disorder
  —Pseudohypoparathyroidism
  —Infiltrative (amyloidosis, sarcoidosis)
- Impaired vitamin D synthesis or action
  —Nutritional malabsorption
  —Renal or liver disease
  —Sepsis
  —Rickets disease
- Calcium complex formation or sequestration
  —Hyperphosphatemia
  —Ethylene glycol, ethylene diaminotetracetatic acid (EDTA), citrate (from transfusion)
  —Pancreatitis, rhabdomyolysis
  —Alkalosis (i.e., hyperventilation)
- Medications
  —Mithramycin, plicamycin, phosphate, calcitonin, bisphosphonates
  —Phenobarbital, dilantin
  —Cisplatinum
  —Cadmium, colchicine
  —Fluoride, citrate
- Malignancies (prostate cancer, breast cancer, lung cancer, chondrosarcoma)

Treatment

INITIAL STABILIZATION

- ABCs
  —Control airway and provide supplemental oxygen as needed
  —Establish intravenous catheter access
  —Cardiac monitor

ED TREATMENT

Acute Management

- Treat symptomatic hypocalcemia as a medical emergency with parenteral calcium administration
- Calcium
  —Administer calcium gluconate 10–20 ml of 10% solution (90 mg of elemental calcium/10 ml ampule intravenously slowly over 10 minutes)
  —Faster IV rates
    -Can cause cardiac dysrhythmias
    -Calcium salts are irritating to veins
  —Intramuscular calcium gluceptate or calcium gluconate if IV access not available
  —Bolus calcium doses increase ionized calcium for only 1–2 hours
    -Must follow by an infusion
- Calcium infusion
  —Calcium gluconate infusion rate = 0.5–2 mg/kg/hr (80 cc of 10% solution = 72 mg in 1000 cc of D5W)
  —Infusion of 15 mg/kg raises serum calcium 2–3 mg/dl
  —Do not mix calcium with bicarbonate or phosphate
    -Precipitates of calcium salts may form
  —Administer cautiously in digitalis patients
    -Can initiate and exacerbate digitalis toxicity
- Response to therapy
  —Individual responses vary
  —Monitor calcium concentrations q 1–4 hrs during therapy
  —Titrate treatment to symptoms or ECG changes
  —Consider hypomagnesemia if the patient fails to respond to calcium therapy
  —Side effects of IV calcium
    -Nausea, vomiting
    -Hypotension
    -Dysrhythmias

Chronic Management

- Oral calcium supplementation
- 1–4 g/day of elemental calcium in divided doses
- Vitamin D
  —Enhances intestinal absorption
  —Initiate when calcium supplementation alone not sufficient to restore calcium levels

MEDICATIONS

CALCIUM	ELEMENTAL CALCIUM PER GRAM	HOW SUPPLIED
IV CALCIUM		
Gluconate	1 g = 90 mg (4.5 mEq)	1 g in 10 ml
Gluceptate (IV/IM)	1 g = 90 mg (4.5 mEq)	1 g in 5 ml
Chloride	1 g = 272 mg (13.6 mEq)	1 g in 10 ml
ORAL CALCIUM		
Glubionate	1 g = 65 mg	18 g/5 ml of syrup
Gluconate	1 g = 90 mg	500–1000 mg tablets
Lactate	1 g = 130 mg	350–1000-mg tablets
Citrate	1 g = 211 mg	950-mg tablets
Carbonate	1 g = 400 mg	350–1500-mg tablets

- Vitamin D preparations
  —Ergocalciferol: 125 μg/day
  —Dihydrotachysterol: 100–400 μg/day
  —Calcifediol: 50–200 μg/day
  —Calcitriol 0.25–1.0 μg/day

PEDIATRIC CONSIDERATIONS

- Initial calcium bolus with 10% calcium gluconate should be 9–18 mg of elemental calcium/kg or 1–2 ml/kg not to exceed 5 ml in premature infants or 10 ml in term infants
- Calcitriol dose in children ranges from 0.1–3 μg/day

Disposition

ADMISSION CRITERIA

- Symptomatic or severe ionized hypocalcemia (<3.2 mg/dl)
- Continuous IV calcium preparations necessary to maintain calcium levels

DISCHARGE CRITERIA

- Asymptomatic hypocalcemia
- Ionized calcium >3.2 mg/dl in healthy patients with no comorbid illness

Miscellaneous

ICD9: 275.4

CORE CONTENT CODE: 4.3.1

SUGGESTED READINGS

Bourk E, Delaney V. Assessment of hypocalcemia and hypercalcemia. Clin Lab Med 1993;13(1):157–181.

Guise TA, Mundy GR. Clinical review 69: Evaluation of hypocalcemia in children and adults. J Clin Endocrinol Metab 1995;80(5):1473–1478.

Tohme JF, Bliezikian JP. Hypocalcemia emergencies. Endocrinol Metab Clin North Am 1993;229(2):363–375.

Zaloga GP. Hypocalcemia in critically ill patients. Crit Care Med 1992;20(2):251–262.

Author: Cherie Terry

Hypoglycemia

Clinical Presentation

SIGNS AND SYMPTOMS

- Adrenergic
  - —Diaphoresis
  - —Anxiety
  - —Tachycardia
  - —Hunger
- Neuroglycopenic
  - —Dizziness
  - —Confusion
  - —Hyperactive or psychotic behavior
  - —Slurred speech
  - —Cranial-nerve palsies
  - —Seizures
  - —Hemiplegia
  - —Decerebrate posturing
- Neonatal presentation
  - —Asymptomatic
  - —Limp
  - —Bradycardia
  - —Irritable
  - —Tremulous
  - —Seizures

MECHANISM/DESCRIPTION

- Deficiency in counterregulatory hormones (glucagon, epinephrine, cortisol, growth hormone) or excessive insulin response
- Fall in serum glucose (<40 mg/dl) stimulates sympathetic catecholamine release

ETIOLOGY

- Increased insulin levels
  - —Overdose of oral hypoglycemic agent or insulin
  - —Sepsis
  - —Insulinoma
- Underproduction of glucose
  - —Alcohol (inhibitory effect on glycogen storage and gluconeogenesis)
  - —Salicylates
  - —β-Blockers
  - —Adrenal insufficiency
  - —Liver disease
  - —Malnutrition
  - —Dehydration
  - —Cerebral edema

PEDIATRIC CONSIDERATIONS

- Infants at greatest risk of hypoglycemia
  - —Mothers with DM
  - —Premature/postmature
  - —Small for gestational age
  - —Intrapartum hypoxia
- Common in critically ill children
- Definitions
  - —<20 mg/dl in preterm infant during first 24 hours of life
  - —<30 mg/dl in newborn
  - —40 mg/dl in infants

Pre-Hospital

CAUTIONS

- Diagnosis with finger stick glucose (Accucheck)
- Oral glucose containing fluids or IV dextrose for hypoglycemia
- Administer thiamine along with dextrose IV to prevent precipitation of Wernicke's encephalopathy

Diagnosis

ESSENTIAL WORKUP

- Diagnosis requires:
  - —Demonstration of neuroglycopenic signs and symptoms as defined above
  - —Lab evidence of hypoglycemia (Accucheck/dextrostix)
  - —Clearing of symptoms following glucose administration

LABORATORY

- Blood glucose
  - —Initial and posttreatment, monitor
- Electrolytes, BUN, Cr
  - —Order if mental status does not improve postglucose administration
- CBC
  - —Order if sepsis present
- Urinalysis

IMAGING/SPECIAL TESTS

- ECG if suspect MI/ischemia due to hypoglycemia
- CXR for
  - —Possible aspiration
  - —Pneumonia as source of sepsis

DIFFERENTIAL DIAGNOSIS

- Neurologic
  - —CVA/TIA
  - —Seizure disorder
- Drug or alcohol intoxication
- Psychosis or depression
- Pediatric considerations
  - —Salicylate ingestion
  - —Reyes' syndrome
  - —Growth hormone deficiency
  - —Ketotic hypoglycemia
  - —Inborn errors of metabolism

Treatment

INITIAL STABILIZATION

- Glucose
  - —Dextrose IVP
  - —Oral glucose in awake patient (with no IV) without risk of aspiration
  - —Glucagon IM if unable to establish IV access
- ABCs with aspiration and seizure precautions

ED TREATMENT

- Administer 50 cc D50W for decreased level of consciousness
  - —Second or third ampule may be necessary
  - —Complications include volume overload and hypokalemia
- Initiate continuous IV infusion of 5–20% glucose solution for persistent mild hypoglycemia or if patient cannot eat
- Administer glucagon
  - —If hypoglycemia refractory to glucose
  - —If IV access delayed
  - —Effective in 10–20 minutes
  - —Ineffective in alcohol-induced hypoglycemia
  - —May repeat twice
- Monitor blood glucose every 2–3 hours and prior to discharge
- Adrenal insufficiency: administer hydrocortisone 100 mg and glucagon 1 mg
- For cases of resistant hypoglycemia due to sulfonylureas administer diazoxide 300 mg IV over 30 minutes every 4 hours PRN
  - —Beware of potent hypotensive effect

MEDICATIONS

- D50W: 1 amp (= 25 g) of 50% dextrose, 1–2 cc/kg (peds: 1–2 ml/kg D25W) IVP
- Diazoxide: 1–3 mg/kg IVP, max 150 mg
- Glucagon: 1–2 mg (peds: <6 yrs: 0.5 mg; >6 yrs: 1.0 mg) IV/IM/SQ
- Hydrocortisone: 100 mg (peds: 1–2 mg/kg) IV
- Oral glucose: 20 g orally equals ~12 oz. nondiet fruit juice, 14 oz. nondiet cola, 2.5 oz. chocolate

PEDIATRIC CONSIDERATIONS

- Children: use D25W 1–2 cc/kg IV or glucagon if unable to achieve IV access
- Infants: D10W IV/intraosseous as needed

Disposition

ADMISSION CRITERIA

- Overdoses of oral hypoglycemic agent or long-acting insulin mandate observation for at least 24 hours
- Failure of neuroglycopenic symptoms to improve after 1 hour suggest neurologic injury, preexisting neurological condition, or another cause for these symptoms
- Recurrent hypoglycemic state in ED
- Older patients may require several days for complete recovery from severe or prolonged hypoglycemia

DISCHARGE CRITERIA

- Discharge mild unintentional insulin over usage if blood glucose normal, symptoms resolved, tolerating oral intake, and can be observed

Miscellaneous

ICD9: 251.2

CORE CONTENT CODE: 4.4.2

SUGGESTED READINGS

Comi RJ. Approach to acute hypoglycemia. Endocrinol Metab Clin North Am 1993;22(2);247–262.

Service FJ. Hypoglycemia. Med Clin North Am 1995;79(1):1–6.

Service FJ. Hypoglycemia disorders. N Engl J Med 1995;27:1144–1150.

Authors: Michelle Ervin; Steven Friedman

Hypoglycemic Agent, Poisoning

Clinical Presentation

SIGNS AND SYMPTOMS

Insulin or Sulfonylureas

- Cause hypoglycemia
  - —Symptoms most often occur when glucose <40–60 mg/dl (may occur at higher concentrations)
  - —Symptoms blunted by β-antagonists
- Facial flushing, tremor, diaphoresis, pallor, piloerection
- Hunger, nausea
- Deep, heavy respirations, apnea, palpitations
- Headache, blurred vision
- Paresthesias, weakness, incoordination
- Anxiety, irritability, bizarre behavior, confusion, stupor, coma, seizures
- Tachycardia, deteriorating to bradycardia late in presentation
- Hypertension
- Hypothermia
- Dysrhythmias: atrial fibrillation, PVCs

Biguanides

- Actions due primarily to lactic acid accumulation
- Nausea, vomiting, abdominal pain
- Agitation, confusion, lethargy, coma
- Kussmaul respirations
- Hypotension, tachycardia

MECHANISM/DESCRIPTION

- Insulin
  - —Enhances glucose uptake from serum into cells; limits the supply of glucose available to the brain (most sensitive to hypoglycemia)
  - —Influences potassium redistribution
- Sulfonylurea agents
  - —Enhance insulin release from β cells and increase sensitivity of peripheral cells to the action of insulin
  - —Enhanced by concurrent use NSAIDs, salicylates, sulfonamides, oral anticoagulants, cimetidine, ethanol, and by hepatic and renal dysfunction
- Biguanide agents
  - —*Antihyperglycemic* agents
  - —Decrease *elevated* serum glucose concentrations, but do not cause hypoglycemia on their own
  - —In the presence of insulin, biguanides
    - -Increase glucose uptake into muscle cells
    - -Decrease glucose absorption from the intestine
    - -Decrease hepatic gluconeogenesis
  - —Promote the formation of lactate from glucose in intestinal cells leading to lactic acidosis with drug accumulation
  - —Do not cause hypoglycemia unless taken in the presence of sulfonylureas, excessive ethanol, or in cases of hepatic dysfunction

ETIOLOGY

- Insulin
- Sulfonylureas (hepatic metabolism)
- Biguanide antihyperglycemic agents: buformin, metformin, phenformin
  - —Enhance glycemic control in Type II Diabetes Mellitus; often used in conjunction with sulfonylureas

PEDIATRIC CONSIDERATIONS

- Neonatal hypoglycemia may occur after maternal use of sulfonylureas during labor
- Susceptible to hypoglycemia after ingestion of 1 sulfonylurea tablet
  - —Precipitates the delayed onset of symptomatic, prolonged hypoglycemia

Pre-Hospital

CAUTIONS

- Hypoglycemia true emergency
  - —Sequelae of hypoglycemia due to the duration of neuroglycopenia
  - —Administer glucose immediately when hypoglycemia suspected or confirmed
  - —Administer glucagon IM if IV access impossible (action delayed and transient)

Diagnosis

ESSENTIAL WORKUP

- Serum glucose concentrations <60 mg/dl diagnostic of hypoglycemia
  - —Symptoms of hypoglycemia may occur at glucose concentrations >60 mg/dl
- Biguanide ingestion or accumulation diagnosis
  - —Anion gap metabolic acidosis due to elevated lactate levels
  - —Absence of tissue hypoperfusion as a cause of lactic acidosis

LABORATORY

- Serum glucose, before and after treatment
- Electrolytes
  - —Check for hypokalemia
  - —Anion gap acidosis
- BUN, Cr
  - —May reveal renal insufficiency, causing drug accumulation
- CBC
  - —Leukocytosis often present in hypoglycemia
  - —Thrombocytopenia reported after biguanide overdose
- Ethanol level
- Lactate level
- Liver function tests
  - —May reveal hepatic dysfunction, causing drug accumulation
- Arterial blood gas
- Assays for immunoreactive insulin and C-peptide levels
  - —Do not correlate with severity of clinical symptoms
  - —Confirm surreptitious self-administration of exogenous insulin if insulin level is high, and C-peptide is low in the setting of hypoglycemia
- Assays for sulfonylureas
  - —Do not correlate with severity of clinical symptoms
  - —Confirm surreptitious drug ingestions when suspected

IMAGING/SPECIAL TESTS

- EKG: sinus tachycardia, PVCs, atrial dysrhythmias
- EEG: diffuse slowing without focal abnormalities
- CT scan: cerebral edema if prolonged hypoglycemia
- CXR: aspiration pneumonia or pulmonary edema

DIFFERENTIAL DIAGNOSIS

- Addison's disease
- Panhypopituitarism
- Sepsis
- Insulinoma
- Neuroendocrine tumors
- Cirrhosis
- Chronic ethanol abuse
- Drug interaction: sulfonylureas with: NSAIDs, oral anticoagulants, salicylates, sulfonamides
- Medications: β-antagonists, ethanol, salicylates, pentamidine

Treatment

INITIAL STABILIZATION

- ABCs
- Administer 50% dextrose IV

ED TREATMENT

- Hypotension
  - —IVF resuscitation
  - —Pressors
    - -May increase lactate production by peripheral tissues
    - -Use cautiously with biguanide induced lactic acidosis
- Neuroglycopenia
  - —May persist shortly after serum glucose corrected
  - —Persistent symptoms requires further dextrose administration
- Hypoglycemia
  - —IV D5W or D10W to maintain euglycemia or mild hyperglycemia
  - —Food
- Activated charcoal for recent or large ingestions of oral agent (sulfonylurea or biguanide)
- Multiple-dose activated charcoal for glipizide; undergoes enterohepatic circulation
- Sodium bicarbonate
  - —Chlorpropamide toxicity
    - -Enhances renal elimination
    - -Alkalinize urine to a pH of 7–8
  - —Biguanide-induced lactic acidosis if pH <7.0
- Benzodiazepines for seizures
- Sulfonylureas overdose with recurrent hypoglycemia; insulin secretion inhibited with
  - —Octreotide
    - -Longer duration and less side effects than diazoxide
  - —Diazoxide
    - -Watch for hypotension
- Sodium dichloroacetate
  - —An *experimental* drug that decreases intracellular lactate production
  - —May be of benefit in biguanide-induced lactic acidosis
- Hemodialysis and hemoperfusion ineffective in sulfonylurea overdose
- Hemodialysis reported beneficial in cases of metformin-induced lactic acidosis to correct acid/base abnormalities and enhance elimination of the drug

MEDICATIONS

- Activated charcoal: 1 g/kg po
- Diazepam (benzodiazepine): 5–10 mg (peds: 0.2–0.5 mg/kg) IV; repeat if necessary
- Dextrose: 50–100 cc D50 (peds: 2 cc/kg of D10 over 1 min) IV; repeat if necessary
- Diazoxide: 200 mg po or 1–3 mg/kg IV (infant: 8–15 mg/kg/24hrs q 8–12 hrs PO/IV; child: 3–8 mg/kg/24hrs q 8 hrs PO/IV)
- Glucagon: 1–2 mg (peds: 0.03–0.1 mg/kg) IM/SC/IV
- Lorazepam (benzodiazepine): 2–6 mg (peds: 0.03–0.05 mg/kg) IV; repeat if necessary
- Octreotide: 50 -100 μg q 8–12 hrs SC/IV
- Sodium bicarbonate: 1–2 mEq/kg IV

Disposition

ADMISSION CRITERIA

- Hypoglycemia due to sulfonylurea agents (may require several days of monitoring) or long-acting insulin preparations
- Hypoglycemia due to these agents in conjunction with ethanol or hepatic or renal dysfunction
- Intentional overdose of sulfonylureas or self-injection of insulin admit for frequent glucose monitoring over 24 hours
- All children with accidental ingestion of sulfonylureas
- Metabolic alterations due to biguanide ingestion or accumulation

DISCHARGE CRITERIA

- Accidental hypoglycemia due to short-acting insulin injection in the setting of dietary insufficiency
- Discharged after glucose correction, and a 4-hour period of observation

Miscellaneous

ICD9: 977.9

CORE CONTENT CODE: 17.2.25

SUGGESTED READINGS

Bailey CJ. Minireview metformin—an update. Gen Pharmacol 1993;24(6):1299–1309.

Boyle PJ, Justice K, Krentz AJ, Nagy RJ, Schade DS. Octreotide reverses hyperinsulinemia and prevents hypoglycemia induced by sulfonylurea overdoses. J Clin Endocrinol Metab 1993;76(3):752–756.

Cook DL. The beta-cell response to oral hypoglycemic agents. Diabetes Res Clin Pract 1995;28(Suppl):S81–S89.

Ellenhorn, MJ. Hypoglycemic agents and insulin; biguanides. In: Ellenhorn MJ, ed. Ellenhorn's medical toxicology: Diagnosis and treatment of human poisoning. 2nd ed. Baltimore: Williams & Wilkins, 1997:721–727.

Moore DF, Wood DF, Volans GN. Features, prevention and management of acute overdose due to antidiabetic drugs. Drug Saf 1993;9(3):218–229.

Author: Sue Farrell

Hypokalemia

Clinical Presentation

SIGNS AND SYMPTOMS

Cardiovascular

- Ventricular dysrhythmias (especially in the setting of heart disease)
- Potentiation of digoxin toxicity

Neuromuscular

- Weakness
  - —Severe weakness (K^+ <2.5)
  - —May progress to paralysis
- Cramps
- Constipation, ileus
- Increased risk of rhabdomyolysis
- Endocrine
  - —Hypokalemia inhibits insulin release
  - —Glucose levels may rise

Renal

- Polyuria (inhibits kidneys' ability to concentrate urine)
- Metabolic alkalosis

MECHANISM/DESCRIPTION

- Increase in the normal intracellular to extracellular potassium gradient
  - —Alters the depolarization threshold for muscles and nerves
  - —Inhibits the termination of action potentials
- Alterations in intracellular potassium directly affect cellular function

ETIOLOGY

Intracellular Shift of Potassium

- Alkalosis
- Insulin (insulin induced hypoglycemia)
- Adrenergic excess
  - —Severe stress (trauma, myocardial infarction, sepsis)
  - —Treatment of asthma
- Hypokalemic periodic paralysis
  - —Familial
  - —Thyrotoxic
  - —Barium poisoning

Renal Losses

- Diuretics (thiazides, loop diuretics, carbonic anhydrase inhibitors)
  - —Usually associated with loss of other cations (Mg^{++}, Ca^{++}, P^{+++}, Na^+)
- Vomiting causes volume depletion and metabolic alkalosis which increases renal losses of potassium
- Renal tubular damage
- Primary renal tubular disorders
- Hyperaldosteronism
  - —Primary
  - —Pseudohyperaldosteronism (licorice ingestion)
- Hypomagnesemia
- DKA

GI Losses

- Diarrhea, vomiting
- Ureterosigmoidostomy
- Villous adenomas
- Laxative abuse
- Intestinal fistulae
- Cystic fibrosis

Poor Intake

- Nutritional
- Eating disorders

Pre-Hospital

N/A

Diagnosis

ESSENTIAL WORKUP

- Serum potassium <3.5 mEq/L

LABORATORY

- Electrolytes, BUN, Cr, glucose
- Calcium
- Urinalysis
  - —Check for myoglobin
  - —Hypokalemia may cause rhabdomyolysis
- Magnesium
  - —Hypomagnesemia may lead to inability to correct hypokalemia
- ABG
  - —Acid-base status

IMAGING/SPECIAL TESTS

- ECG shows
  - —Low voltage T waves
  - —Sagging of the ST segments
  - —U waves
  - —Atrial and ventricular dysrhythmias, especially in patients on digoxin

Parameter for Etiology of Hypokalemia

- Normotensive
  - —urine K^+< 25 mEq/L and serum bicarbonate low or normal: lower GI losses, poor intake
  - —urine K^+< 25 mEq/L and serum bicarbonate high: prior diuretic use
  - —urine K^+ > 25 mEq/L and serum bicarbonate low: renal tubular acidosis, DKA
  - —urine K^+ > 25 mEq/L and serum bicarbonate high: vomiting, current diuretic use, Bartter's syndrome
- Hypertensive: measure plasma renin and plasma aldosterone if renin is low

DIFFERENTIAL DIAGNOSIS

- Intrinsic cardiac disease with arrhythmias

Causes of Muscular Weakness

- Neuromuscular junction disease
  - —Myasthenia gravis
  - —Organophosphate poisoning
  - —Botulism
- Spinal cord disease
- Polyneuropathies
- Primary acute myopathies

Treatment

INITIAL STABILIZATION

- ABCs
- Cardiac monitor
- IV access

ED TREATMENT

- Treat predisposing condition
- Correct volume deficit and acid base disorder

Potassium Replacement

- Because potassium is primarily an intracellular ion, modest hypokalemia can represent significant reductions in total body potassium
  - —At levels above 2.0 mEq/L
    - -Estimate a total potassium deficit of 100–200 mEq for every 1 mEq/L reduction in serum potassium (based on a normal serum pH)
  - —At levels below 2.0 mEq/L
    - -Deficit much higher since a significant portion of exogenous potassium excreted by the kidneys
    - -Total replacement dose required greater than the estimated deficit
- Oral potassium
  - —Preferable to IV therapy whenever possible
  - —Gradual oral repletion effective
  - —Potassium chloride
    - -Oral forms associated with GI upset
    - -Enteric coated forms associated with small bowel ulceration
  - —Use potassium gluconate or citrate in acidotic patients
- IV potassium (KCl)
  - —For serious dysrhythmias or severe weakness
  - —Emergent situations: rates up to 40 mEq/hr (peds: 0.3 mEq/kg/hr)
  - —Less urgent situations: 10–20 mEq/hr
  - —Use central lines for concentrations in excess of 40 mEq/L
  - —Frequent monitoring of potassium levels when large amounts of K^+ are infused
- Increase dietary potassium

Correct Other Electrolyte Abnormalities

- Magnesium
- Chloride
- Calcium

MEDICATIONS

- Oral potassium
  - —Potassium chloride/potassium citrate/potassium gluconate
  - —Available in elixir, soluble preparations, and tablets
  - —Unit doses contain from 10–40 mEq K^+
  - —Replacement dose: adult: 40–100 mEq/d; peds: 3–5 mEq/kg/d
- IV potassium chloride
  - —Emergent situations
    - -Max rate: 40 mEq/hr (peds: 0.3 mEq/kg/hr)
    - -Max concentration via peripheral line: 40 mEq/L
  - —Nonemergent situations
    - -Max rate: 10–20 mEq/hr
- Magnesium sulfate: 1–2 g IV (over minutes when required, or as an infusion)

Disposition

ADMISSION CRITERIA

- Need of IV potassium repletion
- Dysrhythmias
- Serum potassium level <2.5 mEq/L

DISCHARGE CRITERIA

- Able to replete deficiency with oral potassium

Miscellaneous

ICD9 CM: 276.8

CORE CONTENT CODE: 4.3.5

SUGGESTED READINGS

Krishna GG. Hypokalemic states: Current clinical issues. Semin Nephrol 1990;10(6):515–524.

Rodríguez-Soriano J. Potassium homeostasis and its disturbances in children. Pediatr Nephrol 1995;9(3):364–374.

Stedwell RE, Allen KM, Binder LS. Hypokalemic paralyses: A review of the etiologies, pathophysiology, presentation, and therapy. Am J Emerg Med 1992;10:143–148.

Author: Joel Yaphe

Hyponatremia

Clinical Presentation

SIGNS AND SYMPTOMS

Mild: Na^+ >120 mEq/L

- Headache
- Nausea
- Vomiting
- Weakness
- Anorexia
- Muscle cramps
- Rhabdomyolysis

Moderate: Na^+ Between 110–120 mEq/L

- Impaired response to verbal stimuli
- Decreased response to painful stimuli
- Visual/auditory hallucinations
- Bizarre behavior
- Incontinence
- Hyperventilation
- Gait disturbance

Severe: Na^+ <110 mEq/L

- Signs of herniation
  - —Decorticate/decerebrate posturing
- Bradycardia
- Hypertension
- Altered temperature regulation
- Dilated pupils
- Seizure activity
- Respiratory arrest
- Coma/unresponsive

Chronic

- May be asymptomatic

MECHANISM/DESCRIPTION

- Sodium <130 mEq/L
- Most common electrolyte disturbance
  - —2.5% of hospitalized patients

ETIOLOGY

Pseudohyponatremia

- Low-measured serum sodium but normal measured serum osmolarity
- Occurs secondary to the displacement of sodium to aqueous phase of serum
- Seen with elevated lipids or proteins
- Disease examples include
  - —Multiple nephroma
  - —Hyperlipidemia

Hyponatremia with Normal Osmolarity and Fluid Overload

- Inappropriate retention of water
- Disease examples include
  - —CHF
  - —Cirrhosis
  - —Renal failure
  - —Nephrotic syndrome

Hyponatremia with Normal Osmolarity and Evolemia

- Tend to have increased total body water without marked increase no edema
- Purest form of dilutional hyponatremia
- Disease examples include
  - —Endocrine abnormalities
  - —Water intoxication
  - —Mineralocorticoid abnormalities
  - —Postoperative hyponatremia (particularly after TURP)

Hyponatremia with Normal Osmolarity and Hypovolemia

- Deficits in total body water and total body sodium
- Sodium deficits exceed water deficits
- Disease examples include
  - —GI losses
  - —Sweating
  - —Burns
  - —Cystic fibrosis
  - —Salt-wasting nephropathies

Drug-induced

- Drugs may stimulate ADH and cause hyponatremia
  - —Clofibrate
  - —Cyclophosphamide
  - —Carbamazepine
  - —Vincristine
  - —Barbiturates
- Morphine
- Drugs may increase sensitivity to ADH and cause hypotremia
  - —Chlorpropamide
- Tolbutamide
- NSAIDs
- Drugs may stimulate thirst and cause hyponatremia
  - —Tinoridine
  - —Thiothixene
  - —Amitriptyline
  - —Fluphenazine

Hyponatremia with Hyperosmolarity

- Due to excessive osmotically active substances
- Disease examples include
  - —Elevated glucose
    - -Correction factor: for every elevation of glucose of 100 add 1.6 mEq K^+ to sodium valve
  - —Mannitol infusion

PEDIATRIC CONSIDERATIONS

- More prone to water intoxication
- High incidence of iatrogenic hyponatremia

Pre-Hospital

N/A

Diagnosis

ESSENTIAL WORKUP

- Serum sodium level
  - —Recheck sodium to verify not drawn above IV site with hypotonic saline
- Review medications the patient is taking
- Obtain good medical history for possible etiologies

LABORATORY

- Electrolytes, BUN/Cr
- Glucose
  - —Correct sodium value accordingly if severe hyperglycemia
  - —Correction factor: for every elevation of glucose of 100 add 1.6 mEq K to sodium valve

IMAGING/SPECIAL TESTS

- Urine sodium

DIFFERENTIAL DIAGNOSIS

- Pseudohyponatremia due to
  - —Hyperglycemia
  - —Hyperlipidemia
  - —Hyperproteinemia

Treatment

INITIAL STABILIZATION

- ABCs
- Initiate IV fluid with 0.9%NS
- Naloxone, thiamine, D50W (or Accucheck) for altered mental status

ED TREATMENT

- Depends on severity and chronicity of hyponatremia and underlying etiology

Acute Hyponatremia with Severe CNS Symptoms

- Goal
  - —Raise serum sodium by 10 mEq/L or to level >120–125 mEq/L over 6 hours with administration of hypertonic saline
- Sodium requirement
  - —Required sodium = (125-measured serum Na^{+}) × 0.6(body weight in kg)
- 250 ml of 3% or 5% saline solution in adult over 4–6 hours will raise serum sodium by 10–15 mEq/L

Hypovolemic Hyponatremia

- Correct underlying cause
- Replete volume with 0.9%NS IV
- Primary goals to restore
  - —Extracellular fluid
  - —Cardiac output
  - —Organ perfusion

Hypervolemic/Euvolemic Hyponatremia

- Water restriction to less than 1 L per day with high dietary salt intake
- For faster correction of sodium
  - —Administer IV 0.9%NS with loop diuretic (furosemide)
- Maximum rate of correction = 0.5 mEq/L/hr

MEDICATIONS

- Dextrose: D50W 1 amp (50 ml or 25 g) (peds: D25W 2–4 ml/kg) IV
- Furosemide: 1 mg/kg up to 20–40 mg IVP
- Naloxone (narcan): 2 mg (peds: 0.1 mg/kg) IV or IM initial dose
- Thiamine (vitamin B_1): 100 mg (peds: 50 mg) IV or IM

Disposition

ADMISSION CRITERIA

- Symptomatic hyponatremia
- Sodium <120 mEq/L
- Asymptomatic, mild hyponatremia (Na^{+} 120–127 mEq/L), with comorbid factors

DISCHARGE CRITERIA

- Sodium greater than 130 mEq/L and asymptomatic
- Known chronic history of hyponatremia with no acute changes
- Asymptomatic, mild hyponatremia (Na^{+} 120–127 mEq/L) with no comorbid factors; however, must have close outpatient follow-up

Miscellaneous

ICD9: 276.1

CORE CONTENT CODE: 4.3.6

SUGGESTED READINGS

Arieff A. Management of hyponatremia. Br Med J 1993;307:305–308.

Mulloy AL, Caruana RJ. Hyponatremic emergencies. Med Clin North Am 1995;79:155–167.

Schrier R, Briner V. The differential diagnosis of hyponatremia. Hosp Pract 1990;Sept:29–37.

Author: Linda Mueller

Hypoparathyroidism

Clinical Presentation

SIGNS AND SYMPTOMS

- Related to severity, rapidity of onset, and duration of hypocalcemia
- Neuromuscular
  - —Paresthesias (especially circumoral and extremities)
  - —Carpal pedal spasm
  - —Latent spasm elicited by
    - -Chvostek's sign (twitching of circumoral muscles after tapping facial nerve in front of the tragus)
    - -Trousseau's sign (spasm after inflating blood pressure cuff 20 mm above patient's systolic BP for 3–5 minutes)
  - —Laryngospasm/bronchospasm
  - —Blepharospasm
  - —Muscle cramps
  - —Tetany
- Cardiovascular
  - —Prolonged QT interval (due to ST segment prolongation)
  - —Heart block
  - —CHF
  - —Vfib
  - —Vasoconstriction
- Neurologic
  - —Seizures (presenting symptom of one-third with hypoparathyroidism)
  - —Increased ICP with papilledema
  - —Parkinson's syndrome and other extrapyramidal disorders
  - —Myelopathy
- Psychiatric
  - —Impaired memory
  - —Confusion
  - —Hallucinations
  - —Dementia
- General
  - —Weakness
  - —Malaise
- Dermatologic
  - —Brittle hair and nails
  - —Psoriasis
  - —Hyperpigmentation
- Lenticular cataracts

MECHANISM/DESCRIPTION

- Parathyroid hormone (PTH)
  - —Decreases urinary Ca^{++} loss
  - —Increases urinary PO_4 loss
  - —Stimulates vitamin D conversion from 25(OH)-D to $1,25(OH)_2D$ in kidney,
  - —Liberates Ca^{++} and PO_4 from bone
- Calcitonin
  - —Promotes deposition of Ca^{++} and PO_4 into bone (produced primarily in C cells in thyroid)
- Magnesium
  - —Cofactor in production of PTH
  - —Essential for action of PTH in target tissues
- Hypoparathyroidism
  - —Primary failure of the parathyroid gland
- Pseudohypoparathyroidism
  - —Tissue unresponsiveness with elevated PTH levels
  - —Associated with failure of other endocrine systems associated with coupling of c-AMP
  - —Pseudo-pseudohypoparathyroidism—incomplete expression

ETIOLOGY

- Failure of parathyroid gland from
  - —Congenital absence
  - —Autoimmune destruction
  - —Surgical interruption of blood supply or gland removal
  - —Radiation damage
  - —Hypomagnesemia as PTH cofactor
- End organ unresponsiveness to PTH
- DiGeorge's syndrome
  - —Hypoparathyroidism
  - —Thymic dysplasia
  - —Severe immunodeficiency
- Wilson's disease
  - —Destruction of gland due to copper deposition
- Autoimmune polyglandular syndrome type I
  - —Hypoparathyroidism
  - —Adrenal insufficiency
  - —Mucocutaneous candidiasis
- Albright's syndrome (hereditary osteodystrophy)
  - —Short stature
  - —Obesity
  - —Round face
  - —Short neck
  - —Short 4th and 5th metacarpals and metatarsals. (Type I pseudohypoparathyroidism)

PEDIATRIC CONSIDERATIONS

- Neonates/infants
  - —Transient hypoparathyroidism in first year of life
  - —Subnormal intelligence proportional to duration of hypocalcemia
  - —Dental hypoplasia

Pre-Hospital

CAUTIONS

- Administer calcium in hypocalcium induced Vfib in addition to usual ACLS
  - —Hypoparathyroidism
  - —Exposure to hydrofluoric acid or ammonium bifluoride (aluminum wheel cleaner)
- Stridor may herald laryngospasm

Diagnosis

ESSENTIAL WORKUP

- Most common causes of hypocalcemia
  - —Hypoalbuminemia
    - -Total ionized Ca^{++} normal in hypoalbuminemia
    - -Protein bound Ca^{++} low
    - -Laboratory value abnormal, but patient is asymptomatic
  - —Hyperventilation
    - -Ionized Ca^{++}—active form
    - -Alkalosis increases the binding to albumin reducing the ionized Ca^{++}
    - -Symptomatic hypocalcemia in alkalosis with a normal laboratory value
- PTH level
  - —Low in primary hypoparathyroidism and in vitamin D deficiency
  - —Elevated in pseudohypoparathyroidism and hypocalcemia from renal failure

LABORATORY

- Calcium: correct for albumin using formula
  - —Corrected Ca^{++} (mg/dl) = measured Ca^{++} (mg/dl) + 0.8{4.0 − albumin (g/dl)}
- Electrolytes, BUN, Cr, glucose
- Magnesium
- ABG if symptomatic
  - —Elevation of 0.1 pH unit decreases the ionized Ca^{++} by 3–8%
- Phosphorus
  - —Elevated except when hypocalcemia due to vitamin D deficiency

IMAGING/SPECIAL TESTS

- ECG
- Ellsworth-Howard test

DIAGNOSIS	*URINARY CAMP*	*URINARY PHOSPHATE EXCRETION*
Normal	Increased	Increased
Hypoparathyroidism	Increased	Increased
Pseudohypoparathyroidism Type I	No significant increase	No significant increase
Pseudohypoparathyroidism Type II	Increased	No significant increase
Pseudopseudohypoparathyroidism	No significant increase	No significant increase

DIFFERENTIAL DIAGNOSIS

- Causes of hypocalcemia (correct for hypoalbuminemia)
- Hypoparathyroidism
  - —Gland failure
  - —Hypomagnesemia
  - —PTH resistance
- Hypomagnesemia
  - —Lack of magneseium as a cofactor inhibits PTH secretion
- Vitamin D deficiency (low Ca^{++} + low PO_4)
  - —Anticonvulsant use
  - —Liver disease
  - —Resistance to vitamin D
  - —Malabsorption or dietary deficiency
- Renal failure
- Osteoblastic metastases
- Acute hyperphosphatemia
  - —Fleet enemas
  - —Rhabdomyolysis
- Other calcium complexes and uncertain etiology
  - —Pancreatitis
  - —Ammonium bifluoride (tire cleaner spray)
  - —Hydrofluoric acid
  - —Citrated blood
  - —Gram-negative sepsis

PEDIATRIC CONSIDERATIONS

- Suspect hypocalcemia (due to exposure to phosphates or ammonium bifluoride (tire cleaner spray)) in pediatric cardiac arrest of unclear etiology,

Treatment

INITIAL STABILIZATION

- ABCs
  - —Manage airway if laryngospasm
- Administer IV calcium bolus (chloride or gluconate) if unstable cardiac rhythm or tetany
  - —Slow infusion much safer unless patient symptomatic
- Prepare for ventricular dysrhythmias including ventricular fibrillation
- Seizure precautions

ED TREATMENT

- Replete calcium
  - —500–1000 mg elemental Ca^{++} (peds: 100 mg elemental Ca^{++}/kg/24hrs) infused over 6–24 hours with frequent checks of serum Ca^{++} levels
  - —Supplement to lowest possible Ca^{++} level keeping the patient asymptomatic because elevated phosphorus level will precipitate renal stones
- Replace magnesium if low
- Bind phosphorus with
  - —Aluminum hydroxide containing antacids (Maalox, Mylanta, or Gelusil)
  - —Calcium carbonate when concurrent renal failure
- Begin vitamin D supplementation
- Avoid carbonated beverages (high in phosphorus)
- Assess for associated endocrinopathies

MEDICATIONS

- Calcium choride (272 mg elemental Ca^{++}/10 ml amp): 1 amp over 3–5 min IV
- Calcium gluconate (93 mg elemental Ca^{++}/10 ml amp): 1–3 amp over 5–10 min/amp
- Vitamin D: 400 IU/day

Disposition

ADMISSION CRITERIA

- Symptomatic hypocalcemia
- Abnormal EKG
- Inability to take vitamin D or calcium orally
- Corrected calcium <5 mg/dl

DISCHARGE CRITERIA

- Asymptomatic hypocalcemia

Miscellaneous

ICD9: 252.1

CORE CONTENT CODE: 4.6

SUGGESTED READINGS

Andreoli T. Cecil essentials of medicine. 4th ed. Philadelphia: WB Saunders, 1997.

Edmondson S, Almquist TD. Iatrogenic hypocalcemic tetany. Ann Emerg Med 1990;19:938–940.

Fleisher G, Ludwig S. Textbook of pediatric emergency medicine. 3rd ed. Baltimore: Williams & Wilkins, 1993.

Klasner AE. Marked hypocalcemia and ventricular fibrillation in two pediatric patients exposed to a fluoride containing wheel cleaner. Ann Emerg Med 1996;28:713–718.

Noble J, ed. Textbook of primary care medicine. 2d ed. St. Louis: CV Mosby, 1996.

Olinger ML. Disorders of calcium and magnesium. Emerg Med Clin North Am 1989;7:795–822.

Wallach J, ed. Interpretation of diagnostic tests. 6th ed. Boston: Little, Brown and Company, 1996.

Author: Hugh Schuckman

Clinical Presentation

SIGNS AND SYMPTOMS

TEMP °C	*SIGNS/SYMPTOMS*
35	Maximum shivering
34	Amnesia/dysarthria
33	Ataxia/apathy
32	Stuporous
31	Shivering ceases
30	AFib
28	VFib
27	Reflexes/voluntary motion cease
24	Significant hypotension
19	EEG flat
18	Asystole
15.2	Lowest accidental hypothermia survival

Cardiovascular

- Early tachycardia followed by bradycardia
  - —Caused by decreased spontaneous depolarization of pacemaker cells
  - —Refractory to atropine
- Cardiac cycle lengthens resulting in increased intervals
- Osborn J wave = hypothermic hump
  - —Repolarization abnormality seen at the junction of the QRS and ST segments at temperatures less than 32° C
- Core temperature after drop
  - —Decline in a temperature after removal from the cold
  - —Most common during active external rewarming where peripheral vasoconstriction and AV shunting are reversed

Respiratory System

- Progressive respiratory depression with CO_2 retention

Renal System

- Paradoxical large initial diuresis due to
  - —Relative central hypovolemia
  - —Cold-induced defects in distal tubular reabsorption of sodium and water
  - —Renal blood flow depressed 50% at 27–30° C

MECHANISM/DESCRIPTION

- Definition = body temperature <35° C

ETIOLOGY

- Decreased heat production
  - —At age extremes
  - —With endocrine failure and malnutrition
- Impaired thermoregulation
  - —Central CNS conditions affecting the hypothalamus
  - —Spinal cord transection
- Medications/toxins decrease the body's ability to respond to cold stress
- Immersion in cold water and wet clothes increase heat loss
- Shivering increases the metabolic rate

PEDIATRIC CONSIDERATIONS

- Infants have a large body surface to mass ratio and are at greater risk for hypothermia

Pre-Hospital

CONTROVERSIES

- CPR not recommended if
  - —Electrical rhythm present without palpable pulse or blood pressure with short transport time

CAUTIONS

- Prolonged palpation/auscultation for cardiac activity
  - —Apparent cardiovascular collapse may be depressed cardiac output often sufficient to meet metabolic demands

Diagnosis

ESSENTIAL WORKUP

- Accurate core temperature confirms diagnosis

LABORATORY

- ABG
  - —Temperature correction not needed
- CBC
  - —Hematocrit rises due to decreased plasma volume
  - —Leukopenia does not imply absence of infection
- Electrolytes, BUN, Cr
  - —Vary during rewarming; recheck frequently
- PT, PTT, and platelets
  - —Prolonged clotting times with thrombocytopenia common
- Toxicology screen
- Alcohol/drug ingestions—common risk factors

IMAGING/SPECIAL TESTS

- CXR—pneumonia common complication

DIFFERENTIAL DIAGNOSIS

- Environmental
- Sepsis
- Primary CNS disorder

Treatment

INITIAL STABILIZATION

- ABCs
  —Supplemental oxygen
  —Oral and nasotracheal intubation are safe
  —Cardiac monitor
  —Warmed D5.9NS preferred over lactated Ringers
- Remove wet clothing and begin passive external rewarming
- Administer narcan, D50W (or Accucheck), and thiamine with an altered mental status
- Obtain accurate core temperatures using rectal temperature

ED TREATMENT

Cardiac Arrest Resuscitation

- VFib induction occurs with rough handling, chest compressions, hypoxia, and acid/base changes
- CPR is less effective due to decreased chest wall elasticity
- Defibrillation is rarely successful at temperatures <30° C
  —Defibrillate 1-3 times and then again post-rewarming
  —Direct current results in myocardial damage

Arrhythmia Management

- Atrial fibrillation
  —Common below 32° C
  —Usually converts spontaneously with re-warming
- Malignant ventricular arrhythmias
  —Bretylium—drug of choice
  —Avoid lidocaine and procainamide—may increase ventricular fibrillation

Rewarming Techniques

- Faster rewarming rates (1–2° C/hr) generally have better prognosis than slower rewarming rates (<0.5° C/hr)
- Active rewarming is necessary at core temperatures below 32° C
  —Internal thermogenesis (shivering extinguished) insufficient to increase the body temperature
- *Passive external rewarming*
  —Ideal technique for the majority of healthy patients with mild hypothermia
  —Cover the patient with dry insulting material
  —Endogenous thermogenesis must generate an acceptable rate of rewarming
- *Active external rewarming* delivers heat directly to the skin
  —Associated with core temperature after drop
  —Safe in previously healthy young acutely hypothermic victims

Active Core Rewarming Techniques

- *Airway rewarming* (complete humidification at 40–45° C)
  —Administer to all patients
- *Heated IV* (40–42° C)
  —Administer to all patients
  —High flow rates must be maintained to deliver warmed fluid
  —Heat 1 L of crystalloid in a microwave set at high in 2 minutes
- *Heated gastric irrigation* via nasogastric or orogastric tubes
  —Not recommended
  —Low amount of surface area
  —Aspiration risk if the airway not been secured
- *Pleural irrigation* (0.9%NS at 30–42° C)
  —Use in severe hypothermia without cardiac activity
  —One or two chest tubes
  —Contraindicated in patients with a cardiac rhythm because the chest tube may induce VFib
- *Heated peritoneal lavage* (0.9%NS at 40–45° C)
  —Use in unstable hypothermic patients or stable patients with severe hypothermia whose rewarming rates are <1° C/hr
  —One or two catheters
  —Advantageous in patients with an overdose or rhabdomyolysis
- *Hemodialysis*
  —Initiate for patients with drug overdoses or severe electrolyte disturbances
- *Cardiopulmonary bypass*
  —Treatment of choice in severe hypothermia especially for those patients in cardiac arrest
  —Complications include
    -Hemolysis
    -Arterial injury
    -Air embolism
    -Those associated with systemic heparinization

MEDICATIONS

- Bretylium: 5–10 mg/kg IVP
- Dextrose: D50W 1 amp (50 ml or 25 g) (peds: D25W 2–4 ml/kg) IV
- Naloxone (narcan): 2 mg (peds: 0.1 mg/kg) IV or IM initial dose
- Thiamine (vitamin B_1): 100 mg (peds: 50 mg) IV or IM

Disposition

ADMISSION CRITERIA

- Moderate to severe hypothermia (<32° C)
- Young, healthy patients with no comorbid illness who have mild accidental hypothermia (>32° C) that responds well to warming
  —Admit to an observation area
  —Discharge if asymptomatic after 8–12 hours if they remain asymptomatic

DISCHARGE CRITERIA

- Young, healthy patients with no comorbid illness
- Very mild accidental hypothermia (>35° C) that responds well to warming
- Safe, warm environment to go to after discharge

Miscellaneous

ICD9: 991.6

CORE CONTENT CODE: 5.9.2

SUGGESTED READINGS

Britt LD, Dascombe WH, Rodriguez A. New horizons in management of hypothermia and frostbite injury. Surg Clin North Am 1991;71(2):345–370.

Danzl DF. Accidental hypothermia. N Engl J Med 1994;331(26):1756–1760.

Jolly BT, Ghezzi KT. Accidental hypothermia. Emerg Med Clin North Am 1994;10(2):311–327.

Author: Jeffrey Schaider

Hypothyroidism

Clinical Presentation

SIGNS AND SYMPTOMS

Symptoms

- Weakness/fatigue/drowsiness
- Cold intolerance
- Headaches
- Mental status changes
- Myalgias
- Menorrhagia
- Constipation
- Weight gain
- Emotional lability

Signs

- Puffy eyelids
- Sparse pubic, axillary hair
- Absent lateral one-third eyebrows
- Prolonged relaxation phase DTR's
- Yellow tinged/dry skin
- Pallor
- Goiter
- Myxedema—dry, waxy swelling of skin/subcutaneous tissues
- Swelling of hands/feet
- Huskiness of voice
- Galactorrhea

Myxedema Coma

- Extreme form of hypothyroidism (see above)
- Hypothermia
- Bradycardia
- Hypotension
- Coma/altered mental status

MECHANISM/DESCRIPTION

- Results from a deficiency of thyroid hormone
- Primarily due to thyroid disease caused by
  —Autoimmune process
  —Iatrogenic failure
- Pituitary disease or secondary failure accounts for less than 4% of cases
- Usually follows an indolent course with decompensation after specific stress factors
- *Myedema coma* caused by hypothyroidism with hypoxia, hypothermia, hypotension, hypoglycemia, hyponatremia, adrenal insufficiency, drugs (sedative hypnotics)

ETIOLOGY

Primary

- Congenital
- Autoimmune
  —Hypothyroidism
  —Thyroiditis
  —Hashimoto's disease
- Idiopathic
- Iatrogenic
  —Postsurgical
  —External radiation
  —Radioiodine therapy
  —Antithyroid drugs (iodides, lithium)
- Inherited defect: aplasia, hypoplasia, enzymatic defect, ingestion of drugs or goitrogens during pregnancy
- Neoplasm: primary (carcinoma) or secondary infiltration
- Infection: viral (rarely aerobic or anaerobic bacteria)
- Trauma: neck injury

Secondary

- Pituitary tumor
- Infiltrative disease (sarcoid) or tumor
- Trauma

Pre-Hospital

N/A

Diagnosis

ESSENTIAL WORKUP

- Laboratory confirmation of the diagnosis of hypothyroidism/myxedema coma is ususally not possible in the emergency department
- Myxedema coma—life-threatening condition
  —Initiate therapy if a high index of suspicion
- Thyroid function studies
  —Free T_4 (low)
  —High sensitivity TSH (increased)
  —If free T_4 unavailable—total T_4 (decreased) and resin T_3 uptake (increased)
- Electrocardiogram
  —Profound bradycardia

LABORATORY

- CBC
  —Anemia may be noted
- Electrolytes, BUN, Cr, glucose
  —Hyponatremia
  —Hypoglycemia
- AST, LDH, CPK
- Arterial blood gases
  —Hypoxemia/hypercapnia
  —Acidosis
- Search for the underlying etiology

IMAGING/SPECIAL TESTS

- CXR
  —Enlarged heart/CHF
  —Pericardial/pleural effusion
- Echocardiogram for suspected pericardial effusion

DIFFERENTIAL DIAGNOSIS

- Nephrotic syndrome
- Chronic nephritis
- Hypoalbuminemia
- Chronic renal disease
- Sepsis
- Depression
- CHF

Treatment

INITIAL STABILIZATION

- ABCs
  - —Intubation and ventilation may be necessary
- Cardiac monitor
- Blood pressure support
- Supplemental oxygen to meet metabolic needs
- Correct hypothermia
  - —Initiate passive warming measures

ED TREATMENT

- Mild hypothyroidism—oral thyoid replacement as an outpatient

Myxedema coma

- Thyroid hormone replacement
  - —Prompt IV replacement improves survival
  - —l-thyroxine
  - —Use smaller doses of thyroid hormone in the elderly or patients with cardiac disease
- Hydrocortisone to prevent Addisonian crisis
- Dextrose for hypoglycemia
- IV fluid bolus for hypotension
  - —Avoid pressors, if possible, as they may precipitate arrhythmias
  - —Response to pressors is poor until thyoid replacement initiated
  - —Thyroid hormone augments action of pressors
- Correction of the underlying precipitant

MEDICATIONS

- Dextrose: 50–100 cc D50 (peds: 2 cc/kg of D10 over 1 min) IV
- Hydrocortisone: 100 mg (peds: 4 mg/kg) IV
- l-thyroxine: 300–500 μg load IV followed by 50–100 μg IV daily

Disposition

ADMISSION CRITERIA

- Myxedema coma (admit to ICU)

DISCHARGE CRITERIA

- Hypothyroid patients should be referred to a primary care taker for initiation of oral thyroid hormone replacement therapy

Miscellaneous

ICD9: 244.9

CORE CONTENT CODE: 4.9.2

SUGGESTED READINGS

Holmes L, Lakshmanan M. The patient with chronic endocrine disease. In: Herr RD, Cydulka RK, eds. Emergency care of the compromised patient. Philadelphia: Lippincott-Raven, 1994:123–133.

Jordan RM. Myxedema coma. Pathophysiology, therapy, and factors affecting prognosis. Med Clin North Am 1995;79:185–194.

Nicoloff JT, LoPresti JS. Myxedema coma. A form of decompensated hypothyroidism. Endocrinol Metab Clin North Am 1993;22:279–290.

Tsitouras PD. Myxedema coma. Clin Geriatr Med 1995;11:251–258.

Wogan JM. Endocrine disorders. In: Rosen P, et al., eds. Emergency medicine: Concepts and clinical practice. 4th ed. St. Louis: CV Mosby, 1998:2488–2503.

Author: Rita Cydulka

Idiopathic Thrombocytopenic Purpura

Clinical Presentation

SIGNS AND SYMPTOMS

- Bleeding into superficial sites
  - —Skin and mucous membranes = purpura
  - —Genitourinary tract = hematuria
  - —Gastrointestinal = hematemesis, hematochezia, or melena
- Neurologic deficits secondary to intracranial hemorrhage
- Bleeding begins immediately after trauma

MECHANISM/DEFINITION

- Thrombocytopenia without abnormalities in other cell lines or apparent cause for low platelets
- Immune mediated destruction of circulating platelets primarily in the spleen

Acute Idiopathic Thrombocytopenia Purpura (ITP)

- Severe thrombocytopenia following recovery from viral exanthem or upper respiratory illness
- 90% of ITP are pediatric cases
- 90% recover within 3–6 months

Chronic Idiopathic Thrombocytopenia Purpura

- Women aged 20–40 most commonly afflicted
- Caused by autoimmune disorder
- More indolent then acute ITP

Pre-Hospital

N/A

Diagnosis

ESSENTIAL WORKUP

- Diagnosis based on excluding other causes of thrombocytopenia
- Complete history
  - —Assess type of bleeding to differentiate platelet related mucocutaneous bleeding from coagulation disorder which usually cause delayed visceral hematomas
  - —Rule out drug-induced thrombocytopenias
  - —Exclude systemic illnesses as cause of thrombocytopenia
- Directed physical exam excluding other causes of thrombocytopenia
  - —Type of bleeding (mucocutaneous vs. visceral)
  - —Evidence of liver dysfunction, auto immune disorders
  - —Evaluate for signs of thrombosis
  - —Evidence of infection (bacteremia or HIV)
  - —Neurological exam to exclude intracranial hemorrhage

LABORATORY

- CBC/peripheral smear
  - —Results consistent with diagnosis of ITP
    - -Thrombocytopenia
    - -Normal platelet size
    - -Normal red blood cell morphology
    - -Normal white blood cell morphology
- HIV Antibody

IMAGING/SPECIAL TESTS

- Abdominal CT scan or ultrasound for patients with splenomegaly on exam
- Head CT scan for neurologic findings consistent with intracranial bleeding
- Bone marrow aspiration
  - —Not routinely indicated
  - —Indications
    - -Children with persistent thrombocytopenia >6–12 months
    - -Children unresponsive to intravenous immunoglobulin (IV IG)
    - -Adults >60
    - -Patients considering splenectomy

DIFFERENTIAL DIAGNOSIS (OF THROMBOCYTOPENIA)

- Impaired bone marrow production
  - —Bone marrow fibrosis
  - —Bone marrow infiltration with malignant cells
  - —Cytotoxic drugs used in chemotherapy
  - —Congenital bone marrow abnormalities
- Splenic sequestration
  - —As spleen enlarges the fraction of platelets sequestered increases
  - —Common causes
    - -Portal hypertension
    - -Splenic infiltration with tumor
- Accelerated destruction of platelets
  - —Nonimmunologic thrombocytopenia
    - -Vasculitis
    - -Hemolytic uremic syndrome
    - -Thrombotic thrombocytopenic purpura (TTP)
    - -Disseminated intravascular coagulation (DIC)
    - -Cardiac valve abnormalities
  - —Immunologic thrombocytopenia
- Drug-induced thrombocytopenia
  - —Suppress platelet production
    - -Chemotherapeutics
    - -Thiazide diuretics
    - -Ethanol
    - -Estrogen
  - —Cause immunologic platelet destruction
    - -Aspirin
    - -Chlorpropamide
    - -Chloroquine
    - -Gold salts
    - -Insecticides
    - -Sulfa drugs

Treatment

INITIAL STABILIZATION

- ABCs
- Stabilize severe life-threatening bleeding
  - —Intracranial hemorrhage
    - -Airway control
    - -Hyperventilation
    - -Neurosurgery consult
  - —Hemorrhagic shock
    - -Large bore IV lines
    - -Control bleeding with direct pressure if possible
    - -Blood and platelet transfusion
    - -IV glucocorticoids
    - -IV immune globulin

ED TREATMENT

- Initial treatment options for ITP are based on
  - —Degree of thrombocytopenia
  - —Severity of illness
  - —Age
  - —Risk factors for bleeding (hypertension, peptic ulcer disease, vigorous lifestyle)
- Efficacy of specific treatment options demonstrated in terms of platelet recovery time and not in terms of morbidity and mortality

Specific Treatment Options

- High dose oral corticosteroids (suppresses immune response)
- Intravenous immune globulin (IVIG)
  - —Causes temporary phagocytic blockade
  - —Combined with glucocorticoids considered first-line treatment in children
- Splenectomy
  - —Second-line treatment
  - —Inadequate data to make evidence-based recommendations on appropriate indications and timing for emergency and elective splenectomy
  - —Adverse risks
    - -Operative
    - -Fatal bacterial infection
  - —Considered in specific clinical situation
    - -Glucocorticoid therapy unsuccessful
    - -Children with ITP for 1 year, bleeding symptoms, platelet count <10,000
    - -Adults with ITP for 6 weeks, platelet count <10,000
    - -Adults with ITP for 3 months, platelet counts <30,000

MEDICATION

- Collagen absorbable hemostat sponges: apply directly to bleeding surface with pressure 1×2-inch, 3×4-inch sponges
- Intravenous immune globulin: 1 g/kg IV 1-time dose
- Methylprednisolone: 1 g (peds: 30 mg/kg/24 hrs) IV q 8 hrs
- Prednisone: 1–2 mg/kg/d (peds: 4 mg/kg/d) po

Disposition

ADMISSION CRITERIA

- Life-threatening bleeding regardless of platelet count
- Mucus membrane bleeding and platelet count <20,000
- Asymptomatic patient with platelet count <20,000 who may become inaccessible or noncompliant

DISCHARGE CRITERIA

- Asymptomatic patients
- Patients with only minor purpura and platelet count >30,000/mm^3

Miscellaneous

ICD9: 287.2

CORE CONTENT CODE: 7.2.3.1

SUGGESTED READINGS

George JN, et al. Idiopathic thrombocytopenic purpura: A practice guideline developed by explicit methods for the American Society of Hematology. Blood 1996;88(1):3–40.

Handin RI. Disorders of platelet and vessel wall. In: Fauci AS, Braunwald E, Isselbacher KJ, et al. eds. Harrison's principles of internal medicine. 14th ed. New York: McGraw Hill, 1997.

Reid MM. Chronic idiopathic thrombocytopenic purpura: incidence, treatment, and outcome. Arch Dis Child 1995;72(2):125–128.

Author: John McCourt

Initial ED Treatment Options for Patients with ITP

CLINICAL PRESENTATION	*CHILDREN*		*ADULTS*	
	PLATELET >30,000/MM³	*PLATELET <30,000/MM³*	*PLATELET >50,000/MM³*	*PLATELET <50,000/MM³*
Asymptomatic or minor purpura	No treatment	Oral prednisone IVIG	No treatment	Oral prednisone
Mucous membrane bleeding	Topical collagen sponge	Oral prednisone, IVIG; topical collagen Sponge	Topical collagen sponge	Oral prednisone; topical absorbable sponge

Immunosuppression

Clinical Presentation

SIGNS AND SYMPTOMS

- The principle concern is for occult infection
- Fever, altered mental status
- Abdominal pain without peritoneal signs or leukocytosis
- Generalized weakness, malaise
- Meningitis without meningeal signs
- Fever in the neutropenic patient:
  —Single temperature ≥38.3°C or sustained temperature≥38.0°C over 1–2 hours
- Other signs and symptoms dictated by specific diseases

MECHANISM/DESCRIPTION

- Most common sites of infection in neutropenia
  —Lung (25%)
  —Mouth and pharynx (25%)
  —Skin, soft tissue, and intravascular catheters (15%)
  —Perineum and anorectal area (10%)
  —Urinary tract (5%)
  —Nose and sinuses (5%)
  —Gastrointestinal tract (5%)
- The most important bacterial organisms
  —*Escherichia coli*
  —*Klebsiella* species
  —*Pseudomonas aeruginosa*
  —*Staphylococcus epidermidis*
  —α-Hemolytic streptococcal species
  —*Staphylococcus aureus*
- Fungal infections
  —Seen in patients on broad-spectrum antibiotics
  —Persistent fever and neutropenia for >7 days
  —*Aspergillus flavus*
  —*Aspergillus fumigatus*
  —*Candida albicans*
  —*Candida tropicalis*

DEFINITION

- Deficiency in ability to fight infection
  —Congenital (incidence 1:10,000 patients)
    -Antibody (B cell)
    -Cellular (T cell)
    -Combined
    -Phagocytic dysfunction
  —Acquired

ETIOLOGY

- Old age (>75)
  —Decreased antibody and cellular immunity
  —Decreased cough reflex
  —Poor circulation and wound healing
  —Communal living (nosocomial infections)
  —Physiologic responses to infection are blunted
  —Blunted leukocytosis
  —Lack of classic peritoneal signs despite perforated viscus
- Organ transplant recipients
  —Immunosuppressive medications
- Intravenous drug abuse (IVDA)
  —Opiates suppress phagocytosis and bactericidal activity
  —Depressed cellular immunity with methadone and morphine
  —Risk factor for AIDS
- HIV infection (see chapter: HIV/AIDS)
- Diabetes
  —Hyperglycemia causes defective immune function while euglycemia improves it
  —Vascular insufficiency (small and large vessel)
  —Peripheral neuropathy leads to wound neglect
- Malnutrition
  —Homelessness
  —Alcoholism
- Cancer and chemoradiotherapy
  —Neutropenia from chemotherapy or native disease process
    -Defined as absolute neutrophil count (ANC) <500–1000/mm^3
  —Impairment in T cell and B cell function

Pre-Hospital

CAUTIONS

- Observe universal precautions for patient and provider protection
- Patients in septic shock require aggressive resuscitation

Diagnosis

ESSENTIAL WORKUP

- Workup must be tailored to the specific presenting complaint
- CBC, differential, urinalysis, CXR
- Pitfalls in identifying infection with neutropenia
  —Overt signs of inflammation (redness, drainage, swelling) may not be present
  —Peritonitis may not manifest
  —Pyuria can be absent with urinary tract infection
  —Meningitis may be present without CSF pleocytosis (especially cryptococcal meningitis)

LABORATORY

- Obtain cultures
  —Two sets bacterial
  —One fungal culture
  —Cultures from an indwelling central line
  —Urine culture
  —Lumbar puncture if there is suspicion of meningitis (low-grade headache, confusion)

IMAGING/SPECIAL TESTS

- Chest x-ray should be obtained in all patients with fever and immunosuppression
- Sinus CT should be performed if facial pain or swelling is present
- CT, MRI, or radionuclide studies may be indicated to localize site of infection

Treatment

INITIAL STABILIZATION

- Hypotension
  - —Fluid resuscitation; may need 1–2 L NS or more for sepsis with hypotension
  - —Pressors if hypotension unresponsive to fluids
    - -Systolic blood pressure ≥70: Dopamine: 5–20 μg/kg/min
    - -Systolic blood pressure <70: Norepinephrine 0.5–30 μg/min; usual adult dose 2–12 μg/min
- Airway management for ventilatory failure, hypoxia unresponsive to high flow face-mask oxygen
- Cardiac monitor and pulse oximetry

ED TREATMENT

- Start broad-spectrum antimicrobial therapy in the ED after appropriate cultures obtained
- If ANC is less than 100/mm^3, use combination therapy
  - —Aminoglycoside (gentamicin) *plus* extended spectrum penicillin (mezlocillin) or ticarcillin with clavulanate or piperacillin with tazobactam *or*
  - —Aminoglycoside (gentamicin) *plus* an antipseudomonal third-generation cephalosporin (ceftazidime or cefoperazone), *or*
  - —Extended spectrum penicillin (mezlocillin) or ticarcillin with clavulanate, or piperacillin with tazobactam *plus* antipseudomonal third-generation cephalosporin (ceftazidime or cefoperazone)
- If ANC is >100/mm^3, monotherapy is acceptable
  - —Ceftazidime *or* imipenem
  - —For penicillin allergic patients aztreonam *plus* vancomycin
- If anaerobes are suspected (i.e., oral, abdominal, or perianal infection) add clindamycin

MEDICATIONS

- Aztreonam: adult: 2 g IV; peds: 120 mg/kg/day IV div q 6 hrs
- Cefoperazone: adult: 2 g IV; peds: 150 mg/kg/day IV div q 8 hrs
- Ceftazidime: adult: 2 g IV; peds: 150 mg/kg/day IV div q 8 hrs
- Clindamycin: adult: 900 mg IV; peds: 25–40 mg/kg/day IV, IM div q 6 hrs
- Gentamicin: adult: 2–5 mg/kg IV; peds: 5 mg/kg/day IV, IM div q 12 hrs
- Imipenem: adult: 0.5 g IV; peds: safety not established
- Mezlocillin: adult: 3 g IV; peds: safety not established
- Piperacillin/tazobactam: adult: 3.375 g IV; peds: safety not established
- Ticarcillin/clavulanate: adult: 3.1 g IV: peds: safety not established
- Vancomycin: adult: 1 g IV; peds: 40–60 mg/kg/day IV div q 6 hrs

Disposition

ADMISSION CRITERIA

- All febrile patients with neutropenia or organ transplant
- Admit to intensive care if signs of hemodynamic instability
- Admit elderly patients and diabetics with fever and signs of infection
- Admit intravenous drug users with fever, as approximately 20% have serious bacterial infection (pneumonia, endocarditis, bacteremia)

DISCHARGE CRITERIA

- If workup is negative, patient is not neutropenic and is reliable, well appearing, tolerating po liquids, and close follow-up is assured, a trial of outpatient therapy is warranted
- Parenteral antibiotic therapy is given in ED and oral antibiotics as an outpatient. Patient must follow up in 1 day for reevaluation and to check culture results

Miscellaneous

ICD9: 279.2

CORE CONTENT CODE: 8.6.2

SUGGESTED READINGS

Pizzo PA. Management of fever in patients with cancer and treatment-induced neutropenia. N Engl J Med 1993;328:1323.

Rosenberg AS, Brown AE. Infection in the cancer patient. Dis Mon 1993;39:507–569.

Rubin JT, Lotze T. Immune function and dysfunction: A primer for the radiologist. Radiol Clin North Am 1992;30:507.

Schimpff SC. Infections in the cancer patient—diagnosis, prevention and treatment. In: Mandell GL, Bennett JE, Dolin R. Principles and practice of infectious diseases. 4th ed. New York: Churchill Livingstone, 1995:2666–2675.

Sternbach GL. Infections in alcoholic patients. Emerg Med Clin North Am 1990;8:793.

Swenson KK, Rose MA, Ritz L, Murray CL, Adlis SA. Recognition and evaluation of oncology-related symptoms in the emergency department. Ann Emerg Med 1995;26:12.

Author: Mark I. Langdorf

Impetigo

Clinical Presentation

SIGNS AND SYMPTOMS

Classical (Nonbullous) Impetigo

- The result of bacteria entering through traumatic skin portal from scratch, abrasion, or insect bite
- Begins as a single 2–4 mm erythematous macule that may evolve into a vesicle or pustule
- Rupture of the vesicle leaves a *honey-colored* exudative crust
- Highly contagious and may be spread from the original site of infection by scratching
- Mild lymphadenopathy may be seen
- Systemic manifestations are rare

Bullous Impetigo

- Occurs most commonly in the neonate
- Large, superficial, fragile bullae present on the trunk and extremities
- The fragile bullae may have ruptured leaving only a shiny, erythematous base with peeling edges
- Weakness, fever, and diarrhea are common systemic manifestations

Mechanism/Description

Classic Impetigo

- Caused by *Staphylococcus aureus*, Group A β-hemolytic streptococci, or both
- More prevalent in warm climates and warm seasons

Bullous Impetigo

- Caused by *Staphylococcus aureus* alone
- Epidermal separation is caused by a *Staphylococcal* exotoxin

Pre-Hospital

CAUTIONS

- Maintain universal precautions

Diagnosis

ESSENTIAL WORKUP

- The diagnosis is made based on observation of the classic findings. Laboratory and culture confirmation is not necessary unless the diagnosis is in question
- Cultures may be considered in those cases refractory to traditional therapy

DIFFERENTIAL DIAGNOSIS

- Herpes simplex
- Varicella
- Atopic dermatitis
- Contact dermatitis
- Dermatophytosis
- Erysipelas
- Candidiasis
- Scabies
- Pediculosis
- Pemphigus vulgaris
- Bullous pemphigoid
- Thermal burns
- Stevens-Johnson syndrome
- Bullous erythema multiforme

Treatment

INITIAL STABILIZATION

- In healthy children or adults, classic or bullous impetigo is not a life-threatening condition and does not require resuscitative measures

ED TREATMENT

- Small lesions may be treated with topical therapy alone using mupirocin or in conjunction with systemic therapy
- Larger, widespread lesions should be treated with systemic therapy
- Treatment should employ a β-lactamase-resistant penicillin, cephalosporin, or macrolide antimicrobial for 7 days
- Local care should include cleansing, removal of crusts, and application of wet dressings to the affected areas

MEDICATIONS

- All treatment regimens are 7 days
  —Ampicillin/clavulanate: adult: 250 mg po q 8 hrs; peds: 20 mg/kg/day po in divided doses q 8 hrs
  —Azithromycin: adult: 500 mg po day 1; 250 mg po days 2–5; peds: 10 mg/kg po day 1; 5 mg/kg po days 2–5
  —Cephalexin: adult: 500 mg po q 12 hrs; peds: 40 mg/kg/day po in divided doses q 8 hrs Clarithromycin: adult: 250 mg po q 12 hrs; peds: 15 mg/kg/day po q 12 hrs
  —Dicloxacillin: adult: 250 mg po q 6 hrs; peds: 30 mg/kg/day po in divided doses q 6 hrs
  —Erythromycin ethylsuccinate: adult: 250 mg po q 6 hrs; peds: 40 mg/kg/day po in divided doses q 6 hrs
  —Mupirocin (2% ointment): adult and peds: apply topically to affected area 3 times per day

Disposition

ADMISSION CRITERIA

- Admission for impetigo alone is rare
- Patients with disease that is widespread, or refractory to outpatient therapy may require admission
- Toxic, ill-appearing, or immunocompromised patients require admission

DISCHARGE CRITERIA

- Patients should not be toxic appearing
- Patients should be able to comply with the recommended treatment regimen
- Follow-up for reevaluation

Miscellaneous

ICD9: 684

CORE CONTENT CODE: 3.2.1.5

SUGGESTED READINGS

Darmstadt GL, Lane AT. Impetigo: An overview. Pediatr Dermatol 1993;11:4:293–303, 1993.

Shriner DL, Schwartz RA, Janniger CK. Impetigo. Cutis 1995;56:1:30–32.

Author: James L. Larson

Inborn Errors of Metabolism

Clinical Presentation

SIGNS AND SYMPTOMS

- Varies by disease
- Children who initially appear only mildly ill may rapidly decompensate
- Neonates
  —Vomiting
  —Poor feeding
  —Hypotonia or hypertonia
  —Apnea
  —Seizures
  —Coma
  —Jaundice
  —Hypoglycemia
  —Hypothermia
  —Odors in urine/body secretions
- Undiagnosed older children
  —Vomiting with lethargy
  —Unexplained dehydration
  —Diarrhea
  —Headache
  —Ataxia
  —Seizures
  —Recurrent bouts of vomiting
  —Mental retardation
  —Growth failure
  —Intolerance of certain foods
- Physical examination
  —Tachypnea
  —Dermatitis
  —Cataracts
  —Hepatomegaly
  —Splenomegaly
  —Cardiomyopathy
  —Abnormal odor
  —Abnormal facies
  —Altered mental status

MECHANISM/DESCRIPTION

- Clinical manifestations of the individual biochemical disorders are related to the defect involved and the amount and toxicity of the metabolites that accumulate
- Common inherited metabolic diseases include
  —Urea cycle defects
  —Organic acidemias
  —Disorders of amino acid metabolism
  —Defects in fatty acid oxidation
  —Mitochondrial disorders
  —Carbohydrate disorders
  —Mucopolysaccharidoses
  —Sphingolipodoses
  —Peroxisomal disorders

ETIOLOGY

- The classic inherited metabolic diseases are a diverse group of disorders that usually involve a genetic deficiency of an enzyme of an intermediary metabolite, or a deficiency of a membrane transport system
- Most of the metabolic diseases are relatively rare
  —Occurring in 1:100,000–200,000 births
- Over 300 human diseases due to inborn errors of metabolism are now recognized

Pre-Hospital

CAUTIONS

- Careful assessment of the ABCs is essential
- IV glucose infusion takes precedence over fluid boluses unless the patient is in shock
- Avoid lactated Ringer's solution

Diagnosis

ESSENTIAL WORKUP

- Most essential part is thinking of the possible diagnosis
  —Inherited metabolic diseases
    -Often brought to a physician's attention because of neurologic deterioration
    -Often misdiagnosed as sepsis, dehydration, ingestion, or nonaccidental trauma
    -May initially present later in childhood or in adolescence

LABORATORY

- Bedside glucose determination
- Electrolytes, BUN/Cr, glucose
- CBC with differential
- Calcium
- Liver function tests, prothrombin time
- Arterial or venous blood gases
- Uric acid
- Urinalysis
- Ammonia level (free-flowing, placed on ice)
- Quantitative serum amino acids
- Urine organic and amino acids
- Lactate and pyruvate levels (free-flowing, placed on ice)

IMAGING/SPECIAL TESTS

- Blood cultures
- Lumbar puncture
- CXR
- CT head for altered mental status

DIFFERENTIAL DIAGNOSIS

- Sepsis
- Meningitis
- Encephalitis
- Severe dehydration
- Toxic ingestion
- Reye's syndrome
- Hepatic encephalopathy
- Hyperinsulinemia
- Hormonal abnormalities
- Renal failure
- Renal tubular acidosis
- CNS mass lesions
- Nonaccidental trauma

Treatment

INITIAL STABILIZATION

- ABCs
- For altered mental status administer narcan, glucose (or accucheck), and thiamine

ED TREATMENT

Goal of Therapy

- Detoxify/remove existing CNS toxins
- Prevent production of more neurotoxin
- Provide calories to prevent catabolism
- Restore normal acid/base balance
- Identify and treat intercurrent and precipitating illnesses
- Support any failing organ

Specific Measures

- Complete physical examination with strict attention to mental status and hydration status
- Stop all oral intake
  —Amino acid metabolites may be neurotoxic
- Increase urine output to help in removal of some toxins
- Ensure hydration
  —Rehydrate if hypovolemic
- Initiate IV glucose at a rate of 8–10 mg/kg/min to prevent catabolism
  —Corresponds to D10 at 1.5 times maintenance
  —Do not delay glucose infusion to give a "bolus" of isotonic saline; may be given concurrently in a child in shock
  —If a patient is severely hypoglycemic, give IV glucose bolus of D25
- Administer bicarbonate if the pH is < 7.0
  —Initiate dialysis if severe acidosis does not improve quickly
- Treat severe hyperammonemia with dialysis or with ammonia-trapping drugs such as arginine hydrochloride, sodium benzoate, sodium phenylacetate, or sodium phenylbutyrate
  —Dosages vary with disease, and a metabolic physician should be consulted before their use
- Consult a metabolic physician when any child presents with a suspected inherited metabolic disease

MEDICATIONS

- D25: 2–4 cc/kg IV
- Sodium bicarbonate: 1–2 mEq/kg IV

Disposition

ADMISSION CRITERIA

- Infants and children presenting with a new onset of a suspected inherited metabolic disease
- Significant urinary ketones and those not tolerating oral intake will also need admission
- ICU admission for significant altered mental status, severe or persistent acidosis, hypoglycemia which does not resolve quickly with therapy, or hyperammonemia
  —Transfer of these patients to a specialized pediatric center may also be indicated

DISCHARGE CRITERIA

- Normal mental status
- Normal hydration status
- Unremarkable laboratory evaluation
- No evidence of a significant intercurrent illness
- Close follow-up arranged with their primary care physician

Miscellaneous

ICD9: 277.9

CORE CONTENT CODE: N/A

SUGGESTED READINGS

Arens R, Gonzal D, Williams JC, et al. Recurrent apparent life-threatening events during infancy: A manifestation of inborn errors of metabolism. J Pediatr 1993;123(3):415–418.

Goodman SI, Green CL. Metabolic disorders of the newborn. Pediatr Rev 1994;15(9):359–365.

Wappner RS. Biochemical diagnosis of genetic diseases. Pediatr Ann 1993;22(5):282–297.

Author: Joan Bothner

Incompetence, Determination of

Clinical Presentation

SIGNS AND SYMPTOMS

- Inability to make rational decisions about medical treatment

MECHANISM/DESCRIPTION

- Competence
  —Legal term to be defined by a judge
  —In a medical context, refers to a patient's ability to make rational decisions about medical treatment
    -A patient who lacks such ability is said to be incompetent or decisionally incapacitated
- Someone other than the patient must assume responsibility for making medical decisions for patients declared incompetent
  —Depending on circumstances, this role will be assumed by a family member, the physician, or the court

Pre-Hospital

CAUTIONS

- Patients ordinarily have the right to accept or reject treatment as they see fit
  —This right is not absolute
  —Right may be denied if the patient is thought to be incompetent, especially in case of a true emergency
- Rules vary widely from state to state
  —Familiarity with local statutes essential

Diagnosis

ESSENTIAL WORKUP

- Diagnosis is a legal, not a medical, condition
  —Law presumes individuals to be competent until proven otherwise
  —Patient may be declared incompetent only through judicial procedures
- *When the patient's condition necessitates immediate treatment,* physician may be forced to make a presumptive determination of competence without the benefit of judicial decision of legal counsel
- In most states, individuals <18 years old are considered incompetent as a matter of law
  —A parent, guardian, or judge must consent to medical treatment on behalf of the patient
  —Exceptions: when the patient is emancipated or when a true emergency exists
- Incompetence rules vary widely from state to state
  —Familiarity with local statutes essential

Incompetence Evaluation

"Method of Decision" Test

- Most widely accepted by the courts
- Presence of decision test
  —Patient deemed competent so long as the patient makes a decision when one is called for
  —Quality of decision is irrelevant
- Method of decision test
  —Patient deemed competent so long as a reasonable basis exists for reaching the decision
  —Patients who base their decisions on irrelevant issues are considered incompetent
- Nature of decision test
  —Patient is deemed competent so long as the decision seems rational to the examiner
- General incompetence test
  —Patient is deemed competent so long as the patient is fit to function in the world generally, rather than as a patient
  —These conditions render the patient incompetent
    -Intoxication
    -Mental retardation
    -Psychosis

"Sliding Scale" Test

- Uses a variable standard
- As the potential consequences of the patient's decisions become more serious, a more stringent standard of competence is required
  - —A patient demonstrating questionable competence might be allowed to refuse care so long as the associated risk to his health is small
  - —A patient with a life-threatening illness would be allowed to refuse treatment only if clearly competent

LABORATORY

- As appropriate for medical condition
- CBC
  - —For infection
  - —Anemia
- Electrolytes, BUN/Cr, glucose
  - —For ingestion
- Metabolic abnormalities
- Toxicology screen

Treatment

INITIAL STABILIZATION

- Physical restraint
  - —For potentially uncooperative patients and, if the patient's competence is in question, refusal of care would seriously jeopardize the patient's health
- Independent second opinion, psychiatric consult, or consultation with hospital counsel
  - —Useful as a safeguard against liability
  - —Whenever a patient's autonomy is abridged due to incompetence, the reasons must be clearly documented

ED TREATMENT

- No test of competence is valid in all parts of the country
- Practitioners should familiarize themselves with locally accepted standards
- Most competence tests require at a minimum demonstration of the following
  - —Ability to communicate a choice and to maintain that choice long enough for the chosen course of action to be implemented
  - —Ability to understand relevant information
    - -Best evaluated by asking the patient to paraphrase the information provided
  - —Appreciation of the situation and its consequences including comprehension of the following
    - -Nature of the medical condition
    - -Recommended treatment
    - -Treatment alternatives
    - -Risks and benefits of accepting or refusing the proposed treatment
  - —Ability to manipulate information rationally
    - -Patient's conclusion must be logically consistent with the starting premise

Disposition

ADMISSION CRITERIA

- As medically justified

DISCHARGE CRITERIA

- Because forced treatment and the deprivation of decision-making rights represent a serious infringement of the patient's liberty every effort must be made to assist the patient to demonstrate competence

Miscellaneous

ICD9: N/A

CORE CONTENT CODE: N/A

SUGGESTED READINGS

Appelbaum P, Grisso T. Assessing patient's capacities to consent to treatment. N Engl J Med 1988;319(25):1635–638.

Borak J, Veilleux S. Informed consent in emergency settings. Ann Emerg Med 1984;13(9):731–35.

Drane J. Competency to give informed consent. JAMA 1984;252(7):925–27.

Lavoie F. Consent, involuntary treatment, and the use of force in an urban emergency department. Ann Emerg Med 1992;21(1):25–32.

Authors: Jay Weaver; Kathryn Brinsfield

Inflammatory Bowel Disease

Clinical Presentation

SIGNS AND SYMPTOMS

Crohn's Disease

- Any of the clinical correlates of a chronic, inflammatory, fibrostenotic or fistulizing process can be seen

Ulcerative Colitis (UC)

- May begin subtly or as catastrophic illness
- May involve entire colon or be limited to left sided disease or proctitis

MECHANISM/DESCRIPTION

- Idiopathic, chronic, inflammatory disease of the intestines
- Differences between Crohn's and UC
  - —Rectum involved in Crohn's disease and spared in UC
  - —Small bowel not involved in UC
- Similarities between Crohn's and UC
  - —Higher rate of colon cancer with disease >10 years
  - —Pattern of exacerbation/remission
  - —Bimodal age distribution with early peak between teens and early 30s and second peak about age 60
- Crohn's disease clinical pattern
  - —Ileocecal: ~40%
  - —Small bowel: ~30%
  - —Colon: ~25%
  - —Other: ~5%
- UC clinical pattern on presentation
  - —Pancolitis: 30%
    - -Most severe clinical course
  - —Proctitis or proctosigmoiditis: 30%
    - -Relatively mild clinical course
  - —Left-sided colitis (up to splenic flexure): 40%
    - -Between the two in severity

ETIOLOGY

- Unknown
- Two diseases—separate conditions with a common genetic predisposition
- Multifactorial origin involving interplay between
  - —Genetic
  - —Environmental
  - —Immune factors
- Pathogenesis
  - —Gut wall becomes unable to downregulate its immune responses, ultimately resulting in inflammation
- No evidence for etiologic role of infectious agent
- Psychogenic factors play a role in some symptomatic exacerbations

CROHN'S DISEASE

CONSTITUTIONAL

- Low grade fever
- Night sweats
- Weight loss
- Fatigue

GI

- Abdominal pain
  - —Episodic
  - —Periumbilical—may localize to RLQ
  - —Generalized if intestinal involvement more diffuse
  - —Can be localized to a site of intra-abdominal abscess or an area of fistulous involvement
- Diarrhea
  - —Mild loose stool
  - —Rarely more than 4-5/day
  - —Tenesmus, urgency
- Bleeding
  - —Gross blood uncommon
- Nausea/vomiting
  - —Obstruction common with ileocolonic disease
- Mass/tenderness
  - —RLQ mass or tenderness
  - —Generalized tenderness if involvement diffuse
- Tenderness and distension
  - —Consider: obstruction or toxic megacolon

PERIANAL

- Perianal abscess
- Fissure
  - —Characteristically painless
- Fistula
  - —Half of patients with colonic disease
  - —May present prior to other manifestations of illness

EXTRAINTESTINAL

- Renal and gall stone formation
- Peripheral arthralgia/arthritis
  - —Follows disease activity
- Axial arthritis
  - —Ankylosing spondylitis
  - —Sacroilitis
  - —Course not related to underlying disease activity
- Eye
  - —Iritis
  - —Conjunctivitis
- Skin
  - —Erythema nodosum
  - —Pyoderma gangrenosum

ULCERATIVE COLITIS

CONSTITUTIONAL

- Fever
- Weight loss
- Fatigue

GI

- Abdominal pain
  - —More generalized than Crohn's disease
  - —Tender and distended implies toxic dilation
- Diarrhea
  - —Variable, can be severe
  - —With mucus and very bloody
  - —Tenesmus and urgency common
- Bleeding
  - —Common
- Obstruction rare
- Mass
  - —None
  - —Colon can be felt with toxic dilation
- Diminished bowel sounds with toxic megacolon

PERIANAL

- No involvement in ulcerative colitis

EXTRAINTESTINAL

- Renal and gall stone formation
- Peripheral arthralgia/arthritis
  - —Follows disease activity
- Axial arthritis
  - —Ankylosing spondylitis
  - —Sacroilitis
  - —Course not related to underlying disease activity
- Eye
  - —Iritis
  - —Conjunctivitis
- Skin
  - —Erythema nodosum
  - —Pyoderma gangrenosum

PEDIATRIC CONSIDERATIONS

- Can occur in the first few years of life
- Extraintestinal manifestations predominate
  - —May be confused with
    - -Juvenile rheumatoid arthritis
    - -Idiopathic growth failure
    - -Anorexia nervosa

Pre-Hospital

N/A

Diagnosis

ESSENTIAL WORKUP

- May present as initial onset of disease or exacerbation of existing disease
- Maintain high index of suspicion due to subtle presentation of Crohn's disease

LABORATORY

- Nothing diagnostic
- CBC
  - —Anemia secondary to chronic or acute blood loss
- Electrolytes, BUN/Cr, glucose
- Stool examination
  - —Occult blood
  - —Fecal leukocytes may be present
  - —Culture to exclude infectious cause of enteritis
- ESR
  - —Elevated

IMAGING/SPECIAL TESTS

- Plain abdominal films for
  - —Toxic megacolon (>6 cm dilation)
  - —Obstruction
  - —Air in wall of colon (may indicate impending perforation)
  - —Perforation—subdiaphragmatic air or free air outlining liver or gallbladder
- CT abdomen
  - —To distinguish abscess from localized inflammatory mass in Crohn's
- Colonoscopy with biopsy confirms diagnosis of UC
  - —Do not perform with severe symptoms due to perforation risk
  - —Sigmoidoscopy/rectal biopsy/barium enema confirms diagnosis of Crohn's

DIFFERENTIAL DIAGNOSIS

- Infectious enteritis
- Antibiotic associated enteritis (*C. difficile*)
- Appendicitis
- Diverticulitis
- Functional bowel disease
- Diverticulosis
- Lymphoma involving bowel
- Bowel infarction
- Gonococcal or chlamydial proctitis

Treatment

INITIAL STABILIZATION

- IV 0.9%NS volume replacement if dehydrated
- Transfusion if significant blood loss
- NG suction if obstruction or toxic dilatation suspected

ED MANAGEMENT

Indications for Surgical Evaluation

- Free perforation
- Massive, unresponsive hemorrhage
- Toxic dilation
  - —Not an absolute indication for surgical intervention
  - —Intensive medical management with small bowel suction and close radiographic monitoring and surgical consultation
- Walled-off perforation with abscess
  - —Usually not an indication for *emergent* surgery
  - —Careful observation for peritonitis

Medical Therapy

- Treatment usually not initiated unless already established diagnosis
- Refill or restart medications in a patient with known disease
- ED prescribed medical regime usually consists of
  - —Medial regime should be individualized
  - —Steroid (prednisone, budesonide, or hydrocortisone enema, ACTH)
  - —Aminosalicylate (sulfasalazine, asacol, mesalamine)
  - —Antidiarrheal agent (lomotil/imodium)
    - -Not with severe disease if suspect toxic dilation
- Antibiotics (metronidazole) aids in treatment of Crohn's with colon/perineum involvement
- Treat refractory cases with immunosuppressive agents (azathioprine, Cyclosporin A, methotrexate, 6-mercaptopurine)
- Broad spectrum antibiotics for fulminant UC

MEDICATIONS

- ACTH: 80–120 IU/24hrs IM or IV
- Hydrocortisone enema: 60 mg
- Mesalamine enemas: 1–4 g retention enema—retain overnight
- Mesalamine suppositories: 500 mg PR bid
- Mesalamine tablets: (pentasa sustained-release 500 mg; asacol sustained-release 400 mg) 800 mg po TID–1000 mg qid po
- Metronidazole: 250–500 mg (peds: 30 mg/kg/24hrs) po tid
- Prednisone: 40–60 mg po q d
- Sulfasalazine (azulfidine): 500-mg tablets

Disposition

ADMISSION CRITERIA

- Surgical indication
  - —Massive, unresponsive hemorrhage
  - —Perforation
  - —Toxic dilation
  - —Obstruction
- Severe flare-up
  - —Electrolyte imbalance
  - —Severe dehydration
  - —Severe pain
  - —High fever
  - —Significant bleeding

DISCHARGE CRITERIA

- Initial presentation of diarrhea, mild pain, without toxicity with close follow-up
- Mild to moderate exacerbation of known disease without obstruction, severe bleeding, severe pain, dehydration, with close follow-up, on renewed therapy or with addition of prednisone.

Miscellaneous

ICD9: 555.9, 556.9

CORE CONTENT CODE: 1.6.3.2, 1.7.3.1

SUGGESTED READINGS

Janowitz HD. Inflammatory bowel disease; a clinical approach. 2d ed. New York: Oxford University Press, 1994.

Peppercorn MA. Advances in drug therapy for inflammatory bowel disease. Ann Intern Med 1990;112:50–60.

Targan SR, Shanahan F, eds. Inflammatory bowel disease—from bench to bedside. Baltimore: Williams & Wilkins, 1994.

Author: Shayle Miller

Influenza

Clinical Presentation

SIGNS AND SYMPTOMS

- Abrupt onset of high fever: 38°–40°C (100°–104°F)
- Chills, shivering, myalgias, headache, malaise, and anorexia
- Nasal discharge, conjunctivitis, pharyngitis, dry cough
- Elderly may present with high fever, lassitude, and confusion without pulmonary complications

MECHANISM/DESCRIPTION

- Acute, usually self-limited, viral infection
- Transmission: by dispersion in small-particle aerosols created by sneezing, cough, and talking
- Virus deposited on respiratory tract epithelium and absorbed
- Incubation period: 1–2 days
- Duration: 3 days
  —Severity of symptoms in proportion to height of the fever
- Outbreaks usually occur during winter months
- Common complications
  —Primary influenza viral pneumonia
  —Secondary bacterial pneumonia
  —Exacerbations of COPD
  —Rare complications: myositis, myocarditis, pericarditis, and aseptic meningitis
- Key features
  —Epidemic nature of the disease
  —Mortality resulting from pulmonary complications

ETIOLOGY

- Majority caused by three genera of the Orthomyxoviridae family: influenza virus type A, B and C
- Epidemics
  —Every 1–3 years
  —Caused by *antigenic drift*—new variants from minor changes in surface protein
  —Majority of cases occur in 2–3 weeks
  —Duration of the epidemic <6 weeks
- Pandemics
  —Every 10 years
  —Caused by new strains created by *antigenic shift*—major changes in virus structure
- Waterfowl reservoir of influenza virus

PEDIATRIC CONSIDERATIONS

- Children exhibit more lower-respiratory involvement (croup, bronchitis, bronchiolitis, pneumonitis) and higher temperatures than adults
- Myalgias in the calf muscle
- Febrile convulsions occur in approximately 10% of children under 5 with influenza infection
- Reye's syndrome
  —Influenza may be predisposing factor
  —Rare and severe complication
  —Characterized by fatty degeneration of the liver and cerebral edema
  —Symptoms: nausea, vomiting and stupor during convalescence from the viral infection
  —Strong correlation with salicylates: avoid aspirin products in children with influenza

Pre-Hospital

N/A

Diagnosis

ESSENTIAL WORKUP

- Clinical diagnosis based on the signs and symptoms of influenza during the winter months in the setting of an known outbreak

LABORATORY

- CBC
  —WBC: normal to mildly decreased
- Culture of nasopharyngeal swab or aspirate
- Pulse oximetry/ABG for significant pulmonary symptoms

IMAGING/SPECIAL TESTS

- CXR for prominent lower respiratory symptoms
  —Normal (50–90%)
  —Bilateral interstitial infiltration
- Rapid ELISA antigen test

DIFFERENTIAL DIAGNOSIS

- Indistinguishable from most viral infections (URI)
- Bronchitis
- Atypical pneumonia
- Epstein-Barr infection (infectious mononucleosis)

Treatment

INITIAL STABILIZATION

- Aggressive fluid resuscitation, supplemental oxygen, and positive-pressure ventilation as clinical circumstances dictate

ED TREATMENT

- Supportive and symptomatic
  —Antipyretics (acetaminophen or NSAIDs)—avoid aspirin
  —Cough suppressants
  —Rehydration
- Amantidine and rimantidine effective against influenza A
  —Shortens duration of fever/systemic and respiratory symptoms by 1–2 days
  —Accelerates functional recovery
  —Recommended for
    -Pneumonia
    -With severe disease
    -Immunocompromised
    -Patients at high-risk for complications

PREVENTION

- Polyvalent influenza vaccine recommended annually for
  —Adults >65 years
  —High-risk individuals (COPD, cardiovascular disease, immunocompromised, diabetics)
  —Health care workers
- Chemoprophylaxis with amantidine/rimantidine in the following settings
  —Short-term prophylaxis during outbreak of influenza A in high-risk patients who did not receive vaccine
  —In conjunction with vaccine in high-risk patients expected to respond poorly to vaccine, including HIV infections
  —In lieu of vaccine when vaccine is contraindicated in high-risk individuals
  —In individuals providing care for high-risk persons

MEDICATIONS

- Amantadine: 200 mg po initially, then 100 mg po bid for 3–5 d
- Rimantadine: 200 mg po initially, then 100 mg po bid for 3–5 d

Disposition

ADMISSION CRITERIA

- Hypoxia, pneumonia, severe dehydration

DISCHARGE CRITERIA

- Most patients will have a short, self-limited course provided they are able to tolerate fluids and antipyretics

Miscellaneous

ICD9: 487

CORE CONTENT CODE: 9.5.3

SUGGESTED READINGS

Arruda E, Hayden FG. Update on therapy of influenza and rhinovirus infections. Adv Exp Med Biol 1996:394:174–87.

Betts RF. Influenza virus. In: Mandell Gl, Bennett JE, Dolin R, eds. Mandell, Douglas, and Bennett's principles and practice of infectious diseases. 4th ed. New York: Churchill Livingstone 1995.

Nicholson, KG. Clinical features of influenza. Semin Respir Infect 1992;7(1):26–37.

Ryan-Poirier K. Influenza virus infection in children. Adv Pediatr Infect Dis 1995;10:125–56.

Van Voris LP, Newell PM. Antivirals for the chemoprophylaxis and treatment of influenza. Semin Respir Infect 1992;7(1):61–70.

Author: Philip Shayne

Intracerebral Hemorrhage

Clinical Presentation

SIGNS AND SYMPTOMS

- Severe headache, typically sudden in onset
- Hypertension
- Seizures
- Evidence of head injury
- Meningismus; vomiting
- Altered level of consciousness (may be comatose); altered mental status may occur as late as 24–48 hours after head injury
- Variable neurological deficits depending on the site of intracerebral hemorrhage
  —Putamen hemorrhage (35%): contralateral hemiparesis and hemisensory loss, with occasional dysphagia or neglect
  —Lobar hemorrhage (30%): variable signs depending on involved area
  —Cerebellar hemorrhage (15%): vomiting, ataxia, and nystagmus
  —Thalamic hemorrhage (10%): similar to putamen, but may also have eye movement abnormalities
  —Caudate hemorrhage (5%): confusion, memory loss, hemiparesis, gaze paresis
  —Pontine hemorrhage (5%): quadriplegia, pin-point pupils, ataxia, sensorimotor loss

MECHANISM/DESCRIPTION

- Injury occurs primarily from hemorrhage into brain parenchyma leading to compression of brain tissues. Secondary injury results from cerebral edema leading to increased intracranial pressure and the possibility of brain herniation

ETIOLOGY

- Intracerebral hemorrhage can occur spontaneously or secondary to traumatic head injury
  —Uncontrolled or acute hypertension (most common)
  —Vascular malformations (arteriovenous malformation, venous angiomas, and ruptured aneurysms)
  —Neoplasm (particularly melanoma and glioma)
  —Anticoagulant therapy (coumadin, heparin)
  —Thrombolytic agents
  —Illicit drugs (cocaine, amphetamines)
  —Bleeding disorders (hemophilia)
  —Cerebral amyloid angiopathy
  —Traumatic hemorrhage secondary to blunt or penetrating injury

Pre-Hospital

CAUTIONS

- C-spine precautions if head or neck injury is suspected
- Elevation of head with C-spine control
- Initial pre-hospital responder must ascertain the neurologic defect to be able to note progression of symptoms

Diagnosis

ESSENTIAL WORKUP

- Immediate noncontrast head CT (acute hemorrhage appears as a high-density lesion)

LABORATORY

- Check coagulation studies (PT/PTT, INR, platelets)

IMAGING/SPECIAL TESTS

- CT as above
- MRI not indicated because of long scan time and it is difficult or impossible to manage unstable patients in the scanner

DIFFERENTIAL DIAGNOSIS

- The differential diagnosis of mental status change, neuro deficit, headache, etc., is vast and includes
  —Seizure
  —CNS infection
  —CNS mass
  —Electrolyte or acid/base abnormality
  —Intoxication/Wernicke's encephalitis
  —Migraine headache
  —Transient ischemic attack (TIA)
  —Todd's paralysis
  —Air embolism
- The differential diagnosis once bleed is seen on CT is narrowed
  —Spontaneous hemorrhage (hypertensive, AVM, neoplasm, etc.)
  —Traumatic hemorrhage
  —Subarachnoid hemorrhage
  —Subdural hematoma
  —Epidural hematoma

PEDIATRIC CONSIDERATIONS

- Additional differential diagnoses include
  —Moyamoya disease
  —Acute infantile hemiplegia

Treatment

INITIAL STABILIZATION

- ABCs
  - —Patients with depressed level of consciousness should be intubated immediately and mildly hyperventilated.
- Early neurosurgical consultation

ED MANAGEMENT

- Blood pressure management
  - —Must use caution in blood pressure control because acute normalization in the setting of increased intracranial pressure (ICP) could reduce cerebral perfusion to ischemic levels
  - —Only correct hypertension if systolic blood pressure is >200 mm Hg or if diastolic blood pressure is >120 mm Hg
  - —Use nitroprusside, esmolol or labetalol to slowly lower diastolic blood pressure initially by 10%
  - —Normotensive levels should be achieved over 12–24 hours
  - —May use hydralazine as an alternative
- Treatment of elevated intracranial pressure
  - —Hyperventilation to $PaCO_2$ of 35 torr
  - —Fluid restriction; elevate head of bed 30°
  - —Mannitol—osmotic diuresis
  - —Use furosemide as an alternative
  - —Correct coagulopathies if present
  - —Consider anticonvulsants: phenytoin

MEDICATIONS

- Furosemide: 20–40 mg IV may repeat as necessary (peds: 0.5–1.0 mg/kg/dose)
- Esmolol: 0.5–1 mg/kg initial bolus IV followed by 50–150 μg/kg/min infusion
- Hydralazine: 10–40 mg IV may repeat as necessary (peds: 0.1–0.2 mg/kg/dose)
- Labetalol: 20 mg IV may give additional 40–80 mg IV q 10 min to max 300 mg (peds: 0.3–1.0 mg/kg/dose)
- Mannitol: 1 g/kg IV
- Nitroprusside: 0.5 μg/kg/min IV initially and titrate to effect
- Phenytoin: 15–20mg/kg/dose at rate of 40–50 mg/hr (peds: 0.5–1.0 mg/kg/min)

Disposition

ADMISSION CRITERIA

- To the OR if surgical intervention is indicated
- To the ICU if intubated; altered level of consciousness; or on IV infusion for blood pressure control
- Admit to neurological observation unit if normal neurological exam without evidence of progression of bleed, and hemodynamically stable

DISCHARGE CRITERIA

- All patients with intracerebral hemorrhage should be admitted

Miscellaneous

ICD9: 431

CORE CONTENT CODE: 11.1.2

SUGGESTED READINGS

Diringer MH. Intracerebral hemorrhage: pathophysiology and management. Crit Care Med 1993;21(10):1591–1603.

Heiskanen O. Treatment of spontaneous intracerebral and intracerebellar hemorrhage. Stroke 1993;24(12):I-94–I-95.

MacKenzie JM. Intracerebral hemorrhage. J Clin Pathol 1996;49(5):360–364.

Ojemann RG, Heros RC. Spontaneous brain hemorrhage. Stroke 1983;14(4):468–475.

Authors: Paul David; Rebecca Smith-Coggins

Intussusception

Clinical Presentation

SIGNS AND SYMPTOMS

- Classic triad present in less than half of patients
  - —Abdominal pain
  - —Vomiting
  - —Bloody mucoid stools ("currant jelly" stools)
- Irritability
- Repeated screaming attacks accompanied by pallor and drawing up of the legs
  - —Episodes occur in 5–20-minute intervals
- Lethargy or a history of intermittent periods of lethargy
- Fever
- Often patients only have heme-positive stool
- Preceding illness several days or weeks prior to the onset of abdominal pain
  - —Diarrhea
  - —Viral syndrome
  - —Henoch-Schönlein purpura
- A "sausage" mass may be palpated in the right upper-quadrant
- Dependent on the time from onset to diagnosis, peritoneal signs and shock may also be present

MECHANISM/DESCRIPTION

- The invagination of one part of the intestine into the lumen of an immediately adjacent portion
- Greater than 80% involve the ileocecal region
- Often occurs with a pathological lead point
  - —Hypertrophied lymphoid patches in infants
  - —After 2 years of age this is found in only one-third of patients
  - —In children older than 6 years of age, lymphoma is the most common lead point found
  - —Adults almost always have a pathologic lead point
- The most common cause of intestinal obstruction within the first 2 years of life
  - —Most frequently between 5 and 9 months of age
- Epidemiology in the US
  - —The incidence is 2.4 cases per 1000 live births
  - —Male to female predominance of 2:1
  - —Mortality is less than 1%
- Recurrent intussusception occurs in less than 10% of patients
  - —The success of enemas with a recurrent episode appears to approach that of the initial episode
- Morbidity is thought to increase with delayed diagnosis

ETIOLOGY

- Most cases (85%) have no apparent cause
- Predisposing conditions that create a lead point for invagination
  - —Hypertrophied lymphoid patches
  - —Polyps
  - —Meckel's diverticulum
  - —Henoch-Schönlein purpura
  - —Lymphomas
  - —Lipomas
  - —Parasites
  - —Foreign bodies
  - —Adenovirus or rotavirus infection
  - —Small intestine intussusception occurs with celiac disease and cystic fibrosis

Pre-Hospital

CAUTIONS

- Intravenous access
- IV bolus of 20 cc/kg of NS if signs of shock

Diagnosis

ESSENTIAL WORKUP

- The diagnosis is suggested by the history and is proven radiographically
- A guaiac-positive stool may aid in the diagnosis

LABORATORY

- CBC
- Serum electrolytes
- BUN

IMAGING/SPECIAL TESTS

- Plain abdominal radiograph
  - —May aid in excluding intestinal perforation
  - —Minimal gas pattern
  - —Minimal fecal content
  - —Presence of a mass
  - —Paucity of right lower quadrant air
  - —Findings consistent with bowel obstruction
- Ultrasound is highly accurate and presence is rapidly recognizable in children
- Enema
  - —Often both diagnostic and therapeutic
  - —Barium
    - -Standard for diagnosis of intussusception
    - -Characteristic "coiled spring" appearance
  - —Air
    - -Fluoroscopic guidance
    - -Safer as avoids peritoneal contamination of perforation
  - —Water soluble
    - -Safer if risk of perforation
  - —Hydrostatic enemas with ultrasonic guidance
    - -"Crescent in doughnut" sign
  - —Contraindications
    - -Peritonitis
    - -Perforation
    - -Sepsis
    - -Shock

DIFFERENTIAL DIAGNOSIS

- Hirschsprung enterocolitis
- Strangulated hernia
- Trauma
- Gastroenteritis
- Pyelonephritis
- Malrotation/volvulus
- Appendicitis
- Pneumonia
- Inflammatory bowel disease
- Infectious mononucleosis
- Pharyngitis
- Diabetes mellitus
- Anal fissure
- Ulcer disease
- Vascular malformations
- Protein-sensitive enterocolitis
- Polyps
- Henoch-Schönlein purpura
- Hemorrhoids
- Coagulopathy

Treatment

INITIAL STABILIZATION

- Intravenous access and fluid resuscitation
- Nasogastric tube

ED TREATMENT

- Surgical consultation
- Interventional radiography for reduction
  —Barium enemas are 75–80% successful at reduction
  —Recurrences may also be reduced radiographically
- Antibiotics
  —Initiate if evidence of peritonitis or perforation
  —Ampicillin, clindamycin, and gentamycin
- Laparotomy
  —Indications
    -Pathologic lead point
    -Multiple recurrences
    -Signs of shock
    -Perforation
  —Gentle milking of the intussusceptum
    -Resection of any nonviable bowel as well as any lead points may be necessary

MEDICATIONS

- Ampicillin: 100–200 mg/kg q 4 hours IV
- Clindamycin: 30–40 mg/kg q 6 hours IV
- Gentamycin: 5.0–7.5 mg/kg q 8 hours IV

Disposition

ADMISSION CRITERIA

- Patients should be observed for 24–48 hours for complications or reoccurrence
- Patients undergoing surgery

DISCHARGE CRITERIA

- Successful outcomes have been noted with home observation
  —Stable patient
  —Symptomatic relief of abdominal pain during the postreduction period

Miscellaneous

ICD9: 560.0

CORE CONTENT CODE: 13.1.10

SUGGESTED READINGS

Champoux AN, Del Becarro MA, Nazar-Stewart V. Recurrent intussusception: risks and features. Arch Pediatr Adolesc Med 1994;148:474–478.

Fecteau A, Flageole H, Nguyen LT, et al. Recurrent intussusception: safe use of hydrostatic enema. J Pediatr Surg 1996;31(6):859–861.

Stringer MD, Pablot SM, Brererton RJ. Paediatric intussusception. Br J Surg 1992;79:867–876.

Winslow BT, Westfall JM, Nicholas RA. Intussusception. Am Fam Physician. 1996;54(1):213–217.

Author: Charles G. Macias

Iritis

Clinical Presentation

SIGNS AND SYMPTOMS

- Ocular pain, red eye
- Photophobia (consensual)
- Lacrimation
- Decreased visual acuity (usually mild)
- Cells and flare in anterior chamber; hypopyon
- Posterior synechiae (adhesions of iris to the lens)
- Miosis
- Low intraocular pressure (occasionally may be high)
- Injection of perilimbal vessels (ciliary flush)

MECHANISM/DESCRIPTION

- An inflammation of the anterior segment of the uvea—anterior uveitis

ETIOLOGY

- Most cases are idiopathic but may be traumatic or associated with numerous infectious and noninfectious systemic diseases

Noninfectious Systemic Diseases

- Ankylosing spondylitis
- Reiter's syndrome
- Sarcoidosis
- Behçet's disease
- Inflammatory bowel disease
- Juvenile rheumatoid arthritis
- Kawasaki syndrome
- Interstitial nephritis
- IgA nephropathy
- Drug reactions
- Sjögren's syndrome
- Psoriatic arthritis

Infectious

- Viral: rubella, measles, adenovirus, herpes simplex virus, herpes zoster virus, HIV, mumps, varicella, cytomegalovirus
- Bacterial: TB, syphilis, pertussis, brucellosis, Lyme disease, chlamydia, rickettsia, gonorrhea, leprosy
- Fungal

Malignancies

- Leukemia
- Lymphoma
- Malignant melanoma

Other

- Cocaine use
- Exposure to pesticides
- Corneal foreign body
- Blunt trauma

Pre-Hospital

N/A

Diagnosis

ESSENTIAL WORKUP

- History and review of systems—up to 50% may be associated with systemic disease
- Slitlamp exam (SLE)—flare and inflammatory cells in the anterior chamber are diagnostic
  - —Flare is a homogenous fog secondary to protein leakage into aqueous humor
  - —Use short, wide beam to best appreciate cells and flare
  - —Cellular deposits with more severe inflammation
- Intraocular pressure
- If topical anesthesia relieves pain, probably *not* iritis

LABORATORY

- None usually indicated
- Tailored outpatient work up if history, signs and symptoms point strongly to a certain etiology (with referral to ophthalmology, rheumatology or internal medicine)
  - —Ankylosing spondylitis: sacroiliac spine x-rays, ESR, HLA B27
  - —Inflammatory bowel disease: HLA B27, GI consult
  - —Reiter's syndrome: cultures of conjunctiva, urethra, HLA B27, rheumatology consult
  - —Psoriatic arthritis: HLA B27, rheumatology consult
  - —Lyme disease: immunoassays
  - —JRA: ANA, rheumatoid factor, rheumatology consult
  - —Sarcoidosis: ACE, serum lysozyme, PPD, chest x-ray
  - —Sexually transmitted diseases: RPR or VDRL, FTA-ABS, appropriate cultures
  - —TB: PPD, chest x-ray

DIFFERENTIAL DIAGNOSIS

- Conjunctivitis
- Keratitis
- Acute angle-closure glaucoma
- Episcleritis
- Corneal abrasion
- Corneal foreign body

Treatment

INITIAL STABILIZATION

- Goal: reduce inflammation and prevent complications
- Cycloplegic agent
  —Decreases pain, photophobia
  —Prevents development of posterior synechiae

ED MANAGEMENT

- Cycloplegia
- Topical steroids—if indicated
  —Use with caution, in consultation with ophthalmologist
  —May cause significant complications, i.e., progression of HSV keratitis
- Treat secondary glaucoma
- Supportive measures
  —Warm compresses
  —Dark glasses
  —Analgesia
- If specific etiology identified, initiate appropriate management
- Ankylosing spondylitis: systemic antiinflammatory agents, physical therapy
- Inflammatory bowel disease: systemic steroids, sulfadiazine, vitamin A
- Reiter's syndrome: treat urethritis (and sexual contacts)
- Behçet's disease: systemic steroids or immunosuppressive agents
- Infectious causes: appropriate management of underlying infection

MEDICATIONS

- Acetaminophen with codeine: 1 or 2 tabs q 4–6 hrs
- Atropine 1%: 1 gt tid for moderate to severe inflammation (lasts 7–14 days)
- Cyclopentolate 1–2%: 1 gt tid for mild to moderate inflammation (lasts up to 2 days)
- Homatropine 2% or 5%: 1 gt QD tid (lasts up to 3 days)
- Hydrocodone 5–10 mg q 4–6 hrs
- Prednisolone acetate 1%: 1 gt q 1–6 hrs, depending on severity

PEDIATRIC CONSIDERATIONS

- Cycloplegics not recommended in children <6 years
  —May cause systemic anticholinergic toxicity with blurred vision, flushing, tachycardia, hypotension, and hallucinations

Disposition

ADMISSION CRITERIA

- Not indicated unless significant systemic illness

DISCHARGE CRITERIA

- Refer to an ophthalmologist within 24 hours for follow-up care and possible steroid therapy

Miscellaneous

ICD9: 364.3

CORE CONTENT CODE: 6.4.2.4

SUGGESTED READINGS

Bertolini J, Pelucio M. The red eye. Emerg Med Clin North Am 1995;13(3):561–579.

Cullom RD, Chang B. Uveitis. In: Cullen RD, Chang B, eds. The Will's eye manual: Office and emergency room diagnosis and treatment of eye diseases. 2nd ed. Philadelphia: Lippincott-Raven, 1994:351–388.

Lightman S. Uveitis: Management. Lancet 1991;338(14):1501–1503.

Rothenhaus TC, Polis MA. Ocular manifestations of systemic disease. Emerg Med Clin North Am 1995;13(3);607–630.

Author: Mary Stewart

Iron, Poisoning

Clinical Presentation

SIGNS AND SYMPTOMS

- Classically divided into 5 stages (see table)
  - —May present in or skip any one of the stages
  - —Variable time for each stage
  - —Stage I—consistently evident in *significant* exposures

ETIOLOGY

- Elemental iron
  - —Nontoxic <20 mg/kg
  - —Moderate = 20–60 mg/kg
  - —Lethal = 180–300 mg/kg (30–45 tablets in a 10-kg child)
  - —Elemental iron equivalents
    - -Ferrous fumarate = 33%
    - -Ferrous sulfate = 16%
    - -Ferrous gluconate = 12%
    - -Prenatal vitamins vary from 60–90 mg elemental iron/tablet

MECHANISM

- Peak levels
  - —Chewable iron: 4–6 hours
  - —Enteric coated or sustained release—erratic
- Postabsorption: iron redistributes into the tissues and a *fall* in serum iron occurs as the free iron then causes damage at the cellular level
- Injury patterns
  - —Corrosive to the intestinal mucosa, causing damage, profound fluid loss (shock), hemorrhage, and perforations
  - —Liver receives the largest load of iron because of portal venous circulation—has the highest injury
- Free iron
  - —Concentrates in the mitochondria disrupting oxidative-phosphorylation, catalyzes lipid peroxidation, and free radical formation resulting in cell death and increases anaerobic metabolism and acidosis
  - —Causes myocardial depression, venodilation, and cerebral edema
- Hydration of the ferric ($Fe^{+3} + 3\,H_2O \rightarrow Fe(OH)_3 + 3H^+$) adds to acidosis

PEDIATRIC CONSIDERATIONS

- Highest mortality rate among pediatric accidental exposures

Pre-Hospital

- Early recognition of iron exposure essential
- Obtain empty bottles in order to calculate the actual elemental iron exposure dose
- IV fluid resuscitation with 0.9%NS 20 cc/kg bolus for hypotension/shock

Diagnosis

ESSENTIAL WORKUP

- Regardless of laboratory results, acute iron poisoning is a clinical diagnosis

LABORATORY

- Serum iron levels (μg/dl)
  - —Peak absorption between 2–6 hours
  - —4 hours most common time for peak level
  - —Best time to obtain postingestion level controversial
  - —Delayed peak with enteric coated/sustained release
- Electrolytes, BUN/Cr, glucose
  - —Anion gap metabolic acidosis
  - —Hyperglycemia early
  - —Hypoglycemia late
- ABG
  - —Metabolic acidosis
- CBC
  - —Anemia with significant hemorrhage
  - —Leukocytosis
- PTT/PT
  - —Liver function tests
- Lactic acid levels
- Type and Screen if hemorrhage
- TIBC is no longer used as a criteria

IMAGING

- Abdominal radiograph check for
  - —Pills/pill fragments
  - —Perforation

DIFFERENTIAL DIAGNOSIS

- Sepsis
- Acetaminophen toxicity
- Toxic ingestions causing an anion gap acidosis
  - —Salicylate
  - —Cyanide
  - —Methanol
  - —Ethylene glycol
- Mushrooms
- Theophylline toxicity
- GI bleed from other causes (alcoholic liver disease)

Treatment

INITIAL STABILIZATION

- ABCs
  - —Airway if needed
  - —Venous access and volume (normal saline bolus) for hypotension
  - —Cardiac monitor and pulse oximeter
- Narcan, thiamine, dextrose (or Accucheck) if altered mental status

ED TREATMENT

Decontamination

- If the patient has already been vomiting, gastric emptying not useful unless pill fragments seen in the LUQ on KUB. If pills or fragments are seen
  - —Children: ipecac if the child awake and alert
  - —Adults: gastric lavage
- Activated charcoal (unless other toxins ingested), $NaHCO_3$, phospho soda, and oral deferoxamine not recommended
- If pill fragments are not removed with ipecac or lavage
  - —Initiate whole bowel irrigation (WBI) with administration of Go-Lytely (peds: 25 cc/kg/hr; adult: 1–2 L/hr) while monitoring progression with KUBs
  - —Caution with GI bleed
- Endoscopy and gastrostomy to remove adherent particles and/or bezoars

	TIME	SYMPTOMS	
Stage I	0–12 hrs	Profuse GI symptoms	—Abdominal pain —Vomiting and diarrhea (often bloody) —Shock —+/− Hyperglycemia/leukocytosis
Stage II	6–24 hrs	Quiescent Stage	—GI symptoms subside —Hypovolemia —Metabolic acidosis
Stage III	24–72 hrs	Multiple Organ failure	—Decreasing mental status —CVS collapse —Renal failure —Respiratory failure (ARDS)
Stage IV	2–5 days	Hepatic failure	—Hypoglycemia —Coagulopathy —Elevated transaminases/ bilirubin/ammonia
Stage V	Days	Obstructions	—Gastric outlet and small bowel obstructions

Chelation with Deferoxamine (DFO)

- DFO is a highly specific chelator of iron
  - —Only binds the iron in the venous system (not the iron already distributed)
  - —Must be given as soon as possible (<24 hours)
- Administration techniques
  - —Increase IV infusion rate from 0 to 15 mg/kg/hr over 20 minutes monitoring for hypotension
  - —If hypotension occurs, slow rate
  - —IV or IM—IV route preferable
- Goal is to chelate as much iron as soon as possible
  - —Infusion rates as high as 45 mg/kg/hr have been used and tolerated
  - —Disregard the manufacturer's recommendation of maximum daily doses of 6 g in serious iron exposures
- IM DFO challenge test is being replaced with a short course of IV DFO (15 mg/kg/hr)
- Indication for administration
  - —Sustained GI symptoms
  - —Hypotension, lethargy, metabolic acidosis, or shock
  - —Serum iron >500 µg/dl
  - —Serum iron >350 µg/dl *and* pills seen on KUB
  - —Rising serum iron levels
  - —Interpret serum levels cautiously—time since ingestion must be considered
    - -Treatment may be indicated in a patient who presents late, after the distribution stage (>8 hours postingestion) with a serum iron level <350 µg/dl
  - —If serum iron levels not readily available, base treatment decisions on clinical course
- Length of infusion (controversial)
  - —DFO:iron complex causes urine to turn *vin rose* color—suggest continuing the infusion until the urine returns to normal
  - —When no color change is noted, use resolution of signs and symptoms of significant toxicity as a criteria for discontinuing DFO
  - —In severe cases, DFO may need to be discontinued prior to full excretion of the DFO:iron complex to avoid the risks of prolonged treatment
- Controversies
  - —Safety of DFO infusions given for >24 hours
  - —Maximal infusion rates and total amount of DFO given
  - —Serum iron level at which to treat
  - —Endpoint of treatment
  - —Role of extracorporeal elimination
- Contact regional poison centers for moderate to severe iron exposures

Disposition

- Accidental ingestions or ingestions of <20 mg/kg may be monitored at home if brief or no GI symptoms
- Evaluation in the ED warranted in intentional overdoses, or with >20 mg/kg

ADMISSION CRITERIA

- Admit to a well monitored environment if DFO instituted
- ICU admission for shock and lethargy or with high serum iron levels

DISCHARGE CRITERIA

- Asymptomatic after 6 hours of observation
- Mild GI symptoms that have resolved without evidence of metabolic acidosis and serum iron <350 µg/dl

Miscellaneous

ICD9: 964.0

CORE CONTENT CODE: 17.2.27

SUGGESTED READINGS

Ellenhorn MJ, Schoonwald S, Ordog G, Wasserberger J. Iron. In: Ellenhorn MJ, ed. Ellenhorn's medical toxicology. 2d ed. Baltimore: Williams &Wilkins, 1997;1158–1563.

Goldfrank LR. Iron. In: Goldfrank LR, et al., eds. Goldfrank's toxicologic emergencies. 5th ed. Norwalk, CT: Appleton & Lange, 1994;521–534.

Howland MA. Risks of parenteral deferoxamine for acute iron poisoning. J Toxicol Clin Toxicol 1996;34(5);491–496.

Linakis JG, Lacoutrure PG, Woolf A. Iron absorption from chewable vitamins with iron versus iron tablets: Implications for toxicity. Pediatr Emerg Care 1992;8(6):321–324.

Mills KD, Curry SC. Acute iron poisoning. Emerg Med Clin North Am 1994;12(2):397–413.

Tenenbein M. Benefits of parenteral deferoxamine for acute iron poisoning. J Toxicol Clin Toxicol 1996;34(5):485–489.

Author: Kim Sing

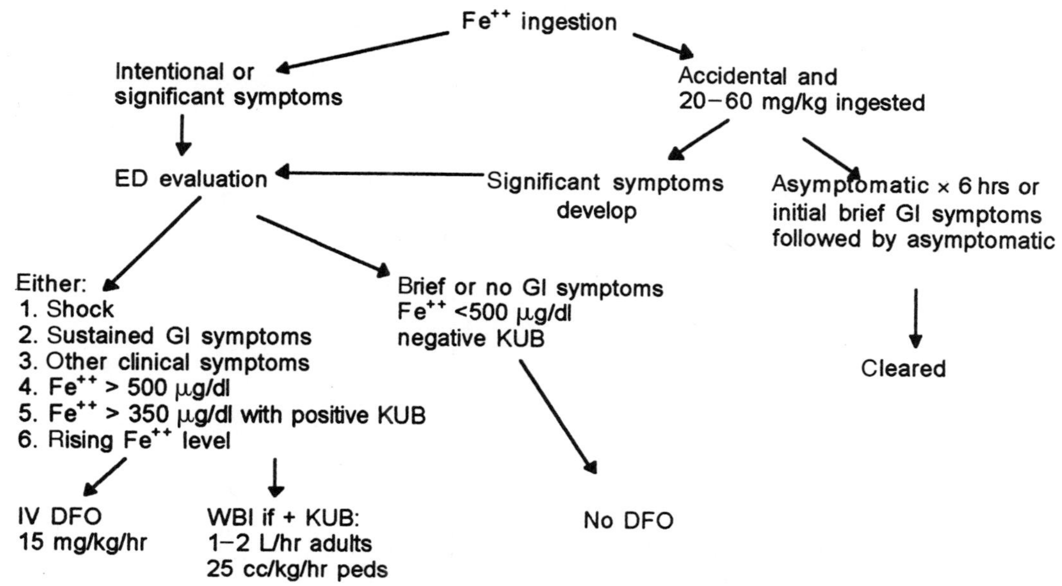

Figure 1.1. Patient Treatment

Irritable Bowel

Clinical Presentation

SIGNS AND SYMPTOMS

- At least 3 months of continuous or recurrent symptoms (Rome criteria)
  —Abdominal pain or discomfort which is
    -Relieved by defecation or
    -Associated with change in stool frequency or consistency
  —Two or more of the following at least 25% of days
    -Altered stool frequency (>3 stools/day or <3 stools/week)
    -Altered stool form (lumpy/hard or loose/watery)
    -Altered stool passage (straining, urgency, or feeling of incomplete evacuation)
    -Passage of mucus
    -Bloating or feeling of abdominal distension
- Other symptoms
  —Postprandial upper abdominal discomfort (dyspepsia)
  —Gastroesophageal reflux
  —Nausea, vomiting,
  —Flatulence
  —Dysmenorrhea
  —Dyspareunia
  —Symptoms tend to be worse about the time of menses
  —Most patients are women under age 40
  —Examination usually unremarkable

MECHANISMS/DESCRIPTION

- Dysfunction of the sensory/perception pathways leading to disordered motility to various stimuli, such as meal or rectal distention
- Altered gut sensation due to lower pain threshold (*visceral hyperalgesia*) for pathophysiologic events and increased awareness of normal GI events
- Altered CNS processing of end organ motor and sensory activity
- Gut irritants such as malabsorbed sugars, food allergen, bile acids, and short chains fatty acids

ETIOLOGY

- Main cause of ED visits with nonspecific abdominal pain
- Dietary factors
  —Some vegetables (e.g., broccoli, cabbage, and legumes), lactose, sorbitol, fructose, aspartame, or tyramine rich products
  —Large meals, fatty, or spicy food causes enhanced gastrocolic reflex
- Bereavement, physical, or sexual abuse in women or during childhood
- Patients adopt the "sick role"; seeking medical attention more than control for non-GI symptoms such as headaches, myalgia, backache, palpitation, and fatigue
- Patients score high on tests of psychoneurotic behavior, and reactions to psychological stress

PEDIATRIC CONSIDERATIONS

- Recurrent abdominal pain, missing many days from school, or chronic nausea

Pre-Hospital

N/A

Diagnosis

ESSENTIAL WORKUP

- Location of abdominal pain, duration, severity, exacerbating factors, associated symptoms, and results of previous work-up and treatments
- Detailed history searching for dietary factors or medications
- Sudden onset of symptoms, peritoneal signs, blood or fat in stool, fever, weight loss, or other systemic symptoms should alert to different etiology
- Avoid excessive investigation, especially for patients under age 40

LABORATORY

- To rule out other disorders
- CBC, ESR, serum albumin, U/A
  —Normal
- Stool studies for leukocytes, ova, and parasites
  —Negative
- Serum calcium, TSH, and giardia antibody

IMAGING/SPECIAL TESTS

- KUB: distention of either of the flexures
- Flexible sigmoidoscopy/biopsy for
  —Rectal bleeding
  —New onset symptoms
  —Atypical features
- Upper GI endoscopy and ultrasound if upper GI symptoms are most bothersome
- Colonoscopy—rarely helpful especially in patients under age 40
- Screen stool for laxative abuse
- Hydrogen breath test if lactose intolerance suspected

DIFFERENTIAL DIAGNOSIS

- Cholelithiasis/cholecystitis
- Acute diverticulitis
- Small bowel obstruction
- Inflammatory bowel disease (IBD)
  - —Family history, tenesmus, rectal bleeding, systemic symptoms, and abnormal lab tests
- Microscopic colitis: watery diarrhea in older patient, and NSAID use
- Endometriosis and PID
  - —Abnormal pelvic examination, or ultrasound
- Infectious diarrhea
  - —Symptoms after recent exposure or travel to endemic area; particularly giardiasis, amebiasis, *Campylobacter* and *yersinia*
- Nonulcer dyspepsia
- Colorectal adenoma or carcinoma: family history or hemoccult positive stool
- Diverticular disease or diverticulitis
  - —Acute onset in older patient with localized tenderness and high WBC
- Intestinal vascular insufficiency in older patients with cardiovascular disease
- Lactose intolerance, and laxative abuse
- Chronic pancreatitis
- Diabetes
- Hypo- or hyperthyroidism
- Psychiatric conditions such as depression, anxiety, panic attacks, hypochondriasis, and somatization

PEDIATRIC CONSIDERATIONS

- Other family members, especially mothers, of children with irritable bowel syndrome (IBS) often have a bowel disease, especially IBS

Treatment

INITIAL STABILIZATION

- 0.9%NS IV 500 cc IV fluid bolus for dehydration with vomiting

ED TREATMENT

- Empathetic approach, and therapeutic physician/patient relationship
- Avoidance of dietary factors, and medications that trigger the symptoms
- Counseling abused patients
- Constipation predominant
  - —Psyllium seeds, polycarbophil, or methylcellulose, and bowel training
  - —If laxative is needed, use warm water enema or oral lactulose, mineral oil, Go-Lytely, or cisapride
- Diarrhea predominant
  - —Loperamide
  - —Cholestyramine—a bile acid binder, anticholinergic agent
- Pain predominant
  - —For postprandial pain use anticholinergic with or without sedative (dicyclomine and hyoscyamine)
  - —For chronic pain use tricyclic antidepressant starting with a small dose
- Flatulence
  - —Activated charcoal may reduce the odor
  - —Simethicone has no effect on abdominal gas
- Selective serotonin reuptake inhibitors (SSRIs)
  - —May improve or worsen IBS—use selectively
- For the difficult to manage case
  - —Benzodiazepine (clonazepam), in small dose, followed by antihistamine (cyproheptadine)
- Lactose intolerance
  - —Lactase capsules: 1–2 po prior to ingesting milk (if unable to avoid dairy products)

MEDICATIONS

- Cisapride: 10–30 mg po tid
- Clonazepam: 0.5 mg po tid
- Cholestyramine: 4 g po tid
- Cyproheptadine: 4 mg po tid
- Dicyclomine: 10–20 mg po qid
- Hyoscyamine: 0.125–0.25 mg po/SL
- Loperamide: 2 mg po q 4 PRN

PEDIATRIC CONSIDERATIONS

- The need for psychological counseling is more frequent in children than adults.

Disposition

ADMISSION CRITERIA

- Suspicion of an emergent abdominal condition
- Severe symptoms with associated psychiatric disorder
- Uncertainty about the diagnosis

DISCHARGE CRITERIA

- Almost all patients managed as outpatients

Miscellaneous

ICD9: 564.1

CORE CONTENT CODE: 1.7.1.1

SUGGESTED READINGS

Almounajed G, Drossman DA. Newer aspects of the irritable bowel syndrome. Prim Care Clin North Am 1996;23:477.

Camilleri M, Prather CM. Irritable bowel syndrome: Mechanisms and practical approach to management. Ann Intern Med 1992;116:1001.

Dromman DA, Whitehead WE, Camilleri M. Irritable bowel syndrome. A review of practice guidelines developed. Gastroenterology 1997;112:2120.

Farthing MSG. Irritable bowel, irritable body or irritable brain? Brit Med J 1995;310:171.

Author: Abbas Zagnoon

Irritable Infant

Clinical Presentation

SIGNS AND SYMPTOMS

General

- Behavior
    - -Degree of irritability
    - -Lethargy
    - -Mental status change
- Fever
- Vital signs
- Hypoxia, cyanosis
- Skin
    - -purpura
    - -petechiae
    - -rashes
- Change in feeding or voiding patterns
    - -Diarrhea
    - -Vomiting
    - -Constipation
- Toxidrome

Nature of Crying

- Onset of crying—sudden or progressive
- Duration/intensity/type
    - -Screaming
    - -Grunting
    - -Whining
    - -High pitched
- Aggravating/alleviating factors
    - -Rocking
    - -Holding
    - -Feeding
    - -Flatulence

MECHANISM/DESCRIPTION

- Most children have some period of the day when they are most irritable, usually toward the evening
    - —Normal infant crying ranges from 1 to 4 hours by 6 weeks of age
- Irritability is relative to normal and the best judge of a change is a parent
- *Colic* is the most common cause of inconsolable crying in infants, occurring in 25% of healthy children
    - —Episodes of screaming accompanied by drawing up knees and passage of flatus
    - —Usually begins at 2–3 weeks and continues through 12 weeks
    - —Diagnosis of exclusion

ETIOLOGY

- DPT immunization
- Medications
    - -New prescriptions
    - -Home remedies
    - -Vitamin use/overdose
- Multiple systemic conditions (see Differential Diagnosis)

Pre-Hospital

- Resuscitate as necessary

Diagnosis

ESSENTIAL WORKUP

- Manage underlying conditions
- Support child and family

LABORATORY

- CBC, urinalysis, chemistries, and cultures as indicated

IMAGING/SPECIAL TESTS

- Fluorescein eye exam
- Chest x-ray to exclude cardiopulmonary disease
- ECG
- Skeletal survey
- Contrast x-ray studies such as barium enema for specific indications

DIFFERENTIAL DIAGNOSIS

- Infection/inflammation
    - —Minor acute infections
        - -Upper respiratory infection,
        - -Otitis media,
        - -Urinary tract infection
    - —Meningitis
    - —Osteomyelitis
    - —Gastroesophageal reflux, esophagitis
- Colic
- Teething
- Parental anxiety
- Intoxication
- Trauma
    - —Foreign body, fracture, tourniquet (hair around digit)
    - —Hematoma—subdural, epidural
    - —Corneal abrasion
    - —Child abuse
    - —Diaper pin, splinter
- Sickle cell crisis
- Deficiency
    - -Malnutriton
    - -Iron deficiency/anemia
- Endocrine/metabolic
- Vascular
- Hypoxia—cardiopulmonary disorder
- Incarcerated hernia, testicular torsion
- Intussusception
- Diphtheria-pertussis-tetanus reaction

Treatment

INITIAL STABILIZATION

- Manage underlying conditions

ED TREATMENT

- Initial evaluation of the child focusing on parent-child interaction and then on potential underlying conditions
- Colic responds to soothing, rhythmic activities, avoiding stimulants (coffee, tea, cola), minimizing daytime sleep
  - —Soy or hydrolyzed casein formula may be transiently beneficial
  - —Parents must reduce stress
  - —No proven pharmacologic therapy
- Support, empathy, close followup
- Prolonged observation of the child is usually appropriate

Disposition

ADMISSION CRITERIA

- Life-threatening underlying condition

DISCHARGE CRITERIA

- No serious condition
- Functional, supportive, and patient family
- Excellent followup is essential

Miscellaneous

ICD9: 799.2

CORE CONTENT CODE: 13.0

SUGGESTED READINGS

Barnett RM. Psychiatric and behavioral disorders. In: Barkin RM, ed. Pediatric emergency medicine. 2d ed. St. Louis: CV Mosby, 1997:954–968.

Hardoin RA, Henslee JA, Christenson CP, Christenson PJ, White M. Colic medication and apparently life-threatening events. Clin Pediatr 1991;30:281–285.

Mullen N. The problem patient—an irritable infant in respiratory distress. Hosp Pract 1984;1:241–245.

Tunnessen WW. Signs and symptoms in pediatrics. 2d ed. Philadelphia: JB Lippincott, 1988.

Author: Laura J. Snyder

Irritant Gas Exposure

Clinical Presentation

SIGNS AND SYMPTOMS

Upper Airway Irritants

- Conjunctival burning and lacrimation
- Nasopharyngeal and oropharyngeal burning and edema
- Mucosal erythema and ulcerations
- Dyspnea, hoarseness, cough, bronchorrhea
- Laryngospasm, stridor, upper airway obstruction

Peripheral Airway and Pulmonary Parenchymal Irritants

- Chest tightness
- Dyspnea
- Cough, tracheobronchitis, bronchoconstriction
- Wheezing, rales
- Pneumonia
- Noncardiogenic pulmonary edema, and ARDS

Other

- Dermal irritation
- Headache
- Nausea
- Vomiting

MECHANISM/DESCRIPTION

- Definition
  - —Caustic: any substance that is in contact with living tissue will cause destruction of tissue by chemical action
  - —Irritant: any substance, not corrosive as defined above, that on immediate, prolonged, or repeated contact with normal living tissue will induce a local inflammatory reaction
- Respiratory irritants: inhaled as gases, fumes, particles, or liquid aerosols
- Inhaled irritants
  - —Pulmonary toxicity determined primarily by its water solubility
  - —Inhaled irritants cause cellular injury through interaction with respiratory mucosal water with the subsequent formation of acids, alkalis, and free radicals
- Inhalation accidents frequently involve a mixture of irritant gases as well as chemical asphyxiants (see chapter: Carbon Monoxide, Poisoning)

ETIOLOGY

- Settings
  - —Industrial settings: chemical manufacturing, mining, plastics, and petroleum industries
  - —Improper use or storage of cleaning chemicals in the home
  - —Fires: toxic gases result of combustion
- *Immediate onset of upper airway inflammation* with highly water soluble irritant gases, or with aerodynamic diameter of >5 mcrm
  - —Ammonia (fertilizers, refrigerants, dyes, plastics, synthetic fibers, cleaning agents)
  - —Sulfur dioxide (fumigation of produce, bleaching, tanning, brewing, and wine making; combustion of coal and smelting of sulfide containing ores)
  - —Hydrogen chloride (formed during combustion of chlorinated hydrocarbons such as polyvinyl chloride)
  - —Acrolein (production of plastics, pharmaceuticals, synthetic fibers; formed during combustion of petroleum products, cellulose, wood, paper)
  - —Formaldehyde (production of plywood, particle board, insulation; combustion product of gas stoves and heaters)
  - —Hydrogen fluoride (combustion of fluorinated hydrocarbons)
- Latent period of minutes to hours before onset of symptoms with irritant gases of intermediate water solubility or aerodynamic diameter of 1–5 mcrm
  - —Chlorine (product of chlorinated chemicals; a bleaching agent)
- Delayed onset of symptoms up to 24 hours after inhalation with irritant gases of poor water solubility or aerodynamic diameter of <1 mcrm (with little or no warning of exposure)
  - —Oxides of nitrogen/nitrogen dioxide (produced in the manufacture of dyes, fertilizers, celluloid; acetylene/electric arc welding and gas blowing; fermentation of nitrogen-rich silage ("Silofillers disease"); combustion of nitrocellulose and polyamides)
  - —Phosgene/carbonyl chloride (arc welding and pesticide production: combustion of chlorinated hydrocarbons, and solvents)
  - —Ozone (produced during arc welding)
  - —Cadmium oxide (oxyacetylene welding and electroplating)

Pre-Hospital

CAUTIONS

- Rescuers should wear appropriate self-contained breathing apparatus, and protective clothing to prevent self-contamination

Diagnosis

ESSENTIAL WORKUP

- History of exposure to irritant gases confirms the diagnosis

LABORATORY

- Arterial blood gas: assess oxygenation, ventilation, and evidence of acidosis (see chapter: Cyanide, Poisoning)
- Carbon monoxide level: if smoke inhalation with concomitant irritant gas inhalation (see chapter: Carbon Monoxide, Poisoning)
- Methemoglobin level: if oxides of nitrogen are suspected
- Serum calcium level: if hydrogen fluoride is suspected

IMAGING/SPECIAL TESTS

- Spirometry: assess clinical evidence of airway narrowing and bronchoconstriction
- CXR: may be negative in cases of upper airway irritants, or *early* assessment of peripheral airway irritants
- Direct laryngoscopy: assess evidence of upper airway edema
- Corneal fluorescein: assess corneal burns
- ECG with significant pulmonary symptoms, in elderly or those with cardiac history

DIFFERENTIAL DIAGNOSIS

- Asthma exacerbation
- Allergic stimuli (pollen)
- Physical stimuli (cold air)
- Bronchitis
- Pneumonia
- Occupational asthma
- Hypersensitivity pneumonitis

Treatment

INITIAL STABILIZATION

- ABCs
  - —Supplemental oxygen—warm humidified oxygen may be more soothing to inflamed tissues
  - —Mechanical airway placement if necessary by oral intubation or nasotracheal intubation over a small bronchoscope
  - —Mechanical ventilation if necessary
  - —CPAP or PEEP if necessary to enhance oxygenation
- Decontaminate by removing clothes and irrigating skin and ocular tissues

ED TREATMENT

- Inhaled nebulized β_2-adrenergic agonists (albuterol) for bronchoconstriction
- Inhaled/IV/ po corticosteroids: beclomethasone, methylprednisolone, prednisone
  - —For cases of severe airway inflammation and bronchospasm
  - —After exposure to oxides of nitrogen and phosgene to limit long-term pulmonary fibrosis and bronchiolitis obliterans
  - —No controlled trials which document the benefit of acute corticosteroids after irritant gas inhalation
  - —Use of inhaled corticosteroids is controversial
- IV diuretics for noncardiogenic pulmonary edema to prevent positive fluid balance
- Nebulized sodium bicarbonate after chlorine gas inhalation
  - —Reported to be of benefit in human case reports and in animals
  - —Not been studied and is not routinely recommended
- Nebulized calcium gluconate after acute hydrogen fluoride inhalation
  - —Has been reported but has not been proven to be of benefit
- Cyanide antidote kit if hydrogen cyanide is suspected. (see chapter: Cyanide, Poisoning)
- Hyperbaric oxygen therapy if carbon monoxide or hydrogen sulfide are suspected

MEDICATIONS

- Albuterol: 0.5 cc (peds: 0.03 cc or 0.15 mg/kg/dose) of 0.5% sol diluted in NS to 3 cc aerosolized
- Beclomethasone: 84 μg (2 puffs) (peds: 42–84 μg) inhaled
- Furosemide: 40 mg (peds: 2 mg/kg/dose) IV
- Bumetanide (bumex): 1–2 mg IV (>18 years old)
- Metaproterenol: 0.3 cc (peds: 0.1–0.3 cc) of 5% sol diluted in NS to 3 cc aerosolized
- Methylprednisolone: 125 mg (peds: 2 mg/kg) IV
- Prednisone: 40–80 mg (1–2 mg/kg/24hrs) po

Disposition

ADMISSION CRITERIA

- ICU admission for intubated patients, or those with significant respiratory difficulty with potential upper airway obstruction or respiratory insufficiency
- Persistently symptomatic with bronchospasm (PEF <50% expected) or oxygen requirement
- Exposure to irritant gases which affect peripheral airways
  - —Delayed pulmonary edema and respiratory failure may occur
- Lower criteria for elderly patients, or those with preexisting COPD

DISCHARGE CRITERIA

- Mild exposures that respond well to supportive care, and have no oxygen requirement or bronchospasm after a 4–6-hour observation period

Miscellaneous

ICD9: 987.9

CORE CONTENT CODE: 17.2.30

SUGGESTED READINGS

Kulling P. Hospital treatments of victims exposed to combustion products. Toxicol Lett 1992;64–65:283–289

Newman-Taylor AJ. Respiratory irritants encountered at work. Thorax 1996;51(5):541–545.

Rorison DG, McPherson SJ. Acute toxic inhalations. Emerg Med Clin North Am 1992;10(2):409–435.

Weiss SM, Lakshminarayan S. Acute inhalation injury. Clin Chest Med 1994;15(1):103–116.

Author: Susan Farrell

Isoniazid, Poisoning

Clinical Presentation

SIGNS AND SYMPTOMS

Acute Toxicity

- Neurologic
  —Altered mental status
  —Seizures
    -Refractory to traditional methods of seizure control
  —Agitation
  —Coma
  —Dizziness
  —Ataxia
  —Hyperreflexia
  —Slurred speech
  —Hallucinations
  —Psychosis
- Gastrointestinal
  —Nausea
  —Vomiting
- Renal
  —Anuria
  —Oliguria
- Cardiovascular
  —Hypotension
  —Tachycardia
  —Shock

Chronic Toxicity

- Neurologic
  —Optic neuritis
  —Psychosis
  —Insomnia
  —Vertigo
- Gastrointestinal hepatitis
  —Liver failure
  —Nausea, vomiting
  —Anorexia

MECHANISM/DESCRIPTION

- Complexes with and inactivates pyridoxine (vitamin B_6) in multiple enzyme systems
- Synthesis of GABA requires pyridoxal phosphate as a cofactor
- Loss of GABA: cause of benzodiazepine refractory seizures
- Blocks conversion of lactate to pyruvate by interfering with NAD
  —Contributes to the profound anion gap acidosis
- Chronic toxicity
  —Interferes with synthesis of nicotinic acid (niacin)
  —Causes syndrome indistinguishable from pellagra (niacin deficiency)
- Structurally similar to the MAO inhibitors
  —Reports of a tyramine-like reaction to INH
  —Palpitations, sweating, flushing, chest tightness, and dyspnea

Pharmacokinetics

- Rapidly absorbed reaching peak levels within 2 hours
- Renally excreted after acetylation in the liver
- Half life <1 hour in fast acetylators, up to 4 hours in slow acetylating individuals

ETIOLOGY

- High risk includes the homeless, HIV infected, alcoholics, and those in the lower socio-economic status populations

Pre-Hospital

CAUTIONS

- Do not induce emesis due to CNS depressant effects/seizures

Diagnosis

ESSENTIAL WORKUP

- Electrolytes, BUN/Cr, glucose
  - —Elevated anion gap acidosis
  - —Hyperglycemia

LABORATORY

- ABG
  - —Severe metabolic acidosis
- CBC
  - —Acute toxicity: leukocytosis, eosinophilia
  - —Chronic toxicity: agranulocytosis, eosinophilia, hemolysis, anemia

IMAGING/SPECIAL TESTS

- CXR
  - —Presence of tuberculous disease increases suspicion for toxicity
  - —For aspiration pneumonia

DIFFERENTIAL DIAGNOSIS

- Toxins
  - —TCA
  - —ASA
  - —Theophylline
  - —Methanol/ethylene glycol
  - —Paraldehyde
  - —Lithium
  - —Carbon monoxide
  - —Cocaine
  - —Agents that cause metabolic acidosis
- CNS
  - —CVA
  - —Intracranial hemorrhage/mass/trauma/abscess
- Hypoglycemia
- Uremia
- Thyrotoxicosis

Treatment

INITIAL STABILIZATION

- ABCs
  - —Supplemental oxygen
  - —Check for gag reflex, intubate if necessary
  - —Cardiac monitor
  - —0.9%NS access
- Narcan, thiamine, D50W (Accucheck) if altered mental status

ED TREATMENT

- B_6 (pyridoxine)
  - —Antidote for INH toxicity
  - —Administer 1 g of pyridoxine for each gram of INH ingested
  - —Administer 5 g (repeat in 20 minutes) for unknown amount of overdose
  - —If insufficient quantity of pyridoxine available, contact other hospital pharmacies and your regional poison control center to obtain more
- Seizure control
  - —Pyridoxine
  - —Benzodiazepine
- Gastric decontamination after stabilization
  - —Gastric lavage for recent ingestions
  - —Activated charcoal
  - —Avoid syrup of ipecac due to acute onset of seizures
- Dialysis
  - —INH poorly protein-bound
  - —Institute if sufficient quantities of pyridoxine unavailable to treat overdose
- Sodium bicarbonate
  - —For severe metabolic acidosis
  - —Acidosis usually resolves spontaneously after elimination of seizures

MEDICATIONS

- Dextrose: D50W 1 amp (50 ml or 25 g) (peds: D25W 2–4 ml/kg) IV
- Diazepam (benzodiazepine): 5–10 mg (peds: 0.2–0.5 mg/kg) IV
- Lorazepam (benzodiazepine): 2–6 mg (peds: 0.03–0.05 mg/kg) IV
- Naloxone (narcan): 2 mg (peds: 0.1 mg/kg) IV or IM initial dose
- Thiamine (vitamin B_1): 100 mg (peds: 50 mg) IV or IM

Disposition

ADMISSION CRITERIA

- ICU admission for moderate to severe toxicity

DISCHARGE CRITERIA

- Asymptomatic or mildly symptomatic after 6-hour observation

Miscellaneous

ICD9: 961.8

CORE CONTENT CODE: 17.2

SUGGESTED READINGS

Ellenhorn MJ, Schoonwald S, Ordog G, Wasserberger J. Isoniazid. In: Ellenhorn MJ, ed. Ellenhorn's medical toxicology. 2d ed. Baltimore: Williams & Wilkins, 1997:240–243.

Wason S, La Coutore PG, Lovejoy, FH. Single high-dose pyridoxine treatment for isoniazid overdose. JAMA 1981;246(10):1102–1104.

Author: Mark Crockett

Isopropanol, Poisoning

Clinical Presentation

SIGNS AND SYMPTOMS

- Usually occur within 30–60 minutes of ingestion

Neurologic

- Lethargy
- Weakness
- Headache
- Inebriation
- Vertigo
- Ataxia
- Apnea
- Coma
- Initial excitation phase seen with ethanol ingestion is absent

Gastrointestinal

- Nausea/vomiting
- Abdominal pain
- Gastritis
- Hematemesis

Cardiovascular

- Hypotension
- Tachycardia
- Myocardial depression
- Peripheral vascular dilatation

Pulmonary

- Respiratory depression
- Hemorrhagic tracheobronchitis

Dermatologic

- Skin irritation
- Burns

Ocular

- Irritation
- Lacrimation

MECHANISM/DESCRIPTION

- CNS depressant effect of isopropanol is 2–3 times as potent as ethanol
- Many products which contain isopropanol also contain methanol, ethylene glycol, and ethanol
- Rapidly absorbed following oral ingestion
- Ketogenic but not does not cause significant acidosis
- Metabolized by alcohol dehydrogenase to acetone (a CNS depressant)
- Acetone eliminated by lung and kidney
- $T_{1/2}$
  —Isopropanol: 3–16 hrs
  —Acetone: 7.5–26 hrs
- Concomitant ethanol ingestion doubles the half-life of isopropanol but not acetone

ETIOLOGY

- Isopropanol (isopropyl alcohol): clear, colorless, volatile liquid with a faint odor of acetone and a bitter taste
- Available as a 70% rubbing alcohol solution
  —May contain a blue dye which was added to inhibit its abuse ("Blue Heaven")
- Found in
  —Various toiletries
  —Disinfectants
  —Window cleaning solutions
  —Paint remover
  —Solvents
  —Jewelry cleaners
  —Detergents
  —Antifreeze
- Typical adult patient: a chronic alcoholic who has been on a drinking binge and recently depleted his ethanol supply
- Rectal administration can cause systemic toxicity

PEDIATRIC CONSIDERATIONS

- Accidental ingestions common <6 years old
- Rubbing alcohol sponge baths may cause toxicity (rare)

Diagnosis

ESSENTIAL WORKUP

- History of ingestion
- Odor of isopropanol or acetone on patient's breath

LABORATORY

- Electrolytes, BUN/Cr, glucose
  —Hypoglycemia occurs
  —Does *not* produce significant acidosis unless accompanied by end organ hypoperfusion
  —Acetone can produce a false elevation of serum Cr
    -When acetone levels exceeds 40 mg/dl, Cr values rise at approximately 1 mg Cr per 100 mg/dl acetone
    -Cr returns to baseline following acetone metabolism
- CBC
  —Decreased Hct with significant hemorrhagic gastritis
- ABG
  —Acidosis rare unless due to hypoperfusion or coingestant
- Urinalysis
  —Ketones present
- Serum osmolality
  —Osmolar gap—difference between measured and calculated osmolality
  —Calculated osmolality = 2 Na^+ BUN/2.8 + glucose/18 + ethanol/4.3
  —Osmolar gap present if measured minus calculated osmolality >10
  —Gap increases by 1 mosm/kg for each 5.9 mg/dl of isopropanol and 5.5 mg/dl of acetone
- Serum ketones present
- Isopropanol level
  —Coma with level >150 mg/dl

IMAGING/SPECIAL TESTS

- CXR: for aspiration pneumonia with AMS and vomiting
- CT head: concomitant head injury occurs

DIFFERENTIAL DIAGNOSIS

- For CNS depression and an elevated osmolar gap includes
  —Ethanol
  —Ethylene glycol
  —Methanol
  —Glycerol
  —Mannitol

PEDIATRIC CONSIDERATIONS

- Prone to hypoglycemia following exposure

Treatment

INITIAL STABILIZATION

- ABCs
  - —Maintain the airway and assist in ventilation if necessary
- Hypotension
  - —Treat initially with 0.9%NS IV fluid bolus
  - —Initiate dopamine or norepinephrine infusion if hypotension persists
  - —PRBC with significant hemorrhagic gastritis
- Narcan, thiamine, dextrose (or Accucheck) if altered mental status

ED TREATMENT

- Primarily supportive therapy—no specific antidote
- Irrigate skin/eyes for dermal or ocular exposure
- Activated charcoal
  - —For coingestants
  - —Large doses can absorb significant amounts of isopropanol
- Do *not* treat with an ethanol infusion or 4-methylpyrazole
- Hemodialysis
  - —Effectively removes isopropanol and acetone
  - —Most managed with supportive care alone
  - —Indications
    - -Hemodynamically instability despite fluid replacement and the use of pressors
    - -Levels >400 mg/dl (associated with severe hypotension and prolonged coma)

MEDICATIONS

- Activated charcoal slurry: 1–2 g/kg up to 90 g po
- Sorbitol: 1–2 g/kg to a max of 150 g (peds >1 yr old: 1–1.5 g/kg as a 35% sol to a max of 50 g) po mixed in the activated charcoal slurry
- Dextrose: D50W 1 amp (50 ml or 25 g) (peds: D25W 2–4 ml/kg) IV
- Naloxone (narcan): 2 mg (peds: 0.1 mg/kg) IV or IM initial dose
- Thiamine (vitamin B_1): 100 mg (peds: 50 mg) IV or IM
- Dopamine: 2–20 μg/kg/min IV

Disposition

ADMISSION CRITERIA

- Moderate to severe isopropanol toxicity (altered mental status, hypotension)

DISCHARGE CRITERIA

- Observe asymptomatic patients following ingestion for 2–4 hours before discharge
- Mild intoxication that resolves over 4–6 hours

Miscellaneous

ICD 9: 980.2

CORE CONTENT CODE: 17.2.2.3

SUGGESTED READINGS

Burkhart KK, Kulig K. The other alcohols methanol, ethylene glycol, and isopropanol. Emerg Med Clin North Am 1990;8(4):913–928.

Ellenhorn MJ, Schoonwald S, Ordog G, Wasserberger J. Isopropyl alcohol. In: Ellenhorn MJ, ed. Ellenhorn's medical toxicology. 2d ed. Baltimore: Williams & Wilkins, 1997:1148–1149.

Goldfrank LR, Flomenbaum NE, Howland MA. Methanol, ethylene glycol, and isopropanol. In: Goldfrank LR, Flomenbaum NE, Hoffman RS, et al., eds. Goldfrank's toxicologic emergencies. 5th ed. Norwalk, CT: Appleton & Lange, 1994;827–846.

Author: Paul Kolecki

Jaundice

Clinical Presentation

SIGNS AND SYMPTOMS

- Cholestasis: pruritus, pale stools, dark urine
- Gallstones or pancreatitis: abdominal pain
- Malignancy: anorexia, weight loss, malaise
- Courvoisier's rule (painless jaundice and a palpable, nontender gallbladder represents malignant common duct obstruction)
- Physical exam
  - —Stigmata of cirrhosis
  - —Palpable gallbladder or right upper quadrant tenderness
  - —Hepatomegaly, splenomegaly
  - —Abdominal mass, evidence of cachexia
  - —Ascites, skin coloration, Kayser-Fleischer rings (Wilson's disease)

MECHANISM/DESCRIPTION

- Yellow pigmentation of tissues and body fluids due to elevated serum bilirubin
- Unconjugated hyperbilirubinemia: unconjugated bilirubin is the direct breakdown product of heme, is water insoluble, and is measured as indirect bilirubin
- Causes include
  - —Hemolytic (excessive production of unconjugated bilirubin)
  - —Hepatic (decreased conjugation of bilirubin, Gilbert's syndrome)
  - —Decreased uptake (i.e., physiologic jaundice)
- Conjugated hyperbilirubinemia
  - —Conjugated bilirubin is water soluble, and is measured as direct bilirubin
  - —In conjugated hyperbilirubinemia, bilirubin is returned to the bloodstream after conjugation in the liver, instead of draining into the bile ducts
  - —Causes include
    - -Hepatocellular dysfunction (i.e., hepatitis, cirrhosis, tumor invasion, toxic injury)
    - -Intrahepatic (nonobstructive) cholestasis
    - -Extrahepatic (obstructive) cholestasis

PEDIATRIC CONSIDERATIONS

- Physiologic jaundice
  - —Full-term infant: bilirubin peaks on the 3rd or 4th day, then steadily decreases by 1 week
  - —Premature newborns: peak occurs at day 5 to 7 and returns to normal over several weeks
  - —Pathologic jaundice appears within the first 24 hours
    - -Characterized by rapidly rising bilirubin, prolonged jaundice, or an elevated direct bilirubin (>2 mg/dl or >20% of total serum bilirubin)
    - -Conjugated hyperbilirubinemia in the newborn never has a physiologic cause and must always be investigated
- Breast milk jaundice
  - —Due to increased enterohepatic circulation
  - —Inhibition of glucuronyl transferase

Pre-Hospital

N/A

Diagnosis

ESSENTIAL WORKUP

- History and physical examination, together with routine laboratory tests, will suggest the diagnosis in approximately 80% of patients with jaundice
- Bilirubin level: unconjugated versus conjugated
  - —Severity may suggest cause of obstruction
    - -Malignancy causes highest levels (10–30 mg/dl)
    - -Choledocholithiasis rarely exceeds 15 mg/dl

LABORATORY

- Alkaline phosphatase
  - —If no bone disease or pregnancy, then elevation suggests impaired biliary tract function
  - —2X: hepatitis and cirrhosis
  - —3X: extrahepatic biliary obstruction (i.e., choledocholithiasis) and intrahepatic cholestasis (i.e., drug-induced and biliary cirrhosis)
- Aminotransferases: Provide evidence of hepatocellular damage
- Alanine aminotransferase (ALT, SGPT): primarily in the liver
- Aspartate aminotransferase (AST, SGOT): liver, heart, kidney, skeletal muscle, and brain
- GGTP (γ-glutamyl transpeptidase): throughout hepatobiliary system, pancreas, heart, kidneys, and lungs
  - —May be the most sensitive indicator of biliary tract disease
- 5′-Nucleotidase: widespread tissue distribution
  - —Confirms hepatic origin of an elevated alkaline phosphatase level
- Albumin: decreased level associated with severe liver disease
- Prothrombin time: prolonged level is an important prognostic indicator in patients with acute hepatitis

IMAGING/SPECIAL TESTS

- Ultrasound: most effective initial imaging technique
  - —Ductal dilatation is a reliable indicator of extrahepatic obstruction
    - -More than 90% effective in identifying cholelithiasis
  - —Tumors of the liver and head of pancreas usually well visualized
  - —Distinguishes solid liver tumors from cystic structures
- Plain radiographs
  - —May show evidence of hepatic and splenic enlargement or biliary calcifications
- Hepatic nuclear scan (HIDA)
  - —Accurate method of diagnosing acute cholecystitis or cystic duct obstruction because the gallbladder cannot be visualized with these agents
- Computed tomography
  - —Superior to ultrasound in detecting pancreatic and intra-abdominal tumors
  - —Can help differentiate fluid-containing structures
- ERCP (endoscopic retrograde cholangiopancreatography)
  - —Diagnostic: stones seen as filling defects within bile duct lumen
  - —Malignancies seen as strictures
- Therapeutic
  - —Extraction of common bile duct stones by insertion of stents to bypass malignant obstructions
  - —Biopsies under direct vision
- Neonatal jaundice workup
  - —Serum bilirubin
- Full-term healthy newborn
  - —Blood group typing of infant and mother, direct Coombs, serum bilirubin
- Premature, ill, or significant jaundice (>15 mg/dl): CBC, reticulocyte count, blood smear, direct bilirubin
- Asian or Greek ethnicity (African-Americans after oxidative agent exposure): G6PD

DIFFERENTIAL DIAGNOSIS

- Prehepatic
  - —Hemolysis (sickle cell, other hemoglobinopathies)
  - —Ineffective erythropoiesis
  - —Drugs
  - —Gilbert's syndrome
  - —Crigler-Najjar syndrome
  - —Prolonged fasting
- Hepatocellular
  - —Hepatitis (infectious, alcoholic, autoimmune, toxin, drug-induced)
  - —Cirrhosis
  - —Postischemia
  - —Hemochromatosis
- Intrahepatic cholestasis
  - —Pregnancy
  - —Drugs
  - —Dubin-Johnson syndrome
  - —Rotor syndrome
  - —Benign recurrent cholestasia
  - —Familial syndromes
  - —Sepsis
  - —Postoperative jaundice
  - —Lymphoma
- Extrahepatic obstruction
  - —Common duct stone
  - —Biliary stricture
  - —Bacterial cholangitis
  - —Sclerosing cholangitis

—Carcinoma (ampulla, gallbladder, pancreas), cholangiosarcoma
—Pancreatitis, pancreatic pseudocyst
—Hemobilia
—Duodenal diverticula
—Ascariasis
—Postlaparoscopic cholecystectomy complications
—Congenital biliary atresia
—Congenital choledochal cyst

PEDIATRIC DIFFERENTIAL DIAGNOSIS

- Intrahepatic cholestasis
  —Cardiovascular (congenital heart disease, congestive heart failure, shock, asphyxia)
  —Metabolic or genetic (α_1-antitrypsin deficiency, trisomy 18 and 21, cystic fibrosis, Gaucher's disease, Niemann-Pick disease, glycogen storage disease type IV)
  —Infectious (bacterial sepsis, CMV, enterovirus, HSV, rubella, syphilis, tuberculosis, varicella, viral hepatitis)
  —Hematologic (severe isoimmune hemolytic disease)

Treatment

INITIAL STABILIZATION

- Isotonic intravenous fluid therapy if dehydrated
- Toxic-appearing patients
  —Supplemental oxygen, cardiac monitoring
  —Nasogastric suction, and bladder catheterization

ED TREATMENT

- For bacterial cholangitis/sepsis obtain blood cultures and administer parenteral antibiotics
  —Ampicillin, gentamicin, and metronidazole *or*
  —Ticarcillin, or piperacillin, and metronidazole *or*
  —Cefoxitin and tobramycin
- Obstructive extrahepatic jaundice
  —Surgical consult
- Choledocholithiasis
  —ERCP papillotomy, balloon or basket retrieval, or open surgery
- Obstructive intrahepatic or nonobstructive jaundice
  —Medical management
    -Withdraw causative drug, ethanol
    -Interferon for chronic hepatitis B and C
    -Penicillamine and phlebotomy for Wilson's disease and hemochromatosis
    -Corticosteroids for chronic hepatitis of autoimmune origin

PEDIATRIC CONSIDERATIONS

- Exchange transfusion
  —Emergent treatment of markedly elevated bilirubin (>20 mg/dl in full-term infants) and for correction of anemia caused by isoimmune hemolytic disease
- Phototherapy: for neonatal jaundice when bilirubin ≥17 mg/dl
  —Measure bilirubin once to twice daily and stop when bilirubin <12 mg/dl
  —Increase fluid intake by 20% during exposure
  —Use eye pads
- Phenobarbital: in sepsis and drug-induced causes; decreases conjugated bilirubin
- Metalloporphyrins: investigational inhibitors of heme oxygenase

MEDICATIONS

- Ampicillin: adult: 2 g IV q 6 hrs; peds: 25 mg/kg IV q 6–8 hrs
- Cefoxitin: adult: 2 g IV q 6 hrs; peds: 40–160 mg/kg/day div q 6–12 hrs
- Gentamicin: adult: 2–5 mg/kg IV q 8 hrs; peds: same
- Metronidazole: adult: 1 g IV q 12 hrs; peds: 30 mg/kg/day div q 12 hrs
- Piperacillin/TZ: adult: 3.375 g IV q 6 hrs; peds: 300 mg/kg/day div q 6 hrs (> 2 mos. age)
- Ticarcillin/CL: adult: 3.1 g IV q 6 hrs; peds: 75–100 mg/kg/day div q 6 hrs
- Tobramycin: adult: 2–5 mg/kg IV q 6hrs; peds: same

Disposition

ADMISSION CRITERIA

- Bacterial cholangitis
- Intractable pain
- Intractable emesis
- Associated pancreatitis

DISCHARGE CRITERIA

- No evidence of infection (evaluate as outpatient)

Miscellaneous

ICD9: 782.4

CORE CONTENT CODE: 22.4.19

SUGGESTED READINGS

Frank BB. Clinical evaluation of jaundice: A guideline of the Patient Care Committee of the American Gastroenterological Association. JAMA 1989;262(21):3031–34.

Lasker MR, Holzman IR. Neonatal jaundice. Postgrad Med 1996;99(3):187–98.

McKnight JT, Jones JE. Jaundice. Am Fam Phys 1992;45(3):1139–48.

Author: Andrew Chang

Jones Fractures

Clinical Presentation

SIGNS AND SYMPTOMS

- Patients often complain of a "sprained ankle"
- Dorsolateral and proximal foot pain is present
- Dependency and weight bearing exacerbate the pain
- Ecchymosis and swelling appear over the proximal and lateral aspect of the dorsal foot
- Point tenderness and even crepitus is palpable soon after the injury
- Plantar palpation of the fifth metatarsal head is painful
- Axial compression of the fifth toe also produces pain at the fracture site

MECHANISM/DESCRIPTION

- Originally described in 1902 by Sir Robert Jones
- Two distinct fracture patterns are described for the proximal fifth metatarsal
  —Avulsion fracture of a variable sized portion of the tuberosity, in the metaphyseal region, at the site of the peroneal brevis insertion or plantar aponeurosis
  —Transverse fracture of the proximal metatarsal within 1.5 cm of the tuberosity, which is the classic Jones fracture
- The Jones fracture is a transverse fracture of the base of the fifth metatarsal at the junction of the metaphysis and the diaphysis, involving the tuberosity
- To establish appropriate treatment and prognosis, it is essential to distinguish between avulsion, proximal midshaft metatarsal, and Jones fractures
- If not recognized and treated appropriately, Jones fractures can result in delayed union or nonunion, which does not occur with avulsion or simple midshaft metatarsal fractures

ETIOLOGY

- Often seen in adult runners, walkers, dancers, hikers, and jumping athletes
- Sudden inversion of the foot is a common cause
- An indirect mechanism of twisting the forefoot results in a fractured proximal metatarsal
- Occasionally, direct blunt force to the dorsolateral aspect of the foot causes fracture
- There is some evidence to suggest that a stress fracture can precede a Jones fracture

Pre-Hospital

- Pre-hospital care includes immobilization of the foot/ankle complex, as well as cold therapy to the point of maximal tenderness
- Lights and siren (Code 3) transportation of patients with isolated distal extremity injuries with a normal neurovascular examination is unnecessary

Diagnosis

ESSENTIAL WORKUP

- Anterior-posterior (AP), lateral, and oblique radiographs are the mainstay for diagnoses

DIFFERENTIAL DIAGNOSIS

- Avulsion or midshaft fractures of the fifth metatarsal
- Cuboid or cuneiform fractures
- Lateral ankle ligament injury

Treatment

INITIAL STABILIZATION

- Cold therapy and analgesics upon presentation
- Radiographs of the foot

ED TREATMENT

- Immobilization with a posterior splint or short leg cast
- Nonweight-bearing crutch-walking instructions

MEDICATIONS

- Opiates and/or nonsteroidal anti-inflammatory analgesics for pain management

Disposition

- Discharge from the emergency department with crutches and analgesics
- Close orthopedic follow-up for the application of a short leg cast if not done in the emergency department and ongoing management in the event of delayed or nonunion of the fracture

Miscellaneous

ICD9: 825.25

CORE CONTENT CODE: 18.4.13.1.2

SUGGESTED READINGS

Dameron TB. Fractures and anatomic variations of the proximal portion of the fifth metatarsal. J Bone Joint Surg 1975;57:788.

Kavanaugh JH, Brower TD, Mann RV. The Jones fracture revisited. J Bone Joint Surg 1978;60A:776–782.

Simon RR, Koenigsknecht SJ. Metatarsal fractures. In: Simon RR, et al., eds. Emergency orthopedics: The extremities. 2d ed. Norwalk, CT: Appleton and Lange, 1995:333–335.

Author: Vincent P. Verdile

Kaposi's Sarcoma

Clinical Presentation

SIGNS AND SYMPTOMS

- Classical and African forms
  - —Multiple firm, reddish brown or bluish plaques and nodules that may ulcerate
  - —Tumors may appear simultaneously anywhere on skin surface or mucus membranes
  - —10% show visceral involvement
  - —Lesions most common on lower extremities where often associated with lymphedema
- Epidemic HIV-associated form
  - —Skin lesions may be obscure, initially resembling insect bites, bruises, or cigarette burns
  - —Initially form slightly raised, oval or elongated, poorly demarcated lesions ranging in color from pink to reddish-brown to blue
  - —May occur as macules, papules, plaques, or nodules
  - —Most common on trunk, head, and neck
  - —Mucus membrane and visceral involvement common
  - —Widespread dissemination to the gastrointestinal tract, lung, liver, spleen, lymph nodes, and other organs may occur
  - —Gastrointestinal involvement may cause bleeding
  - —Pulmonary involvement may cause shortness of breath

MECHANISM/DESCRIPTION

- A multicentric neoplasm consisting of multiple vascular nodules appearing in the skin, mucus membranes, and viscera
- Course ranges from indolent, with only mild skin or lymph node involvement, to fulminant, with extensive cutaneous and visceral involvement
- Risk factors
  - —Classical form: most commonly in elderly North American and European men of Mediterranean or eastern European Jewish ancestry
  - —African (endemic) form: young black adult males and prepubescent children in sub-Saharan Africa
  - —Epidemic form in HIV infected individuals (male:female ratio is 50:1)
  - —Also iatrogenic immunosuppressed form most commonly in renal transplant patients

Pre-Hospital

N/A

Diagnosis

ESSENTIAL WORKUP

- Diagnosis is made by biopsy of a suspicious lesion or lymph node although rarely done in the ED

IMAGING/SPECIAL TESTS

- Chest x-ray may show pulmonary nodules
- Body CT may demonstrate visceral involvement

DIFFERENTIAL DIAGNOSIS

- Clinical differential diagnosis of Kaposi's sarcoma (KS) is extensive and includes many benign or malignant vascular or nonvascular skin lesions

Treatment

INITIAL STABILIZATION

- No specific considerations
- Patients with HIV may have serious underlying diseases that need stabilization

ED TREATMENT

- Treatment of complications of visceral involvement, e.g., gastrointestinal bleeding, or obstruction, or pulmonary involvement
- Consultation with an oncologist
- Local therapy: radiation
  —Classical and African KS: localized lesions that are large, painful, ulcerated, invasive, or associated with significant lymphedema should be treated with radiation therapy
  —Epidemic HIV-associated KS: painful, disfiguring, or cosmetically disturbing cutaneous lesions or oropharyngeal lesions causing dysphagia, airway obstruction, pain, ulceration, hemorrhage, or cosmetic disfigurement may be treated with radiation therapy
- Systemic therapy: chemotherapy
  —Classical KS recalcitrant to local radiotherapy may respond to intralesional or systemic chemotherapy
  —African and epidemic HIV-associated KS may respond to a variety of single agent or multiagent chemotherapy regimens

MEDICATIONS

- No specific medications

Disposition

ADMISSION CRITERIA

- Patients with KS do not need admission solely for the KS lesions
- Severe underlying disease or complication of KS such as GI bleeding, bowel obstruction, or hypoxia may require admission

DISCHARGE CRITERIA

- Patients with uncomplicated KS may be discharged with appropriate referral

Miscellaneous

ICD9: 176.9

CORE CONTENT CODE: 3.7.2

SUGGESTED READINGS

Fauci AS, Lane HC. Human immunodeficiency virus disease: AIDS and related disorders. In: Isselbacher KJ, Braunwald E, Wilson JD, et al., eds. Harrison's principles of internal medicine. New York: McGraw Hill, 1994:1604–1605.

Martin RW, Hood AF, Farmer ER. Kaposi sarcoma. Medicine 1993;72:245–261.

Safai B, Schwartz JJ. Kaposi's sarcoma and the acquired immunodeficiency syndrome. In: DeVita VT, Hellman S, Rosenberg SA, eds. AIDS: Etiology, diagnosis, treatment, and prevention. Philadelphia: JB Lippincott, 1992:209–223.

Tirelli U, Franceschi S, Carbone A. Malignant tumours in patients with HIV infection. Br Med J 1994;308:1148–1153.

Author: Glenn Hebel

Kawasaki Disease

Clinical Presentation

SIGNS AND SYMPTOMS

- Also known as *mucocutaneous lymph node syndrome*
- Symptoms are generally described in three phases

Acute Febrile Phase (0–2 Weeks)

- Fever
  —Unresponsive to antibiotics or antipyretics
- Cervical adenopathy
  —Anterior and often greater than 1.5 cm in diameter
- Bulbar conjunctivitis
  —Bilateral, nonexudative
- Mucocutaneous changes
  —Erythema of lips
  —Strawberry tongue
- Cutaneous changes
  —Polymorphous rash
  —Diaper area in patients <2 years of age

Subacute Phase (2–4 Weeks)

- Desquamation—initially periungual
- Thrombocytosis
- Cardiac
  —Pancarditis
  —Coronary artery aneurysms
  —Myocardial infarction (most common cause of death)
  —Valvular insufficiency
  —Congestive heart failure
  —Pericardial effusion
  —Dysrhythmias
- Acalculous cholecystitis/*hydrops gallbladder*
- Right upper-quadrant abdominal pain
- Palpable mass in RUQ

Recovery or Convalescent Phase (Months to Years)

- Regression or recurrence of cardiovascular manifestations

MECHANISM/DESCRIPTION

- Multisystem vasculitis with greatest predilection for coronary arteries
- Peak incidence between 1 and 2 years of age, with cases before the age of 3 months uncommon

ETIOLOGY

- Unknown cause; infectious vs. immune response
- Japanese and Korean ancestry appear to be at greatest risk

Pre-Hospital

N/A

Diagnosis

ESSENTIAL WORKUP

- Clinical diagnosis
- Fulfill at least 5 of 6 clinical criteria (adapted from CDC guidelines)
  —Fever for ≥5 days, and
  —4 of these 5
    -Bilateral conjunctival infection usually with limbal sparing
    -Oropharyngeal mucous membrane changes including, erythematous or fissured lips, strawberry tongue and infected pharynx
    -Peripheral extremity changes with erythema or edema of hands and feet, or periungual desquamation
    -Polymorphous rash which is primarily truncal
    -Cervical lymphadenopathy which is often unilateral and 1.5 cm in diameter
- Atypical cases not fulfilling diagnostic criteria may be seen
  —Especially in children less than 6 months of age

LABORATORY

- Findings are usually nonspecific
- CBC shows
  —Anemia
  —Thrombocytopenia
  —Polymorphonuclear leukocytosis
- Erythrocyte sedimentation rate and C-reactive protein elevated
- Urinalysis
  —Sterile pyuria
- Liver function tests
  —Elevated transaminase and bilirubin
- ECG
  —ST-segment changes
  —Increased QTc
  —Low voltage
  —Nonspecific abnormalities

IMAGING/SPECIAL TESTS

- Echocardiogram
  —Most sensitive screening test for identifying proximal coronary artery aneurysms
  —80–90% sensitivity
- Angiography
  —Use in select cases to diagnose peripheral coronary artery pathology

DIFFERENTIAL DIAGNOSIS

- Viral infections
  —Rubella
  —Rubeola
  —Ebstein-Barr virus
  —Adenovirus
  —Enterovirus
- Bacterial infections
  —Toxic shock syndrome
  —Scarlet fever
  —Rickettsial disease
  —Rocky Mountain Spotted Fever
  —Juvenile rheumatoid arthritis
- Drug reactions
  —Erythema multiforme
  —Stevens-Johnson's Syndrome
- Mercury vapor poisoning

Treatment

INITIAL STABILIZATION

- ABCs with particular focus to cardiovascular system

ED TREATMENT

- Initiate aspirin and intravenous γ-globulin (IVGG) therapy when diagnostic criteria met
  - —Monitor salicylate levels
  - —Risk of Reye's syndrome
  - —Early administration of IVGG decreases risk of coronary artery aneurysm
- Cardiology consultation for atypical or incomplete cases
- Treat myocardial infarction as in adults, including early administration of thrombolytic therapy
- Steroids contraindicated

MEDICATIONS

- Aspirin: 50–100mg/kg/24hrs q 6 hrs then 3–10 mg/kg/24hrs
- IVGG: 2 g/kg over 10–12 hours

Disposition

ADMISSION CRITERIA

- Admit patients fulfilling clinical criteria to the pediatric service with cardiology consultation
- Low admission threshold for patients who appear ill yet do not meet all the diagnostic criteria
  - —Many of these patients will subsequently be found to have Kawasaki's disease, or are toxic from another etiology

DISCHARGE CRITERIA

- Patients not fulfilling criteria who appear nontoxic with close follow-up

Miscellaneous

ICD9: 446.1

CORE CONTENT CODE: 13.11.2

SUGGESTED READINGS

Bell D, et al. Kawasaki syndrome: Description of two outbreaks in the United States. N Engl J Med 1981;304:1568–1575.

Kawasaki T, et al. A new infantile acute febrile mucocutaneous lymph node syndrome (MLNS) prevailing in Japan. Pediatrics 1974;54:271–276.

Melish M. Kawasaki syndrome. Pediatr Rev 1996;17:153–162.

Newburger J, et al. A single intravenous infusion of gamma globulin as compared with four infusions in the treatment of acute Kawasaki syndrome. N Engl J Med 1991;324:1633–1639.

Authors: Robert Davis; Robert Sidman

Knee Dislocation

Clinical Presentation

SIGNS AND SYMPTOMS

- Vascular injury to popliteal artery is the primary concern in this injury
- Grossly deformed knee
- Grossly unstable knee in anterior/posterior plane, or on varus/valgus stress
  - —Anterior and posterior cruciate ligament, and collateral ligament injury
- Lack of distal pulses
- Signs of distal ischemia
  - —Pallor, paresthesias, pain, paralysis
- Unequal temperature of lower extremities

ETIOLOGY

- High energy injuries such as MVA, auto versus pedestrian, and athletic injuries
  - —Football most common

MECHANISM/DESCRIPTION

- Defined by the position of the tibia in relationship to the distal femur
- *Anterior dislocation*
  - —Most common dislocation, accounts for 60%
  - —Hyperextension of the knee
  - —Rupture of the posterior capsule at 30°
  - —Rupture of the posterior cruciate ligament (PCL) and popliteal artery (PA) occurs at 50°
- *Posterior dislocation*
  - —Direct blow to the anterior tibia with the knee flexed at 90°
  - —Anterior cruciate ligament (ACL) is usually spared
- *Medial dislocation*
  - —Varus stress causing tear to ACL, PCL and lateral collateral ligament (LCL)
- *Lateral dislocation*
  - —Valgus stress causing tear to ACL, PCL and medial collateral ligament (MCL)
- *Popliteal artery injury*
  - —PA injury occurs in 33% of dislocations
  - —If vascular injury is not reversed within 6–8 hours, amputation rate approaches 90%
  - —Anterior dislocations place traction on the PA and cause contusion or intimal injury which may result in delayed thrombosis
  - —Posterior dislocations cause direct intimal fracture or transection of the artery with immediate thrombosis
- *Peroneal nerve injury*
  - —Less common than arterial injury
    - -If present, must rule out concomitant arterial insult
  - —Characterized by hypesthesia at first web space and lack of dorsiflexion of the foot
  - —Poor prognosis for recovery
  - —Medial dislocations cause injury by traction to the nerve
  - —Rotatory injuries have a high incidence of traction and transection

Pre-Hospital

CAUTIONS

- Documentation of pulses and motor response is essential
- Splint in slight flexion to prevent traction or compression of the popliteal artery

Diagnosis

ESSENTIAL WORKUP

- Complete and careful physical exam including
  - —*Pulses*—by palpation, Doppler, ankle-brachial pressure indexes, and distal perfusion
  - —*Neurologic*—sensation to the first web space and great toe, movement of the toes, dorsiflexion of the foot
- Knee x-rays
- Repeat examination if any closed reduction is attempted
- Arterial imaging if any signs of limb ischemia exist

IMAGING/SPECIAL TESTS

- AP and lateral plain X-rays
- Angiogram is indicated for any patient with poor distal perfusion, pulse return after reduction, abnormal pulses, signs of peroneal nerve injury, and ischemic symptoms despite normal pulse

DIFFERENTIAL DIAGNOSIS

- Tibial plateau fracture
- Supracondylar femoral fracture

Treatment

INITIAL STABILIZATION

- ABCs especially since this occurs most frequently in the multiply injured patient
- Fluid resuscitation as hypotension may alter distal pulses and perfusion
- Closed reduction must be performed immediately for any limb ischemia
- Early surgical consultation in an open injury or a high suspicion of arterial injury

ED TREATMENT

- Closed reduction by longitudinal traction and lifting femur into normal alignment without placing pressure on the popliteal artery
- Posterior leg splint in 15° of flexion at knee
- IV analgesia for patient comfort
- Vascular and orthopedic surgical consultation for open injury, evidence of popliteal artery injury, or unable to reduce dislocation

Disposition

ADMISSION CRITERIA

- All patients with knee dislocation require admission for either arterial injury repair or observation of limb perfusion

Miscellaneous

ICD9: 836.50

CORE CONTENT CODE: 18.4.13.2.4

SUGGESTED READINGS

Ghalambor N, Vangsness CT. Traumatic dislocation of the knee: A review of the literature. Bull Hosp J Dis 1995;54(1):19–24.

Kendell RW, Taylor DC, Salvian AJ, et al. The role of arteriography in assessing vascular injuries associated with dislocations of the knee. J Trauma 1993;35(6):875–878.

Stewart C. Knee injuries: Diagnosis and repair. EM Med Reports 1997;18(1):1–12.

Treiman GS, Yellin AE, Weaver FA, et al. Examination of the patient with a knee dislocation: The case for selective arteriography. Arch Surg 1992;127(9):1056–1062.

Authors: Kelly Anne Foley; Francis Counselman

Labor

Clinical Presentation

SIGNS AND SYMPTOMS

- Symptoms of labor include intermittent low abdominal pain with or without low back pain occurring regularly at least every 5 minutes and lasting 30–60 seconds
- Preterm labor is labor of sufficient frequency and intensity to bring about changes in dilation or effacement of the cervix before 37 weeks gestational age
- Labor is not associated with vaginal bleeding, and any patient with third trimester abdominal pain or vaginal bleeding should raise suspicion of placenta previa or placental abruption
- The sudden release of clear fluid from the vagina or a feeling of constant perineal wetness can represent rupture of membranes. This is not always associated with labor but often leads to onset of labor

MECHANISM/DESCRIPTION

- Labor is the physiologic process that brings about changes in the cervix to allow passage of the fetus through the birth canal. Labor is divided into three stages
- Stage 1: From the onset of uterine contractions to the time of full dilation of the cervix
  —Stage 1 is further divided into a latent and active phase
    -The *latent phase* is a time of uterine contraction with little change in cervical dilation or effacement
    -This is followed by the *active phase* where the cervix shows more rapid changes. The active phase generally begins around the time of cervical dilation of 3–4 cm
- Stage 2: From the onset of complete cervical dilation to the time of delivery of the infant
- Stage 3: From the time of delivery of the baby to the time of placental delivery
- The length of labor varies in nulliparous versus multiparous patients, and a general framework for progress of labor is provided in the table

	LENGTH OF LABOR			
STAGE OF LABOR	*MEAN*	*MEDIAN*	*MODE*	*LIMIT*
Nulliparous				
1st stage (hr)	14.4	12.3	9.5	
Latent phase (hr)	8.6	7.5	6.0	20
Active phase (hr)	4.9	4.0	3.0	12
Maximum slope (cm/hr)	3.0	2.7	1.5	1.2
2nd stage (hr)	1.0	0.8	0.6	2.5
Parous				
1st stage (hr)	7.7	6.5	5.1	
Latent phase (hr)	5.3	4.5	3.5	14
Active phase (hr)	2.2	1.8	1.5	5.2
Maximum slope (cm/hr)	5.7	5.2	4.5	1.5
2nd stage (hr)	0.2	0.2	0.1	0.8

- The "Three P's" of labor
  —Powers (uterine contractions)
  —Passageway (the bony pelvis and soft tissue)
  —Passenger (fetus)
- Problems with any of these three factors such as uterine dysfunction, cephalopelvic disproportion, or fetal malposition, can cause an abnormal progression of labor

ETIOLOGY

- Premature labor occurs in 8–10% of pregnancies. Approximately 30–40% of premature labor is due to uterine, cervical, or urinary tract infections
- Premature rupture of membranes is defined as the rupture of the amniotic/chorionic membranes at least 2 hours before the onset of labor in a patient earlier than 37 weeks gestational age. This occurs in only 3% of pregnancies, but accounts for 30–40% of all premature births

Pre-Hospital

- EMS personnel should place patients in labor on oxygen and in the left lateral recumbent position to maximize delivery of oxygen to the uterus
- In cases of hospital transfer of the high-risk obstetric patient, maternal transport before delivery has been shown to be quicker, easier, more cost-effective, and results in lower infant morbidity and mortality than the transfer of the neonate after delivery
- Air transport of high-risk obstetric patients has been shown to be beneficial and cost-effective
- Patients in labor who are transported by aircraft should have high-flow oxygen available in the event of cabin decompression at high altitudes
- Need special training, monitoring of EMS personnel

Diagnosis

ESSENTIAL WORKUP

- All patients presenting in possible labor should have an *immediate pelvic exam* to assess dilation, effacement of the cervix, and the possibility of imminent delivery
- A bimanual pelvic exam should not be done in the third trimester patient with vaginal bleeding until ultrasound can be done to assess for placenta previa or placental abruption
- Suspected rupture of membranes should have a sterile speculum exam with visual examination of the cervix and collection of fluid from the vaginal area
  - —The presence of ferning when the fluid is allowed to dry on a slide and examined under a microscope, the presence of *pooling* of fluid in the vagina, and the *change of color of litmus paper* from yellow to blue is suggestive of rupture of membranes
- Patients with preterm labor and with cervical changes should have urinalysis with culture and cervical cultures
- Fetal monitoring should be initiated

LABORATORY

- If patient is in labor, CBC, type, and screen should be sent; urinalysis for proteinuria
- In patients with no prenatal care, obtain Rh factor and antibody screen
- Cervical cultures and urine culture in patients with preterm labor

IMAGING/SPECIAL TESTS

- Not generally needed
- Third-trimester patients with abdominal pain and vaginal bleeding should have emergent ultrasound to evaluate for placenta previa or abruption

DIFFERENTIAL DIAGNOSIS

- Braxton-Hicks contractions are irregular uterine contractions without associated cervical changes
- Round uterine ligament pain, musculoskeletal back pain
- Other common causes of abdominal pain such as appendicitis, etc

Treatment

INITIAL STABILIZATION

- If delivery is imminent (presenting part visible), prepare for immediate vaginal delivery in the ED (see chapter on Delivery)

ED TREATMENT

- Unless delivery is imminent, patient should be sent directly to labor and delivery unit
- If transport to Labor and Delivery will be delayed, or if transfer to another facility is necessary, these steps should be taken
  - —IV hydration with 1 L of normal saline or D5LR over 30–60 minutes
  - —Maternal monitoring and, if available, fetal monitoring
  - —If labor needs to be arrested (premature fetus), begin a tocolytic such as the β-agonist terbutaline or $MgSO_4$
    - -Magnesium toxicity is suggested by loss of deep tendon reflexes
    - -High doses of magnesium can cause cardiac arrhythmias and respiratory depression

MEDICATIONS

- Magnesium sulfate: 4–6 g IV over 30 min, followed by 2–6 g/hr
- Terbutaline: 0.25 mg subcutaneously; may repeat same dose in 30 min

Disposition

ADMISSION CRITERIA

- All patients in labor who are not at risk for imminent delivery should be admitted to a labor and delivery department
- Preterm patients in labor demand immediate obstetric consultation and should be admitted to a labor and delivery department for further treatment

Miscellaneous

ICD9: 650.0

CORE CONTENT CODE: 12.4

SUGGESTED READINGS

Elliott JP, O'Keefe DF, Freeman RK. Helicopter transportation of patients with obstetric emergencies in an urban area. Am J Obstet Gynecol 1982;143:157–162

Gianopoulos JG. Emergency complications of labor and delivery. Emerg Med Clin North Am 1994;12:201–217

Parer T. Effects of hypoxia on the mother and fetus with emphasis on maternal air transport. Am J Obstet Gynecol 1982;142:957–961

Authors: S. Brent Barnes; James S. Walker

Labyrinthitis

Clinical Presentation

SIGNS AND SYMPTOMS

- Vertigo of sudden onset
- Peaks in 2–4 hours
- Intense spinning sensation
- Nausea
- Diaphoresis
- Nystagmus or oscillopsia
- The nystagmus extinguishes with repeated testing
- Symptoms may occur in clusters over days to weeks
- Accompanying hearing loss may be inconsistent
- The vertigo is usually positional
- By definition, there are no other focal neurologic abnormalities

MECHANISM/DESCRIPTION

- Labyrinthitis is characterized by peripheral vertigo and decreased hearing
- The "labyrinth" of the inner ear is composed of two parts
  - —*Bony labyrinth* in the petrous part of the temporal bone
  - —*Membranous labyrinth* within the bony cavities
- Space between labyrinths is filled with *perilymphatic fluid*
- Membranous labyrinth itself is filled with *endolymph*
- Primary function of the labyrinth is maintenance of equilibrium

ETIOLOGY

- Change in the volume of perilymph or inflammation
- Viral infection
- Measles and mumps
- Rarely by extension of bacterial infection from otitis media, mastoiditis, or meningitis
- Trauma that results in a perilymphatic leak
- Allergic and toxic
- *Meniere's disease*
- Increased volume of endolymph (endolymphatic hydrops)
- Disabling vertigo results
- Idiopathic

Pre-Hospital

- Nausea and vomiting may be profuse
- IV hydration is often necessary
- Vertigo can be a symptom of stroke
- Prompt transport to ED is essential
- Protect patient from falling
- Monitor for dysrhythmia

Diagnosis

ESSENTIAL WORKUP

- Thorough history and neurologic examination
- Stroke may present with
  - —Acute onset of dizziness/vertigo
  - —Focal neurologic abnormalities (other than decreased hearing or abnormal eye movements)
- History of previous similar symptoms
- Recent upper respiratory tract infection
- *Hallpike maneuver*
  - —Patient's head supported
  - —Assuming a supine position from a sitting position with the head neutral
  - —Repeat with head turned 45° left and right
  - —Observe for vertigo and nystagmus
  - —Patients with peripheral vertigo will have a brief latency period before vertigo and nystagmus begin
- Orthostatic vital signs
- Rapid glucose determination
- Exclude central vertiginous symptoms
  - —Less intense vertigo
  - —No positional component
  - —Nonfatigable nystagmus
  - —Gradual onset of symptoms
  - —Cranial nerve abnormalities other than CN VIII and nystagmus
  - —Central vertigo is an indication for immediate CT scanning

LABORATORY

- ECG and cardiac monitoring to evaluate for possible dysrhythmia

IMAGING/SPECIAL TESTS

- Head CT urgently if suspect central cause of vertigo
- MRI (typically nonurgent) demonstrates pathology in the posterior fossa better

DIFFERENTIAL DIAGNOSIS

- Benign positional vertigo
- Meniere's disease
- Orthostatic hypotension
- Cholesteatoma
- Vestibular neuronitis
- Perforated tympanic membrane
- Perilymphatic fistula
- Labyrinthine trauma
- Ototoxic drugs
- Cerumen impaction
- Cerebellopontine angle tumor
- Postconcussive dizziness
- Benign paroxysmal vertigo of childhood

Treatment

INITIAL STABILIZATION

- IV hydration with isotonic fluid
- Benzodiazepines, antiemetics intravenously
- Discharge with meclizine or benzodiazepine orally

MEDICATIONS

- Droperidol: 0.625–2.5 mg IV/IM
- Diazepam: 2–10 mg IV
- Lorazepam: 0.5–2 mg IV
- Meclizine: 25 mg po tid

Disposition

ADMISSION CRITERIA

- Patients suspected of acute stroke
- Patients who do not respond to therapy should be observed and possibly admitted for a neurologic consultation
- Patients with central cause of vertigo requiring urgent intervention

DISCHARGE CRITERIA

- Patients with peripheral vertigo, an otherwise normal neurologic examination, and satisfactory response to ED therapy can be discharged home
- Recurrent bouts of acute labyrinthitis over several weeks are typical
- Patients should avoid driving, operating dangerous equipment, and working at heights until attacks resolve and sedating treatments successfully withdrawn
- The elderly and infirm should observe fall precautions
- Neurology or otolaryngology referral should be arranged

Miscellaneous

ICD9: 386.9; 386.1; 386.2; 386.30

CORE CONTENT CODE: 6.1.3

SUGGESTED READINGS

Adams RD, Victor M, Ropper AH. Deafness, dizziness, and disorders of equilibrium. In: Adams RD, Victor M, Ropper AH, eds. Principles of neurology. 6th ed. New York: McGraw-Hill, 1997:284–310.

Caplan LR. Management of acute peripheral vestibular disorders. Eur Neurol 1993;33:337–44.

Edwards FJ. Overcoming the diagnostic challenges of dizziness, vertigo, and syncope. Emergency Medicine Reports. Atlanta: American Health Consultants, January 10, 1994.

Author: Charles V. Pollack

Laceration Management

Clinical Presentation

SIGNS AND SYMPTOMS

- Lacerations may be accompanied by
  - —Bleeding
  - —Tissue foreign bodies
  - —Hematoma
  - —Pain or numbness
  - —Loss of motor function
  - —Diminished pulses, delayed capillary refill

MECHANISM/DESCRIPTION

- A laceration is a disruption in skin integrity most often resulting from trauma
- May be single or multiple layered

Pre-Hospital

CAUTIONS

- Obtain hemostasis, or control of bleeding with direct pressure
- Unkink any flaps of skin whose blood supply may be strangulated
- Universal precautions

PEDIATRIC CONSIDERATIONS

- Assess for possible nonaccidental trauma

Diagnosis

ESSENTIAL WORKUP

- Mechanism and circumstances of injury
- Time of injury
- History of foreign body (glass, splinter, teeth)
  - —Avoid digital exploration if the object is believed to be sharp
- Tetanus immunization
- Comorbid condition that may impede wound healing
- Evaluate nerve and motor function
- Document associated neurovascular injury
- Assess presence of devitalized tissue, debris from foreign materials, bone or joint violation

LABORATORY

N/A

IMAGING/SPECIAL TESTS

Evaluation for possible foreign bodies

- Plain radiography
  - —Soft tissue views may aid in visualization
  - —Objects with the same density as soft tissue may not be seen (wood, plants)
- Ultrasonography

DIFFERENTIAL DIAGNOSIS

- Skin avulsion
- Contusion
- Abrasion

Treatment

INITIAL STABILIZATION

- ABCs
- Control of hemostasis

ED TREATMENT

Time of Onset

- Lacerations may be closed primarily up to 8 hours old in areas of poorer circulation
- Lacerations may be closed up to 12 hours old in areas of normal circulation
- On face, lacerations may be closed up to 24 hours if clean and well irrigated
- If not closed, wound may heal by secondary intention, or delayed primary closure (DPC) in 3–5 days

Analgesia and Conscious Sedation

- Adequate analgesia is crucial for good wound management
- Conscious sedation may be required (see chapter: Conscious Sedation/Rapid Sequence Intubation)

Local Anesthetics

- Topical
  - —TAC (tetracaine, adrenaline, cocaine)
  - —EMLA ("eutectic mixture," lidocaine, prilocaine)
- Local/regional
  - —Lidocaine, bupivacaine
  - —Epinephrine will cause vasoconstriction and improve duration of action
    - -Avoid in the penis, digits, toes, ears, eyelids, skin flaps (necrosis), and severely contaminated wounds (impairs defense)
  - —For patient comfort, inject slowly with small gauge needle; buffer every 9 cc of 1% lidocaine with 1 cc 8.4% sodium bicarbonate

Exploration and Removal of Foreign Body

- Indications for removal of a foreign body include
  - —Potential or actual injury to tendons, nerves, vasculature
  - —Toxic substance, or reactive agent
  - —Continued pain

Irrigation and Debridement

- Clean surrounding skin with an antiseptic solution (betadine)
  - —Do not use antiseptic solution within the wound itself as it may impair healing
- Scrub with a fine-pore sponge only if significant contamination, or particulate matter
- Irrigation with 200 cc or more of NS
  - —Optimal pressure (5–8 psi) generated with 30 cc syringe through 18–20-gauge needle
  - —Débride devitalized tissue

Wound Repair
- Universal precautions
- Wounds that cannot be cleaned adequately should heal by secondary intention, or DPC
- Reapproximate all anatomic borders carefully (skin-vermilion border of lip, etc.)

Simple Layered Closure
- Simple interrupted sutures
  —Avoid in lacerations under tension
- Horizontal mattress sutures (running or interrupted)
  —Edematous finger and hand wounds
  —Ideal in skin flaps where edges at risk for necrosis
- Vertical mattress
  —For wounds under greater tension

Multiple Layered Closure
- Closes deep tissue dead space
- Lessens tension at the epidermal level, improves cosmetic result
- Buried interrupted absorbable suture, simple or running nonabsorbable sutures for epidermis

Dressing
- Dress wound with antibiotic ointment and nonadherent semiporous dressing
- Inform patient about scarring and risk of infection, use of sunscreen

Antimicrobial Agents
- Uncomplicated lacerations do not need antibiotic prophylaxis
- Lacerations with high likelihood of infection
  —Human bite to hand (see chapter: Hand Infection)
  —Contaminated with dirt, bodily fluids, feces
    -Polymicrobial, enteric prophylaxis
- Tetanus immunization

MEDICATIONS
- See chapter: Conscious Sedation/Rapid Sequence Intubation
- Tetanus (Td adults, DT peds): 0.5 cc IM

Local Anesthetics
- Topical, applied directly to wound with cotton, gauze
  —TAC (0.5% tetracaine, (1:2000) adrenaline, (11.8% cocaine)): apply for 20 min
  —EMLA ("eutectic mixture," 5% lidocaine and prilocaine): apply for 60 min
- Injected

(*See table below*)

MATERIALS
Suture Materials
Absorbable
- For use in mucous membranes and buried muscle/fascial layer closures
  —Natural—dissolve <1 week, poor tensile strength, local inflammation
    -Plain catgut
    -Chromic
    -Fast absorbing gut for certain facial lacerations where cosmesis is important
  —Synthetic braided—tensile strength diminishing over 1 month, mild inflammation
    -Polyglycolic acid (dexon)
    -Polyglactin 910 (vicryl)
  —Synthetic monofilament-tensile strength 70% at 1 month, inflammation degree unknown
    -Polydioxanone (PDS)
    -Polyglyconate (maxon)

Nonabsorbable
- Greatest tensile strength
  —Monofilament
    -Nylon (ethilon, dermalon)
    -Polypropylene (prolene)
    -Polybutester (novofil): can stretch with wound edema
    -Polyethylene, stainless steel
  —Multifilament
    -Cotton
    -Silk (local inflammation)

Needle types
- Cutting (cuticular and plastic) are most often used in outpatient wound repair

Staples
- For linear lacerations of scalp, torso, extremities
- Avoid in hands, face, and areas requiring CT or MRI

Adhesive Tapes (Steri-Strips)
- For lacerations that are clean, small, and under minimal tension
- Avoid in wounds that have potential to become very swollen
- Pretreat wound edges with tincture of benzoin to improve adhesion

Tissue Adhesives
- Good cosmetic results have been achieved in simple lacerations with low skin tension
- An alternative to sutures/staples especially in children, if adhesive is available

LOCAL/REGIONAL	MAXIMUM DOSE (MG/KG)	DURATION (HOURS)
Lidocaine	4.5	1.5–3.5
Bupivacaine	2	3–10

Disposition

ADMISSION CRITERIA
- Few lacerations by themselves necessitate admission unless they require significant debridement, ongoing intravenous antibiotics, or are complicated by extensive wound care issues or comorbid processes (head injury, abdominal trauma)

DISCHARGE CRITERIA
- Wounds at risk for infection or poor healing requiring a wound check within 48 hours
- Time of suture removal dependent upon location and peripheral perfusion
  —Scalp: 7–10 days
  —Face: 3–5 days
  —Oral: 7 days
  —Neck: 4–6 days
  —Abdomen, back, chest, hands, feet: 7–10 days
  —Upper extremity: 7–10 days
  —Lower extremity: 10–14 days

PEDIATRIC CONSIDERATIONS
- If it is unsafe for a child to return home if nonaccidental trauma is suspected

Miscellaneous

ICD9: 998.2

CORE CONTENT CODE: 18.4.17.2

SUGGESTED READINGS
Chisolm C, Howell JM. Soft tissue emergencies. Emerg Med Clin North Am 1992;10(4):665–705.

Roberts PA, Lamacraft G. Techniques to reduce the discomfort of pediatric laceration repair. MJA 1996;164(1):32–35.

Edich RF, Rodeheover GT, Thacker JG. Wound preparation. In: Tintinalli JE, Ruiz E, Krome RL, eds. Emergency medicine a comprehensive study guide. 4th ed. New York: McGraw Hill, 1996:279–283.

Author: Gordon Chew

Laryngitis

Clinical Presentation

SIGNS AND SYMPTOMS

- Hoarseness
- Abnormal sounding voice
- Throat tickling
- Feeling of throat rawness
- Constant urge to clear the throat
- Cough
- Fever
- Malaise
- Dysphagia
- Regional lymphadenopathy

MECHANISM/DESCRIPTION

- Inflammation of the mucosa of the larynx
- Peaks parallel epidemics of individual viruses
- Most common during late fall, winter, early spring

ETIOLOGY

- Viral upper respiratory tract infections are the most common cause
  - —Influenza A
  - —Influenza B
  - —Parainfluenza
  - —Adenovirus
  - —Coxsackievirus
  - —Adenovirus
  - —Respiratory syncytial virus
  - —Measles
- Bacaterial infections occur in 10% of cases
  - —*ß-Hemolytic streptococcus*
  - —*Streptococcus pneumoniae*
  - —*Hemophilus influenzae*
  - —Diphtheria
  - —*Moraxella catarrhalis*
  - —Tuberculosis
  - —Syphilis
  - —Leprosy
- Fungal infections
  - —Histoplasmosis
  - —Blastomycosis
  - —Candidiasis
- Allergic
- Autoimmune
- Idiopathic

Pre-Hospital

- Supportive care and ambulance transport are not generally indicated

CAUTIONS

- If there are signs of respiratory distress, epiglottitis should be suspected
  - —Transport sitting up
  - —Provide supplemental oxygen
  - —Intubation may be difficult or impossible and should only be attempted in patients in extremis

Diagnosis

ESSENTIAL WORKUP

- Acute laryngitis
  - —In the majority of cases, the history and inspection of the throat suffice to distinguish between viral and bacterial laryngitis
- Chronic laryngitis
  - —The workup should be directed towards chronic infections and tumors
  - —Visualization of the larynx should be performed
  - —The patient should be referred to ENT for biopsy
  - —Visualization of nodules indicate the need to admit to rule out tuberculosis

LABORATORY

- Blood tests are not generally indicated
  - —An elevated WBC is not a reliable way to distinguish between bacterial and viral illness
- Throat culture
  - —Indicated when throat inspection suggests a bacterial infection

IMAGING/SPECIAL TESTS

- Soft tissue neck films
  - —Rarely indicated as direct laryngoscopy provides a more comprehensive assessment
- Direct laryngoscopy
  - —Red, inflamed vocal cords, with rounded edges
  - —Occasionally hemorrhage or exudate
  - —Demonstration of laryngeal pseudomembrane to distinguishing diphtheria from other infectious forms of laryngitis
  - —This procedure is mainly used to rule out epiglottitis

DIFFERENTIAL DIAGNOSIS

- Epiglottitis
- Excessive use of voice
- Caustic ingestion or inhalation
- Esophageal reflux
- Vocal nodules
- Laryngeal malignancy
- Thyroid malignancy

Treatment

INITIAL STABILIZATION

- Stabilization is only required if the patient show signs of respiratory distress
  —The patient should be managed for epiglottitis
  —Supplemental oxygen via a nonrebreathing mask
  —Orotracheal intubation when time permits in the OR
  —The neck should be prepped and the equipment ready for a surgical airway

ED TREATMENT

- Antibiotics should be administered only for bacterial infection
  —Oral penicillin for streptococcal infections
  —Erythromycin for *M. catarrhalis*
- Steroids may aid in decreasing the time to resolution of symptoms

MEDICATIONS

- Penicillin V: 250 mg qid po
- Erythromycin: 250 mg qid po

Disposition

ADMISSION CRITERIA

- Tuberculosis laryngitis
  —Highly contagious requiring isolation

DISCHARGE CRITERIA

- Voice rest
- Steam inhalations or cool-mist humidifier
- Increase fluid intake
- Analgesics
- Avoid smoking
- Refer patients with chronic laryngitis to otolaryngologist

Miscellaneous

ICD9: 464.0; 476.0

CORE CONTENT CODE: 6.3.3.2.3

SUGGESTED READINGS

Ballenger JI, Snow JB, eds. Otorhinolaryngology head and neck surgery. 15th ed. Philadelphia: Williams & Wilkins, 1996.

Klassen TP. Recent advances in the treatment of bronchiolitis and laryngitis. Pediatr Clin North Am 1997;44:249–56.

Author: Richard Wolfe

Larynx Fracture

Clinical Presentation

SIGNS AND SYMPTOMS

- Neck emphysema
- Dyspnea
- Stridor
- Loss of normal cartilaginous landmarks of neck
- Dysphonia
- Hematoma

MECHANISM/DESCRIPTION

- Disruption of any of the nine cartilaginous structures (epiglottis, thyroid, arytenoid, cricoid, corniculate, and cuneiform cartilages) joined by ligaments and muscles, which comprise the airway passage between the pharynx and trachea

ETIOLOGY

- Blunt trauma to neck associated with MVA, assaults, or recreational activities
  —"Clothesline" injury is a classic mechanism (victim struck in neck by cord, wire, branch, etc., hung across path of travel)

Pre-Hospital

CAUTIONS

- Aggressive airway management is necessary: oxygen, suction
- Cervical spine immobilization

Diagnosis

ESSENTIAL WORKUP

- X-rays
  —Neck (soft tissue lateral)
  —Cervical spine and chest—identifies bony and soft tissue injuries
- CT scan of neck soft tissue—defines location of soft tissue, cartilage, and bony injuries
- Fiberoptic endoscopy—allows visualization of injuries involving the airway, vocal cords

LABORATORY

- Arterial blood gas—identifies hypoxia, hypercarbia
- Hematocrit—follow serially to identify vascular injury with resultant blood loss
- Type and cross—preparation for transfusion as needed

IMAGING/SPECIAL TESTS

- Arteriography—definitive test to identify vascular injuries
- Surgical exploration

DIFFERENTIAL DIAGNOSIS

- Associated Injuries
  —Hyoid fracture
  —Thyroid cartilage disruption
  —Carotid artery injury
  —Phrenic nerve injury
  —Cervical spine injury
  —Hypoxic cerebral injury
  —Airway edema
  —Aspiration pneumonitis
  —Air embolism

PEDIATRIC CONSIDERATIONS

- Structures of the neck are more cartilaginous and mobile than in adults. Thus, pediatric patients are more resistant to injuries. However, because of the relatively smaller airway diameter rapid airway compromise can occur with relatively little edema of the soft tissues

Treatment

INITIAL STABILIZATION

- Airway management is of primary concern
  - —Severe injuries of the larynx may require operative management
  - —Early intubation to preclude respiratory embarrassment
  - —Cricothyrotomy may be necessary if severe maxillofacial injuries are present
  - —*Avoid* cricothyrotomy if a hematoma is seen over the cricothyroid membrane or if there is evidence of cricotracheal disruption
  - —Emergent tracheostomy may be the only option to secure an airway

ED TREATMENT

- Supplemental humidified oxygen
- Elevate head of bed to decrease cerebral and neck soft tissue edema
- IV access
- Consider ICP monitoring if there is evidence of severe hypoxic cerebral injury
- Consult otolaryngologist for surgical evaluation
- Consider use of positive-end expiratory pressure and volume-controlled ventilation for severe pulmonary injury associated with ARDS or aspiration pneumonitis

MEDICATIONS

Laryngeal Injury with Subcutaneous Emphysema

- Assume that the mucosa of the upper airway have communicated with the deep tissue of the neck
  - —Clindamycin: adult: 600 mg IV; peds: 10 mg/kg/dose q 8 hrs

Laryngeal Edema

- Consider steroids
  - —Dexamethasone: adult: 4 mg IV; peds: 0.25–0.5 mg/kg/dose IV

Disposition

ADMISSION CRITERIA

- Patients with true laryngeal injuries must be admitted to a monitored setting for observation and airway management
  - —Prepare for emergent surgical correction of laryngeal defect
- Patients with suspected laryngeal injury or highly suspicious mechanism must be admitted to a monitored setting for observation

DISCHARGE CRITERIA

- Patients that have been ruled out for serious laryngeal injury by objective testing and who have no evidence of airway edema or compromise after an appropriate period of observation in the ED (usually no less than 6 hours) can be considered for discharge. If there is any doubt, admit to a monitored setting

Miscellaneous

ICD9: 959.09

CORE CONTENT CODE: 18.4.9, 18.4.9.4

SUGGESTED READINGS

Kadish H, et al. Blunt pediatric laryngotracheal trauma: Case reports and review of the literature. Am J Emerg Med 1994;12:207–211.

Minard G, et al. Laryngeal trauma. Am Surg 1992;58:181–187.

Yen PT, et al. Clinical analysis of external laryngeal trauma. J Laryngol Otol 1993;108:221–225.

Author: Catherine M. Hurt

Le Fort Fracture

Clinical Presentation

SIGNS AND SYMPTOMS

- Facial injury with massive swelling and ecchymosis
- Airway obstruction may be present
- Dyspnea (especially when supine), malocclusion, vision disturbance (diplopia)
- Facial lengthening or flattening, periorbital ecchymosis (raccoon's eyes)
- CSF rhinorrhea, facial hemorrhage/epistaxis
- Facial anesthesia, midface mobility upon traction, open bite
- Frequently associated with multisystem injury (especially head and C-spine)

MECHANISM/DESCRIPTION

- Maxillofacial fractures caused by high-energy blunt trauma to the midface
  —The most common causes include motor vehicle accidents, physical assault, and domestic violence
- Upon traction of the maxillary arch/hard palate you should find
  —Le Fort I: Movement of the hard palate and maxillary dentition only
  —Le Fort II: Movement of the hard palate, maxillary dentition, and the nose
  —Le Fort III: Movement of the entire midface including orbital rims (inferior and lateral aspects)

PEDIATRIC CONSIDERATIONS

- Maxillofacial fractures occur less frequently in children
  —Because of the smaller facial skeleton there is a higher incidence of skull fractures and head trauma compared to midface injuries
  —Le Fort fractures are particularly uncommon in young children. By ages 10–12, as facial morphology becomes adultlike, more mid- and lower facial fractures are seen
  —Be suspicious of child abuse or family violence as possible causes of midfacial injuries, especially in children under 6

Pre-Hospital

CAUTIONS

- Airway management
  —Airway compromise is common
  —Bag valve mask (BVM) ventilation may be difficult
  —Avoid nasotracheal intubation
- Strict cervical spine precautions
- Multisystem injury is likely with high-energy trauma

Diagnosis

ESSENTIAL WORKUP

- Evaluate the patency of the airway and need for immediate airway control
- Le Fort fractures can be diagnosed by careful intraoral examination and the pattern of facial movement
  —If fracture fragments are impacted, there may be little or no midface mobility
  —Carefully evaluate the patient for CSF rhinorrhea and malocclusion

IMAGING/SPECIAL TESTS

- Facial imaging may be delayed for 24–72 hours in patients requiring care of other life-threatening conditions
- *Computed tomography* is the diagnostic standard for defining midface fractures
- *Conventional radiographs* may be used as a screening test. The occipitomental (Waters) and lateral views of the skull may reveal bony fracture/asymmetry, subcutaneous emphysema, or layering of blood in the maxillary sinuses

DIFFERENTIAL DIAGNOSIS

- Le Fort fracture classification
  —Le Fort I: transverse (horizontal) fracture/palate facial dysjunction
  —Le Fort II: pyramidal dysjunction
  —Le Fort III: craniofacial dysjunction
  —Le Fort IV: involves the frontal bone in addition to a Le Fort III maxillary fracture
- Different grade Le Fort fractures may be found on opposite sides of the face

PEDIATRIC CONSIDERATIONS

- Young children are often frightened and in pain. Through kindness, patience, and distraction cooperation can be gained
- Sedation may be required to perform a thorough exam after ruling out head injury
- Incomplete (greenstick) fractures with minimal or no displacement can occur
- Be cognizant of possible child abuse and evaluate for prior nonaccidental trauma, if appropriate

Treatment

INITIAL STABILIZATION

- Aggressive airway control is paramount
- Orally suction patients to minimize aspiration of blood, saliva, and stomach contents
- Remove any foreign matter or teeth from the airway
- After cervical spine clearance, stable and alert patients may be allowed to sit up and suction themselves
- When airway management is needed, *rapid sequence induction* is recommended to maximize airway control and minimize rise of ICP in patients with head injuries
  —If there is concern that paralysis will result in loss of airway tone and inability to intubate because of subsequent distortion of airway anatomy in patients with severe facial injuries, oral intubation under sedation with midazolam, etomidate, droperidol, or ketamine is an option
- *Emergency cricothyroidotomy* may be necessary if orotracheal intubation is unsuccessful. Recall that BVM ventilation may be difficult due to loss of bony support and altered anatomy
- *Nasotracheal intubation* is not recommended in patients with midface trauma because of the lack of success and danger of intracranial placement

ED TREATMENT

- *Cervical spine:* Due to the risk of cervical spine injury in patients with head and maxillofacial trauma, it is imperative that radiographic clearance of the cervical spine is obtained
- *Hemorrhage control:* Direct pressure should be applied to areas of bleeding and nasal packing (anterior and posterior) may be necessary for epistaxis. In some cases, manual reduction of the midface may be required to control intractable hemorrhage. Although blood loss from facial bleeding may be significant, it is rarely a primary cause of hemorrhagic shock
- Early consultation with oral maxillofacial or plastic surgeon
- Analgesics, antibiotics, and tetanus prophylaxis

MEDICATIONS

SEDATIVE/ANALGESICS*	ADULT DOSE (MG/KG IV)	PEDIATRIC DOSE (MG/KG IV)
Diazepam	0.1–0.2	0.1–0.2
Droperidol	2.5 mg aliquots	1–1.5 mg aliquots
Etomidate	0.2–0.3	0.2–0.3
Fentanyl	2–10 ugm	2–3 ugm
Ketamine	2	1–2
Meperidine	1–2	1–2
Midazolam	0.1	0.15
Morphine sulfate	0.1–0.2	0.1–0.2

* All of these sedatives/analgesics should be titrated to effect

DEFASCICULATING DRUG	ADULT DOSE (MG/KG IV)	PEDIATRIC DOSE (MG/KG IV)
Vecuronium	0.01	0.01
PARALYTIC AGENTS		
Pancuronium	0.1–0.15	0.1–0.15
Rocuronium	0.6	0.6
Succinylcholine	1.5	1.5–2
Vecuronium	0.1–0.3	0.1–0.3

PEDIATRIC CONSIDERATIONS

- Surgical cricothyroidotomy should not be considered in children under age 10
  —Needle cricothyroidotomy with jet ventilation may be attempted if intubation attempts fail
- There is a higher incidence of multiple injuries in children, especially head trauma, skull fractures, and orthopedic injuries
- Cervical spine injuries tend to involve upper levels more commonly in children. Also, spinal cord injury without radiographic abnormality (SCIWORA syndrome) may be seen
- Definitive repair of pediatric facial fractures should not be delayed for more than 3–4 days. The facial bones heal rapidly and delayed repair may result in malunion and cosmetic deformity

Disposition

ADMISSION CRITERIA

- All patients are admitted for ORIF of maxillofacial injuries
- Patients should be admitted to an intensive care unit setting

DISCHARGE CRITERIA

N/A

Miscellaneous

ICD9: 802.4

CORE CONTENT CODE: 18.4.4.3

SUGGESTED READINGS

Colucciello SA, Sternbach G, Walker SB. The treacherous and complex spectrum of maxillofacial trauma: Etiologies, evaluation, and emergency stabilization. Emerg Med Rep 1995;16;7:59–69.

Hehmann RJ, Sargent LA. Maxillary fractures. Trauma Q 1992;9:67–75.

Hunter JG. Pediatric maxillofacial trauma. Pediatr Clin North Am 1992;39:1127–1143.

Le Fort R. Experimental study of fractures of the upper jaw. Rev Chir de Paris 1901;23:208, 360, 479. Reprinted in Plast Reconstr Surg 1972;50:497, 600.

Author: Raymond A. Viducich

Lead, Poisoning

Clinical Presentation

SIGNS AND SYMPTOMS

- Subacute or chronic intoxication is more common than acute intoxication

Constitutional

- Malaise
- Fatigue
- Metallic taste

Gastrointestinal

- Nausea/vomiting
- Abdominal pain
- Milky emesis (due to lead chloride)
- Black stools (due to lead sulfite)
- Constipation
- Intestinal spasms (lead colic)
- Gingival pigmentation
  - —Dark bluish-black discoloration of gingiva at the dental border

Neurologic

- Insomnia
- Irritability
- Vertigo
- Ataxia
- Headache
- Memory loss
- Peripheral neuropathy
  - —Wrist drop
  - —Paresthesias
- Visual disturbances
- Encephalopathy
  - —Confusion
  - —Delirium
  - —Convulsions
  - —Coma
  - —Papilledema

Renal

- Interstitial nephropathy
- Proteinuria
- Hematuria
- Cast cells
- Nuclear inclusion bodies (lead-protein complexes)

Hematologic

- Basophilic stippling
- Hypochromic/microcytic anemia
- Karyorrhexis (rupture of RBC nucleus)

Dermatologic

- Ashen color
- Retinal stippling
- Lead lines (deposition of lead sulfide along gingival border)

MECHANISM/DESCRIPTION

- Binds to sulfhydryl groups of proteins and enzymes altering their structure and function
- Interferes with calcium transport, synthesis and release of neurotransmitters, and activity of protein kinase C
- Organic lead much more toxic than inorganic lead
- Intoxication after single oral ingestion rare
- Children absorb ~50% of dietary load; adults 10%
- Half-life in bone is 30 years

ETIOLOGY

- Common sources of exposure include
  - —Lead storage batteries
  - —Pigments
  - —Ceramics
  - —Glass
  - —Moonshine whiskey
  - —Solder
  - —Paint (predominately house paint sold prior to the early 1970s)

PEDIATRIC CONSIDERATIONS

- Toxic neurologic effects more common than in adults
- 25% of affected children with CNS involvement die
  - —40% of survivors have permanent defects
- Chronic exposure results in decreased intelligence and impaired neurobehavioral development
- Greater level of deposition in bone

Pre-Hospital

CAUTIONS

- Secure ABCs
- Remove patient from exposure
- Treat seizures with benzodiazepines, barbiturates, or other appropriate anticonvulsants
- Treat coma with glucose, thiamine, narcan, oxygen

Diagnosis

ESSENTIAL WORKUP

- Lead level

LABORATORY

- CBC
  - —Anemia (microcytic or normocytic)
  - —Basophilic stippling of erythrocytes
- Electrolytes, BUN/Cr, glucose
  - —Increased BUN/Cr
- Urinalysis
  - —Proteinuria
  - —Hematuria
  - —Cast cells
  - —Nuclear inclusion bodies (lead-protein complexes)

Lead Level

- Store whole blood lead sample in lead free tubes or tubes containing heparin or EDTA
- Level <10 μg/dl
  - —Normal
- Level 10–25 μg/dl
  - —Decreased intelligence and impaired neurobehavioral development in young children
  - —No affect in adults
- Level 25–60 μg/dl
  - —Headache, irritability, neuropsychiatric effects
  - —Subclinical anemia
- Level 60–80 μg/dl
  - —Gastrointestinal symptoms
  - —Subclinical renal effects
- Level >80 μg/dl
  - —Abdominal pain
  - —Nephropathy
- Level >100 μg/dl
  - —Neuropathy and encephalopathy

IMAGING/SPECIAL TESTS

- Abdominal radiograph
  - —For acute ingestion
  - —Lead radiopaque
- Free erythrocyte protoporphyrin
  - —Elevation reflects lead-induced inhibition of heme synthesis
  - —Affects actively forming and not mature erythrocytes and therefore lags lead exposure by few weeks
  - —Nonspecific and may also occur with iron deficiency
- Urinary lead excretion
  - —Increases and decreases more rapidly than blood levels
- CT scan of the head/lumbar puncture for altered mental status if indicated

DIFFERENTIAL DIAGNOSIS

- Encephalopathy (hepatic, toxic, etc.)
- Arsenic and mercury toxicity
- Cyclic antidepressant poisoning
- Intracerebral hemorrhage
- Sickle cell crisis
- Hepatic porphyrias
- Pancreatitis
- Peptic ulcer disease
- Gastroenteritis

Treatment

INITIAL STABILIZATION

- Secure ABCs and monitoring
- Control seizures with benzodiazepines, phenytoin, or barbiturates
- D50W (or Accucheck), thiamine, narcan; oxygen if altered mental status

ED TREATMENT

Decontamination

- Acute oral ingestion
  - —Gastric lavage if recent (<1–2 hours) ingestion
  - —Activated charcoal
  - —Whole bowel irrigation (if lead-containing material visible on x-ray after initial treatment)
- Dermal exposure
  - —If stable, decontaminate in the ED decontamination room prior to further evaluation

Chelation Therapy

- Encephalopathy—administer
  - —Dimercaprol (BAL) 4 mg/kg IM
  - —Calcium EDTA 75 mg/kg/24hrs continuous infusion
- Severely symptomatic without encephalopathy (level >70 μg/dl)
  - —Dimercaprol (BAL) 12 mg/kg/24hrs
  - —Calcium EDTA 50 mg/kg/24hrs continuous infusion 4 hours after BAL administration
- Moderately symptomatic (level between 45 and 70 μg/dl)—options
  - —Oral DMSA (succimer) 10 mg/kg q 8 hrs for 5 days then q 12 hrs for 14 days or
  - —Calcium EDTA 25 mg/kg/24hrs infusion
- Asymptomatic children with elevated levels >45 μg/dl-treat with oral DMSA (succimer) 10 mg/kg q 8 hrs for 5 days then q 12 hrs for 14 days
- Asymptomatic children with level between 25 and 45 μg/dl
  - —Aggressive environmental intervention
  - —Follow-up lead level
  - —Oral chelation with DMSA or d-penicillamine (30 mg/kg/day) if levels remain elevated
- Asymptomatic children with levels <25 μg/dl
  - —Aggressive environmental intervention
  - —Follow-up lead level
- Asymptomatic adults
  - —Remove from exposure and observe
  - —If level is >80 μg/dl, administer oral DMSA (succimer) 10 mg/kg q 8 hrs for 5 days then q 12 hrs for 14 days

Disposition

ADMISSION CRITERIA

- All symptomatic patients
- Lead level >60 μg/dl
- IV chelation therapy

DISCHARGE CRITERIA

- Level <60 μg/dl and minimal symptoms or asymptomatic

Miscellaneous

ICD9: 984.9

CORE CONTENT CODE: 17.2.21

SUGGESTED READINGS

Casey R, et al. Longitudinal assessment for lead poisoning. Clin Pediatr 1996;35(2):58–61.

Ellenhorn MJ, Schoonwald S, Ordog G, Wasserberger J. Lead. In: Ellenhorn's medical toxicology. 2d ed. Baltimore: Williams & Wilkins, 1997:1563–1578.

Nadig R. Lead. In: Goldfrank's toxicologic emergencies. 5th ed. Norwalk, CT: Appleton & Lange, 1994:1029–1050.

Authors: Yat Leung; Lisandro Irizarry

Legg-Calvé-Perthes Disease

Clinical Presentation

SIGNS AND SYMPTOMS

- Insidious onset
- Limp
  - —Presenting symptom in most cases
  - —Initially slight
  - —Gradually becomes more pronounced
  - —Motion becomes limited in all directions, especially abduction and rotation
- Vague ache in the groin
  - —Radiates to the medial thigh and inner aspect of the knee
  - —Aggravated by activity
  - —Relieved by rest
- Joint stiffness
- Tenderness over the anterior aspect of the joint
- Muscle spasm
  - —Common complaint in the early stages of the disease
- Shortening of the affected limb and muscle atrophy
  - —Late in the course of the disease

MECHANISM/DESCRIPTION

- Avascular necrosis of the femoral head occurring in children
- Repeated episodes of infarction and ensuing abnormalities have been implicated
- The condition results in necrosis of the head and all or part of the epiphysis
- This disorder is usually self-limited
  - —The femoral head undergoes aseptic necrosis and replacement
  - —Resulting in flattening of the femoral head (coxa plana)
  - —A variable amount of permanent deformity and restricted motion usually result
- Predominates in boys with a ratio of 5:1
- Most common between the ages of 4 and 12 years
  - —The majority of patients are less than 7 years of age
- The condition is unilateral in 85% of cases and bilateral in 15%
- Children with short stature are at increased risk for the disease

ETIOLOGY

- Vascular disturbance of unknown etiology

Pre-Hospital

N/A

Diagnosis

ESSENTIAL WORKUP

- Obtain hip films on children presenting with a limp
- If normal, these children still require orthopedic referral for further studies of etiology of limp
  - —Must always exclude hip-threatening septic arthritis

LABORATORY

- CBC
  - —An elevated WBC is often used to determine the need for arthrocentesis of the hip
  - —Poor discrimination of this test suggests this does not help distinguish a septic joint
- ESR
  - —Values >20 mm/hr

IMAGING/SPECIAL TESTS

- Hip radiographs
  - —Early findings
    - -Joint space widening
    - -A subchondral lucent area
    - -Prominence of the soft tissues over the capsule
    - -Minimal joint effusion
    - -The femoral head may be laterally shifted slightly in the acetabulum
  - —A few weeks later
    - -The femoral head appears more dense than the rest of the bone
    - -Fragmentation of the femoral head
- Technetium-99
  - —Obtain if hip films are non diagnostic to distinguish from transient synovitis
    - -Shows changes earlier than hip films
    - -Early diagnosis is needed to maximize outcome
    - -Low uptake in the femoral head
- Magnetic resonance imaging
  - —Low signal density in the femoral head

DIFFERENTIAL DIAGNOSIS

- Unilateral involvement
  - —Toxic synovitis
  - —Septic arthritis
  - —Osteomyelitis
  - —Juvenile rheumatoid arthritis
  - —Rheumatic fever
  - —Tuberculosis
  - —Transient synovitis
  - —Tumors
    - -Eosinophilic granuloma
    - -Osteoid osteoma
    - -Chondroblastoma
    - -Lymphoma
- Bilateral involvement
  - —Bone dysplasias
  - —Hypothyroidism

Treatment

INITIAL STABILIZATION

N/A

ED TREATMENT

- Pain management
  - —NSAID
  - —Muscle relaxants
- Orthopedic consultation to select definitive management
  - —Goals
    - -Restoration of range of motion is the first step
    - -Containment of the femoral head
  - —Avoidance of weight-bearing with the use of crutches
  - —Orthotic bracelike device
    - -Loss of range of motion
    - -Advanced disease
  - —Petrie cast
  - —Traction for a few days to several weeks
    - -At home or in the hospital
    - -Affords relief from spasm
    - -Maintaining the hips in abduction and mild internal rotation
  - —Exercise program
  - —Surgical osteotomy
    - -Loss of range of motion of the hip
    - -Major involvement of the lateral pillar
    - -Unable to tolerate a brace

MEDICATIONS

- Diazepam: 0.1–0.2 mg/kg/dose (max 5 mg) po q 6–8 hrs PRN muscle spasm
- Ibuprofen: 10–15 mg/kg/dose po q 6–8 hrs PRN pain

Disposition

ADMISSION CRITERIA

- Need for admission is rare
  - —Significant pain with ambulation
  - —Severe limitation in range of motion
  - —Muscle spasm
  - —Family situation
    - -Bedrest is not possible
    - -Traction cannot be arranged as an outpatient

DISCHARGE CRITERIA

- Adequate pain control provided
- Orthopedic follow-up arranged

Miscellaneous

ICD9: 732.1

CORE CONTENT CODE: 13.6.1

SUGGESTED READINGS

DeLee JC, Drez D. Orthopaedic sports medicine. Vol 2. Philadelphia: WB Saunders, 1994:1083.

Herring JA. The treatment of Legg-Calvé-Perthes disease. Current concepts review. J Bone Joint Surg 1994;76(3):448–458.

Tachdjian MO. Pediatric orthopedics. Vol 2. Philadelphia: WB Saunders, 1990:933–1003.

Author: Lydia Ciarallo

Leukemia

Clinical Presentation

SIGNS AND SYMPTOMS

Chronic Myelogenous Leukemia (CML)

- Asymptomatic
- Fatigue
- Weight loss
- Left upper-quadrant pain/tenderness
- Splenomegaly (most common)
- Later stage
  - —Headaches
  - —Bone pain
  - —Arthralgias
  - —Fever
  - —Leukotactic symptoms
    - -Dyspnea
    - -Drowsiness
    - -Confusion

Chronic Lymphocytic Leukemia (CLL)

- Asymptomatic
- Fatigue
- Lethargy
- Weight loss
- Lymphadenopathy
- Splenomegaly
- Hepatomegaly

Acute Lymphocytic Leukemia (ALL)/Acute Myelogenous Leukemia (AML)

- Fatigue
- Pallor
- Headache
- Angina
- CHF
- Easy bleeding (thrombocytopenia)
  - —Petechiae
  - —Ecchymosis
  - —Epistaxis
  - —Hemorrhage
- Infections (granulocytopenic)
- Organ involvement with advanced ALL
  - —Lymphadenopathy
  - —Hepatomegaly
  - —Splenomegaly
  - —Leukemic meningitis
    - -Headache
    - -Nausea
    - -Seizures

MECHANISM/DESCRIPTION

- Neoplasms of white blood cells that have undergone a malignant transformation
- Hyperleukocytosis
  - —Occurs with WBC >100,000/mm^3
  - —Leads to occlusions of small vessels primarily in brain or lungs
  - —Present with confusion, stupor or shortness of breath

CML

- Overproduction of granulocytic WBCs (neutrophils)
  - —Neutrophil function preserved
- Thrombocytosis
- Basophilia
- Philadelphia chromosome present in bone marrow of >95%

CLL

- Most common leukemia in adults
- Overproduction of monoclonal lymphocytes
- Cells accumulate in lymph nodes, bone marrow, liver, spleen

Acute Leukemias

- Proliferation of undifferentiated immature cells
  - —AML—immature myeloid cells
  - —ALL—immature lymphoid cells (blasts)
- Rapidly fatal

ETIOLOGY

- Cause unknown
- Familial clustering in CLL
- Increased incidence of AML, ALL, and CML with ionizing radiation

PEDIATRIC CONSIDERATIONS

- Usually have ALL
  - —Most common pediatric cancer
- 60–80% remission in those who are standard risk
- Better overall prognosis
- May develop leukostasis at lower levels

Pre-Hospital

N/A

Diagnosis

ESSENTIAL WORKUP

- CBC/platelets
  - —CML
    - -WBC range 10,000–1 million/mm^3
    - -Neutrophils predominate
    - -Thrombocytosis in 50%
  - —CLL
    - -Absolute lymphocytosis >5000
    - -WBC range 40,000–150,000/mm^3
  - —Acute leukemia (AML/ALL)
    - -Anemia
    - -Thrombocytopenia
    - -Elevation/depression of WBC

LABORATORY

- Electrolytes, BUN, Cr, glucose
- Uric acid level
  - —Frequently elevated especially in ALL
- Lactate dehydrogenase
  - —Increased in acute leukemias
- Coagulation profile
  - —PT, PTT, fibrinogen, fibrin-split products
  - —If disseminated, suspect intravascular coagulation
- Blood/urine cultures if fever
- ABG/pulse oximetry for shortness of breath

IMAGING/SPECIAL TESTS

- Bone marrow biopsy
  - —Required to make diagnosis
  - —CML—hypercellular with myeloid hyperplasia
  - —CLL—lymphocytosis (30–100%)
  - —Acute leukemia—hypercellular with blast cells which replace normal marrow
- Leukocyte alkaline phosphatase test
  - —Decreased in neutrophils in CML
- Ph1 chromosome present in CML
- CXR

DIFFERENTIAL DIAGNOSIS

CML

- Lymphoma
- Myeloproliferative syndromes
- Systemic lupus erythematosus
- Infection—bacterial, fungal, mycobacterial

CLL

- Pertussis
- Infectious lymphocytosis
- Cytomegalovirus
- Epstein-Barr virus mononucleosis
- Hepatitis
- Rubella

Acute Leukemia

- Aplastic anemia
- Leukemoid reactions to infections

Treatment

INITIAL STABILIZATION

- 100% oxygen for hypoxia/shortness of breath
- IV access with 0.9%NS
- Initiate platelet transfusion for severe bleeding from thrombocytopenia
- Begin broad spectrum antibiotics for fever and granulocytopenia
- Treat disseminated intravascular coagulation (see disseminated intravascular coagulation chapter)

ED TREATMENT

- Treat leukostasis
  - —Rehydrate with 500 cc bolus (20 cc/kg) IV 0.9%NS
  - —Administer acetazolamide to alkalinize urine
  - —Initiate allopurinol
  - —Arrange for leukapheresis
  - —Whole-brain radiation for CNS affects
  - —Administer hydroxyurea 3 g/m^2 for 2–3 days
- Transfuse PRBC for symptomatic anemia
  - —May require irradiated, filtered, and HLA-type specific blood

Post-ED Therapy

- CLL
  - —Chemotherapy
  - —Prednisone for immune-mediated thrombocytopenia
  - —Radiation to localized nodular masses/enlarge spleen
- CML
  - —Interferon therapy
  - —Chemotherapy
  - —Bone marrow transplantation
- ALL
  - —Chemotherapy
  - —CNS prophylaxis with intrathecal methotrexate/cranial radiation
  - —Bone marrow transplantation
- AML
  - —Chemotherapy
  - —Bone marrow transplantation

Disposition

ADMISSION CRITERIA

- Newly diagnosed leukemia with
  - —Symptomatic anemia
  - —WBC >30,000
  - —Thrombocytopenia
- ICU admission for unstable patients with DIC, blast crisis, or bleeding

DISCHARGE CRITERIA

- Asymptomatic patients without significant laboratory abnormalities

Miscellaneous

ICD9: 208.9

CORE CONTENT CODE: 7.7.1, 13.4.4

SUGGESTED READINGS

Applebaum FR. The acute leukemias. In: Bennet JC, Plum F, et al., eds. Cecil's textbook of medicine. 20th ed. Philadelphia: WB Saunders, 1996:936–940.

Baer M. Management of unusual presentations of acute leukemia. Hematol Oncol Clin North Am 1993;7(1):275–292.

Keating MJ. The chronic leukemias. In: Bennet JC, Plum F, et al., eds. Cecil's textbook of medicine. 20th ed. Philadelphia: WB Saunders, 1996:925–935.

Koeffler P. Syndromes of acute nonlymphocytic leukemias. Ann Intern Med 1987;107(7):48–58.

Wade J. Management of infection in patients with acute leukemia. Hematol Oncol Clin North Am 1993;7(1):297–315.

Author: Linda Mueller

Lightning Injuries

Clinical Presentation

SIGNS AND SYMPTOMS

Cardiorespiratory

- Cardiac asystole
  - —Due to direct current injury
  - —May resolve spontaneously as the heart's intrinsic automaticity resumes
- Respiratory arrest
  - —Due to paralysis of medullary respiratory center
  - —May persist longer than cardiac asystole and lead to hypoxic induced VFib
- Acute myocardial infarction rare
- Shock
  - —Neurogenic (spinal injury)
  - —Hypovolemic (trauma)
- Mottled or cold extremities
  - —Due to autonomic vasomotor instability
  - —Usually resolves spontaneously in a few hours

Neurological Injuries

- Confusion
- Memory defects
- Alteration of level of consciousness (>70% of cases)
- Flaccid motor paralysis
- Seizures
- Fixed dilated pupils due either to serious head injury or autonomic dysfunction

Traumatic Injuries

- Blunt trauma
  - —To the head or spine
  - —Fractures, dislocations, muscle tears, and compartment syndromes
- Ruptured tympanic membrane with ossicular disruption (up to 50%)
- Burns
  - —Discrete entrance and exit wounds uncommon
  - —Thermal burns due to evaporation of water on skin, ignited clothing, heated metal objects (buckles/jewelry)
- Feathering (fernlike pattern) "burns"
  - —Cutaneous imprints from electron showers that track over skin
  - —Pathognomonic of lightning injury
  - —Resolve within 24 hours

Ophthalmologic Injuries

- Cataracts occur days to years postinjury
- Corneal lesions
- Intraocular hemorrhages
- Retinal detachment

MECHANISM/DESCRIPTION

- Due to the brief duration (1–100 msec) of lightning
  - —Current passes over the skin rather than through the body (flashover)
  - —Deep tissue injuries are rare
- Mechanisms of injury
  - —Direct strike—strikes victim directly
  - —Splash injury—moves from object to victim of lesser resistance to current flow
  - —Ground strike—current moves through ground and may injure multiple victims
  - —Blunt injury due to direct explosive effect
  - —Thermal burning

Pre-Hospital

CONTROVERSIES

- Field triage should rapidly focus on providing ventilatory support to unconscious victim(s) or those in cardiopulmonary arrest
  - —Prevents reversible asystolic cardiac arrest from degenerating into hypoxic induced VFib
- Conscious victims are at lower risk of imminent demise

CAUTIONS

- Spine immobilization for
  - —Cardiopulmonary arrest (suspected trauma)
  - —Significant mechanical trauma
  - —Suspected loss of consciousness at any time
- Cover superficial burns with sterile saline dressings
- Immobilize injured extremities
- Rapid extrication prevents exposure to repeat lightning strikes

Diagnosis

ESSENTIAL WORKUP

- Confirmatory history from bystanders or rescuers of the circumstances of the injury

LABORATORY

- CBC for baseline Hct
- Urinalysis for myoglobin
- Electrolytes for acidosis
- BUN, Cr for baseline renal function
- CK and CKMb fraction for muscle/cardiac damage

IMAGING/SPECIAL TESTS

- CXR
- C-spine radiograph
- CT head for altered mental status or significant head trauma
- ECG should be performed in all cases
  - —Nonspecific ST changes common
  - —Acute myocardial infarction rare

DIFFERENTIAL DIAGNOSIS

- Consider lightning strike in unwitnessed falls, cardiac arrests, or unexplained coma in an outdoor setting
- Other causes of coma, cardiac dysrhythmia, or trauma
  - —Hypoglycemia
  - —Intoxication
  - —Drug overdose
  - —Cardiovascular disease
  - —CVA

Treatment

INITIAL STABILIZATION

- ABCs
- Standard ACLS measures for cardiac arrest
- Diligent primary and secondary survey for traumatic injuries
  - —Maintain cervical spine precautions until cleared
- Treat altered mental status with glucose, naloxone, or thiamine as indicated
- Hypotension requires volume expansion and pressor agents

ED TREATMENT

- IV access for medication administration
- Volume expansion
  - —Do not follow burn treatment formulas as flashover burns are rarely the cause of fluid loss
  - —Occult deep burn injury is rare when compared to other types of electrical current injury
  - —Titrate volume administration to urine output—fluid-loading may be dangerous with head injuries
- Clean and dress burns
- Tetanus prophylaxis
- Treat myoglobinuria with
  - —Diuretics, such as furosemide or mannitol,
  - —Alkalinization of urine to a pH $\geq$7.45
  - —Maintain urine output with IV fluid administration
- Compartment syndrome
  - —Must be distinguished from vasospasm, autonomic dysfunction, and paralysis which are usually self-limited phenomena
  - —Delay fasciotomy if possible because it will rarely be necessary

MEDICATIONS

- Furosemide: 1 mg/kg IV slow bolus q 6 hrs
- Mannitol: 0.5 mg/kg IV, repeat PRN
- Sodium bicarbonate: 1 amp IVP (peds: 1 mEq/kg) followed by 2–3 amps/L of D5W IV fluid

Disposition

ADMISSION CRITERIA

- Seriously injured and postcardiac arrest victims
- History of change in mental status/altered level of consciousness
- Myoglobinuria
- Acidosis
- History dysrhythmias or ECG changes
  - —May not resolve spontaneously
  - —24–48-hour observation period to identify potentially unstable cases

DISCHARGE CRITERIA

- Asymptomatic patients with no injuries
- Close follow-up due to the risk of delayed sequelae

Miscellaneous

ICD9: 994.0

CORE CONTENT CODE: 5.4

SUGGESTED READINGS

Browne BJ, Gaasch WR. Lightening Emerg Med Clin North Am 1992;10:2:211–230.

Cooper MA. Lightning injuries. In: Rosen P, Barkin R, Danzl D, et al., eds. Emergency medicine: Concepts and clinical practice. 4th ed. St. Louis: CV Mosby, 1998:1010–1022.

Cooper MA, Andrew CJ. Lightning injuries. In: Auerbach P, ed. Wilderness medicine. St. Louis: CV Mosby, 1995:261–290.

Lichtenberg R, et al. Cardiovascular effects of lightning strikes. J Am Coll Cardiol 1993;21(2):531–536.

Author: Paul Arnold

Lisfranc Fracture

Clinical Presentation

SIGNS AND SYMPTOMS

- Pain, swelling, forefoot hematoma
- Shortening of the foot in anteroposterior plane
- Widening of the foot
- Pathologic movement of the tarsometatarsal joint

MECHANISM/DESCRIPTION

- Direct crush injury to dorsum of foot (e.g., falling object, foot under car tire)
- Indirect injury (e.g., fall, kicking a door with foot plantar flexed, motor vehicle crash with foot plantar flexed against pedal)
- Tarsometatarsal joint (Lisfranc joint) fracture-dislocation
  - —Homolateral—all metatarsals are displaced in the same direction
  - —Isolated—one or two metatarsals are displaced from the others
  - —Divergent—medial displacement of the first metatarsal and lateral displacement of the other four metatarsals

Pre-Hospital

N/A

Diagnosis

ESSENTIAL WORKUP

- Physical examination with specific attention to skin integrity, gross deformity, and neurovascular status
- Three-view foot radiographs: AP, 30° internal oblique, lateral
  - —On AP radiograph look for widening and an associated fracture fragment between the bases of the first and second metatarsals
  - —Minor fracture-dislocations may be overlooked on radiographs (20% of cases)

IMAGING/SPECIAL TESTS

- For subtle injuries, weight-bearing lateral radiographs of both feet are helpful in identifying a flattened longitudinal arch

Treatment

INITIAL STABILIZATION

- In cases of major trauma, assess for other more life-threatening injuries first
- Assess for ischemia distal to the fracture-dislocation
- Ice, elevation, and immobilization in a bulky splint
- Early orthopedic consultation
- Appropriate pain management

ED TREATMENT

- Closed reduction and casting is often inadequate
- Anatomic reduction with surgical fixation provides optimal outcome
- Measure compartment pressures if associated with crush injury

MEDICATIONS

- Morphine sulfate: adult: 2–10 mg IV/IM titrated to pain control; peds: 0.1 mg/kg IV
- Fentanyl: 50–250 μg IV titrated to pain control
- Meperidine: 25–100 mg IV/IM titrated to pain control

Disposition

ADMISSION CRITERIA

- Concomitant potentially life-threatening injuries
- Open fracture
- Evidence of compartment syndrome or neurovascular compromise

DISCHARGE CRITERIA

- Isolated Lisfranc fracture-dislocation without neurovascular compromise or compartment syndrome and only after evaluation by an orthopedic surgeon

Miscellaneous

ICD9: 825.20

CORE CONTENT CODE: 18.4.13.2.2

SUGGESTED READINGS

Arntz CT, Veith RG, Hansen ST. Fracture and fracture-dislocations of the tarsometatarsal joint. J Bone Joint Surg 1988;70A:173–181.

Faciszewski T, Burks RT, Manaster BJ. Subtle injuries of the Lisfranc joint. J Bone Joint Surg 1990;72A:1519–1522.

Goossens M, De Stoop N. Lisfranc's fracture-dislocations: Etiology, radiology, and results of treatment: A review of 20 cases. Clin Orthop 1983;176:154–162.

Karasick D. Fractures and dislocations of the foot. Semin Roentgen 1994;29:152–175.

Myerson M. The diagnosis and treatment of injuries to the Lisfranc joint complex. Orthop Clin North Am 1989;20:655–664.

Author: Peter C. Ferrera

Lithium, Poisoning

Clinical Presentation

SIGNS AND SYMPTOMS

Acute Toxicity

Neurologic

- Most common
- Mild
  - —Weakness
  - —Fatigue
  - —Fine tremor
  - —Dizziness
- Moderate
  - —Ataxia
  - —Slurred speech
  - —Blurred vision
  - —Profound weakness
  - —Coarse tremor
  - —Fasciculations
  - —Hyperreflexia
  - —Choreoathetoid movements
- Severe
  - —Confusion
  - —Coma
  - —Seizure

Gastrointestinal

- Nausea/vomiting
- Diarrhea
- Abdominal pain

Cardiac

- Prolonged QT, ST/T wave abnormalities
- T wave flattening *most common* ECG abnormality
- Serious arrhythmia (rare)

Chronic Toxicity

Renal

- Nephrogenic diabetes insipidus
- Direct cellular damage

Dermatologic

- Dermatitis
- Ulcers

Endocrine

- Hyper/hypothyroidism

Hematologic

- Leukocytosis
- Aplastic anemia

MECHANISM/DESCRIPTION

- Oral absorption
  - —Regular release: peak serum levels 2–4 hours
  - —Sustained release: peak serum levels 4–12 hours
- Half-life of 24 hours
- Elimination
  - —*Not* metabolized
  - —Excreted unchanged by the kidneys
  - —Reabsorbed in the *proximal* tubules by sodium transport mechanism
- Therapeutic and toxic indices
  - —Therapeutic and toxic effects occur *only* when lithium is intracellular
  - —Narrow therapeutic window
    - -0.6–1.2 mEq/L (post-intra/extracellular equilibration)

ETIOLOGY

- Conditions that increase risk of lithium toxicity
  - —Acute conditions
    - -Dehydration (decreases renal filtration and increases reabsorption)
    - -Intentional overdose
  - —Chronic conditions
    - -Hypertension
    - -Diabetes mellitus
    - -Renal failure
    - -Congestive heart failure
    - -Advanced age
    - -Dose change
    - -Drug interactions
    - -Lithium therapy
    - -Low salt diet
- Drug interactions with lithium
  - —Increase serum lithium levels (decrease renal clearance)
    - -NSAIDs
    - -Thiazides
    - -ACE inhibitors
    - -Dilantin
  - —Potentiate lithium effects
    - -Tricyclic antidepressants
    - -Phenothiazines

Pre-Hospital

CAUTIONS

- Transport all medications to hospital suspected in acute ingestions

Diagnosis

ESSENTIAL WORKUP

- Lithium level
  - —Repeat q 4 hrs
- Stratify patient into one of three categories to interpret lithium level and predict toxicity
  - —Acute toxicity
    - -Intentional overdose in a patient not previously taking lithium
    - -Poor correlation between lithium level and symptoms as intracellular distribution has not yet occurred and toxic levels occur in asymptomatic patients
    - -Lithium level >4 mEq/L is toxic as clearance is slow and complications are inevitable
  - —Acute on chronic toxicity
    - -Intentional or accidental overdose in a patient on lithium therapy
    - -Lithium level >3 mEq/L usually associated with symptoms
  - —Chronic toxicity
    - -Patients on lithium therapy who progressively develop toxicity secondary to factors other than acute ingestion
    - -Strong correlation between lithium level and symptoms
    - -Lithium level >1.5 mEq/L may be toxic

LABORATORY

- Electrolytes, BUN/Cr, glucose for electrolytes disturbances/renal function
- Aspirin and APAP levels in all acute ingestions
- U/A
  - —Specific gravity

DIFFERENTIAL DIAGNOSIS

- Consider lithium toxicity with altered mental status and fasciculations
- Endocrine: hypoglycemia
- Toxicologic
  - —Organophosphates
  - —Cholinergic substances
  - —Heavy metal poisoning
  - —Neuroleptic overdose
  - —Black widow/scorpion envenomation
  - —Strychnine poisoning

Treatment

INITIAL STABILIZATION

- ABCs
- Secure IV access with 0.9%NS
- Cardiac monitor
- Naloxone, thiamine, dextrose (or Accucheck) if altered mental status
- Administer diazepam for seizures

ED TREATMENT

Prevent Absorption

- Syrup of ipecac
  - —Not recommended due to aspiration risk secondary to potential for change in mental status
- Gastric lavage if patient presents within 1 hour of acute ingestion
- Charcoal
  - —Lithium poorly absorbed by charcoal
  - —Give 1 dose of activated charcoal with sorbitol if possibility of coingestion exists
- Whole-bowel irrigation
  - —Polyethylene glycol solution (PEG/GoLitely)
  - —Flushes out toxin
  - —Administer until rectal effluent is clear
  - —Contraindications
    - -Bowel obstruction or perforation
    - -Ileus
    - -Unprotected airway in obtunded or seizing patient

Enhance Elimination

- Saline diuresis
  - —Rapidly correct any preexisting fluid deficit with 0.9%NS
  - —Saline hydration promotes filtration and decreases proximal tubule reabsorption of lithium
  - —Maintain urine output between 100–200 cc/hr
  - —Limited value once GFR maximized
- Loop, thiazide, and osmotic diuretics not recommended
  - —Dehydration may result
  - —No direct effect on renal reabsorption as lithium reabsorbed in proximal tubules
- Kayexalate (sodium polystyrene sulfonate) not recommended
  - —Complications include hypokalemia and sodium overload

Dialysis

- Peritoneal dialysis not recommended secondary to iatrogenic complications
- Hemodialysis
  - —Best method for augmenting elimination
  - —Consider in chronic lithium therapy or in sustained release ingestions as complications are more likely to develop
  - —Definitive indications for hemodialysis
    - -Presence of moderate to severe neurological abnormalities
    - -Lithium level >4 mEq/L
    - -Renal failure
    - -Ventricular arrhythmia/cardiogenic shock
  - —Continue until serum lithium level <1 mEq/L
  - —Repeat dialysis for patients on chronic lithium therapy due to rebound effect (redistribution of intracellular lithium)
  - —Reduces the potential for developing permanent neurological sequelae with chronic toxicity

Supportive care

- Correct electrolyte abnormalities
- Continuous cardiac monitoring
- Maintain well-hydrated state
- Observe for neurological changes

MEDICATIONS

- Activated charcoal: 1 g/kg po
- Dextrose: D50 1 amp (25 g) (peds: D25W 4 ml/kg) IV
- Diazepam: 5 mg (peds: 0.2–0.4 mg/kg) IV q 5 min until seizures controlled
- Naloxone: 2 mg (peds: 0.1 mg/kg) IV/ET
- Polyethylene glycol: 2 L/hr (peds: 2 cc/kg/hr) PO/NGT
- Sorbitol 70% solution: 30 cc (peds: 2 ml/kg) PO/NGT
- Thiamine: 100 mg IV

Disposition

ADMISSION CRITERIA

- Symptomatic
- Requiring hemodialysis
- Lithium level unchanged, increased, or greater than 2 mEq/L despite ED intervention
- Psychiatric consultation for intentional ingestion

DISCHARGE CRITERIA

- Decreasing lithium levels q 4 hrs in an *asymptomatic* patient *and*
- Most recent serum lithium level <2 mEq/L

Miscellaneous

ICD9: 985.8

CORE CONTENT CODE: 17.2.7.1

SUGGESTED READINGS

Belanger DR, Tierney MG, Dickinson G. Effect of sodium polystyrene sulfonate on lithium bioavailability. Ann Emerg Med 1992;21:1312–1315.

Bosse GM, Arnold TC. Overdose with sustained release lithium preparation. J Emerg Med 1992;10:719–721.

Jaeger A, Kopferschmitt SJ. Toxicokinetics of lithium treated by hemodialysis. Clin Toxicol 1986;23:501.

Smith SW, Ling LJ, Halstenson C. Whole-bowel irrigation as a treatment for acute lithium overdose. Ann Emerg Med 1991;20:536–539.

Tomaszewski C, Musso C, Pearson JR, Kulig K, Marx JA. Lithium absorption prevented by sodium polystyrene sulfonate in volunteers. Ann Emerg Med 1992;21:1308–1311.

Author: Saul Melman

Low Back Pain

Clinical Presentation

SIGNS AND SYMPTOMS

- Musculoligamentous
  - —Poorly localized and dull back/gluteal pain without radiation past the knee
  - —Usually there are no objective neurologic signs
  - —Back spasm is a variable and poorly reproducible finding
- Sciatica
  - —Sharp, shooting, well-localized pain
  - —Leg complaints often greater than back
  - —May present with
    - -Asymmetric deep tendon reflexes
    - -Decreased sensation in a dermatomal distribution
    - -Objective weakness
- Massive central disc herniation (cauda equina syndrome)
  - —Decreased perineal sensation
  - —Urinary retention
  - —Fecal incontinence
- Infectious processes
  - —Fever
  - —Localized percussion tenderness of the vertebral bodies
- Bony lesion or vascular etiology
  - —Continuous pain that does not change with rest

MECHANISM/DESCRIPTION

- Low back pain (LBP)
  - —Refers to pain in the area between the lower rib cage and the gluteal folds, often with radiation into the thighs
- Sciatica
  - —Pain in the distribution of the lower lumbar spinal roots
  - —Often accompanied by neurosensory and motor deficits
- Pain classification
  - —Acute if 0–6 weeks
  - —Subacute if 6–12 weeks
  - —Chronic if >12 weeks

ETIOLOGY

- Nonspecific musculoligamentous source (great majority)
- Herniation of the nucleus pulposus
- Degenerative joints or disks
- Spinal stenosis
- Anatomic abnormalities—especially spondylolisthesis
- Fractures from trauma and osteoporosis
- Underlying systemic diseases
  - —Neoplasm
  - —Infections
  - —Vascular
  - —Renal

Pre-Hospital

CAUTIONS

- Trauma patients with acute back pain should be immobilized on a backboard until an unstable fracture can be ruled out

Diagnosis

ESSENTIAL WORKUP

- Thorough history and physical including detailed neurologic and vascular examination
- No specific tests are needed for uncomplicated musculoligamentous or sciatic pain without complicating factors

LABORATORY

- Urinalysis for suspected
  - —Urinary tract infection
  - —Pyelonephritis
  - —Prostatitis

IMAGING AND ADDITIONAL TESTS

- Lumbosacral radiograph for
  - —Significant trauma
  - —Age >50
  - —History or signs/symptoms of cancer
  - —Fever
  - —Intravenous drug user
  - —Pain at rest
  - —Suspicion of ankylosing spondylitis
  - —Pain that does improve after 4 weeks
- MRI for
  - —Suspicion of abscess
  - —Rapidly progressing neurologic symptoms or urinary retention or fecal incontinence associated with back pain
- ESR
  - —Very sensitive for infectious etiologies
  - —May be used in screening if suspicion exists
- Abdominal CT/ultrasound for suspicion of abdominal aortic aneurysm

DIFFERENTIAL DIAGNOSIS

- Spinal origins
  - —Musculoligamentous
  - —Discogenic
  - —Fracture
  - —Spondylolisthesis
  - —Ankylosing spondylitis
  - —Osteomyelitis
  - —Epidural abscess/hematoma
  - —Neoplasm
- Nonspinal causes
  - —Abdominal aortic aneurysm
  - —Prostatitis
  - —Urinary tract infection
  - —Abdominal neoplasm
  - —Renal colic

Treatment

INITIAL STABILIZATION

- IV fluid resuscitation if hypotension/leaking abdominal aortic aneurysm

ED TREATMENT

- Acute uncomplicated back pain
  —*Short course* of bed rest: 24–48 hours followed by early mobilization
  —Return to regular activity within limits

MEDICATIONS

- Nonsteroidal anti-inflammatory agents
  —Treatment of choice
  —No agent has definitive benefits over others
  —Recommend using cost and dosing schedules as guide
- Muscle relaxants helpful
  —Cyclobenzaprine
  —Metaxalone
  —Methocarbamol
- Limited course of narcotic analgesics for severe pain not relieved by anti-inflammatory agents
- Spinal manipulation
  —A short course (<2 weeks) of may be helpful in acute low back pain without sciatica
- Physical therapy/exercise
  —No clear consensus for indications
  —May be helpful in preventing further episodes
- Expected recovery to pain-free state
  —33%: within 1 week
  —75%: within 3 weeks
  —90%: within 2 months

MEDICATIONS

- Acetaminophen: 650–1000 mg po every 4–6 hrs
- Cyclobenzaprine: 10 mg po 3 times a day
- Hydrocodone/acetaminophen: 5/500 mg po every 4–6 hrs
- Ibuprofen: 600–800 mg po every 6–8 hrs
- Metaxalone: 800 mg po every 6–8 hrs
- Methocarbamol: 1000–1500 mg po every 6 hrs
- Naproxen: 250–500 mg po every 12 hrs
- Oxycodone/acetaminophen: 5/500 mg po every 4–6 hrs

Disposition

ADMISSION CRITERIA

- Severe pain with inability to ambulate
- Progressive neurologic deficits
- Signs of cauda equina syndrome
- Evidence of infectious or neoplastic etiologies

DISCHARGE CRITERIA

- Uncomplicated presentation with ability to control pain and ambulate

Miscellaneous

ICD9: 724.2

CORE CONTENT CODE: 10.3.4

SUGGESTED READINGS

Deyo RA, Rainville J, Kent DL. What can the history and physical tell us about low back pain? JAMA 1992;268:760–765.

Frymoyer JW. Back pain and sciatica. N Engl J Med 1988;318:291–299.

Malmivaara A, Hakkinen U, Aro T, et al. The treatment of acute low back pain—bed rest, exercises, or ordinary activity? N Engl J Med 1995;332:351–355.

Author: Eric Legome

Ludwig's Angina

Clinical Presentation

SIGNS AND SYMPTOMS

- Neck pain
- Tongue elevation and protrusion
- Trismus
  - —Makes mouth examination difficult
- Dysphonia
- Odynophagia
- Stridor
- Anxiety
- Salivary incontinence
- Fever
- Tachypnea and tachycardia
- The patient will prefer sitting/"sniffing" position
- Submandibular area will be hard, "woody," and painful

MECHANISM/DESCRIPTION

- Ludwig's angina is a life-threatening infection of the floor of the mouth
- First described by von Ludwig in 1936
- Mortality exceeded 50% in the preantibiotic era
- Most deaths due to respiratory obstruction (asphyxiation)
- Improved dental care and antibiotics have made this a rare condition
- Rapidly spreading gangrenous cellulitis and necrotizing fasciitis of the submaxillary, sublingual, and submandibular spaces
- Four cardinal aspects are
  - —Bilateral involvement of more than one deep-tissue space
  - —Gangrene with serosanguineous, putrid infiltration but little or no frank pus
  - —Involvement of connective tissue, fasciae, and muscles, but not glandular structures
  - —Spread by fascial space continuity rather than by lymphatics
- The brawny, painful induration of the suprahyoid region of the neck results in a woody edema of the floor of the mouth, forcing the tongue and soft tissues superiorly and posteriorly
- Rapid respiratory obstruction (asphyxia) can occur

ETIOLOGY

- Dental in origin in 50–90% of reported cases
- Most commonly from the second or third mandibular molars
- Less common sources
  - —IV drug injections into neck veins
  - —Mandibular fractures
  - —Oral lacerations
  - —Sialadenitis
  - —Tongue piercing
- Invariably polymicrobial, consisting of oral flora
  - —Most common pathogens
    - -*Streptococcus viridans*
    - -*Staphylococcus aureus*
    - -*Staphylococcus epidermidis*
    - -Anaerobes: most commonly *Bacteroides* species

Pre-Hospital

- Transport in sitting position
- Early, aggressive airway protection is paramount

Diagnosis

ESSENTIAL WORKUP

- The diagnosis is apparent from the history and physical examination

LABORATORY

- White blood cell count (to gauge systemic response)
- Blood cultures

IMAGING/SPECIAL TESTS

- Soft tissue films of the neck
- Presence of gas
- CT scan of neck or MRI will detect intrathoracic involvement/abscess
- Panorex view
- Dental origin
- Chest x-ray
- Intrathoracic extension

DIFFERENTIAL DIAGNOSIS

- Cellulitis
- Peritonsillar abscess
- Salivary gland abscess
- Lymphadenitis
- Angioneurotic edema
- Lingual carcinoma
- Sublingual hematoma formation following anticoagulation

Treatment

INITIAL STABILIZATION

- Airway compromise is the primary concern
- Oral endotracheal intubation may be difficult due to altered anatomy and trismus
- Administration of paralyzing agents may result in loss of supporting structures maintaining a patent airway
  —Loss of visualization of the airway may occur
- *Sedation-assisted orotracheal intubation is preferred*
  —Ultrashort barbiturate (etomidate, thiopental) should be used
  —If adequate relaxation has not occurred, paralytics may be necessary
- Blind nasotracheal intubation should be avoided
  —Distorted anatomy
  —May induce bleeding or rupture a pharyngeal abscess
- Fiberoptic intubation has been proven useful
- Cricothyrotomy is not contraindicated but may be difficult due to swollen tissues

ED TREATMENT

- Institute antibiotic therapy in the ED
- Broad spectrum for anaerobic/polymicrobial infection
- Penicillin, gentamicin, metronidazole, Cefoxitin, Clindamycin, Ticarcillin/clavulanate, Piperacillin/tazobactam, Ampicillin/sulbactam
- Steroids are of no proven benefit
- If mediastinitis, or necrotizing fasciitis of the chest wall develop hyperbaric oxygen therapy is an important adjunct

MEDICATIONS

- Antibiotics
  —Ampicillin/SB: 3 g IV q 6 hrs
  —Cefoxitin: 2 g IV q 6 hrs
  —Clindamycin: 900 mg IV q 6 hrs
  —Gentamicin: 2–5 mg/kg IV q 8 hrs
  —Metronidazole: 500 mg IV q 6 hrs
  —Penicillin G: 2–4 million units IV q 4 hrs
  —Piperacillin/TZ: 3.375 g IV q 6 hrs
  —Ticarcillin/CL: 3.1 g IV q 6 hrs
- Sedatives
  —Etomidate: 0.2 mg/kg IV
  —Thiopental: 3–5 mg/kg IV

Disposition

ADMISSION CRITERIA

- All patients are admitted
- Admit to an ICU or monitored setting as airway compromise can occur rapidly

DISCHARGE CRITERIA

N/A

Miscellaneous

ICD9: 528.3

CORE CONTENT CODE: 6.3.4

SUGGESTED READINGS

Ferrera PC, Busino LJ, Snyder HS. Uncommon complications of odontogenic infections. Am J Emerg Med 1996;14(3):317–22.

Ruiz CC, Labaio DR, Vilas IY, Paniagua J. Thoracic complications of deeply situated serious neck infections. J Craniomaxillofac Surg 1993;21:76–81.

Spitalnic SJ, Sucov A. Ludwig's angina: case report and review. J Emerg Med 1995;13(4):499–503.

Weiss L, Finkelstein JA, Storrow AB. Fever and neck pain. Ludwig's angina. Acad Emerg Med 1995;2(9):835, 843–844.

Author: Paul Blackburn

Lumbar Spine Fracture

Clinical Presentation

SIGNS AND SYMPTOMS

- Pain in lumbar region
- Ecchymosis or deformity overlying lumbar region, localized spinal tenderness, palpable deformity, paraspinal muscle spasm
- Increased interspinous distance by palpation
- "Step-off" (anterior or posterior displacement of spinous process) by palpation
- Neurologic deficits referable to lumbar spinal nerves
  - —Loss of bladder control
  - —Motor: hip flexion (L1–L4), leg extension (L3, L4), ankle dorsiflexion (L4, L5), toe extension (L5)
  - —Sensory: inguinal crease (L1), medial thigh (L2–L3), knee (L4), lateral calf (L5)
  - —Reflexes: knee jerk (L2–L4)
- Pain may be masked by associated injuries (e.g., pelvis, calcaneal fractures)
- Multiple injury trauma patients with altered mental status have unreliable exam

ETIOLOGY

- Blunt trauma with axial distraction, axial compression or translational forces applied to lumbar region
- Fall from height landing on the feet (associated calcaneal fractures) or on the buttocks
- Motor vehicle accident

PEDIATRIC CONSIDERATIONS

- Rare reports of child abuse presenting as lower extremity flaccid paralysis due to lumbar spine fracture
- Spinal cord terminates at L3 in newborn and recedes to T12 by adulthood; direct cord damage possible in children with high lumbar fractures
- *End plate avulsion fractures:* adolescent injury usually at L4–L5 or L5–S1 level. Ligament pulls off vertebral body end plate. Associated neurologic findings usually resolve with excision of end plate fracture

Pre-Hospital

CAUTIONS

- It is difficult to determine if an injury is stable in the field, suspected spinal injuries should be immobilized to prevent further injury

Diagnosis

ESSENTIAL WORKUP

- Lumbar radiographs (described below)
- Careful neurologic examination including assessment of rectal tone, postvoid residual urinary catheterization, bulbocavernosus and cremasteric reflexes

LABORATORY

- Standard trauma labs as indicated

IMAGING/SPECIAL TESTS

- Lumbar radiography with minimum of AP and lateral views
  - —Characteristics of *unstable* fractures include: widening of interspinous, interlaminar or interpedicular distance, kyphosis >20°, translation >2 mm, vertebral body height loss >50%, or articular process fracture
- Radiographs may not diagnose burst fractures in 25% of cases
- If a fracture is identified, entire spine should be imaged
- Spinous process fracture, transverse process fracture, simple transverse sacral fracture require lumbar *flexion/extension films* if neurologically intact and stable injury
- CT should be performed for further evaluation of suspected fractures or fractures identified on plain films to assess spinal cord integrity

MECHANISM/DESCRIPTION

FRACTURE TYPE	CHARACTERISTICS	ASSOCIATED FINDINGS	EXAM
Flexion compression			
A. Wedge compression	<50% anterior compression of the vertebral body, stable injury	(−) ligamentous injury	(−)neurologic deficit
B. Burst fracture	vertebral body fracture with retropulsion of bone into the neural canal	(−) kyphosis on lateral x-ray	(+)/(−)neurologic deficit
		(+) posterior ligamentous injury (+) kyphosis on lateral x-ray (+) anterior compression, lower extremities, calcaneal fractures	
Flexion distraction: "Lap Belt Injury"		*Abdominal injuries likely*	
A. Chance fracture	purely bony injury, fracture line thru spinous process, pedicles, and vertebral body	(−) kyphosis on lateral x-ray	(−) neurological deficit
B. Facet dislocation	mostly soft tissue injury, no fracture	(+) complete disruption of posterior ligaments and intervertebral disc	(+) neurological deficit
Flexion rotation	unstable injury		(+) neurological deficit
Extension	unstable, uncommon	disruption of anterior longitudinal ligament and intervertebral disc	neurologic sequelae rare but possible
Shear injuries: "Translational Injuries"	(+) anterior, posterior, +/or lateral translation of superior vertebral segment over the inferior segment	(+) complete ligamentous disruption	(+) neurological deficit
Simple fractures	isolated *spinous process fracture*	(−) ligamentous disruption	(−) neurological deficit
	isolated *transverse process* fracture	(−) ligamentous disruption	(−/+) neurological deficit; rare isolated root injury

DIFFERENTIAL DIAGNOSIS

- Contusion
- Pathologic fracture (metastatic cancer)
- Osteoporosis
- Pelvic fracture
- Traumatic herniated disc
- Low posterior rib fracture
- Tuberculous spondylitis (Pott's Disease)
- Ankylosing spondylitis
- Osteogenesis Imperfecta (pediatric)
- Congenital scoliosis with hemivertebra (mistaken for lateral wedge fracture)
- Child abuse

Treatment

INITIAL STABILIZATION

- Immobilization while tending to immediate life-threatening conditions
- ABCs of trauma care

ED TREATMENT

- Maintain spinal immobilization
- High-dose steroid protocol for any neurologic deficit
- Consultation with orthopedic spine, or neurosurgery service
- Appropriate analgesia
- The following "stable" injuries may be treated conservatively if the CT confirms stability of injury and patient is neurologically intact
  —Isolated spinous process, transverse process fracture, chance fractures, anterior wedge compression (<50%) fracture, and "stable" burst fractures
- Total contact orthotic devices may be useful, limited activities, sleep prone, avoid pillows and soft mattresses which may worsen deformity

MEDICATIONS

- Narcotic pain medication in absence of contraindications
- *High-dose steroid protocol*
  —Methylprednisolone 30 mg/kg IV load over 1 hour, then 5.4 mg/kg per hour for the next 23 hours. Initiate in ED within 8 hours of injury

Disposition

ADMISSION CRITERIA

- Patients with traumatic lumbar fractures should be admitted for stabilization procedures, parenteral pain control, management of possible ileus and evaluation for associated injuries

DISCHARGE CRITERIA

- Neurologically intact patients with stable nontraumatic fractures evaluated in conjunction with spine surgeon
- Patients with simple compression (wedge) fractures with no neurologic deficit may be considered for outpatient management if adequate pain control and appropriate follow up can be arranged
- Simple transverse sacral fracture, isolated spinous process fracture, isolated transverse process fracture may also be considered for outpatient management
- The patient must be neurologically intact with a stable living situation and the CT scan and flexion/extension films must confirm fracture stability

Miscellaneous

ICD9: 805.4

CORE CONTENT CODE: 18.4.3.1.3

SUGGESTED READINGS

Campana BA. Soft tissue injuries and back pain. In: Rosen P, Barkin R, eds. Emergency medicine: concepts and clinical practice. 4th ed. St. Louis: CV Mosby, 1998:878–905.

Denis F. Spinal instability as defined by the three-column spine concept in acute spinal trauma. Clin Orthop 1984;189:65–76.

Gabos P, Tuten H, Leet A, Stanton R. Fracture-dislocation of the lumbar spine in an abused child. Pediatrics 1998;101(3):473–477.

Hockenberger RS, Kirshenbaum KJ, Doris PE. Spinal injuries. In: Rosen P, Barkin R, eds. Emergency medicine: concepts and clinical practice. 4th ed. St Louis: CV Mosby, 1998:462–505.

Krueger MA, Green DA, Hoyt D, Garfin SR. Overlooked spine injuries associated with lumbar process fractures. Clin Orthop 1996;327:191–195.

Petersilge C, Emery S. Thoracolumbar burst fracture: evaluating stability. Semin Ultrasound CT MR 1996;17(2):105–113.

Savitsky E, Votey S. Emergency department approach to acute thoracolumbar spine injury. J Emerg Med 1997;15:49–60.

Authors: Bret Ginther; Teresa Carlin

Lunate Dislocation

Clinical Presentation

SIGNS AND SYMPTOMS

- Pain in the wrist
- Mass or swelling in the wrist, most prominent dorsally

MECHANISM/DESCRIPTION

- Fall from height; violent palmar or dorsiflexion of the hand
- Dislocation of the lunate relative to the radius and distal row of metacarpals
- Disruption of the radiocarpal ligament

Pre-Hospital

- Consider other injuries
- Dress open wounds
- Immobilization in neutral position
- Elevation; cold to reduce swelling
- Age-appropriate social management

Diagnosis

ESSENTIAL WORKUP

- Exam including two-point discrimination; clinical exam is frequently not helpful
  - —In volar dislocations of the lunate, injury to the median nerve occurs in the carpal tunnel
  - —Pay special attention to assessing skin integrity and neurovascular status
- Radiographs as outlined below

IMAGING/SPECIAL TESTS

- Radiographic imaging to include three views of the wrist
  - —On a lateral radiograph the lunate appears either dorsal or volar to its normal position in relationship to the radius and the distal row of metacarpals
  - —In volar dislocations, the lunate is frequently tilted with the opening of the "cup" toward the palm (spilled teacup sign)
- Some authorities recommend specialized views of the wrist

DIFFERENTIAL DIAGNOSIS

- Lunate fracture
- Lunate dislocation
- Scapholunate dissociation
- Scaphoid fracture

PEDIATRIC CONSIDERATIONS

- X-ray can be difficult to interpret unless full ossification is present

Treatment

INITIAL STABILIZATION

- Immobilize in position of comfort with a volar or sugar-tong splint

ED TREATMENT

- Identify multiple trauma or other injuries
- Contact a hand surgeon for reduction and possible operative intervention
- These dislocations can be difficult to manually reduce and frequently need open reduction

MEDICATIONS

- Pain control pending definitive management

PEDIATRIC CONSIDERATIONS

- Wrists are rarely sprained in children and the x-ray is difficult to interpret
- Although serious injury is unusual, children with wrist pain should be splinted and referred for ongoing evaluation of possible fractures

Disposition

ADMISSION CRITERIA

- Dislocations should be reduced immediately, therefore, patients usually are admitted at the contact point for definitive orthopedic care
- Open fracture, presence of multiple trauma, or other more serious injuries mandates admission

DISCHARGE CRITERIA

- Closed fractures that have been adequately reduced in the ED may be appropriately immobilized and discharged with orthopedic follow-up

Miscellaneous

ICD9: 833.00

CORE CONTENT CODE: 18.4.12.2.3.1

SUGGESTED READINGS

American Society for Surgery of the Hand. The hand: Primary care of common problems. 2d ed. New York: Churchill Livingston, 1990: pp 637–649.

Eisenhauer MA. Forearm & wrist. In: Rosen P, et al., eds. Emergency medicine: Concepts and clinical practice. 4th ed. St. Louis: Mosby-Year Book, 1998:669–689.

Simon RR, Slobodkin D. In: American College of Emergency Physicians. Emergency medicine: A comprehensive study guide. 4th ed. New York McGraw Hill, 1996:1217–1226.

Uehara DT. The hand in emergency medicine. Emerg Clin North Am 1993;11(3). 781–96.

Author: John MacKay

Lyme Disease

Clinical Presentation

SIGNS AND SYMPTOMS

Stage I (Early)

- Onset a few days to a month after tick bite
- 30–50% of patients recall tick bite
- Erythema chronicum migrans (ECM)
  - —Pathognomonic finding
  - —Maculopapular, irregular expanding annular lesion
    - -Single or multiple
  - —Central clearing with red outer border
  - —Diameter >5 cm
- Regional adenopathy
- Low grade, intermittent fever
- Headache
- Myalgia
- Arthralgias
- Fatigue
- Malaise

Stage II (Secondary, Disseminated)

- Days to weeks after tick bite
- Intermittent and fluctuating symptoms with eventual disappearance
- Triad of aseptic meningitis, cranial neuritis and radiculoneuritis
  - —Facial (Bell's) palsy the most common cranial neuritis
  - —May present without rash
  - —Prognosis generally good
- Cardiac
  - —Tachycardia
  - —Bradycardia
  - —Atrioventricular block
  - —Myopericarditis

Stage III (Tertiary, Late)

- Onset greater than 1 year after disease onset
- Acrodermatitis chronica atrophicans
  - —Extensor surfaces of extremities, especially lower leg
  - —Initial edematous infiltration evolving to atrophic lesions
  - —Resembles scleroderma
- Arthritis
  - —Brief arthritis attacks
  - —Monoarthritis
  - —Oligoarthritis
  - —Occasionally migratory
  - —Most common joints (descending order)
    - -Knee
    - -Shoulder
    - -Elbow

Other

- Gastrointestinal
  - —Hepatitis
  - —Right upper-quadrant pain
- Ocular
  - —Keratitis
  - —Uveitis
  - —Iritis
  - —Optic neuritis
- Jarisch-Herxheimer reaction
  - —Worsening of symptoms a few hours after treatment initiated
  - —More common in patients with multiple ECM lesions
- Babesiosis occurs simultaneously in endemic areas

Persistent Lyme Disease

- Articular and neurologic symptoms despite treatment

Recurrent Lyme Disease

- Relapse despite treatment
- Second episodes less severe

ETIOLOGY

- Most common tick-borne illness in North America
- Endemic in northeastern, upper midwestern, and western states
- Peak between April and November; 80–90% in the summer months
- Spirochete *Borrelia burdorferi* introduced by *Ixodes* tick
  - —*I. dammini* (deer tick) the most common
- <50% of patients recall tick bite
- Pathogenesis—combination of
  - —Organism induced local inflammation
  - —Cytokine release
  - —Autoimmunity

PEDIATRIC CONSIDERATIONS

- More likely than adults to be febrile
- Only 50% of children with arthralgias have a history of ECM
- Facial palsy accompanied by aseptic meningitis in one-third
- Asymptomatic cardiac involvement with abnormal ECGs
- Appropriately treated children have excellent prognosis for unimpaired cognitive functioning
- Untreated children may have keratitis, joint pain, or chronic encephalopathy

Pre-Hospital

N/A

Diagnosis

ESSENTIAL WORKUP

- Clinical diagnosis
  - —Presence of ECM obviates serologic tests
- Careful search for tick
- Lumbar puncture when meningeal signs
- Arthrocentesis for acute arthritis
- ECG

LABORATORY

- CBC
  - —Leukocytosis
  - —Anemia
  - —Thrombocytopenia
- ESR
  - —>30 mm/hr
  - —Most common laboratory abnormality
- Electrolytes, BUN/Cr, glucose
- Liver function tests
  - —Elevated liver enzymes (GGT most common)
- Culture
  - —Low yield
  - —Not indicated
- CSF
  - —Pleocytosis
  - —Elevated protein
  - —Obtain CSF spirochete antibodies

IMAGING/SPECIAL TESTS

- Serology
  - —Obtain ELISA, IFA, and western blot when disease suggested without ECM lesion
- Polymerase chain reaction assay
  - —Highly specific and sensitive
  - —Not available for routine use
- Joint fluid
  - —Cryoglobulin increased five-fold compared with serum
- Joint films may show soft tissue, cartilaginous, osseous changes

DIFFERENTIAL DIAGNOSIS

- Other tick-borne illnesses
  - —Deer tick usually larger (1 cm) than Ixodid ticks(1–2 mm)
  - —Rocky Mountain spotted fever
  - —Tularemia
  - —Relapsing fever
  - —Colorado tick fever
  - —Tick-bite paralysis

- Rheumatic fever
  - —Rash of erythema marginatum
  - —Temporomandibular joint arthritis more common than in Lyme
  - —Valvular involvement rather than heart block
  - —Chorea may be isolated finding
- Viral meningitis
- Syphilis
- Septic arthritis
- Parvovirus B19 infection—polyarticular arthritis
- Infectious endocarditis
- Juvenile rheumatoid arthritis
- Reiter's syndrome
- Brown recluse spider bite
- Fibromyalgia
- Chronic fatigue syndrome

Treatment

INITIAL STABILIZATION

- 500 cc (20 ml/kg) 0.9%NS IV fluid bolus fluids for dehydration
- IV access for neurologic and cardiac involvement
- Cardiac monitoring
- Temporary pacemaker for heart block

ED TREATMENT

- Remove tick
  - —Disinfect site
  - —With blunt instrument grasp tick close to skin and pull upward with gentle pressure
- Administer
  - —Aspirin as adjunctive therapy for cardiac involvement
  - —NSAIDs for arthritis and arthralgias

Stage I

- Amoxicillin, doxycycline, or cefuroxime (21 days)
- Azithromycin (14–21 days)
- Parenteral therapy in pregnant patients

Stage II

- Oral therapy for isolated Bell's palsy and mild involvement
  - —Amoxicillin with probenecid (30 days) or doxycycline (avoid if pregnant or <9 years old) (10–21 days)
- Parenteral therapy for more severe involvement (meningitis, carditis, severe arthritis)
  - —Ceftriaxone, cefotaxime (14–21 days), or penicillin G (14–28 days)

Stage III

- Parenteral therapy
  - —Penicillin G, cefotaxime (14–21 days), or ceftriaxone (14–28 days)

MEDICATIONS

- Amoxicillin: 500 mg (peds: 40 mg/kg/24hrs) po tid
- Aspirin: 80–100 mg/kg/day (peds: 50–100 mg/kg/day in 6 divided doses) po
- Azithromycin: 500 mg po q day
- Cefotaxime: 2 g (peds: 100–150 mg/kg/24hrs) IV q 8 hrs
- Ceftriaxone: 2 g (peds: 100 mg/kg/24hrs) IV q day
- Doxycycline: 200 mg po BID x 3 days, then 100 mg po bid for 21–28 days
- Penicillin G: 20–24 mIU IV divided q 4–6 hrs
- Probenecid 500mg po tid

Disposition

ADMISSION CRITERIA

- Meningoencephalitis
- Telemetry/ICU admission for carditis

DISCHARGE CRITERIA

- Patients treated with oral therapy

Miscellaneous

ICD9: 88.81

CORE CONTENT CODE: 9.1.10.2

SUGGESTED READINGS

Asch ES, Bujak DI, Weiss M, et al. Lyme disease: An infectious and post-infectious syndrome. J Rheumatol 1994;121:157–162.

Sigal LH. Current recommendations for the treatment of Lyme disease. Drugs 1992;43:683–699.

Steere AC. Lyme disease. N Eng J Med 1989;321:586–596.

Author: Moses Lee

Lymphadenitis

Clinical Presentation

SIGNS AND SYMPTOMS

- Painful swelling, inflammation/infection of lymph nodes
- Commonly presents simultaneously with acute cellulitis or abscess
- Axillary lymphadenitis
  —Fever, axillary pain, and acute lymphedema of arms and chest

MECHANISM/DESCRIPTION

- Lymph nodes may be swollen and tender as part of the systemic response to infection as they become engorged with normal lymphocytes and macrophages. Infection in a distal extremity often results in painful tender adenopathy proximally
- Acute suppurative lymphadenitis may occur after pharyngeal or skin infection

ETIOLOGY

- Most frequently caused by bacterial infection
- Most common organisms
  —Group A β-hemolytic Streptococcus
  —*Staphylococcus aureus*

PEDIATRIC CONSIDERATIONS

- No unique considerations

Pre-Hospital

N/A

Diagnosis

ESSENTIAL WORKUP

- Lymphadenitis is a *clinical diagnosis,* often part of a larger syndrome (cellulitis)
- Physical examination to reveal infectious source

LABORATORY

- White blood cell count is not essential
  —Possible leukocytosis with left shift or normal

IMAGING/SPECIAL TESTS

- None

DIFFERENTIAL DIAGNOSIS

- Systemic infections
  —Cat scratch disease
  —Fungal or parasitic nodular lymphangitis
  —HIV
- Drug reaction
- Phenytoin
- Allopurinol
- Silicone implants
- Malignancy
- Rheumatologic disorders
- Systemic lupus erythematosus
- Rheumatoid arthritis
- Sarcoidosis
- Amyloidosis
- Serum sickness

PEDIATRIC CONSIDERATIONS

- Acute unilateral cervical suppurative lymphadenitis
  —Most common under age 6 years
  —Group A streptococci in 75%

Treatment

INITIAL STABILIZATION

- Insure ABCs and hemodynamic stability

ED TREATMENT

- Antibiotics based on suspected pathogen
  - —Oral first-generation cephalosporins or dicloxacillin well-tolerated, 7–10 days
  - —Erythromycin if penicillin and cephalosporin allergic
  - —Other agents based on concurrent or primary infection source
  - —Refer to Cellulitis and Lymphangitis sections
  - —Parenteral cefazolin in ED may produce adequate blood levels sooner and probenecid orally may prolong duration
- Drainage of abscesses if present
- Elevation
- Application of moist heat
- Analgesics

MEDICATIONS

- Cefazolin: adult: 1–2 g IV/IM; peds: 50–100 mg/kg/day IV div q 6–8 hrs
- Cephalexin: adult: 250–500 mg po qid; peds: 25–50 mg/kg/day po div qid
- Dicloxacillin: adult: 125–500 mg po qid; peds: 12.5–25 mg/kg/day po div q 6 hrs
- Erythromycin: adult: 250–500 mg po qid or 333 mg po tid; peds: Erythromycin ethyl succinate 30–50 mg/kg/day po divided qid
- Probenecid: adult: 1 g po; peds: 25 mg/kg po, not in children <2 years old

Disposition

ADMISSION CRITERIA

- Toxic appearing
- History of immune suppression
- Concurrent chronic medical illnesses
- Unable to take oral medications
- Unreliable patients

DISCHARGE CRITERIA

- Mild infection in a nontoxic-appearing patient
- Able to take oral antibiotics
- No history of immune suppression or concurrent medical problems
- Has adequate follow-up within 24–48 hours

Miscellaneous

OTHER CONSIDERATIONS

- If not found in the context of an acute infection, and not quick to resolve with a course of antibiotics, evaluate for more serious underlying causes (malignancy, etc.)

ICD9: 683

CORE CONTENT CODE: 3.2.1

SUGGESTED READINGS

Boyce JM. Severe streptococcal axillary lymphadenitis. N Engl J Med 1990;323:655–658.

Henry PH, Longo DL. Enlargement of the lymph nodes and spleen. In: Fauci AS, Braunwald E, Isselbacher KJ, et al., eds. Harrisons's principles of internal medicine. 14th ed. New York: McGraw Hill, 1998:345–351.

Swartz MN. Lymphadenitis and lymphangitis. In: Mandell GE, Bennett JE, Dolin R, eds. Mandell, Douglas and Bennett's principles and practice of infectious diseases. 4th ed. New York: Churchill Livingstone, 1995:936–942.

Author: John F. Mahoney

Lymphangitis

Clinical Presentation

SIGNS AND SYMPTOMS

Acute Lymphangitis

- Warm, tender erythematous streaks develop and extend proximally from a source of infection
- Regional lymph nodes often become enlarged and tender (lymphadenitis)
- Systemic manifestations
  —Fever
  —Rigors
  —Tachycardia
  —Headache

Chronic (Nodular) Lymphangitis

- Erythematous nodule, chancriform ulcer, or wartlike lesion develops in the subcutaneous tissue at the inoculation site
- Often presents without pain or evidence of systemic infection
- Multiple lesions possible along lymphatic chain

MECHANISM/DESCRIPTION

- Lymphangitis is an *infection of the lymphatics* that drain a focus of inflammation
- Histologically, the lymphatic vessels are dilated and filled with lymphocytes and histiocytes. The inflammation frequently extends into the perilymphatic tissues and may lead to cellulitis or abscess formation

ETIOLOGY

Acute Lymphangitis

- Likely caused by bacterial infection
- Most common organisms
  —Group A β-hemolytic streptococcus and *Staphylococcus aureus*
- Other organisms
  —*Pasteurella multocida*
  —*Nocardia brasiliensis*
  —*Nocardia asteroides*

Chronic Lymphangitis

- Usually caused by mycotic, mycobacterial and filarial infections
- *Sporothrix schenckii* (most common cause of chronic lymphangitis in U.S.)
  —Inoculation occurs while gardening
  —Organism is present on some plants and in sphagnum moss
  —Multiple subcutaneous nodules appear along the course of the lymphatic vessels
  —Typical antibiotics and local treatment fail to cure the lesion
- *Mycobacterium marinum*
  —Atypical mycobacterium
  —Grows optimally at 25–32°C in fish tanks and swimming pools
  —May produce a chronic nodular, single wart-like or ulcerative lesion at the site of an abrasion
  —Additional lesions may appear in a distribution similar to sporotrichosis
- *Mycobacterium kansasii*
- *Wuchereria bancrofti (filariasis)*

Pre-Hospital

- No specific considerations

Diagnosis

ESSENTIAL WORKUP

- Examination findings
  —Peripheral infection or traumatic injury, accompanied by fever and erythematous streaks proceeding towards regional lymph nodes, indicates lymphangitis
- Directed at discovering the source of the infection

LABORATORY

- White blood count (WBC) is often elevated
- Gram stain and culture obtained from the source lesion may focus antimicrobial selection
- If sporotrichosis or *M. marinum* infection is suspected, the diagnosis should be confirmed by culture of the organism from the wound
- In uncomplicated lymphangitis blood culture is not necessary

IMAGING/SPECIAL TESTS

- Imaging not commonly performed
- Plain x-ray may reveal abscess formation, subcutaneous gas, or foreign bodies if these are suspected

DIFFERENTIAL DIAGNOSIS

- Thrombophlebitis
- Differentiation from lymphangitis
  —Absence of an initial traumatic or infectious focus
  —No regional lymphadenopathy

PEDIATRIC CONSIDERATIONS

- *Haemophilus influenzae* may cause cellulitis in children that have not been vaccinated

Treatment

INITIAL STABILIZATION

- Ensure adequate ABCs and hemodynamic stability

ED TREATMENT

- Antimicrobial therapy should be initiated with first dose in the ED
- To cover both staphylococcus and Group A β-hemolytic streptococcus in acute lymphangitis, a penicillinase-resistant penicillin or first-generation cephalosporin is recommended
  - —First-generation cephalosporins are well tolerated with regard to GI side effects
  - —Penicillin may be used when the etiologic agent is known to be Group A β-hemolytic streptococcus
  - —There are many acceptable alternatives listed in medication section below
- Sporotrichosis
  - —Itraconazole or saturated solution of potassium iodide (SSKI)
- *Mycobacterium marinum*
  - —Antimicrobial therapy is usually reserved for more severe infections
  - —Localized granulomas are usually excised
  - —Limited data on what combination of agents should be employed
  - —Rifampin and ethambutol may be the best choice
- Heat and extremity elevation are also useful adjuncts

MEDICATIONS

- Amoxicillin clavulanate: adult: 500–875 mg po bid or 250–500 mg po tid; peds: 45 mg/kg/day po bid or 40 mg/kg/day po tid
- Azithromycin: adult: 500 mg po day 1; 250 mg po days 2–5 days; peds: 10 mg/kg po day 1; 5 mg/kg po days 2–5
- Cephalexin: adult: 250 mg po qid or 500 mg po bid; peds: 25–50 mg/kg/day po divided qid
- Dicloxacillin: adult: 125–500 mg po qid; peds: 12.5–25 mg/kg/day po divided q 6 hrs
- Erythromycin base: adult: 250–500 mg po qid or 333 mg po tid; peds: EES 40 mg/kg/day po qid
- Itraconazole: adult: 100–200 mg po QD, continue at maximal dose until lesions resolve (6–12 weeks); peds: safety or dose not established
- Nafcillin: adult: 1–2 g IV/IM q 4 hrs, 250–500 mg po q 4–6 hrs; peds: 100–200 mg/kg/24hrs IV divided q 6 hrs
- Penicillin VK: adult: 250–500 mg po qid; peds: 25–50 mg/kg/day po divided qid
- SSKI: adult: 5–10 drops po tid increase to 40–50 po tid; peds: 5–10 drops po tid increase to 25–40 po tid, continue at maximal dose until lesions resolve (6–12 weeks)

Disposition

ADMISSION CRITERIA

- Toxic appearing
- History of immune suppression
- Concurrent chronic medical illnesses
- Unable to take oral medications
- Unreliable patients

DISCHARGE CRITERIA

- Mild infection in a nontoxic-appearing patient
- Able to take oral antibiotics
- No history of immune suppression or concurrent medical problems
- Adequate follow-up within 24–48 hours

Miscellaneous

ICD9: 457.2, 682.9

CORE CONTENT CODE: 3.2.1.2

SUGGESTED READINGS

Kostman JR, DiNubile MJ. Nodular lymphangitis: A distinctive but often unrecognized syndrome. Ann Intern Med 1993;118(11):883–888.

Rex JH. Sporotrichosis. In: Mandell GE, Bennett JE, Dolin R, eds. Mandell, Douglas and Bennett's principles and practice of infectious diseases. 4th ed. New York: Churchill Livingstone, 1995:2321–2323.

Swartz MN. Lymphadenitis and lymphangitis. In: Mandell GE, Bennett JE, Dolin R, eds. Mandell, Douglas and Bennett's principles and practice of infectious diseases. 4th ed. New York: Churchill Livingstone, 1995:942–943.

Authors: Owen T. Traynor; John F. Mahoney

Lymphogranuloma Venereum

Clinical Presentation

SIGNS AND SYMPTOMS

Primary genital lesions

- Painless genital papule, vesicle, or ulcer
- Develops 3–30 days after sexual exposure to *chlamydia trachomatis*
- Lesion often goes unnoticed

Inguinal Adenopathy

- Large inguinal lymph nodes, called buboes, develop days to weeks after primary genital lesions
- Adenopathy is unilateral in two-thirds of cases
- Buboes above and below inguinal ligament produces characteristic "groove sign" in less than one-third of patients
- Buboes may rupture, forming chronic sinus tracts
- Anal receptive patients may develop hemorrhagic proctitis
- Systemic symptoms may include fever, myalgias, headache, meningismus, nausea, and vomiting

Chronic Complications

- Genital strictures, chronic fistulae, and elephantiasis of the ipsilateral leg

ETIOLOGY

Chlamydia trachomatis (lymphogranuloma venereum (LGV))

Pre-Hospital

- No specific considerations

Diagnosis

ESSENTIAL WORKUP

- Thorough history and physical examination

LABORATORY

- Culture of bubo aspirate is specific but expensive and impractical
- Serologic testing for LGV complement fixation is indirect evidence of current or past infection
- Standard chlamydia DNA probes *do not* test for the LGV strain

DIFFERENTIAL DIAGNOSIS

- Genital herpes
- Syphilis
- Chancroid
- Granuloma inguinale

Treatment

INITIAL STABILIZATION

- Patients are typically well appearing and do not need aggressive early interventions

ED TREATMENT

- Start antibiotics in suspected cases
- CDC recommendations: doxycycline
- Alternative antibiotics: erythromycin, or sulfisoxazole
- Needle aspiration of suppurative nodes to prevent chronic sinus drainage from spontaneous rupture; use 18-gauge needle through lateral intact skin
- Incision and drainage of buboes is contraindicated

MEDICATIONS

- CDC recommendations
  —Doxycycline: 100 mg po bid × 21 days
- Alternative antibiotics
  —Erythromycin: 500 mg po qid × 21 days *or*
  —Sulfisoxazole: 500 mg po qid × 21 days

Disposition

ADMISSION CRITERIA

- Hospitalization is rarely required unless there is serious underlying infection

DISCHARGE CRITERIA

- Immunocompetent patient without systemic involvement
- Outpatient follow-up is required to confirm diagnosis and cure

Miscellaneous

ICD9: 099.1

CORE CONTENT CODE: 19.4

SUGGESTED READINGS

Ernst AA, Marvez-Valls E, Martin DH. Incision and drainage versus aspiration of fluctuant buboes in the emergency department during an epidemic of chancroid. Sex Transm Dis 1995;22(4):217–220.

Goens JL, Schwartz RA, DeWolf K. Mucocutaneous manifestations of chancroid, lymphogranuloma venereum and granuloma inguinale. Am Fam Physician 1994;49(2):415–415.

Van Dyck E, Piot P. Laboratory techniques in the investigation of chancroid, lymphogranuloma venereum and donovanosis. Genitourin Med 1992;68(2):130–133.

Authors: Yvette Calderon; Paul Gennis

Maisonneuve Fracture

Clinical Presentation

SIGNS AND SYMPTOMS

- Pain and swelling on the medial aspect of ankle with ecchymosis
- Pain along entire lower leg or both ankle and leg pain
- Inability to bear weight on affected extremity
- Valgus deformity of the ankle due to talar shift
- Bony tenderness over the proximal fibula and the medial malleolus

MECHANISM/DESCRIPTION

- Complex of a medial malleolus avulsion fracture or deltoid ligament tear, disruption of the tibiofibular syndesmosis, and an oblique fracture of the proximal fibula
- External rotation of the adducted or inverted foot. Usually patient's foot is planted and body internally rotates relative to the ankle joint
- Pankovich described five stages of production
  - —Rupture of the anterior—inferior tibiofibular ligament
  - —Fracture of the posterior malleolus of the tibia or rupture of the posterior tibiofibular ligament
  - —Rupture of the anteromedial capsule
  - —Oblique fracture of the proximal fibula
  - —Fracture of the medial malleolus or rupture of the deltoid ligament

Pre-Hospital

CAUTIONS

- The proximal component of the fracture can result in injury to the common peroneal nerve as it wraps around the fibular head if the lower extremity, including the knee, is inadequately immobilized

Diagnosis

ESSENTIAL WORKUP

Physical Examination

- Consider this fracture type in all ankle injuries/fractures and palpate the proximal fibula for tenderness
- Careful evaluation of distal neurovascular status
  - —The peroneal nerve is at risk for injury as it wraps around the fibular head. Test the anterior tibialis and extensor hallucis longus by dorsiflexing the foot and big toe

Radiography

- Anteroposterior, lateral, and mortise (leg internally rotated 20°) views of the ankle
- Anteroposterior and lateral views of the proximal fibula

IMAGING/SPECIAL TESTS

- Stress view the ankle with external rotation to evaluate the stability of the syndesmotic ligaments and the deltoid ligament; these views, however, are frequently not necessary to delineate the fracture

DIFFERENTIAL DIAGNOSIS

- Ankle sprain
- Ankle dislocation

Treatment

INITIAL STABILIZATION

- Immediate reduction of significant deformity if vascular compromise is evident
- Splinting
- Ice
- Elevation

ED TREATMENT

- Analgesia
- Placement in bulky splint
- Long leg cast for those patients without evidence of a medial malleolus fracture and with a normal medial joint space
- Orthopedic consultation in the emergency department is advisable because these injuries typically are unstable and may require operative fix

Disposition

ADMISSION CRITERIA

- Open fracture
- Inadequate closed reduction
- Large amount of swelling to observe for the development of compartment syndrome
- Early operative fixation necessary

DISCHARGE CRITERIA

- Reliable patient
- Good alignment is maintained after reduction
- Early orthopedic follow-up
- Must be nonweight-bearing on crutches or platform walker

Miscellaneous

ICD9: 827.0

CORE CONTENT CODE: 18.4.13.1.5

SUGGESTED READINGS

Geissler WB, Tsao AK. Fractures and injuries of the ankle. In: Rockwood CA, Green DP, Bucholz RW, Heckman JD, eds. Rockwood and Green's fractures in adults. 4th ed. New York: Lippincott Raven, 1996:2201–2258.

Pankovich AM. Maisonneuve fracture of the fibula. J Bone Joint Surg 1976;58A:337–342.

Authors: Joseph Rabinovich; Stacy Nunberg

Malaria

Clinical Presentation

SIGNS AND SYMPTOMS

General

- Malaise
- Chills
- Fever
  - —Classic malaria paroxysm
    - -15 minutes to 1 hour of chills
    - -Followed by 2–6 hours of nondiaphoretic fever up to 39–42°C
    - -Profuse diaphoresis followed by defervescence
    - -Pattern every 48 hours (vivax and ovale) or every 72 hours (falciparum)
  - —Fever pattern may be varied
- Orthostatic hypotension
- Myalgias/arthralgias

Hematology

- Hemolysis
  - —"Blackwater fever"—named from the dark color of the urine partially due to hemolysis in overwhelming falciparum infections
- Jaundice
- Splenomegaly
  - —More common in chronic infections
  - —May cause splenic rupture

CNS

- Headache
- Mental status changes
- Coma
- Seizures

GI

- Emesis
- Diarrhea
- Abdominal pain

Pulmonary

- Shortness of breath
- Rales
- Pulmonary edema

MECHANISM/DESCRIPTION

- Protozoan infection transmitted through the anopheles mosquito
- Incubation period 8–16 days
- Periodicity of disease due to life cycle of protozoan
  - —Exoerythrocytic phase: immature sporozoites migrate to liver where they rapidly multiply into mature parasites (merozoites)
  - —Erythrocytic phase: mature parasites released into circulation and invade RBC
  - —Replication within RBC followed 48–72 hours later by RBC lysis and release of merozoites into ciruclation which repeat cycle
  - —Fever corresponds to RBC lysis
- Plasmodium falciparum
  - —Usually presents as an acute, overwhelming infection
  - —Able to infect red cells of all ages
    - -Results in greater degree of hemolysis and anemia
  - —Causes widespread capillary obstruction
    - -Results in end organ hypoxia and dysfunction
- More moderate infection in people who are on or who have recently stopped prophylaxis with an agent to which the falciparum is resistant
- Plasmodium vivax and ovale
  - —May present with an acute febrile illness
  - —Dormant liver stages (hypnozoites) that may cause relapse 6–11 months after the initial infection
- Plasmodium malariae
  - —May persist in the blood stream at low levels up to 30 years

ETIOLOGY

- Transmission usually occurs from the bite of infected female anopheles mosquito
- North American transmission possible
  - —Anopheles mosquitoes on the east and west coasts of the United States
  - —Transmission may also occur through infected blood products and shared needles
- *P. falciparium* antibiotic resistance
  - —Chloroquine sensitive in Carribean, Central America, and Middle East
  - —Pyrimethamine-sulfadoxine resistance in South America, Africa, southern and southeast Asia, and Indonesia
  - —Mefloquine resistance in southeast Asia

PEDIATRIC CONSIDERATIONS

- Sickle cell trait protective
- Cerebral malaria more common in children

Pre-Hospital

N/A

Diagnosis

ESSENTIAL WORKUP

- Oil emersion light microscopy of a thick smear Giemsa stain
  - —Demonstrates intraerythrocytic malaria parasites
- Only high degrees of parasitemia will be evident on a standard CBC smear

LABORATORY

- CBC for anemia/thrombocytopenia
- Electrolytes, BUN/Cr, glucose for
  - —Renal failure
  - —Hypoglycemia
  - —Lactic acidosis
- Urinalysis
- Liver function tests

IMAGING/SPECIAL TESTS

- CXR
- IFA, ELISA, or DNA probes
  - —Differentiates the type of plasmodium present
  - —5–7% will have mixed infections
- Lumbar puncture/CSF analysis
  - —Performed to distinguish cerebral malaria from meningitis
  - —CSF lactate/protein elevated with malaria
  - —CSF pleocytosis/hypoglycemia absent with malaria

DIFFERENTIAL DIAGNOSIS

- Meningitis
- Encephalitis
- Stroke
- Acute renal failure
- Acute hemolytic anemia
- Sepsis
- Hepatitis
- Viral diarrheal illness
- Hypoglycemic coma
- Heat stroke

Treatment

INITIAL STABILIZATION

- ABCs
- 0.9%NS fluid bolus for hypotension
- Immediate cooling if temperature >40° C
  - —Acetaminophen
  - —Mist/cool air fans
- Narcan, D50W (or Accucheck), and thiamine if altered mental status

ED TREATMENT

- Dependent on identifying the type of malaria present
- *P. vivax, P. ovale* malariae and nonchloroquine-resistant falciparum
  - —Treated with oral chloroquine in both adults and children
    - -Chloroquine—safe in pregnant women
  - —Chloroquine-sensitive falciparum include Central America, Caribbean, and Middle East
  - —Eradicate persistent hypnozoites in vivax and ovale with primaquine beginning after completion of course of chloroquine
- Chloroquine-resistant falciparum infection—PO treatment options
  - —Quinine plus
    - -Tetracycline or doxycycline (avoid in pregnant women and children <8 years old)
    - -Clindamycin (use in pregnant women and children <8 years old)
    - -Pyrimethamine-sulfadoxine
  - —Mefloquine—safety unproven in pregnancy
- IV treatment for severe malaria
  - —Quinidine (rotary isomer of quinine)
  - —Quinine
    - -Not readily available in the United States
    - -Known abortifacient
- Exchange transfusions
  - —Rapidly removes parasitic RBCs, toxins, and red cell debris replacing them with fresh plasma and RBCs
  - —Efficacy not proven in randomized trials
  - —Consider in seriously ill with *P. falciparum* parasitemias >10%
- Steroids not recommended for cerebral malaria
  - —Dexamethasone worsens both duration of coma and prognosis
- Supportive therapy for complications
- Chemoprophylaxis
  - —Chloroquine
    - -Drug of choice for travel to areas without chloroquine resistance
    - -300 mg po q week
    - -Begin 2 weeks prior to departure and continue for 4 weeks after return
  - —Mefloquine
    - -For chloroquine-resistant areas
    - -250 mg po q week
    - -Begin 2 weeks prior to departure and continue for 4 weeks after return
  - —Doxycycline
    - -For chloroquine/mefloquine-resistant areas
    - -100 mg po q day
    - -Continue for 4 weeks after return
  - —Terminal prophylaxis with 14-day course of primaquine after completing chemoprophylaxis to prevent relapse from hypnozoites of *P. vivax* or *P. ovale*

MEDICATIONS

- Acetaminophen: 1 g (ped: 15–20 mg/kg) po
- Chloroquine: 600-mg base initially (1000 mg of chloroquine phosphate) followed by an additional 300-mg base (500-mg tablet) 6 hrs later and again on days 2 and 3 (peds: 10 mg/kg base po, followed by 5 mg/kg base 6 hrs later and on days 2 and 3)
- Clindamycin: 900 mg (peds: 20–40 mg/kg/24hrs) po tid for 3 days beginning on the third day of quinine therapy
- Dextrose: D50W 1 amp (50 ml or 25 g) (peds: D25W 2–4 ml/kg) IV
- Doxycycline: 100 mg po bid for 7 days
- Mefloquine: 1250-mg single dose (peds: 25-mg/kg single dose)
- Naloxone (narcan): 2 mg (peds: 0.1 mg/kg) IV or IM initial dose
- Primaquine phosphate: 15-mg base (peds: 0.3-mg base/kg/24hrs) po for 14 days
- Pyramethamine-sulfadoxine (fansidar): 3 tablets po on last day of quinine treatment
- Quinidine gluconate: 10 mg/kg loading dose (max 600 mg) in normal saline infused slowly over 1–2 hrs, followed by continuous infusion of 0.02 mg/kg/min until patient is able to begin oral therapy
- Quinine: 650 mg po tid for 3–7 days
- Quinine dihydrochloride: 20 mg salt/kg loading dose in 5% dextrose over 4 hrs, followed by 10 mg salt/kg over 2–4 hours every 8 hrs (max 1800 mg/day) until patient is able to begin oral treatment
- Tetracycline: 250 mg qid for 7 days
- Thiamine (vitamin B_1): 100 mg (peds: 50 mg) IV or IM

Disposition

ADMISSION CRITERIA

- ICU admission for severe *P. falciparum* infection
- Suspected acute *P. falciparum* infection
- Severe dehydration
- Inability to tolerate oral solution/medication
- >3% of RBC containing parasites

DISCHARGE CRITERIA

- Non-*P. falicparium* infection
- Able to tolerate oral medications

Miscellaneous

ICD9: 84.6

CORE CONTENT CODE: 9.3.1

SUGGESTED READINGS

Hoffman SL. Diagnosis, treatment, and prevention of malaria. Med Clin North Am 1992;76(6);1327–1355.

Stanley J. Malaria. Emerg Med Clin North Am. 1997;15:113–155.

Strickland GT. Fever in the returned traveler. Med Clin North Am 1992;76(6);1375–1391.

White NJ. The treatment of malaria. N Engl J Med 1996;335:800–806.

Author: Kathryn Brinsfield

Malgaigne Fracture

Clinical Presentation

SIGNS AND SYMPTOMS

- Gross pelvic instability, often with anterior iliac crest displaced or mobile
- Shortening of the legs from migration of the hemipelvis
- Ecchymoses, swelling, abrasions, and open wounds involving the hips, groin, buttocks, perineum, pelvis
- Severe pain on pelvic movement, tilt, and compression
- Often presents in the setting of multiple trauma
- Evidence of perineal, urethral, rectal, and vaginal injuries
- See chapter: Hemorrhagic Shock
  - —Tachycardia, hypotension, narrowed pulse pressure
  - —Altered mental status, cool and pale extremities

MECHANISM/DESCRIPTION

- Malgaigne fracture indicates that significant forces were applied to the pelvic bones
- Vertical shear forces result in anterior and posterior disruption of the hemipelvis
- Most commonly, these fractures occur as result of motor vehicle accidents (MVA)—pedestrian struck by automobile—or falls from great heights
- As many as 20% of all MVA fatalities have associated Malgaigne fracture
- These fractures are among the most unstable pelvic fractures with displacement or potential displacement of the entire hemipelvis
- Associated injuries that must be sought
  - —*Pelvic hemorrhage and hemorrhagic shock*
  - —Intra-abdominal
  - —Genitourinary and urinary tract
  - —Gynecologic injuries including uterine and vaginal
  - —Neurologic
  - —Major vessel

ETIOLOGY

- The Malgaigne fracture is a Type III pelvic fracture involving at least 2 breaks in the continuity of the pelvic ring
- Both anterior and posterior disruption with real or potential displacement of the intervening fragments or hemipelvis

PEDIATRIC CONSIDERATIONS

- Children can have proportionately greater blood loss with pelvic fractures
- The possibility of nonaccidental trauma should always be considered

Pre-Hospital

CONTROVERSIES

- Use of the Pneumatic Anti-Shock Garment (PASG) is an alternative in victims suspected of having a pelvic fracture, particularly when faced with a prolonged transport time or hemodynamically instability

CAUTIONS

- Aggressive fluid resuscitation must occur before deflation of the PASG abdominal compartment if it has been used

Diagnosis

ESSENTIAL WORKUP

- *Pelvic radiology* is the most valuable initial diagnostic test
- A single AP view of the pelvis should be done early for any major trauma victim
  - —Most Malgaigne fractures will be seen on the AP view of the pelvis
- An *inlet projection* (30° caudal angulation) allows visualization of posterior pelvis and may aid in the assessment of posterior displacement
- Other radiographic signs suggesting the presence of a Malgaigne fracture include
  - —Pubic symphysis disruption with diastasis greater than 15 mm
  - —Symphysis disruption associated with overlapping of the pubis
  - —Symphysis disruption associated with unilateral fracture of both rami
  - —Bilateral breaks of both pelvic rami or markedly displaced unilateral fractures of both rami
  - —A vertical fracture of the sacrum (these fractures rarely occur as isolated pelvic fractures)
  - —Asymmetry of iliac wings
  - —Avulsion of the ischial spine or L5 transverse process associated with hemipelvis migration

LABORATORY

- Type and crossmatch for blood
- Hemoglobin/hematocrit, platelet count, and coagulation studies (PT/PTT)

IMAGING/SPECIAL TESTS

- CT scan further delineates Malgaigne fracture and *retroperitoneal hematoma*
- MRI scan may be indicated when there is evidence of neurologic injury
- *Abdominal ultrasound (US)* or *Diagnostic peritoneal lavage (DPL)* are rapid bedside evaluations for intraperitoneal hemorrhage
  - —There is a high mortality rate in victims with Malgaigne fractures who undergo celiotomy; caution must be exercised to avoid false positive results
  - —In the setting of Malgaigne fracture, the supraumbilical open approach for DPL should be used

DIFFERENTIAL DIAGNOSIS

- Other Type III pelvic fractures (straddle fracture, open book fracture, severe multiple pelvic fractures)
- Intra-abdominal injury and hemorrhage

Treatment

INITIAL STABILIZATION

- ABCs of trauma
  - —Aggressive airway management
  - —Avoid using lower extremity IV sites
  - —Aggressive resuscitation with blood or crystalloid, O-negative or type-specific blood if hemodynamically unstable
  - —Immobilize the pelvis to prevent further injury and decrease bleeding
    - -Pneumatic anti-shock garment (PASG): use in ED is controversial but allows rapid pelvic immobilization and pelvic compression to slow bleeding
    - -External fixator: requires more time to place than PASG but "splints" pelvis in a similar manner. Contraindicated in severely comminuted Malgaigne pelvic fracture
    - -Placement of a stabilization device should not interfere with further workup and care (DPL, etc.)

ED TREATMENT

- Immediate trauma surgery and orthopedics consultation; patient should be NPO
- Pelvic hemorrhage
  - —Angiography and selective vessel embolization; particularly for small vessel arterial bleeding
  - —Direct operative control of pelvic bleeding; most likely necessary for large vessels
- Prioritization of studies: CT, angiography, or surgery
  - —In the hemodynamically *unstable* patient, a rapidly performed US or DPL can determine treatment course with minimal delay. If the US or DPL aspirate is positive, the patient should go for celiotomy with external pelvic fixation followed by selective angiography
  - —If the US or DPL is negative, the patient should go to angiography
  - —If the US or DPL is positive by cell count only, the patient should go to angiography with external fixation first, then to celiotomy
  - —In the hemodynamically *stable* patient, the patient can go to CT scan for evaluation of the abdomen, pelvis, and retroperitoneum

MEDICATIONS

- Crystalloid fluids: normal saline or lactated ringers: adult: IV bolus 2 L; peds: 20 cc/kg
- Blood products: crossmatched, type specific, or O-negative: adult: 4–6 IU; peds: 10cc/kg

Disposition

ADMISSION CRITERIA

- All patients with Malgaigne fractures should be admitted given the magnitude of the insult, the instability of the fracture, and the likelihood of pelvic hemorrhage and concomitant injury
- Patients should be admitted to an ICU or monitored setting

DISCHARGE CRITERIA

- No patients with an acute Malgaigne fracture should be discharged from the ED

Miscellaneous

ICD9: 808.43, 808.8

CORE CONTENT CODE:18.4.15.4

SUGGESTED READINGS

Berger JJ, Britt LD. Pelvic fracture hemorrhage. Current strategies in diagnosis and management. Surg Annu 1995;27:107–112.

Cryer H, Miller F, Evers B. Pelvic fracture classification: Correlation with hemorrhage. J Trauma 1988;28:973–980.

Cwinn AA. Pelvis and hip. In: Rosen P, et al., eds: Emergency medicine: Concepts and clinical practice. 4th ed. St. Louis: CV Mosby, 1998:739–762.

Evers M, Cryer H, Miller F. Pelvic fracture hemorrhage: Priorities in management. Arch Surg 1989;124:424.

Jerrard DA. Pelvic fractures. Emerg Med Clin North Am 1993;11(1):147–163.

Author: Theodore C. Chan

Mallet Finger

Clinical Presentation

SIGNS AND SYMPTOMS

- The only symptom is pain in the DIP joint area
- Physical signs include inability to fully extend the distal phalanx, pain and swelling at the dorsal DIP joint

MECHANISM/DESCRIPTION

- A mallet finger is caused by forced flexion of the distal interphalangeal joint of a finger. This injury can be of bony or tendinous origin
  - —Usually it consists of a closed fracture of the dorsal base of the distal phalanx with the extensor tendon holding the proximal fragment, allowing the rest of the distal phalanx to have unopposed flexor motion
  - —The alternate mechanism is a rupture of the extensor tendon at its insertion on the phalanx

ETIOLOGY

- The most frequent cause of the injury is a ball striking a fully extended digit, causing the forced flexion

PEDIATRIC CONSIDERATIONS

- Diagnosis of the fracture may be more difficult in children due to lack of calcification of the fracture fragment. The physical exam is unchanged

Pre-Hospital

N/A

Diagnosis

ESSENTIAL WORKUP

- A complete history, physical exam of the hand, and an x-ray series of the digit are required

LABORATORY

- None necessary

IMAGING/SPECIAL TESTS

- No additional tests are needed

DIFFERENTIAL DIAGNOSIS

- Fracture and/or dislocation of the body of the phalanx
- Open laceration of the extensor tendon

Treatment

INITIAL STABILIZATION

- Ice; immobilization of affected joint as outlined below

ED TREATMENT

- Elevation, rest, and intermittent application of ice are appropriate for all hand injuries. The injured joint (DIP) should be placed in extension and splinted
  —Hyperextension of DIP should be avoided to prevent blanching of dorsal skin and subsequent skin breakdown with prolonged immobilization
  —The splint may be on the dorsal or volar surface, or a combination, but should be appropriately padded as it must remain in place for a full 8 weeks

MEDICATIONS

- Analgesics may be necessary, but narcotics are usually not indicated

PEDIATRIC CONSIDERATIONS

- Even if the fracture fragment cannot be seen on x-ray, the physical findings are so definitive that treatment should be instituted

Disposition

ADMISSION CRITERIA

N/A

DISCHARGE CRITERIA

- Patients may be managed as outpatients in an appropriate splint with orthopedist follow-up within a week

Miscellaneous

ICD9: 736.1

CORE CONTENT CODE: 18.4.12.1

SUGGESTED READINGS

American Society for Surgery of the Hand. The hand: Examination and diagnosis. 2d ed. New York: Churchill Livingston, 1983:505–600.

American Society for Surgery of the Hand. The hand: Primary care of common problems. 2d ed. New York: Churchill Livingston, 1990:637–649.

Antosia RE, Lyn E: The Hand. In: Rosen P, et al. Emergency medicine: Concepts and clinical practice. 4th ed. St. Louis: Mosby-Year Book, 1998:625–668.

Uehara DT. The hand in emergency medicine. Emerg Clin North Am 1993;11(3) 781–96.

Author: Matthew Walsh

Mallory-Weiss Syndrome

Clinical Presentation

SIGNS AND SYMPTOMS

- Multiple bouts of vomiting and retching followed by hematemesis
  - —Majority of bleeding spontaneously resolves
- Also occurs after
  - —Seizures
  - —Forceful coughing/laughing
  - —Lifting
  - —Straining
  - —Blunt abdominal trauma
  - —Childbirth
- Abdominal pain
  - —Found in the presence of gastritis, esophagitis, or gastric ulcer disease

MECHANISM/DESCRIPTION

- Intraluminal mucosal tear of the distal esophagus
- Sudden increase in intra-abdominal pressure causes mucosal tear in the distal esophagus or gastric cardia
- Bleeding is arterial and ranges from mild to moderate
- Cause of bleeding may be related to underlying pathology; "mushrooming" of the stomach into the esophagus during retching has been observed endoscopically

ETIOLOGY

- Often found in those who consume alcohol especially after a recent binge
- Patients with hiatal hernia appear to be at increased risk

PEDIATRIC CONSIDERATIONS

- Rarely found in children

Pre-Hospital

CAUTIONS

- Airway control
  - —100% oxygen or intubate if unresponsive or airway patency in jeopardy
- Initiate one or two large-bore intravenous (IV) catheters if hemodynamically unstable or massive hemorrhage
  - —Lactated ringer's (LR) solution or 0.9%NS
  - —1 L bolus (20 cc/kg) if hypotensive
- Trendelenburg position if hypotensive

Diagnosis

ESSENTIAL WORKUP

- Spun Hct
- CBC
- PT/PTT
- Rectal exam for occult blood in stool

LABORATORY

- Electrolytes, BUN/Cr, glucose
- Amylase/lipase if abdominal pain
- Type and cross
  - —At least 4 units of packed red blood cells (PRBC's) if bleeding is severe

IMAGING/SPECIAL TESTS

- ECG in elderly or those with cardiac history
- Upright CXR for free air from esophageal or gastric perforation
- Endoscopy (esophagogastroscopy)
  - —Procedure of choice to locate, identify, and treat the source of bleeding

DIFFERENTIAL DIAGNOSIS

- Nasopharyngeal bleeding
- Hemoptysis
- Esophageal rupture (Boerhaave's syndrome)
- Esophagitis
- Gastritis
- Duodenitis
- Ulcer disease
- Varices
- Carcinoma
- Vascular-enteric fistula

Treatment

INITIAL STABILIZATION

- ABCs
  - —Intravenous access with at least one large-bore catheter; more if unstable
  - —Central catheter placement if unstable for more efficient delivery of fluids and monitoring of central venous pressure
  - —IV fluids of either 0.9%NS (or LR) at 250 cc/hr if stable; wide open if hemodynamically unstable
  - —Dopamine for persistent hypotension unresponsive to aggressive fluid resuscitation
- Large-bore Ewald tube placement
  - —Safe
  - —Will not aggravate Mallory-Weiss tear
  - —Lavage blood from stomach with water while the patient is on side in Trendelenburg position
- Transfuse O-negative red blood cells immediately if hypotensive and not responsive to 2 L of crystalloid
- Most bleeding from Mallory-Weiss syndrome stops spontaneously with conservative therapy

ED TREATMENT

- Transfuse packed red blood cells if unstable or lowering Hct with continued hemorrhage
- Bladder catheter to monitor urine output
- Monitor fluid status closely
- With continuing hemorrhage, arrange for immediate endoscopy
  - —Control bleeding endoscopically via coagulation techniques and application of blood-clotting agents
- Administer intravenous vasopressin in massive bleeding and unavailable endoscopy
- Intra-arterial vasopressin infusion or arterial embolization in persistent/unresponsive hemorrhage
- Surgery—last but definitive treatment modality employing techniques to oversew the bleeding site or perform a gastrectomy
- Sengstaken-Blakemore Tubes
  - —Avoid because of potential for complications (especially in the presence of hiatal hernia)
  - —May use as last effort when other modalities have failed with mixed results
- Antacids and H_2 blockers unnecessary

MEDICATIONS

- Dopamine: 2–20 μg/kg min IVPB
- Vasopressin: 0.2–0.4 IU/min IVPB titrating up to 0.9 IU/min as necessary

Disposition

ADMISSION CRITERIA

- ICU admission for
  - —Continued or massive hemorrhage
  - —Hemodynamic instability
  - —Extreme age
  - —Poor underlying medical condition
  - —Complications
- General floor admission if always stable with minimal bleed that has since cleared

DISCHARGE CRITERIA

- History of minimal bleed that has stopped
- Hemodynamically stable
- Normal/stable hematocrit
- Negative or trace heme-positive stool
- Negative or trace gastric aspirate

Miscellaneous

ICD9: 530.7

CORE CONTENT CODE: 1.1.2.4

SUGGESTED READINGS

Bubrick MP, et al. Mallory-Weiss syndrome: Analysis of fifty-nine cases. Surgery 1980;88(3);400–405.

Hastings PR, et al. Mallory-Weiss syndrome: Review of 69 cases. Am J Surg 1981;142(5);560–562.

Michel L, et al. Mallory-Weiss syndrome: Evolution of diagnostic and therapeutic patterns over two decades. Ann Surg 1980;192(6);716–721.

Sugawa C, et al. Mallory-Weiss syndrome: A study of 224 patients. Am J Surg 1983;145(1);30–33.

Author: Dino Rumero

Malrotation

Clinical Presentation

SIGNS AND SYMPTOMS

- Neonates
  - —Bilious emesis
  - —Constipation
  - —Bloody stools
  - —Abdominal distension
  - —Difficulty feeding
  - —Poor weight gain
- Older than 1 year
  - —Abdominal pain followed by bilious emesis
- Older children and adolescents
  - —Chronic vomiting
  - —Intermittent colicky abdominal pain
  - —Diarrhea
  - —Hematemesis
  - —Constipation
  - —Many children (50–75%) may not exhibit abnormal *physical* findings at the time of presentation
  - —Symptoms in adults are vague and nonspecific

MECHANISM/DESCRIPTION

- Usually found in combination with other congenital anomalies (70%)
- When associated with volvulus, it is typically the patient's only surgical problem
- Other associated gastrointestinal anomalies include
  - —Duodenal atresia/web
  - —Meckel's diverticulum
  - —Intussusception
  - —Gastroesophageal reflux
  - —Omphalocele or gastroschisis
  - —Congenital diaphragmatic hernia
  - —Hirschsprung's disease

ETIOLOGY

- When embryonic development does not proceed normally
  - —Duodenojejunal junction remains right of midline
  - —Cecum remains in the upper left abdomen with abnormal mesenteric attachments

Pre-Hospital

CAUTIONS

- Volume and electrolyte replacement needed in patients with severe emesis or significant dehydration

Diagnosis

ESSENTIAL WORKUP

- Diagnosis is suggested by history and delineated by radiography

LABORATORY

- Electrolytes, BUN/Cr, glucose
  - —Assessment of severity of emesis
  - —Hypoglycemia in infants with poor feeding and emesis
- CBC
- Urinalysis

IMAGING/SPECIAL TESTS

- Plain abdominal x-rays
  - —Diagnostic in fewer than 30%
  - —May suggest volvulus if there is evidence of
    - -Duodenal obstruction (requiring no further studies)
    - -Gastric distention with paucity of intraluminal gas distally
    - -Generalized distention of small bowel loops
  - —Upright films in the neonate
    - -Triangular gas shadows in the right upper quadrant from the liver edge overlying the air-filled duodenum
- Upper GI contrast studies
  - —95% sensitive and 86% accurate
  - —Findings
    - -Absence of the ligament of Treitz
    - -Dilatation of the proximal duodenum with a termination in a conical or beak shape
    - -Spiral or corkscrew appearance of the duodenum, proximal jejunum on the right side of the abdomen (although readily displaced in neonates), or thickening of small bowel folds
- Contrast enema
  - —If obstruction equivocal
    - -Evaluates for position of the cecum
    - -More than 20% false-negative
- Sonography
- CT scan
- MRI
- Angiography ("barber pole sign")

DIFFERENTIAL DIAGNOSIS

- Early life
  - —Midgut volvulus
  - —Hirschsprung's disease
  - —Necrotizing enterocolitis
- Children—acute abdominal pain with peritoneal signs
  - —Intussusception
  - —Appendicitis
  - —Overwhelming sepsis
- Older children and adults—vague abdominal pain
  - —Irritable bowel syndrome
  - —Peptic ulcer disease
  - —Biliary and pancreatic disease
  - —Psychiatric disorders

Treatment

INITIAL STABILIZATION

- ABCs
- 0.9% IV fluid bolus for shock, overwhelming sepsis or significant dehydration
- Initiate antibiotic for signs of sepsis

ED TREATMENT

- Surgical correction when associated with midgut volvulus for
  —Detorsion of the volvulus
  —Restoration of intestinal perfusion
  —Resection of obviously necrotic areas
  —Replacement of long segments with questionable vascular integrity back into the abdominal cavity for return celiotomy in 36 hours

Disposition

ADMISSION CRITERIA

- Patients requiring surgery
- Significant dehydration
- Shock
- Sepsis
- Acute abdomen

DISCHARGE CRITERIA

- Outpatient evaluation of the stable patient
- Surgical evaluation

Miscellaneous

ICD9: 751.4

CORE CONTENT CODE: 13.1.12

SUGGESTED READINGS

Ford EG, Senac Mo, Srikanth MS, Weitzman JJ. Malrotation of the intestine in children. Ann Surg 1992;215(2):172–78.

Maxson RT, Franklin PA, Wagner CW. Malrotation in the older child: surgical management, treatment, and outcome. Am Surg 1995;61(2):135–38.

Messineo A, MacMillan JH, Palder SB, Filler RM. Clinical factors affecting mortality in children with malrotation of the intestine. J Pediatr Surg 1992;27(10):1343–345.

Torres AM, Ziegler MM. Malrotation of the intestine. World J Surg 1993;17(3):326–31.

Author: Charles G. Macias

Mandibular Fracture

Clinical Presentation

SIGNS AND SYMPTOMS:

- Patient complaints include
  - —Facial asymmetry, deformity, dysphagia, and mandibular pain
  - —Malocclusion, decreased range of motion of the temporomandibular joint, or a grating sound conducted to the ear with movement of the mandible

MECHANISM/DESCRIPTION

- Fracture of the mandible is usually due to a direct force
- The most common area to be fractured is the angle, followed by the condyle, molar, and mental regions
- Because of its thickness the mandibular symphysis is rarely fractured

ETIOLOGY

- The mandible is the third most common facial fracture following nasal and zygomatic fractures
- Fractures usually result from a direct force applied to the mandible by motor vehicle accidents, personal violence, contact sports, or industrial accidents
- Patients are often intoxicated and unable to give a clear history of events

Pre-Hospital

CAUTIONS:

- First priority is to protect the airway as severe fractures of facial structures may result in airway obstruction from lack of glossal supporting structures, blood clots, loose teeth, dentures, or bony fragments
- Protect the C-spine

Diagnosis

ESSENTIAL WORKUP:

Physical Examination

- Inspect the maxillofacial area for obvious deformity including areas of ecchymosis or swelling
- Loose, fractured, or missing teeth, gross malalignment of teeth, separation of tooth interspaces, and ecchymosis or hematoma of the floor of the mouth
- Step-off, bony disruption, or point tenderness with palpation along the entire length of the mandible
- Protrusion or lateral excursion of the jaw. Interference with normal mandibular function including decreased range of motion or deviation of the mandible with opening
  - —The examiner should be able to insert three fingers between the mandible and maxilla
  - —Mandible fracture is also suggested by inability of the patient to break a tongue depressor placed between the teeth and forced downward
- Paresthesia of the lower lip or gums strongly indicates a mandibular fracture with secondary damage to the inferior alveolar nerve
- Inability of the examiner to note motion of the mandibular condyles when palpated through the external ear canals with motion of the jaw is highly suggestive of a mandibular fracture

IMAGING/SPECIAL TESTS

- Plain films including an AP, bilateral obliques, and a Townes view should be obtained
  - —Mandibular views are best for evaluating the condyles and neck of mandible
- Dental panoramic view should be obtained
  - —Panorex best evaluates the symphysis and body
- If condylar fracture is still suspect and not noted on initial radiographs, obtain CT of the condyles in the coronal plane
- Multiple fractures are noted in greater than 50% because of the ringlike structure of the mandible

DIFFERENTIAL DIAGNOSIS

- Contusions
- Dislocation of the mandible may also result from blunt trauma. If a single condyle is dislocated, the jaw will deviate away from the side of the dislocation. If fractured, the jaw will deviate towards the fractured side
- Isolated dental trauma may have a similar presentation

Treatment

INITIAL STABILIZATION:

- 20–40% of patients with mandibular fractures have associated injuries and emergency treatment is directed towards immediate, potentially lethal injuries such as airway obstruction, aspiration, major hemorrhage, cervical spine or cord injury, and intracranial injury
- Airway must be protected as intraoral edema and hematoma, bony fragments, loose teeth, broken dentures, and loss of tongue support may compromise the airway
- C-spine precautions must be maintained
- If intubation is to be performed, an oral tracheal tube should be placed
- If oral intubation cannot be performed secondary to extent of injuries, a blind nasotracheal intubation should be performed unless associated facial injuries are present, in which case cricothyrotomy is indicated

ED TREATMENT:

- With the exception of condylar fractures many mandibular fractures are associated with mucosal, gingival, or tooth socket disruption, and should be considered open fractures
  - —Patients should receive antibiotics such as penicillin or erythromycin to cover intraoral anaerobic pathogens
- Tetanus prophylaxis if appropriate
- Definitive care usually consists of reduction and fixation by wiring upper and lower teeth in occlusion for 4–6 weeks
  - —This may not be possible initially due to patient instability or local edema
  - —Linear, nondisplaced or greenstick fractures may be treated with soft diet without wiring
- If *mandible dislocation* is present, bilateral downward pressure while the jaw is open is placed on the occlusal surface of the posterior lower teeth while grasping the mandible
  - —The goal is to free the condyle from its anterior position to the eminence
  - —Reduction is facilitated by muscle relaxants (diazepam or midazolam), or anesthetic injection of mastication muscles
  - —A bite block should be used or examiner's fingers should be wrapped in gauze to prevent injury

MEDICATIONS

- Diazepam: adult: 10 mg IV; peds: 0.1–0.2 mg/kg/dose IV
- Midazolam: adult: 2–5 mg IV; peds: safety not established but 0.02–0.05 mg/kg/dose have been used
- Penicillin: adult: 500mg po qid; peds: 25–50 mg/kg/24hrs divided q 6 hrs po
- Erythromycin: adult: 500mg po qid; peds: 30–50 mg/kg/24hrs divided q 6–8 hrs po

PEDIATRIC CONSIDERATIONS

- Mandibular fractures are uncommon in children <6 years of age. When they do occur, they are usually greenstick fractures and can be managed with soft diet alone. The parents should be informed that because any fracture of the mandible has the potential to damage permanent teeth and cause facial asymmetry, long-term follow-up with a specialty consultant is advisable

Disposition

ADMISSION CRITERIA

- Those fractures in which there is significant displacement or associated dental trauma, or those fractures that are thought to be open, require urgent specialty consultation for admission
- The severity of associated trauma may indicate admission
- Any patient with the potential for airway compromise, including oropharyngeal edema or bilateral mandibular body fractures, should be admitted
- An unreliable patient with nondisplaced fractures should be admitted for definitive fixation
- In the pediatric population, if the mechanism of injury is not appropriate to the injuries seen, pediatric or child protective services consultation should be obtained

DISCHARGE CRITERIA

- Relatively asymptomatic patients with nondisplaced, closed fractures may be discharged on analgesics and a soft diet. They should be referred to an otorhinolaryngologist or an oral maxillofacial surgeon within 1–2 days

Miscellaneous

ICD9: 802.20

CORE CONTENT CODE: 18.4.4.2

SUGGESTED READINGS

Alonso LL, Purcell TB. Accuracy of the tongue blade test in patients with suspected mandibular fracture. J Emerg Med 1995;13:297–304.

Busuito MJ, Smith DJ, Robson MC. Mandibular fractures in an urban trauma center. J Trauma 1986;26:826–829.

Luyk NH, Ferguson JW. The diagnosis and initial management of the fractured mandible. Am J Emerg Med 1991;9:352–359.

Shepherd, S. Maxillofacial trauma: Evaluation and management by the emergency physician. Emerg Med Clin North Am 1987;5(2):371–392.

Authors: Anthony J. Musielewicz; David W. Munter

Marine Envenomation

Clinical Presentation

SIGNS AND SYMPTOMS

Sponges

- Itching and burning a few hours after contact
- Local joint swelling and soft tissue edema
- Fever
- Malaise
- Dizziness
- Nausea
- Muscle cramps
- In severe cases, desquamation in 10 days to 2 months

Coelenterates (Cnidaria—"Jellyfish")

- Mild envenomation
  —Immediate stinging sensation
  —Pruritus
  —Paresthesia
  —Throbbing
  —Blistering/local edema/wheal formation
- Moderate/severe
  —Neurologic
    -Malaise
    -Headache
    -Vertigo/ataxia
    -Paralysis
    -Delirium
    -Seizures
  —Cardiovascular
    -Anaphylaxis
    -Hemolysis
    -Hypotension
    -Arrhythmias
  —Respiratory
    -Bronchospasm
    -Laryngeal edema
    -Pulmonary edema
    -Respiratory failure
  —Musculoskeletal
    -Muscle cramps or spasm
    -Arthralgias
  —Gastrointestinal
    -Nausea, vomiting, diarrhea
    -Dysphagia
    -Hypersalivation
  —Ophthalmologic
    -Conjunctivitis
    -Corneal ulcers
    -Elevated intraocular pressure

Echinodermata

Starfish

- Immediate pain
- Bleeding
- Mild edema

Sea urchins

- Intense pain and severe local muscle aches
- Nausea, vomiting
- Paresthesias, hypotension, or respiratory distress with multiple stings

Sea Cucumbers

- Mild contact dermatitis
- Corneal and conjunctival involvement
  —Severe reactions can lead to blindness

Mollusks

Cone Shells

- Puncture wounds similar to wasp stings
- Sharp burning and stinging
- Paresthesias indicate severe envenomation
- Can evolve into muscular paralysis and respiratory failure, dysphagia, syncope, DIC

Stingrays

- Puncture wounds or jagged lacerations
- Local, intense pain, edema, bleeding; necrosis if severe
- Nausea, vomiting, diarrhea
- Diaphoresis
- Headache
- Tachycardia
- Seizures
- Paralysis
- Hypotension
- Arrhythmias

Scorpionfish

- Intense local pain for 6–12 hours
- Erythema may progress to cellulitis
- Headache
- Nausea, vomiting, diarrhea
- Pallor
- Delirium
- Seizures
- Fever
- Hypertension

Catfish

- Local pain, ischemic appearance progressing to erythema
- Swelling, bleeding, and edema
- Local muscle spasms
- Diaphoresis
- Neuropathy

Sea Snakes

- Bite initially causes very little pain
- Pin-like pairs of fang marks
- Onset from 5 minutes to 6 hours
- Muscle pain, lower extremity paralysis, arthralgias
- Trismus, blurred vision, dysphagia, drowsiness
- Severe signs include
  —Ascending paralysis
  —Aspiration
  —Coma
  —Renal and liver failure
- 25% mortality if untreated

MECHANISM/DESCRIPTION

- Sponges
  —Contain sharp spicules with irritants that cause a pruritic dermatitis
- Coelenterates (Cnidaria—"Jellyfish")
  —Contain stinging cells known as nematocysts on their tentacles
  —Fluid filled cysts eject a sharp, hollow thread-tube upon contact
  —Thread-tube penetrates skin and envenomates victim
  —Box-jellyfish can kill within 30 seconds
- Starfish
  —Very sharp, rigid spines are coated with a slimy venom
- Sea urchins
  —Hollow, sharp spines filled with various toxins
- Sea cucumbers
  —Hollow tentacles secrete holothurin, a liquid toxin
- Cone shells
  —Venom injected through a dartlike, detachable tooth
  —Active peptides interfere with neuromuscular transmission
  —Presents with puncture wounds similar to wasp stings
- Stingrays
  —Most common cause of human marine envenomations
  —Tapered spines attached to tail inject venom into victim
- Scorpionfish
  —Lionfish usually mild; stonefish can be a life threat
  —Sharp spines along dorsum and pelvis of fish
  —Often stepped on inadvertently
  —Neurotoxic venom
- Catfish
  —Dorsal and pectoral spines contain venom glands
- Sea snakes
  —Hollow fangs with associated venom glands
  —Highly neurotoxic venom blocks neuromuscular transmission

Diagnosis

ESSENTIAL WORKUP

- Careful history/repeat evaluation of wound sites
- Soft-tissue radiographs to detect foreign body

LABORATORY

- CBC
- Electrolytes, BUN/Cr, glucose
- Liver function test
- Urinalysis
- Arterial blood gases if severe symptoms

Treatment

INITIAL STABILIZATION

- ABCs
- Establish IV access with 0.9%NS

ED TREATMENT

General

- Tetanus prophylaxis
- Prepared for anaphylaxis reactions and intubation
- Corticosteroids for severe local reactions
- Narcotic analgesia for severe pain
- Antibiotic prophylaxis for
  —Large lacerations or burns
  —Deep puncture wounds
  —Grossly contaminated wounds
  —Elderly or chronically ill
- Antibiotic choices
  —Trimethoprim-sulfamethoxazole (bactrim)
  —Tetracycline
  —Ciprofloxacin
  —Third-generation cephalosporin

Sponges

- Gently dry skin and remove spicule
  —Adhesive tape may aid in removal
- 5% vinegar (or 40–70% isopropyl alcohol) soaks qid for 10–30 minutes

Coelenterates (Cnidaria—"Jellyfish")

- Rinse wound with saltwater or seawater
  —Hypotonic solutions trigger more nematocysts
- Do not rub skin—may trigger more nematocysts
- Inactivate toxin with 30-minute soak of 5% vinegar
- Remove remaining nematocysts with razor
- Apply topical anesthetics once nematocysts removed
- Box-jellyfish stings (Australia)—emergent cases
  —Administer chironex antivenin
  —1 ampule (20,000 units) IV diluted 1:5 with crystalloid

Echinodermata

Starfish

- Immerse in nonscalding hot water for pain relief
- Irrigate and explore of all puncture wounds

Sea Urchins

- Immerse in nonscalding hot water for pain relief
- Removal of any remaining spines

Sea Cucumbers

- Immerse in nonscalding hot water for pain relief
- 5% acetic acid soaks
- Ocular involvement
  —Proparacaine for pain
  —Copious irrigation with normal saline
  —Careful slitlamp exam

Mollusks

Cone shells

- Hot water immersion for pain relief
- Be prepared for cardiac or respiratory support

Stingrays

- Copious irrigation with removal of any visible spines
- Local suction is controversial
- Hot water soaks for pain relief
- Narcotics for pain control
- High incidence of bacterial infection-consider prophylactic antibiotics

Scorpionfish

- Hot water soaks for pain relief and venom inactivation
- Copious irrigation, removal of any visible spines
- Local lidocaine or regional block for severe pain
- Surgical exploration for deep penetration/foreign bodies
- Stonefish antivenin for severe envenomations
  —May cause serum sickness
  —One 2 ml ampule diluted in 50 ml saline IV slow

Catfish

- Hot water soaks for pain relief and venom inactivation
- Copious irrigation, removal of any visible spines
- Consider local lidocaine, regional block, or narcotics for severe pain
- Surgical exploration for deep penetration/foreign bodies
- Leave puncture wounds open to heal
- Consider prophylactic antibiotics for hand, foot, or deep wounds

Sea Snakes

- Immobilize bitten extremity
- Apply pressure bandage for venous occlusion (pre-hospital)
- Keep victim warm and still
- Polyvalent sea snake antivenin reduces mortality to 3%
  —May require 3–10 ampules (1000 units each)
  —Prepare early for assisted ventilation

MEDICATIONS

- Cefixime: 400 mg (peds: 8 mg/kg/24hrs) po q day
- Ciprofloxacin: 500 mg po bid
- Tetracycline: 500 mg po qid
- Trimethoprim-sulfamethoxazole (bactrim DS): 1 tablet (peds: 5 mg liquid (40/200 per 5 ml)/10 kg/dose) po bid

Disposition

ADMISSION CRITERIA

- Significant signs of systemic involvement

DISCHARGE CRITERIA

- No signs of systemic illness after 8 hours of observation
- Wound check within 48 hours

Miscellaneous

ICD9: 989.5

CORE CONTENT CODE: 5.10.3

SUGGESTED READINGS

Aldred B, Erickson T, Lioscomb J. Lionfish envenomations in an urban wilderness. Wilderness Environ Med 1996;4:291–296.

Bowman MA, Herman BE. Marine envenomations. In: Strange G, Ahreno W, Lelyveld S, et al, eds. Pediatric emergency medicine. New York: McGraw Hill. 1996:599–600.

McKinistry DM. Catfish stings in the United States: Case report and review. J Wilderness Med 1993;4:293.

Authors: Adam Black; Timothy Erickson

Mastitis

Clinical Presentation

SIGNS AND SYMPTOMS

- Fever usually >39°C
- Chills, rigors, malaise
- Tachycardia
- Breast pain, induration, erythema, warmth; usually unilateral
- Onset typically 2–3 weeks to months postpartum while breastfeeding
- Rare during first postpartum week

ETIOLOGY

- *Staphylococcus aureus* most common
- Coagulase-negative staphylococcus, streptococcus species, *Escherichia coli, H. influenza*

Pre-Hospital

N/A

Diagnosis

ESSENTIAL WORKUP

- Physical examination with special attention to detecting abscess
  —Purulent nipple discharge with palpation

LABORATORY

- Breast milk culture usually not required

IMAGING/SPECIAL TESTS

None required

DIFFERENTIAL DIAGNOSIS

- Breast engorgement: transient fever <39°C of duration 4–16 hours appearing 48–72 hours postpartum with bilateral nonerythematous bilateral engorgement
- Carcinoma (inflammatory)
- Cyst, tumor
- Abscess formation

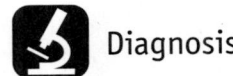

Treatment

INITIAL STABILIZATION

- No specific stabilization

ED TREATMENT

- Outpatient oral antibiotics for 10 days
  - —β-lactamase-resistant penicillin, e.g., dicloxacillin (dynapen)
  - —First-generation cephalosporin, e.g., cephalexin (keflex)
  - —Erythromycin if penicillin allergic
- Surgical consultation if evidence of abscess

MEDICATIONS

- Cephalexin: 500 mg every 6 hours po
- Dicloxacillin: 250 mg every 6 hours po
- Erythromycin: 500 mg every 6 hours po

Disposition

ADMISSION CRITERIA

- Incision and drainage under general anesthesia may be necessary and require admission
- Immunocompromised or evidence of septicemia

DISCHARGE CRITERIA

- The vast majority of patients may be managed in the outpatient setting
- Most symptoms resolve within 48 hours of therapy

Miscellaneous

- In simple mastitis, breastfeeding may be continued, including using the affected breast
  - —Gently massage to enhance drainage
  - —Counsel that this will not harm baby
- Breast support, ice packs, and analgesia for comfort
- In frank abscess, discontinue breastfeeding until purulent discharge resolves

ICD9: 611.0

CORE CONTENT CODE: 12.8.4

SUGGESTED READINGS

Calhoun BC, Brost B. Emergency management of sudden puerperal fever. Obstet Gyn Clin North Am 1995;22(2):357–367

Hansen WF, Hansen AR. Problems in pregnancy. In: Tintinalli J, et al, eds. Emergency medicine: A comprehensive study guide. 4th ed. New York: McGraw Hill, 1996

Author: Marco Coppola

Mastoiditis

Clinical Presentation

SIGNS AND SYMPTOMS

- Symptoms
  - —Ear pain
  - —Otorrhea
  - —Headache
  - —Hearing loss
  - —History of fever or irritability in a child
  - —History of recurrent otitis media
- Signs
  - —Tenderness over the mastoid
  - —Lateral and inferior displacement of the auricle
  - —Red fluctuant mass behind pinna, loss of the postauricular crease
  - —Tympanic membrane abnormalities consistent with a severe otitis media

MECHANISM/DESCRIPTION

- Middle ear and the mastoid air cells are contiguous
- Mastoiditis: inflammation and infection of the mastoid air cells caused by acute purulent otitis media
  - —All otitis media accompanied by some degree of mastoiditis- not usually clinically significant
- Acute mastoid osteomyelitis due to infection of the mastoid air cells leads to destruction of the mastoid trabeculae
  - —May progress to severe head and neck complications if untreated
- Acute mastoiditis
  - —Inflammatory changes of the mastoid
  - —Usually secondary to contamination with infectious material trapped in the mastoid by inflammatory obstruction of the communication between the middle ear and the mastoid air cells
  - —Occurs to some degree with every case of otitis media
- Masked mastoiditis
  - —Mastoid infection which lingers after an acute otitis media has been treated
  - —May progress to acute or coalescent mastoiditis
- Coalescent mastoiditis
  - —Destruction of the trabeculae and honeycombing due to osteomyelitis
- Chronic mastoiditis
  - —Infection lasting more than 3 months

COMPLICATIONS

- Bezold's abscess
  - —Extension of infection to soft tissue of neck after erosion through the mastoid tip
- Gradenigo's syndrome
  - —Erosion of the medial temporal bone causing otorrhea, retro-orbital pain, and CN VI paralysis
- Subperiosteal abscess
- Subdural empyema
  - —Extension of infection to CNS with empyema around the tentorium

ETIOLOGY

- Common isolates
  - —*S. pneumoniae*
  - —*H. influenzae*
  - —*Streptococcal viridans*
  - —Gram negative bacteria most common with chronic mastoiditis
    - -Bacteroides
    - -Pseudomonas pyocyanea
    - -Proteus mirabilis
  - —Mycobacterium tuberculosis—rare cause of acute or chronic mastoiditis
- Prevalence is equal in males and females

PEDIATRIC CONSIDERATIONS

- More frequently seen in the pediatric population

Pre-Hospital

N/A

Diagnosis

ESSENTIAL WORKUP

- Mastoid plain radiographs
  - —May reveal opacification of the mastoid air cells or coalescence
  - —Low sensitivity
- CT Scan
  - —Can determine presence and extent of destruction of trabeculae as well as evaluate for the complications

LABORATORY

- CBC
  - —Leukocytosis
- Cultures of drainage
  - —If spontaneous drainage present or after surgical drainage
- Blood culture

IMAGING/SPECIAL TESTS

- MRI
  - —If intracranial involvement suspected but not confirmed by CT
- Lumbar puncture/CSF evaluation for signs of meningitis

DIFFERENTIAL DIAGNOSIS

- Otitis media
- Cellulitis
- External otitis media
- Scalp infection with inflammation of posterior auricular nodes
- Rubella—posterior auricular node enlargement
- Trauma to pinna or postauricular area

Treatment

INITIAL STABILIZATION

- Airway management for signs of airway compromise
- 0.9%NS IV fluid bolus for hypotension/volume depletion

ED TREATMENT

- Otolaryngologist consult for surgical drainage
  - —Drainage is the definitive therapy for acute or coalescent mastoiditis
  - —Emergent drainage if the patient is toxic appearing
  - —Types of surgical procedures
    - -Myringotomy drainage and tympanostomy tube placement
    - -Mastoidectomy and drainage for severe extension
- Initiate IV antibiotics—options
  - —Semisynthetic penicillins (unasyn, timentin) with chloramphenicol
  - —third-generation cephalosporins (ceftriaxone, cefotaxime)
  - —Imipenem
- Administer pain medications
  - —NSAIDs
  - —Oral or parenteral narcotics

MEDICATIONS

- Ampicillin sulbactam (unasyn): 1.5–3 g IV q 6 hrs
- Cefotaxime: 1–2 g (peds: 50–180 mg/kg/24hrs) IV q 4–6 hrs
- Ceftriaxone: 1–2 g (peds: 50–75 mg/kg/24hrs) IV q 12–24 hrs
- Chloramphenicol: 50–100 mg/kg/24hrs IV/PO q 6 hrs
- Imipenem: 250 mg–1 g IV q 6–8 hrs
- Ticarcillin clavulanate (timentin): 3.1 g IV q 4–6 hrs

Disposition

ADMISSION CRITERIA

- Clinical suspicion of acute or coalescent mastoiditis
- Toxic appearing

DISCHARGE CRITERIA

- No patient with acute or coalescent mastoiditis should be discharged

Miscellaneous

ICD9: 383.00, 383.9, 383.1

CORE CONTENT CODE: 6.5.1

SUGGESTED READINGS

Biter CN, Kluka EA, Steele RW. Mastoiditis in children. Clin Pediatr 1996;35(8):391–395.

Bluestone CD, et al., eds. Pediatric otolaryngology. 2d ed. Philadelphia: WB Saunders, 1990:521–527.

Gliklich RE, Eavey RD, Iannuzzi RA, Camacho AE. A contemporary analysis of acute mastoiditis. Arch Otolaryngol Head Neck Surg 1996;122(2):135–139.

Nadol JB, Eavey RD. Acute and chronic mastoiditis: Clinical presentation, diagnosis, and management. Curr Clin Top Infect Dis 1995;15:204–229.

Peacock WF. Otolaryngologic emergencies. In: Tintinalli, JE, et al., eds. Emergency medicine: A comprehensive study guide. 4th ed. New York: McGraw Hill, 1996:1069–1070.

Pfaff JA, Moore GA. Ear, nose, and throat emergencies. In: Rosen P, Barkin R, Danzl D, et al., eds. Emergency medicine: Concepts and clinical practice. 4th ed. St. Louis: CV Mosby, 1998:2720–2729.

Authors: Michael Simmons; Nicole DuVal

Measles

Clinical Presentation

SIGNS AND SYMPTOMS

Classic Presentation Sequence

- 10-day asymptomatic period postexposure (incubation period) followed by
- 1–2 days of mild respiratory illness followed by
  —Fever (up to 40° C)
  —Cough (often brassy)
  —Coryza, conjunctivitis
  —Nausea
  —*Koplik's spots*—minute whitish, gray spots on buccal mucosa and conjunctivae
- 1–2 days later rash develops
  —Starts at hairline and behind ears
  —Spreads from head to feet
  —Initially pale, subsequently maculopapular
  —Discrete lesions become confluent
  —Clearing begins after 3–4 days
  —Desquamation may occur as rash fades

Respiratory

- Laryngotracheobronchitis occurs in <2 years old
- Pneumonia rare

Cardiovascular

- Transient, occurs infrequently, and is generally of no clinical significance
  —Myocarditis
  —Pericarditis
  —Conduction defects

Hematopoietic System

- Rare hemorrhagic form seen most commonly in Third World countries
- Thrombocytopenic purpura may follow a course of measles

Central Nervous System

- Encephalitis
  —May occur at any time in the course of illness
  —Rare (~0.1%)
  —Symptoms include irritability, seizures, lethargy, coma, ataxia
- Subacute sclerosing panencephalitis (SSPE)
  —Insidious, progressive cerebral dysfunction
  —Develops weeks to years after infection (very rare)
  —Manifestations include personality change, intellectual deterioration, myoclonic jerks, dyskinesias, visual loss, coma, and inevitably death

MECHANISM/DESCRIPTION

- Exceptionally contagious viral infection spread by large respiratory droplets
- Enters host through upper respiratory passages

ETIOLOGY

- Humans are only known reservoir for measles virus
- Most commonly encountered in children
- Outbreaks occur in nonimmune adults

Pre-Hospital

CAUTIONS

- Pre-hospital care workers, if nonimmunized, should be cautioned about the risks of disease transmission
- Pregnant pre-hospital personnel should be advised of the risk of premature birth and spontaneous abortion if they are infected

Diagnosis

ESSENTIAL WORKUP

- Clinical diagnosis
- A history of prodromal symptoms of a URI, followed by coryza, conjunctivitis, and Koplik's spots with subsequent appearance of a maculopapular rash, is sufficient to make the diagnosis

LABORATORY

- Viral cultures technically difficult, impractical
- Antibody testing possible, but unnecessary

IMAGING/SPECIAL TESTS

- CXR for suspected pneumonia
- Lumbar puncture/CSF analysis for suspected encephalitis

DIFFERENTIAL DIAGNOSIS

- Rubella
  —No conjunctivitis or cough
  —Fine rash of short duration
- Scarlet fever
  —Rash occurs 12–14 hours postonset of fever
  —Rash diffuse with sandpaper texture
- Roseola
  —High fever
  —Rash appears after temperature falls
- Erythema infectiosum (fifth disease)
  —No prodrome/no fever
  —Red flushed cheeks/circumoral pallor
  —Maculopapular rash with lacelike appearance when fading
- Enterovirus
  —No respiratory symptoms
- Mucocutaneous lymph node syndrome (Kawasaki's disease)
  —Rash involves palms/soles
  —Dryness/erythema of lips, mouth, tongue, conjunctive
- Drug reactions

Treatment

- Mainstay is prevention
  —Vaccine two dose schedule prophylaxis at 12–15 months and school entry or older

INITIAL STABILIZATION

- ABCs for complicated cases
  —Pneumonia
  —Encephalitis
- Antipyretics (acetaminophen/ibuprofen)

ED TREATMENT

- IV/oral rehydration when indicated
- Confirm diagnosis
- Isolate suspect cases and minimize contacts
- Postexposure prophylaxis for at risk contacts
  —Live measles vaccine if less than 72 hours postexposure (avoid if severe febrile illness, immune deficient, pregnant, or neomycin allergy)
  —Immune globulin prevents illness if given less than 6 days postexposure

MEDICATIONS

- Acetaminophen: 650 mg (peds: 15 mg/kg) po q 4–6 hrs
- Ibuprofen: 400–600 mg (peds: 20mg/kg/24hrs) po q 6–8 hrs
- Immune globulin: 0.25 ml/kg to maximum 15 ml IM

Disposition

ADMISSION CRITERIA

- Severe pneumonia
- Encephalitis
- SSPE
- Immunocompromised hosts
  —AIDS
  —Immunosuppressive therapy
- Admit to respiratory isolation

DISCHARGE CRITERIA

- All other patients
- Contagious
  —From 1–2 days before symptoms (2–5 days before rash) and up to 4 days after onset of rash
  —Immunocompromised patients contagious for the duration of illness

Miscellaneous

ICD9: 55.9

CORE CONTENT CODE: 13.12.4.2

SUGGESTED READINGS

Atkinson WL, Kaplan JM, Clover R. Measles: Virology epidemiology, disease, and prevention. Immunization in medical education. Am J Prev Med 1994;10(Supp):22–30.

Katz M. Clinical spectrum of measles. Curr Top Microbiol Immunol 1995;191:1–12.

Author: Isser Dubinsky

Meckel's Diverticulum

Clinical Presentation

SIGNS AND SYMPTOMS

Common Presenting Sequelae/Complications

- Obstruction
- Intussusception
- Diverticulitis
- Hemorrhage
- Volvulus

Gastrointestinal

- Abdominal pain
  - —Location depends on cause
  - —"Appendicitis-like"
- Vomiting
- Changes in bowel movements
- Hematochezia
- Melena
- Peritonitis and septic shock (late complications)

General

- Fever
- Malaise
- Weakness
- Fatigue

Cardiovascular

- Tachycardia (due to pain or blood loss)
- Hypotension and shock (due to bleeding)

MECHANISM/DESCRIPTION

- Most common congenital abnormality of the gastrointestinal tract
- Remanant of the omphalomesenteric duct, which usually regresses by the 7th week of gestation
- Ileal diverticula
  - —50% contain normal ileal mucosa
  - —50% contain either gastric, duodenal, colonic, or pancreatic mucosa
- "Rule of Two"
  - —Male-Female ratio 2:1
  - —Average length 2 inches
  - —Approximately 2 feet from the ileocecal valve
- Complications
  - —Obstruction and diverticulitis in adults
  - —Hemorrhage and obstruction in children
- Obstruction
  - —Diverticulum attached to the umbilicus, abdominal wall or other viscera, or is free and unattached
  - —Intussusception—diverticulum is the leading edge
  - —Volvulus—persistent fibrous band leads to bowel rotation
- Diverticulitis
  - —Opening obstructed
  - —Bacterial infection follows
  - —Presents like appendicitis (most common preoperative diagnosis with Meckels's diverticulum)

PEDIATRIC CONSIDERATIONS

- Present under the age of 5 with episodic painless rectal bleeding
- Brisk and bright red bleeding
- Most common ectopic: gastric tissue
  - —Gastric secretions lead to erosions and bleeding

Pre-Hospital

CAUTIONS

- High mortality associated with Meckel's diverticulum is due to a lack of recognition of presenting features, potential for hypotension, and complications
- Transport all patients with rectal bleeding or abdominal pain for evaluation
- IV access with 0.9%NS because patients can become hypotensive and require fluid resuscitation

Diagnosis

ESSENTIAL WORKUP

- Meckel's diverticulum causes a variety of signs and symptoms
  - —Consider in any patient with abdominal pain or rectal bleeding
- History/physical narrow diagnosis but will not give findings specific to Meckel's diverticulum
- Rectal exam mandatory
- Nasogastric tube placement
  - —Most common cause of lower GI bleeding is upper GI bleeding

LABORATORY

- CBC
  - —Decreased Hct due to acute bleeding
  - —Meckel's diverticulum rarely a cause of chronic anemia
  - —Leukocytosis with diverticulitis/gangrene/perforation
- Electrolytes, BUN/Cr, glucose
- Type and screen when significant GI bleeding

IMAGING/SPECIAL TESTS

- Abdominal radiographs
  - —No value in diagnosing Meckel's diverticulum
  - —Eliminates other causes of abdominal pain or GI bleeding
- Technetium-99m pertechnetate radioisotope scan
  - —Noninvasive scan that identifies Meckel's diverticulum containing gastric mucosa
  - —90% accurate in children
  - —Positive predictive value only 60% in adults
- Small bowel enteroclysis
  - —Barium/methyl cellulose introduced through NG tube into distal duodenum or proximal jejunum
  - —Radiologist looks for diverticulum
  - —Increases the ability to detect Meckel's diverticulum in adults
- Barium enema
  - —Introduces fluid into distal small bowel
  - —Look for diverticulum
- Angiogram for further evaluation of Meckel's diverticulum if radioisotope scan and enteroclysis normal
- EKG
  - —Eliminate myocardial ischemic causes of abdominal pain
  - —When significant blood loss

DIFFERENTIAL DIAGNOSIS

Abdominal Pain

- Appendicitis
- Volvulus
- Bowel obstruction
- Diverticulitis
- Adhesions
- Internal hernias
- Intussusception

Bleeding

- Intussusception
- Upper GI bleeding
- Diverticulosis
- Hemorrhoids
- Inflammatory bowel disease
- Pseudomembranous colitis
- Polyps

PEDIATRIC CONSIDERATIONS

- Abdominal pain: intussusception, volvulus, atresia, strictures, malrotation, adhesions
- Bleeding: milk allergy, gastroenteritis, intussusception, Henoch-Schönlein purpura, volvulus, hemolytic uremic syndrome, anal fissures, polyps

Treatment

INITIAL STABILIZATION

- ABCs
- Fluid resuscitation with 0.9%NS in 20 cc/kg bolus amounts
- Cardiac monitoring in older patients

ED TREATMENT

- Stabilization followed by early surgical evaluation
- Hypotension
  —Aggressive fluid resuscitation
  —PRBC transfusion with brisk rectal bleeding (more common in children)
  —Pressors for septic shock
- NG tube
- Foley
- Preoperative antibiotics

MEDICATIONS

- Ampicillin sulbactam (unasyn): 3 g (peds: 100–200 mg ampicillin/kg/24hrs) q 8 hrs IV
- Cefoxitin (mefoxin): 1–2 g (peds: 100–160 mg/kg/24hrs) IV q 6 hrs
- Dopamine: 2–20 μg/kg/min IV

Disposition

ADMISSION CRITERIA

- Presumptive diagnosis of Meckel's diverticulum with diverticulitis, obstruction, intussusception, hemorrhage, or volvulus requires admission and surgical evaluation

DISCHARGE CRITERIA

- None

Miscellaneous

ICD 9: 751.0

CORE CONTENT CODE: 13.1.13

SUGGESTED READINGS

Bono MJ. Lower gastrointestinal tract bleeding. Emerg Med Clin North Am 1996;14:547–556.

Cullen JJ, Kelly KA. Current management of Meckel's diverticulum. Adv Surg 1996;29:207–214.

Schwartz MW, ed. The 5-minute pediatric consult. Baltimore: Williams & Wilkins, 1997;478–479.

Turgeon DK, Barnett JL. Meckel's diverticulum. Am J Gastroenterol 1990;85(7):777–781.

Author: David Hale

Medial Collateral Ligament Strain

Clinical Presentation

SIGNS AND SYMPTOMS

- Tearing sensation and immediate pain medial aspect of knee
  - —Medial pain and tenderness may be more pronounced with partial tears than with complete tears
- Localized swelling
  - —Hemarthrosis signifies tear of capsular portion of medial collateral ligament (MCL) or cruciate injury
- Variable ability to weight-bear
  - —May be able to bear weight with complete tear
  - —Often describe buckling sensation on weight bearing
- Additional findings with involvement of other ligaments

MECHANISM/DESCRIPTION

- Most commonly injured knee ligament
- Direct trauma to lateral knee
- Most common: valgus stress with external rotary component on flexed knee
  - —From catching a ski tip
  - —Side tackle (football)
- When accompanied by other ligament injury
  - —Hyperextension with external rotation (ACL and PCL injured first)
  - —Anterior stress (ACL injured first)

PEDIATRIC CONSIDERATIONS

- MCL attaches distal to tibial epiphysis and proximal to femoral epiphysis
- MCL injury *infrequent* prior to growth plate closure (<14 years old)
- MCL injury may accompany underlying fracture
- Most injuries due to direct trauma producing valgus stress (sports, auto-pedestrian)

Pre-Hospital

CAUTIONS

- Evaluate for knee dislocation
- Document neurovascular status
- MCL injury may be overlooked in the multiple trauma victim
- Immobilize in slight flexion

Diagnosis

ESSENTIAL WORKUP

Complete knee examination

- Palpate medial femoral condyle (MCL most commonly tears there)
- *Valgus stress testing:* MCL injury causes joint instability more commonly than LCL injury; complete tears will reveal instability but may have little swelling or pain
  - —*In flexion:* grasp lateral aspect of knee and abduct while externally rotating at ankle with knee in 30° of flexion
    - -Joint laxity
    - -Mild: severe partial or complete MCL tear
    - -Moderate: complete MCL tear, possible ACL tear
    - -Marked: complete MCL and ACL tear, possible PCL tear
  - —*In extension:* same as above but with knee extended
    - -Joint laxity: complete MCL rupture +/− ACL and PCL tear
- *Note*
  - -Underlying fracture should be ruled out prior to stress test
  - -Reexam in 24 hours may be necessary if severe muscle spasm and ligamentous pain present
  - -Intra-articular instillation of anesthetic and analgesic may be required to perform adequate exam
- Classification of ligament injuries (sprains)
  - —Grade 1: stretched fibers without tear; firm end point on stress testing
  - —Grade 2: fibers tear without complete rupture; firm end point on stress testing
  - —Grade 3: complete rupture; no fixed end point on stress testing

LABORATORY

- Aspiration of joint effusion may be therapeutic (relieve pain) and diagnostic (cruciate tears result in hemarthrosis)

IMAGING/SPECIAL TESTS

- Standard radiographs give no clues to MCL tears but can reveal fractures, effusions, tendon calcifications and foreign bodies
  - —Views: AP, lateral, oblique, notch view
  - —Fat-fluid level is pathognomonic of fracture
- MRI used by consultant for diagnosis of other intra-articular disorders
- Arthroscopy used by consultant for diagnosis and repair of meniscal and cruciate injuries

DIFFERENTIAL DIAGNOSIS

- Meniscal, other ligament injuries, and fractures may be concomitant
- *Hip injury* may present with knee pain
- Arthritis (rheumatoid, osteo, septic), cellulitis, bursitis

PEDIATRIC CONSIDERATIONS

- Examine hip and obtain radiograph if any concern for hip pathology (especially slipped capital femoral epiphysis)
- Epiphyseal plate tenderness may signify nondisplaced Salter I fracture

Treatment

INITIAL STABILIZATION

- Maintain joint immobilization in neutral position or position of comfort by pre-hospital personnel

ED TREATMENT

- Grade I or II: intermittent ice, elevation, rest, crutches, compression (splint or knee immobilizer)
- Grade III: as I or II but require definitive orthopedic referral
- Joint aspiration of large hemarthrosis may help relieve pain

MEDICATIONS

- Nonsteroidal anti-inflammatory agents recommended
- Narcotic analgesics as needed
- Joint installation of anesthetic (e.g., marcaine) with an analgesic (e.g., morphine) may be required for severe pain

Disposition

ADMISSION CRITERIA

- To manage severe associated injuries

DISCHARGE CRITERIA

- Patients are usually discharged if no other associated injuries require admission
- Ensure compliance with splinting and adequate follow-up

Miscellaneous

ICD9: 844.1

CORE CONTENT CODE: 18.4.14.3

SUGGESTED READINGS

Sherk HH. Injuries of the knee. In Fleisher GR, Ludwig, eds. Textbook of Pediatric Emergency Medicine. 3rd ed. Baltimore: Williams & Wilkins, 1993:1091–1093.

Simon R, Koenigsknecht SJ. The knee. In: Emergency orthopedics: The extremities. 3rd ed. Stamford, CT: Appleton & Lange, 1996:437–470.

Smith BW, Green GA. Acute knee injuries Part II: Diagnosis and treatment. Am Fam Physician 1995;51:799–806.

Stewart C. Knee injuries: Diagnosis and repair. Emerg Med Reports 1997;18(1):1–12.

Author: Richard A. Craven

Medial Meniscus Injury

Clinical Presentation

SIGNS AND SYMPTOMS

- Patients usually present within 24 hours of an acute injury
- A sensation of "giving way" with ambulation occurs
- Another common historical feature is hearing or feeling a "pop"
- The inability to fully extend a "locked" knee results from *pseudo* or *true* locking
- Progressive pain with the *gradual* development of an effusion usually within 6–12 hours

MECHANISM/DESCRIPTION

- Medial meniscal tears are among the most common orthopedic injuries seen in adult emergency department patients
- Usually a disease of young active adults, but the geriatric knee has a predisposition to injury as well
- Sudden rotatory motion of the knee without the normal compensatory rotation that is required of the tibia
  —Those patients with an aged meniscus may recall nothing more than a simple twist or rising from a squat

ETIOLOGY

- The medial meniscus is injured more frequently owing to its relative immobility. There are several factors that increase the propensity for meniscal injuries
  —Congenital discoid meniscus, weakness of the surrounding musculature, and ligamentous laxity
- Meniscal injuries often accompany ligamentous injuries to the knee especially injuries to the deep medial collateral ligament
- Meniscal tears are the result of violent stretching or a crushing force between the femoral and tibial condyles
  —With knee flexion the femur rotates internally on the fixed tibia, displacing the medial meniscus toward the center of the joint
  —With rapid forceful extension, the meniscus may be trapped centrally, resulting in peripheral segment stretching or tear
  —Extension of the tear results in a free segment that may become displaced into the joint resulting in joint locking

PEDIATRIC CONSIDERATIONS

- Rarely occurs in children under age 10, especially with open epiphyses
- Most pediatric cases occur as a result of direct trauma

Pre-Hospital

CAUTIONS

- Immediate application of ice packs
- Immobilization in a position of comfort
- Careful neurovascular examination

Diagnosis

ESSENTIAL WORKUP

- Physical examination with special attention to joint line pain, tenderness and locking
  —Muscle spasm following the development of a painful effusion commonly causes *pseudo locking* with *true locking* occurring only in 30%
  —Limitation of the last few degrees of extension is among the most common clinical findings
  —Provocative tests which should be deferred until severe pain resolves include
    –McMurray's test, Apley compression test, Payr's sign, Bragard's sign, and Steinman's signs

IMAGING/SPECIAL TESTS

- Plain x-rays usually reveal little more than effusion though are recommended to rule out bony abnormalities
- Diagnostic accuracy of MRI is over 98%
- Arthrography has an accuracy of 95% though as an invasive procedure is less commonly performed

LABORATORY

- No specific tests are useful unless suspicion for septic effusion/arthritis exists; arthrocentesis will reveal increased WBC and protein, and decreased glucose and viscosity
  —Lack of hemarthrotic effusion aid diagnosis

DIFFERENTIAL DIAGNOSIS

- Osteochondral fractures, rupture of the cruciate ligament, and a loose body should be considered in the true "locked" knee
- Other ligamentous injuries
- Consider rheumatoid and gouty effusions in those with minor mechanisms of injury
- Infectious effusions should be considered in those at-risk

Treatment

INITIAL STABILIZATION

- Application of ice packs decreases pain and inflammation

ED TREATMENT

- Aspiration of large effusions followed by placement of a bulky dressing may afford considerable relief
- Reduction of the locked joint should be performed within the first 24 hours after injury
  —Hanging extremity off the edge of the table with the knee in 90° of flexion may facilitate reduction. Gentle rotation of the tibia performed after a period of rest in the above position, with careful traction along the axis of the leg, usually results in reduction
- Definitive treatment usually performed with arthroscopic surgery though minor insults may be effectively rehabilitated with physical therapy
- Stabilization in position of comfort
- Analgesia
- Early orthopedic referral
- Nonweight-bearing knee immobilizer or compressive wrap as needed for comfort

MEDICATIONS

- Appropriate analgesic and anti-inflammatory agents
- Ibuprofen: adult: 400–600 mg po q 6 hrs; peds: 5–10 mg/kg/dose q 6 hrs

Disposition

ADMISSION CRITERIA

- Intractable pain suggestive of complex disease
- High risk of consequential injuries in the unassisted elderly who are sent home

DISCHARGE CRITERIA

- Patients capable of following a structured discharge plan

Miscellaneous

ICD9: 959.7

CORE CONTENT CODE: 18.4.14.2

SUGGESTED READINGS

Rosen P, et al., eds. Emergency medicine: Concepts and clinical practice. 4th ed. St. Louis: CV Mosby, 1997.

Simon R, Koeingsknecht SJ. The knee. In: Emergency orthopedics: The extremities. 3rd ed. Stamford, CT: Appleton & Lange, 1996:437–470.

Smith BW, Green GA. Acute knee injuries. Part II: Diagnosis and treatment. Am Fam Physician 1995;51:799–806.

Stewart C. Knee injuries: Diagnosis and repair. Emerg Med Rep 1997;18(1):1–12.

Authors: Charles Graffeo; Francis Counselman

Megacolon, Aganglionic

Clinical Presentation

SIGNS AND SYMPTOMS

- Also known as congenital aganglionosis (CA) or Hirschsprung's disease
- Three presentations of CA
  - —Infancy
    - -Abdominal distention
    - -Poor feeding
    - -Vomiting
    - -Constipation (60% do not pass meconium within 48 hours)
    - -Intestinal obstruction
  - —In childhood with chronic constipation
  - —Enterocolitis at any age
- Bowel movements frequently require rectal stimulation or enemas
- Stools are thin shaped
- Encopresis and diarrhea are uncommon
- Absence of inciting factors for functional constipation (i.e., fissures, diet)
- Enterocolitis
  - —Fever
  - —Decreased activity (toxic child)
  - —Abdominal distention
  - —Bloody, foul smelling diarrhea
- Possible palpable colon on the left
- Occult blood may be from enterocolitis or from fissures (constipation)

ETIOLOGY

- Caused by the absence of ganglions in the distal bowel
  - —Creates functional obstruction to passage of stool
- Failure of neural crest cells to migrate or to differentiate into parasympathetic Meissner's (submucosal) and Auerbach's (myenteric) ganglions
- CA begins at the internal anal sphincter and involves the rectosigmoid colon (75% of cases)
- CA may extend to all of the colon and small bowel
- Aganglionic segment chronically contracts, forming an obstruction to the passage of stool
  - —Proximal colon distends to hold stool that has not passed
  - —Stimulation of the anus allows passage of stool
  - —Toxic megacolon may develop

Epidemiology

- CA occurs in 1:5000 live births
- 4:1 male to female ratio
- 8% of CA have positive family history; 5–12% of siblings may have CA
- 20% have other miscellaneous congenital anomalies (i.e., Down's syndrome)

Pre-Hospital

- Infants may be dehydrated and hypoglycemic

Diagnosis

ESSENTIAL WORKUP

- Abdominal x-rays
  - —Enlarged stool filled colon
  - —Transition zone into a narrowed rectosigmoid segment
  - —In neonates, films will commonly show a distal obstructive pattern
  - —In children, with chronic constipation films may show only large amounts of stool
  - —In children, with enterocolitis bowel wall edema or *pneumatosis intestinales* may be present

LABORATORY

- CBC, electrolytes, glucose, urinalysis, blood culture if toxic

IMAGING/SPECIAL TESTS

- Barium enema
  - —Dilated colon proximal to the contracted aganglionic colon
  - —Presence of colonic contrast 24 hours after the enema is suggestive for CA
- Rectal manometry may differentiate CA from constipation (90% sensitive)
- Rectal biopsy makes the definitive diagnosis by the lack of ganglion cells

DIFFERENTIAL DIAGNOSIS

Infants

- Meconium ileus or meconium plug
- Sepsis
- Intestinal or anal atresia or hypoplasia
- Malrotation with volvulus
- Necrotizing enterocolitis
- Functional constipation

Children

- Functional constipation
- Toxic
  - —Opiates, anticholinergics
- Infectious
  - —Botulism, trypanosoma cruzi acquired aganglionic colon
- Metabolic or endocrine
  - —Hypothyroid/ parathyroid, electrolyte abnormality
- Structural
  - —Spinal cord defects, abdominal masses

Treatment

INITIAL STABILIZATION

- Ill-appearing children
  - —Oxygen 100%
  - —Cardiac and oximetry monitoring
  - —IV normal saline
    - -Initial bolus 10–20 cc/kg

ED TREATMENT

- Infants should be managed for bowel obstruction
- Consultation with a pediatric surgeon, pediatric gastroenterology
- Stable children
  - —Workup may be done as an outpatient
  - —Definitive treatment is resection of the aganglionic section of bowel
  - —Return to normal bowel function is the usual result
    - -Enterocolitis may still occur

MEDICATIONS

- When the child is toxic or has enterocolitis then use triple IV antibiotic coverage
  - -Ampicillin: 50 mg/kg q 8–12 hrs
  - -Gentamicin: 2.5 mg/kg q 6–12 hrs
  - -Flagyl: 7.5 mg/kg q 12–48 hrs

Disposition

ADMISSION CRITERIA

- Infants and neonates presenting with bowel obstruction
- Enterocolitis
- Ill-appearing infants should be admitted to the PICU/NICU
- If pediatric surgery is not available, transfer to a pediatric tertiary care center

DISCHARGE CRITERIA

- Older children with constipation
- Well-hydrated and taking oral fluid
- Responsible parents

Miscellaneous

ICD9: 751.31

CORE CONTENT CODE: 13.1.1

SUGGESTED READINGS

Kays DW. Surgical conditions of the neonatal intestinal tract. Clin Perinatol 1996;23:353–75.

Rudolph C, Benaroch L. Hirschsprung disease. Pediatr Rev 1995;16:5–11.

Schnaufer L, Mahboubi S. Abdominal emergencies. In: Fleisher GR, et al., eds. Pediatric emergency medicine. 3rd ed. Baltimore: William & Wilkins, 1993;1307–1336.

Skinner MA. Hirschsprung disease. Curr Prob Surg 1996;399–460.

Author: Sally Santen

Melanoma

Clinical Presentation

SIGNS AND SYMPTOMS

- Cutaneous melanoma
  - —Presents as a pigmented skin lesion
  - —Differentiation from a pigmented mole (nevus) is key
  - —Features of a pigmented lesion suggestive of melanoma: the *abcd* of melanoma
    - -*A*symmetry (not regularly round or oval)
    - -*B*order irregularity (notched, scalloped, or poorly defined borders)
    - -*C*olor variegation (shades or combinations of brown, tan, red, white, or blue/black)
    - -*D*iameter greater than 6 mm
  - —Although all pigmented lesions change in size, shape, and color over time, melanomas do so rapidly (weeks to months)
  - —Cutaneous melanoma rarely symptomatic itself except for localized irritation if ulcerated or large
- Metastatic melanoma
  - —Presenting features are related to organ systems involved
  - —Most common initial spread is through lymphatic channels to produce local, then regional, lymphadenopathy
  - —Melanomas will eventually spread if left untreated; this may take weeks to years
  - —Preferred visceral sites of hematogenous spread
    - -Liver: abdominal pain or mass, liver function abnormalities
    - -Lung: shortness of breath or chest pain
    - -Bone: musculoskeletal pain
    - -Brain: headache, altered central nervous system function

MECHANISM/DESCRIPTION

- A malignancy of pigmented (melanin-producing) cells
- Risk factors
  - —Acute, intense exposure to sunlight, especially exposure that causes sunburn, is strongly linked to the development of melanoma
  - —Evidence that sunburn early in life carries a higher risk of later melanoma remains limited
  - —20% of the world's melanomas are in black Africans and in Asians and are not clearly associated with sun exposure
  - —No clear relation established between diet, alcohol, or vitamin a, beta-carotene, or related compounds and the development of melanoma
  - —Additional risk factors in adults: sun-sensitive skin type, multiple common melanocytic nevi, atypical nevi, immunosuppression, family history of melanoma, and a history of nonmelanocytic skin cancer (i.e., Basal cell or squamous cell carcinoma)

PEDIATRIC CONSIDERATIONS

- Melanoma rare under age 14; this age group contributes only 0.3–0.4% of all melanomas
- Risk factors for childhood melanoma: giant congenital melanocytic nevi, atypical mole syndrome, xeroderma pigmentosum, and immunodeficiency states

Pre-Hospital

- No specific pre-hospital considerations

Diagnosis

ESSENTIAL WORKUP

- Although rarely an ED consideration, the diagnosis of primary cutaneous melanoma is made by a properly performed excisional biopsy of a suspicious lesion
- Diagnosis and staging
  - —For patients with localized primary cutaneous melanoma the most important prognostic factor is tumor thickness
  - —Staging system
    - -Stages I and II represent primary localized disease
    - -Stage III involves regional lymph node or in-transit disease
    - -Stage IV involves distant metastatic disease

LABORATORY

- The only specific laboratory tests of value are liver enzyme and liver function tests in patients with suspected metastatic disease

IMAGING/SPECIAL TESTS

- Chest x-ray may show pulmonary involvement
- Head or body CT may show visceral involvement

DIFFERENTIAL DIAGNOSIS

- Common acquired nevus, atypical (dysplastic) nevus, actinic keratosis, pigmented basal cell carcinoma, squamous cell carcinoma

Treatment

INITIAL STABILIZATION

- Not generally required unless hemorrhage from visceral metastasis occurs

ED TREATMENT

- Only specific ED treatment necessary is treatment of the possible complications of visceral involvement

GENERAL TREATMENT

- Early detection and prompt excision of melanoma give the patient the best chance of cure
- Surgical treatment may require regional lymph node dissection
- Adjuvant therapy involves single- or multiple-agent chemotherapy

MEDICATIONS

None

Disposition

ADMISSION CRITERIA

- Admission criteria for the patient with melanoma usually depend on general principles involving the overall state of the patient and the presence of any complications of visceral metastatic disease, not on the melanoma lesions themselves

DISCHARGE CRITERIA

- Nearly all patients can be managed as outpatients with appropriate primary care or dermatology follow-up for biopsy and definitive management

Miscellaneous

ICD9: 172.9

CORE CONTENT CODE: 3.7.3

SUGGESTED READINGS

Marks R. An overview of skin cancers: Incidence and causation. Cancer 1995;75:607–612.

NIH Consensus Development Panel on Early Melanoma. Diagnosis and treatment of early melanoma. JAMA 1992;268:1314–1319.

Rivers JK. Melanoma. Lancet 1996;347:803–807.

Sober AJ, Koh HK. Melanoma and other pigmented skin lesions. In: Isselbacher KJ, Braunwald E, Wilson JD, et al., eds. Harrison's principles of internal medicine. New York: McGraw Hill, 1994:1867–1871.

Author: Glenn Hebel

Ménière's Disease

Clinical Presentation

SIGNS AND SYMPTOMS

- Unilateral ear fullness and pressure
- Decreased hearing
- Tinnitus
- Vertigo
  —Intense and whirling in nature
  —Reaching maximum intensity within minutes, slowly subsides over several hours
- Horizontal nystagmus, often with a rotational component
- Nausea and vomiting
- Patient preferentially lies with the affected ear up and avoids looking toward the normal side because doing so exaggerates the nystagmus and dizziness

MECHANISM/DESCRIPTION

- Estimated to affect approximately 0.1% U.S. population
- Affects male and females equally
- May develop at any age
  —Peak incidence between the ages of 20 and 50 years
  —Classically unilateral, but may be bilateral in up to 40% of cases
  —Characterized by *recurrent,* intermittent attacks of rotatory vertigo, deafness, tinnitus, and a sensation of aural pressure
  —Attacks occur with little or no warning
  —Persist from 5 minutes to several hours
  —Close clustering of attacks may occur
  —Hearing loss is progressive over time, sensorineural in nature, and initially involves lower frequencies

ETIOLOGY

- Endolymphatic hydrops
  —Progressive dilation of the endolymphatic space
  —Thought to be overproduction or reduced absorption of endolymphatic fluid
  —Therapy directed at decreasing production or enhancing drainage of endolymph

Pre-Hospital

- Vertigo and neurologic symptoms can represent a stroke
  —Rapid transport to ED
- Protect patient from falling
- Maintain a position of comfort
- Intravenous isotonic fluid for patients with active vomiting
- Monitor for dysrhythmia

Diagnosis

ESSENTIAL WORKUP

- Complete history and neurologic exam
- Patients with central vertigo or focal neurologic findings need neuroimaging
  —Focal findings include new unilateral hearing loss

LABORATORY

- None routinely helpful

IMAGING/SPECIAL TESTS

- Computed tomography or magnetic resonance imaging
  —Indicated for any patient with focal neurologic deficit or central vertigo
  —The most important diagnosis to exclude is acoustic neuroma
- Patients with Ménière's disease ultimately require audiometry and ENG testing, but these studies are not necessary to the ED evaluation

DIFFERENTIAL DIAGNOSIS

- Otologic
  —Chronic suppurative otitis media
  —Benign positional vertigo
  —Acoustic neuroma
  —Vestibular neuronitis
  —Otosclerosis
  —Otic capsule dysplasia
- Systemic
  —Vertebrobasilar insufficiency, or stroke
  —Basilar migraine
  —Epilepsy
  —Multiple sclerosis
  —Paget's disease
  —Thyroid disease
  —Autoimmune disorders
  —Syphilis

Treatment

INITIAL STABILIZATION

- IV hydration with isotonic fluid
- Antiemetics, benzodiazepines

ED TREATMENT

- Supportive therapy

MEDICATIONS

- Symptomatic
  —Diazepam: 5–10 mg PO/IV/PR
  —Droperidol: 0.625–2.5 mg IV/IM
  —Lorazepam: 0.5–2.0 mg PO/IV/IM
  —Meclizine: 25 mg po q 8 hrs
  —Promethazine: 10–25 mg PO/IV/IM/PR
- Therapeutic (patients with established diagnosis of Ménière's disease)
  —Acetazolamide: 250 mg po
  —Furosemide: 20 mg po
  —Triamterene: 100 mg po

Disposition

ADMISSION CRITERIA

- Central cause of vertigo
- Patients refractory to ED therapy

DISCHARGE CRITERIA

- Patients with normal neurologic examination
- Symptoms adequately controlled in ED
- Refer to neurology or ENT for outpatient audiometry and electronystagmography (ENG) testing
- Recurrent attacks are typical
- Restrict sodium, tobacco, caffeine, and alcohol intake
- Avoid driving, operating dangerous equipment, and working at heights until attacks have resolved and sedating medications have been withdrawn

Miscellaneous

ICD9: 388.31, 386.00, 386.10, 386.20

CORE CONTENT CODE: 6.1.5

SUGGESTED READINGS

Baloh RW, Jacobson KM. Neurotology. Neurol Clin 1996;14:85–101.

Knox GW, McPherson A. Ménière's disease: Differential diagnosis and treatment. Am Fam Phys 1997;55:4:1185–90.

Saeed SR, Birzgalis AR, Ramsden RT. Ménière's disease. Br J Hosp Med 1994;51:603–12.

Authors: Paul G. Flatley; Charles V. Pollack, Jr.

Meningitis

Clinical Presentation

SIGNS AND SYMPTOMS

- "Classic Triad" present in two-thirds of adults (rare in infants)
  - —Fever
  - —Stiff neck
  - —Alteration in mental status
- Headache
- Photophobia
- Meningeal irritation: nuchal rigidity, Kernig's and Brudzinski's signs
- Alterations in CNS function: altered mental status, focal CNS abnormalities, seizures
- Increased intracranial pressure: cranial nerve palsies, papilledema
- Evidence of associated infection: rash (meningococcal); pneumonia; ear, nose, or throat (ENT) infection
- AIDS patients: present with less striking symptoms
  - —Chronic headache
  - —Isolated fevers

ETIOLOGY

Infectious Agents

- Bacterial
  - —Neonates: Group B *streptococcus, Listeria monocytogenes,* Gram-negative bacilli
  - —Children: *Haemophilus influenzae* (less common due to immunization), *Neisseria meningitidis, Streptococcus pneumoniae*
  - —Adults: above agents plus syphilis, staphylococci
  - —Elderly: Gram-negative bacilli, *Listeria*
- Viral
- Fungal (usually immunocompromised hosts): *Cryptococcus neoformans, Coccidioides immitis, Histoplasma capsulatum, Aspergillus, Candida* species

Noninfectious Etiologies

- Chemical: drugs or toxic exposure
- Autoimmune
- Neoplastic

AIDS Patients

- Primary HIV meningitis
- Opportunistic infections
  - —Mycobacteria
  - —Fungal

MECHANISM/DESCRIPTION

- Inflammatory changes of meninges
- Infection
  - —Hematogenous spread from
    - -Colonized sites (ENT source)
    - -Acutely infected source (pneumonia, osteomyelitis, endocarditis)
    - -Nosocomial (e.g., colonized intravascular catheter)
  - —Direct extension from
    - -Basilar skull fracture with CNS leak
    - -CSF shunt
    - -Mastoiditis or sinusitis with bony destruction
- Inflammatory response due to microorganism products (endotoxin, teichoic acid)

PEDIATRIC CONSIDERATIONS

- Typical signs and symptoms less common
  - —Small children present with nonspecific symptoms: irritability, vomiting, dehydration
    - -Age <6 months: meningismus in 27%
    - -Age <12 months: meningismus in 72%
    - -Age >12 months: meningismus in 93%
- Differentiate febrile seizure from meningitis
  - —Meningitis does not present as uncomplicated febrile seizure
  - —Typical uncomplicated febrile seizure
    - -Generalized
    - -Self-limited, single seizure
    - -Short postictal period
    - -Child returns to normal behavior
  - —Perform LP if
    - -Taking antibiotics to rule out partially treated meningitis
    - -Complicated seizure
    - -Ill appearing
    - -<12 months old

Pre-Hospital

- Administer prophylactic antibiotics for family members and health care workers with close personal contact with patients known to have *N. meningitidis*

Diagnosis

ESSENTIAL WORKUP

- Lumbar puncture
  - —For suspicion of meningitis in absence of contraindications (increased intracranial pressure with mass lesion, soft tissue infection overlying puncture site; anticoagulation – relative contraindication)
- CSF analysis
  - —Culture is considered Gold Standard
  - —Leukocyte count >6 WBC/cc
    - -Highly sensitive for meningitis
    - -Not accurate in immunocompromised patients (AIDS)
    - -If bloody LP, number of WBCs introduced can be estimated by this formula:

WBCs introduced = (peripheral WBC) × (RBC in CSF)/(peripheral RBC count)

  - —Gram stain
    - -80% sensitive for bacterial meningitis
    - -Use to guide antibiotic therapy after initial empiric treatment
  - —Protein
  - —Glucose
  - —Culture
  - —Latex agglutination
    - -Best if performed on CSF, urine, and blood simultaneously
    - -Detects antigens from specific bacteria (streptococcus, *H. influenzae, E. coli*) and serotypes
    - -Useful in identifying organism in patients with prior antibiotic therapy
    - -Does not rule out presence of bacterial infection
  - —Cryptococcal detection
    - -Cryptococcal antigen
      - *Sensitive for detection of organism in CSF
      - *Chronically elevated in immunocompromised patients undergoing suppressive therapy after episode of cryptococcal meningitis
    - -India Ink: 50% sensitive for cryptococcal meningitis
  - —Special neonatal (<1 month) considerations
    - -Normal leukocyte count up to 25 WBC/mm^3
    - -Normal protein up to 120–170 mg/dl

Typical Cerebrospinal Fluid Findings

TYPE OF INFECTION	*LEUKOCYTE COUNT*	*LEUKOCYTE DIFFERENTIAL*	*GLUCOSE*	*PROTEIN MG/DL*
Bacterial	1000–20,000	Mostly PMNs	<40% of serum	>200
Viral	10–1000	Initial mostly PMNs; late (>24 hrs) lymphs	Elevated	<200
Fungal	<500	Lymphocytes	Low	>200
Tuberculous	100–400	Lymphocytes or PMNs (27% of cases)	Low or normal	Normal or elevated

LABORATORY

- CBC
  - —WBC and differential—not sensitive enough to rule out meningitis
- Electrolytes, BUN/Cr, glucose
  - —Serum/CSF glucose comparison
  - —Metabolic acidosis
- Urinalysis
- Blood/urine/CSF cultures

IMAGING/SPECIAL TESTS

- CT Scanning
  - —Routine CT before LP not necessary
  - —Indicated with coma, focal neurologic deficits, evidence of increased intracranial pressure, and immunocompromised host
- CXR: may demonstrate source of infection (TB, pneumonia)

DIFFERENTIAL DIAGNOSIS

- Meningitis—various forms
  - —Infectious: bacterial, viral, fungal, parasitic
  - —Noninfectious: chemical, autoimmune, neoplastic
- Febrile seizure
- Other diseases causing similar presentations including CSF pleocytosis
  - —Empyema: ventricular, subdural
  - —Abscess: spinal, epidural, brain
  - —Endocarditis with embolism
  - —Venous sinus thrombophlebitis
  - —Encephalitis

Treatment

INITIAL STABILIZATION

- ABCs
- IV rehydration for hypotension
- Early, empiric antibiotics as soon as diagnosis suspected

ED TREATMENT

Antibiotics

- Do not delay IV antibiotics for LP
- Penetrance of antibiotics delayed and unlikely to affect culture results for 2–3 hours
- Antibiotic resistance
  - —Especially a problem with penicillin resistant pneumococci
  - —Consider adding vancomycin if *Streptococcal pneumoniae* is a possible organism

Steroid Therapy

- In children
  - —Dexamethasone therapy reduces auditory and other neurologic sequelae if *H. influenzae* is causative organism
  - —No proven benefit with other organisms
- In adults
  - —No clear benefit
  - —Some recommend in cases of increased ICP (very controversial; not supported by clinical research)

MEDICATIONS

- Ceftriaxone: 2 g (peds: 50–100 mg/kg) q 12 hrs IV
- Ceftazidime: 2 g (peds: 50–100 mg/kg) q 8 hrs IV
- Ampicillin: 2 g q 4 hrs (peds: 100 mg/kg q 8 hrs) IV
- Vancomycin: 1 g q 12 hrs (peds: 10–15 mg/kg q 6 hrs) IV
- Tobramycin: 1 mg/kg q 8 hrs or 5 mg/kg q 24 hrs (peds: 2–2.5 mg/kg q 8 hrs) IV
- Gentamicin: 1 mg/kg q 8 hrs or 5 mg/kg q 24 hrs (peds: 2–2.5 mg/kg q 8 hrs) IV
- Dexamethasone: 4–10 mg (peds: 0.15 mg/kg q 6 hrs, beginning shortly before or simultaneous with first dose of antibiotics) IV for 4 days

Disposition

ADMISSION CRITERIA

- Known or suspected bacterial or fungal source
- Indeterminate CSF studies in patient already receiving antibiotics
- Immunocompromised host
- Viral meningitis with uncontrolled pain or toxic appearance

DISCHARGE CRITERIA

- Clear viral source of meningitis
  - —Well-controlled symptoms
  - —Nontoxic appearance

Miscellaneous

ICD9: 320, 047.9

CORE CONTENT CODE: 11.4.3

SUGGESTED READINGS

Durand ML, Calderwood SB, et al. Acute bacterial meningitis in adults: A review of 493 episodes. N Engl J Med 1993;328:21–28.

Greenlee JE. Approach to diagnosis of meningitis: Cerebrospinal fluid evaluation. Infect Dis Clin North Am 1990;4:583–598.

Quagliarello VJ, Scheld WM. Treatment of bacterial meningitis. N Engl J Med 1997;10:708–716.

Tunkel AR, Scheld WM. Acute bacterial meningitis. Curr Clin Top Infect Dis 1996;16:215–239.

Author: Howard Blumstein

Empiric Antibiotic Selection for Bacterial Infection

CLINICAL SCENARIO	LIKELY PATHOGENS	ANTIBIOTIC THERAPY
Neonate	Group B Streptococci *L. monocytogenes* Gram-negative enteric bacilli	Ampicillin plus either broad spectrum cephalosporin* or aminoglycoside
Age 3 months to 50 years	*S. pneumoniae* *N. meninginitis* *H. influenzae*	Broad spectrum cephalosporin* plus Vancomycin (if high incidence of resistant *S. pneumoniae*)
Age over 50 years	*S. pneumoniae* *L. monocytogenes* Gram-negative enteric bacilli	Ampicillin plus broad spectrum cephalosporin*
Immune impaired	*L. monocytogenes* Gram-negative enteric bacilli	Ampicillin plus ceftazidime
Head trauma, CSF shunt, neurosurgery	Staphylococcal organisms Gram-negative enteric bacilli	Vancomycin Ceftazidime

* Broad spectrum cephalosporin (usually ceftriaxone; cefotaxime in children <1 month); consider ceftazidime if *pseudomonas* is clinical consideration

Meningococcemia

Clinical Presentation

SIGNS AND SYMPTOMS

"Mild" Meningococcemia (Most Common)

- Preceded by URI
- Fever, chills, myalgias/arthralgias, malaise
- Often self-limited, resolving in several days
- Can progress to meningitis or overwhelming sepsis without meningitis

Overwhelming Meningococcal Sepsis (10%)

- High fatality rate
- Sudden onset of illness and rapid progression of clinical course
- Initial presentation
  —Mild tachycardia
  —Mild tachypnea
  —Mild hypotension
- Fever, chills, vomiting, headache, rash, muscle tenderness
- Toxic appearing
- Rash—combination of
  —Purpura
    -May later exhibit coalescence, necrosis/sloughing of the involved skin (*purpura fulminans*)
  —Petechiae (over skin, mucous membranes, conjunctivae)
  —Macules
  —Papules (scrapings of papules demonstrate the organism on Gram stain)
- Deteriorate quickly over several hours
  —Hypotension/shock
  —Acidosis
  —ARDS
  —DIC
- Meningitis may or may not be present
- Waterhouse-Friderichsen syndrome
  —Bilateral hemorrhagic destruction of adrenal glands
- Acute renal failure
  —From prolonged hypotension (low renal perfusion causing acute tubular necrosis)

Chronic Meningococcemia (Uncommon)

- Well appearing
- Recurrent fevers, chills, arthralgias over weeks to months
- Intermittent rash—alone or in combination of
  —Purpura
  —Petechiae
  —Macules
  —Papules
- Splenomegaly (20%)
- Meningococcal meningitis (25%)
  —Headache
  —Fever
  —Neck stiffness
  —Confusion
  —Lethargy
  —Obtundation

Septic Arthritis

- Occurs during active meningococcemia
- Multiple joints involved
- Joint pain, redness, swelling, effusion, fever, chills
- Extremely limited or no range of motion

Other Meningococcal Infections

- Occur with meningococcal infection elsewhere
- Conjunctivitis—may occur alone
- Sinusitis
- Panophthalmitis
- Urethritis
- Salpingitis
- Prostatitis
- Pneumonia
- Pericarditis

MECHANISM/DESCRIPTION

- Acquired from close contact with an infected individual, or an asymptomatic carrier by inhalation of airborne nasopharyngeal droplets carrying the bacteria
- Bacteria attach to and enter nasopharyngeal epithelial cells
- Bacteria spread from the nasopharynx through the bloodstream via entry of vascular endothelium
- Majority of circulating meningococci eliminated by the spleen—some penetrate endothelial cells at other sites to cause infection (meninges, synovium, conjunctivae)
- Meningococci produce an endotoxin
  —Involved in pathogenesis of the skin, adrenal manifestations, and vascular collapse
- Human oro/nasopharynx—only reservoir
- Carrier usually has developed immunity to serotype-specific antibody (not immune to *all* serotypes)
  —Age $<$5 years: 1% carrier rate
  —Age 20–40 years: 30–40% carrier rate
  —Lower rate of immunity in children, which is reflected by the higher rates of infection
- Most common in winter and spring

ETIOLOGY

- *Neisseria meningitidis*
  —Serotypes A, B, C, D, H, I, K, L, X, Y, Z, 29E, and W135
  —Serotype B most common
  —$>$95% of infections caused by A, B, C, Y, and W135
- Available vaccines offer protection against serotypes A, C, Y, W135

Pre-Hospital

CAUTIONS

- Postexposure prophylactic antibiotics for prehospital personnel in close contact with patient

Diagnosis

ESSENTIAL WORKUP

- Suspect diagnosis in setting of dramatic clinical presentation
- Gram stain and culture of
  —Peripheral blood, CSF, sputum, urine, joint aspirate, or petechial/papular scrapings
  —Gram stain: intra- or extracellular Gram-negative diplococci

LABORATORY

- CBC
  —Elevated WBC initially, later may be suppressed
  —Decreased platelet count when large areas of purpura/petechiae
- Electrolytes, BUN, Cr, glucose
- ABG for acidosis, hypoxia
- Fibrinogen levels, fibrin degradation products, PT, and PTT if DIC suspected
- Throat/nasopharyngeal swab
  —Positive swab does not establish the diagnosis of meningococcemia
- Analysis of buffy coat layer of peripheral blood for bacteria if sepsis is suspected
- Blood culture
  —Often negative with chronic meningococcemia
  —Positive in mild and overwhelming meningococcemia

IMAGING/SPECIAL TESTS

- CXR
  —If pneumonia suspected
  —For the source of meningococcal sepsis
  —To rule out ARDS

DIFFERENTIAL DIAGNOSIS

- Viral exanthem
- Vasculitis
- Mycoplasma
- Rocky Mountain Spotted Fever

Treatment

INITIAL STABILIZATION

Overwhelming Meningococcal Sepsis

- ABCs—immediate endotracheal intubation for severe acidosis, hypoxia, or decreased mental status
  - —Hyperventilate to treat acidosis (target pCO_2 approximately 25)
- Treat hypotension
  - —0.9% NS bolus of 20 cc/kg; cautious rehydration with ARDS, CHF
  - —Begin dopamine or norepinephrine (epinephrine if no response) if hypotensive after 2 L of IVF
- Narcan, thiamine, dextrose (Accucheck) for altered mental status
- Initiate IV antibiotics
  - —First line: high-dose penicillin or third-generation cephalosporin
  - —Second line: ampicillin
  - —Third line: chloramphenicol

ED TREATMENT

Overwhelming Meningococcal Sepsis

- Severe acidosis (pH <7.0–7.1 or serum HCO_3 <8–10)
  - —Administer IV $NaHCO_3$ along with hyperventilation
- Insert Foley catheter to monitor urine output
- Place in respiratory isolation
- High-dose steroids
  - —To protect against cranial nerve injury in the setting of ongoing infection (controversial)
  - —Administer with adrenal gland injury
- DIC treatment
  - —Administer fresh frozen plasma and platelet transfusions
  - —Heparin not indicated unless significant thrombotic complications evident clinically (e.g., cyanosis and coolness of digits, low urine output despite adequate volume status, and BP)

Mild Meningococcemia

- Initiate IV antibiotics immediately
- Admission in respiratory isolation

Prophylaxis Options for Close Contacts

- Rifampin
- Single-dose ceftriaxone
- Single-dose ciprofloxacin

MEDICATIONS

- Ampicillin: 2–3 g (peds: 200 mg/kg/24hrs) IV q 6 hrs
- Cefotaxime: 2 g (peds: 200 mg/kg/24hrs) IV q 6–8 hrs
- Ceftriaxone: 2 g (peds: 80–100 mg/kg/24hrs) IV q 12 hrs
- Chloramphenicol: 50–100 mg/kg/24hrs IV q 6 hrs
- Ciprofloxacin: 500 mg po
- Dopamine: 5–20 µg/kg/min IV titrate to BP
- Epinephrine: 2–10 µg/min IV titrate to BP
- Heparin: 3000–5000 IU (peds: 80 IU/kg) IV bolus followed by 600–1000 IU/hr (peds: 18 IU/kg/hr) IV drip
- Hydrocortisone (solu-cortef): 100 mg (peds: 2 mg/kg) bolus IV
- Norepinephrine: 0.5–30 µg/min IV titrate to BP
- Penicillin G: 6 mIU (peds: 250,000 IU/kg/24hrs) IV q 6 hrs
  - —Prophylaxis: 250 mg (peds: 25–37.5 mg/kg) IM single dose
- Rifampin: 600 mg (peds: 5–10 mg/kg) po bid for 2 days
- Sodium bicarbonate: 2–5 mEq/kg (peds: 0.5–1.0 mEq/kg) IV over 30 min to 4 hrs

Disposition

ADMISSION CRITERIA

- ICU admission for overwhelming sepsis with respiratory isolation
- Respiratory isolation admission for mild meningococcemia

DISCHARGE CRITERIA

- Prophylaxis for close patient contacts

Miscellaneous

ICD9: 36.2

CORE CONTENT CODE: 9.1.6

SUGGESTED READINGS

Giraud T, et al. Adult overwhelming meningococcal purpura. Arch Intern Med 1991;151:310–316.

Guidelines for control of meningococcal disease. Can J Infect Cont 1994;9(2):41–46.

Mok Q, Butt W. The outcome of children admitted to intensive care with meningococcal septicaemia. Intensive Care Med 1996;22:259–263.

Van Deuren M. et al. Plasma and whole blood exchange in meningococcal sepsis. Clin Infect Dis 1992;15:424–430.

Author: Murtaza Galamhussein

Clinical Presentation

SIGNS AND SYMPTOMS

- Naturally occurring mercury is converted into three primary forms each with its own toxicological effects

Elemental Mercury

- Classic triad
  —Tremor
  —Neuropsychiatric disturbance (erethism)
  —Gingivostomatitis
- Acrodynia
  —Idiosyncratic, occurs mainly in children
  —Painful extremities
  —Pink discoloration with desquamation ("pink disease")

Inorganic Salts

- Gastrointestinal
  —Abrupt onset of abdominal pain and hemorrhagic gastroenteritis
  —Sore throat
  —Nausea/vomiting
  —Gingivostomatitis
  —Diarrhea
- Acute tubular necrosis in a few days
- Metallic taste
- Acrodynia in chronic exposures

Organic Mercury

- CNS
  —Primarily affect
  —Paresthesias
  —Ataxia
  —Visual field constriction
  —Dysarthria
  —Hearing loss
  —Mental deterioration
  —Paralysis
  —Death
- Symptom onset several weeks after exposure

Inhalation Exposure

- Initial phase (first few days)
  —Fever
  —Chills
  —Muscle aches
  —Dry mouth/throat
  —Headache
- Intermediate phase (2 weeks postexposure)
  —CNS, respiratory, GI, urologic symptoms develop
  —Noncardiogenic pulmonary edema
  —Acute renal failure
  —Seizures
- Late phase
  —Respiratory, GI, urologic symptoms resolve
  —CNS symptoms persist

MECHANISM/DESCRIPTION

- Reacts with sulfhydryl groups causing enzyme inhibition and alterations in cellular membranes
- Binds to phosphoryl, carboxyl, amide, and amine groups of enzymes

ETIOLOGY

- Manufacturing of chlorine and caustic soda, diuretics, antibacterial agents, antiseptics, thermometers, batteries, fossil fuels, plastics, paints, and pigments
- Contaminated seafood
- Dental exposure

Pre-Hospital

- Remove from toxin exposure
- For altered mental status: dextrose, thiamine, narcan, oxygen

Diagnosis

ESSENTIAL WORKUP

- As per patient complaint and clinical condition
  —Abdominal pain, gastrointestinal bleeding
    -CBC
    -Electrolytes, BUN/Cr, glucose
    -PT/PTT
    -Amylase
    -LFTs
    -Abdominal x-rays
  —Tremors, neuropsychiatric effects
    -CBC
    -Electrolytes, BUN/Cr, glucose
    -Toxicology screen
    -Head CT scan
    -Consider lumbar puncture

LABORATORY

Elemental and Inorganic Mercury

- Normal urine levels $<10\ \mu g/L$
- Neurologic effects occur with chronic urine levels $>100–200\ \mu g/L$

Organic Mercury

- Whole blood levels $>200\ \mu g/L$ associated with symptoms
- Organic mercury concentrated in RBC's
  —Compare RBC content to plasma (inorganic) content to help determine which form of mercury is involved

IMAGING/SPECIAL TESTS

- CXR for noncardiogenic pulmonary edema
- Abdominal radiograph for presence of mercury with intentional oral ingestion

DIFFERENTIAL DIAGNOSIS

- Multisystem involvement often confused with other heavy metal intoxications
- CVA
- Parkinson's disease
- Peptic ulcer disease
- Gastrointestinal bleeding
- Pancreatitis
- Shock
- Sepsis

Treatment

INITIAL STABILIZATION

- Secure ABCs and monitoring
- IV 0.9%NS IV fluid resuscitation if hypotension
  - —Blood transfusion for significant GI hemorrhage
- Narcan, D50W (or Accucheck), thiamine for altered mental status

ED TREATMENT

Elemental Mercury

- For inhalation exposure, observe closely for several hours for the development of noncardiogenic pulmonary edema
- Ingestion of elemental mercury passes through the normal intestinal tract with minimal absorption
- Chelate with oral DMSA (dimercaprol succinic acid)
  - —Enhances urinary mercury excretion
- Avoid BAL (dimercaprol) since it may cause redistribution of mercury to brain

Inorganic Salt Ingestion

- Administer activated charcoal
- Perform gastric lavage for recent ingestion as indicated
- Do not induce emesis because of risk of serious caustic injury
- Aggressive 0.9%NS IV fluid resuscitation/blood products for gastrointestinal bleeding and hypovolemic shock
  - —Hydrate and maintain urine output
- Chelate with BAL
  - —Early administration may avert severe renal injury
- Oral DMSA efficacy limited secondary to severe gastrointestinal symptomatology

Organic Mercury

- Perform gastric lavage and administer activated charcoal
- Provide symptomatic care as needed
- Chelate with oral DMSA
  - —Help decrease tissue levels
- Avoid BAL administration

MEDICATIONS

- DMSA (dimercaprol succinic acid): 10 mg/kg po q 8 hrs for 5 days then q 12 hrs for 2 weeks
- BAL (dimercaprol): 3 mg/kg IM q 4–6 hrs for 2 days then q 12 hrs for 7–10 days
- Dextrose: D50W 1 amp (50 ml or 25 g) (peds: D25W 2–4 ml/kg) IV
- Naloxone (narcan): 2 mg (peds: 0.1 mg/kg) IV or IM initial dose
- Thiamine (vitamin B_1): 100 mg (peds: 50 mg) IV or IM

Disposition

ADMISSION CRITERIA

- Symptomatic patients

DISCHARGE CRITERIA

- Asymptomatic patients with history of ingestion of elemental mercury and an intact intestinal tract
- Patients with a history of inhalational exposure to elemental mercury who remain asymptomatic after several hours of observation

Miscellaneous

ICD9: 985.0

CORE CONTENT: 17.2.21

SUGGESTED READINGS

Agency for Toxic Substance and Disease Registry. Mercury toxicity. Am Fam Physician 1992;46(6):1731–1741.

Ellenhorn MJ, Schoonwald S, Ordog G, Wasserberger J. Mercury. In: Ellenhorn's medical toxicology. 2d ed. Baltimore: Williams & Wilkins, 1997:1588–1602.

Sue YJ. Mercury. In: Goldfrank LR, Flombaum NA, Lewin RG, eds. Goldfrank's toxicologic emergencies. 5th ed. Norwalk, CT: Appleton & Lange, 1994:1051–1062.

Authors: Yat Leung; Lisandro Irizarry

Mesenteric Ischemia

Clinical Presentation

SIGNS AND SYMPTOMS

Abdominal Pain

- Moderate to severe pain with *minimal* or *no tenderness* initially on physical exam
  —Generally diffuse, poorly localized, and constant
- Onset variable
  —Acute onset with embolic source
  —Hours to days onset with thrombosis causing occlusion
- Abdominal tenderness—late finding after bowel infarction or rupture has occurred

Other Symptoms

- Nausea, vomiting (75%), diarrhea (often guaiac-positive)
- Frank GI bleeding as the bowel becomes gangrenous and mucosa sloughed off
- Evidence of systemic toxicity, which worsens as time progresses
  —Tachycardia
  —Tachypnea
  —Hypotension
  —Fever
  —Altered mental status
- Evidence of a possible embolic source—AFib

MECHANISM/DESCRIPTION

- Most commonly caused by a thromboembolus (usually from the heart) to the superior mesenteric artery (SMA)
- 15–25% caused by primary thrombosis of the SMA in an area of preexisting atherosclerosis
- Less frequently caused by "low flow states": patients in an ICU setting and hypotensive for an extended period are rarely seen in the ED

ETIOLOGY

- >50 years of age with
  —Valvular or atherosclerotic heart disease
  —Dysrhythmias
  —H/O myocardial infarction
  —Chronic congestive heart failure
  —Previous embolic phenomena
  —Hypotension or hypovolemia
- Mortality is 85%—can be reduced to 50% with prompt diagnosis and treatment

Pre-Hospital

CAUTIONS

- Cardiac monitor for dysrhythmia

Diagnosis

ESSENTIAL WORKUP

- Plain abdominal films to exclude other disease
- Selective angiography confirms diagnosis

LABORATORY

- *Normal lab values do not rule out the diagnosis*
  —CBC
  —Leukocytosis and/or left shift in >50%
  —Elevated hematocrit initially due to hemoconcentration
  —Decreased hematocrit later due to GI bleeding
- ABG
  —Acidosis later in course
- Electrolytes, BUN, Cr, glucose
  —Anion gap (lactic acidosis) worsening as bowel ischemia and necrosis progresses
- Serum lactate
  —Elevated as disease progresses
- Serum amylase
  —Modest elevation (1–2 times normal)
  —Not reliable indicator
- Urinalysis

IMAGING/SPECIAL TESTS

- Plain films
  —Cannot be used to "exclude" mesenteric ischemia
  —Initially: normal
  —Late in the course: bowel-wall thickening and thumbprinting; gas in the portal system or bowel wall
- Selective angiography (Gold Standard)
  —Catheter is placed into the SMA and dye infused
  —Abrupt cutoff suggests an embolic obstruction
  —Tapered occlusion suggests a thrombus
- ECG
  —Myocardial ischemia in differential
  —Dysrhythmia as etiology
- CT nonspecific; excludes other causes of abdominal pain
  —Bowel-wall thickening, thumbprinting
  —Late in the course the thrombus or embolus may be identified

DIFFERENTIAL DIAGNOSIS

- Abdominal aortic aneurysm
- Aortic dissection
- Myocardial infarction
- Perforated duodenal ulcer
- Cholelithiasis
- Urolithiasis
- Bowel obstruction
- Sepsis
- Splenic vein thrombosis
- Pancreatitis

Treatment

INITIAL STABILIZATION

- ABCs
- 100% oxygen; intubate if severe respiratory compromise
- Resuscitate
  - —Cardiac monitor
  - —Insert two IVs
  - —Use lactated Ringers if potassium not elevated
  - —Type and cross; transfuse if necessary
  - —Insert Foley to record and follow urine output
  - —NG tube
- Maximize cardiac status
  - —Treat arrhythmias, congestive heart failure, hypotension, hypovolemia, anemia;
  - —Consider blood transfusion to aid in oxygen delivery if ischemia present on EKG
- *Avoid* the use of pressor agents (dopamine or norepinephrine)—worsen bowel ischemia
- Swan-Ganz catheter may be necessary to achieve optimal cardiac performance

ED TREATMENT

- Obtain surgical consult as soon as diagnosis is suspected
- NPO
- Perform angiogram as soon as possible to confirm the diagnosis and define arterial anatomy
- Consultant may choose to use intra-arterial papaverine
  - —Vasodilator
  - —30–60 mg bolus then 30–60 mg/hr infusion through the angiography catheter directly into the SMA to relieve mesenteric vasoconstriction pre- and postoperatively
  - —Limits the extent of bowel infarction
- Preoperative antibiotics (cefoxitin or gentamicin plus either clindamycin or metronidazole)
- Definitive management includes arteriotomy and embolectomy, or thrombectomy with a bypass procedure if there is underlying atherosclerosis, plus resection of necrotic bowel

MEDICATIONS

- Cefoxitin (mefoxin): 1–2 g (peds: 100–160 mg/kg/24hrs) IV q 6 hrs
- Gentamicin: 1.5 mg/kg IV load
- Clindamycin: 900 mg (peds: 25–40 mg/kg/24hrs) IV q 8 hrs
- Metronidazole: 1.0 g (peds: 15 mg/kg) load followed by 500 mg (7.5 mg/kg) IV q 6 hrs

Disposition

ADMISSION CRITERIA

- Admit suspected mesenteric ischemia in ICU or directly to angiography and the operating room

DISCHARGE CRITERIA

- Exclude mesenteric ischemia prior to discharge

Miscellaneous

ICD 9: 557.1

ICD9: 1.6.2.1

SUGGESTED READINGS

Kaleya RN, Boley SJ. Acute mesenteric ischemia. Crit Care Clin 1995;11(2):479–511.
Moore WM Jr, Hollier LH. Mesenteric artery occlusive disease. Cardiol Clin 1991;9(3):535–541.

Reinus JF, Brandt LJ, Boley SJ. Ischemic diseases of the bowel. Gastroenterol Clin North Am 1990;19(2):319–343.

Walker JS, Dire DJ. Vascular abdominal emergencies. Emerg Med Clin North Am 1996;14(3):571–592.

Author: Paula Ward

Metacarpal Injuries

Clinical Presentation

SIGNS AND SYMPTOMS

- Pain at the site of injury
- Deformity at the site of injury
- Malalignment of the distal tip of the finger on flexion indicates rotational deformity
  - —Lines drawn down the longitudinal axis of each ray in flexion normally should converge on the scaphoid volarly
- Limitation of movement secondary to pain and anatomic deformity
- A special category of injury is the direct blow of a closed fist against a human tooth
  - —The concern here is violation of the MCP joint, or metacarpal fracture, by the tooth and subsequent infection with oral flora

MECHANISM/DESCRIPTION

- Most of these are caused by crush injuries or by a direct blow with the hand to an object
- The most common is the "Boxer's Fracture" of the distal 5th metacarpal neck

PEDIATRIC CONSIDERATIONS

- These fractures are rare in children who do not possess the strength to strike an object hard enough to cause the fracture

Pre-Hospital

CAUTIONS

- These injuries should be splinted in a position of comfort. Patients often feel their symptoms are not serious because they have little pain, but all patients with hand injuries seen by pre-hospital personnel should be seen by a physician

Diagnosis

ESSENTIAL WORKUP

- A careful history and complete physical exam should be accompanied by a full x-ray series of the affected hand
- Examination should pay specific attention to skin integrity

IMAGING/SPECIAL TESTS

- Special radiographic views of the proximal metacarpals and the carpal-metacarpal joints may be necessary for patients with a suggestive physical exam and no definite fracture on a standard three-view series

DIFFERENTIAL DIAGNOSIS

- Fracture of the metacarpal may be accompanied by dislocation of adjacent phalanges or carpal bones

Treatment

INITIAL STABILIZATION

- Other more serious injuries should be treated first
- Immobilize hand pending evaluation

ED TREATMENT

- Elevation, rest, and intermittent application of ice are appropriate treatment for all hand injuries
- Boxer's fractures may have volar flexion of the distal fragment
  - —Reduction should be attempted for volar angulation of 40° or more
  - —Fractures of the 4th and 5th metacarpal that are stable and with no significant rotational component are treated with a padded ulnar gutter splint
- Fractures of the index and middle metacarpals are more difficult to stabilize and should have early orthopedic consultation
- Dislocations should be reduced immediately and splinted
- Appropriate splinting position for the MCP joint is the intrinsic plus, or "cobra," position
  - —MCP joint as close to 90° of flexion as possible
  - —PIP and DIP joints in extension
- Antibiotics for oral flora should be started early for any open injuries to the metacarpals suspicious for injury against a tooth

MEDICATIONS

- Mild analgesics may be necessary, but narcotics are usually not indicated
- Augmentin 875/125 mg po tid for prophylaxis in bite wounds

PEDIATRIC CONSIDERATIONS

- Even if the fracture fragment cannot be seen on x-ray the physical findings are so definitive that treatment should be instituted

Disposition

ADMISSION CRITERIA

- Open fractures or dislocations require urgent surgical intervention and should be admitted. All thumb metacarpal fractures or dislocations should be seen by an orthopedist or hand surgeon due to the special importance of the thumb in all activities of the hand.
- Simultaneous infection from human bite wound requires prompt orthopedic consultation, admission for irrigation, debridement, and intravenous antibiotics

DISCHARGE CRITERIA

- Patients with a stable fracture in a good splint may be discharged for early orthopedic follow-up
- Metacarpal-carpal dislocations are usually unstable enough to require surgery even if reduction is achieved, but this may be semi-urgent rather than emergent
- If a metacarpal fracture produces impaired range of motion or malalignment of the finger, the patient will require surgical repair in the first several days postinjury

Miscellaneous

ICD9: 815.00, 834.01, 833.05

CORE CONTENT CODE: 18.4.12.1.2, 18.4.12.2.4.1

SUGGESTED READINGS

American Society for Surgery of the Hand. The hand: Examination and diagnosis. 2d ed. New York: Churchill Livingston, 1983.

American Society for Surgery of the Hand. The hand: Primary care of common problems. 2d ed. New York: Churchill Livingston, 1990.

Antosia RE, Lyn E. The hand. In: Rosen P, et al. Emergency medicine: Concepts and clinical practice. 4th ed. St. Louis: Mosby-Year Book 1998:625–668.

Uehara DT. The hand in emergency medicine. Emerg Clin North Am 1993;11(3):585–600.

Author: Matthew Walsh

Metatarsal Injuries

Clinical Presentation

SIGNS AND SYMPTOMS

- Pain over dorsum of foot, increases with dependency and weight-bearing
- Swelling, ecchymosis
- Pain with axial compression of effected toe

MECHANISM/DESCRIPTION

Fractures

- Direct injury, e.g., heavy object dropped onto foot
- Indirect forces, e.g., body twisting with toes fixed
  —Produces spiral fractures
- Stress fractures

Dislocations—First Metatarsophalangeal Joint

- Compared to sprains, relatively rare because of strong ligamentous support
- High energy forces; usually not isolated injuries
- Dorsal dislocation most common; obvious on physical examination (dorsal displacement, shortening)

Dislocations—Other Metatarsophalangeal Joints

- Axial load; unprotected toes
- Lateral displacement more common than medial

PEDIATRIC CONSIDERATIONS

- Salter-Harris type 1 injuries may present with bony tenderness at epiphysis

Pre-Hospital

CAUTIONS

- Splinting, ice, elevation
- Address other associated injuries

Diagnosis

ESSENTIAL WORKUP

- Foot x-rays (see next section)

IMAGING/SPECIAL TESTS

- Standard radiographs, anteroposterior, oblique, lateral
- Bone scan if suspect stress fractures
- Computed tomography or magnetic resonance imaging if suspect occult injury

DIFFERENTIAL DIAGNOSIS

- Soft tissue injury
- Other fracture or dislocation (e.g., Lisfranc)

Treatment

INITIAL STABILIZATION

- Assess for other more life-threatening injuries first in cases of major trauma
- Assess for ischemia distal to the fracture-dislocation
- Ice, elevation

ED TREATMENT

Fractures

- Posterior splint, nonweight-bearing
- Ambulatory assistance
  - —Cane, crutches
- Orthopedic referral
  - —Nondisplaced or 2nd–4th displaced only in the frontal plane
    - -Short-leg walking cast for 2–4 weeks
  - —Dorsal or plantar displacement and medial displacement of 1st or lateral displacement of 5th
    - -Closed reduction
    - -Open reduction if closed reduction fails

Dislocations

- Reduction, traction
  - —Finger traps with weights may be used on toes as well
  - —After adequate analgesia or sedation is achieved, reduction can be accomplished by gentle manipulation
- Orthopedic referral
  - —Short leg-walking cast for 3–4 weeks
  - —For reduction if unable to reduce

MEDICATIONS

- Analgesics (opioids or NSAIDs)
- Digital or hematoma block may facilitate reduction of dislocations

Disposition

ADMISSION CRITERIA

- Need for open reduction, internal fixation
- Open (compound) injuries
- As dictated by associated injuries or circumstances

DISCHARGE CRITERIA

- Vast majority of patients can be discharged with orthopedic follow-up

Miscellaneous

ICD9: 825.25, 838.04

CORE CONTENT CODE: 18.4.13.1.2, 18.4.13.2.1

SUGGESTED READINGS

Heckman JD. Fractures and dislocations of the foot. In: Rockwood CA, Green DP, Bucholz RW, Heckman JD, eds. Rockwood and Green's fractures in adults. 4th ed. New York: Lippincott-Raven, 1996:2267– 2405.

O'Malley MJ, Hamilton WG, Munyak J. Fractures of the distal shaft of the fifth metatarsal. "dancer's fracture." Am J Sports Med 1996;24(2):240–243.

Simon RS, Koeningsknecht SJ. Metatarsal fractures. In Simon RS, Koeningsknecht SJ, eds. Emergency orthopedics: The extremities. 2d ed. Norwalk, CT: Appleton & Lange, 1987:285–287.

Author: Joel M. Bartfield

Methanol, Poisoning

Clinical Presentation

SIGNS AND SYMPTOMS

Gastrointestinal

- Anorexia
- Nausea/vomiting
- Abdominal pain

Central Nervous System

- Headache
- Dizziness
- Confusion
- Inebriation
- Coma
- Seizures

Ophthalmologic

- Blurry vision
- Photophobia
- "Snow fields"
- Mydriasis
- Blindness
- Optic disc
  —Hyperemia or pallor
  —Papilledema

MECHANISM/DESCRIPTION

- Colorless, volatile liquid
- Absorbed in 30–60 minutes
- Metabolized by the liver
- Half-life 12 hours
- Methanol
  —Inebriating
  —Nontoxic
  —Metabolites (formaldehyde and formic acid) produce toxic effects
- Formic acid level determines degree of acidosis, visual symptoms, and mortality
- Formic acid–directly toxic to retinal and optic nerve tissue
- Methanol metabolism
  —Methanol converted to formaldehyde by the liver enzyme alcohol dehydrogenase
  —Formaldehyde then rapidly converted to formic acid
  —Formic acid degraded into carbon dioxide and water by a folate-dependent mechanism
  —Steps 1 and 3 are rate-limiting steps

ETIOLOGY

Common Sources of Methanol

- Wood alcohol
- Windshield washer fluid
- Antifreeze
- Formalin
- Gasoline ("gasohol")
- Paint solvents
- Household cleaners

Pre-Hospital

CAUTIONS

- Transport all substances that the patient may have ingested

Diagnosis

ESSENTIAL WORKUP

- History of all substances ingested
- Inquire about visual symptoms
- Thorough funduscopic examination
- Drawn *simultaneously*
  —ABG
  —Serum methanol, ethylene glycol, and ethanol levels
  —Electrolytes, BUN, Cr, and glucose
  —Measured serum osmolality (by freezing point depression)

LABORATORY

- Calculate anion gap = $(Na^+) - (Cl^- + HCO_3^-)$
  —Normal = 8–12
- Determine osmol gap
  —Osmol gap = measured osmolality − calculated osmolarity
    -Calculated osmolarity = $2(Na^+)$ + glucose/18 + BUN/2.8 + ethanol (in mg/dl)/4.6
    ->10 increased
  —Osmol gap
    -Screens for toxic alcohols
    -Primarily affected by methanol, not methanol metabolites
    -Increased early in poisoning and normalizes as methanol metabolized
    -Most sensitive early in poisoning
    -Normal osmol gap does *not* rule out methanol ingestion
- Toxic alcohol levels *confirm* methanol poisoning
- Ethanol level
  —Determines the amount of ethanol bolus necessary to attain a therapeutic level
- Urinalysis
  —Envelope-shaped oxalate crystals
    -Insensitive but specific finding in ethylene glycol poisoning
  —Ketones
    -Due to isopropyl alcohol ingestion, starvation or DKA
- Serum iron, salicylate, and acetaminophen level

IMAGING/SPECIAL TESTS

- Wood's lamp inspection of urine and/or gastric contents
  —Detects the presence of fluorescein, a common antifreeze additive (usually ethylene glycol)
  —Insensitive but specific marker of antifreeze ingestion

DIFFERENTIAL DIAGNOSIS

- Increased osmol gap: *ME DIE A*
  —*M*ethanol
  —*E*thanol
  —*D*iuretics (mannitol, glycerin, sorbitol)
  —*I*sopropyl alcohol
  —*E*thylene glycol
  —*A*cetone, ammonia
- Elevated anion gap metabolic acidosis: *ACAT MUDPILES*
  —*A*lcoholic ketoacidosis
  —*C*yanide, CO, H_2S, others
  —*A*SA, other salicylates
  —*T*oluene
  —*Methanol*, metformin
  —*U*remia
  —*D*iabetic ketoacidosis
  —*P*araldehyde, phenformin
  —*I*ron, INH
  —*L*actic acidosis from other causes
  —*E*thylene glycol
  —*S*tarvation ketosis

Treatment

INITIAL STABILIZATION

- ABCs
- Dextrose (or Accucheck), naloxone, and thiamine for altered mental status

ED TREATMENT

Prevent Further Methanol Absorption

- Gastric lavage if the patient presents within 1 hour of ingestion or if the patient's clinical condition mandates endotracheal intubation
- Ipecac-induced emesis not recommended
- Activated charcoal
  - —For potential coingestants
  - —Poorly adsorbs methanol

Prevent Methanol Conversion to Toxic Metabolites

- Ethanol therapy
  - —Initiate before the methanol level returns if a potentially toxic ingestion is highly suspected or confirmed by history
  - —Ethanol has greater affinity than methanol for alcohol dehydrogenase
    - -Slows metabolism to formaldehyde and formic acid by competitive inhibition
  - —Indications for ethanol therapy
    - -Intention methanol ingestion
    - -Accidental methanol ingestion of greater than a sip
    - -Altered mental status or visual symptoms associated with an unexplained osmol gap or elevated anion gap metabolic acidosis
  - —Therapeutic range = 100–150 mg/dl
  - —Continue until the methanol level is zero
- 4-Methylpyrazole (4-MP, antizol)
  - —Competitive inhibitor of alcohol dehydrogenase
  - —FDA approval for use in ethylene glycol poisoning
  - —Used in Europe for methanol and ethylene glycol toxicity
  - —Expensive alternative to ethanol infusion
  - —Advantages over ethanol infusion
    - -No need for continuous infusion
    - -No inebriation/CNS depression

Enhance Elimination of Methanol and Its Toxic Metabolites

- Hemodialysis
  - —Decreases the elimination half-life of methanol to 2.5 hours
  - —Removes formaldehyde and formic acid
  - —Indications
    - -Ingestion of >1 cc/kg of 100% methanol
    - -Ophthalmologic manifestations
    - -Severe acidosis unresponsive to bicarbonate therapy
    - -Persistent electrolyte or fluid imbalance
    - -Renal insufficiency
    - -Serum methanol level >25 mg/dl
  - —Continue hemodialysis until methanol level approaches zero
- Folic acid and folinic acid (leucovorin)
  - —Folic acid: cofactor required for the conversion of formic acid to carbon dioxide and water
  - —Folinic acid: activated form of folic acid, used only for the initial dose
  - —Supplemental folate important in malnourished individuals (alcoholics)

Correct Secondary Disorders, Especially Acid/Base Abnormalities

- Sodium bicarbonate for severe acidosis (pH <7.1)

MEDICATIONS

- Ethanol—IV
  - —10% ethanol in D5W
  - —Loading dose: 10 ml/kg over 30–60 min
  - —Maintenance infusion rates
    - -Nonalcoholic patient: 1–1.2 ml/kg/hr
    - -Alcoholic patient: 1.5–2 ml/kg/hr
    - -During hemodialysis: 3–4 ml/kg/hr
- Ethanol—oral
  - —40% ethanol solution (80 proof liquor) via NGT
  - —Loading dose: 2.5 ml/kg
  - —Maintenance dosing
    - -Nonalcoholic patient: 0.3 ml/kg/hr
    - -Alcoholic patient: 0.5 ml/kg/hr
    - -During hemodialysis: 1 ml/kg/hr
- Folic acid: 50 mg IVP q 4 hrs for 24 hrs
- Folinic acid: 1–2 mg/kg IV
- 4-Methylpyrazole
  - —Loading dose: 15 mg/kg slow infusion over 30 min
  - —Maintenance dosing: 10 mg/kg q 12 hrs for 4 doses, then 15 mg/kg q 12 hrs
  - —Increased dosing during dialysis
- Sodium bicarbonate: 1 mEq/kg IV
- Thiamine: 100 mg IVP

Disposition

ADMISSION CRITERIA

- Significant methanol ingestion even if initially asymptomatic
- ICU admission for seriously ill patients
- Transfer to another facility if hemodialysis is indicated but not readily available

DISCHARGE CRITERIA

- Asymptomatic patient with isolated methanol ingestion if the serum methanol level is undetectable

Miscellaneous

ICD9: 980.1

CORE CONTENT CODE: 17.2.2.4

SUGGESTED READINGS

Burkhart KK, Kulig KW. The other alcohols: Methanol, ethylene glycol and isopropanol. Emerg Med Clin North Am 1990;8(4):913–928.

Jacobsen D, McMartin KE. Antidotes for methanol and ethylene glycol poisonings. J Toxicol Clin Toxicol 1997;35(2):127–143.

Jacobsen D, McMartin KE. Methanol and ethylene glycol poisonings: Mechanisms of toxicity, clinical course, diagnosis and treatment. Med Toxicol 1986;1:309–334.

Authors: Saul Melman; Jeffrey Schlab; Theodore Torn

Methemoglobinemia

Clinical Presentation

SIGNS AND SYMPTOMS

- "Chocolate cyanosis" unaffected by supplemental oxygen
  - —1.5 g methemoglobin/dl blood necessary to produce cyanosis
- Tissue hypoxia
  - —Syncope
  - —Altered mental status
  - —Chest pain
  - —Dysrhythmias
  - —Dyspnea
- Brown-red blood color
  - —Unchanged by bubbling oxygen through it

MECHANISM/DESCRIPTION

- Methemoglobin
  - —Produced normally in small amounts through aberrant oxygen dissociation from hemoglobin
  - —Detoxified by RBC NADH-methemoglobin (cytochrome b_5) reductase
- Normal deoxyhemoglobin contains heme with Fe in the +2 state
- Methemoglobin contains heme with Fe in the +3 (oxidized) state
  - —Cannot reversibly bind oxygen
- Methemoglobin (like carboxyhemoglobin)
  - —Decreases total oxygen carrying capacity, producing a functional anemia
  - —Shifts the hemoglobin oxygen-dissociation curve to the left
  - —Distorts the sigmoid shape of the hemoglobin oxygen-dissociation curve
- Congenital methemoglobin occurs in patients with
  - —Heterozygous hemoglobin M and other abnormal hemoglobins
  - —Homozygous NADH-methemoglobin (cytochrome b_5) reductase deficiency
- Acquired methemoglobinemia results from oxidant stress on red blood cells
  - —Some methemoglobin-inducing agents are direct oxidants (e.g., nitrites)
  - —Many substances produce oxidant injury to the RBC through their N-hydroxylamine metabolites
    - -Methemoglobinemia may be delayed relative to initial substance exposure
- Many methemoglobin-inducing agents also cause Heintz body hemolytic anemia
  - —Due to oxidant injury of RBC proteins
  - —G-6-PD deficient patients have a higher incidence of such hemolytic anemia
- Methemoglobinemia may serve as a marker for genetic abnormalities
  - —Heterozygous NADH-methemoglobin (cytochrome b_5) reductase deficiency

ETIOLOGY

- Dyes
  - —Aniline dyes
  - —Methylene blue in excess may itself cause methemoglobinemia and hemolytic anemia
- Antiparasitic drugs
  - —Dapsone
  - —Primaquine
- Local anesthetics
  - —Benzocaine
  - —Lidocaine
  - —Prilocaine
- Analgesics
  - —Phenazopyridine (pyridium)
  - —Phenacetin
- Antibiotics
  - —Nitrofurantoin
  - —Sulfones
  - —Sulfonamides
- Nitrates/nitrites
  - —Nitrites (NO_2)
  - —Nitrates (NO_3); e.g., nitroglycerine, via metabolic conversion to nitrites
  - —Nitric oxide (NO)
- Others
  - —Metoclopramide
  - —Naphthalene (mothballs)
  - —Paraquat (a herbicide)
  - —Arsine gas (AsH_3)
  - —Chlorates ($-ClO_4$)
  - —Phenols (e.g., dinitrophenol, hydroquinone)

PEDIATRIC CONSIDERATIONS

- Neonates and younger infants have an increased susceptibility to develop methemoglobinemia

Pre-Hospital

CAUTIONS

- Bring to the hospital all substances the patient may have ingested
- Question witnesses and observe the scene for household products and other potential coingestants
  - —Document and relay findings to emergency medical staff
  - —At commercial or industrial sites of exposure obtain relevant Material Safety Data Sheets (MSDS) if readily available to identify commercial or chemical products

Diagnosis

ESSENTIAL WORKUP

- Thorough history
  - —Exposure to a methemoglobin-inducing agent
  - —All substances ingested and the time(s) of ingestion
  - —G-6-PD deficiency
  - —Conditions vulnerable to impaired oxygen delivery (e.g., coronary artery disease)
- Physical exam
  - —Emphasis on mental status and cardiovascular findings
  - —Icterus or dark-colored urine with accompanying hemolytic anemia
- Pulse oximetry
  - —Methemoglobinemia interferes with pulse oximetry hemoglobin oxygen saturation measurement
    - -Saturation decreases to approximately 85% with increasingly more severe methemoglobinemia
    - -Saturation is not accurate and should not be used to guide management
- Methemoglobin level by co-oximetry is reported as % of total hemoglobin
- ABG by co-oximetry
  - —Hemoglobin oxygen saturation
    - -Accurately measured only by co-oximetry
    - -Falsely elevated by nonco-oximetry methods in patients with methemoglobinemia
- ECG

LABORATORY

- CBC with manual differential count and smear analysis for evidence of hemolytic anemia
- Urinalysis for blood versus intact RBCs to detect presence of free hemoglobin in urine
- Enzyme activity studies or hemoglobin electrophoresis if indicated
- Salicylate and acetaminophen levels for patients with suicidal ingestions
- Pregnancy test

DIFFERENTIAL DIAGNOSIS

- Blue discoloration
  - —Hypoxia
  - —Sulfhemoglobinemia
  - —Cyanide poisoning
  - —Hydrogen sulfide poisoning
  - —Excess methylene blue administration
  - —Tellurium toxicity
  - —Skin contact/staining with blue dye

Treatment

INITIAL STABILIZATION

- ABCs
  - —Administer oxygen by nonrebreather for shortness of breath/chest pain/altered mental status
- Treat based on the patient's condition and not on a specific methemoglobin level

ED TREATMENT

- Decontamination if indicated with activated charcoal for oral ingestions
- Methylene blue
  - —To reverse methemoglobinemia in symptomatic patients
  - —Avoid if possible in patients with G-6-PD deficiency because it may induce more severe hemolysis
  - —Repeat doses of methylene blue in patients with ongoing absorption or production of methemoglobin-inducing agents
- RBC transfusion
  - —May be necessary to increase blood oxygen carrying capacity
  - —Especially if hemolytic anemia is present
- Exchange transfusion
  - —Especially with neonates/infants
- Hyperbaric oxygen therapy
  - —Increases oxygen delivery to tissues by mass effect, independent of hemoglobin
  - —Use in life-threatening methemoglobinemia if immediately available
- Treatment of other toxin-induced problems

MEDICATIONS

- Activated charcoal: 1 g/kg po or per NGT
- Methylene blue: 1–2 mg/kg IVP over 5 min

Disposition

ADMISSION CRITERIA

- Admit all patients with serious symptomatic acquired methemoglobinemia for observation
  - —To evaluate for return of treated methemoglobinemia and development of delayed hemolysis

DISCHARGE CRITERIA

- Known congenital methemoglobinemia if asymptomatic and without significant change in usual methemoglobin level
- Mild, asymptomatic acquired methemoglobinemia if on chronic, stable therapy with a known methemoglobin-inducing agent (e.g., dapsone) with close follow-up
- Mild, asymptomatic acquired methemoglobinemia may be discharged if successfully treated after 4–6 hours observation and no return of methemoglobinemia

Miscellaneous

ICD9: 289.7

CORE CONTENT CODE: 17.2.32

SUGGESTED READINGS

Coleman MD, Coleman NA. Drug-induced methemoglobinemia. Treatment issues. Drug Saf 1996;14(6):394–405.

Curry SC. Methemoglobinemia. Ann Emerg Med 1982;11:214.

Author: Theodore Toerne

Migraine Headache

Clinical Presentation

SIGNS AND SYMPTOMS

- *Common migraine*
  - —Unheralded onset of headache that is recurrent, throbbing, and frequently unilateral
  - —Usually associated with photophobia, phonophobia, nausea, anorexia, and vomiting
- *Classic migraine:* common migraine, which is preceded by a prodrome; usually visual symptoms such as bright lights or jagged lines
- *Complicated migraine:* migraine headache with associated neurologic symptoms such as numbness, weakness, paralysis, or aphasia

MECHANISM/DESCRIPTION

- The prevailing theory is that a migraine begins with intracranial artery vasoconstriction, which results in reduced cerebral blood flow. This produces the *aura,* the type of which is dependent on the area of reduced flow
  - —This is followed by a rebound vasodilation of the arteries during which the headache occurs
  - —The arterial dilation gives rise to pain

ETIOLOGY

- Idiopathic
- May be precipitated by chocolate, cheese, nuts, alcohol, sulfites, MSG, stress, tension, or puberty
- There is a family history of migraines in 60%
- Affects 5–15% of the population (women 3 times more than men)

PEDIATRIC CONSIDERATIONS

- Migraines do present in the pediatric age group, but are less common
- The typical pediatric patient is a prepubertal female with a strong family history of migraine

Pre-Hospital

CAUTIONS

- It is important to recognize life-threatening causes of headache and transport rapidly
  - —Sudden onset of symptoms, altered mental status, neck stiffness, fever, or neurologic deficits are useful signs that suggest a more serious cause of headache
  - —Prior history of similar headache, absence of above symptoms, or strong family history is more suggestive of migraine
- Allow patients with migraine headache to be in a calm, dark environment

Diagnosis

ESSENTIAL WORKUP

- An accurate history and physical exam should confirm the diagnosis
- Patients with new onset of headache syndrome need an objective evaluation to rule out more serious causes of severe headaches
  - —Complete neurologic examination
  - —CT or MRI of the head
  - —Lumbar puncture
  - —If the patient can be assured of close follow-up, imaging studies and LP can be done as an outpatient if the clinical presentation does not suggest a life-threatening cause of headache

LABORATORY

- Not needed for classic migraine or established migraines with typical symptoms
- Lumbar puncture if suspect meningitis, intracranial hemorrhage, or pseudotumor cerebri
- ESR if suspect temporal arteritis
- Carbon monoxide (CO) level if there is history or suspicion of CO exposure

IMAGING/SPECIAL TESTS

- CT scan or MRI to rule out intracranial hemorrhage or tumor

DIFFERENTIAL DIAGNOSIS

- Meningitis
- Subarachnoid/intracranial hemorrhage
- Cerebral ischemia
- Hypertension
- Brain tumor
- Arteriovenous malformation
- Dental cause
- Temporal mandibular joint (TMJ) syndrome
- Pseudotumor cerebri
- Temporal arteritis

Treatment

INITIAL STABILIZATION

- ABCs
- Patients with evidence of increased intracranial pressure may need rapid sequence intubation and therapeutic hyperventilation

ED TREATMENT

- Abortive therapy and pain management are the primary issues for patients in which life-threatening causes of headache have been ruled out
- Generally, abortive therapy options such as sumatriptan should be attempted first
- Narcotic pain medications may be administered as rescue therapy
- Intravenous saline hydration is often a helpful adjunct for migraine headaches

MEDICATIONS

- Abortive therapy in ED
  —Ergot alkaloids: DHE 1 mg IM or IV, then repeat in 1 hr if necessary
  —Metoclopramide: 10 mg IV
  —NSAIDs: ketorolac 15–30 mg IM/IV
  —Prochlorperazine: 10mg IV
  —Sumatriptan: 6 mg SQ, may repeat in 1 hr (max of 2 doses per 24 hrs)
- Rescue pain medication
  —Meperidine: 25–100 mg IM/IV per dose
  —Morphine: 2–10 mg I/IV per dose
- Prophylactic therapy
  —β-blockers: propranolol 40 mg po bid
  —Ca^{++} channel blockers: verapamil 40 mg po tid
  —Cyclic antidepressants: amitriptyline 25 mg po tid

Disposition

ADMISSION CRITERIA

- Severe intractable headache pain
- Intractable vomiting, electrolyte imbalance, or inability to take oral food or fluid
- Suicidal ideation secondary to unremitting headache

DISCHARGE CRITERIA

- Patients with moderate to complete pain relief and a confident diagnosis of migraine

Miscellaneous

ICD9: 346.90

CORE CONTENT CODE: 11.10

SUGGESTED READINGS

Goadsby PJ, Olesen J. Diagnosis and management of migraine. Br Med J 1996;312(7041):1279–1283.

Noack H, Rothrock JF. Migraine: Definitions, mechanisms, and treatment. So Med J 1996;89(8):762–769.

Silberstein SD, Lipton RB. Overview of diagnosis and treatment of migraine. Neurology 1994;44(Suppl 7):S6–16.

Singer HS. Migraine headaches in children. Pediatr Rev 1994;15(3):94–101; quiz 101.

Spierings EL. Symptomatology and pathogenesis of migraine. J Pediatr Gastroenterol Nutr 1995;21(Suppl 1):S37–S41.

Authors: George Kondylis; Gary Johnson

Mitral Valve Prolapse

Clinical Presentation

SIGNS AND SYMPTOMS

- Palpitations
  —Usually ventricular premature beats or PSVT
- Chest pain
- Dyspnea and fatigue
- Early to midsystolic click
- Mid or late systolic murmur
  —Standing the patient or, valsalva causes the click to move closer to S1
  —May bring out previously unheard click
  —Squatting will move the click closer to S2
- Scoliosis
- Pectus excavatum
- Narrow anterior-posterior diameter of the chest
- Arachnodactyly

MECHANISM/DESCRIPTION

- Prolapse of the mitral valve leaflets into the left atrium during systole
  —Produces nonejection click heard at the apex
- Occurs in two phenotypic patterns
  —Anatomic form
    -Thickened, billowing mitral leaflets
  —Functional form
    -Dynamic systolic expansion of the mitral annulus
- Familial occurrence
- Marfan's syndrome
- Von Willebrand's syndrome
- Duchenne's muscular dystrophy

PEDIATRIC CONSIDERATIONS

- Dysrhythmias, sudden death and bacterial endocarditis have been reported

Pre-Hospital

CAUTIONS

- MVP may be associated with preexcitation syndromes
  —Supraventricular tachydysrhythmias may worsen with treatment that blocks conduction through the A-V node
- Bradycardia associated with A-V block may be resistant to atropine and require isoproterenol or cardiac pacing

Diagnosis

ESSENTIAL WORKUP

- Electrocardiogram
  —Usually normal
  —Occasionally ST-T wave depression and inversion in leads III and aVF
  —Premature atrial and ventricular contractions

LABORATORY

- CBC
- Thyroid function tests
- Serum potassium and magnesium

IMAGING/SPECIAL TESTS

- Chest x-ray
  —Typically normal
  —May show skeletal abnormalities
  —If mitral regurgitation is present, may show both left atrial and ventricular enlargement
  —Calcification of the mitral annulus in patients with Marfan's syndrome
- Holter monitor
- Echocardiogram
  —Most useful for defining MVP
- Exercise stress test
  —Indicated for patients with chest pain syndromes
- Myocardial perfusion scintigraphy
- Cardiac catheterization

DIFFERENTIAL DIAGNOSIS

- Anemia
- Thyrotoxicosis
- Pregnancy
- Myocardial infarction/ischemia
- Hypertrophic cardiomyopathy with obstruction
- Papillary muscle dysfunction
- Hypokalemia, hypomagnesemia
- Valvular heart disease
- Pheochromocytoma
- Anxiety/panic disorder
- Stress
- Menopause

PEDIATRIC CONSIDERATIONS

- Toxin/drug ingestion, otherwise same as above

Treatment

INITIAL STABILIZATION

- Intravenous access, oxygen, cardiac monitor, pulse oximetry
- Treat dysrhythmias if present

ED TREATMENT

- Reassurance and explanation of the disease
- Search for underlying causes as listed above
- Patients with tachycardia or severely symptomatic often respond to β blockers
- Patients do require endocarditis prophylaxis for minor procedures

MEDICATIONS

- Propranolol 1–10 mg IV load, then 3 mg/hr; 80–640 mg/d po

PEDIATRIC CONSIDERATIONS

- Full activity for asymptomatic and uncomplicated MVP

Disposition

ADMISSION CRITERIA

- Severe mitral regurgitation
- Severe chest pain with ischemic symptoms
- Syncope or near syncope
- Life-threatening dysrhythmias
- Cerebral ischemic events, including TIA

DISCHARGE CRITERIA

- Asymptomatic
- No laboratory abnormalities
- No significant mitral regurgitation or dysrhythmias

Miscellaneous

ICD9: 424.0

CORE CONTENT CODE: 2.6.2.2

SUGGESTED READINGS

Devereux RB. Mitral valve prolapse. Am J Med 1979;67:729.

Greenwood RD. Mitral valve prolapse in children. West J Med 1986;144:375.

Hanson EW, Neerhurt RK, Lynch III. Mitral valve prolapse. Anesthesiology 1996;85:178.

Savage DD, Devereus RB, Garrison RJ, et al. Mitral valve prolapse in the general population. 2. Clinical features: The Framingham Study. Am Heart J 1983;106:577.

Savage DD, Levy D, Garrison RJ, et al. Mitral valve prolapse in the general population. 3. Dysrhythmias: The Framingham Study. Am Heart J 1983;106:582.

Author: Liudvikas Jagminus

Molluscum Contagiosum

Clinical Presentation

SIGNS AND SYMPTOMS

- Lesions are smooth-surfaced, firm spherical papules, 3–5 mm in diameter
- May be flesh-colored, white, translucent, or light-yellow in color
- Distinctive central umbilication in 25%
- Distribution in children: face, trunk, and extremities. Healthy adults: genitals and lower abdomen; occasionally perioral; rarely on palms and soles
- Molluscum contagiosum (MC) is commonly seen with HIV infection causing atypical involvement of face, neck, and trunk, lesions to 1.5 cm, and a progressive course
- Occasional intraocular or periocular involvement presenting as trachoma or chronic follicular conjunctivitis
- Incubation period: 14–50 days
- Patients are usually asymptomatic, with occasional pruritus or tenderness
- 10–25% of patients may have eczematous reaction surrounding the lesions
- Untreated lesions in immunocompetent hosts usually resolve within several months, but can last up to 5 years

ETIOLOGY

- MC is caused by a double-stranded DNA poxvirus
- Transmission in children is by direct skin-to-skin contact or fomites
- Transmission in adults is most often by sexual contact

Pre-Hospital

- Maintain universal precautions

Diagnosis

ESSENTIAL WORKUP

- History and careful skin examination
- Skin biopsy for confirmation. Lesions may mimic many other dermatologic conditions

DIFFERENTIAL DIAGNOSIS

- Basal cell carcinoma, histiocytoma, keratoacanthoma, intradermal nevus
- Darier's disease, nevoxanthoendothelioma, syringoma, epithelial nevi, sebaceous adenoma
- Atopic dermatitis, dermatitis herpetiformis, mycosis fungoides, Jessner's lymphocytic infiltration

Treatment

INITIAL STABILIZATION

- Not applicable in routine cases

ED TREATMENT

- Treatment is aimed at destruction or removal of viral-infected epithelial cells and is indicated to prevent autoinoculation and transmission
- Curettage after local anesthesia with EMLA or ethyl chloride is the first line of therapy and is effective in children and adults
- Podophyllin, trichloroacetic acid, cantharidin, and tretinoin used topically are all effective
- Cryotherapy with liquid nitrogen is also effective
- Griseofulvin and methisazone orally for extensive disease have given mixed results
- No therapy has been effective in halting progression in HIV-infected patients
- Examine sexual partners for MC and other sexually transmitted diseases
- Reexamine treated patients after 6 weeks for recurrence

MEDICATIONS

- Cantharidin 0.9% solution with equal parts acetone and flexible collodion: apply topically 1–3 treatments q 7 days or until resolution
- Podophyllin (podofilox 0.5%): apply topically q 12 hrs for 3 days, withhold for 4 days. Repeat 1 week cycle up to 4 times until resolved
- Trichloroacetic acid (50–80%): apply and cover with bandage 5–6 days
- Tretinoin 0.1%: topically q 12 hrs for 10 days or until resolution of lesions

PEDIATRIC CONSIDERATIONS

- For painless therapy in children use topical EMLA (lidocaine/prilocaine cream) 1 hour prior to curettage or use cantharidin, a painless blister inducing agent

Disposition

ADMISSION CRITERIA

- Widespread disease with extensive superinfection in an immunocompromised host

DISCHARGE CRITERIA

- Patients without extensive superinfection may be safely treated as outpatients

Miscellaneous

ICD9: 078.0

CORE CONTENT CODE: 3.2.4.4

SUGGESTED READINGS

Epstein WL. Molluscum contagiosum. Semin Dermatol 1992;11:184–189.

Gottlieb SL, Myskowski PL. Molluscum Contagiosum Int J of Dermatology. 1994;33(7):453–61.

Gottlieb S, Myskowski P. Review: Molluscum contagiosum. Intern J Dermatol 1994;33(7)453–61.

Stone M, Lynch P. Viral warts. In: Sams et al, eds. Principals and practice of dermatology. 2d ed. New York: Churchill Livingstone, 1996:133–135.

Author: Guy Tarleton

Monoamine Oxidase Inhibitor, Poisoning

Clinical Presentation

SIGNS AND SYMPTOMS

Monoamine Oxidase Inhibitor (MAOI) Overdose

- Delayed onset (12 hours)
- Initial hypertension with headache
- Delayed cardiovascular collapse
- Neurologic
  - —Nystagmus
  - —Hyperreflexia
  - —Tremor
  - —Myoclonus
  - —Seizures
- Neuroleptic malignant syndrome (NMS)-like complex
  - —Elevated temperature with diaphoresis
  - —Rigidity
  - —Autonomic instability
  - —Altered mental status
  - —Associated complications
    - -Rhabdomyolysis
    - -Renal failure
    - -DIC
    - -ARDS

MAOI Hypertensive Crisis Syndrome

- Hypertension
- Tachycardia or bradycardia
- Hyperthermia
- Headache, usually occipital
- Altered mental status
- Intracranial hemorrhage
- Seizures

Serotonin Syndrome (SS)

- Loosely-described syndrome
- Due to increased CNS serotonin
- Dysfunction in three general physioanatomic areas
  - —Cognitive-behavorial
  - —Autonomic nervous system
  - —Neuromuscular
- Severe SS
  - —May resemble neuroleptic malignant syndrome (NMS)
  - —Differences between SS and NMS
    - -Types of precipitating agents
    - -Onset: several hours (SS) vs. days (NMS)
    - -Syndrome resolution: hours (SS) vs. days (NMS)
    - -Laboratory abnormalities: uncommon (SS) vs. common (NMS)
    - -Hyperreflexia: common (SS) vs. rare (NMS)
    - -Myoclonus: common (SS) vs. rare (NMS)

ETIOLOGY

MAOI Physiology/Pharmacology

- MAOI pharmacologic actions
  - —Disruption of equilibrium between endogenous monoamine synthesis and degradation resulting in
    - -Increased neural norepinephrine levels
    - -Down-regulation of several receptor types
  - —Inhibition of irreversible (noncompetitive) enzyme
  - —Inhibition of other B6-containing enzymes
- Monoamine oxidase (MAO): principal inactivator of neural bioactive amines
  - —MAO A
    - -Present in the gut and liver
    - -Protects against dietary bioactive amines
  - —MAO B
    - -Present in neuron terminals and platelets
    - -Sympathomimetic amines: type of bioactive amines

MAOI Overdose

- Toxicopharmacology poorly understood
- MAO inhibitors
  - —Amphetaminelike in structure
  - —Initially produce an indirect sympathomimetic effect
  - —Later produce a sympatholytic response

MAOI Hypertensive Crisis Syndrome

- Results from impaired norepinephrine degradation, combined with massive norepinephrine release precipitated by exposure to an indirect- or mixed-acting sympathomimetic agent
- Common precipitants: tyramine, cocaine, amphetamines

Serotonin Syndrome

- Commonly results from exposure to combinations of agents which affect serotonin metabolism or action
- Mechanisms/agents
  - —Increased serotonin synthesis
    - -Tryptophan
  - —Increased serotonin release
    - -Indirect- and mixed-acting sympathomimetic agents
    - -Dopamine receptor agonist
  - —Decreased serotonin reuptake
    - -Selective serotonin reuptake inhibitors (SSRIs)
    - -Tricyclic antidepressants
    - -Newer antidepressants: trazodone, nefazodone, venlafaxine
    - -Meperidine, dextromethorphan, tramadol
  - —Direct serotonin receptor agonist
    - -Buspirone, sumatriptan, LSD
  - —Decreased serotonin breakdown
    - -MAOIs
  - —Increased nonspecific serotonin activity
    - -Lithium
- SSRIs
  - —Frequently prescribed drugs
  - —Consider serotonin syndrome with multiple poorly described symptoms

PEDIATRIC CONSIDERATIONS

- Serious toxicity after minimal MAOI exposure

Pre-Hospital

CAUTIONS

- Transport all substances the patient may have ingested or used
- Question witnesses and observe the scene for household products and other potential coingestants

Monoamine Oxidase Inhibitor, Poisoning

Diagnosis

ESSENTIAL WORKUP

- History of ingested substances
- Rectal temperature monitoring as indicated
- Blood pressure/cardiac monitoring

LABORATORY

- No laboratory or ancillary tests for
  - —Mild, clinically uncomplicated hypertensive syndromes
  - —Mild, clinically uncomplicated serotonin syndrome
- DIC
  - —CBC
  - —PT/PTT
  - —Fibrin-split products
- Rhabdomyolysis
  - —Electrolytes, BUN/Cr, glucose
  - —Urinalysis
  - —CPK
  - —Myoglobin
- Acetaminophen levels on all patients with suicidal ingestion

IMAGING/SPECIAL TESTS

- ECG for all patients with suicidal ingestions
- CXR for fever and hypoxemia
- Head CT and LP for altered mental status with fever

DIFFERENTIAL DIAGNOSIS

Hyperthermia

- Infection
- Hyperthyroidism
- Heat stroke
- Anatomic thalamic dysfunction
- Neuroleptic malignant syndrome
- Malignant hyperthermia
- Malignant catatonia
- Ethanol or drug withdrawal
- Anticholinergic toxicity
- Sympathomimetic overdose
- Cocaine-associated delirium/rhabdomyolysis
- Salicylate toxicity
- Theophylline toxicity
- Nicotine toxicity

Hypertension

- Hypoglycemia
- Carcinoid syndrome
- Pheochromocytoma
- Accelerated renovascular hypertension
- Ethanol or drug withdrawal
- Sympathomimetic toxicity

Treatment

INITIAL STABILIZATION

- ABCs
- 0.9%NS IV access
- Dextrose (or Accucheck), naloxone, and thiamine for altered mental status

ED TREATMENT

- GI decontamination
  - —Gastric lavage if within *1 hour* of ingestion or if clinical condition mandates endotracheal intubation
  - —Administer activated charcoal
- Hyperthermia
  - —Aggressive control via mist/fan evaporation cooling
- Severe, malignant hypertension
  - —Nitroprusside or phentolamine
  - —Phentolamine contraindicated in MAOI overdose
- Hypotension
  - —Initially with 0.9%NS IV 1–2 L fluid bolus
  - —If no response, administer norepinephrine
  - —Dopamine theoretically contraindicated
- Arrhythmias (premorbid sign in MAOI overdose)
  - —Treat with lidocaine or procainamide
  - —Bretylium contraindicated
- Seizures
  - —Benzodiazepines (initial)
  - —Barbiturates
  - —Pyridoxine for refractory seizures
- Rigidity
  - —Lorazapam
  - —Paralysis with vercuonium, endotracheal intubation and mechanical ventilation
- ARDS
  - —Oxygen
  - —Intubation and PEEP as indicated
- DIC
  - —Fresh frozen plasma
  - —Platelet
  - —Whole-blood transfusions
- Rhabdomyolysis
  - —Urinary alkalinization with sodium bicarbonate bolus and infusion
- Specific treatment for serotonin syndrome
  - —Human data limited to case reports and series
  - —Nonselective serotonin antagonists
    - -Cyproheptadine

MEDICATIONS

- Activated charcoal: 1–2 g/kg po
- Cyproheptadine: 4–8 mg PO/per NGT q 1–4 hrs until therapeutic response; maximum daily dose: 0.5 mg/kg
- Dextrose: D50W 1–2 amp (50–100 ml or 25–50 g) (peds: D25W 2–4 ml/kg) IVP
- Diazepam: 5–10 mg (peds: 0.1mg/kg) increments IVP
- Lidocaine: bolus 1–3 mg/kg IVP, infusion: 1–4 mg/min (peds: 20–50 μg/kg/min) IV
- Lorazepam: 1–2 mg increments IVP
- Nitroprusside: 0.3–10 μg/kg/min IV
- Norepinephrine: 2–4 μg/min IV
- Phentolamine: 5 mg (peds: 1 mg) increments IVP
- Phenylephrine: adult bolus: 50 μg IVP; infusion: 40–180 μg/min IV
- Procainamide: 20 mg/min IV to arrhythmia suppression, hypotension, QRS >100 ms or 18 mg/kg
- Pyridoxine: 70 mg/kg IV at 0.5 g/min
- Sodium bicarbonate: bolus: 1–2 mEq/kg IVP; adult infusion: 3 amp sodium bicarbonate in 1000 cc D5W at 2–3 cc/kg/hr IV
- Vecuronium: 0.1 mg/kg IVP

Disposition

ADMISSION CRITERIA

- All MAOI overdose patients require admission to a monitored unit for 24 hours
- ICU admission for seriously ill patients

DISCHARGE CRITERIA

- Resolved mild hypertensive syndrome or resolved mild serotonin syndrome
  - —Discharge after several hours of ED observation

Miscellaneous

ICD9: 969

CORE CONTENT CODE 17.2.7.2

SUGGESTED READINGS

Brent J. Monoamine oxidase inhibitors and the serotonin syndrome. In: Haddad LM, Shannon MW, Winchester JF, eds. Clinical management of poisoning and drug overdose. 3rd ed. Philadelphia: WB Saunders, 1998:452–464.

Mills KC. Serotonin syndrome: A clinical update. Crit Care Clin 1997;13(4):763–783.

Author: Theodore Toerne

Mononucleosis

Clinical Presentation

SIGNS AND SYMPTOMS

Symptoms

- Slow in onset over a few days
- Fever
- Headaches
- Malaise/arthralgias/myalgias
- Sore throat

Signs

- Exudative discharge on tonsils and pharynx (mimic streptococcal pharyngitis)
- Edematous pharynx
- Lymphadenopathy
- Hepatomegaly (hepatitis is the most common complication)
- Splenomegaly (30–40%)
  —Splenic rupture occurs rarely when splenic enlargement significant
- Rash (<10%)
  —Nonspecific maculopapular
  —Can be precipitated by treatment with ampicillin

Complications (Rare)

- Meningitis
- Encephalitis
- Transverse myelitis
- Guillain-Barré syndrome
- Cranial and peripheral nerve palsies

MECHANISM/DESCRIPTION

- Subclinical infection in childhood (asymptomatic <2 years old)
- More symptomatic in adolescents and adults
- 4–6 week incubation period
- Transmitted by *close* contact between susceptible (EBV antibody-negative) individuals and symptomatic or carrier (asymptomatic) individuals
- Fever and sore throat resolve in 10–21 days
- 10–20% experience persistent malaise and fatigue for several weeks or months

ETIOLOGY

- Epstein-Barr virus (EBV)
  —Herpes virus
  —Infects only humans
  —By age 35 vast majority of people have had EBV infection
- Virus infects and replicates in cells of the oropharynx (causing cytolysis and virus shedding) and then B-lymphocytes (causing B-cell proliferation)
- Previously infected individuals may shed the virus intermittently from the oropharynx for many months or years
- Virus shedding is more frequent and in greater numbers of virion particles in immunocompromised patients
- Reactivation of EBV after primary infection is subclinical

Pre-Hospital

N/A

Diagnosis

ESSENTIAL WORKUP

- Monospot test positive in first month
- Bacterial throat culture
  —Excludes concomitant β-hemolytic streptococcal infection (common association)

LABORATORY

- CBC
  —Atypical lymphocytosis (larger than normal lymphocytes, containing eccentrically placed and lobulated nuclei, and vacuolated cytoplasm)
  —Hematological complications: anemia, neutropenia, and thrombocytopenia
- Liver function tests
  —Elevated transaminases up to 3 times normal found in 80–85%
- Heterophil antibody test
  —IgM antibodies that bind antigens of horse, beef, and sheep red blood cells
  —Rise (positive test) between the 2nd and 3rd week of symptoms
  —Negative test possible in the first week
  —>95% sensitive/specific in adolescents and adults
  —Produced by less than 40–50% of children infected at age <5 years
- EBV titers
  —Use in heterophil antibody negative/equivocal individuals to make diagnosis

IMAGING/SPECIAL TESTS

- CT abdomen for splenic rupture when severe abdominal pain/hypotension

DIFFERENTIAL DIAGNOSIS

- Other viral or bacterial pharyngitis
  —Difficult to distinguish from Group A β-hemolytic streptococcal infection
- Superimposed bacterial pharyngitis on primary EBV infection
- Cytomegalovirus
  —Causes syndrome with atypical lymphocytes and hepatosplenomegaly but no heterophil antibodies
- *Toxoplasma gondii*
- HIV
- Hepatitis A, B, and C

Treatment

INITIAL STABILIZATION

- ABCs if patient unstable
- IV hydration/stabilization if splenic rupture

ED TREATMENT

- Supportive therapy
  —Hydration (oral/IV)
  —Analgesics/antipyretics
- Steroids (methylprednisolone)
  —Not administered routinely
  —Indicated if pharyngeal/tonsillar edema significant enough to cause airway compromise
  —Not indicated for EBV-induced neurologic complications or hepatitis
- No effective antiviral treatment available
- Avoid
  —Ampicillin due to associated rash
  —Contact sports due to possible splenic rupture for 6–8 weeks
  —Aspirin due to associated Reyes syndrome

MEDICATIONS

- Methylprednisolone (solu-medrol): 80–125 mg (peds: 2 mg/kg) IV
- Prednisone: 40 mg (peds: 1 mg/kg) q day for 4 days

Disposition

ADMISSION CRITERIA

- Significant pharyngeal or tonsillar edema to indicate potential airway compromise
- Neurologic or severe hematologic/hepatic complications
- Inability to take po

DISCHARGE CRITERIA

- No airway compromise
- Mild hematologic complications or mild hepatitis
- Able to tolerate oral fluids

Miscellaneous

ICD9: 075 INFECTIOUS MONONUCLEOSIS

CORE CONTENT CODE: 9.5.2

SUGGESTED READINGS

Bailey RE. Diagnosis and treatment of infectious mononucleosis. Am Fam Physician 1994;49(4):879–885.

Straus SE, moderator. Epstein-Barr virus infections: Biology, pathogenesis, and management. Ann Intern Med 1993;118(1):45–58.

Tynell E. Acyclovir and prednisolone treatment of acute infectious mononucleosis: A multicenter, double-blind, placebo-controlled study. J Infect Dis 1996;174:324–331.

Author: Murtaza Galamhussein

Multiple Myeloma

Clinical Presentation

SIGNS AND SYMPTOMS

- Bone pain predominates (with secondary disuse or neurologic sequelae)
  - —Ribs/sternum
  - —Spine
  - —Clavicle
  - —Skull
  - —Shoulder
  - —Hip
- Constitutional symptoms
  - —Anemia
  - —Weakness
  - —Fatigue
  - —Recurrent infection
  - —Weight loss
- Asymptomatic (20%)
  - —Multiple myeloma (MM) found on follow-up of routine blood screening
- Multiple bouts of sepsis secondary to the encapsulated organisms (*Streptococcus pneumoniae, H. influenzae,* and *S. aureus*)

MECHANISM/DESCRIPTION

- Normal cells transform into myeloma cells at the hematopoietic stem cell level
- Pathologic derangements
  - —Tumor cells within marrow lead to bone destruction and cytopenias
  - —Immunodeficiency develops secondary to suppression of normal immune functions
  - —Myeloma proteins lead to hyperviscosity and amyloidosis
  - —Multifactorial renal failure
- Plasma cells secretions activate osteoclasts leading to
  - —Bone lysis, pathologic fractures, and neurologic impairment
  - —Hypercalcemia (exacerbated by impaired renal function)
- Anemia due to marrow infiltration and renal insufficiency
- Immunocompromised due to
  - —Decrease in the number of normal immunoglobulins
  - —Qualitative and quantitative defects in T and B cell subsets
  - —Granulocytopenia
  - —Decreased cell-mediated immunity
- Hyperviscosity secondary to protein accumulation
  - —Leads to high output congestive heart failure
- Myeloma light chains accumulate in the renal epithelial cells and destroy the entire nephron

ETIOLOGY

- Incidence: 4 cases per 100,000 population
  - —1% of all cancers
  - —15% of all hematopoietic malignancies
  - —10,000 deaths per year
- Mean age at diagnosis is 62 years

PEDIATRIC CONSIDERATIONS

- MM is rarely seen in children

Pre-Hospital

CAUTIONS

- Patients with MM who present with back pain or neurologic symptoms
  - —Presume to have a pathologic spinal fracture
  - —Immobilize appropriately

Diagnosis

ESSENTIAL WORKUP

- Official diagnosis requires
  - —Demonstrating pathologic cells in the bone marrow
  - —Monoclonal gammopathy on electrophoresis
  - —Clinical signs such as anemia, renal insufficiency, or lytic bone lesions
- Complications
  - —Pathologic fractures
  - —Hypercalcemia
  - —Renal failure
  - —Recurrent infection
  - —Anemia
  - —Spinal cord compression (10% of all MM patients)

LABORATORY

- CBC
  - —Normochromic, normocytic anemia
  - —Thrombocytopenia
  - —Leukocytosis
- Rouleux formation on peripheral blood smear
- Electrolytes, BUN, Cr, glucose
  - —Renal insufficiency
- Serum calcium
  - —Hypercalcemia due to bone resorption
- Urinalysis
  - —Dipstick selects for albumin and not light chain proteinuria
  - —False-negative screening urinalysis for protein common
- Elevated ESR

IMAGING/SPECIAL TESTS

- Plain radiographs demonstrate
  - —Lytic bone lesions
  - —Pathological fractures
- Urinary and serum electrophoresis: show a monoclonal protein spike
- Technicum pyrophosphate bone scan
  - —Lights up bone deposition
  - —False-negative scan with MM due to an uncoupling of bone absorption and deposition which results in a negative bone scan even when lytic lesions present
- Bone marrow biopsy: increase in plasma cells

DIFFERENTIAL DIAGNOSIS

- Monoclonal gammopathy
- Chronic lymphocytic leukemia
- Non-Hodgkin's lymphoma
- Waldenstrom's macroglobulinemia
- Bone marrow plasmacytosis includes collagen vascular disease, cirrhosis, immune complex disease, viral illness, papular mucinosis

Treatment

INITIAL STABILIZATION

- Recognition and treatment of
  - —Hypercalcemia
  - —Renal failure
  - —Sepsis
  - —Spinal cord compression

ED TREATMENT

- Analgesics mainstay of therapy in ED
- Splint pathological fracture; immobilize pathological spine fractures
- Chemotherapy—administer on inpatient/outpatient basis
  - —Early or asymptomatic stages do not need treatment
  - —Melphalan and prednisone combination chemotherapy the most common treatment; symptom relief and decrease in M protein levels in up to 70% of patients
- Prolonged melphalan use may lead to a secondary leukemia

Disposition

ADMISSION CRITERIA

- Refractory pain requiring systemic analgesics
- Life-threatening complications of MM including acute renal failure, hypercalcemia, sepsis, spinal cord compression, hyperviscosity, and cardiac tamponade

DISCHARGE CRITERIA

- Pain controlled with oral analgesics

Miscellaneous

ICD9: 203.0

CORE CONTENT CODE: 7.7.4

SUGGESTED READINGS

Alexanian R, Dimopoulos M. The treatment of multiple myeloma. N Engl J Med 1994;330:484–489.

Duffy TP. The many pitfalls in the diagnosis of myeloma. N Engl J Med 1992;326:394–396.

Dunbar CE, Nienhuis AW. Multiple myeloma. New approaches to therapy. JAMA 1993;269:2412–2416.

Kyle RA. Newer approaches to the management of multiple myeloma. Cancer 1993;72:489–494.

Author: Nicholas Jouriles

Multiple Sclerosis

Clinical Presentation

SIGNS AND SYMPTOMS

- Initial attacks of multiple sclerosis (MS) usually represent a single lesion, are abrupt in onset, and are seen in characteristic patterns (in order of decreasing frequency)
  - —Optic neuritis (pain exacerbated by eye movement progressing to visual loss)
  - —Paresthesias (or a sensory level) in one limb
  - —Limb (usually leg) weakness
  - —Diplopia
    - -Internuclear ophthalmoplegia is a lesion of the medial longitudinal fasciculus that results in unilateral or bilateral paralysis of adduction of the eye on horizontal gaze. This produces diplopia
  - —Trigeminal neuralgia
  - —Urinary retention
  - —Vertigo
  - —Acute onset of motor and sensory findings at a specific spinal cord level often associated with bladder or bowel incontinence is indicative of transverse myelitis. This can be an early manifestation of MS
- Symptoms typically develop abruptly (minute to hours) and last 6–8 weeks
- Most common in young women of northern European descent, increased risk in 1st degree relatives
  - —Peak age:30 years
  - —Female:Male ratio = 2:1
- Pain is an uncommon symptom in MS (exception: trigeminal neuralgia, early optic neuritis)

MECHANISM/DESCRIPTION

- Recurrent episodes of demyelinization in the CNS cause signs and symptoms that depend upon the location of the lesions. MS occurs in distinct patterns
- *Relapsing recurring multiple sclerosis:* 2 or more episodes lasting ≥24 hours separated by ≥1 month
- *Primary progressive multiple sclerosis:* slow or stepwise progression over at least 6 months
- *Secondary progressive multiple sclerosis:* initial exacerbations and remissions followed by slow progression over at least 6 months
- *Stable multiple sclerosis:* no progression (without treatment) over at least 18 months

ETIOLOGY

MS is a chronic demyelinating disease of the CNS. The etiology is not well understood

- Presumed to be a T-cell mediated autoimmune disease
- There is evidence for a viral "trigger"
- Plaques in the white matter: characterized by an infiltrate of T cells and macrophages
- Persons of northern European origin most often affected (in US)
- Increased prevalence is seen moving away from equator

Diagnosis

ESSENTIAL WORKUP

The initial diagnosis is based on history and physical exam (outlined above). Definite diagnosis will not be made in ED; diagnosis requires observation over time and confirmatory testing

- Physical exam: focus on "hard" neurologic signs such as afferent pupillary defect, internuclear ophthalmoplegia, a sensory level, sphincter disturbance (transverse myelitis), etc. The physical exam should reveal *objective* evidence of neurologic dysfunction
- MRI is sensitive but not specific; may see plaques
- LP may reveal oligoclonal bands on CSF electrophoresis

DIFFERENTIAL DIAGNOSIS

Most signs and symptoms are focal; diffuse symptoms (seizures, syncope, and dementia) are seldom due to MS

- Systemic lupus erythematosus: CNS involvement usually in setting of known disease; usually nonfocal
- Sarcoid: CNS manifestations usually with known disease and lung involvement; nonfocal
- Lyme disease: may mimic MS; seek history of rash and tick exposure in geographic areas of high risk. Lyme titers may aid in diagnosis
- Psychiatric illness: diagnosis of exclusion
- Postinfectious or postimmunization demyelination: may mimic MS; usually in children
- MS unlikely in patients with
  - —normal neurologic exam
  - —Abrupt hemiparesis
  - —Aphasia
  - —Pain predominates
  - —Very brief symptoms (seconds to minutes)
  - —Age <10 or >50 years

Treatment

INITIAL STABILIZATION

- Fever in MS patients should be treated aggressively as it can worsen neurologic manifestations of MS

ED TREATMENT

- Acute optic neuritis or transverse myelitis: high-dose parenteral steroids
- Treatment of exacerbations: high-dose IV methylprednisolone (up to 1 g/day) or other parenteral corticosteroid regimen
- Symptomatic treatment
  —Spasticity: baclofen
  —Tremor: clonazepam
  —Urinary symptoms: treat infection; self-catheterization for increased PVR; oxybutynin may promote continence between catheterizations
  —Trigeminal neuralgia: carbamazepine
  —Fatigue, general weakness: no specific treatment

MEDICATIONS

- Baclofen: 10 mg po tid initially, may increase to 25 mg tid
- Carbamazepine: 100 mg po bid to 200 mg qid
- Clonazepam: 0.5 mg/day po, increase in 0.5 mg increments and up to 3 times a day
- Oxybutynin: 5 mg po bid or tid
- Methylprednisolone: 1 g IV

Disposition

ADMISSION CRITERIA

- Acute exacerbation which requires IV therapy
- Patients unable to care for themselves due to the severity of their illness or for whom another condition requiring inpatient treatment cannot be effectively ruled out

DISCHARGE CRITERIA

- *Suspected MS:* patients may be referred for outpatient evaluation if their general condition permits and other serious conditions requiring admission have been effectively ruled out
- *Complication of known MS:* discharge if effective outpatient treatment available for the condition

Miscellaneous

ICD9: 340

CORE CONTENT CODE: 11.3.1

SUGGESTED READINGS

Antel JP, ed. Multiple sclerosis. Neurol Clin 1995;13(1):1–228.

Brod SA, Lindsey JW, Wolinsky JS. Multiple sclerosis: Clinical presentation, diagnosis, and treatment. Am Fam Physician 1996;54(4):1301–1311.

Rolak LA. The diagnosis of multiple sclerosis. Neurol Clin 1996;14(2):27–43.

Weinshaker BG. Epidemiology of multiple sclerosis. Neurol Clin 1996;14(2);291–306.

van Oosten BW, Truyen L, Barkhof F, Polman CH. Multiple sclerosis therapy a practical guide. Drugs 1995;49(2);200–212.

Authors: Timothy VanDuzer; Richard S. Krause

Mumps

Clinical Presentation

SIGNS AND SYMPTOMS

Incubation Period

- 12–25 days
- Virus enters respiratory tract and cervical lymph nodes

Prodrome

- 1–3 days
- Malaise, anorexia, chills, fever, sore throat, tender jaw
  - —May not always occur

Active Illness

- 1–7 days
- Parotid gland
  - —Sudden enlargement
  - —Pain and tenderness
  - —No warmth or erythema of overlying skin
  - —Swelling may extend to submaxillary, sublingual glands, or to presternal area
  - —Bilateral in two-thirds of cases
- Fever/malaise
- Headache
- Anorexia
- Earache
- Difficulty with eating, swallowing, talking
- Contagious for 9 days after onset swelling

Epididymoorchitis

- Orchitis in 20–30%
  - —May be sole manifestation of illness
  - —Bilateral in 3–17%
- Accompanied by recrudescence with fever, chills, headache, nausea, vomiting
- Testicle painful, swollen, tender
- Epididymitis may occur alone
- Resolves over 3–7 days
- Approximately 50% develop atrophic testicles
- Bilateral atrophic testicles results in diminished sperm count
  - —Infertility rare

Pancreatitis

- Incidence 5%
- Fever, nausea, vomiting, epigastric pain
- May be accompanied by pseudocyst formation and shock
- May occur without any other manifestations of mumps

CNS

- Aseptic meningitis
  - —Incidence 10%
  - —Develops 3–10 days after parotitis
  - —Generally benign
- Rare complications
  - —Encephalitis
  - —Transverse myelitis
  - —Cerebellar ataxia
  - —Guillain-Barré syndrome
  - —Deafness/hearing loss

Other

- Glandular tissue involvement, including lacrimal, breast, thyroid, thymus, ovaries
- Ocular including optic neuritis, keratitis, iritis, conjunctivitis, episcleritis (usually resolve with no sequelae)
- Myocarditis
- Glomerulonephritis
- Hepatitis
- Thrombocytopenic purpura
- Polyarthritis

ETIOLOGY

- Caused by paramyxovirus, a single-strand RNA virus
- Tends to occur in spring
- Rare before age 2; approximately one-third of cases >16 years
- 25% of cases subclinical

PEDIATRIC CONSIDERATIONS

- Systemic symptoms often absent in children
- Nonimmunized children should be immunized
- May increase risk of spontaneous abortion if contracted in first trimester
- No evidence of effects on offspring exposed in early pregnancy

Pre-Hospital

CAUTIONS

- Pre-hospital care workers exposed to mumps should be advised of potential risks

Diagnosis

ESSENTIAL WORKUP

- Clinical diagnosis
- No lab tests are required

LABORATORY

- CSF evaluation when meningitis suspected
- Amylase
  - —Hyperamylasemia occurs secondary to parotitis
  - —Diagnosis of pancreatitis difficult
- Viral isolation
  - —Provides definitive diagnosis
  - —From blood, throat swabs, salivary gland secretions, CSF, or urine
  - —Not indicated unless need to confirm diagnosis in absence of parotitis
- Immunofluorescence studies
  - —Rapid detection
  - —Not indicated unless need to confirm diagnosis in absence of parotitis
- ELISA testing determines acute infection or susceptibility

DIFFERENTIAL DIAGNOSIS

- Bacterial parotitis
  - —*Staphylococcus aureus*
  - —Usually occurs in older or disabled
  - —Glands warm, tender
  - —WBC elevated
- Calculus parotitis
  - —Stone may be palpable
  - —Sialogram will reveal stone
- Drug reactions
  - —Iodides
  - —Guanethidine
  - —Phenothiazines
  - —Heavy metals
  - —Thiouracil
- Cervical adenitis
- Tumors
  - —More indolent course
  - —Older persons affected
- Testicular torsion
- Bacterial epididymitis

Treatment

INITIAL STABILIZATION

- IV fluids for vomiting/dehydration

ED TREATMENT

- Supportive and symptomatic therapy
- Antipyretics/analgesia
  - —Acetaminophen, NSAIDs
  - —Narcotics required for severe pain
- Orchitis
  - —Ice packs to scrotum reduce pain
  - —Scrotal support
- Prevention with live, attenuated vaccine
  - —Confers 75–95% protection
  - —Administer after 1 year of age

Disposition

ADMISSION CRITERIA

- Severe pancreatitis
- Encephalitis
- Isolate any inpatients
- Seriously ill for support care

DISCHARGE CRITERIA

- Virtually all patients
- Contagious until approximately 9 days after onset of pain

Miscellaneous

ICD9: 72.9

CORE CONTENT CODE: 9.5.4

SUGGESTED READINGS

Ray CG. Harrison's principles of internal medicine. 13th ed. New York: McGraw Hill, 1997:830–832.

Pomeroy C, Jordan MC. Infectious diseases. 5th ed. Philadelphia: JB Lippincott, 1994:829–834.

Author: Isser Dubinsky

Munchausen's Syndrome

Clinical Presentation

SIGNS AND SYMPTOMS

- Chronic factitious illness
- Present to emergency departments (EDs) with an apparent acute illness
- Plausible but dramatic case history
- Escalating demands for diagnostic testing and therapeutic interventions
- Presentations may involve any organ system
  —Gastrointestinal common
  —Bleeding/anemia from self-phlebotomy or abuse of anticoagulants
  —Feigned seizures or loss of consciousness
  —Self-induced wounds, multiple scars
  —Chest pain
  —Self-administration of insulin, thyroxine, or epinephrine
  —Evidence of infection from injection of sputum or feces
  —Factitious fever from manipulation of thermometers
- Psychiatric
  —Hostile and evasive
  —Numerous medical reports, hospital cards, insurance forms, etc
  —Evidence of multiple hospital admissions
  —Pseudologia fantastica (the telling of tall tales)
  —Masochistic acceptance of painful procedures
  —Uses medical jargon
  —Paucity of verifiable history
  —Absence of close interpersonal relationships
  —History of sadistic and rejecting parents, chronic childhood illness
  —Employment in a medically related field

PEDIATRIC CONSIDERATIONS

- Munchausen's syndrome by proxy
  —A form of child abuse
  —Parent presents a misleading history or induces illness in order to obtain medical attention

Pre-Hospital

N/A

Diagnosis

ESSENTIAL WORKUP

- Diagnosis is suggested by recognizing above patterns of behavior
- Direct observation may reveal the method of the deception (e.g., vials of insulin and syringes)
- Obtain records from other hospitals
- Calls to family members provide evidence of similar presentations in the past

LABORATORY

- Testing the stool for phenolphthalein to detect laxative abuse
- Determination of exogenous insulin administration with C3 peptide

IMAGING/SPECIAL TESTS

N/A

DIFFERENTIAL DIAGNOSIS

- True physical illness
- Comorbid illness
- Intentionally produced illness (e.g., septicemia from self-injection of saliva)
- Illness that is the unintentional result of self-destructive acts or surgical interventions
  —Small bowel obstruction
- Malingering
  —Clear-cut secondary gain
- Conversion disorder
  —Blindness, hemiparesis, seizures
  —Symptoms are not consciously produced
- Somatization disorder
  —Multiple somatic complaints
  —Multiple organ system involvement
  —Symptoms are not intentionally produced

Treatment

INITIAL STABILIZATION

- Treat obvious threats to life or limb
  —Hypoglycemia, bleeding, wounds, etc.

ED TREATMENT

- Satisfactory outcome is rare
- Psychiatric intervention
  —Individual and group therapy
  —Behavior modification
  —Blacklisting of identified patients
- Report cases of Munchausen's syndrome by proxy to child protective services and insure child has a safe environment
- Attention to the physician's own emotional reaction

Disposition

ADMISSION CRITERIA

- Admission is often required to stabilize and evaluate serious physical illness
- Psychiatric admission is useful but seldom accepted by the patient

DISCHARGE CRITERIA

- Medically stable
- Not considered a continued threat to harm self
- Appropriate medical and psychiatric followup arranged

Miscellaneous

ICD9: 301.51

CORE CONTENT CODE: 14.5.1

SUGGESTED READINGS

Folks DG. Munchausen's syndrome and other factitious disorders. Neurol Clin 1995;13(2):267–81.

Jones RM. Factitious disorders. In: Kaplan HI, Sadock BJ, eds. Comprehensive textbook of psychiatry. 6th ed. Baltimore: Williams & Wilkins, 1995:1271–79.

Stern TA. Munchausen's syndrome revisited. Psychosomatics 1980;21:329–36.

Stern TA. Malingering, factitious illness, and somatization. In: Hyman SE, ed. Manual of psychiatric emergencies. 3rd ed. Boston: Little Brown, 1994:265–76.

Authors: Joshua F. Boverman; Theodore A. Stern

Clinical Presentation

SIGNS AND SYMPTOMS (GROUPED BY TOXIN)

Amanitin/Phalloidin

- Nausea
- Vomiting
- Abdominal cramps
- Bloody diarrhea
- Clinical course
  - —Onset of symptoms 6–36 hours
  - —Transient latent phase may last 2 days
  - —Can progress to hepatic or renal failure and death in 4–7 days
  - —Most lethal mushroom toxins

Orellanine

- Nausea
- Headache
- Sweating
- Chills
- Low-back pain
- Thirst
- Clinical course
  - —May progress to oliguria and acute renal failure
  - —Markedly delayed onset of symptoms (2–14 days)

Ibotenic Acid/Muscimol

- Anticholinergic symptoms include
  - —Hallucinations
  - —Dysarthria
  - —Ataxia
  - —Muscle cramps
  - —Vomiting
  - —Seizures
  - —Coma
- Clinical course
  - —Relatively rapid onset of 30–60 minutes

Gyromitrin

- First 6 hours
  - —Abdominal cramps
  - —Vomiting
  - —Watery diarrhea
- Later symptoms
  - —Weakness
  - —Cyanosis
  - —Confusion
  - —Seizures
  - —Coma

Muscarine

- Cholinergic symptoms include
  - —Miosis
  - —Salivation
  - —Lacrimation
  - —Sweating
  - —Flushed skin
  - —Nausea
  - —Bradycardia
  - —Bronchoconstriction
- Onset usually within 1 hour (may be delayed)

Coprine

- Disulfram-like reaction when combined with alcohol
  - —Flushing
  - —Sweating
  - —Nausea
  - —Vomiting
  - —Palpitations
  - —Chest pain
- Begins minutes after combining this toxin with ethanol

Psilocin/Psilocybin

- Visual hallucinations
- Alteration of perception
- Nausea
- Mydriasis
- Tachycardia
- Fever and seizures in children

Gastric Irritants

- Group of toxins that cause nausea, vomiting, and watery diarrhea
- Onset 30 minutes to 2 hours

MECHANISM/DESCRIPTION

Amanitin/Phalloidin

- Species
  - —Amanita phalloides ("death cap")
  - —Amanita virosa/verna ("destroying angel")
  - —Gallerina marginata; Gallerina venenata
- Mechanism
  - —Cyclopeptide toxins inhibit RNA polymerase 2
  - —Which kills GI epithelium, hepatocytes, nephrocytes

Orellanine

- Species
  - —Cortinarius (several species)
- Mechanism
  - —Direct renal toxicity

Ibotenic Acid/Muscimol

- Species
  - —Amanita pantherina ("the panther")
  - —Amanita muscaria ("fly agaric")
- Mechanism
  - —GABA agonists

Gyromitrin

- Species
  - —Gyromitra esculenta ("false morels")
  - —Other Gyromitra species
- Mechanism
  - —Inhibits pyridoxal phosphate
  - —Damage to RBCs, hepatocytes, neurons

Muscarine

- Species
  - —Inocybe (several species)
  - —Clitocybe (several species)
- Mechanism
  - —Parasympathomimetic

Coprine

- Species
  - —Coprinus atramentarius ("inky caps")
- Mechanism
  - —Blocks acetaldehyde dehydrogenase

Psilocin/Psilocybin

- Species
  - —Psilocybe and Panaeolus species as well as others
- Mechanism
  - —Similar structure to LSD

Gastric Irritants

- Many various mushrooms including those normally considered edible

Pre-Hospital

CAUTIONS

- Bring any unconsumed mushrooms or mushroom pieces to the hospital to aid in diagnosis
  - —Refrigerate specimens if possible

Diagnosis

ESSENTIAL WORKUP

- Mushroom description
  - —< 3% of cases result in an exact mushroom identification
- Careful H&P
  - —Special detail to the timing of symptom onset

LABORATORY

- CBC
- PT/PTT
- Electrolytes, BUN/Cr, glucose
- U/A
- Liver function tests

DIFFERENTIAL DIAGNOSIS

- Symptoms with a late onset (>6 hours) indicate the more lethal toxins
- Always entertain the possibility of multiple species ingestion
- Combination with ETOH may suggest coprine
- Consider other illicit drugs with visual hallucinations
- Fertilizers, insecticides, fungicides, etc., if in a public place

Treatment

INITIAL STABILIZATION

- ABCs
- Establish IV 0.9%NS
- Monitor
- Naloxone, D50W (or Accucheck) and thiamine for altered mental status

ED TREATMENT

General

- Decontamination
  - —Activated charcoal (20–50 g) superior to ipecac
    - -Particularly with delayed presentation
  - —Induce vomiting only if
    - -Patients have not yet vomited
    - -Normal mental and respiratory status
    - -Not undergoing hallucinations
    - -Syrup of ipecac
- Fluid rehydration and electrolyte replacement as necessary
- Call local poison control center and ask for mycologist
- Obtain specimens (vomitus if needed) for identification

Toxin-Specific Therapy

Amanitin/Phalloidin

- Ewald oral gastric tube aspiration of mushroom fragments
- Administer charcoal every 2–4 hours
- Hypoglycemia and elevated PT
  - —Signs of liver failure
  - —Administer FFP and vitamin K for coagulation disorders with active bleeding
- Liver transplant for severe hepatic necrosis
- Consider high-dose penicillin G or silibinin (controversial)

Orellanine

- Closely monitor BUN/Cr, electrolytes, and urine output
- Lasix contraindicated
  - —Accelerates nephrotoxicity in rats
- Diuresis with alkalinization of urine with $NaHCO_3$
- Hemodialysis/renal transplant may be needed

Ibotenic Acid/Muscimol

- Usually self-limited toxicity
- Provide supportive care
- Monitor for hypotension
- Treat severe anticholinergic symptoms with physostigmine

Gyromitrin

- Administer pyridoxine in severely symptomatic patients
- Treat seizure with benzodiazepines
- Treat liver dysfunctions as outlined in *Amanitin/Phalloidin* group
- Dialysis for renal failure

Muscarinic

- Administer atropine in severe cases

Coprine

- Self-limited toxicity
- Avoid syrup of ipecac (contains alcohol)
- Propranolol for cardiac dysrhythmias

Psylocin/Psilocybin

- Self-limited toxicity
- Dark, quiet room and reassurance
- Do not induce emesis if hallucinating,
- External cooling measures if needed in children

GI Irritants

- When poisoning from the above groups not suspected
  - —Administer acetominophen and antiemetics
  - —Supportive care
- Monitor LFT's in cases where cyclopeptide containing mushrooms are suspected

MEDICATIONS

- Activated charcoal slurry: 1–2 g/kg up to 90 g po
- Atropine: 0.5 mg (peds: 0.02 mg/kg) IV repeat 0.5–1.0 mg IV (peds: 0.04 mg/kg) q 10 min if secretions recur to maximum 1 mg/kg in children and 2 mg/kg in adults
- Dextrose: D50W 1 amp (50 ml or 25 g) (peds: D25W 2–4 ml/kg) IV
- Diazepam (benzodiazepine): 5–10 mg (peds: 0.2–0.5 mg/kg) IV
- Ipecac: 30 ml (peds: 15 ml for children <12 yrs) po
- Lorazepam (benzodiazepine): 2–6 mg (peds: 0.03–0.05 mg/kg) IV
- Naloxone (narcan): 2 mg (peds: 0.1 mg/kg) IV or IM initial dose
- Physostigmine: 0.5–2 mg IM/IV in adults
- Propranolol: 1 mg (peds: 0.01–0.1 mg/kg) IV
- Pyridoxine: 25 mg/kg over 30 min
- Sorbitol: 1–2 g/kg to a max of 150 g (peds: >1 yr: 1–1.5 g/kg as a 35% solution to a max of 50 g) po mixed in the activated charcoal slurry
- Thiamine (vitamin B_1): 100 mg (peds: 50 mg) IV or IM

Disposition

ADMISSION CRITERIA

- All symptomatic patients
  - —Protracted vomiting, dehydration, liver or renal toxicity, or seizures
- Transfer to a tertiary medical center for early signs of renal or hepatic failure
- Infants and young children found with mushrooms
  - —Assume ingestion
- ICU admission for known ingestion of an amanitin-containing mushroom
  - —Early liver service consultation

DISCHARGE CRITERIA

- Asymptomatic during 6–8 hours with 24 hours of close home observation available

Miscellaneous

ICD9: 988.1

CORE CONTENT CODE: 17.2.35

SUGGESTED READINGS

Jacobs J, Von Behren J, Kreutzer R. Serious mushroom poisonings in California requiring hospital admission, 1990 through 1994. West J Med 1996;165(5):283–288.

McPartland JM, Vilgalys RJ, Cubeta MA. Mushroom poisoning. Am Fam Physician 1997;55(5):1797–1800, 1805–1809, 1811–1812.

Pinson CW, Bradley AL. A primer for clinicians on mushroom poisoning in the West. West J Med 1996;165(5):318–319.

O'Donnel M, Fleming S. The renal pathology of mushroom poisoning. Histopathology 1997;30(3):280–282.

Authors: Adam Black; Timothy Erickson

Myasthenia Gravis

Clinical Presentation

SIGNS AND SYMPTOMS

- Myasthenia gravis (MG) is the most common disease of neuromuscular transmission
- Fluctuating symptoms of muscle weakness are characteristic
- Weakness is worse with repeated or sustained muscular activity, improvement is noted after rest (30 minutes)
- Often progressive with generalized weakness developing in 85% patients
- Respiratory or oropharyngeal involvement are the two most dangerous symptoms, as these can lead to *myasthenic crisis* (respiratory failure and aspiration)
- Most common initial symptom (70%) is ocular dysfunction
  - —Ptosis, and diplopia with sustained directional gaze
  - —Decreased strength in the ability to keep the eye shut against resistance is universal
  - —Ocular symptoms are usually worse with reading, aggravated by bright light
  - —MG never affects the pupil
- Oropharyngeal weakness is the initial manifestation in 17% of patients
  - —Voice change, especially after prolonged speech, fluidity of speech preserved
  - —Difficulty chewing/swallowing
  - —Flattened smile
- Extremity weakness is initial manifestation in 10% of patients
  - —Weakness in a proximal distribution
  - —Neck flexors/extensors, deltoids, diaphragm and wrist extensors
  - —No associated sensory, ataxic or areflexic findings
  - —Fatigue/weakness noted to worsen as the day progresses
- Myasthenic crisis occurs when respiratory or bulbar weakness is severe enough to mandate mechanical ventilation or a feeding tube
  - —Nasal regurgitation of fluid with swallow or cough indicates bulbar weakness

MECHANISM/DESCRIPTION

- Incidence 2–10 per 10,000. Approximately 25,000 cases per year
- Bimodal age distribution with early peak in second and third decade, and late peak in sixth to seventh decade
- No pattern of classic genetic inheritance, but inherited factors do predispose
  - —Family members of patients with MG are 1000 times more likely to develop MG themselves
- Autoimmune mediated attack against the acetylcholine (Ach) receptors on the motor end plate at the neuromuscular junction (NMJ)
- In MG, the concentration of Ach receptors are reduced, so for a given release of Ach the sum of the miniature end plate potential (MEEPs) will be less resulting in the failure to trigger action potentials
- When neuromuscular transmission fails at many junctions, the contraction of the entire muscle is affected manifesting clinically as weakness, the hallmark of MG

ETIOLOGY

- Thymus is considered to be the immunologic origin of MG
  - —Thymoma (15%) or thymic hyperplasia (85%)
- Secondary triggers
  - —Illness/infection
  - —Emotional distress
  - —Thyroid dysfunction
  - —Fever
  - —Pregnancy/menses
  - —Neuromuscular blocking agents, aminoglycosides, Class IA antiarrhythmics, cholinergic drugs
  - —Steroid therapy
  - —Surgery

PEDIATRIC CONSIDERATIONS

- Neonatal MG can affect 10–20% of infants whose mothers have MG
- Hypotonia, poor suck/feeding, weak cry usually within the first 48 hours of life

Diagnosis

ESSENTIAL WORKUP

- Workup should be directed at uncovering secondary triggers
- ABG to assess respiratory status

LABORATORY

- CXR, electrolytes
- Thyroid function tests
- Ach receptor antibodies

IMAGING/SPECIAL TESTS

- Electromyography; repetitive nerve stimulation will show a progressively decremental response
- Assay for Ach receptor antibodies (100% specific)

DIFFERENTIAL DIAGNOSIS

- CVA/TIA
- Thyroid dysfunction
- Polymyositis
- Muscular dystrophy
- Lambert-Eaton syndrome
- Guillain-Barré syndrome
- Botulism
- Progressive external ophthalmoplegia
- Metabolic derangement

Treatment

INITIAL STABILIZATION

- Initial treatment should focus on airway assessment and stabilization
- Patients with respiratory decompensation should be intubated immediately
- Signs of respiratory decompensation
  - —Severe hypoxia (pO_2 <50)
  - —Tachypnea >30
  - —Hypercarbia (PCO_2 >50) and respiratory acidosis (pH <7.25)
  - —Poor patient appearance, decreased breath sounds, paradoxical respiratory movements
  - —Vital capacity <15 ml/kg
  - —Inability to protect airway
- Neuromuscular blocking drugs should be avoided unless absolutely necessary
  - —Nondepolarizing agents can produce extremely long lasting neuromuscular blockade
  - —Succinylcholine may require doses far greater than normally used
  - —Versed, thiopental, etomidate as alternatives

Myasthenic Crisis

- May need emergent plasmapheresis
- Intravenous immunoglobulin when plasmapheresis contraindicated
- Anticholinesterase treatment should be started in ED
- Neurology consult should be obtained

ED TREATMENT

Tensilon Test

- Tensilon (an acetylcholinesterase inhibitor) prevents the degradation of Ach, resulting in more powerful muscle contraction
- Transiently improved strength in an objectively weak muscle is considered a positive test
- Onset is <30 seconds, duration of effect is <5 minutes
- It can be difficult to distinguish myasthenic from treatment crisis
  - —Excess effect of anticholinergic medications can cause weakness
  - —Be prepared to manage the airway if patient's respiratory effort worsens after Tensilon test

Ice Pack Test

- Neuromuscular transmission is improved with cooling due to inhibition of acetylcholinesterase
- Place an ice filled glove on the affected eye for 2 minutes, improvement of the ptosis is considered a positive test

Anticholinesterase Treatment

- Pyridostigmine
- Onset at 30 minutes, peaks at 2 hours
- Dosing adjustment based on clinical effect and can vary widely from patient to patient

Immunosuppressive Therapy

- Steroids and immunosuppressive drugs have no role in acute management

Thymectomy is definitive treatment

MEDICATIONS

- Tensilon
  - —2 mg test-dose given IVP
  - —Occasional hypersensitivity reaction seen and manifested as bradycardia or bronchospasm; follow-up dose of 5–8 mg IV can be given if no change noted after 1 minute
  - —Pediatric dose: test dose of 0.03 mg/kg IV; follow-up dose not to exceed combined total of 0.15 mg/kg
- Pyridostigmine
  - —Initial dosing 30 mg po tid/qid
  - —Pediatric dose: 1 mg/kg po

Disposition

ADMISSION CRITERIA

- Myasthenic or impending crisis should be admitted to the ICU
- Myasthenic patients presenting with worsening symptoms should be admitted
- All patients with weakness, respiratory or bulbar symptoms should be admitted
- New onset myasthenic symptoms should be admitted

DISCHARGE CRITERIA

- Myasthenic patients with mild ptosis, intermittent diplopia, who feel that their symptoms are improving can be discharged home on anticholinesterase drugs with follow-up

Miscellaneous

ICD9: 358.0

CORE CONTENT CODE: 11.5.2

SUGGESTED READINGS

Drachman DB. Myasthenia gravis. N Engl J Med 1994;330(25):1797–1810.

Oosterhuis HJ, Kuks JB. Myasthenia gravis and myasthenic syndromes. Curr Opin Neurol Neurosurg 1992;5(5):638–644.

Pourmand R. Recognizing and managing the myasthenic crisis. Emerg Med 1995;28(9):74–80.

Sanders DB, Scoppetta C. The treatment of patients with myasthenia gravis. Neurol Clin 1994;12(2):343–368.

Author: Paul File

Myocardial Contusion

Clinical Presentation

SIGNS AND SYMPTOMS

- The clinical picture is varied and nonspecific—from excruciating chest pain and shock to subtle ECG changes without clinical symptoms
- Most common sign is tachycardia out of proportion to the degree of trauma or blood loss. Friction rub may rarely occur
- Retrosternal angina-like chest pain unrelieved by nitroglycerin, often delayed up to 24 hours. May respond to oxygen
- Evidence of significant thoracic trauma such as contusions, abrasions, palpable crepitus, or visible flail segments should heighten suspicion
- Other associated abdominal, skeletal, or central nervous systems injuries may mask the signs and symptoms of myocardial contusion

MECHANISM/DESCRIPTION

- The heart may be compressed between the sternum and vertebrae, swing forward and strike the sternum during deceleration, or be damaged by abdominal viscera upwardly displaced by force on the abdomen
- Pathologically characterized by a discrete and well-demarcated area of hemorrhage
  —Usually subendocardial
  —May extend in a pyramidal transmural fashion
  —Most commonly the anterior wall of the right ventricle or atrium is involved
- Coronary artery occlusion from intimal tearing or adjacent hemorrhage and edema may rarely occur
- Reported complications include life-threatening dysrhythmias, conduction abnormalities, congestive heart failure, cardiogenic shock, hemopericardium with tamponade, late cardiac rupture, valvular rupture, intraventricular thrombi, thromboembolic phenomena, coronary artery occlusion, ventricular aneurysms, and constrictive pericarditis

ETIOLOGY

- Caused by blunt trauma to the chest, most commonly in high-speed deceleration accidents
  —May occur in accidents with speeds as low as 20–35 mph
- Also seen in auto-pedestrian injuries, falls, and after prolonged closed chest cardiac massage
- Always consider when multisystem blunt trauma is present
  —Other severe injuries may distract from possible cardiac contusion

Pre-Hospital

CAUTIONS

- Pre-hospital personnel must accurately convey information to emergency department personnel concerning the mechanism of injury, motor vehicle status, steering wheel and dashboard damage, use of restraint devices, vehicle speed, and patient position

Diagnosis

ESSENTIAL WORKUP

- No single diagnostic study or Gold Standard (other than autopsy findings!) confirms the presence of myocardial contusion
- Recent meta-analysis suggests that only abnormal ECG and CPK-MB correlate directly with complications requiring treatment
- ECG is the best initial screening tool
  —Most common rhythm is sinus tachycardia (70%), but almost any may occur
- A negative ECG doesn't rule out significant myocardial damage
- Echocardiography should be performed on all patients with any ECG changes or elevated CPK-MB

LABORATORY

- Sensitivity of CK-MB isoenzymes varies from 11% to 85%
  —Specificity decreased in multiple trauma
- CPK-MB levels should be sent on all patients being admitted
- Currently experimental, cardiac troponin and myoglobin show promise for definitive diagnosis

IMAGING/SPECIAL TESTS

- Plain radiography: detects associated injuries such as pulmonary contusion, rib or sternal fractures (particularly important), acute pulmonary edema with normal-sized heart secondary to cardiac decompensation
- Echocardiography: detects wall motion abnormalities; effusions, allows direct visualization of cardiac chambers and valves; will not visualize small contusions
- Radionuclide angiography: sensitive; detects wall motion abnormalities; allows differentiation between right and left ventricles but is limited in visualizing small areas
- Thallium-201 scintigraphy: sensitive and specific to left ventricular injury but unable to evaluate the right ventricle
- Technetium pyrophosphate scan: lacks sensitivity and requires patient transfer

DIFFERENTIAL DIAGNOSIS

- Cardiac rupture
- Tamponade
- Valvular damage
- Other traumatic chest wall injury
- Angina or myocardial infarction

Treatment

INITIAL STABILIZATION

- All patients require oxygen, intravenous access, and cardiac monitoring
- The priorities of trauma care take precedence

ED TREATMENT

- Dysrhythmias may be treated with the same pharmacologic agents as nontraumatic dysrhythmias
  —SVT: adenosine or verapamil if patient is not hypovolemic
  —Bradycardia: atropine, pacing
  —Ventricular dysrhythmias: electrical conversion, lidocaine, procainamide, bretylium
  —Cardiac arrest: epinephrine, atropine, etc
  —Rapid atrial fibrillation or flutter: digoxin or diltiazem, if patient not hypotensive
- Prophylactic treatment of dysrhythmias is not indicated
- In cardiogenic shock caused by myocardial contusion, judicious fluid administration, inotropic support (dopamine or dobutamine), and intra-aortic balloon counterpulsation may be necessary

MEDICATIONS

- Adenosine: 6 mg rapid IVP, may repeat 12 mg q 1–2 min × 2 if no response; peds: 0.1–0.2 mg/kg
- Atropine: 0.5–1.0 mg IV/ET; peds: 0.02 mg/kg/dose IV, minimum 0.1 mg
- Bretylium: initial 5 mg/kg IV, repeat 10 mg/kg if needed; infusion is 1–3 mg/min
- Digoxin: load 0.25 mg IV q 6 hrs up to 1 mg; peds: 0.02 mg/kg IV load then 0.01 mg/kg IV q 6 hrs × 2
- Diltiazem: 0.25 mg/kg (adult and peds) or 20 mg IV (adult) over 2 min; may rebolus 0.35 mg/kg 15 min later
- Dobutamine: 2–15 μg/kg/min (adult and peds)
- Dopamine: 2–20 g/kg/min (adult and peds)
- Epinephrine: 1 mg IV/ET for cardiac arrest (1:10,000 solution); peds: 0.01 mg/kg IV
- Lidocaine: load 1 mg/kg IV then 0.5 mg/kg q 8–10 min to max 3 mg/kg; infusion in adults: 1–4 mg/min; peds: 20–50 μg/kg/min IV
- Procainamide: 100 mg IV q 10 min or 20 mg/min up to 17 mg/kg
- Verapamil: 0.1–0.3 mg/kg up to 5–10 mg IV over 2 min

Disposition

Numerous studies show that adverse outcomes, particularly dysrhythmias, are uncommon but generally occur within the first 24 hours. There is no single test or combination of tests that will accurately predict which patients can be discharged safely from the ED, therefore, all patients in whom there is evidence of myocardial contusion or in whom the diagnosis is seriously being entertained should be admitted

ADMISSION CRITERIA

- Any patient with ECG abnormalities, hemodynamic instability, or other studies suggestive of cardiac contusion must be admitted to a monitored unit for close observation and work up

DISCHARGE CRITERIA

- Patients that are asymptomatic, with no ECG abnormalities, or dysrhythmia may be discharged after a 4–6-hour ED observation period. Obtaining radionuclide angiography may assist in safely discharging patients

Miscellaneous

ICD9: 861.01

CORE CONTENT CODE: 18.4.10.7

SUGGESTED READINGS

Cachecho R, Grindlinger GA, Lee VW. The clinical significance of myocardial contusion. J Trauma 1992;33(1):68–71.

Jackimczyk K. Blunt chest trauma. Emerg Med Clin North Am 1993;11(1):85–88.

Maenza RL, Seaberg D, D'Amico F. A meta-analysis of blunt cardiac trauma: Ending myocardial confusion. Am J Emerg Med 1996;14(3):237–241.

Markovchick V, Wolfe R. Cardiovascular trauma. In: Rosen P, et al., eds. Emergency medicine: Concepts and clinical practice. 4th ed. St. Louis: CV Mosby, 1998: 527–545.

Wilson RF. Thoracic trauma. In: Tintinalli J, et al., eds. Emergency medicine: A comprehensive study guide. 4th ed. New York: McGraw Hill, 1996.

Author: Robert S. Hamilton

Myocardial Infarction

Clinical Presentation

SIGNS AND SYMPTOMS

- Chest pain
  —Substernal squeezing tight or pressure like
  —Not usually pleuritic
  —Not reproducible by chest wall palpation
  —May radiate to the arms or jaw
- Dyspnea
- Diaphoresis
- Nausea or vomiting
- MI may occur without chest pain, especially in diabetics and elderly
  —Dyspnea, syncope, weakness, diaphoresis, or confusion
- Symptoms normally last longer than 30 minutes
- Symptoms may occur at rest or during exertion
- Often a prodrome of crescendo angina
- Stigmata of hyperlipidemia (i.e., xanthelasmas)
- Complications of acute MI
  —Murmur associated with papillary muscle dysfunction
  —Signs of congestive heart failure

MECHANISM/DESCRIPTION

- Each year in the United States, 350,000 patients with acute MI suffer cardiac arrest and death before reaching a hospital
- Myocardial damage due to ischemia
  —Myocardial oxygen demand exceeding supply
  —Interruption of coronary blood flow from rupture of an atherosclerotic intimal plaque
  —Formation of local occluding thrombus
- Risk factors for atherosclerotic coronary artery disease (CAD)
  —Family history of CAD in a first-degree relative less than age 55
  —Cigarette smoking
  —Hypertension
  —Hypercholesterolemia
  —Diabetes mellitus
  —Male sex
- Less common causes of MI
  —Sympathomimetic drug use (i.e., cocaine)
  —Coronary vasospasm
  —Intraluminal thrombus due to coagulopathy
  —Congenital anomalies
  —Coronary arteritis
  —Coronary artery trauma
  —Coronary artery gas embolus
  —Severe anemia, or hypotension
  —Carbon monoxide poisoning
  —Thyroid storm

Pre-Hospital

- Transmit 12-lead ECG to receiving hospital if available

CONTROVERSIES

- Do not administer thrombolytics or heparin if aortic dissection is suspected

Diagnosis

ESSENTIAL WORKUP

- ECG
  —ST segment elevation (in transmural MI)
  —ST depression (in ischemia)
  —T-wave inversion (in non-Q-wave MI)
  —Inferior wall MI in leads II, III, and aVF
  —Lateral wall MI in leads I, aVL, and V4–V6
  —Anterior wall MI in the precordial leads (V1–V6)
  —Posterior wall MI with tall R waves and ST depression in V1, V2
  —New left bundle branch block
  —Over 50% of MI will have abnormal but nondiagnostic ECG
  —A normal ECG does not preclude the diagnosis of MI
- Chest x-ray
  —Congestive heart failure
    -Cardiomegaly
    -Cephalization of pulmonary vasculature
    -Fluid in septal lines
    -Alveolar fluid
- Serum creatinine phosphokinase-MB fraction (CPK-MB) level
  —Elevated up to12 hours after acute MI
  —A single normal CK-MB does not exclude MI
- Serum troponin level
  —Elevated within 3–6 hours
  —Will be elevated for several days after an MI

LABORATORY

- CBC may reveal underlying anemia
- Electrolytes
- Coagulation studies

IMAGING/SPECIAL TESTS

- Two-dimensional echocardiography
- Segmental akinesis or hypokinesis
- Pericardial effusion
- Measure left ventricular ejection fraction
- Saddle pulmonary embolism or aortic dissection (transesophageal)
- Right-sided ECG in inferior wall MI
  —Diagnose right ventricular involvement
  —Q pattern in rV1
  —ST or T changes in rV4
- Radionuclide (technetium, thallium) scans
- Exercise stress testing if MI ruled out
- Cardiac catheterization
  —Diagnostic
  —Therapeutic (angioplasty)

DIFFERENTIAL DIAGNOSIS

- Pulmonary embolus
- Aortic dissection
- Pneumothorax
- Esophageal rupture
- Pneumonia
- Mitral valve prolapse
- Pericarditis
- Esophagitis
- Esophageal spasm
- Peptic ulcer disease
- Musculoskeletal chest pain
- Panic disorder, anxiety state, and stress related

Treatment

INITIAL STABILIZATION

- Cardiac monitor, IV access, oxygen administered
- Continuous blood pressure monitoring and pulse oximetry
- If blood pressure is >90–100 mm Hg systolic, administer nitroglycerin
- Aspirin 80–325 mg po
- If heart rate >50–60 and no hypotension or CHF, administer IV β-blocker (e.g., metoprolol)
- Intravenous heparin
- Morphine sulfate IV for adjunct ischemic pain control
- If patient is in cardiogenic shock, treat as appropriate (see congestive hear failure chapter)
- Angiotensin converting enzyme (ACE) *inhibitors* may effect a small decrease in mortality when given acutely
- Supraventricular tachydysrhythmia
  - —Adenosine, diltiazem, or procainamide
  - —Premature atrial complexes do not warrant treatment
  - —If hemodynamic compromise present, cardioversion may be necessary
  - —Refractory atrial flutter may be managed with overdrive pacing
- Ventricular dysrhythmias
  - —Lidocaine bolus followed by infusion
  - —Lidocaine should not be used prophylactically
  - —Lidocaine should not be used to treat reperfusion dysrhythmias
    - -Accelerated idioventricular rhythm
  - —Magnesium sulfate is indicated for refractory ventricular dysrhythmias
  - —Cardioversion/defibrillation may be necessary if hemodynamically unstable
- Bradydysrhythmia associated with hypotension should be treated with atropine or external pacing
- Conduction disturbances
  - —First-degree AV block and Mobitz I (Wenckebach)
    - -Self-limited and do not require treatment
  - —Mobitz II, complete heart block, new RBBB in anterior MI, RBBB plus LAFB or LPFB, LBBB plus first-degree AV block require pacing

ED TREATMENT

- Reperfusion therapy
  - —Thrombolytic therapy within 30–60 minutes
  - —Immediate cardiac catheterization/angioplasty if available within 60 minutes

MEDICATIONS

- Adenosine: 6 mg IV push, repeat 12 mg IV push × 2 doses
- Aspirin: 80–325 mg po
- Atropine: 0.5–1 g IV max 0.3 mg/kg total dose
- Diltiazem: 10–20 mg IV over 2 min
- Heparin: 5000–7500 unit bolus, 1000 units per hour
- Lidocaine: 1.5 mg/kg bolus, infusion of 2–4 mg/kg/min
- Metoprolol: 5 mg IV q 5 min × 3 doses
- Morphine: 2 mg IV
- Magnesium: 2 g bolus IV
- Nitroglycerin: 0.3–0.4 mg SL q 5 min × 3 doses; nitropaste: 1–2 inches to chest wall; intravenous: 10–20 μg/min, titrate to 200 μg/min or systolic BP <90
- Procainamide: 50 mg/min IV infusion to total of 1 g; stop if hypotension, QRS widening occurs

Disposition

ADMISSION CRITERIA

- All patients with acute MI should be admitted to a coronary care unit
- They should not be transferred to another hospital unless the current facility cannot offer definitive care
- Transfers should be made in an ACLS-equipped ambulance

DISCHARGE CRITERIA

- Only patients ruled out for MI by appropriate protocol should be discharged for outpatient work-up

Miscellaneous

ICD9: 410.0

CORE CONTENT CODE: 2.2.6

SUGGESTED READINGS

Collins R, et al. Aspirin, heparin, and fibrinolytic therapy in suspected acute myocardial infarction. N Engl J Med 1997;336:12.

Lau J, et al. Cumulative meta-analysis of therapeutic trials for myocardial infarction. N Engl J Med 1992;327:4.

Niemann JT. Ischemic heart disease, angina pectoris, and myocardial infarction. In: Harwood-Nuss, ed. The clinical practice of emergency medicine. 2nd ed. Ch. 129. Philadelphia: Lippincott-Raven Publishers, 1996.

Scott IL, Pigman EC, Gordon GG, Silverstein S. Ischemic Heart Disease. In: Rosen, Barkin, Braen, et al., eds. Emergency medicine: concepts and clinical practice. 3rd ed. Ch. 69. St. Louis: C.V. Mosby-Year Book, 1992.

Authors: Liese Schwarz; Robert Woolard

Myocarditis

Clinical Presentation

SIGNS AND SYMPTOMS

- Decreased exercise tolerance
- Fatigue
- Dyspnea
- Palpitations
- Chest discomfort
- Increased jugular venous pulsation
- Decreased pulse pressure
- Fever
- Cyanosis
- Hypotension, tachycardia
- S1 heart sound may be muffled
- Diastolic murmurs are unusual
- In fulminant disease, signs and symptoms of acute congestive heart failure
  —Rales, JVD, peripheral edema, and hepatomegaly

MECHANISM/DESCRIPTION

- Inflammatory disease of the myocardium
- Often results in cardiac dysfunction and heart failure
- History: 40% of patients report recent viral illness

ETIOLOGY

Infectious

- Viral
  —Enteroviruses (coxsackie B)
  —Adenovirus
  —Herpesvirus (including CMV)
  —Hepatitis C
  —Influenza
  —HIV
- Bacteria
  —Diphtheria
  —Meningococcus
  —Mycoplasma
  —Group A streptococcus
- Protozoa
  —*Treponema cruzi* (Chagas disease)
    -Most common cause of heart failure and myocarditis worldwide
    -20 million persons infected
    -Central and South America
- Spirochetes *(Borrelia)* and rickettsial diseases in the U.S.

Noninfectious

- Drugs
  —Chemotherapeutic agents (anthracyclines)
  —Radiation
  —Hypersensitivity
    -Sulfamethoxazole, sulfadiazine and penicillins
  —Heavy metals
  —Venoms
- Autoimmune disorders
  —SLE
  —Wegener's granulomatosis
  —Kawasaki's disease
- Sarcoidosis
- Peripartum cardiomyopathy
  —Last month of pregnancy to 5 month postpartum period
- Cardiac rejection

Pre-Hospital

- Standard protocol for management of CHF/pulmonary edema

Diagnosis

ESSENTIAL WORKUP

- ECG
  —Transient, nonspecific ST-T wave changes
  —Atrial and ventricular dysrhythmias
  —Heart block and conduction defects common
    -20% of patients have left bundle branch block
- Chest X-ray
  —Normal or may demonstrate cardiomegaly, pulmonary edema

LABORATORY

- CBC, ESR
- CPK/MB and LDH
- Cardiac Troponin-I
- Viral titers; cultures rarely positive
- Mycoplasma, antistreptolysin titers
- Hepatitis panels
- Monospot testing
- CMV serology
- Peripheral blood cultures

IMAGING/SPECIAL TESTS

- Echocardiography
  —Emergent study for fulminant cases
  —Ventricular wall motion abnormalities
  —Left ventricular dilatation or increased wall thickness
  —Left ventricular thrombus (15% of patients)
  —Abnormal systolic and diastolic filling
  —Right ventricular enlargement and dysfunction carries a poor prognosis
- Gallium-67- and Indium-111-labeled antimyosin antibody scans
  —Indicate cardiac inflammation and myocyte necrosis
- Endomyocardial biopsy
  —Appropriate in heart transplant patients
  —Polymerase chain reaction amplification of viral genome in endomyocardial tissue

DIFFERENTIAL DIAGNOSIS

- Acute myocardial infarction
- Acute and chronic pulmonary embolus
- Pericarditis
- Adrenal insufficiency
- Severe hypo- and hyperthyroidism
- Sepsis
- Environmental challenges
  —Hyperpyrexia, hypothermia
  —Toxin-mediated disease

Treatment

INITIAL STABILIZATION

- Same as for acute CHF/pulmonary edema (see "Congestive Heart Failure")
- Treat dysrhythmias if present
- Transvenous pacing for symptomatic heart block

ED TREATMENT

- ACE inhibitors (captopril)
  - —Reduce afterload and inflammation
- Digoxin
  - —CHF or atrial fibrillation
- Diuretics (furosemide, bumetanide)
- Immunosuppressive therapy (e.g., cyclosporine, prednisone) are of unproved benefit except in patients with immune mediated disease (e.g., SLE)
- Hyperimmunoglobulin therapy improves cardiac function in cytomegalovirus-associated myopericarditis
- Nonsteroidal anti-inflammatory medicines contraindicated in early and acute phase myocarditis as they increase myocardial damage
- Heparin and warfarin decrease risk of thromboembolic events in patients with depressed LV function or intracardiac thrombus
- Cardiac transplantation
  - —Five-year mortality or the need for cardiac transplantation is 56%
  - —Approximately 20–33% of patients recover completely

MEDICATIONS

- Bumetanide: 0.5–1.0 mg IV/dose
- Captopril (po)
  - —Neonates: 0.025–0.1 mg/dose qid
  - —Infants: 0.15–0.3 mg/kg/dose (max = 6 mg/kg)
  - —Children: 0.5–1.0 mg/kg/24 hrs
  - —Adults: initial dose 6.25 mg; can titrate to 50 mg/dose
- Digoxin
  - —Infants: 12.5–20.0 μg/kg IV/PO
  - —2–10 years old: 7.5–15.0 μg/kg IV
- Furosemide: 1 mg/kg/dose

PEDIATRIC CONSIDERATIONS

- IVIG is an effective treatment option in pediatric viral myocarditis
  - —Improved left ventricle function and trend toward better survival

Disposition

ADMISSION CRITERIA

- Symptomatic patients with myocarditis should be admitted
- Congestive heart failure, dysrhythmia, embolic events, cardiogenic shock
  - —Admit to ICU setting

DISCHARGE CRITERIA

- Asymptomatic patient with no evidence of dysrhythmia or cardiac dysfunction

Miscellaneous

ICD9: 429.0

CORE CONTENT CODE: 13.2.3.3

SUGGESTED READINGS

Brown CA, O'Connell JB. Myocarditis and idiopathic dilated cardiomyopathy. Am J Med 1995;99(3):309–14.

Gajarski RJ, Towbin JA. Recent advances in the etiology, diagnosis and treatment of myocarditis and cardiomyopathies in children. Curr Opin Pediatr 1995;7(5):587–94.

Kontos CD, Hess ML. Myocarditis: overcoming obstacles to diagnosis. J Crit Illness 1994;9(1):28–37.

Maisch B, et al. Immunosuppressive treatment for myocarditis and dilated cardiomyopathy. Eur Heart J 1995;16(Suppl O): 153–61.

Mason JW, et al. A clinical trial of immunosuppressive therapy for myocarditis. N Engl J Med 1995;333(5):269–75.

Wynne J, Braunwald E. The cardiomyopathies and myocarditises. In: Braunwald E, ed. Heart disease. 5th ed. Philadelphia: WB Saunders, 1997.

Author: William Binder; Liudvikas Jagminis

Nasal Fracture

Clinical Presentation

SIGNS AND SYMPTOMS

- Nasal deformity, asymmetry, swelling, or ecchymosis
- Epistaxis: possibly due to septal or turbinate laceration
- Periorbital ecchymosis ("raccoon eyes") from damage to branches of ethmoidal artery, may indicate naso-frontoethmoid complex injury
- Palpable sharp edges, depressions, or other irregularities suggest nasal fracture
- Crepitus or mobility of skeletal parts on palpation indicates a fracture
- *Septal hematoma:* a bluish fluid-filled sac overlying the nasal septum. This is critical to detect
- Flattening of the nasal root and widening of the inter canthal distance (telecanthus) is indicative of naso-frontoethmoid complex injury
- Clear rhinorrhea indicates possible CSF leak—rhinorrhea may be delayed in presentation
- Loss of sense of smell suggests significant injury
- Tear duct injuries may be present with abnormal tearing
- Associated eye injuries including subconjunctival hemorrhage, hyphema, and retinal detachments may be present

MECHANISM/DESCRIPTION

- Fractures of the nasal skeleton are the most common body fractures
- Most nasal fractures are the result of blunt trauma, frequently from motor vehicle accidents, sports injuries, and altercations
- Lateral forces are more likely to cause displacement than are straight-on blows
- History of trauma with significant force, loss of consciousness, or findings of facial bone injury, frontal bone crepitus, or CSF leak suggests associated injuries

PEDIATRIC CONSIDERATIONS

- Always consider child abuse a potential mechanism of injury
- Fractures are rare in children; nasal injuries in children are more likely to be cartilaginous
- Significant injuries in children are not always fully appreciated

Pre-Hospital

CAUTIONS

- Management of the airway takes precedence
- Nasotracheal intubation is contraindicated
- Consider orotracheal intubation or cricothyroidotomy if definitive airway control is needed
- C-spine precautions are indicated if there is associated trauma

Diagnosis

ESSENTIAL WORKUP

- Physical examination with visual inspection and palpation are most important
- It is critical to identify a *septal hematoma*
- Examine closely for telecanthus: inter canthal width greater than 30–35 mm or wider than the width of one eye may indicate a naso-frontoethmoid fracture
- Evaluate the nasolacrimal duct for patency by instilling fluorescein into the eye and looking for fluorescein at the entrance of the lacrimal duct into the nasopharynx under the inferior turbinate (absence implying a duct injury)
- Eyelash "traction test" is simply done by grasping the eyelashes on one eyelid with one's fingers and pulling laterally. If the eyelid margin does not become taut or "bowstring" then the medial portion of the tendon has been disrupted. The test is performed on both the upper and lower eyelids as it is possible for only one portion of the tendon to be selectively injured

IMAGING/SPECIAL TESTS

- Radiographs are rarely indicated as they normally do not alter the initial management
  - —Patients with associated facial bone deformity, crepitus, or tenderness may require radiographs
- CT is the test of choice if facial bone fractures or depressed skull fractures are suspected

DIFFERENTIAL DIAGNOSIS

- Nasal fractures may be associated with other facial injuries such as orbital, frontal sinus, maxillary sinus, or cribriform plate fractures, and these more serious injuries must be ruled out
- A naso-frontoethmoid fracture will have frontal crepitus and may have associated telecanthus or obstruction of the naso-lacrimal duct

Treatment

INITIAL STABILIZATION

- Airway: orotracheal intubation or cricothyroidotomy. Nasotracheal intubation is contraindicated
- C-Spine precautions are indicated if there are associated injuries

ED TREATMENT

- Abrasions and lacerations—proper cleansing of facial wounds is essential. Lacerations may be sutured
- Bleeding: usually stops spontaneously. Packing may be required on rare occasions
- Displaced fractures do not need reduction in the ED unless airway compromise is present
  - —It is preferable to let the swelling go down and reduce in 3–5 days
- *Septal hematoma* must be drained immediately in the ED
  - —Anesthetize with topical cocaine or lidocaine and vascular constriction with neosynephrine
  - —Attempt to aspirate with an 18–20 gauge needle on a 3-ml syringe
  - —Rolling a cotton swab down the septum may facilitate the drainage
  - —Holding the mucosa down against the cartilage must be done to prevent reaccumulation of hematoma
    - –This can be done by vaseline gauze packing
    - –Both nares should be packed to ensure adequate pressure. The packing is left in place for 3–5 days or until follow up with ENT
    - –Prophylactic antibiotics are prescribed

MEDICATIONS

- Antibiotics if packing placed
- Amoxicillin/clavulanate adult: 500 mg bid (peds: 40 mg/kg/day bid) *or*
- Trimethoprim/sulfamethoxazole: adult DS bid; peds: 40 mg/kg/day sulfamethoxazole
- Cocaine: topical 4%
- Lidocaine: 1–2% without epinephrine
- Neosynephrine nasal spray

Disposition

ADMISSION CRITERIA

- Most nasal fractures do not require admission
- Admit those with nasoethmoid fractures or those with more significant craniofacial injuries

DISCHARGE CRITERIA

- No evidence of significant head, neck, or other injuries
- Follow up with ENT, plastic surgery, or OMF surgeon in 3–5 days for fracture reduction or follow up
  - —Patients with septal hematoma should follow up in 24 hours for reevaluation after drainage
- Return for signs of clear rhinorrhea, difficulty breathing, fever, or signs associated with head injury

PEDIATRIC CONSIDERATIONS

- Follow-up with specialist sooner since fibrous union begins in only 3–4 days
- Consider contacting Child Protective Services if any suspicion of abuse (i.e., history does not fit injury)

Miscellaneous

ICD9: 802.0

CORE CONTENT CODE: 18.4.4.4

SUGGESTED READINGS

Altreuter RW. Nasal Trauma. Emerg Med Clin North Am 1987;5(2):293–298.

Fedok FG. Comprehensive management of naso-ethmoid—orbital injuries. J Craniomaxillofac Surg 1995;1(4):36–48.

Holt GR, Holt JE. Naso-ethmoid complex injuries. Otolaryngol Clin North Am 1985;18(1):87–98.

Renner GJ. Management of nasal fractures. Otolaryngol Clin North Am 1991;24(1):195–212.

Authors: Adam R. Saperston; David W. Munter

Nausea

Clinical Presentation

SIGNS AND SYMPTOMS

- Sensation of the imminent desire to vomit
  —May be experienced in the abdomen, epigastrium, or pharynx
- Often accompanied by autonomic signs and symptoms
  —Anorexia
  —Diaphoresis
  —Hypersalivation
  —Skin pallor
  —Tachycardia
  —Bradycardia
- Findings suggestive of the underlying etiology
  —Fever
  —Diarrhea
  —Abdominal pain
  —Headache
  —Vertigo
  —Neurologic signs
  —Nystagmus
    -CNS disorders
    -Glaucoma
    -Vertigo
  —Decreased, high pitched, or absent bowel sounds
  —Abdominal bruit

MECHANISM/DESCRIPTION

- Derived from the Greek word for sea sickness
- Gastrointestinal
  —The stomach normally has 3 contractions per minute
  —Delayed gastric emptying or a rapid increase in gastric contractions triggers changes in gastric tone and stimulates nausea via the central nervous system
    -Withdrawal of vagal tone
    -Increase in epinephrine levels
    -Significant increase in CNS vasopressin levels
- CNS
  —Many of the specific mechanisms for CNS induced nausea have not been elucidated
  —Elevated ICP or inflamed meninges are common causes
- Medication and toxins
  —Mediated through dopamine receptors in the area postrema
  —The precise mechanisms are unknown
  —Chemotherapy-induced nausea is related in part to increased serotonin release

ETIOLOGY

- Gastrointestinal
  —Gastroenteritis
  —Gastritis
  —Peptic ulcer disease
  —Bowel obstruction
  —Pancreatitis
  —Biliary colic
  —Cholecystitis
  —Hepatitis
  —GI carcinoma
  —Gastroparesis
  —Appendicitis
  —Peritonitis
- Metabolic/endocrine
  —Ketoacidosis (alcoholic and diabetic)
  —Thyrotoxicosis
  —Uremia
  —Metabolic alkalosis
  —Adrenal insufficiency
  —Hyperparathyroidism
- Toxicologic
  —Nearly any drug or ingestion can cause vomiting
  —Most common offenders
    -Antibiotics
    -Opioids
    -NSAIDs
    -Anti-immunologics including chemotherapeutic agents
    -Digoxin
    -Ethanol
    -Anticholinergics
- Neurologic
  —CNS mass
  —CNS bleeding
  —Cerebral edema
  —Hydrocephalus
  —Meningitis
  —Encephalitis
  —Concussion
  —Vascular headaches
- Vascular
  —Myocardial or mesenteric infarction or ischemia
  —Torsion of ovary or testicle
- Ophthalmologic
  —Glaucoma
  —Postsurgical
- ENT
  —Labyrinthus
  —Ménière's disease
  —Other peripheral vertigo
- Psychiatric
  —Bulimia
  —Anxiety disorder
- Other
  —Nephrolithiasis
  —Pregnancy (normal or ectopic)
  —Motion sickness

Pre-Hospital

CAUTIONS

- Transport and monitor if the patient has chest pain or cardiac risk factors
- Most often ambulance transport and field interventions are not warranted for nausea alone

Diagnosis

ESSENTIAL WORKUP

- Directed by the history and physical examination
- Use the characteristics of associated pain to separate CNS from gastrointestinal workup
- The contents of the vomitus
  —Undigested food suggests a gastric disorder
  —The presence of bilious or feculent material suggests bowel obstruction
  —Hematemesis suggests peptic diseases or mucosal lacerations
- Relationship to meals
  —5–30 minutes after meals: gastroparesis
  —30–60 minutes after meals: cholecystitis or pancreatitis
- Nausea reduced after eating
  —Esophagitis
  —Gastritis
  —Peptic ulcer disease

LABORATORY

- Urinalysis
  —Inexpensive way to assess dehydration
  —Nephrolithiasis or pyelonephritis may present with minimal flank pain
  —Urine β-HCG
  —Indicated in all women of child bearing age presenting with nausea or vomiting
- Serum glucose and electrolytes
  —Patients in DKA with new onset diabetes may present with nausea and vomiting
- Serum lipase
  —More accurate in detecting pancreatitis than the serum amylase
  —Indicated only if pancreatitis is suggested by the clinical assessment
- Liver function tests and hepatitis profile
  —Hepatitis may first present as nausea alone
  —Generally not needed during the ED evaluation
  —Should be ordered when associated with jaundice

IMAGING/SPECIAL TESTS

- EKG
  - —Presence of chest pain, shortness of breath, or cardiac risk factors should lead to a workup for myocardial ischemia
- KUB and upright abdominal radiographs
  - —Indicated in the presence of abdominal distention, decreased bowel sounds, or abdominal pain associated with prior abdominal surgery
- Ultrasound of the gallbladder, pancreas, and liver
  - —Indicated if right-upper quadrant tenderness or jaundice is present
- Upper endoscopy
  - —Indicated as an outpatient to evaluate patients with chronic nausea
- Head CT Scan
  - —Indicated in the presence of headache or neurological findings
  - —Noncontrast CT during the ED visit to rule out hemorrhage
  - —Contrast studies for tumors and metastasis can be done as an outpatient

DIFFERENTIAL DIAGNOSIS

- Life threats must be ruled out in the ED
  - —Acute myocardial infarction
  - —Vascular torsion
  - —CNS bleed or infection
  - —Drug intoxication
  - —Acute angle-closure glaucoma
  - —Ectopic pregnancy
  - —Peritonitis
  - —Appendicitis
  - —GI bleeding
  - —Intestinal obstruction

Treatment

INITIAL STABILIZATION

- Intravenous access
- Supplemental oxygen

ED TREATMENT

- Fluid resuscitate hypovolemic patients with isotonic crystalloid
- Decompress stomach with nasogastric or orogastric tube if bowel obstruction is present
- Administration of antiemetic medication
  - —Neuroleptic agents
    - -Droperidol, prochlorperazine
    - -Parenteral agents of choice for ED treatment of nausea
    - -Prochlorperazine suppositories are good first-line agents for the outpatient management
    - -Warn of possible dystonic reaction with these medications
  - —Benzamides
  - —Cisapride, metoclopramide
  - —Indicated for reflux esophagitis and gastroparesis
  - —First-line agents in the outpatient management of diabetics with intractable nausea
  - —Antihistamines
    - -Promethazine
    - -Indicated primarily for nausea induced by motion disorder or vertigo
  - —Ondansetron
    - -Chemotherapy or postoperative nausea

MEDICATIONS

- Prochlorperazine: 5–10 mg IV/IM or 25 mg PR
- Cisapride: 10 mg po qid
- Droperidol: 0.625–2.5 mg IV/IM
- Metoclopramide: 10 mg IV/IM
- Ondansetron: 4–32 mg IV
- Promethazine: 25–50 mg IV/IM/PR
- Trimethobenzamide: 200 mg IM/PR

Disposition

ADMISSION CRITERIA

- Serious underlying etiologies
- Benign etiologies for intractable vomiting or inability to take po fluids

DISCHARGE CRITERIA

- Benign etiologies that respond to treatment and patients who are able to take adequate po fluid
- Close followup, especially in elderly or pediatric patients
- Small volumes of liquid meals such as soups should be ingested hourly
- As nausea resolves, complex starches such as noodles, pastas, potatoes, and rice
- Avoid fatty foods and red meats
- 4–6 small meals each day

Miscellaneous

ICD9: 787.0

CORE CONTENT CODE: N/A

SUGGESTED READINGS

Sternbach G. Vomiting. In: Harwood-Nuss A, et al. (eds). The clinical practice of emergency medicine. Philadelphia: J.B. Lippincott, 1991.

Author: Myles Greenberg

Near Drowning

Clinical Presentation

SIGNS AND SYMPTOMS

Cardiovascular

- Cardiopulmonary arrest: apneic and pulseless
- Cyanosis

Pulmonary

- Dyspnea
- Cough
- Copious pulmonary secretions

CNS

- Loss of consciousness
- Hypoxic-induced cerebral injury
- Cerebral edema

Other

- Evidence of trauma
  - —Cervical spine injury
- Hypothermia

MECHANISM/DESCRIPTION

Definitions

- Drowning
  - —Death by suffocation after submersion in a liquid
  - —Death within 24 hours of the accident
- Near drowning
  - —Survival, or at least temporary survival, following a submersion accident
  - —Survival beyond 24 hours

Stages of Drowning

- Stage I
  - —Unexpected submersion with struggle
  - —Aspiration of small amount of water
  - —Laryngospasm
- Stage II
  - —Increased hypoxia and panic
  - —Large volume of water swallowed
- Stage III
  - —Wet drowning (85–90% of cases)
    - -Laryngospasm relaxes due to persistent hypoxia
    - -Aspiration
  - —Dry drowning (10–15% of cases)
  - —Aspiration of small amount of water
  - —Further laryngospasm
  - —Severe hypoxia leading to seizure or death

Physiologic Responses

- Saltwater drowning
  - —Protein-rich fluid pulled into the alveoli causing pulmonary edema and hypoxia
  - —Reduced circulating blood volume with elevated hemoglobin and sodium
- Freshwater drowning
  - —Affects surface-tension properties of surfactant making the alveoli unstable
    - -Collapse or atelectasis of alveoli
    - -Intrapulmonary shunting and hypoxia
  - —Hypotonic fluid absorbed quickly into the circulation and redistributed into the body
    - -Hemodilution and fluid overload
    - -Reduced hemoglobin and serum electrolytes
    - -Lysis of red cells leads to hyperkalemia

Pathophysiology

- Aspiration
  - —Small volume of water usually aspirated
    - -Significant electrolyte changes uncommon
    - -Grossly contaminated water increases risk of pulmonary infection
- Hypoxemia
  - —Metabolic lactic acidosis
  - —Multisystem organ dysfunction
    - -Myocardial dysfunction
    - -Coagulation abnormalities (DIC)
    - -Renal failure
    - -CNS dysfunction

PEDIATRIC CONSIDERATIONS

- Hypothermia
  - —More common in young children due to larger body surface to mass ratio and less subcutaneous fat
  - —Decreases the metabolic rate
  - —Survival and full recovery possible after prolonged submersion in cold water (record: 66 minutes)
- Diving reflex
  - —Young children may be more susceptible
  - —Potentiated by fear
  - —Triggered by submersion of face in cold water
  - —Bradycardia ensues with redistribution of blood flow to the heart and brain

Pre-Hospital

CAUTIONS

- Attention to ABCs
- Avoid further aspiration
- Apply cricoid pressure during bag-to-mask ventilation until airway is secured by intubation
- Strict C-spine precautions
- 90% survival with appropriate intervention at the scene

CONTROVERSIES

- Abdominal thrusts to remove water
  - —Not appropriate to "remove water from the lungs"
  - —Increased risk of aspiration
  - —Only useful if foreign body lodged in airway

Diagnosis

ESSENTIAL WORKUP

- Diagnosis made from information gathered at the scene from witnesses or from EMS personnel
- Rectal temperature for hypothermia

LABORATORY

- Arterial blood gas
  —Temperature correction not necessary
- CBC
- Electrolytes, BUN, Cr, glucose
  —Usually normal
  —Hyperkalemia
  —Hyper- or hyponatremia
- Alcohol and toxicology screen
  —Especially in young adults

IMAGING/SPECIAL TESTS

- CXR
  —Bilateral fluffy infiltrates
  —Localized infiltrate
  —May be normal initially
- Cervical spine series
- ECG

DIFFERENTIAL DIAGNOSIS

- Consider reason for submersion
  —Dysrhythmia
  —Myocardial infarction
  —Seizure
  —Syncope
  —Trauma

PEDIATRIC CONSIDERATIONS

- Consider child abuse/neglect
  —Especially infants in bathtub near-drowning

Treatment

INITIAL STABILIZATION

- ABCs
- Remove wet clothing
- Obtain accurate core temperature
  —Initiate rewarming (see chapter: Hypothermia)

ED TREATMENT

- Correct hypoxemia
  —Titrate to oxygen saturation
  —Intubate and provide mechanical ventilation with positive end-expiratory pressure to maintain oxygenation
- Evaluate and treat traumatic injuries
- Correct acidosis
  —Administer sodium bicarbonate if pH <7.1
- Cardiopulmonary arrest
  —Initiate ACLS measures
  —Continue rewarming efforts
  —Continue resuscitation until core temperature >32°C, or until spontaneous pulse and respirations return
- Importance of admission
  —Pulmonary edema may develop as long as 12 hours later
  —Delayed neurologic abnormalities

MEDICATIONS (PER ACLS PROTOCOLS)

- Atropine: 1 mg (peds: 0.02 mg/kg) IV
- Epinephrine: 1 mg (peds: 0.01 mg/kg) IV
- Sodium bicarbonate: 1 mEq/kg IV
- Lidocaine: 1 mg/kg IV

PEDIATRIC CONSIDERATIONS

- Hypothermia may be protective
  —Aggressive rewarming
  —Aggressive resuscitation
- Evaluate for child abuse/neglect
  —Social service consult
- Prevention is key to treatment
  —Supervision around all water environments
  —Empty pails and buckets of water
  —Fences around pools

Disposition

ADMISSION CRITERIA

- ICU
  —Patients who required CPR or artificial ventilation
  —Abnormal chest radiograph
  —ABG abnormalities
- Admit observation status
  —Submersion for >1 minute
  —History of cyanosis or apnea
  —Patients who required brief assisted ventilation

DISCHARGE CRITERIA

- Questionable history of submersion
  —Observe in ED for 6–8 hours
  —No signs or symptoms of respiratory distress or change in neurologic status
- Discharge to reliable home
- Instruction include close follow-up of respiratory and neurologic status

Miscellaneous

ICD9: 994.1

CORE CONTENT CODE: 5.3

SUGGESTED READINGS

DeNicola LK, Falk JL, Swanson ME, Gayle MO, Kissoon N. Submersion injuries in children and adults. Crit Care Clin 1997;13:477–502.

Fields AI. Near-drowning in the pediatric population. Crit Care Clin 1992;8:113–129.

Lavelle JM, Shaw KN, Seidl T, Ludwig S. Ten-year review of pediatric bathtub near-drowning: Evaluation for child abuse and neglect. Ann Emerg Med 1995;25:344–348.

Olshaker JS. Near drowning. Emerg Med Clin North Am 1992;10:339–349.

Quan L, Wentz KR, Gore EJ, Copass MK. Outcome and predictors of outcome in pediatric submersion victims receiving prehospital care in King County, Washington. Pediatrics 1990;86:586–593.

Author: Janet Poponick

Neck Injury by Strangulation/Hanging

Clinical Presentation

SIGNS AND SYMPTOMS

Airway Disruption

- Neck ecchymosis or emphysema, dyspnea, dysphonia, stridor, loss of normal cartilaginous landmarks

Neurologic Injury

- Hoarseness, dysphagia, decreased level of consciousness, neurologic deficit

Vascular Injuries

- Expanding hematoma, pulse deficits, bruits, evidence of cerebral infarction, petechiae

Cervical Spine Injury

- Respiratory arrest, paralysis

MECHANISM/DESCRIPTION

Strangulation

- Ligature: cord used to compress structures of the neck
- Manual: use of physical force to compress structures of neck
- Postural: victim's neck lies over an object with weight of body applying pressure to neck

Hanging

- Complete: victim's feet are suspended off the ground
- Incomplete: any position when feet are not freely suspended
  - —Typical: point of suspension is placed centrally over the occiput
  - —Atypical: point of suspension not centrally placed over the occiput

ETIOLOGY

Strangulation or Hanging

- Suicide, homicide, accidental
  - —Neck pressure results in venous obstruction causing cerebral hypoxia and then death
  - —Pressure on neck structures may cause airway, soft tissue, and vascular injuries
  - —Rarely may cause cervical spine injury
    - -Fracture of the neural arch of C2; the "hangman's fracture"
- Judicial
  - —Victim dropped a distance that is proportional to their weight
  - —Forceful distraction of head from torso results in decapitation type injury

Pre-Hospital

CAUTIONS

- Early and aggressive airway management: oxygen, suction, intubation
- Cervical spine immobilization

Diagnosis

ESSENTIAL WORKUP

- X-ray: neck (soft tissue), c-spine, and chest; evaluate for evidence of bony and soft tissue injury, subcutaneous emphysema as well as aspiration pneumonitis
- CT scan of the neck: further defines soft tissue injuries

LABORATORY

- Arterial blood gas (ABG): evaluate for evidence of hypoxia
- Hematocrit: check for evidence of significant blood loss
- Type and cross: prepare for transfusion as required by vascular disruption

IMAGING/SPECIAL TESTS

- Fiberoptic endoscopy: allows direct visualization for evaluation of endolaryngeal injury; may aid in intubation
- Arteriography: definitive evaluation for potential vascular injuries
- Surgical exploration

DIFFERENTIAL DIAGNOSIS

Associated Injuries

- Larynx fracture
- Hyoid fracture: most commonly seen in manual strangulation
- Thyroid cartilage disruption
  - —Most commonly an anterior vertical fracture from thyroid cartilage notch to cricothyroid membrane
- Vascular disruption: arterial or venous
- Phrenic nerve injury
- Cervical spine injury
  - —Fracture of the neural arch of C2; the "hangman's fracture"
- Hypoxic cerebral injury
- Airway edema
- Aspiration pneumonitis
- Air embolism
  - —Consider when subcutaneous air and vascular injuries are present

PEDIATRIC CONSIDERATIONS

- Structures of the neck are more cartilaginous and mobile than in adults. Thus, pediatric patients are more resistant to crush and fracture injuries; however because of the relatively smaller airway diameter rapid airway compromise can occur with relatively little edema of the soft tissues.

Treatment

INITIAL STABILIZATION

- Early and aggressive airway management, with cervical spine precautions, is paramount.
  - —Early intubation to preclude respiratory embarrassment
  - —Severe injuries of the larynx may require operative management
- Patient may require emergent tracheostomy
- Cricothyrotomy if severe maxillofacial injuries are present
  - —*Avoid* cricothyrotomy if a hematoma is seen over cricothyroid membrane or evidence of cricotracheal disruption—arrange for emergent tracheostomy (see chapter: Larynx Fracture).
- Supplemental humidified oxygen
- Control bleeding with application of direct pressure—do *not* explore in the emergency department.

ED TREATMENT

- IV access
- Consult otolaryngologist in the management of neck soft tissue injuries
- Elevate head of bed to decrease edema
- Consider ICP monitoring if there is evidence of severe hypoxic cerebral injury
- Consider use of positive end expiratory pressure and volume cycled ventilation in cases of severe pulmonary dysfunction associated with ARDS or aspiration pneumonitis

MEDICATIONS

For Hypoxic Brain Injury

- Dilantin: adult: 1 g IV; peds: 15 mg/kg IV
- Mannitol: adult and peds: 1 g/kg IV
- Steroids: controversial

For Neck Injury With Subcutaneous Emphysema

- Assume that the mucosa of the upper airway communicates with the deep tissues of the neck and administer antibiotics
  - —Clindamycin: 600 mg IV; peds: 10 mg/kg/dose IV q 8 hrs

For Laryngeal Edema

- Steroids may be useful
  - —Dexamethasone: adult: 4 mg IV; peds: 0.25–0.5 mg/kg/dose IV

Disposition

ADMISSION CRITERIA

- All patients with significant strangulation or hanging injuries must be admitted to a monitored setting to observe for airway compromise
- Prepare for emergent surgical correction of laryngeal defect

DISCHARGE CRITERIA

- Only patients proven not to have strangulation or hanging injuries may be discharged after appropriate observation in the ED for the development of any airway compromise or mental status changes

Miscellaneous

ICD9: 959.09

CORE CONTENT CODE: 18.4.8, 18.4.9

SUGGESTED READINGS

Aufderheide TP, et al. Emergency airway management in hanging victims. Ann Emerg Med 1994;24:879–884.

Campbell W, et al. Neck trauma. In: Rosen P, et al., eds. Emergency medicine: Concepts and clinical practice. 4th ed. St. Louis: Mosby-Year Book, 1998.

Hanigan WC, et al. Strangulation injuries in children. Part 2. Cerebrovascular hemodynamics. J Trauma 1996;40(1):73–77.

Sabo RA, et al. Strangulation injuries in children. Part 1. Clinical analysis. J Trauma 1996;40(1):68–72.

Ubelaker DH. Hyoid bone and strangulation. J Forensic Sci 1992;37:1216–1222.

Author: Catherine M. Hurt

Neck Trauma, Blunt, Anterior

Clinical Presentation

SIGNS AND SYMPTOMS

- The presentation of blunt anterior neck trauma varies depending on the mechanism of injury and the structures involved
- Vascular injury
  —Hemorrhage, ecchymosis, edema
  —Loss of character of lateral neck profile
  —Carotid bruit
  —Neurologic deficits (often delayed)
- Laryngotracheal injury
  —Voice changes, hoarseness, aphonia
  —Dyspnea, inspiratory stridor, labored breathing
  —Subcutaneous emphysema, tenderness to palpation
- Pharyngoesophageal injury
  —Dysphagia, odynophagia
  —Tenderness to palpation
  —Infection, sepsis (delayed presentation)
- Neurologic injury
  —Central or peripheral nervous system deficits

MECHANISM/DESCRIPTION

- Many injuries may result from blunt anterior neck trauma
  —Fracture of the thyroid cartilage, vocal cord disruption, or dislocation of airway cartilages
  —Hematoma of the larynx or trachea, or complete tracheal transection at the junction with the cricoid cartilage
  —Pharyngoesophageal injury results from hematoma or perforation of the pharynx or esophagus and usually occurs in conjunction with laryngotracheal injury
    -Presentation is often delayed, and injury may only be detected when infection develops
  —Vascular injuries involving the carotid artery include intramural hematoma, intimal tear, thrombosis, and pseudoaneurysm
    -Injury may result in ischemic or thromboembolic events
  —Nervous system injury includes damage to the recurrent laryngeal nerve or injury to the stellate ganglion resulting in *Horner's syndrome*
  —Cervical spine injury may occur with blunt neck injury

ETIOLOGY

- Motor vehicle accidents
  —Unrestrained occupants involved in frontal collisions may strike neck on the dashboard or steering wheel
  —The shoulder harness can also cause shearing injury to the anterior neck
  —Assault
    -Blows from fists, weapons, or other objects to the anterior neck
  —"Clothesline injury" is seen when motorcycle, snowmobile, or all-terrain vehicle drivers strike neck on a cord or wire suspended between two objects

PEDIATRIC CONSIDERATIONS

- The head is proportionally larger in children, increasing the risk of acceleration-deceleration injury to the neck

Pre-Hospital

- The airway must be vigilantly monitored as edema or expanding hematoma can progress to airway compromise
- Early oral intubation is indicated for clinical signs of respiratory distress such as stridor, air hunger, or labored breathing, or if an expanding neck hematoma is present

CAUTIONS

- Blind nasotracheal intubation should be avoided because of potential rupture of an expanding hematoma and is difficult to perform because of distortion of anatomy

Diagnosis

ESSENTIAL WORKUP

- Inspection of the neck for distortion of anatomy, auscultation for carotid bruits, and palpation to detect tenderness or subcutaneous emphysema
- A neurologic exam should be performed to detect evidence of an ischemic event, spinal cord injury, or peripheral nerve damage
- Cervical spine radiographs
- Chest radiograph to rule out associated injury to the thorax

LABORATORY

- Type and crossmatch
- Baseline CBC and chemistry panel

IMAGING/SPECIAL TESTS

- Computed tomography may be used in the stable patient to evaluate laryngotracheal injury and delineate cartilage disruption
- Angiography
  - —Considered the Gold Standard to evaluate arterial injury
  - —Indicated in the presence of a carotid bruit, large hematoma, CVA with normal head CT scan or suspected occult vascular injury
- Carotid duplex ultrasound is a noninvasive, rapid screening test for arterial injury
- Endoscopy to detect internal soft tissue defects in the larynx and trachea
- Esophagram or rigid esophagoscopy to rule out pharyngoesophageal injury when odynophagia, hematemesis, or subcutaneous emphysema are present

DIFFERENTIAL DIAGNOSIS

- Vascular injury
- Laryngotracheal injury
- Pharyngoesophageal injury
- Peripheral or central nervous system injury
- Cervical spine injury
- Associated head or thoracic trauma

Treatment

INITIAL STABILIZATION

Airway Management with C-spine Control

- Immediate intubation indicated for patients with signs of airway compromise
  - —Orotracheal intubation is the method of choice
- Cricothyroidotomy may be needed if oral intubation fails
- Emergency tracheostomy is preferred in blunt upper airway trauma because cricothyroidotomy may worsen an injury below the level of the cricoid
- Care should be taken to avoid puncturing a neck hematoma during invasive procedures
- Bleeding into the pharynx can be tamponaded by packing the throat with heavy gauze after the airway is secured by intubation
- Unstable patients should go directly to the operating room

ED TREATMENT

- Surgical consultation should be obtained for patients with recurrent symptoms, angiographic evidence of vascular injury, or suspected tracheal or esophageal injury
- Once the airway is secured, laryngeal injuries do not require immediate surgical repair
  - —The patient should be placed on voice rest, humidified air, and be given prophylactic antibiotics
- Tracheal injury requires prompt surgical repair
- Extensive pharyngeal lacerations and esophageal injuries require immediate surgical repair
- Asymptomatic patients with arterial injury may be observed and do well without intervention
  - —Surgery is indicated for patients with recurrent symptoms or angiographic progression of disease

MEDICATIONS

- *Prophylactic antibiotics* recommended in the presence of laryngotracheal or pharyngoesophageal injury
- Cefoxitin: adult: 2 g IV q 8 hrs; peds: 80–160 mg/kg/day IM/IV div q 6 hrs *or*
- Clindamycin: adult: 600–900 mg IV q 8 hrs; peds: 25–40 mg/kg/day IV div q 6–8 hrs *or*
- Penicillin G: adult: 24 million IU/day div q 4–6 hrs; peds: 150,000–250,000 IU/kg/day div q 4–6 hrs *plus*
- Metronidazole: adult: 1 g load then 500 mg IV q 6 hrs; peds: 30 mg/kg/day IV div q 12 hrs

Disposition

ADMISSION CRITERIA

- Patients who are symptomatic, have abnormal studies, or significant blunt trauma mechanism must be admitted and observed for at least 24 hours
- Patients with suspicion of airway or vascular injury must be admitted to the ICU

DISCHARGE CRITERIA

- Only patients with the most trivial injuries who have negative studies may be discharged from the ED following thorough evaluation

Miscellaneous

ICD9: 959.09

CORE CONTENT CODE: 18.4.8

SUGGESTED READINGS

Camnitz PS, Shepherd SM, Henderson RA. Acute blunt laryngeal and tracheal trauma. Am J Emerg Med 1987;5(2):157.

Fuhrman GM, Stieg FH, Buerk CA. Blunt laryngeal trauma. J Trauma 1990;30:87.

Jorden RC. Neck Trauma. In: Rosen P, et al., eds. Emergency medicine: Concepts and clinical practice. 4th ed. St. Louis: CV Mosby, 1998;505–513.

Author: Tamaki Kimbro

Neck Trauma, Penetrating, Anterior

Clinical Presentation

SIGNS AND SYMPTOMS

- Signs and symptoms vary depending on the specific structures injured
- Vascular injury
  - —Active hemorrhage or hematoma
  - —Tracheal deviation, loss of normal anatomic landmarks
  - —Pulse deficits in upper extremities
  - —Thrills or bruits in neck
- Laryngotracheal injury
  - —Respiratory distress
  - —Hoarseness, voice changes
  - —Hemoptysis
  - —Neck pain or tenderness
  - —Crepitance
- Pharyngoesophageal injury
  - —Dysphagia
  - —Odynophagia
  - —Hematemesis
- Neurologic injury
  - —Central or peripheral nervous system deficits

MECHANISM/DESCRIPTION

- Penetrating neck trauma is defined as a wound that penetrates the platysma muscle
- The neck is divided into *three zones* based on superficial landmarks
  - —Zone I extends from the top of the sternum to the sternal notch or cricoid cartilage
    - -Penetrating trauma in this zone carries the highest mortality due to injury to thoracic structures
  - —Zone II extends from the sternal notch or cricoid cartilage to the angle of the mandible
    - -The majority of penetrating neck wounds occur in this zone
    - -Zone II wounds have a lower mortality because hemorrhage can be controlled with direct pressure and structures are easily accessible for surgical exploration
  - —Zone III extends from the cephalad to the angle of the mandible

ETIOLOGY

- Gunshot wounds
- Stab wounds
- Miscellaneous (glass shards, metal fragments)

PEDIATRIC CONSIDERATIONS

- In the pediatric patient, the larynx is located higher in the neck and receives better protection from the mandible and hyoid bone

Pre-Hospital

- Frequent suctioning to clear airway of blood, secretions, or vomitus
- Lateral decubitus or prone positioning may be required to prevent aspiration
- The airway must be vigilantly monitored as edema or expanding hematoma can progress to airway compromise
- Early oral intubation is indicated for clinical signs of respiratory distress, such as stridor, air hunger, or labored breathing, or if an expanding neck hematoma is present

CAUTIONS

- Nasotracheal intubation should be avoided because of potential rupture of an expanding hematoma and is difficult to perform because of distortion of anatomy
- Occlusive dressings should be applied to lacerations over major veins to prevent air embolism

Diagnosis

ESSENTIAL WORKUP

- Careful examination of the wound to determine the extent of injury and if it penetrates the platysma
  - —Wounds should never be blindly probed as this may result in uncontrolled hemorrhage
- Lateral neck radiograph to evaluate soft tissue injury and detect foreign bodies
- Chest radiograph to detect hemopneumothorax, mediastinal air, or bleeding that extends into the upper mediastinum

LABORATORY

- Type and crossmatch
- Baseline CBC and chemistry panel

IMAGING/SPECIAL TESTS

- Angiography
  - —Considered the Gold Standard to evaluate arterial injury
  - —Indicated for penetrating wounds in Zone I or Zone III
- Color duplex ultrasound is a noninvasive, rapid screening test for arterial injury
- Bronchoscopy can be helpful to evaluate tracheal injury but it may increase airway edema and is difficult in patients with respiratory distress
- Esophagram with gastrografin or dilute barium
  - —Low sensitivity
  - —Combine with esophagoscopy to exclude injury
  - —Indications
    - -wound approaches/crosser midline
    - -subcutaneous air
- Esophagoscopy to evaluate for esophageal injury

DIFFERENTIAL DIAGNOSIS

- Vascular injury
- Pharyngoesophageal injury
- Laryngotracheal injury
- Peripheral or central nervous system injury
- Cervical spine injury
- Associated head or thoracic trauma

Treatment

INITIAL STABILIZATION

Airway management with C-spine Control

- Patients who are comatose or in respiratory distress require immediate intubation
- Stable patients without evidence of respiratory distress may be aggressively managed with prophylactic intubation or closely observed with airway equipment at the bedside
- Orotracheal intubation with rapid sequence induction or sedation is the method of choice for securing the airway in penetrating neck trauma
- Nasotracheal intubation is contraindicated with apnea, severe facial injury, or airway distortion because of the risk of puncturing an expanding hematoma
- Endoscopic intubation is contraindicated with active bleeding that may obscure the scope
- Percutaneous transtracheal ventilation may be useful when oral or nasotracheal intubation fails
  —Leaves the airway unprotected and is contraindicated in cases of upper airway obstruction as it may cause barotrauma
  —Cricothyroidotomy, tracheostomy, or intubation via a penetrating wound may be required in cases of severe facial injury, laryngotracheal injury, or uncontrolled upper airway hemorrhage

Breathing

- Zone I injury can cause pneumothorax or subclavian vein injury and hemothorax, requiring needle decompression and tube thoracostomy

Circulation

- External hemorrhage should be controlled with direct pressure. Blind clamping of vessels is contraindicated due to the risk of further neurovascular injury
- Patients with uncontrollable bleeding or hemodynamic instability must go directly to the operating room
- Following intubation, the throat can be packed with heavy gauze to tamponade the bleeding
- Tube thoracostomy for bleeding into the chest

ED TREATMENT

- Nasogastric tube should not be placed due to risk of rupturing a pharyngeal hematoma
- Prophylactic antibiotics are recommended (cefoxitin, clindamycin, penicillin G plus metronidazole)
- Surgical consult for all wounds that penetrate the platysma muscle
- There is controversy in mandatory versus selective surgical exploration in stable patients
  —Mandatory approach
  -Surgical exploration is indicated in all cases of penetrating neck trauma because significant injury may not manifest outward signs or symptoms
  —Selective approach
  -Surgical exploration for specific indications including expanding or pulsatile hematoma, active bleeding, absence of peripheral pulses, hemoptysis, Horner's syndrome, bruit, subcutaneous emphysema, respiratory distress, or air bubbling through a wound
- Tetanus prophylaxis

MEDICATIONS

- Cefoxitin: adult: 2 g IV q 8 hrs; peds: 80–160 mg/kg/day IM/IV div q 6 hrs *or*
- Clindamycin: adult: 600–900 mg IV q 8 hrs; peds: 25–40 mg/kg/day IV div q 6–8 hrs *or*
- Penicillin G: adult: 24 million IU/day div q 4–6 hrs; peds: 150,000–250,000 IU/kg/day div q 4–6 hrs *plus*
- Metronidazole: adult: 1 g load then 500 mg IV q 6 hrs; peds: 30 mg/kg/day IV div q 12 hrs

Disposition

ADMISSION CRITERIA

- All patients with penetrating neck trauma should be admitted and observed for at least 24 hours
- Observation must take place in a facility capable of providing definitive surgical care
- Patients with suspicion of airway or vascular injury must be admitted to the ICU

DISCHARGE CRITERIA

- Asymptomatic patients who have negative studies may be discharged after at least 24 hours of observation

Miscellaneous

ICD9: 959.09

CORE CONTENT CODE: 18.4.8.2

SUGGESTED READINGS

Carducci B, Lowe RA, Dalsey W. Penetrating neck trauma: Consensus and controversies. Ann Emerg Med 1986;15:208.

Jorden RC. Neck trauma. In: Rosen P, et al., eds. Emergency medicine: Concepts and clinical practice. 4th ed. St. Louis: CV Mosby, 1998:505–513.

Roon AJ, Christensen N. Evaluation and treatment of penetrating cervical injuries. J Trauma 1979;19:391.

Author: Tamaki Kimbro

Necrotizing Soft Tissue Infections

Clinical Presentation

SIGNS AND SYMPTOMS

- Rapid progression of pain and swelling of involved area
- Pain out of proportion to physical findings
- In first 24 hours: rapid development of local swelling, heat, erythema and tenderness
- 24–48 hours: purple and blue discoloration, blisters and bullae develop
- Necrosis of fascia and fat produces a watery, thin, foul-smelling fluid
- Systemic toxicity with fever, tachycardia, and depressed mentation

MECHANISM/DESCRIPTION

- Necrotizing soft-tissue infections are usually caused by toxin-producing, virulent bacteria, characterized by widespread fascial and muscle necrosis with relative sparing of the skin
- Crepitant anaerobic cellulitis: necrotic soft tissue infection with abundant connective tissue gas
- Progressive bacterial gangrene: slowly progressive erosion affecting the total thickness of skin but not involving deep fascia
- Nonclostridial myonecrosis (synergistic necrotizing cellulitis): aggressive soft tissue infection of skin, muscle, subcutaneous tissue and fascia
- Necrotizing fasciitis: a progressive, rapidly spreading, infection with extensive dissection and necrosis of the superficial and deep fascia
- Fournier's gangrene: a mixed aerobic-anaerobic soft tissue necrotizing fasciitis of the skin of the scrotum and penis in males and the vulvar and perianal skin in women

ETIOLOGY

- Conditions that lead to the development of necrotizing soft tissue infections include
  - —Local tissue trauma with bacterial invasion
  - —Local ischemia and reduced host defenses: occurs more frequently in diabetics, alcoholics, immunosuppressed patients, IV drug users, and patients with peripheral vascular disease
- Polymicrobial etiology including
  - —Group A β-hemolytic streptococcus; Group B streptococcus, staphylococci, enterococci, bacillus, pseudomonas, Enterobacter, Bacteroides, clostridium, and vibrio species

PEDIATRIC CONSIDERATIONS

- Neonates: omphalitis and circumcision are predisposing factors
- Children: surgery, trauma, varicella, and congenital and acquired immunodeficiencies are major factors for the development of necrotizing fasciitis. Group A β-hemolytic streptococcal necrotizing fasciitis as a complication of varicella has been reported

Pre-Hospital

N/A

Diagnosis

ESSENTIAL WORKUP

- Diagnosis can be difficult
- Careful examination for the above signs and symptoms in high risk patients
- Necrotizing soft tissue infections must be suspected in patients who appear very ill and have pain out of proportion to physical findings

LABORATORY

- CBC with differential, electrolytes, BUN, and creatinine
- Calcium level: hypocalcemia can develop from extensive fat necrosis
- Aerobic and anaerobic cultures of wound or tissue biopsy

IMAGING/SPECIAL TESTS

- X-rays to detect soft-tissue gas
- CT scan to delineate extent of spread of the infection

DIFFERENTIAL DIAGNOSIS

- Cellulitis
- Gas gangrene

Treatment

INITIAL STABILIZATION

- ABCs
  - —Control airway as needed.
  - —Supplemental oxygen, monitor, evaluate for acid-base disturbances
    - -Intravenous access, central venous pressure line may be needed.
  - —Aggressive volume expansion including crystalloid, plasma, packed red blood cells, and albumin

ED TREATMENT

- Antibiotics: broad coverage of aerobic Gram-positive and Gram-negative organisms and anaerobes
  - —Penicillin or cephalosporin, an aminoglycoside, and anaerobic coverage with either clindamycin or metronidazole
- Surgical consultation
  - —Early debridement of all necrotic tissue with fasciotomy and drainage of fascial planes is paramount
- Hyperbaric oxygen as an adjunct
  - —Early transfer to hyperbaric facility may result in greater tissue salvage
- Observe for major complication including ARDS, renal failure, myocardial irritability, and DIC

MEDICATIONS

- Ceftriaxone: adult: 2.0 g q 12 hrs IV; peds: 100 mg/kg/dose
- Clindamycin: adult: 900 mg q 8 hrs IV load; peds: 40 mg/kg/day divided q 6 hrs
- Gentamicin: adult and peds: 2.0 mg/kg IV load
- Metronidazole: adult: 500 mg IV load; peds: safety not established
- Penicillin G: adult: 24 million IU/day divided q 4–6 hrs IV; peds: 250,000 IU/day IV divided q 4 hrs

Disposition

ADMISSION CRITERIA

- All patients with a necrotizing soft tissue infection *must be admitted* for surgical debridement and IV antibiotics. Early hyperbaric oxygen therapy is an important adjunct

DISCHARGE CRITERIA

None

Miscellaneous

ICD9: 709.8

CORE CONTENT CODE: 10.6.1

SUGGESTED READINGS

Bakker DJ. Aerobic/anaerobic soft tissue infections and hyperbaric oxygen as adjunct. In: Kindwall EP, ed. Hyperbaric medicine practice. Best Publishing, Flagstaff, AZ 1994:395–418.

Barton LL, Jeck DT, Vaidya VU. Necrotizing fasciitis in children: Report of two cases and review of the literature. Arch Pediatr Adolesc Med 1996;150(1):105–108.

Green RJ, Dafoe, DC, Tafin TA. Necrotizing fasciitis. Chest 1996;110(1):219–229.

Author: Karen Van Hoesen

Needle Stick

Clinical Presentation

SIGNS AND SYMPTOMS

- History of exposure to blood or body fluid
- Mechanisms of exposure
  - —Percutaneous
  - —Mucous Membrane
  - —Skin

MECHANISM/DESCRIPTION

- Risk of seroconversion from a single needle-stick injury without prior immunization
  - —Hepatitis B (HBV): 6–30% from HB_sAg positive source, 27–43% in HB_eAg positive source
  - —Hepatitis C (HCV): 2.7%–10%
  - —HIV: 0.004% (1 in 250)
- The CDC reports 8700 HBV infections annually with >400 requiring hospitalization and approximately 200 dying
- Estimated 150,000–170,000 new HCV infections annually
- There are 37 documented HIV seroconversions in health care workers as of December 1993 with an additional 75 possible occupational infections.

ETIOLOGY

- How infectious are various bodily fluids for HIV?
  - —10–5000 ppm: plasma/serum
  - —10–1000 ppm: CSF
  - —10–50 ppm: semen
  - —<1: vaginal secretions, urine, saliva, tears, breast milk
- Factors affecting risk include
  - —Viral load, actual injection volume, type and size of needle, portal of entry (depth of inoculation), duration of contact, level of disease in source patient, host susceptibility, barriers (e.g., through gloves, etc.)

PEDIATRIC CONSIDERATIONS

N/A

Pre-Hospital

CAUTIONS

- Pre-hospital personnel should always maintain universal precautions to prevent needle stick or other body fluid exposure
- Patients with exposure should be evaluated for prophylactic therapy

Diagnosis

ESSENTIAL WORKUP

- Direct and immediate referral from ED triage to occupational health office when available to assure strictest confidentiality in laboratory testing and treatment
- In the ED after hours patients with needle-stick exposure must be triaged with high priority as time is of the essence in the initiation of prophylactic therapy
- Female recipients of body fluid exposure that are considering antiviral therapy must have serum or urine pregnancy testing
- Immunization history

LABORATORY

- To be done with occupational health if possible
  - —Baseline serology for HIV, hepatitis B, hepatitis C
  - —Assess adequacy of hepatitis-B vaccination
  - —Obtaining consent from source patient for HIV, HB_sAg, HCV

IMAGING/SPECIAL TESTS

- Not applicable unless there is a concern for retained tissue foreign body

DIFFERENTIAL DIAGNOSIS

- Principally concerned with transmission of HBV, HCV, and HIV

Treatment

INITIAL STABILIZATION

- Copious cleaning, wound care
- Direct and immediate referral to occupational health when available to assure strictest confidentiality in laboratory testing and treatment.

ED TREATMENT

- Tetanus prophylaxis if necessary
- If referral to occupational health unavailable initiate prophylactic therapy in ED
- HIV
  —Antiretroviral prophylaxis with 3-drug regimen: zidovudine, lamivudine, indinavir after consideration of risks and benefit
  —Safer sex advice
  —Counseling
- HBV
  —Known HB_sAg positive source
    -Complete vaccination confirmed by titer: no Rx
    -Incomplete vaccination: hepatitis B vaccine booster
    -Unvaccinated: HBIG ASAP, begin vaccine series
    -Nonresponder to Vaccine: HBIG ASAP, repeat in 30 days
    -Unknown responder to vaccine with inadequate titer: HBIG ASAP, vaccine booster
  —Known HB_sAg Neg source
    -Vaccinated: no Rx
    -Unvaccinated: Hepatitis B vaccine series
  —Unknown source
    -Complete vaccination confirmed by titer: no Rx
    -Incomplete vaccination: Hepatitis B vaccine booster
    -Unvaccinated: begin vaccine series
    -Nonresponder to vaccine: HBIG ASAP, repeat in 30 days if high-risk exposure
    -Unknown responder to vaccine with inadequate titer: vaccine booster
  —HCV
  —Use of immunoglobulins inconclusive

MEDICATIONS

- Zidovudine (AZT, ZDV): 200 mg po tid
- Lamivudine (3TC): 150 mg po bid
- Indinavir (saquinavir, IDV): 800 mg po tid
- Preferably initiated 1–2 hours postexposure
- Side effects
  —Zidovudine: GI sx, headache, fatigue, myalgias, marrow suppression
  —Lamivudine: GI sx, headache, fatigue, neuropathy, congestion, cough (caution with TMP/SMX)
  —Indinavir: nephrolithiasis, hyperbilirubinemia, elevated LFTs (caution with nonsedating antihistamines)
- Pregnancy factors
- Zidovudine: safe 2nd, 3rd trimester; unknown risk 1st trimester
- Lamivudine: unknown risk, class C
- Indinavir: unknown risk, class C

Hepatitis

- Hepatitis B immune globulin: 0.06 ml/kg IM
- Hepatitis B booster: unit dose vial

Disposition

ADMISSION CRITERIA

- Isolated needle stick or body fluid exposures need not be admitted

DISCHARGE CRITERIA

- Patients can be managed as outpatients with appropriate follow-up in occupational medicine clinic.

Miscellaneous

Prevention

- Avoid recapping of needles; if necessary, use one-handed technique
- Wear gloves: can decrease amount of blood exposure by 50%
- Consider double gloving
- Follow body substance isolation protocols
- Hepatitis B vaccination

ICD9: 998.2

CORE CONTENT CODE: 18.4.17.5

SUGGESTED READINGS

Berry AJ, Greene ES. The risk of needle-stick injuries and needle-stick-transmitted diseases in the practice of anesthesiology. Anesthesiology 1992;77:1007–1021.

Centers for Disease Control. Update: Provisional Public Health Service recommendations for chemoprophylaxis after occupational exposure to HIV. MMWR 1996;45(22):468–472.

Fraser VJ, Powderly WG. Risks of HIV infection in the health care setting. Ann Rev Med 1995;46:203–11.

Henderson, DK. Risk for exposures to and infection with HIV among health care providers in the emergency department. Emerg Med Clin North Am 1995;13(1):199–211.

Author: Gordon Chew

Neonatal Jaundice

Clinical Presentation

SIGNS AND SYMPTOMS

- Visible yellowing of the skin or sclerae in the newborn infant
  —Correlates with serum bilirubin levels in excess of 5–8 mg/dl
- Jaundice
  —Increasing levels of bilirubin affect skin color from the face downward in term infants
    -Face—bilirubin levels of 6–8 mg/dl
    -Feet—bilirubin levels of 12–15mg/dl
- Physical examination clues to some etiologies
  —Sepsis
    -Lethargy
    -Fever or hypothermia
    -Poor tone
    -Respiratory problems
  —Hemolysis
    -Splenomegaly
  —Birth trauma
    -Cephalohematoma
  —Polycythemia
    -Ruddy complexion

MECHANISM/DESCRIPTION

- All newborns have bilirubin levels above the adult normal level of 1.5 mg/dl during the first week of life, and approximately 50% are jaundiced to the naked eye
  —In the vast majority of newborns, this represents physiologic jaundice and is not pathologic
- Serum bilirubin levels may rise to dangerous levels, require therapy, and the hyperbilirubinemia may be caused by pathologic conditions
- Risk factors for prolonged or elevated physiologic jaundice
  —Prematurity
  —Asian or Native American race
  —Breast feeding
- Further evaluation is recommended for those newborns with jaundice that
  —Occurs in the first 24 hours of life
  —Persists beyond the first week of life
  —Peak bilirubin levels >13–15 mg/dl
  —Jaundice that consists of >10% or 2 mg/dl conjugated bilirubin
- Bilirubin levels over 20mg/dl
  —Associated with kernicterus, a pathologic condition characterized by staining of CNS tissues and neuronal death in infants with hemolytic disease

ETIOLOGY

Unconjugated Hyperbilirubinemia

- Physiologic jaundice
  —Common
  —Rise in bilirubin from 1.5 mg/dl in cord blood to a mean of 6.5 mg/dl on day 3, followed by a gradual decline to normal adult levels by day 10 or 12 of life
  —Unknown etiology
  —Contributing factors include
    -Increased production of bilirubin due to increased red cell mass and decreased red cell life
    -Increased enterohepatic circulation due to absence of gut flora which in the adult reduce conjugated bilirubin to poorly absorbed urobilinogen
    -Diminished binding of bilirubin to albumin and intracellular bilirubin binding protein
    -Patency of the ductus venosus that allows bilirubin to bypass hepatic conjugation
- Hemolytic disease
  —ABO, Rh, or minor blood group incompatibility
- Red cell abnormalities
  —Hereditary spherocytosis
  —G6PD deficiency
- Birth trauma
  —Increased bilirubin load due to resolving cephalohematoma
- Polycythemia
  —Due to maternal-fetal transfusion
  —Fetal-fetal transfusion
  —Infants of diabetic mothers
- Defective hepatic conjugation
  —Crigler-Najjar syndrome (congenital absence of glucuronyl transferase leading to lifelong unconjugated hyperbilirubinemia)
  —Gilbert syndrome (familial partial defect in glucuronyl transferase activity)
  —Lucy-Driscoll syndrome (severe unconjugated hyperbilirubinemia thought to be due to inhibition of infant's glucuronyl transferase by unidentified maternal serum factors)
- Sepsis
- Congenital hypothyroidism
- Breast feeding
  —Breast feeding jaundice—prolongation and exaggeration of physiologic jaundice thought to be due to inadequate delivery of breast milk to the infant in the first week of life
  —Breast milk jaundice—prolonged (up to 8 weeks) elevation of unconjugated bilirubin in some breast-fed infants thought to be due to factors in breast milk that inhibit hepatic conjugation of bilirubin

Conjugated Hyperbilirubinemia

—Due to failure of hepatic excretion of conjugated bilirubin
—Causes include neonatal hepatitis, congenital biliary atresia, extrahepatic biliary obstruction, shock liver from neonatal asphyxia, neonatal hemosiderosis

Pre-Hospital

N/A

Diagnosis

ESSENTIAL WORKUP

- Clinical diagnosis
- Conjugated and unconjugated bilirubin levels

LABORATORY

- Maternal blood type
- Infant blood type
- CBC
- Reticulocyte count
- Microscopic examination of blood smear
- Direct Coombs test on cord blood
  —Routinely done in infants of all type O mothers in most hospitals

IMAGING/SPECIAL TESTS

- Further workup is directed at suspected cause
- Red cell enzyme assay
- Liver function tests
- Sepsis evaluation
- Evaluation for obstructive liver disease for direct hyperbilirubinemia

Treatment

INITIAL STABILIZATION

- 0.9%NS 20 cc/kg, bolus for signs of dehydration

ED TREATMENT

- Indications for phototherapy
  —Bilirubin levels of >15, 18, 20, and 22 mg/dl at 24, 48, 72, and >72 hours of life, respectively
- Indications for exchange transfusions
  —Bilirubin levels >20 mg/dl in the first 24 hours and >30 mg/dl at any other time
- Treat comorbid illness (sepsis, liver dysfunction, polycythemia, hypothyroidism, etc.)
- Reassurance for physiologic jaundice
- Daily bilirubin levels for infants with borderline bilirubin levels until a decline is documented
- Breast feeding and breast milk jaundice
  —Most infants can continue to breast feed
  —2–3-day cessation of breast feeding recommended for those infants with breast milk jaundice and levels approaching the need for therapy

Disposition

ADMISSION CRITERIA

- Infants requiring phototherapy
- Evidence of significant anemia, sepsis, dehydration, or evidence of obstructive liver disease that may require hospitalization for diagnostic evaluation
- ICU admission for infants requiring exchange transfusion

DISCHARGE CRITERIA

- Stable infant with adequate follow-up in the absence of evidence of serious disease

Miscellaneous

ICD9: 774.6

CORE CONTENT CODE: 13.4.3

SUGGESTED READINGS

Gartner LM. Neonatal jaundice. Pediatr Rev 1994;15:422–432.

Martinez JC. Hyperbilirubinemia in the breast-fed newborn: A controlled trial of four interventions. Pediatrics 1993;91:470–473.

Author: David Magilner

Neonatal Sepsis

Clinical Presentation

SIGNS AND SYMPTOMS

- Parental concerns
  - —"Just not acting right"
  - —Feeding poorly
  - —Decreased number of wet diapers or just more sleepy than usual
  - —Irritable
  - —Vomiting
- Toxic-appearing infant
- Fever or hypothermia
- Infants are irritable and difficult to console
- Obtundation with episodes of apnea and bradycardia
- Tachypnea
- Tachycardic
- Cool, mottled to pale, ashen, or frankly cyanotic skin
- Pulses may be difficult to palpate
- Prolonged capillary refill time
- Abdominal distention
- Jaundice
- Bruising or prolonged bleeding

MECHANISM/DESCRIPTION

- Life-threatening infection of the newborn
- Early onset: the first few days after birth
- Late onset: from the second to fourth weeks of life
- Less commonly occurring as late as two months of age
- Overwhelming bacterial, or, in some instances, viral or fungal infection
- Commonly caused by organisms present in the maternal perineal flora
- Sepsis syndrome in the neonate
  - —Septic shock
  - —Hypoglycemia
  - —Seizures
  - —Disseminated intravascular coagulation
  - —If untreated, cardiovascular collapse and death
- Occurs in 3–5 newborns per 1000 live births
- Risk factors
  - —Prematurity
  - —Prolonged rupture of membranes
  - —Maternal history of recent fever
  - —Chorioamnionitis
  - —Urinary tract infection
  - —Foul lochia
  - —Intrapartum asphyxia
  - —Intravascular catheters
  - —Uterine tenderness
  - —Fetal tachycardia (>180 beats/minute)
  - —Male sex
  - —Developmental or congenital immune defects
  - —Galactosemia
  - —Administration of intramuscular iron
  - —Congenital anomalies
  - —Omphalitis
  - —Second twin of an infected twin

ETIOLOGY

- Bacterial
  - —Group B or D streptococcus
  - —*Escherichia coli*
  - —*Listeria monocytogenes*
  - —*Haemophilus* sp
  - —*Staphylococcus aureus*
- Viral
  - —Enterovirus
  - —Herpes simplex is common viral etiology
- Low birth weight and chronically hospitalized infants
  - —Candida species
  - —Coagulase-negative staphylococci

Pre-Hospital

CAUTIONS

- Ventilatory support if obtunded or apneic
- Intravenous access

Diagnosis

ESSENTIAL WORKUP

- Neutrophilia and neutropenia are needed to determine treatment in borderline cases
- Determine a source for the infection
- Identify metabolic abnormalities

LABORATORY

- Bedside glucose determination
- Complete blood count
  - —Severe neutropenia or neutrophilia
  - —Immature band forms
  - —Toxic granulations
  - —Thrombocytopenia
- Urinalysis
- Cultures as soon as the diagnosis is entertained
  - —Blood
  - —Urine
  - —Stool
  - —CSF
- Lumbar puncture (if patient condition allows)
  - —May be delayed 6–12 hours in unstable patients
  - —Cell count
  - —Glucose
  - —Protein
  - —Culture
- Serum glucose needed to exclude hypoglycemia
- Arterial blood gas
  - —Metabolic acidosis is common
- Electrolytes and calcium
  - —Hyponatremia
  - —Hypocalcemia
- DIC panel
  - —Coagulopathy is a late complication
  - —Monitor PT, PTT, and fibrinogen-split products

IMAGING/SPECIAL TESTS

- Chest radiograph to rule out pneumonia

DIFFERENTIAL DIAGNOSIS

- Heart disease
  - —Hypoplastic left heart syndrome
  - —Myocarditis
- Congenital adrenal hyperplasia
- Metabolic disorders
  - —Hypoglycemia
  - —Adrenal insufficiency
  - —Organic acidoses
  - —Urea cycle disorder
  - —Salicylate toxicity
- Intussusception
- Child abuse
- Intracranial hemorrhage
- Neonatal jaundice
- Perinatal asphyxia
- Hematologic emergencies
  - —Neonatal purpura fulminans
  - —Severe anemia
  - —Methemoglobinemia
  - —Malignancies

Treatment

INITIAL STABILIZATION

- Airway management indicated if obtundation or apneic spells
- Intravenous access
- If evidence of shock, administer fluids and pressors as needed

ED TREATMENT

- Implement treatment for neonatal sepsis if any of the following are present
  - —Overt signs and symptoms
  - —Any symptoms with an abnormal white count
  - —Premature delivery with any symptoms
- Administer antibiotics
  - —Ampicillin and gentamycin
  - —Add oxacillin if the patient's condition continues to deteriorate
  - —Cefotaxime may be substituted for gentamycin
- Colloid or blood for shock (10 cc/kg over 2 hours)

MEDICATIONS

- Ampicillin: 100 mg/kg/day q 12 hrs IV/IM
- Cefotaxime: 100 mg/kg/day q 12 hrs IV/IM
- Gentamycin: 5 mg/kg/day q 12 hrs IV/IM; <7 days of age: 7.5 mg/kg/day q 8 hrs IV/IM
- Oxacillin: 75 mg/kg/day q 12 hrs IV/IM

Disposition

ADMISSION CRITERIA

- All patients with suspected sepsis are admitted to the hospital for supportive care, IV antibiotic therapy, and close monitoring

DISCHARGE CRITERIA

N/A

Miscellaneous

ICD9: 771; 790.7

CORE CONTENT CODE: 13.16.3

SUGGESTED READINGS

Anderson MR, Blumer JL. Advances in the therapy for sepsis in children. Ped Clin North Am 1997;44:179–205.

Gotoff SP. Neonatal sepsis and meningitis. In: Nelson VE, Behrman RE, Kliegman RM, Arvin AM, eds. Nelson's textbook of pediatrics. 15th ed. Philadelphia: W.B. Saunders, 1996:528–37.

Jafari HS, McCracken GH. Sepsis and septic shock: A review for clinicians. Pediatr Infect Dis J 1992;1:739–48.

Selbst SM. Septic-appearing infant. In: Fleisher GR, Ludwig S, eds. Textbook of pediatric emergency medicine. 3rd ed. Baltimore: Williams & Wilkins, 1993:456–63.

Vesikari T, Janas M, Gronroos P, et al. Neonatal septicemia. Arch Dis Child 1985;60:542–46.

Author: Mark Roback

Nephritic Syndrome

See Glomerulonephritis chapter for glomerulonephritis due to primary renal disease and systemic diseases

Clinical Presentation

SIGNS AND SYMPTOMS

- Hematuria
  - —Abrupt onset with red blood cell casts
  - —Gross hematuria in 30–40%
- Hypertension
- Edema
  - —Periorbital edema
  - —Generalized edema more common in infants
- Azotemia
- Infection source: upper respiratory tract or skin in post streptococcal glomerulonephritis (PSGN)
- Congestive heart failure
  - —40% occurrence in patients over 60 years old
  - —Rare in children
- Renal failure in elderly
- Arthritis, arthralgias, and various skin rashes: seen occasionally in PSGN
- Nonspecific manifestations
  - —Malaise
  - —Weakness
  - —Anorexia
  - —Nausea/vomiting

MECHANISM/DESCRIPTION

- Acute glomerulonephritis (AGN) associated with
  - —Abrupt onset of hematuria with red blood cell casts
  - —Mild proteinuria
  - —Edema, hypertension, azotemia
- Exact mechanism of AGN unclear
  - —Combination of autoimmune reactivity to specific antigens at renal glomeruli
- Diffuse inflammatory changes occur in the glomeruli

ETIOLOGY

Infectious Causes of Acute Nephritic Syndrome

Poststreptococcal Glomerulonephritis

- Occurs between the ages of 2–12 years old
- Preceded by infection: upper respiratory tract (pharynx) > cutaneous infections > all other sources
- Latent period between infection and onset of nephritis
  - —6–10 days in pharyngeal infection
  - —2 weeks in cutaneous infection
- Prognosis
  - —Evidence of nephrosis indicates a more serious long-term prognosis
  - —End-stage renal disease occurs <5%
  - —Rapidly progressive glomerulonephritis (RPGN) occurs <1%
  - —Epidemic outbreaks associated with good prognosis
  - —Sporadic cases associated with progression of renal disease in 50%
- Most cases resolve spontaneously
  - —Signs and symptoms typically resolve 1 week after onset of nephritis
  - —Urine abnormalities resolve over months

Hepatitis Virus-Related Glomerular Disease

- Hepatitis carrier state associated mainly with membranous GN in children, ages 2–12
- Hypertension present in 25% of children, 45% in adults
- Two-thirds of children remit 3 years after diagnosis.
- Adults with hepatitis tend to have progressive course leading to eventual renal failure.

Human Immunodeficiency Virus-Associated Nephropathy (HIV-AN)

- Main presentation
  - —Proteinuria (nephrotic range) with varying degrees of renal insufficiency
  - —No hematuria present
  - —No hypertension present
- >50% of HIV-AN are asymptomatic carriers of HIV
- Focal segmental glomerulosclerosis most common nephropathy
- Acute edema and renal failure can occur in patients without previous renal disease
- Despite dialysis, endstage renal failure occurs in 4–6 months resulting in death within 1 year in most patients

Infectious Endocarditis (IE)

- Gross or microscopic hematuria, mild proteinuria, and azotemia
- Risk groups: parenteral drug abusers and patients with prosthetic valves
- Antibiotic treatment of IE results in resolution of GN

Visceral Infections

- Involving pulmonary, intra-abdominal, cutaneous or infected vascular prosthesis, leading to GN
- Typically severe infection present for months
- Syphilis, leprosy, schistosomiasis, and quartan malaria can also cause GN

Pre-Hospital

N/A

Diagnosis

ESSENTIAL WORKUP

- Urinalysis to detect
  - —Hematuria, proteinuria, and red blood cell casts
  - —Red blood cell casts diagnostic of an active glomerular inflammation

LABORATORY

- CBC for
  - —Anemia (seen in more chronic cases of GN or other systemic disease)
  - —Acute leukocytosis (indicates infectious process)
- Electrolytes, BUN, Cr, glucose
  - —Baseline for renal function
  - —Check for hyperkalemia
- Serum albumin
  - —Indicator of severity of proteinuria
- Cultures
  - —Throat, skin, urine, blood
  - —As clinically suspected for infection source

IMAGING/SPECIAL TESTS

- KUB film—normal or enlarged kidneys
- CXR: normal or slightly enlarged heart +/− pulmonary edema
- Renal biopsy
  - —Generally not done since acute PSGN resolves completely in less than 2 weeks.
  - —Recommended if atypical features of PSGN, persistent abnormal complement levels, persistent hypertension, and proteinuria >3 g/day

Special Diagnostic Tests

- Serum complement level (C3, CH_{50}): decreased in IE, shunt nephritis and PSGN
- Streptococcal exoenzymes
  - —Antistreptolysin (ASO), antistreptokinase (ASK), antideoxyribonuclease B (ADNase B), Antinicotinyl adenine dinucleotidase (ANADase), and antihyaluronidase (AH)
  - —ASO more reactive in pharyngeal infections
  - —ADNase B, ANADase, and AH more reactive in cutaneous infections
  - —ASK elevated in recent hemolytic streptococcus infections
- 24-hour urine protein collection
  - —Proteinuria present initially in 5% of children, 20% adults with PSGN

DIFFERENTIAL DIAGNOSIS

(See chapter: Glomerulonephritis, for further information on types of GN)

- Renal
  —Primary glomerular disease
- Systemic
  —Goodpasture's syndrome
  —Vasculitis
  —Henoch Schönlein purpura
- Other (rare): hemolytic uremic syndrome, thrombotic thrombocytopenic purpura, acute hypersensitivity interstitial nephritis, Guillain-Barré, DPT vaccine, serum sickness

Treatment

INITIAL STABILIZATION

- ABCs

ED TREATMENT

- Antibiotics for streptococcal infection
  —Penicillin (erythromycin if penicillin allergic)
  —Prophylactic antibiotics to siblings of PSGN patients
- Restriction of salt and water intake
- Administer loop diuretics (furosemide)
- Treat pulmonary edema
  —Oxygen
  —Morphine
  —Loop diuretics
  —Digitalis not effective
- Lower blood pressure for hypertensive emergency
  —Nitroprusside
  —Diazoxide
- Dialysis for
  —Severe hyperkalemia
  —Fluid overload
  —Uremia

MEDICATIONS

- Erythromycin: 250 mg (peds: 30–50 mg/kg/24hrs) po q 6 hrs for 7–10 days
- Furosemide: 20–100 mg (peds: 1 mg/kg/dose)
- Penicillin
  —Benzathine penicillin: 1.2 million units (peds: 0.6 million units for <30 kg) IM
  —Penicillin: 2 million units po q 6 hrs for 7–10 days
- Diazoxide: 1–3 mg/kg IV, max 150 mg, repeat q 15 min
- Nitroprusside: 0.5–10 μg/kg/min IV
- Morphine sulfate: 2–4 mg (peds: 0.1 mg/kg/dose; max 15 mg/dose) IV q 5 min

Disposition

ADMISSION CRITERIA

- Evidence of infectious cause for GN
- Oliguria, anuria
- Uremia
- Acute renal failure
- Hyperkalemia
- Hypertension
- Congestive heart failure

DISCHARGE CRITERIA

- Mild cases of clinical nephritis in healthy patients with
  —No comorbid illness
  —Strict supervision/monitoring of symptoms, diet, urine output, and medication
  —Close follow-up

Miscellaneous

ICD9: 583.9

CORE CONTENT CODE: 15.3.1

SUGGESTED READINGS

Kirpal SC, Sakhuja V. Glomerulonephritis due to other infections. In: Massry SG, Glassock RJ, eds. Textbook of nephrology. Chap. 41. 3rd ed. Baltimore: Williams & Wilkins, 1995:703–710.

Korbet SM, Schwartz MM. Human immunodeficiency virus infection and nephrotic syndrome. Am J Kidney Dis 1992;20:97–103.

Montseny J, Meyrier A, Kleinknecht D, Callard P. The current spectrum of infectious glomerulonephritis: Experience with 76 patients and review of the literature. Medicine. 1995;74(2):63–73.

Rodriguez-Iturbe B. Poststreptococcal glomerulonephritis. In: Massry SG, Glassock RJ, eds. Textbook of nephrology. Chap. 41. 3rd ed. Baltimore: Williams & Wilkins, 1995:698–703.

Author: Shirley Lee

Nephrotic Syndrome

Clinical Presentation

SIGNS AND SYMPTOMS

- Proteinuria
- Edema
  - —Mild pitting edema to generalized anasarca with ascites
- Hyperlipidemia
- Lipiduria (fatty casts and oval fat bodies in urine)
- Postural hypotension/syncope/shock
- Hypertension
- Hematuria
  - —Microscopic or gross hematuria (secondary to renal vein thrombosis)
  - —Flank pain (rare)
- Tachypnea, tachycardia, +/− hypotension
  - —Acute onset: suggests pulmonary embolus (secondary to renal or deep vein thrombosis due to hypercoagulable state in nephrotic disease)
  - —Chronic or exertional tachypnea due to
    - -Pulmonary edema (due to severe hypoalbuminemia)
    - -Pleural effusions
    - -Increased respiratory effort due to diaphragm motion restriction secondary to ascites
- Bone fractures (due to underlying osteomalacic bone disease)

MECHANISM/DESCRIPTION

Definition

- Proteinuria >3.5 g/day
- Serum albumin <3.0 g/dl
- Peripheral edema
- Hyperlipidemia (fasting cholesterol >200 mg/dl)
- Glomerular basement
  - —Membrane altered by
    - -Immune complexes
    - -Nephrotoxic antibodies
    - -Nonimmune mechanisms
  - —Resulting in
    - -Increased filtration and excretion of albumin and large proteins into Bowman's capsule

Pathophysiology

- Edema due to hypoalbuminemia
- Hyperlipidemia due to hepatic lipoprotein synthesis stimulated by decreased plasma oncotic pressure
- Postural hypotension, syncope, and shock due to severe hypoalbuminemia with plasma volume reduction
- Hypertension, in association with abnormal urinalysis or decrease renal function, indicates
  - —GN
  - —Diabetes mellitus
  - —Connective tissue disease

ETIOLOGY

- Primary pathologies (percentage of occurrence in adults)
  - —Minimal change disease: 22% (75% primary nephrotic disease in children)
  - —Membranous glomerulonephritis: 20%
  - —Focal segmental glomerulosclerosis: 12%
  - —Membranoproliferative glomerulonephritis: 10%
  - —Miscellaneous proliferative glomerulonephropathies: 16%
- Secondary pathologies
  - —Accounts for 20% of causes of nephrotic syndrome
  - —History usually suggestive for coexisting disease
  - —Diseases present initially as a nephritic process, with progression to nephrotic syndrome

Pre-Hospital

N/A

Diagnosis

ESSENTIAL WORKUP

- Urinalysis
  - —Dipstick protein-positive
    - -Urine specific gravity >1.025 lowers the diagnostic significance of proteinuria
  - —Microscopic analysis for urinary casts and the presence of cellular elements
    - -Oval fat bodies
    - -Free lipid droplets

LABORATORY

- CBC
  - —Anemia common in renal disease and in other diseases that cause proteinuria
  - —Leukocytosis: infection
  - —Leukopenia: neoplastic disease
- Serum albumin: <3 g/dl
- Serum total protein: <6 g/dl
- Creatinine, BUN: elevated in renal insufficiency
- Lipid profile: elevated total cholesterol, LDL, and VLDL
- Serum calcium: lowered

IMAGING/SPECIAL TESTS

- Renal ultrasound
  - —Not helpful
  - —Utilized in suspected secondary causes of nephrotic syndrome
- Renal biopsy
  - —Definitive test for patients who do not respond to a short course of corticosteroids
  - —Helpful in SLE (several forms of nephritis—help specify target therapy)
  - —Not done with long-standing diabetes, uncontrolled hypertension, bleeding disorders, or shrunken kidneys

Specific Lab Tests

- Used to identify systemic disorders
- See chapter: Glomerulonephritis, for review of laboratory tests

DIFFERENTIAL DIAGNOSIS

Proteinuria Due to Other Causes

- Renal Parenchymal disease
  - —Chronic renal disease
  - —Mechanical nephropathy (obstruction/reflux)
  - —Orthostatic proteinuria
  - —Acute pyelonephritis
  - —Sickle cell disease
- Other causes
  - —Congestive heart failure
  - —Essential hypertension
  - —Acute febrile illness
  - —Pregnancy
  - —Severe obesity

Treatment

INITIAL STABILIZATION

- ABCs
  - —Supplemental oxygen if respiratory distress
  - —IV fluids
    - -Slow rehydration for decreased blood pressure or orthostatic hypotension due to decreased intravascular volume
    - -Active rehydration in the presence of severe hypotension, shock

ED TREATMENT

- Control edema
  - —Loop diuretic (furosemide): titrate dose until response seen
  - —Supplement diuresis with low-dose metolazone
  - —Goal: slow diuresis
    - -Aggressive diuresis can precipitate acute renal failure due to intravascular volume depletion, prerenal azotemia, and even renal ischemia.
  - —No improvement in potentiating furosemide diuresis with intravenous albumin

Post-ED Treatment

- Glucocorticosteroids: mainstay of treatment for primary nephrotic syndrome
- Protein restriction
  - —0.8 g/kg daily of ideal body weight
  - —Protein loading increases urinary protein excretion and worsens hypoalbuminemia
- Cholesterol lowering agents/dietary manipulation (bile acid resin, lovastatin)
- ACE inhibitor/calcium channel blocker: reduces proteinuria in diabetic nephropathy only
- Cytotoxic agents/cyclosporine: second line in glomerulonephritis treatment, especially in recurrent remissions despite adequate steroid trials
- Recombinant erythropoietin: useful in erythropoietin deficient anemias due to nephrotic syndrome

MEDICATIONS

- Furosemide: 20–100 mg (peds: 1 mg/kg/dose; max 6 mg/kg) IV; max: 2 mg/kg/day
- Metolazone (zaroxolyn): 5–20 mg/day

Disposition

ADMISSION CRITERIA

- Moderate to severe heart failure, ascites, respiratory compromise
- Signs of comorbid illness, e.g., undiagnosed malignancy, poorly controlled diabetes, immunocompromised host
- Acute renal failure
- Evidence of thromboembolic event

DISCHARGE CRITERIA

- Patients with no comorbid disease who present with a history and physical compatibility with primary glomerulonephritis, normal vital signs, and normal blood work
- Close follow-up with a nephrologist or general internist for further evaluation and treatment mandatory

Miscellaneous

ICD9: 581.9

CORE CONTENT CODE: 15.3.2

SUGGESTED READINGS

Carome MA, Moore J. Nephrotic syndrome in adults: A diagnostic and management challenge. Postgrad Med 1992;2:209–220.

Glassock RJ, Brenner BM. The major glomerulopathies. In: Wilson et al., eds. Harrison's principles of internal medicine. Chaps. 240, 241. 13th ed. McGraw Hill, New York, NY 1995:1295–1313.

Glassock RJ, Cohen AH. The primary glomerulopathies. Dis Mon 1996;42(6):329–383.

Howard AD, et al. Routine serologic tests in the differential diagnosis of the adult nephrotic syndrome. Am J Kidney Dis 1990;15:24–30.

Author: Shirley Lee

Neuroleptic Malignant Syndrome

Clinical Presentation

SIGNS AND SYMPTOMS

- Life-threatening condition
- Hallmarks of the disease
  - —Hyperthermia (temperature may be as high as 106–107°F, 41°C)
  - —Altered level of consciousness
  - —Skeletal muscle rigidity, "lead pipe rigidity"
  - —Autonomic instability (tachycardia, labile blood pressure)

MECHANISM/DESCRIPTION

- May develop anytime during therapy with neuroleptics—from a few days to many years after initiating treatment
- Muscular rigidity may result from dopamine antagonism in the nigrostriatal pathway and hyperthermia due to blockage of hypothalamic thermoregulation

ETIOLOGY

- Rare complication of treatment with neuroleptic drugs such as phenothiazines, butyrophenones, and thiothixene
- Occurs in approximately 1.0% of patients treated with neuroleptics (especially haloperidol)
- Has been associated with withdrawal from dopamine agonists in Parkinson's disease

Pre-Hospital

CAUTIONS

- Ventilation may be difficult due to chest wall rigidity
- Cool the patient, and treat seizures if they occur
- Check fingerstick glucose
- Paralysis with a nondepolarizing neuromuscular blocker is preferable to succinylcholine

Diagnosis

ESSENTIAL WORKUP

- An accurate history (especially current medications) and physical exam confirm the diagnosis
- CPK, WBC determination, and LFTs

LABORATORY

- Electrolytes, glucose, BUN, creatinine, PT/PTT, urine (for myoglobin)
- Lumbar puncture is usually normal

IMAGING/SPECIAL TESTS

- CT scan, EEG if the cause of altered level of consciousness is unclear

DIFFERENTIAL DIAGNOSIS

- Meningitis, encephalitis, sepsis
- Malignant hyperthermia, severe dystonic reaction
- Tetanus
- Heat stroke
- Strychnine poisoning
- Vascular CNS event
- Fatal catatonia
- Thyrotoxicosis
- Rabies
- Central anticholinergic toxicity

Treatment

INITIAL STABILIZATION

- ABCs, IV, O_2, cardiac monitor
- Immediate intravenous benzodiazepines (diazepam, lorazepam), may require repeated large doses
- If symptoms are not controlled within a few minutes *rapid sequence intubation* and *neuromuscular blockade* is necessary
  - —Nondepolarizing neuromuscular blockers (vecuronium, rocuronium, pancuronium) are preferable to succinylcholine
- Measure to control hyperthermia
  - —Ice packs, mist and fan, cooling blankets, etc.
- Aggressive IV fluid therapy with lactated ringers or normal saline

ED TREATMENT

- Relief of muscle rigidity
  - —Bromocriptine is a dopamine agonist that may play a role in longer term management
  - —Dantrolene is a direct skeletal muscle relaxant that may play a role in longer term management
  - —Neither bromocriptine or dantrolene have rapid onset and have not been demonstrated to alter outcome
- Discontinue neuroleptics
- Recognize complications (rhabdomyolysis, respiratory failure, acute renal failure), mortality can be as high as 20%

MEDICATIONS

- Bromocriptine: adult: 20–30 mg/day po; peds: dose not established
- Dantrolene: adult/peds: 1–2.5 mg/kg IV
- Diazepam: adult: 5–10 mg IV; peds: 0.2–0.5 mg/kg/dose (titrate to effect)
- Lorazepam: adult: 2–4 mg IV; peds: safety not established (titrate to effect)
- Pancuronium: adult/peds: 0.1–0.15 mg/kg
- Rocuronium: adult/peds: 0.6 mg/kg
- Vecuronium: adult/peds: 0.1–0.3 mg/kg

Disposition

ADMISSION CRITERIA

- All patients should be admitted to an ICU

DISCHARGE CRITERIA

- No patients with a diagnosis of NMS should be discharged

Miscellaneous

ICD9: 333.92

CORE CONTENT CODE: 22.2.6.3

SUGGESTED READINGS

Caroff SN, Mann SC. Neuroleptic malignant syndrome. Med Clin North Am 1993;77(1):185–202.

Ebadi M, Srinivasan SK. Pathogenesis, prevention, and treatment of neuroleptic-induced movement disorders. Pharmacol Rev 1995;47(4):575–604.

Heiman-Patterson TD. Neuroleptic malignant syndrome and malignant hyperthermia. Important issues for the medical consultant. Med Clin North Am 1993;77(2):477–492.

Authors: George Kondylis; Gary Johnson

Noncardiogenic Pulmonary Edema

Clinical Presentation

- Noncardiogenic pulmonary edema (NCPE) was first described by William Osler in 1889 in a patient "poisoned" by morphine. Approximately 250,000 cases occur each year in the United States

SIGNS AND SYMPTOMS

- Tachycardia is characteristically seen secondary to decreasing PO_2 levels
- Scattered rhonchi and rales
- Dyspnea, tachypnea, and cyanosis may appear
- Pink, frothy sputum
- The stigmata of left- and right-sided heart failure will *not* be found

MECHANISM/DESCRIPTION

- Functional disruption of the capillary-alveolar membrane from a noncardiac source
- Diffuse injury to either the alveolar epithelium or to the vascular endothelium
- Pulmonary parenchymal changes mimic CHF
  - —Cephalad redistribution of blood flow, pulmonary effusions, and cardiomegaly do *not* develop
- Typically, onset of this edema is within 1–2 hours of noxious insult

ETIOLOGY

- Cause of capillary leak or alveolar membrane damage is uncertain
- Proposed mechanisms include hypoxia, immunologic effects, or direct toxic effects
- Major causes
  - —Smoke inhalation
  - —Salicylate intoxication
  - —Toxic gas inhalation
  - —Transfusion reaction
  - —Near drowning
  - —DIC
  - —High-altitude pulmonary edema (HAPE)
  - —Radiation pneumonitis
  - —Narcotic abuse
  - —Uremia
  - —Cardiopulmonary bypass
  - —Major trauma
  - —Aspiration
  - —Bacterial pneumonia

Pre-Hospital

- Patent airway and adequate oxygenation are main concerns
- Patients will not typically respond to usual measures to treat CHF

Diagnosis

ESSENTIAL WORKUP

- Chest x-ray
- Radiologic findings may include
  - —Classic butterfly pattern of pulmonary edema
  - —Unilateral patchy infiltrates resembling pneumonia
  - —Lack of cardiomegaly
- Arterial blood gas

LABORATORY

- Electrolytes, BUN, creatinine
- Electrocardiogram

IMAGING/SPECIAL TESTS

- Echocardiogram may help identify normal cardiac function and ejection fraction

DIFFERENTIAL DIAGNOSIS

- Cardiogenic pulmonary edema
- COPD exacerbation
- Pulmonary embolus
- Restrictive lung disease

Treatment

INITIAL STABILIZATION

- Supplemental oxygen (high flow oxygen)
- Intravenous catheter
- Continuous cardiac monitor
- Continuous pulse oximetry

ED TREATMENT

- The treatment of NCPE is supportive
- NCPE associated with drug overdose usually responds to high flow O_2
- Diuretics are *not* used
- Removal of trigger that may have caused NCPE
  —Noxious gas
  —Having patient descend from elevation in cases of HAPE
- Noninvasive ventilatory support (Bi-PAP, CPAP) may be used if immediately available
  —Measure blood gases frequently
  —If unable to provide adequate oxygenation or ventilation, intubation is required
  —Useful in NCPE caused by drug overdose
- Endotracheal intubation is often necessary
  —Positive end-expiratory pressure (PEEP) of 5–10 cm H_2O
    -NCPE of a neurogenic etiology has a worsened prognosis when PEEP is employed
  —Improved oxygenation
  —Decrease work of breathing
  —To reduce the likelihood of atelectasis, tidal volumes should be on order of 12–15 ml/kg
  —Initially place on 100% O_2
    -Measure PO_2 and decrease FIO_2 accordingly
- Steroids and cyclooxygenase inhibitors have not been proven effective

Disposition

ADMISSION CRITERIA

- All symptomatic patients should be admitted to the intensive care unit
  —Symptoms may worsen at any point for up to three days after noxious insult

DISCHARGE CRITERIA

- Asymptomatic patients (especially narcotic overdose, high-altitude pulmonary edema or aspiration)
  —Observe in ED for 6–12 hours and then discharge with close follow up scheduled if no evidence of pulmonary edema is present and adequate oxygenation is demonstrated

Miscellaneous

ICD9: 518.4

CORE CONTENT CODE 16.5

SUGGESTED READINGS

Brillman JC, Eliastam M. Adult respiratory distress syndrome. In: Harwood-Nuss A, Linden C, Luten R, Sternbach G, Wolfson A, eds. The clinical practice of emergency medicine. Philadelphia: JB Lippincott, 1991.

Macias DJ, Brillman JC. Adult respiratory distress syndrome. In: Harwood-Nuss A, Linden C, Luten R, Sternbach G, Wolfson A, eds. The clinical practice of emergency medicine. 2nd Edition. Philadelphia: JB Lippincott 1996. pp 640–643.

Author: David Jerrard

Nonsteroidal Anti-inflammatory Drugs, Poisoning

Clinical Presentation

SIGNS AND SYMPTOMS

Gastrointestinal

- Nausea
- Vomiting
- Epigastric pain

CNS

- Drowsiness
- Dizziness
- Lethargy
- Seizures

Cardiovascular

- Hypotension
- Tachycardia

Pulmonary

- Eosinophilic pneumonia
- Apnea
- Hyperventilation

Renal

- Acute renal failure
- Acute tubular necrosis
- Acute interstitial nephritis

Liver

- Hepatocellular injury
- Cholestatic jaundice

Metabolic

- Mild, short lived metabolic acidosis

MECHANISM/DESCRIPTION

- Inhibit cyclooxygenase that blocks the conversion of arachidonic acid to prostaglandin
- Typically, ingestion of a nonsteroidal anti-inflammatory drug (NSAID) is benign
- Fatalities reported with large ingestions
- Greater potential for toxicity with underlying CHF or renal failure
  —NSAIDs cause sodium and water retention and decrease renal blood flow

PEDIATRIC CONSIDERATIONS

- Piroxicam, naproxen, ketoprofen and mefenamic acid have caused seizures in children

Pre-Hospital

CAUTIONS

- Collect prescription bottles/medications for identification in ED

Diagnosis

ESSENTIAL WORKUP

- Generally, NSAID ingestion results only in mild toxicity
- Exact identification of drug helpful
  —Subtle toxicologic differences amongst the NSAIDs

LABORATORY

- Electrolytes, BUN/Cr, glucose
  —Baseline renal function
  —Check for metabolic acidosis
- CBC
- ABG for large overdoses
- PT/PTT
- Urinalysis
  —False-positive bilirubin/ketone dipstick with etodolac ingestion
- NSAID difficult to detect on toxicology screens
- Plasma ibuprofen levels
  —Minimal utility
  —Nomogram for ibuprofen has a poor predictive value

DIFFERENTIAL DIAGNOSIS

- Agents causing metabolic acidosis, altered mental status, and GI irritation
  —Salicylates
  —INH
  —Ethylene glycol
  —Methanol
  —Isopropanol

Treatment

INITIAL STABILIZATION

- ABCs
- Naloxone, thiamine, dextrose (or Accucheck) for altered mental status

ED TREATMENT

- Supportive care and gastrointestinal decontamination
- Gastric lavage
  - —If the patient presents within 1 hour post ingestion with an intact gag reflex
  - —If no gag reflex is present: protected airway with a cuffed endotracheal tube prior to lavage
- Avoid syrup of ipecac since NSAIDs may cause CNS depression and seizures in the overdose setting
- Administer activated charcoal and sorbitol early (after lavage completion)
- Extracorporeal methods to enhance elimination are not beneficial due to high degree of plasma protein binding

MEDICATIONS

- Activated charcoal slurry: 1–2 g/kg up to 90 g po
- Dextrose: D50W 1 amp (50 ml or 25 g) (peds: D25W 2–4 ml/kg) IV
- Naloxone (narcan): 2 mg (peds: 0.1 mg/kg) IV or IM initial dose
- Sorbitol: 1–2 g/kg to a max of 100 g (peds: >1 year old: 1–1.5 g/kg as a 35% solution to a max of 50 g) po mixed in the activated charcoal slurry only use for first dose
- Thiamine (vitamin B_1): 100 mg (peds: 50 mg) IV or IM

Disposition

ADMISSION CRITERIA

- Protracted vomiting, hematemesis
- CNS depression, seizure activity
- Metabolic acidosis
- CHF, hypotension, hypertension
- Renal failure

DISCHARGE CRITERIA

- Nontoxic ingestion in a patient who is asymptomatic 6–8 hours postingestion

Miscellaneous

ICD9: 965.6

CORE CONTENT CODE: 17.2.38

SUGGESTED READINGS

Ellenhorn MJ, Schonwald S, Ordog G, Wasserberger J. Nonsteroidal antiinflamatory drugs. In: Ellenhorn MJ, ed. Ellenhorn's medical toxicology. 2d ed. Baltimore: Williams & Wilkins, 1997:196–206.

Le HT, Bosse GM, Tsai YY. Ibuprofen overdose complicated by renal failure, adult respiratory distress syndrome, and metabolic acidosis. Clin Toxicol 1994; 32:315–320.

Smolinske SC, Hall AH, Vandenburg SA, et al. Toxic effects of nonsteroidal anti-inflammatory drugs in overdose. Drug Saf 1990;5:252.

Zuckerman GB, Uy CC. Shock, metabolic acidosis, and coma following ibuprofen overdose in a child. Ann Pharmacother 1995;29:869–871.

Author: Michele Kanter

Nursemaid's Elbow

Clinical Presentation

SIGNS AND SYMPTOMS

- Nonuse of the arm
- Elbow kept in a flexed position while maintaining the forearm close to the trunk
- Pain on flexion of the elbow
- Pain with wrist supination or pronation
- Point tenderness usually not elicited
- Minimal to no swelling

MECHANISM/DESCRIPTION

- Most common injury of the upper extremity in children <5 years of age
  —History of a sharp pull on a partially pronated forearm
  —History of a fall in which the forearm or elbow is pinned between the ground and the child's torso
- Subluxation of the radial head
  —Symptom-complex is a result of a tear or upward sliding of the mobile annular ligament
  —Radial head slips through this aperture and the ligament, capsule, or synovium becomes trapped between the radial head and the capitellum

Pre-Hospital

CAUTIONS

- Place ice on the injured elbow to alleviate some of the pain immediately following injury and to prevent swelling
- Immobilize in a sling or splint to facilitate transport and prevent further injury
- Assess distal neurovascular status

Diagnosis

ESSENTIAL WORKUP

- Clinical diagnosis
  —Usually no doubt as to the diagnosis when the mechanism of injury, arm positioning, and examination are classic
- Radiographs
  —No radiographic abnormalities associated with this injury
  —Not routinely indicated
  —Obtained if
    -Point tenderness
    -Soft tissue swelling
    -Deformity
    -Ecchymosis of the elbow
    -Reduction techniques unsuccessful

LABORATORY

N/A

DIFFERENTIAL DIAGNOSIS

- Humeral condyle fracture
- Intercondylar fracture
- Radial head fracture

Treatment

INITIAL STABILIZATION

- Assess distal motor, sensory, and vascular function

ED TREATMENT

- Reduction technique
  - —Place thumb over the child's radial head
  - —Grasp child's hand
  - —Begin with the elbow in extension and the forearm in pronation
  - —Perform following three maneuvers swiftly
    - -Downward pressure of the radial head by the physician's thumb
    - -Passive full *supination* of the forearm
    - -Passive full *flexion* of the elbow
  - —Occurrence of a palpable click is common, although not necessary, to have achieved a successful reduction
  - —Child may cry out in pain during the initial reduction but is frequently pain-free and using arm soon thereafter
- Second reduction attempt if the child continues to not use arm 15–20 minutes after a reduction attempt
- Radiographic studies indicated if the second reduction attempt unsuccessful
- Perform postreduction neurovascular assessment
- Patient instructions
  - —Place arm in a sling if not completely functional at discharge
  - —Inform parents not to pull or lift the child up by the hand, wrist, or forearm
  - —Warn family of the increased incidence of recurrence until the child reaches 5–6 years of age
  - —Spontaneous recurrent radial head subluxation may occur in a small group of patients

MEDICATIONS

- Acetaminophen: 15 mg/kg po q 4 hrs

Disposition

ADMISSION CRITERIA

- None

DISCHARGE CRITERIA

- Regain full, unrestricted use of the arm
- Orthopedic followup for any injury of the elbow with a radiologic abnormality

Miscellaneous

ICD9: 832.0

CORE CONTENT CODE: 18.4.12.2.2.1

SUGGESTED READINGS

Christoph R. Musculoskeletal disorders in children. In: Tintinalli JE, et al., eds. Emergency medicine: a comprehensive study guide. 4th ed. New York: McGraw Hill, 1996:673–685.

Salter R, Zaltz C. Anatomic investigations of the mechanism of injury and pathologic anatomy of "pulled elbow" in young children. Clin Orthop 1971;77:141.

Schunk J. Radial head subluxation: epidemiology and treatment of 87 episodes. Ann Emerg Med 1990;19:1019–1023.

Authors: William Sabina, Daniel L. Savitt

Oculomotor Nerve Palsy

Clinical Presentation

SIGNS AND SYMPTOMS

- Complete
  - —Diplopia, with involved eye deviated laterally and downward
  - —Mydriasis of the involved eye
- Partial
  - —Diplopia with involved eye deviated laterally and downward
  - —Reactive midpoint pupil of the involved eye

ETIOLOGY

- Intracranial or orbital tumor
- Aneurysm (particularly posterior communicating artery)
- Trauma
- Intracranial hemorrhage
- Diabetes mellitus
- Migraine headache
- Infection, meningitis
- Arteriovenous malformation or fistula
- Cavernous sinus thrombosis
- Neuropathy (myasthenia gravis, Guillain-Barré, etc.)
- Collagen vascular diseases (sarcoidosis, etc.)

MECHANISM/DESCRIPTION

- Complete oculomotor nerve palsy
  - —Compressive lesions such as aneurysms or tumors, etc.
  - —Brainstem herniation with compression of the third cranial nerve by the temporal lobe (i.e., increased intracranial pressure)
- Incomplete oculomotor nerve palsy
  - —Vascular infarction of the vasa nervorum of the third cranial nerve

PEDIATRIC CONSIDERATIONS

- Trauma is the most common cause of acquired oculomotor nerve palsies
- Congenital oculomotor nerve palsy should be considered in the differential of the pediatric patient. Other causes such as diabetes, posterior communicating artery aneurysms, metastatic tumor, and pituitary lesions are less common than in the adult population

Pre-Hospital

- Without associated trauma, there are no specific pre-hospital care issues

Diagnosis

ESSENTIAL WORKUP

- History is of utmost importance in determination of etiology and aid in focusing the examination and required workup. Important historical elements include
  - —History of long standing diabetes mellitus
  - —Head trauma, either recent or distant
  - —Unintentional weight loss
  - —Recent infection involving the upper respiratory tract, eyes, or ears
  - —Severe headache (classical "thunder-clap," or chronic and worsening)
  - —Constitutional symptoms: nausea, vomiting, fever, etc.
- Ophthalmologic examination
  - —Extraocular movements
  - —Exophthalmus
  - —Funduscopic examination to demonstrate papilledema
  - —Direct and consensual pupillary reaction

LABORATORY

- CBC with differential, ESR to rule-out infection and malignancy
- ANA, rheumatoid factor, to rule out vasculitis
- Lumbar puncture

IMAGING/SPECIAL TESTS

- CT/MRI of brain, orbit, sinuses
- Doppler imaging for arteriovenous malformations, dural sinus thrombosis
- Cerebral arteriogram rarely useful as most aneurysms are seen on CT or MRI

Treatment

INITIAL STABILIZATION

- Initial stabilization of the posttraumatic patient with oculomotor nerve palsy should concentrate on the underlying traumatic condition in an effort to preserve life
- ABCs
- Any patient with evidence of herniation should have the following measures to control intracranial pressure
  - —Intubation using rapid sequence induction and hyperventilation to a PCO_2 in the low 30s
  - —Elevate the head of the bed 30°
  - —Mannitol, furosemide

ED TREATMENT

- Crucial to differentiate between aneurysm and other compressive lesions early in the emergency department evaluation
  - —Differentiation between partial and complete oculomotor nerve palsy guides focus of treatment in the emergency department

MEDICATIONS

- Depending on the etiology of oculomotor nerve palsy, specific medication regimens should be administered as appropriate
  - —Aneurysm: control of severe hypertension with nitroprusside, decrease intracranial pressure with intubation, mannitol, furosemide, etc.
  - —Intracranial tumor: control increasing intracranial pressure with intubation, mannitol, and furosemide
    - -Decrease inflammation and edema with intravenous steroids
  - —Meningitis: rapid administration of intravenous antibiotics, intravenous steroids may be useful to decrease inflammatory response and edema
  - —Vasculitis and collagen vascular diseases: decrease inflammatory cell infiltration with intravenous steroids
  - —Neuropathy: myasthenia gravis–edrophonium chloride test, Guillain-Barré and others are often a diagnosis of exclusion
- Ceftriaxone: adult: 1–2 g IV; peds: 50–100 mg/kg IV
- Dexamethasone: adult: 10 mg IV; peds: 0.15–0.5 mg/kg IV single dose in ED
- Edrophonium Cl: adult: 5–8 mg IV; peds: 0.15 mg/kg IV, 1/10 test dose is given first
- Furosemide: adult/peds: 1 mg/kg IV
- Mannitol: adult/peds: 1 g/kg IV
- Methylprednisolone: adult/peds: 1–2 mg/kg IV single dose in ED

Disposition

ADMISSION CRITERIA

- Complete oculomotor nerve palsy of any etiology requires admission and emergency neurosurgical evaluation
- Incomplete oculomotor nerve palsy with abnormal CT or MRI, abnormal laboratory studies, or other focal neurologic or constitutional symptoms

DISCHARGE CRITERIA

- Incomplete oculomotor nerve palsy with negative CT or MRI, normal laboratory studies, and otherwise asymptomatic can be referred for urgent outpatient neurological evaluation

Miscellaneous

ICD9: 378.81

CORE CONTENT CODE: 11.2.3

SUGGESTED READINGS

Henry G, Little N. Neurological emergencies: a symptom oriented approach. New York: McGraw Hill, 1985.

Ing EB, Sullivan TJ, Clarke MP, Buncic JR. Oculomotor nerve palsies in children. J Pediatr Ophthalmol Strabismus 1992;29(6):331–336.

Kodsi SR, Younge BR. Acquired oculomotor, trochlear, and abducent cranial nerve palsies in pediatric patients. Am J Ophthalmol 1992;114(5):568–574.

Richards BW, Jones FR Jr, Younge BR. Causes and prognosis in 4,278 cases of paralysis of the oculomotor, trochlear, and abducens cranial nerves. Am J Ophthalmol 1992;113(5):489–496.

Sammuels MA. Manual of neurologic therapeutics with essentials of diagnosis. 2d ed. Boston: Little, Brown and Company, 1982.

Tiffin PA, MacEwen CJ, Craig EA, Clayton G. Acquired palsy of the oculomotor, trochlear, and abducens nerves. Eye 1996;10(Pt 3):377–384.

Author: James M. Leaming

Opiate, Poisoning

Clinical Presentation

SIGNS AND SYMPTOMS

CNS

- CNS depression
- Coma
- Increased intracranial pressure
- Seizures

Gastrointestinal

- Nausea
- Vomiting
- Constipation

Cardiovascular

- Hypotension
- Bradycardia
- Palpitations

Pulmonary

- Respiratory depression
- Bronchospasm
- Pulmonary edema
- Apnea

Other

- Miosis
- Hypothermia
- Urinary retention

Withdrawal

- Hypertension
- Tachycardia
- Tachypnea
- Abdominal cramps
- Diarrhea
- Piloerection

MECHANISM/DESCRIPTION

- Analgesics for moderate to severe pain
- Physical and psychological dependence occur
- Histamine release may occur
- Peak plasma levels
  —1–2 hours po
  —0.5–1 hour IM
- Serious toxicity with concomitant ingestion of CNS depressants
  —Alcohol
  —Benzodiazepines
  —Barbiturates
- Street preparations of narcotic analogues may contain adulterants
  —Cocaine
  —PCP
  —Strychnine
  —Dextromethorphan
  —Quinine

Pre-Hospital

CAUTIONS

- Do not induce emesis due to risk of CNS depression and aspiration
- Provide respiratory support
- Administer naloxone

ETIOLOGY

- Bind to μ, κ, and Δ opiate receptors in the brain and spinal cord inhibiting ascending pain pathways

Diagnosis

ESSENTIAL WORKUP

- Monitor vital signs and pulmonary status with significant exposure
  —Pulse oximetry or arterial blood gases
  —CXR if persistent hypoxia or possible aspiration

LABORATORY

- Plasma opiate levels not clinically useful
  —Treatment based upon clinical presentation—not level

DIFFERENTIAL DIAGNOSIS

- Clonidine overdose
- Barbiturate overdose
- Benzodiazepine overdose

PEDIATRIC CONSIDERATIONS

- Neonatal withdrawal
  —Infants born to addicted mothers
  —Onset: 12–72 hours after birth
  —Irritability, tremors, poor feeding, and dehydration
- Diphenoxylate (lomotil): toxicity—more severe in children than adults and often fatal

Treatment

INITIAL STABILIZATION

- ABCs
  - —Airway control essential
  - —Administer supplemental oxygen
- Administer naloxone (thiamine, glucose/Accucheck)
  - —Reverses both coma and cardiopulmonary depression in opiate overdoses
  - —Intubate if naloxone does not reverse respiratory depression

ED TREATMENT

Naloxone Administration

- High doses of naloxone (10–20 mg) required to reverse the effects of propoxyphene, methadone, and fentanyl
- Administer repeat doses, which reversed symptoms, as needed every 20–60 minutes
- Initiate an infusion of two-thirds the naloxone dose needed to reverse symptoms; may be given every hour

Decontamination

- Perform gastric lavage in recent large ingestion
- Administer activated charcoal and cathartic after lavage
- Administer whole bowel irrigation with polyethylene glycol for asymptomatic body packers
- Multidose activated charcoal for
  - —Propoxyphene and diphenoxylate overdoses
  - —Body packers or body stuffers with retained packets

Complications

- Treat hypotension with 0.9%NS IV fluid bolus and naloxone
  - —Initiate dopamine for resistant hypotension
- Treat seizures with diazepam
  - —Administer either phenobarbital or phenytoin for persistent seizures
- Treat opiate withdrawal with clonidine or methadone

MEDICATIONS

- Activated charcoal: 1–2 g/kg for initial dose and 0.5 g/ kg for subsequent doses
- Clonidine: 6 µg/kg acutely, then 10–17 µg/kg/day for 10 days po; 0.1–0.2 mg/kg/day transdermal patch
- Diazepam: 5–10 mg (peds: 0.2–0.5 mg/kg) IV q 10–15 min
- Dopamine: 2–20 mg/kg/min with titration to effect
- Methadone: 15–40 mg/day
- Naloxone: 0.4–2 mg (peds: 0.1 mg/kg; neonatal: 10–30 µg/kg) IV
- Phenobarbital: 15–20 mg/kg IV
- Phenytoin: 15–20 mg/kg IV
- Polyethylene glycol: 15–60 ml/kg/hour till clear rectal effluent and passage of packets
- Sorbitol: 1–2 g/kg only use with first dose of charcoal

Disposition

ADMISSION CRITERIA

- Symptomatic after oral overdose
- Requiring repeat naloxone dosing/infusion to reverse symptoms
- Children <5 years old postdiphenoxylate ingestion should be observed for 24 hours

DISCHARGE CRITERIA

- Asymptomatic 6 hours after oral overdose
- Asymptomatic 4 hours after naloxone administration

Miscellaneous

ICD9: 850.0, 850.1, 850.2

CORE CONTENT CODE: 17.2.40

SUGGESTED READINGS

Ellenhorn MJ, Schonwald S, Ordog G, Wasserberger J. The opiates. In: Ellenhorn MJ, ed. Ellenhorn's medical toxicology. Baltimore: Williams & Wilkins, 1997:405–447.

Ford M, Hoffman RS, Goldfrank LR. Opioids and designer drugs. Emerg Med Clin North Am 1990;8:495–511.

Goldfrank LR, Weisman RS. Opioids. In: Goldfrank LR, Weisman RS, Flomenbaum NE, et al., eds. Goldfrank's toxicologic emergencies. East Norwalk, CT: Appleton and Lange, 1994:769–786.

Author: Robert June

Opportunistic Infections

Clinical Presentation

SIGNS AND SYMPTOMS

- Presentation of a patient with an opportunistic infection varies with the site of the infection
- Can present with subtle signs with rapid deterioration
  - —Signs such as fever must lead to a full evaluation of the patient
  - —Thorough physical examination critical to search for site of infection
- Signs of systemic inflammatory response syndrome
  - —Temperature >38°C or <36°C
  - —HR >90 beats/min
  - —RR >20 breaths/min or PCO_2 <32 mm Hg
  - —WBC >12K
- Septic shock
- New or worsening fatigue
- Confusion
- Pulmonary
  - —Cough
  - —Congestion
  - —Rales
  - —Egophony
  - —Tachypnea
- Genitourinary
  - —Dysuria
  - —Frequency
  - —Retention
- Gastrointestinal
  - —Vomiting
  - —Diarrhea
  - —Blood in stool
- Cardiovascular
  - —New murmur
  - —Hypotension
  - —Tachycardia
- Physical exam
  - —Inspect skin and mucosa carefully for a portal of entry
  - —Examine oral mucosa and perianal area for erythema and palpate for tenderness or crepitus
    - -Tumor invasion or cytotoxic drug effects on the alimentary canal allow gut flora to invade and cause local or systemic effects

MECHANISM/DESCRIPTION

- Opportunistic infection occurs when the host suffers a decrease in resistance against normally nonpathogenic organisms
- Type of immunocompromise predicts the type of infection that will occur
  - —Cell-mediated deficiency
  - —Neutrophil impairment/depletion
- Causes of cell-mediated deficiency
  - —Hematological malignancies
    - -Leukemia
    - -Multiple myeloma
    - -Lymphoma
  - —High-dose glucocorticoid therapy
    - -Cytotoxic drugs
    - -Cyclosporine
    - -Methotrexate
    - -Cisplatin
    - -Azathioprine
    - -6-Mercaptopurine
    - -Hydroxyurea
  - —Radiation Therapy
  - —Viral infections
    - -CMV
    - -HIV
  - —Antilymphocyte globulins
    - -Autoimmune disorders
    - -Rheumatic diseases
- Causes of neutrophil impairment/depletion
  - —Cytotoxic drugs
  - —Aplastic anemia
  - —Drug reactions
    - -Dapsone
    - -Chloramphenicol
    - -Penicillin
    - -Procainamide
  - —Neoplastic invasion of the marrow
    - -Multiple myeloma
  - —Chemicals
    - -Benzene
    - -Arsenic
  - —Vitamin deficiency
    - -B_{12}
    - -Folic acid
- Cell-mediated dysfunction associated with intracellular organisms infections
  - —Legionella
  - —Salmonella
  - —Mycobacteria
  - —Nocardia
- Neutrophil disorders associated with
  - —Staphylococcus
  - —α-Hemolytic streptococcus
  - —Enteric organisms
  - —Anaerobes

Pre-Hospital

N/A

Diagnosis

ESSENTIAL WORKUP

- Full workup indicated due to impaired immunity
  - —Signs of infection in the immunocompromised patient may not be present

LABORATORY

- Cultures (aerobic, anaerobic, fungal, viral as indicated)
  - —Urine
  - —Blood
  - —Wound
  - —Fecal
- CBC with differential
  - —Neutropenia or leukocytosis
- Urinalysis for presence of WBC, nitrite, leukocyte esterase
- Electrolytes, BUN/Cr, glucose
  - —Anion gap acidosis suggests severe infection
- ABG for hypoxia/acidosis
- Lactate level
  - —Elevated value suggestive of serious infection
- PT/PTT for evidence of disseminated intravascular coagulation
- CSF analysis if signs of CNS infection

IMAGING/SPECIAL TESTS

- CXR

Treatment

INITIAL STABILIZATION

- ABCs
- Initiate IV 0.9%NS
  —500 cc bolus for hypotension
- Oxygen
- Cardiac monitor for unstable vital signs
- Early initiation of antibiotic therapy

ED TREATMENT

- Strict isolation
- Antibiotics
  —Combination of expanded spectrum penicillin (mezlocillin, ticarcillin, piperacillin) and aminoglycoside (amikacin, tobramycin) is most common
  —Expanded spectrum penicillin and a third-generation cephalosporin (ceftazidime, cefoperazone) if aminoglycoside contraindicated
  —Vancomycin is not recommended as part of initial therapy unless there is a high incidence of methicillin-resistant organisms in the area
  —Antifungals (amphotericin B, fluconazole) if patient is on adequate antibiotics for 1 week

MEDICATIONS

- Amikacin: 15 mg/kg/24 hrs (peds: 15–30 mg/kg/24 hrs) IV q 8 hrs
- Amphotericin B: 0.25 mg/kg IV q d
- Cefoperazone: 2–4 g q 12 hrs IV
- Ceftazidime: 1–2 g (peds: 100–150mg/kg/24 hrs) IV q 8–12 hrs
- Fluconazole: 400 mg first dose then 200–400 mg IV q d (peds: 3–6 mg/kg/24 hrs IV q 12 hrs)
- Mezlocillin: 3 g (peds: 200–300 mg/kg/24 hrs) q 4 hrs over 30 min
- Piperacillin: 3 g q 4 hrs over 30 min
- Ticarcillin: 3 g (peds: 200–300 mg/kg/24 hrs) IV q 4 hrs over 30 min
- Tobramycin: 3–5 mg/kg/24 hrs (peds: 6–8mg/kg/24 hrs) IV q 8 hrs
- Vancomycin: 1–2 g IV q 12 hrs (peds: 10–50 mg/kg/24 hrs IV q 6 hrs)

Disposition

ADMISSION CRITERIA

- Suspected or confirmed systemic infection

DISCHARGE CRITERIA

- Systemic infection excluded

Miscellaneous

ICD9: N/A

CORE CONTENT CODE: N/A

SUGGESTED READINGS

Daar ES, Meyer RD. Bacterial and fungal infections. Med Clin North Am 1992;17(1): 173–195.

Giamarellou H. Empiric therapy for infections in the febrile, neutropenic, compromised host. Med Clin North Am 1992;79 (3): 559–578.

Pizzo PA. The compromised host. In: Bennett, JC et al., eds. Cecil's textbook of medicine. Philadelphia: WB Saunders, 1996:908–915.

Author: Andrzej Dmowski

Optic Artery Occlusion

Clinical Presentation

SIGNS AND SYMPTOMS

- Sudden painless monocular loss of vision
- "Count fingers" or "light perception" visual acuity (90%)
- Partial field defects
  - —If only a branch of the central retinal artery (CRA) involved
- Normal visual acuity (rare)
  - —If the macula spared by anomalous circulation from the choroid (a cilioretinal vessel)
- Prior episodes of sudden temporary visual loss
  - —Lasts a few seconds to minutes (amaurosis fugax)
  - —Caused by transient embolic phenomena or decreased ocular blood flow

Retinal Appearance

- Emboli visualized within the vascular tree of the retina
  - —Appears as glinting white or yellow flecks within the vessels
- Ischemic edema visible within 15–20 minutes of occlusion
- Affected arteries empty or showing dark red stationary or barely pulsatile segmented rouleaux ("boxcaring")
- Within 1–2 hours
  - —Opacification of the usually transparent infarcting retinal nerve layer occurs
  - —"Cherry-red spot" remaining over the fovea (only area where there is very thin retina allowing the vascular choroid to show through)

MECHANISM/DESCRIPTION

- Central retinal artery
  - —First branch of the ophthalmic artery that arises from the internal carotid artery
  - —Retinal arteries are not innervated, but instead depend on autoregulation (e.g. response to resistance-pressure and PCO_2) for dilatation and constriction
- Ischemic injury results from obstruction of blood flow by any embolus or thrombus small enough to enter the ophthalmic artery and large enough to block the retinal artery (or one of its branches)
- Unlike cerebral neural tissue that is completely destroyed within 10 minutes of complete ischemia, the nerve layer of the retina may remain viable for up to 2 hours due to the dual circulation of the retina, with the separate choroidal blood flow nourishing the sensitive outer layer of the retina while the inner half is anoxic

ETIOLOGY

- Cause
  - —Embolic phenomena (majority)
  - —Thrombosis
  - —Spasm (postulated but unproven)
- Embolic events related to
  - —Atherosclerotic disease (majority)
  - —Valvular heart disease
  - —Atrial myxoma
  - —Dissection of the ophthalmic artery in the region of the cribriform plate (rare)
- Thrombosis occurs with
  - —Giant cell (temporal) arteritis
  - —Disseminated lupus erythematosus
  - —Other collagen vascular diseases (polyarteritis nodosa)
  - —Risk factors for thrombotic events
    - -Oral contraceptives
    - -Polycythemia vera
    - -Sickle cell disease
    - -Syphilis
    - -Behçet's syndrome
    - -Migraine

Pre-Hospital

N/A

Diagnosis

ESSENTIAL WORKUP

- Accurate funduscopy essential
- Diagnosis made by comparison of the retinas of the two eyes, looking for
  - —Unilateral diffuse pallor
  - —Macular "cherry-red spot"
  - —Focal or diffuse attenuation of the retinal arterioles
  - —"Boxcaring" the nonmobile or barely pulsatile segmental rouleaux within the retinal vessels
- Do not delay treatment while waiting for laboratory results

LABORATORY

- CBC with differential and platelet count
- PT/PTT
- Electrolytes, BUN/Cr, glucose
- ESR for giant cell arteritis (in patients >55 years old)
- ANA
- Rheumatoid factor
- RPR
- Hemoglobin electrophoresis
- Serum protein electrophoresis

IMAGING/SPECIAL TESTS

- Carotid artery evaluation by ultrasound and Doppler
- Cardiac evaluation
  - —ECG
  - —Echocardiography
  - —Holter monitoring
- Fluorescein angiography or electroretinography to confirm the diagnosis

DIFFERENTIAL DIAGNOSIS

- Acute ophthalmic artery occlusion (treatment is the same as for central retinal artery occlusion (CRAO)
- Arteritic ischemic optic neuropathy
- Other causes of "cherry-red spot" (e.g., Tay-Sachs disease)
- Recent inadvertent intraocular injection of gentamicin

PEDIATRIC CONSIDERATIONS

- Cause in young patients: embolism from valvular heart disease

Treatment

INITIAL STABILIZATION

- Initiate treatment *as soon as the diagnosis is made and before the workup proceeds* if the CRAO is <24 hours old
  - —Only immediate treatment may help to salvage or restore sight to the affected eye

ED TREATMENT

- Immediate massage of the globe of the eye
  - —Apply digital pressure to the eye (a few seconds on and off) to dislodge the embolus or thrombus from a larger to a smaller less important vessel
  - —Perform for only 1–2 minutes, as any effect will be noticeable within that time
- Increase CO_2 to dilate the retinal vessels
  - —Initiate rebreathing the patient's own exhalation into a paper bag
  - —Administer carbogen (95% oxygen, 5% carbon dioxide) q 10 min q 1–2 hrs
- Urgent ophthalmologic consultation
- Anterior chamber paracentesis with 25-gauge needle
- Administer carbonic anhydrase inhibitor (acetazolamide) or topical β-blockers (timolol) to lower intraocular pressure

MEDICATIONS

- Acetazolamide: 500 mg IV
- Timolol 0.25–1.0%: 1 drop to eye

Disposition

ADMISSION CRITERIA

- Acute central retinal artery occlusion for workup for source of embolic phenomena or thrombosis

DISCHARGE CRITERIA

- Chronic retinal artery occlusion with no evidence of active disease, can be worked up as an outpatient

Miscellaneous

ICD9: 362.30

CORE CONTENT CODE: 6.4.3.5.1

SUGGESTED READINGS

Feinberg AW. The evaluation of amaurosis fugax. Hosp Pract 1992;27:47–57.

Newell FW. The retina. In: Newell FW, ed. Ophthalmology, principles and concepts. 7th ed. St. Louis: CV Mosby, 1992.

Younge BR. The significance of retinal emboli. J Clin Neurophthalmol 1989;9(3):190–194.

Author: Evan Liu

Optic Neuritis

Clinical Presentation

SIGNS AND SYMPTOMS

- Visual loss occurring over days (rarely over hours)
  - —Adults usually unilateral
  - —Bilateral visual loss more common in children
- Retrobulbar pain: increased with movement of the affected eye
- Light, color vision, and depth perception loss more pronounced than visual acuity loss
- Afferent pupillary defect occurring in unilateral cases
- Visual field defects
  - —Central scotoma
- Funduscopic exam usually reveals either
  - —Swollen (papillitis) or normal disc
- Uhthoff's sign
  - —Visual deficit occurring with exercise or increased body temperature
  - —Unusual sign which is seen occasionally

MECHANISM/DESCRIPTION

- Inflammatory process of the optic nerve, characterized by myelin destruction
- Grouped by site of inflammation
  - —Papillitis: inflammation of the optic disc
  - —Retrobulbar neuritis: inflammation of the optic nerve proximal to the globe

ETIOLOGY

- Between ages 15 and 45 years
- Idiopathic
  - —Most common
  - —Single isolated events
- Multiple sclerosis
  - —20–50% of patients with optic neuritis
- Viral infections
  - —Chicken pox
  - —Measles
  - —Mononucleosis
  - —Herpes zoster
  - —Encephalitis
- Granulomatous inflammation
  - —Tuberculosis
  - —Syphilis
  - —Sarcoidosis
  - —Cryptococcal infection
- Systemic lupus erythematosus
- HIV
  - —Cytomegalovirus
  - —*Cryptococcus*
- Lyme disease
- Contiguous inflammation of meninges, orbit, sinuses, and intraocular inflammation
- Postviral optic neuritis
  - —Usually occurs 4–6 weeks following a nonspecific viral illness
- Drug induced
  - —Ethambutol
  - —Tamoxifen

Pre-Hospital

N/A

Diagnosis

ESSENTIAL WORKUP

- History
  - —Age
  - —Speed of onset of symptoms
  - —Associated symptoms
  - —Previous episodes
- Check blood pressure
- Complete ophthalmologic and neurologic examination, especially assessment of
  - —Pupillary function
  - —Color vision (Ishihara color plates)
  - —Evaluation of the vitreous for cells
  - —Dilated retinal exam

LABORATORY

- CBC
- ESR
- RPR, FTA-ABS
- Lyme titre
- ANA
- PPD testing

IMAGING/SPECIAL TESTS

- CXR for tuberculosis
- CT scan or MRI of brain and orbits
  - —Inflammation of the retrobulbar optic nerve during the acute phase may appear as enlargement, thus falsely raising the issue of an optic nerve mass
  - —Visual field testing (preferably automated testing, such as Octopus or Humphrey)

DIFFERENTIAL DIAGNOSIS

- Acute papilledema
- Ischemic optic neuropathy
- Severe systemic hypertension
- Intracranial tumor compressing the afferent visual pathway
- Orbital mass compressing the optic nerve
- Toxic or metabolic neuropathy
  - —Heavy metal poisoning
  - —Anemia
  - —Malnutrition
  - —Alcohols
  - —Chloroquine
  - —INH
- Leber's hereditary optic atrophy

Treatment

INITIAL STABILIZATION

N/A

ED TREATMENT

- Early ophthalmologic and neurologic consultations
- Avoid prednisone, ACTH, and other corticosteroids
  —Steroid therapy may worsen the course of optic neuritis
  —Probably not helpful in the treatment of multiple sclerosis

Disposition

ADMISSION CRITERIA

- Bilateral vision loss
- If other sources of acute vision loss cannot be ruled out

DISCHARGE CRITERIA

- Good home support systems
- No other medical or social reason for admission
- Unilateral visual impairment

Miscellaneous

ICD9: 377.3

CORE CONTENT CODE: 6.4.3.2

SUGGESTED READINGS

Beck RW, Clery PA, Trobe JD, et.al. The effect of corticosteroids for acute optic neuritis on the subsequent development of multiple sclerosis. N Engl J Med 1993;329:1764.

Optic Neuritis Study Group. The clinical profile of optic neuritis: Experience of the optic neuritis treatment trial. Arch Ophthalmol 1991;109:1673.

Purvin VA, Van Dyk HJL. Optic neuritis. In: Fraunfelder FT. Current ocular therapy. 4th ed. Philadelphia: WB Saunders, 1995.

Rothenhous TC, Polis MA. Ocular manifestations of systemic disease. Emerg Med Clin North Am 1995;13:607–630.

Author: Evan Liu

Orbital Cellulitis

Clinical Presentation

SIGNS AND SYMPTOMS

- Painful, red, warm, swollen eye (unilateral 95%)
- Typically ill-appearing on presentation
- Fever
- Headache
- Blurred or double vision
- Conjunctival injection
- Chemosis
- Clinically distinguished from preseptal cellulitis by
  —Restricted painful extraocular muscle movement
  —Proptosis
  —Visual impairment
  —Afferent pupillary defect
- Anatomically distinguished from preseptal cellulitis by
  —Tissue involvement deep to the orbital septum
- Associated complications
  —Ophthalmoplegia
    -Due to toxic myopathy and soft tissue edema
  —Intraorbital periosteal abscess
  —Meningitis
  —Brain abscess
  —Septic cavernous sinus thrombosis
  —Visual loss
    -Toxic or compressive ischemic optic nerve dysfunction
    -Optic neuritis
    -Retinal venous congestion
  —Abnormal pupillary response
    -Suggests involvement of the orbital apex
  —Orbital osteomyelitis
  —Bacteremia/septicemia

ETIOLOGY

- Occurs secondary to extension from an adjacent structure
  —Sinusitis
  —Dental abscess
  —Periorbital cellulitis
  —Retained foreign body in the orbit
  —Lacrimal apparatus
    -Dacryoadenitis
    -Dacryocystitis
  —Orbital fracture
  —Postoperative infection
  —Hematogenous spread from a remote source
- Most common organisms
  —*Streptococcus* pneumonia
  —*Staphylococcus aureus*
  —*Streptococcus pyogenes*
  —Bacteroides
  —Gram-negative
    -Associated with trauma
  —Gonococcus extending from conjunctivitis and dacryoadenitis
  —*Hemophilus influenza* (children)
- Cerebro-rhino-orbital phycomycosis (CROP) (mucormycosis)
  —Life-threatening disease presenting with orbital cellulitis
    -Rapidly fatal in 75%
  —Etiology fungal most commonly *Rhizopus sp.* and less often *Mucor sp.*
  —80% diabetics with a recent episode of DKA
  —Predisposing factor: severe metabolic acidosis
  —Begins in the paranasal sinuses
  —Proliferates in the blood vessel walls causing thrombosis and necrosis
    -Bloody nasal discharge
    -Frequently evidence of necrosis of the palate and nasal mucosa at presentation
  —May present with multiple cranial nerve palsies
  —Toxic appearance
  —All age groups
  —High level of suspicion in immunocompromised patients

PEDIATRIC CONSIDERATIONS

- With *Hemophilus influenza B:* high risk of associated bacteremia and meningitis
  —Less common with vaccine
  —Periorbital swelling classically has a violaceous hue (also seen with pneumococcus)
- Difficult to assess visual acuity in this age group
  —Pay close attention to pupillary abnormalities as a sign of orbital apex involvement

Pre-Hospital

N/A

Diagnosis

ESSENTIAL WORKUP

- High suspicion with periorbital pain, swelling, and fever
  —Elevated temperature, headache, proptosis, and painful restricted extraocular movements increase likelihood
- Identify likely precipitating infectious source
- Look for altered mental status, meningismus or visual loss which suggest CNS penetration
- Identify associated medical problems that would render them immunocompromised with a higher morbidity and mortality

LABORATORY

- Supportive but not diagnostic
- Serum glucose in adults
  —To identify occult diabetes
- CBC
  —Elevated WBC with left shift
- Blood cultures
  —Identify organism
- Gram's stain and culture of any drainage
  —Chocolate agar plate when gonorrhea suspected

IMAGING/SPECIAL TESTS

- Lumbar puncture/CSF analysis—controversial
  —Indicated in all patients with signs and symptoms suggestive of meningitis
  —Consider with patients at high risk for *Hemophilus influenza B* as causative organism due to high risk of associated bacteremia and meningitis
    -Age <4 years
    -Toxic in appearance
    -Non-HiB vaccinated at the onset of infection
- Cultures of conjunctival and nasopharyngeal swab specimens: not indicated
- Plain radiographs
  —Little value and not indicated
- Orbital and sinus CT scan
  —Identifies extent of involvement and source
    -Sinusitis
    -Orbital cellulitis
    -Subperiosteal abscess formation
    -Orbital abscess
    -Presence of an orbital foreign body
    -Proptosis
  —Best if obtained with and without contrast
  —Axial and coronal views necessary

DIFFERENTIAL DIAGNOSIS

- Periorbital cellulitis
- Dacryoadenitis
- Retrobulbar hemorrhage
- Cavernous sinus thrombosis
- Cranial nerve palsy
- Inflammatory orbital pseudotumor
- Orbital rhabdomyosarcoma
- Leukemia or lymphoma with orbital involvement
- Dermoid cyst
- Subperiosteal hematoma
- Graves disease
- Hordeolum

PEDIATRIC CONSIDERATIONS

- High fever (≥39°C), toxic appearance and elevated WBC (>15,000)
  - —Suggests bacteremia making Hemophilus or Pneumococcus the likely causative agent
  - —Determine *Hemophilus influenza B* vaccine status
  - —Higher risk of hemophilus infection if child has not completed two vaccinations prior to onset of infection

Treatment

INITIAL STABILIZATION

- IV access
- Early antibiotic therapy after appropriate cultures

ED TREATMENT

- Ophthalmologic or ENT consultation
- IV antibiotic therapy
  - —Coverage for Gram-positive, Gram-negative and anaerobic organisms seen in sinusitis
  - —Must have good CSF penetration
  - —Children: ceftriaxone and vancomycin
  - —Adults: ceftriaxone and vancomycin/nafcillin
  - —Add metronidazole if anaerobic infection suspected (trauma, foreign body, or bite)
  - —Substitute gentamicin for ceftriaxone in cephalosporin/penicillin allergic patient
- Incision, drainage, and debridement
  - —When Bacteroides is the causative organism
    - -Both surgical debridement and specific antibiotic therapy necessary to achieve a cure
  - —Surgically remove retained foreign bodies
  - —Appropriate consultation to ophthalmology or ENT
- Tetanus toxoid if indicated
- Ophthalmic antibiotic ointment and lubricating drops if proptosis leaves the cornea exposed
- Cerebro-Rhino-Orbital Phycomycosis (CROP)
  - —Amphotericin B intravenous in the highest tolerated doses
  - —Topical amphotericin B (1 mg/ml) irrigation or nasal packing
  - —Local debridement

MEDICATIONS

- Ceftriaxone: 1–2 g (peds: 100 mg/kg/24hrs) IV q 12–24 hr
- Gentamicin: 5 mg/kg IV q 24 hrs
- Erythromycin ophthalmic ointment: applied q 4 hrs to lower lid cul de sac
- Lacri-Lube: 2 drops q 2–4 hrs PRN
- Metronidazole: 15 mg/kg IV load then 7.5 mg/kg q 6 hrs.
- Nafcillin: 1–2 g IV q 4 hrs
- Vancomycin: 1 g (peds: 40 mg/kg/24hrs) q 12 hrs IV

Disposition

ADMISSION CRITERIA

- Orbital cellulitis
- Ill-appearing patients with periorbital cellulitis in whom the risk of deep penetration is high

DISCHARGE CRITERIA

- None with orbital cellulitis

Miscellaneous

ICD9: 376.01

CORE CONTENT CODE: 6.4.4.2

SUGGESTED READINGS

Anonymous. Orbital disease. Int Ophthalmol Clin 1992;32(3):1–205.

Ciarallo LR, Rowe PC. Lumbar puncture in children with periorbital and orbital cellulitis. J Pediatr 1993;122(3):355–359.

Danter EM, Jolly BT. Pediatric ophthalmology. Emerg Med Clin North Am 1995;13(3):669–680.

Lessner A, Stern GA. Preseptal and orbital cellulitis. Infect Dis Clin North Am 1992;6(4):933–952.

Powell KR. Orbital and periorbital cellulitis. Pediatr Rev 1995;16(5):163–167.

Tole DM, Anderton LC. Orbital cellulitis demands early recognition, urgent admission and aggressive management. J Accid Emerg Med 1995;12(2):151–153.

Williams SR, Carruth JA. Orbital infection secondary to sinusitis in children: Diagnosis and management. Clin Otolaryngol 1992;17(6):550–557.

Author: Shari Schabowski

Organophosphate, Poisoning

Clinical Presentation

SIGNS AND SYMPTOMS

- Classic presentation: SLUDGE (salivation, lacrimation, urination, defecation, GI upset, emesis)
- Chronic intermittent exposure—nonspecific symptoms
  —Weakness
  —Fatigue
  —Malaise
  —Anorexia

Mild Exposure

- Visual
  —Miosis
  —Decreased visual acuity
- CNS
  —Headache
  —Dizziness
  —Tremors of tongue and eyelids
  —Anxiety
  —Weakness
- GI
  —Anorexia

Moderate Exposure

- CNS
  —Muscle fasciculation followed by flaccid paralysis
  —Respiratory muscle weakness
  —Incoordination
- GI
  —Nausea
  —Vomiting
  —Abdominal cramps
- Exocrine glands
  —Salivation
  —Lacrimation

Severe Exposure

- Visual
  —Pinpoint nonreactive pupils
- Respiratory
  —Respiratory difficulty
  —Pulmonary edema
- Cardiovascular
  —Bradycardia
  —Heart block
- CNS
  —Convulsion
  —Coma
  —No sphincter tone
- GI
  —Diarrhea

Muscarinic Manifestations

- Respiratory
  —Chest tightness, wheezing, dyspnea, increased bronchial secretion, cough, pulmonary edema, cyanosis
- GI
  —Nausea, vomiting, abdominal tightness and cramps, diarrhea,
  —tenesmus, fecal incontinence
- Exocrine glands
  —Increased sweating, salivation, lacrimation
- Pupils
  —Miosis, occasionally unequal
- Ciliary body
  —Blurred vision
- Bladder
  —Frequency, urinary incontinence

Nicotinic Manifestations

- Striated muscle
  —Muscular twitching, fasciculation, cramping, weakness including respiratory muscles
- Sympathetic ganglia
  —Pallor, tachycardia, hypertension
- CNS
  —Anxiety, restlessness, tremors, depression, ataxia, weakness, coma without reflexes, seizures, Cheyne-Stokes respiration

MECHANISM/DESCRIPTION

- Organophosphate insecticides are irreversible cholinesterase inhibitors
- Cholinesterase breaks down acetylcholine when it is released at the synapse in preganglionic junctions of parasympathetic, sympathetic, and myoneural junction, and the postganglionic junction of the parasympathetic and some sympathetic nervous system
- Organophosphate insecticides cause inhibition of cholinesterase, causing an overproduction of acetylcholine
- Acetylcholine accumulation causes an overstimulation of central and peripheral nervous system

PEDIATRIC CONSIDERATIONS

- SLUDGE symptoms difficult to differentiate in children <3 years old
- Common symptoms: miosis, salivation, and muscle weakness
- Seizures found in 25% (3% of adults)

Pre-Hospital

CAUTIONS

- Maintain airway and oxygenate
- Avoid direct contact with the toxin
- Decontaminate skin with dermal exposure
  —Remove clothing
  —Flush exposed skin

Diagnosis

ESSENTIAL WORKUP

- Inquire about possible exposure, occupation, recent insecticide in home, mislabeled or poorly stored insecticides
- Look for parasympathetic and CNS signs with muscle weakness or paralysis

LABORATORY

- RBC and serum cholinesterase levels to confirm diagnosis
  —RBC (true) cholinesterase level corresponds to synaptic level
  —Serum (pseudo) cholinesterase level found in the plasma
  —Cholinesterase levels
    -Latent exposure: more than 50% of normal value
    -Mild exposure: 20–50% of normal value
    -Moderate exposure: 10–20% of normal value
    -Severe exposure: less than 10% of normal value
  —Do not wait for cholinesterase results before administering treatment
- CBC
- Electrolytes, glucose, BUN, Cr
- ABG when respiratory symptoms

IMAGING/SPECIAL TESTS

- CXR if respiratory difficulty is present
- ECG
  —Dysrhythmias
  —Bradycardia
  —Tachycardia
  —Heart block
  —ST-T wave abnormalities
  —Prolonged QTc interval
- CT scan head for altered mental status when diagnosis uncertain

DIFFERENTIAL DIAGNOSIS

MILD TO MODERATE EXPOSURE

- Gastroenteritis
- Asthma
- Venomous arthropods bite (black widow, scorpion)
- Nonspecific viral syndrome
- Progressive peripheral neuropathy (Guillain-Barré Syndrome)
- Carbon monoxide

Severe Exposure

- Narcotic overdose
- Coma and miosis
  —PCP, meprobamate, phenothiazine, clonidine
  —Muscarinic containing mushrooms—cholinergic crisis without nicotinic symptoms
  —Nicotinic poisoning

- Metabolic and infectious
  - —Ketoacidosis, sepsis, meningitis, encephalitis
  - —Hypoglycemia
  - —Reye's syndrome
- Neurologic
  - —CVA
  - —Subdural or epidural hematoma
  - —Postictal state

Treatment

INITIAL STABILIZATION

- ABCs
  - —Maintain airway and oxygenate
  - —For unstable airway, intubate, and ventilate
  - —IV access with D5W 0.9%NS
- Altered mental status: administer thiamine, glucose, and narcan

ED TREATMENT

Atropine

- Blocks acetylcholine at muscarinic receptor sites
- No effect on nicotinic receptors
- Goal of therapy: maintain atropinization
  - —Mydriasis
  - —Flush, dry mouth
  - —Tachycardia
- Administer 1 mg IV if organophosphate poisoning suspected
  - —No clinical response (tachycardia, dry mouth, flushing) should confirm the suspicion of organophosphate poisoning
- Dose: 1–4 mg IV q 5 min (peds: 0.05–0.2 mg/kg)
  - —Can be administered IM every 15 minutes until IV access obtained
- Common failure in therapy: not maintaining atropinization

Pralidoxime (2-PAM)

- Cholinesterase regenerator and reverses the cholinergic effects on nicotinic receptors
- Not indicated in carbamate poisoning
  - —Controversy: believed that pralidoxime can worsen carbamate toxicity
  - —Theory—not proved
  - —Carbamate is reversible and symptoms last for 8 hours

Supportive Care

- Dermal decontamination: remove clothes and flush skin with water
- Gastric lavage
  - —Gastric emptying should be done with continuous suction via a nasogastric tube
  - —Handle contents with care, and avoid coming in direct contact with it to prevent exposure
- Respiratory difficulty
  - —Frequent respiratory secretion suction required
  - —Treat bronchospasm with atropine and not bronchodilators
  - —Intubate and ventilate if necessary

MEDICATIONS

- Atropine: 1–4 mg (peds: 0.05–0.2 mg/kg) IV q 5 min
- Dextrose: D50W 1 amp (25 g) of 50% dextrose (peds: 2–4 ml/kg D25W) IVP
- Naloxone (narcan): 2 mg (peds: 0.1 mg/kg) IV or IM initial dose
- Pralidoxime: 1–2 g (peds: 20–40 mg/kg) over 15–20 min IV; repeat in 2 hrs, then 8–10 hrs later

Disposition

ADMISSION CRITERIA

- ICU admission for mild, moderate, or severe exposure confirmed with a response to atropine

DISCHARGE CRITERIA

- Asymptomatic for 6 hours after exposure

Miscellaneous

ICD9: 989.3

CORE CONTENT CODE: 17.2.39

SUGGESTED READINGS

Chuang FR, Jang SW, et al. QTc prolongation indicates a poor prognosis in patients with organophosphate poisoning. Am J Emerg Med 1996;14:451–453.

Mackey CL. Anticholinesterase insecticide poisoning. Heart Lung 1982;11:479–484.

Tafuri J, Toberts J. Organophosphate poisoning. Ann Emerg Med 1987;16:193–202.

Zwiener RJ, Ginsburg CM. Organophosphate and carbamate poisoning in infants and children. Pediatrics 1988;81:121–126.

Author: Karyn Cole

Osgood-Schlatter Disease

Clinical Presentation

SIGNS AND SYMPTOMS

- Pain and swelling over the tibial tuberosity
  —May be bilateral
- Quadriceps use against resistance aggravates pain during climbing of steps or kneeling

MECHANISM/DESCRIPTION

- Secondary to incomplete separation of the cartilaginous link between the patellar tendon and the tibia
  —Separation interrupts the blood supply
  —Results in aseptic necrosis fragmentation and eventually new bone formation
- Fusion of the tubercle to the tibia occurs by 18 years of age
  —Eliminates any further symptoms

ETIOLOGY

- Typically seen in adolescents during a growth spurt

Pre-Hospital

N/A

Diagnosis

ESSENTIAL WORKUP

- Clinical diagnosis
  —Typically pain, swelling, and tenderness localized over the tibial tubercle

LABORATORY

N/A

IMAGING/SPECIAL TESTS

- Knee radiographs to exclude other causes of knee pain

DIFFERENTIAL DIAGNOSIS

- Fracture
- Legg-Calve-Perthes disease
  —Referred hip pain
- Osteochondritis desiccans
- Osteomyelitis
- Osseous malignancy
- Patellofemoral dysfunction
- Sinding-Larsen-Johannson syndrome
- Slipped-capital femoral epiphysis
  —Referred hip pain
- Stress fracture
- Tendinitis or bursitis around the knee

Treatment

INITIAL STABILIZATION

- Place leg in position of comfort
- Splint if necessary to minimize pain

ED TREATMENT

- Mainstay of therapy
  - —Nonsteroidal anti-inflammatory agents
  - —Rest
  - —Ice to the affected area 3 times per day
  - —Compress the painful area with an elastic bandage
  - —Elevate the leg
- Mild cases
  - —Avoid forceful knee extension as during running, jumping, or long walks
- Severe cases
  - —Cylinder casting for 4–6 weeks

MEDICATIONS

- Ibuprofen: 400–800 mg po q 8 hrs

Disposition

ADMISSION CRITERIA

None

DISCHARGE CRITERIA

- Discharge all patients

Miscellaneous

ICD9: 732.4

CORE CONTENT CODE: 13.6.7

SUGGESTED READINGS

Micheli LJ, Fehlandt AF. Overuse injuries to tendons and apophyses in children and adolescents. Clin Sports Med 1992;11:713–726.

Peck DM. Apophyseal injuries in the young adult. Am Fam Physician 1995;51(8):1891–1895.

Smith JB. Knee problems in children. Pediatr Clinic North Am 1986;33:1439–1456.

Author: Lydia Ciarallo

Osteogenesis Imperfecta

Clinical Presentation

SIGNS AND SYMPTOMS

- Osteogenesis imperfecta refers to multiple heritable defects that lead to brittle bones and are often associated with other connective tissue abnormalities

Bones

- Multiple recurrent fractures (especially in long bones) are the hallmark of this disease
- Fractures may be present at birth or may recur in the elderly
- All bones are affected to some extent (see Imaging/Special Tests)

Eyes

- Blue sclera are another hallmark of the disease
- No visual changes are reported

Ears

- Hearing loss usually begins in adolescence; over 90% of patients have some deficit by age 30 years
- Hearing loss is generally sensorineural, although some middle ear pathology can be demonstrated

Other

- Yellow-brown or blue-gray discoloration and abnormal shape of teeth
- Shares several features with Ehlers-Danlos syndrome: loose joints, valve problems, and vascular abnormalities
- Thyroid abnormalities may be seen
- Extreme cases may result in perinatal death

MECHANISM/DESCRIPTION

- Inherited abnormality of procollagen amino acid sequence
- Bone hypomineralization and incomplete ossification result in brittle bones
- Abnormal collagen affects all connective tissue to varying degrees
- The time course is variable, with most cases involving fractures during childhood followed by improvement in adolescence and early adulthood

ETIOLOGY

- Procollagen defects result in bone and connective tissue matrix abnormalities
- Defects in different sites on the procollagen protein chain result in more severe forms
- Defects are inherited, either autosomal recessive (generally milder) or autosomal dominant (more severe)
- Lethal cases involve sporadic or new mutations
- Ehlers-Danlos syndrome involves mutations of the same procollagen protein in a different location

PEDIATRIC CONSIDERATIONS

- Most cases involve pathologic fractures during childhood
- Multiple fractures often initiate evaluation for abuse, but should also consider pathologic fractures

Pre-Hospital

Pre-Hospital personnel should obtain information about mechanism or social factors that point towards pathologic fracture versus nonaccidental trauma

Diagnosis

ESSENTIAL WORKUP

- Diagnosis is usually made as a combination of clinical findings with radiographs
- History of repeated fractures or fractures with unimpressive mechanism
- Thorough search for other tender areas and evaluation of eyes, teeth, and joints is crucial for diagnosis
- Careful examination of neurovascular status distal to fracture

IMAGING/SPECIAL TESTS

- Radiographs of fracture sites may reveal osteopenia (usually mild), crumpled long bones ("accordion femora"), or incomplete ossification at physes
- Skeletal survey is mandatory, especially in children
- Skull films may show "wormian" appearance of irregular ossification
- "Popcornlike" deposits on long-bone ends is a poor prognostic finding
- Formal audiologic testing as an outpatient is needed in older patients

LABORATORY

- Evaluate for metabolic derangements such as hyperparathyroidism, vitamin C or D deficiencies, and calcium/phosphate abnormalities
- DNA studies may be indicated for familial analysis, prenatal testing, and genetic counseling
- Tissue biopsy is controversial but may help differentiate from tumors

DIFFERENTIAL DIAGNOSIS

- Nonaccidental trauma in children
- Ehlers-Danlos syndrome
- Hypophosphatasia
- Achondroplasia
- Scurvy
- Congenital syphilis
- Celiac disease

Treatment

INITIAL STABILIZATION

- ABCs of trauma come first, depending on the mechanism of injury
- Fracture immobilization/splinting

ED TREATMENT

- Specific fracture management dictated by type and location of injury
- Orthopedic consultation regarding the need for traction or internal fixation (open versus external)
- No specific treatment for osteogenesis imperfecta exists at present

MEDICATIONS

- Pain medications as indicated
- Elderly females may benefit from calcium (1–1.5 g/day) and estrogen replacement (0.625 mg/day)

Disposition

ADMISSION CRITERIA

- Admission is determined by multiple trauma or operative needs for fracture repair
- Pediatric patients may need admission to investigate the possibility of nonaccidental trauma

DISCHARGE CRITERIA

- Patients may be considered for outpatient management if isolated fracture present and appropriate home resources are available
- Most patients should be discharged with orthopedic and primary physician follow-up

Miscellaneous

ICD9: 756.51

CORE CONTENT CODE: 10.1.2

SUGGESTED READINGS

Chandrasoma P, Taylor CR. Concise pathology. East Norwalk: Appleton & Lange, 1991.

McKusick VA. Heritable disorders of connective tissue. 4th ed. St. Louis: CV Mosby, 1972.

Prockop DJ. Heritable disorders of connective tissue. In: Wilson JD, et al., eds. Harrison's principles of internal medicine. 12th ed. New York: McGraw Hill, 1991:1860 Wilson JD.

Sillence DO. Osteogenesis imperfecta: An expanding panorama of variance. Clin Orthop 1981;Sep (159):11–25.

Author: Daniel Davis

Osteomyelitis

Clinical Presentation

SIGNS AND SYMPTOMS

- Pain can be localized, deep, dull, and throbbing
- Chills and fever though may be absent
- Malaise
- Nausea, vomiting
- Tenderness and warmth to palpation
- Edema
- Erythema, drainage of sinus tract can be present due to chronic infection
- Reluctance to use extremity
- Antalgic gait or reluctance to walk

MECHANISM/DESCRIPTION

- Osteomyelitis (OM) is an infection of bone with ongoing inflammatory destruction and apposition of bone. It is usually bacterial in origin but fungal osteomyelitis does exist

ETIOLOGY

Hematogenous OM

- Infection caused by seeding of bacteria to bone from a remote site of infection
- Often after bacteremia in prepubertal children and the elderly
- Neonates: *S. aureus,* Enterobacteriaceae, and Group A & B Streptococci
- Children: *S. aureus,* Group A Streptococci, *H. Influenza,* Enterobacteriaceae
  - —*Salmonella* is the most common organism found in children with *sickle cell disease*
- Adults: *S. aureus,* occasionally Enterobacteriaceae, *Pseudomonas,* Gram-negative rods
- Illicit drug users: *Candida* and *Pseudomonas*
- Prolonged neutropenia: *Candida*

Hematogenous Vertebral OM

- Uncommon
- Most prevalent in adults >45 years of age
- Commonly involves the disk and vertebra above and below
- Often history of long-term urinary catheter placement or intravenous drug use
- *Pseudomonas* or Candida
- Lumbar vertebrae involved, followed by thoracic, then cervical

Direct or Contiguous OM

- Organism(s) directly seeded in bone due to trauma; spread from an adjacent site of infection or from surgery
- More common in adults and adolescents
- *S. aureus,* Enterobacteriaceae, Pseudomonas
- Normal vascularity
  - —*S. aureus* and *S. epidermis,* Gram-negative bacilli, and anaerobic organisms
- Vascular insufficiency/diabetes
  - —Small bones of feet are common sites
  - —Infection develops due to minor trauma, infected nail beds, cellulitis, or skin ulceration
  - —Polymicrobial infection is common, including anaerobes
- Puncture wound through a tennis shoe causes infection due to *S. aureus, Pseudomonas*

Chronic OM

- Osteomyelitis that persists or recurs regardless of the initial insult
- Most distinguishing characteristic is necrotic bone

Pre-Hospital

N/A

Diagnosis

- The standard for diagnosis is microbiologic and histopathologic exam of the bone
- Polymorphonuclear cells are highly suggestive of osteomyelitis
- Positive culture of the bone for bacterial pathogen confirms the diagnosis

ESSENTIAL WORKUP

- CBC; WBC count may be elevated but frequently is normal
- ESR is usually elevated
- Blood cultures
- X-rays
- Culture from bone biopsy
  - —Culture of sinus or drainage from wound can be misleading

IMAGING/SPECIAL TESTS

- X-rays
  - —Initially can be normal
  - —Deep soft tissue swelling may be evident
  - —At 10–12 days, bone lysis and periosteal elevation may be detectable
  - —40–50% of focal bone loss is needed to detect a lucency on X-rays
- Bone scan
  - —^{99}Tc-methylene diphosphonate
  - —Increase in bone metabolic activity
  - —Highly sensitive but less specific than MRI
  - —Bone scan abnormal after 1–2 days of symptoms
- Leukocyte scintigraphy
  - —^{111}In-labeled white blood cells
  - —More specific but less sensitive than bone scan
  - —Difficult to distinguish bone inflammation from soft tissue inflammation
- Computer tomography (CT)
  - —Often reveals bone edema, cortical destruction, periosteal reaction, joint surface damage and soft tissue involvement when plain films are not helpful
  - —Needle-guided biopsies
  - —Useful in vertebral osteomyelitis
- Magnetic resonance imaging (MRI)
  - —Reveals bone edema, cortical destruction, periosteal reaction, joint surface damage, and soft tissue involvement when plane films are not helpful
  - —Effective in early detection
  - —Diagnosis of osteomyelitis may be evident by MRI before scintigraphy
  - —Best for identifying spinal infection
  - —Rapidly replacing CT

DIFFERENTIAL DIAGNOSIS

- Cellulitis
- Paronychia
- Felon
- Bursitis
- Extremity fracture
- Mechanical back pain
- Toxic synovitis
- Septic arthritis
- Spinal epidural abscess

PEDIATRIC CONSIDERATIONS

- 70–85% of children have a fever >38.5°C
- Neonates commonly afebrile
- Only 31% of children will have leukocytosis
- Blood cultures are positive in 50% of cases
- Growth plate infection can lead to asymmetric limb length and limb deformity

Treatment

INITIAL STABILIZATION

- Emergent stabilization only if septic

ED TREATMENT

- Empirical antibiotic treatment should be initiated in the emergency department and cultures should guide subsequent antibiotic regimen
- Antibiotic regimen depends on patient's age and the organism cultured
- Orthopedic and infectious disease consultation
- Surgical intervention may be needed to optimize treatment (e.g., infected fracture, extensive bone necrosis)
- Parenteral antibiotic treatment for 4–6 weeks

Hematogenous OM

- Neonate–4 years: penicillinase-resistant synthetic penicillin (e.g., nafcillin) plus a third-generation cephalosporin; alternative: vancomycin plus a third-generation cephalosporin
- 4 years–adult: penicillinase-resistant synthetic penicillin and third-generation cephalosporin if stain is Gram-negative bacilli; alternatives: vancomycin *or* clindamycin plus a third-generation cephalosporin if Gram-negative bacilli are present on stain
- Adult: penicillinase-resistant synthetic penicillin *or* cefazolin; alternative: Vancomycin
- Sickle cell anemia with OM *(S. aureus* and salmonella): fluoroquinolone antibiotic (*not* in children); alternative: third-generation cephalosporin (e.g., ceftriaxone)
- Postnail puncture through a tennis shoe: ceftazidime; alternative: ciprofloxacin
- Posttraumatic OM: nafcillin plus ciprofloxacin; alternatives: vancomycin plus third-generation cephalosporin with antipseudomonal activity

PEDIATRIC CONSIDERATIONS

- Children with hematogenous OM may undergo short course of intravenous antibiotics and then be changed to oral antibiotics for an additional 1–2 months

MEDICATIONS

DRUG	ADULT DOSE	PEDIATRIC DOSE
Cefazolin	2 g IV q 8 hrs	20 mg/kg IV q 8 hrs
Ceftazidime	2 g IV q 8 hrs	150 mg/kg/day divided q 8 hrs (maximum 6 g/d)
Ceftriaxone	2 g IV qd	75 mg/kg/day IV given once per day
Ciprofloxacin	200–400 mg IV q 12 hrs	Contraindicated
Nafcillin	1–2 g IV/IM q 4 hrs	100–200 mg/kg/day divided q 6 hrs

Disposition

ADMISSION CRITERIA

- Patients with acute osteomyelitis should be admitted for parenteral antibiotics

DISCHARGE CRITERIA

- Selected patients with subacute or chronic OM may be considered for outpatient management if home health care resources and home parenteral antibiotics can be arranged

Miscellaneous

ICD9: 730.20

CORE CONTENT CODE: 10.1.3

SUGGESTED READINGS

Hass DW, McAndrew MP. Bacterial osteomyelitis in adults: Evolving considerations in diagnosis and treatment. Am J Med 1996;101(5):550–561.

Jaramillo D, Treves ST, Kasser JR. Osteomyelitis and septic arthritis in children: Appropriate use of imaging to guide treatment. AJR Am J Roentgenol 1995;165:399–403.

Lew DP, Waldvogel FA. Osteomyelitis: Current concepts. N Engl J Med 1997;336:99–107.

Maguire JH. Osteomyelitis and infections of prosthetic joints. In Isselbacher KJ, Braunwald E, Wilson JD, Martin JB, Fauci AS, Kasper DL, eds. Harrison's principles of internal medicine. 13th ed. New York: McGraw Hill, 1994:358–360.

Authors: Boris Lubavin; Federico Vaca

Osteoporosis

Clinical Presentation

SIGNS AND SYMPTOMS

- Usually asymptomatic until pathologic fractures occur
- Fractures with insignificant mechanism or recurrent fractures are hallmark
- Vertebral column most commonly involved
- Multiple compression fractures of vertebral column often lead to kyphosis and scoliosis
- Hip fractures (femoral neck and intertrochanteric fractures) also common

MECHANISM/DESCRIPTION

- Overall decrease in skeletal mass, generally diffuse
- Trabecular bone (especially vertebrae and femur) affected more commonly and earlier
- Disease begins in adolescence, but fractures do not usually manifest until age 50 or greater
- Females affected much more commonly than males, especially postmenopause

ETIOLOGY

- Overall increase in resorption over formation of new bone
- Advanced age is most important risk factor
- Inadequate dietary calcium important factor, especially early in life
- Sedentary lifestyle is risk factor (weight-bearing on bone favors new bone formation)
- Decreases in estrogen with menopause is a key factor in women
- Other causes include long-term steroid use, alcoholism, methotrexate
- May be a familial or hereditary factor as well

PEDIATRIC CONSIDERATIONS

- Although disease appears to start in adolescence, pediatric patients are asymptomatic

Pre-Hospital

CAUTIONS

- Obtain pre-hospital information on mechanism to help diagnose pathologic nature of fracture
- Avoid aggressive manipulation or movement of patient as this may exacerbate bony injury

Diagnosis

ESSENTIAL WORKUP

- Fracture without significant mechanism and identification of risk factors is most important
- Careful neurovascular examination distal to femur or other extremity fracture
- Rectal tone and postvoid residual determination should be done in patients with vertebral fractures
- Radiographs of suspected fracture may show osteopenia (late finding in disease)
- Spine films may show old compression fractures
- CT scan should be performed to better evaluate vertebral fractures
  - —Retropulsion, spinal canal compromise is not always apparent on plain films
  - —Make sure CT cuts extend a full level above and below injuries identified on spine x-rays

LABORATORY

- Serum chemistries, such as calcium, parathyroid hormone, alkaline phosphatase, may help differentiate between illnesses listed above

IMAGING/SPECIAL TESTS

- Plain films can identify fractures; however, the age of each fracture may be difficult to determine
- Bone scan or computerized tomography help determine the age of fractures, especially in the spine
- Newer bone density determinations can provide prognostic information and help guide therapy

DIFFERENTIAL DIAGNOSIS

- Multiple myeloma or other metastatic tumor
- Osteogenesis imperfecta (usually apparent in childhood)
- Hyperparathyroidism
- Other demineralizing bone diseases

Treatment

INITIAL STABILIZATION

- Immobolize fractures

ED TREATMENT

- Fractures are treated with the expectation of delayed or incomplete healing
- Prevention is far more effective than treatment
- Long-term therapy is beneficial (see Medications)
- Use of orthotic back braces and vests should be arranged in conjunction with orthopedic spine specialists
- Exercise is also helpful
- Balance must be achieved between osteoporosis risk and steroid or methotrexate therapy

MEDICATIONS

- Alendronate: 10mg/day
- Estrogen: 0.625 mg/day (with or without medroxyprogesterone) for virtually all postmenopausal women
- Calcium supplementation (often with vitamin D): 1–1.5 g/day
- Calcitonin: 0.5 mg/day SQ of human, 100 IU/day SQ of salmon
- Etidronate: 400 mg/day for 2-week cycles every 15 weeks
- Sodium fluoride: 25 mg bid with calcium

PEDIATRIC CONSIDERATIONS

- Ensure adequate calcium in diet from early age

Disposition

ADMISSION CRITERIA

- As per normal orthopedic protocols, with special considerations for age and social situation
- Compression fractures are generally stable, but the possibility of a burst fracture with cord compression must be ruled out
- Any cervical fracture or fracture with neurologic symptoms requires admission with emergent consultation with neurosurgery or orthopedics
- Admission may be necessary for pain control and because of decreased ambulation

DISCHARGE CRITERIA

- As per normal orthopedic protocols, with special considerations for age and social situation
- Patients with minimal injuries, able to care for themselves at home, or with appropriate assistance, and adequate po pain control may be discharged with orthopedic spine follow-up

Miscellaneous

ICD9: 733.00

CORE CONTENT CODE: 10.1.6

SUGGESTED READINGS

Chandrasoma P, Taylor CR. Concise pathology. East Norwalk: Appleton & Lange, 1991.

Krane SM, Holick MF. Metabolic bone disease. In: Wilson JD, et al., eds. Harrison's principles of internal medicine. 12th ed. New York: McGraw Hill, 1991:1921.

Prestwood KM, Kenny AM. Osteoporosis: pathogenesis diagnosis, and treatment in older adults. Clin in Geriatric Med. 1988 Aug; 14(3):577–99.

Raisz LG. Local and systemic factors in the pathogenesis of osteoporosis. N Engl J Med 1988;318:818–828.

Author: Daniel Davis

Otitis Externa

Clinical Presentation

SIGNS AND SYMPTOMS

- Itching of the external ear canal is usually the first symptom
- Pain in ear or with motion of pinna/tragus
- Swollen, erythematous external ear canal
- Ear drainage
  - —Cheesy white or gray green exudate
- Decreased auditory acuity
- Clogged sensation in ear
- Pain/swelling in preauricular area

Malignant Otitis Externa

- Pain, tenderness, swelling in periauricular area
- Headache
- Otorrhea
- Cranial nerve palsy
  - —Facial nerve most affected

MECHANISM/DESCRIPTION

- Inflammation or infection of the auricle, auditory canal, or external surface of the tympanic membrane
  - —Spares the middle ear
- Also called "swimmer's ear" due to the usual history of recent swimming
  - —Occasional cases after normal bathing
- Predisposing factors include
  - —History of ear surgery or TM perforation
  - —Narrow or abnormal canal
  - —Humidity
  - —Allergy
  - —Trauma
  - —Abnormal cerumen production
- Malignant otitis externa
  - —Occurs in adults with diabetes mellitus
  - —Necrotizing external otitis
  - —Caused by *P. aeruginosa*
  - —Infection starts at ear canal and progresses through periauricular tissue toward base of skull

ETIOLOGY

- Often precipitated by an abrasion of the ear canal or maceration of the skin from persisting water or excessive dryness
- Multiple organisms, but particularly *P. aeruginosa,* play a role in this disease

Pre-Hospital

N/A

Diagnosis

ESSENTIAL WORKUP

- Clinical diagnosis with typical signs/symptoms
  - —Otoscopic examination

LABORATORY

- None usually indicated except when possibility of malignant otitis externa
  - —In elderly, diabetic, or other immunocompromised patients with otorrhea and intense ear pain
  - —Signs of systemic toxicity, or local spread of infection should be checked
- WBC
- ESR
- Cultures

DIFFERENTIAL DIAGNOSIS

- Malignant otitis externa
- Otitis media
- Folliculitis from obstruction of sebaceous glands
- Otic foreign bodies
- Herpes zoster infection of the geniculate ganglion
- Parotitis
- Periauricular adenitis
- Mastoiditis
- Dental abscess
- Sinusitis
- Tonsillitis
- Pharyngitis
- Temporomandibular joint pain

Treatment

ED TREATMENT

- Clean external ear canal
  - —Remove the inflammatory debris by gentle curettage with a cotton-tipped wire applicator
  - —Occasional suction with a Fraser suction tip may be necessary
- Insert a cotton or gauze wick 10–12 mm into the canal after cleansing, if the ear canal is very edematous
- Antibiotics
  - —Topical
    - -Antiseptic, anti-inflammatory, and drying otic drops
    - -Eliminates the pathogenic bacteria and allows for rapid healing of the canal
    - -Either acetic acid solutions such as domeboro-otic or a combination of antibiotics and corticosteroids such as cortisporin applied in 4 drops qid
    - -Use suspensions and not solutions with suspected tympanic membrane perforation
  - —Oral
    - -For concurrent otitis media: Amoxicillin, Bactrim DS
    - -Strongly consider when the tympanic membrane cannot be visualized
    - -Treat diabetics and other immunocompromised patients with oral ciprofloxacin and follow closely for symptoms of malignant otitis externa
- Prophylaxis
  - —Apply rubbing alcohol or acetic acid (2%) to keep the external ear canal dry and prevent recurrence of infection
- Proven or suspected malignant otitis externa
  - —Initiate parenteral antibiotics such as a third-generation cephalosporin or an antipseudomonal penicillin
- Complications
  - —Chronic use of antibiotics/corticosteroids may lead to overgrowth of fungi such as aspergillus in the ear canal
  - —Toxicity
  - —Meningitis
  - —Facial palsy
  - —Local spread of infection leading to necrotizing otitis externa
  - —Osteomyelitis
  - —Malignant otitis externa
    - -Requires immediate admission and treatment with intravenous antibiotics (ciprofloxacin or aminoglycoside/semisynthetic penicillin)
    - -CT/MRI to exclude osteomyelitis
- Patient instructions
  - —Avoid swimming and keep ears completely dry for 3–4 weeks
  - —Apply medications as directed

—Return if worse pain, fever, hearing loss develops, or if there is any change in mental or neurological status
—Follow up if symptoms are not improved within 2–3 days

MEDICATIONS

- Amoxicillin: 500 mg (peds: 40 mg/kg/24 hrs) po tid
- Ciprofloxacin: 500 mg po or 400 mg IV bid
- Corticosporin otic (hydrocortisone 1%, polymyxin + neomycin) suspension: 4 drops to ear canal qid
- Domeboro otic (2% acetic acid): 4–6 drops q 4–6 hrs
- Trimethoprim/sulfamethoxazole (bactrim DS or suspension): 1 tablet (peds: 5 ml suspension per 10 kg per dose) po bid

Disposition

ADMISSION CRITERIA

- Malignant otitis externa
- Significant involvement of the pinna
- Signs of systemic illness

DISCHARGE CRITERIA

- Most patients who are on topical antibiotics
- Close followup for patients at risk for otitis externa
- ENT followup for worsening of symptoms or failure of initial management

Miscellaneous

ICD9: 380.10

CORE CONTENT CODE: 6.1.6

SUGGESTED READINGS

Severance H Jr. Acute otitis externa. In: Harwood-Nuss AL, Linden CH, et al, eds. The clinical practice of emergency medicine. 2d ed. Philadelphia: Lippincott-Raven, 1996:112–115.

Stair T. Otolaryngologic disorders. In: Rosen P, Barkin R, et al., eds. Emergency medicine: concepts and clinical practice. 4th ed. St. Louis: CV Mosby, 1992: 2460–2469.

Author: Assaad J. Sayah

Otitis Media

Clinical Presentation

SIGNS AND SYMPTOMS

General

- Fever
- Irritability
- Rhinitis
- Vomiting, diarrhea

Otolaryngologic

- Ear pain
- Pulling at ear
- Tympanic membrane
  - —Full visualization essential
  - —Increased vascularity, erythema, purulence
  - —Obscured landmarks—bony, light reflex
  - —Pneumatic otoscopy—mobility, bulging, retracted
- Vertigo, tinnitus
- Exclude associated illnesses

Complications

- Persistent, recurrent otitis media
- Perforated tympanic membrane
- Serous otitis media
- Conductive hearing loss
- Facial nerve injury
- Mastoiditis
- Cholesteatoma
- Meningitis, subdural empyema, venous sinus thrombosis

MECHANISM/DESCRIPTION

- Usually associated with upper respiratory tract infection
- Blockage of eustachian tube because of sharp angle and size
- Predisposing factors
  - —Deficient mucous, cilia, or antibodies
  - —Intubation, especially nasotracheal
  - —American Indians, Eskimos
  - —Down's syndrome

ETIOLOGY

- Usually infectious
- Viral: parainfluenza, respiratory syncytial virus, influenza, adenovirus
- Bacterial: *S. pneumoniae, Branhamella catarrhalis, H. Influenzae,* group A streptococcus
- *Mycoplasma pneumoniae*

Pre-Hospital

- Assess for associated conditions

Diagnosis

ESSENTIAL WORKUP

- Exclude associated conditions
- Otoscopic examination for appearance and mobility of membrane

LABORATORY

- Cultures unhelpful unless done by tympanocentesis

IMAGING/SPECIAL TESTS

- CT Scan of head/sinuses if associated infection is considered
- Tympanocentesis—indications
  - —Severe pain or toxicity
  - —Failure of antimicrobial therapy
  - —Suspicion of suppurative complication
  - —Sick neonate
  - —Immunocompromised patient
- Tympanometry and acoustic otoscopy may be useful with difficult examinations

DIFFERENTIAL DIAGNOSIS

- Infection
  - —External otitis media
  - —Mastoiditis
  - —Dental abscess
  - —Peritonsillar abscess
  - —Sinusitis
  - —Lymphadenitis
  - —Parotitis
  - —Meningitis
- Trauma
  - —Perforation of the tympanic membrane
  - —Foreign body in ear
  - —Barotrauma
  - —Instrumentation
- Serous otitis media or eustachian tube dysfunction
- Impacted ear cerumen
- Impacted third molar
- Temporomandibular joint dysfunction

Treatment

INITIAL STABILIZATION

- Evaluate and manage associated conditions

ED TREATMENT

- After evaluation antibiotics are usually initiated for 10–14 days
- Considerations should include recurrent nature of otitis media, lack of clinical response, and resistance patterns in community
- Parenteral antibiotics indicated in febrile toxic children <1 year of age or with immunocompromise
- Antihistamines and decongestants have no proven efficacy

MEDICATIONS

- Amoxicillin: 40 mg/kg/day po tid
- Trimethoprim (TMP)-sulfamethoxazole: 8 mg TMP/kg/day po bid
- Cefaclor: 50 mg/kg/day po tid
- Amoxicillin-clavulanic acid: 50 mg AMX/kg/day po tid

Disposition

ADMISSION CRITERIA

- Febrile toxic children who are
  —<1 year of age, immunocompromised
  —Moderately or severely dehydrated
  —Unable to tolerate oral fluids or medications
  —Suspected or proven associated significant infection
  —Suspected abuse
  —Unreliable caretaker

DISCHARGE CRITERIA

- Children without any of the above criteria
- Followup in 10–14 days to assure resolution or earlier if:
  —child does not get better in 24–48 hours
  —There is any progression of signs or symptoms
  —New problems develop including a rash
  —Any concerns arise

Miscellaneous

ICD9: 382.9

CORE CONTENT CODE: 13.7.6, 6.1.8

SUGGESTED READINGS

Barkin RM. Acute otitis media. In: Barkin RM, Rosen P. Emergency pediatrics. 5th ed. St. Louis: CV Mosby, 1999:545–548.

Koranyi K. Otitis media and mastoiditis. In: Harwood-Nuss A, et al., eds. The clinical practice of emergency medicine. 2d ed. Philadelphia: Lippincott-Raven, 1996: 545–548.

Severance H. Acute otitis media in adults. In: Harwood-Nuss A, et al., eds. The clinical practice of emergency medicine. 2d ed. Philadelphia: Lippincott-Raven, 1996: 545–548.

Author: Assaad J. Sayah

Otologic Trauma

Clinical Presentation

SIGNS AND SYMPTOMS

- Bleeding, deformed, swollen, or erythematous ear
- Laceration or hematoma may be present

MECHANISM/DESCRIPTION

- Blunt trauma or shearing forces cause a subperiosteal hematoma
  —Cartilage is separated from the perichondrium
  —Cartilage has no intrinsic blood supply and relies on the perichondrium
  —A subperiosteal hematoma deprives the cartilage of nutrients, potentially resulting in necrosis, and predisposing to infection
  —The risk of infection is increased if the overlying skin is penetrated or lacerated
  —Recurrent or untreated injuries may lead to cauliflower ear
- Ear lacerations and dog bites can expose ear cartilage
  —Infection or erosion may result if the injury is not treated properly

Pre-Hospital

- Transport an avulsed auricle in a cold solution not in direct contact with ice
- Wrap first with moist gauze and place in plastic bag

Diagnosis

ESSENTIAL WORKUP

- History and physical examination including tetanus status
- Otoscopic examination of the external canal and tympanic membrane should be performed
- Hearing loss may require a further audiologic workup
- Examine for concomitant head trauma

LABORATORY

- Wound cultures may be considered in bite wounds or other grossly infected wounds

DIFFERENTIAL DIAGNOSIS

- Infection of the ear
- Hemangioma

Treatment

INITIAL STABILIZATION

- ABCs of trauma care
- Cover exposed cartilage with sterile dressings
- Manage avulsed parts as in pre-hospital section

ED TREATMENT

Hematoma

- To prevent permanent deformity, complete evacuation of the subperichondrial hematoma is necessary
  —Reapproximation of the perichondrium to the cartilage must be performed
  —*Needle aspiration*
    –A 20-gauge needle with syringe is inserted and the hematoma is milked until completely evacuated
    –A pressure dressing is then applied
    –The ear needs to be reexamined frequently to detect reaccumulation of hematoma
    –Reaspiration is necessary if fluid reaccumulates
  —*Incision* is a more effective treatment, especially for larger hematomas
    –It may be performed if the hematoma is less than 7 days old
    –Anesthetize the overlying skin with 1% lidocaine (no epinephrine)
    –A circumferential auricular block may also be used
    –With a No. 15 scalpel incise the skin at the edge of the hematoma along the natural skin folds
    –Evacuate the hematoma and irrigate the cavity
    –Close the incision with 6–0 chromic interrupted sutures
    –A pressure dressing or dental roles sutured into position over the area is needed to prevent reaccumulation of blood
    –The dental rolls should be left in place for 7–10 days
  —Antistaphylococcal antibiotics for 10 days are needed because of possible chondritis
    –Hematomas over 7 days old need surgical referral because new perichondrial growth must be débrided to prevent auricular deformity

Laceration

- Cover exposed cartilage and minimize wound hematoma
- Débride jagged or devitalized cartilage and skin
- If the skin cannot be stretched to cover the defect additional cartilage along the wound margin can be removed
- Reapproximate major landmarks of the pinna using 4–0 or 5–0 absorbable sutures

- Sutures tear through cartilage, so the perichondrium should be included in the stitch
- In through and through lacerations, first reapproximate the posterior surface and then the anterior surface
  - —Use 5–0 or 6–0 nonabsorbable synthetic sutures, joining the landmarks point by point
  - —Evert the wound at the helical rim to avoid notching
  - —A lacerated ear that has been sutured needs a compression dressing
- Tetanus status needs to be addressed

Dog Bites

- Bites that are clean, less than 5 hours old, and not from human bite can be closed primarily in the same manner as other ear lacerations and with the placement of a compressive dressing
- Highly contaminated, severely contused, old injuries (longer than 24 hours), and dog bites older than 5 hours need to be treated open because of the high risk of infection
  - —Dress with sterile, compressive dressing
- Tetanus status and rabies prevention should be addressed
- All patients should receive prophylactic antibiotics for 10 days (augmentin)
- For human bites, consult plastic surgery or ENT specialist

MEDICATIONS

- For hematomas, nonhuman bite lacerations, and dog bites: antistaphylococcal antibiotics for 7–10 days
- Augmentin (amoxicillin-clavulanate): adult: 875/125 mg po tid; peds: 40 mg/kg/day po divided tid

PEDIATRIC CONSIDERATIONS

- Ear trauma suggests possibility of nonaccidental trauma

Disposition

ADMISSION CRITERIA

- Associated serious head trauma
- Severe cosmetic defects requiring operative repair
- Need for intravenous antibiotics
- Unable to take po antibiotics
- Immunosuppressed persons with serious infections, perichondritis, or chondritis

DISCHARGE CRITERIA

- Able to take po antibiotics and appropriate follow-up for wound check

Miscellaneous

ICD9: 959.09

CORE CONTENT CODE: 18.4.7

SUGGESTED READINGS

Clemons JE, Severeid LR. Trauma. In: Cummings C, et al. Otolaryngology—Head and neck surgery. 2d ed. St. Louis: Mosby-Year Book, 1993.

Gilmer PA. Trauma of the auricle. In: Bailey BJ, et al. Head and neck surgery—Otolaryngology. Philadelphia: JB Lippincott, 1993.

Lammers RL, Trott AT. Methods of wound closure. In: Roberts JR, Hedges JR, eds. Clinical procedures in emergency medicine. 3rd ed. Philadelphia: WB Saunders, 1998.

Manthey DE, Harrison BP. Otolaryngologic procedures. In: Roberts JR, Hedges JR, eds. Clinical procedures in emergency medicine. 3rd ed. Philadelphia: WB Saunders, 1998.

Potsic WP, Cotton RT, Handler SD. Surgical pediatric otolaryngology. New York: Thieme Medical Publishers, 1997.

Stucker FJ, et al. Management of animal and human bites in the head and neck. Arch Otolaryngol Head Neck Surg 1990;116:789–793.

Weber EJ, Callaham M. Animal bites and rabies. In: Rosen P, et al., eds. Emergency medicine: Concepts and clinical practice. 4th ed. St. Louis: Mosby-Year Book, 1998.

Author: Tim J. Wells

Ovarian Cyst/Torsion

Clinical Presentation

SIGNS AND SYMPTOMS

Ovarian Cyst

- Sudden, sharp, unilateral pelvic pain
- Onset often with exercise, intercourse, trauma, or pelvic exam
- Abdominal tenderness, adnexal tenderness, adnexal mass, peritoneal signs
- Fever rare
- Hemorrhagic shock if large ovarian vessel torn, hemoperitoneum, dizziness, orthostasis, syncope (usually from a corpus luteal cyst rupture)

Adnexal Torsion

- Sudden, sharp, unilateral, constant pain is typical, but may have a dull ache with sharp exacerbations if torsion is intermittent
  —Pain generally increases with time but may subside
- Onset is often with exercise or intercourse
- Nausea, vomiting, apprehension
- Occasionally will have abnormal vaginal bleeding and UTI symptoms
- Usually afebrile but may have low grade fever, tachycardia
- Exam ranges from mild lower abdominal pain with localized rebound tenderness to frank peritonitis
- Large adnexal mass is most important finding

ETIOLOGY

Ovarian Cyst

- Cysts are generally asymptomatic until complicated by hemorrhage, torsion, rupture, or infection. Follicular cysts are by far the most common; however, corpus luteal cysts are more clinically significant
- Rupture of a follicular cyst during ovulation causes mittelschmerz, pain is secondary to rupture of cyst and a small leakage of blood
- Rupture of a corpus luteum cyst is similar to mittelschmerz except pain occurs just before menses begins, usually days 20–26 of menstrual cycle
- Hemorrhage into a cyst distends capsule and also may cause pain without rupture

Adnexal Torsion

- Twisting of the vascular pedicle of an ovary, fallopian tube, or para-tubal cyst, causes ischemia. Occlusion of lymphatics and venous drainage lead to rapid enlargement. Risk factors for torsion include
  —Intrinsic factors: ovarian cyst, tumor, hydrosalpinx, pyosalpinx
  —Extrinsic factors: pelvic adhesions, tubal ligation, masses, trauma

Pre-Hospital

- Patients with acute pelvic pain may become hemodynamically unstable so intravenous access is essential

Diagnosis

ESSENTIAL WORKUP

- Pregnancy test is essential to rule out an ectopic pregnancy
- Rapid hemoglobin determination

LABORATORY

- Complete blood count to evaluate hematocrit and white blood cell count
  —Leukocytosis is uncommon with cysts and common with torsion
- Urinalysis may be useful in patients with UTI symptoms
- Type and cross PRBCs for patients with significant hemorrhage

IMAGING/SPECIAL TESTS

- Ultrasonography will often reveal evidence of torsion or precipitating pathology as well as demonstrate ovarian cysts
- Adnexal cystic masses less than 8 cm in premenopausal women are generally benign and should be reevaluated at the end of menstruation
- Culdocentesis is usually negative but may yield serosanguineous fluid, hematocrit >15% suggests significant hemoperitoneum

SPECIAL CONSIDERATIONS

- Anticoagulated patients are at increased risk of having a hemorrhagic corpus luteal cyst and of having a significant bleed from a ruptured cyst. These patients also may have a significant bleed secondary to ovulation or "mittelschmerz"

DIFFERENTIAL DIAGNOSIS

- In addition to adnexal torsion and ruptured ovarian cyst, the differential diagnosis for acute pelvic pain includes the following
  —Ectopic pregnancy
  —Appendicitis
  —Tuboovarian abscess
  —Ruptured endometrioma ("chocolate cyst")
- The differential diagnosis of an adnexal mass also includes
  —Benign tumors (Teratoma or "dermoid cyst" most common)
  —Malignant tumors
  —Polycystic ovaries

Treatment

INITIAL STABILIZATION

- ABCs
  - —Patients in shock should receive supplemental oxygen and intubation as indicated for respiratory failure
  - —Intravenous access and volume replacement with normal saline or lactated ringers solution or blood transfusion when indicated

ED TREATMENT

Follicular Cyst

- Uncomplicated rupture of a serous cyst needs only analgesics and observation

Adnexal torsion

- Immediate admission to the OR

MEDICATIONS

- Acetaminophen: adult: 325–650 mg q 4 hrs; peds: 15 mg/kg (max 650 mg) po q 4 hrs
- Ibuprofen: adult: 400–600 mg po q 6 hrs; peds: 5–10 mg/kg/dose po q 6 hrs
- Morphine sulfate: adult: 2–4 mg IV q 5 min; peds: 0.1 mg/kg/dose q 5 min (max 15 mg)

Disposition

ADMISSION CRITERIA

- Culdocentesis fluid hematocrit >15%
- Significant hemorrhage ascertained by serial hematocrits, orthostasis, culdocentesis, or evidence of shock
- All patients with torsion need admission for emergent surgery

DISCHARGE CRITERIA

- Stable patients with a ruptured follicular cyst and those with a ruptured corpus luteal cyst without a coagulopathy and without evidence of significant hemorrhage can be discharged with close follow-up with a gynecologist

Miscellaneous

ICD9: 620.2, 620.5

CORE CURRICULUM CODE: 19.1.1.1, 19.1.1.2

SUGGESTED READINGS

Baker EB, Copas PR. Adnexal torsion: A clinical dilemma. J Reprod Med 1995;40:447–449.

Bernardus RE, et al. Torsion of the fallopian tube: Some considerations on its etiology. Obstet Gynecol 1984;64:675–78.

Tanos, Scheaher JG. Ovarian cysts: a clinical dilemma. Gynecol Endocrinol. 1994: Mar 8(1): 59-67.

Author: Kyan J. Berger

Clinical Presentation

SIGNS AND SYMPTOMS

Paget's disease involves the resorption of normal bone and its replacement with fibrous and sclerotic tissue. It is also known as osteitis deformans

- Usually focal, involvement frequency is (most frequent to least frequent): pelvis; femur; skull; tibia; spine; flat bones
- Many patients are asymptomatic with the disease discovered by incidental radiographs or elevated alkaline phosphatase levels
- *Acute (resorptive/osteolytic) phase*
  - —*Pathologic fractures*
  - —Pain from acute lysis, pathologic fracture, or resultant arthritis
  - —Hypercalcemia or *renal stones*
  - —*Hypervascularity* may result in significant bleeding complications and hematoma formation if affected bone is fractured
  - —With widespread disease, increased vascularity and blood flow may result in *high-output cardiac failure*
- *Secondary (sclerotic/osteoplastic) phase*
  - —Long bone involvement may present with swelling or deformity and resultant gait abnormality
  - —Skull involvement may lead to headaches or abnormal skull contours (change in hat size)
  - —Severe skull or spine involvement may result in CNS compression
  - —Hearing loss may result from nerve compression or ossicle involvement
  - —Sarcoma occurs in less than 1% of patients

MECHANISM/DESCRIPTION

- Occurs in approximately 3% of patients over age 40 years
- Starts with resorptive or osteolytic phase during which osteoclasts remove otherwise healthy bone
- Hypervascularity begins in the resorptive phase and predisposes to hematoma formation
- Eventually resorbed bone is replaced by irregular, dense, disorganized trabecular bone in the sclerotic or osteoplastic phase
- Rarely malignant transformation occurs
  - —*Osteosarcoma* is the malignancy of concern
  - —Usually malignant transformation occurs in no more than 1%

ETIOLOGY

- Unknown
- Possibly represents vascular hyperplasia with subsequent inflammation
- Presence of nucleocapsids from measles, canine distemper, or respiratory syncytial virus may implicate a viral etiology
- Familial or genetic component

PEDIATRIC CONSIDERATIONS

- Generally not seen in children

Pre-Hospital

- Pre-hospital personnel should obtain information about mechanism of injury or social factors that suggest pathologic fracture
- Adequate immobilization can limit excessive bleeding around fracture site

Diagnosis

ESSENTIAL WORKUP

- Diagnosis usually suggested by radiographs
- During resorptive phase, lytic lesions are often not seen, except in skull where lesions are well-demarcated ("osteoporosis circumscripta")
- Bowing of long bones may occur with resorption and strength loss
- New bone appears initially as irregular and spotty, then later as homogeneous and dense ("ivory pattern")
- Excess bone may lay along stress lines leading to cortical irregularities
- A thorough neurologic exam must be documented due to possibility of hematoma formation and mass effect, especially with vertebral or pelvis involvement

IMAGING/SPECIAL TESTS

- CT or MRI define margins and help evaluate for neoplasm or hematoma
  - —Spiral CT is becoming the imaging modality of choice to detect renal calculi
- Bone scan is most sensitive for diagnosis of Paget's
- Radionuclide scans (Technetium-99m, Gallium-67) may help guide subsequent therapy by assessing response to current therapy

LABORATORY

- Alkaline phosphatase is the most dramatic marker of disease activity (especially resorptive phase) with any elevation abnormal, but it is most useful to monitor disease activity over time
- Calcium and phosphate levels should be checked as well, but are usually normal
- ECG if suspect hypercalcemia or high output cardiac failure as well as a CXR
- Increased bone formation may be indicated by urine hydroxyproline, serum osteocalcin, or procollagen fragments
- Alterations in parathyroid hormone (PTH) levels occur as secondary changes during the resorptive/osteolytic phase (low PTH) and the sclerotic/osteoplastic phase (high PTH)

DIFFERENTIAL DIAGNOSIS

- Primary hyperparathyroidism
- Multiple myeloma
- Hodgkin variants
- Acromegaly
- Osteosarcoma

Treatment

INITIAL STABILIZATION

- ABCs are always indicated first, depending upon mechanism of injury
- High-output cardiac failure should be treated as indicated in Congestive Heart Failure chapter
- Prompt immobilization of fractures will limit excessive bleeding around fracture site

ED TREATMENT

- Analgesia for the pain of lytic lesions, fractures, or arthritis includes aspirin, indomethacin, narcotics
- High-dose prednisone can suppress disease
- Fracture treatment is often more conservative, due to difficulties with bleeding during operative repair
- Orthopedic referral for severe arthritis and definitive fracture management
- Hypercalcemia may be treated with IV fluids, lasix, calcitonin, inorganic phosphate, etidronate, mitramycin
- Long-term chemotherapy may provide temporary or prolonged remission
- CNS compression requires emergent neurosurgical consultation and possible decompression

MEDICATIONS

- Alendronate: 40mg/day for 6 months
- Calcitonin: 0.5 mg/day SQ of human, 100 IU/day SQ of salmon
- Etidronate: 400 mg/day for 6-month cycles
- Furosemide (lasix): 20–80 mg IV for hypercalcemia
- Inorganic phosphate
- Chemotherapy with plicamycin/mitramycin, dactinomycin, diphosphonate

Disposition

ADMISSION CRITERIA

- Admission as indicated for major trauma or injury, or excessive bleeding
- Orthopedic procedures
- Hypercalcemia
- CNS compressive symptoms

DISCHARGE CRITERIA

- No evidence of significant bleeding, neurologic compromise, or hypercalcemia, and adequate pain control
- Appropriate fracture immobilization and orthopedic follow-up

Miscellaneous

ICD9: 731.0

CORE CONTENT CODE: 10.1.9

SUGGESTED READINGS

Chandrasoma P, Taylor CR. Concise pathology. East Norwalk, CT: Appleton & Lange, 1991.

Favus M. Primer on the metabolic bone diseases and disorders of mineral metabolism. Kelseyville CA: American Society for Bone and Mineral Research, 1990.

Krane SM. Paget's disease of bone. In: Wilson JD, et al., eds. Harrison's principles of internal medicine. 12th ed. New York: McGraw Hill, 1991:1860 Wilson JD.

Ryan WG. Parathyroid hormone, calcitonin, vitamin D, minerals, and metabolic bone diseases. In: Bone RC, Rosen RL, eds. Quick reference to internal medicine. New York: Igaku-Shoin, 1994:1329 Bone RC, Rosen RL.

Singer FR, Wallach S. Paget's disease of bone: Clinical assessment, present and future therapy. New York: Elsevier, 1991.

Author: Daniel Davis

Pancreatic Pseudocyst

Clinical Presentation

SIGNS AND SYMPTOMS

SIGN/SYMPTOM:	FREQUENCY
Abdominal pain	86%
Nausea/vomiting	72%
Palpable mass	49%
Weight loss	35%
Pleural effusion	15%
Jaundice	13%
Ascites	11%
Internal hemorrhage	7%

Gastrointestinal

- In chronic pancreatitis, pseudocyst heralded by change in typical pain pattern
- Symptoms reflecting structural compression by pseudocyst
  —Nausea, vomiting, weight loss—duodenal or gastric outlet obstruction
  —Jaundice—common bile duct compression

Respiratory

- Left lung pleural effusion common

Cardiac

- Commonly occurs with pseudocyst rupture or hemorrhage
- Tachycardia
- Hypotension
- Shock (depending on fluid losses)

Infected Pseudocyst

- Fever
- Chills
- Leukocytosis

Pseudocyst Hemorrhage

- Hypotension
- Expanding abdominal mass
- Usually erodes into splenic or gastroduodenal arteries

Ruptured Pseudocyst

- Abdominal rigidity; severe pain
  —Occurs when cyst ruptures into peritoneal cavity

MECHANISM/DESCRIPTION

- A cystic collection of fluid with a high content of pancreatic enzymes lacking a true epithelial lining
- Localized in parenchyma of pancreas or adjacent abdominal spaces (lesser peritoneal sac)

ETIOLOGY

- Ethanol abuse and biliary disease account for majority of cases
- 45 years is average age at diagnosis
- Occurs more frequently in men than in women
- Complication in 2% of acute pancreatitis; up to 10% of chronic pancreatitis

PEDIATRIC CONSIDERATIONS

- Etiology secondary to congenital malformations

Pre-Hospital

N/A

Diagnosis

ESSENTIAL WORKUP

- Laboratory tests of little help
  —Useful to anticipate complications

LABORATORY

- Amylase
  —Normal value in up to 50% of pseudocysts
- CBC
  —Leukocytosis suggests infected pseudocyst
  —Low Hct with pseudocyst hemorrhage
- Electrolytes, BUN, Cr, glucose
  —Hypocalcemia
  —Hypokalemia with extensive fluid losses
  —Hypomagnesemia with underlying ethanol abuse
  —Hyperglycemia

IMAGING/SPECIAL TESTS

- CT scan
  —Imaging test of choice
  —Indicated for all cases of newly suspected pseudocyst
- Ultrasound
  —Useful for follow-up of previously diagnosed pseudocyst to assess pseudocyst dimensions
- Angiography
  —Helpful in cases of pseudocyst hemorrhage
  —Usually impractical due to instability of patient

DIFFERENTIAL DIAGNOSIS

- Pancreatic abscess
- Neoplastic pancreatic cysts
- Perforated ulcer
- Ruptured abdominal aortic aneurysm (pseudocyst hemorrhage)
- Myocardial infarction
- Biliary colic
- Intestinal obstruction

Treatment

INITIAL STABILIZATION

- ABCs
  - —Supplemental oxygen
  - —Cardiac monitor
  - —0.9%NS IV fluids

ED TREATMENT

- Fluid resuscitation
  - —Fluid losses may necessitate large fluid volumes
  - —Continuously assess vitals, urine output, and electrolytes to ensure rapid and adequate replacement of intravascular volume
  - —Consider CVP monitoring in elderly
- Correct electrolytes abnormalities (hypocalcemia, hypokalemia, hypomagnesemia)
- Blood products
  - —Transfuse immediately in cases of pseudocyst hemorrhage pending definitive surgical treatment
- Analgesia (meperidine)
- Nasogastric suction if intractable nausea/vomiting
- Antiemetics (prochlorperazine)
- Surgical consultation
  - —Emergent surgical consultation mandatory in cases of suspected ruptured pseudocyst or pseudocyst hemorrhage as definitive treatment is emergent laparotomy
  - —Surgical treatment options(pseudocyst >5 cm)
    - -Observation (no acute intervention)
    - -Surgical excision is only possible in few cases
    - -External drainage in critically ill or when cyst wall is immature (reoccurrence rate 20%)
    - -Internal drainage is preferred method in most patients
    - -Percutaneous drainage
    - -Endoscopic drainage

MEDICATIONS

- Calcium gluconate 10%: 10 ml IV over 15–20 min
- Magnesium sulfate: 16 mEq (2 g) in 50 ml D5W over 20 min
- Meperidine (demerol): 25–50 mg IV; 50–75 mg IM q 3–4 hrs
- Potassium chloride: 10 mEq/hr IV
- Prochlorperazine: 5–10 mg IV

Disposition

ADMISSION CRITERIA

- All newly diagnosed pseudocysts >5 cm
- Pseudocysts <5 cm if symptoms of acute pancreatitis
- Previously known pseudocysts if cyst is increasing in size compared to old studies
- Hemodynamic instability
- Severe abdominal pain
- Fever/infected pseudocyst

DISCHARGE CRITERIA

- Refer stable, asymptomatic patient with pseudocyst less than 5 cm for urgent surgical clinic follow-up

Miscellaneous

ICD9: 577.2

CORE CONTENT CODE: 1.4.1.3

SUGGESTED READINGS

Aguilar M, Jones RS, Sanfey H. Pseudocysts of the pancreas: A review of 97 cases. Am Surg 1994;60(9):661–668.

Reber H, Cryer, H. Local complications of pancreatitis including pseudocyst and ascites. In: Valenzuela J, et al., eds. Medical and surgical diseases of the pancreas. New York: Igaku-Shoin, 1991: 73–85.

Maule W, Reber H. Diagnosis and management of pancreatic pseudocysts, pancreatic ascites, and pancreatic fistulas. In: Go V, et al., eds. The pancreas. New York: Raven Press, 1993:71–78.

Author: Trevor Lewis

Pancreatic Trauma

Clinical Presentation

SIGNS AND SYMPTOMS

- Epigastric pain, often out of proportion to physical exam and vital signs
- Soft tissue contusion in upper abdomen
- Injury to lower ribs or costal cartilage
- Acute abdomen, often associated with other intra-abdominal injuries
- Hypotension

MECHANISM/DESCRIPTION

- Most common mechanism is penetrating trauma
- Blunt trauma
  - —Direct epigastric blow compressing pancreas against the vertebral column
  - —Steering wheel or bicycle handlebars to abdomen

PEDIATRIC CONSIDERATIONS

- Due to smaller body, trauma affects proportionately larger areas leading to multisystem injuries
- Children have less protective muscle and subcutaneous tissue
- Bicycle accidents with trauma from the handlebars can cause significant pancreatic injury
- Children will less often present with hypotension as symptom
- Evaluate for possible child abuse

Pre-Hospital

CAUTIONS

- The extent of pancreatic injury may not be apparent on initial evaluation
- Transport to closest, appropriate facility or trauma center

Diagnosis

ESSENTIAL WORKUP

- Concise history, details of incident especially important for blunt trauma
- Physical examination
  - —Inspection for abrasions, contusions, penetrating wounds—must log roll patient for full inspection
  - —Auscultation for presence or absence of bowel sounds
  - —Palpation to determine location and severity of pain, presence of guarding, and rebound tenderness
  - —Rectal examination for occult blood, vaginal, and penile exam as for all trauma patients
  - —Serial physical examinations for unidentified injuries

LABORATORY

- Blood type, screen, or crossmatch
- Hematocrit, white blood cell count with differential
- Amylase is not a reliable indicator of pancreatic trauma
  - —Serial levels may increase sensitivity but specificity is still poor
  - —Elevated amylase may be an early indicator of potential pancreatic injury
  - —Normal amylase does not rule out pancreatic injury
- Lipase
- Urinalysis
- Pregnancy test
- Alcohol and drug screening if indicated
- PT/PTT, BUN, and creatinine

IMAGING/SPECIAL TESTS

Note: All imaging tests may miss pancreatic injury
- C-spine, CXR, and pelvis films as for all blunt trauma patients
- Ultrasound
- CT scan with IV and oral contrast
- DPL to identify intraperitoneal injuries, check fluid for amylase level
- ERCP is useful for patients with persistent hyperamylasemia or unexplained abdominal symptoms

DIFFERENTIAL DIAGNOSIS

- 90% of pancreatic injuries are associated with injuries to adjacent structures: liver, stomach, major arteries and veins, spleen, kidney, duodenum, colon, small bowel, common bile duct, and gallbladder

Treatment

INITIAL STABILIZATION (ATLS PROTOCOL)

- Primary survey
- Secure airway, supplemental oxygen, intubation as needed
- 2 large-bore IVs, fluid resuscitation with crystalloid followed by blood products as needed
- Control of external hemorrhage
- Identify and manage life-threatening injuries
- Cardiac monitoring
- Urinary catheter to monitor volume status
- Nasogastric catheter to reduce stomach distention and decrease aspiration risk
- Monitor vital signs

ED TREATMENT

- Secondary survey—total patient evaluation
- Oxygenation and ventilation
- Fluid resuscitation and hemodynamic monitoring is essential in patients with pancreatic injuries
- Constant reevaluation of clinical status
- Pain management is warranted after appropriate trauma surgery evaluation
- Antibiotic treatment for penetrating trauma, and intraabdominal injury that will require operative intervention

MEDICATIONS

Penetrating trauma: tetanus prophylaxis and broad spectrum antibiotic therapy

—Must cover for colonic bacteria: aerobic (*E. coli, Enterobacter, Klebsiella, Enterococcus*), and anaerobic organisms (*Bacteroides fragilis, Clostridia, Peptostreptococcus*)
—Cefotetan: 2 g IV (peds: 20 mg/kg IV) + Gentamicin: 2 mg/kg IV *or*
—Cefoxitin: 2 g IV (peds: 40mg/kg IV) + Gentamicin: 2 mg/kg IV *or*
—Ceftriaxone: 1–2 g IV (peds: 50mg/kg/dose IV) + Flagyl: 15 mg/kg IV *or*
—Clindamycin: 600 mg IV (peds: mg/kg IV) + Gentamicin 2 mg/kg IV

Disposition

ADMISSION CRITERIA

- All patients with pancreatic injuries must be admitted
- Abdominal pain after blunt trauma requires serial examinations and observation for 24 hours
- Intoxicated trauma patient requires admission and serial examinations for unidentified injury

DISCHARGE CRITERIA

- Only for very minor trauma and with no evidence of pancreatic or any other intra-abdominal injury

Miscellaneous

ICD9: 863.84

CORE CONTENT CODE: 18.4.11.3

SUGGESTED READINGS

American College of Surgeons Committee on Trauma. Advanced trauma life support course [Manual]. Chicago: American College of Surgeons, 1993.

Emmick RH Jr., Peterson SR. Evaluation of pancreatic injury after blunt abdominal trauma. Ann Emerg Med 1996;27(5):658–661.

Fabian TC. Prevention of infections following penetrating abdominal trauma. Am J Surg 1993;165(Suppl 2A):14S–19S.

Jurkovich J. Injury to the duodenum and pancreas. In: Feliciano DV, Mattox KL, Moore EE, eds. Trauma. 3rd ed. Norwalk, CT: Appleton & Lange, 1996:473–494.

Ney A, Hollerman JJ, Anderson R. Abdominal trauma. In: Tintinalli J, et al., eds. Emergency medicine: A comprehensive study guide. 4th ed. New York: McGraw Hill, 1996:1182–1188.

Author: Beth Anne DeGennaro

Pancreatitis

Clinical Presentation

SIGNS AND SYMPTOMS

SIGN/SYMPTOM:	FREQUENCY
Abdominal pain	95–100%
Epigastric tenderness	95–100%
Nausea and vomiting	70–90%
Low grade fever	70–85%
Hypotension	20–40%
Altered mental status	20–35%
Grey Turner/Cullen's sign	<5%
Subcutaneous fat necrosis	<1%

Gastrointestinal

- Severe, persistent epigastric pain radiating to back
  —Colicky pain or rebound tenderness suggest nonpancreatic source
- Bowel sounds usually decreased or absent
- Cullen's sign
  —Bluish discoloration at umbilicus secondary to hemorrhagic pancreatitis
- Grey Turner's sign
  —Bluish discoloration at flank secondary to hemorrhagic pancreatitis

Respiratory

- Pleuritic chest pain
- Dyspnea
- Lung exam
  —Left pleural effusion (most common)
  —Atelectasis
  —Pulmonary edema
- Hypoxemia (30%)

Cardiac

- Tachycardia
- Hypotension
- Shock

Neurologic

- Irritability
- Confusion
- Coma
- Chvostek and Trousseau signs are rare despite laboratory evidence of hypocalcemia

Ranson's Criteria

- Indicators of morbidity and mortality
  —0–2 criteria: 2% mortality
  —3–4 criteria: 15% mortality
  —5–6 criteria: 40% mortality
  —7–8 criteria: 100% mortality
- Criteria on admission
  —Age >55 years
  —White blood cell count >16,000 IU/L
  —Blood glucose >200 mg/d
  —Serum LDH >350 IU/L
  —SGOT >250 IU/dL
- Criteria during first 48 hours
  —Hematocrit fall >10%
  —BUN increase >8 mg/dl
  —Arterial PO_2 <60 mm Hg
  —Base deficit >4 mEq/L
  —Estimated fluid sequestration >6 liters

MECHANISM/DESCRIPTION

- Inflammation of the pancreas due to activation, interstitial liberation, and digestion of the gland by its own enzymes
- Acute pancreatitis
  —Exocrine and endocrine function of the gland impaired for weeks to months
  —Glandular function will return to normal
- Chronic pancreatitis
  —Exocrine and endocrine function progressively deteriorate with resultant steatorrhea and malabsorption
  —Dysfunction progressive and irreversible

ETIOLOGY

- Gallstones and alcohol abuse most common etiologies of *acute pancreatitis* (75%)
- Alcohol abuse accounts for 70–80% of *chronic pancreatitis*

ACUTE	CHRONIC
Biliary tract disease	Chronic alcoholism
Chronic alcoholism	Obstruction pancreatic duct
Obstruction pancreatic duct	Tropical
Ischemia	Hereditary
Drugs	Shwachman's disease
Infectious	Enterokinase deficiency
Postoperative	Enzyme deficiency
Post ERCP	Idiopathic
Metabolic diseases	Hyperlipidemia
After renal transplant	
Scorpion venom	
Penetrating peptic ulcer	
Hereditary	
Idiopathic	

PEDIATRIC CONSIDERATIONS

- Etiology mainly viral, trauma, and drugs
- Pancreas well-imaged with ultrasound

Pre-Hospital

N/A

Diagnosis

ESSENTIAL WORKUP

- Laboratory tests confirm physical diagnosis

LABORATORY

- Amylase
  —Rise within 6 hours of pain onset
  —>5 times upper limit is highly specific for pancreatitis
  —>1000 IU suggests biliary pancreatitis
  —May be normal during acute inflammation due to significant preexisting pancreatic destruction
  —Secreted from a variety of sources
- Lipase
  —More reliable indicator of pancreatitis than amylase
- Electrolytes, BUN, Cr, glucose
  —Hypokalemia occurs with extensive fluid losses
  —Hyperglycemia
- CBC
  —Increased Hct with fluid losses
  —Decreased Hct with retroperitoneal hemorrhage
  —WBC >12,000 unusual
- Calcium/magnesium
  —Hypocalcemia signifies significant pancreatic injury
  —Hypomagnesemia occurs with underlying alcohol abuse
- Liver function tests
  —Useful for prognostic indicators and if suspected biliary etiology
- Pregnancy test
- Arterial blood gas
  —Indicated if hypoxic (assess PO_2) or toxic appearing (assess base deficit)

IMAGING/SPECIAL TESTS

- EKG
  —Assess electrolyte imbalances, ischemia
- Abdominal series
  —Excludes free air
  —May visualize pancreatic calcifications
  —Most common finding is isolated dilated bowel loop (sentinel loop) near pancreas
- CXR for
  —Pleural effusion
  —Atelectasis
  —Infiltrate
- Ultrasound indicated if gallstone pancreatitis suspected
- Abdominal CT Scan indicated acutely if
  —High risk pancreatitis (>3 Ranson's criteria)
  —Hemorrhagic pancreatitis
  —Suspicion of pseudocyst

DIFFERENTIAL DIAGNOSIS

- Mesenteric ischemia/infarction
- Myocardial infarction
- Biliary colic
- Perforated ulcer
- Pneumonia
- Ruptured aortic aneurysm
- Ectopic pregnancy

Treatment

INITIAL STABILIZATION

- ABCs
  —Supplemental oxygen
  —Cardiac monitor
  —Intravenous fluids

ED TREATMENT

- Airway management
  —Pulmonary complaints necessitate supplemental oxygen
  —Endotracheal intubation for ARDS or severe encephalopathy
- Fluid resuscitation
  —Large fluid volumes (up to 5–6 L in first 24 hours) due to fluid losses
  —Continuously assess vitals, urine output, and electrolytes to ensure rapid and adequate replacement of intravascular volume
  —Consider CVP monitoring in elderly and when fluid overload is a concern
- Correct electrolyte abnormalities if present
  —Hypocalcemia (calcium gluconate)
  —Hypokalemia occurs with extensive fluid losses
  —Hypomagnesemia occurs with underlying alcohol abuse
- Blood products
  —In hemorrhagic pancreatitis, transfuse hematocrit to a level of 30%
  —Fresh frozen plasma and platelets if coagulopathic and bleeding
- Analgesia
  —Meperidine is drug of choice
  —Morphine not recommended due to contraction of Sphincter of Oddi
- Nasogastric suction
  —Not useful in cases of mild pancreatitis
  —Beneficial in severe pancreatitis or intractable nausea and vomiting
- Antiemetics
- Antibiotics not routinely indicated

MEDICATIONS

- Calcium gluconate 10%: 10 ml IV over 15–20 min
- Meperidine (demerol): 25–50 mg IV 50–75 mg IM q 3–4 hrs
- Magnesium sulfate: 16 mEq (2 g) in 50 ml D5W over 20 min
- Potassium chloride: 10 mEq/hr IV
- Prochlorperazine: 5–10 mg IV

Disposition

ADMISSION CRITERIA

- Acute pancreatitis with significant pain, nausea, vomiting
- ICU admission for hemorrhagic/necrotizing pancreatitis

DISCHARGE CRITERIA

- Mild acute pancreatitis without evidence of biliary tract disease and able to tolerate oral fluids
- Chronic pancreatitis with minimal abdominal pain and able to tolerate oral fluids

Miscellaneous

ICD9: 577.0, 577.1

CORE CONTENT CODE: 1.4.1.1

SUGGESTED READINGS

Folsch UR, Loser C. A concept of treatment in acute pancreatitis: Results of controlled trials and future developments. Hepatogastroenterology 1993;40(6):569–573.

Go V, et al., eds. The pancreas. New York: Raven Press, 1993:575–635.

Heinisch A, Scholmerich J, Leser H. Diagnostic approach to acute pancreatitis: Diagnosis, assessment of etiology and prognosis. Hepatogastroenterology 1993;40(6):531–537.

Valenzuela J, et al, eds. Medical and surgical diseases of the pancreas. New York: Igaku-Shoin, 1993:23–72.

Author: Trevor Lewis

Panic Attacks

Clinical Presentation

SIGNS AND SYMPTOMS

- Characteristic, acute episodes of physical symptoms and intense fear that rapidly peak within 10 minutes and resolve in about 20 minutes

Physical Symptoms

- Multiple systems suggest autonomic arousal
- Cardiac
  - —Palpitations
  - —Tachycardia
  - —Chest pain
- Respiratory
  - —Shortness of breath
  - —Smothering
  - —Choking
- Neurologic
  - —Tremor
  - —Dizziness
  - —Lightheadedness
  - —Feeling faint
  - —Numbness
  - —Tingling
  - —Sweating
  - —Chills
  - —Flushing
  - —Feelings of unreality or detachment
- Gastrointestinal
  - —Nausea
  - —Cramps
  - —Abdominal pain

Intense Fears

- Automatic, stereotypic
- Imminent death
- Humiliation
- Loss of control—"going crazy"

MECHANISM/DESCRIPTION

- Limbic system, norepinephrine release, other neurotransmitters (e.g., serotonin) implicated

Panic Disorder

- Recurrent, unexpected panic attacks with one or more months of persistent
  - —Concerns about having another attack
  - —Worry about the implications or consequences of the attacks
  - —Behavioral change, such as phobic avoidance, related to the attacks
- Episodic, recurrent, or chronic; frequently comorbid with depression, substance abuse, disability, suicidal tendency

ETIOLOGY

- Probably genetic
- Risk factors
  - —Family history of panic or anxiety
  - —Childhood shyness or separation anxiety
  - —Major life events in year preceding onset
- May develop in the course of predisposing physical illness or cocaine abuse
  - —May persist after the illness or substance use has resolved

Pre-Hospital

N/A

Diagnosis

ESSENTIAL WORKUP

- Clinical diagnosis—history should include
  - —Known medical conditions
  - —All medications, including over-the-counter
  - —Recreational drugs/alcohol use
  - —Caffeine consumption
  - —Age at onset
  - —Family history of panic, anxiety
  - —Initiating life events
  - —Childhood antecedents
  - —Resultant avoidance
  - —Response to previous medication trials
- Thorough physical and neurological exam

LABORATORY

- Toxicology screen
- ECG
  - —Over 40
  - —Cardiac symptoms
- CBC
- Electrolytes, BUN/Cr, glucose
- TSH

IMAGING/SPECIAL TESTS

- Echocardiogram for suspected mitral valve prolapse
- Sleep deprived EEG if seizure suspected

DIFFERENTIAL DIAGNOSIS

- Consider organic causes if
  - —Panic presents late in life
  - —No childhood antecedents or family history
  - —No initiating life events
  - —Without avoidance or significant fear
  - —With a history of poor response to previous trials of anti-panic or antidepressant medication
- Medications
  - —Neuroleptics (akathisia)
  - —Bronchodilators
  - —Digitalis
  - —Anticholinergic agents
  - —Diet pills
- Respiratory
  - —COPD
  - —Pulmonary embolus
- Cardiovascular
  - —Angina
  - —Arrhythmia
  - —Anemia
  - —Mitral valve prolapse (MVP) may be comorbid with panic
- Substances
  - —Stimulant abuse
  - —Withdrawal (alcohol, sedative-hypnotics)
  - —Excessive caffeine intake
- Endocrine
  - —Hyperthyroidism
  - —Hypoglycemia
  - —Parathyroid disorders
  - —Pheochromocytoma

- Neurologic
  —Complex partial, or limbic seizures (fear, physical symptoms, perceptual distortions)
  —TIA
- Psychiatric
  —Other anxiety, stress, or phobic disorders; e.g., obsessive-compulsive disorder, post-traumatic stress disorder, or social phobia

Treatment

INITIAL STABILIZATION

- Be calm and reassuring
- Most panic attacks resolve within 20–30 minutes without any treatment
- Fear may trigger another panic attack

ED TREATMENT

- High-potency benzodiazepines
  —Drugs of choice
    -Alprazolam, clonazepam, lorazepam
  —Clonazepam
    -Slow for emergency use
    -Long-acting without rapid onset/offset phenomena
    -Best choice in this class for maintenance therapy of recurrent panic attacks
  —Alprazolam
    -Rapid onset
    -Rebound anxiety occurs due to short duration and rapid offset
    -May lead to escalating doses with continued use
  —Lorazepam
    -Quick onset
    -Advantage of sublingual use
    -Longer effect and less abrupt offset than alprazolam
  —Avoid low-potency benzodiazepines
    -Diazepam
    -Chlordiazepoxide
- Treat recurrent panic attacks and panic disorder with SSRI, TCA, or MAOI antidepressants, with or without clonazepam
  —Will not work immediately
  —Do not need to be started emergently
- Discharge therapy
  —Several clonazepam tablets in case of repeated attacks
    -Do not prescribe alprazolam—withdrawal may trigger further attacks
  —Psychopharmacological and *cognitive behavioral therapy* evaluation for repeated attacks, or interepisode fear or avoidance, for evaluation

MEDICATIONS

- Alprazolam: 0.5 mg po
- Clonazepam: 0.5 mg po in the ED; 0.25–0.5 mg po bid for initial outpatient therapy
- Lorazepam: l mg po or SL

Disposition

ADMISSION CRITERIA

- As medically indicated to rule out organic cause (e.g., MI)
- Meets criteria for psychiatric admission (suicidal, homicidal)

DISCHARGE CRITERIA

- Majority of panic attacks do not require inpatient level of care

Miscellaneous

ICD9: 300.01

CORE CONTENT CODE: 14.3.2

SUGGESTED READINGS

Ballenger JC. Panic disorder in the medical setting. J Clin Psychiatry 1997;58(Suppl 2):13–17.

Craske MG, Brown TA, Barlow DH. Behavioral treatment of panic disorder a two-year follow-up. Behav Ther 1991;22:289–304.

Jeffereson JW. Antidepressants in panic disorder. J Clin Psychiatry 1997;58(Suppl 2):20–24.

Kierman GL, Weissman MM, Ouellette R, et al. Panic attacks in the community: social morbidity and health care utilization. JAMA 1991;265:742–746.

Tesar GE, Rosenbaum JF, Pollack MH, et al. Double-blind, placebo-controlled comparison of clonazepam and alprazolam for panic disorder. J Clin Psychiatry 1991;52:69–76.

Author: B.J. Beck

Paraphimosis

Clinical Presentation

SIGNS AND SYMPTOMS

- Retracted foreskin
- Pain
- Swollen, edematous glans
- Local cellulitis
- Necrosis of glans in untreated cases

MECHANISM/DESCRIPTION

- Paraphimosis is a *urologic emergency!*
- It is the entrapment of the retracted foreskin proximal to the penile glans, which leads to lymphatic congestion, venous obstruction, and which may result in arterial compromise to the glans

ETIOLOGY

- There are a number of conditions of the foreskin that may predispose to paraphimosis including
  —Phimosis
  —Inflammation
  —Trauma
- Paraphimosis is commonly *iatrogenic,* from failure to replace the foreskin following examination, catheterization, or cleaning

Pre-Hospital

CAUTIONS

- Patients should be transported promptly; *do not* attempt reduction in the field
- Pre-hospital personnel can be advised to apply an ice pack to the glans with adequate protection of the skin

Diagnosis

ESSENTIAL WORKUP

- Paraphimosis is a clinical diagnosis with the pathognomonic clinical findings described above
- Examination should include a search for constricting foreign bodies
- Treatment must not be delayed pending diagnostic laboratory or radiographic studies

IMAGING/SPECIAL TESTS

- If history suggests penile foreign body, x-rays may be obtained once the vascular compromise has been relieved

DIFFERENTIAL DIAGNOSIS

- Foreign bodies constricting the penile shaft may mimic paraphimosis. These include
  —Hair tourniquets
  —Wire, string, or other material used for sexual enhancement or punishment
- Balanoposthitis
- Trauma (zipper injuries)
- Acute idiopathic penile edema

Treatment

INITIAL STABILIZATION

- Ice can be applied to the glans while preparing to reduce the prepuce. Use the thumb of a glove as an ice-filled condom to aid in direct application
- The incarcerated foreskin must be released as soon as possible to prevent ischemia and necrosis of the glans
- The pain associated with reduction techniques must be managed with conscious sedation, adequate analgesia, and local anesthesia

ED TREATMENT

- Rolled gauze or an elastic wrap may be applied to aid in reducing edema of the glans
- Attempt manual reduction by gentle, steady traction on the foreskin with downward pressure on the glans
- Decrease in glans edema has been obtained with the "puncture" technique, making one or more holes in the swollen foreskin with a small sterile needle, allowing expression of edema fluid. This requires adequate analgesia or anesthesia
- Failure of these techniques or the development of ischemia necessitates a dorsal longitudinal slit in the foreskin
- Urologic consultation is required for subsequent circumcision to prevent recurrence

MEDICATIONS

- See conscious sedation chapter
- Appropriate analgesics or anesthetics as required

Disposition

ADMISSION CRITERIA

- Necrosis or cellulitis of the penis

DISCHARGE CRITERIA

- Successful reduction with relief of symptoms
- Close urologic follow-up

Miscellaneous

ICD9: 605

CORE CONTENT CODE: 19.2.2.1, 13.13.2.2

SUGGESTED READINGS

Barone JG, Fleisher MH. Treatment of paraphimosis using the "puncture" technique. Pediatr Emerg Care 1993;9(5):298–299.

Pontari MA. Phimosis and paraphimosis. In: Seidman EJ, Hanno PM, eds. Current urologic therapy. 3rd ed. Philadelphia: WB Saunders, 1994:392–7.

Raveenthwan, V. Reduction of paraphimosis: a technique based on pathophysiology. Br J of Surg. 1996 Sep;83(9):1247.

Super DM. Phimosis. In: Hoekelman R, et al., eds. Primary pediatric care. St. Louis: CV Mosby, 1987:1232–4.

Authors: Lorne Sherman; Joseph LaMantia

Parkinson's Disease

Clinical Presentation

SIGNS AND SYMPTOMS

- "Pill-rolling" resting tremor
- "Cog-wheel" rigidity due to increased muscular tone
- Stooped posture and instability of posture
- Stiffness and slowness of movement
- "Masked face" appearance
- Depression and dementia
- Sudden change in baseline motor function or mental status in a patient with Parkinson's disease may be the only indication of systemic disease such as infection

ETIOLOGY

- Sporadic or idiopathic, degenerative
- Type A encephalitis of von Economo
- CNS viral infections
- Vascular infarction
- Intoxications
  - —Phenothiazine
  - —Butyrophenones
  - —Metoclopramide
  - —Illicit drugs
  - —Carbon monoxide (bilateral infarctions of the globus pallidus)
  - —Manganese

MECHANISM/DESCRIPTION

- Gradually progressive disorder of middle or late life
- Aggregates of melanin-containing nerve cells in the brain stem (substantia nigra locus ceruleus)
- Reactive gliosis with nerve cell loss
- Lewy bodies (eosinophilic intracytoplasmic inclusions)
- *Decreased dopamine* in the caudate nucleus and putamen
- Accelerated *cortical atrophy*
- Can begin unilaterally, but generalizes to symmetrical

PEDIATRIC CONSIDERATIONS

- The earliest variants of Parkinson's disease have been found in patients 20 years of age or older

Pre-Hospital

- There are no particular pre-hospital care issues

Diagnosis

ESSENTIAL WORKUP

- *History* is of primary importance as diagnosis is made based on clinical findings
- Important historical information includes
  - —Onset of symptom, whether gradual or sudden
  - —History of encephalitis, herpes virus infection, or carbon monoxide exposure
- In patients with established Parkinson's disease, sudden change in baseline motor function or mental status should prompt workup for infectious process such as urinary tract infection

LABORATORY

- There are no specific or recommended laboratory studies necessary to confirm the diagnosis of Parkinson's disease
- Nonidiopathic Parkinson's disease may require directed laboratory studies relative to the specific disease process
- Urinalysis, CBC, and other appropriate workup for occult infection in patients with established disease

IMAGING/SPECIAL TESTS

- CT scan/MRI are not required to diagnose Parkinson's disease, but are often elements of evaluation for dementia
- CXR may be indicated for any signs of respiratory infection

Treatment

ED TREATMENT

- Treatment with antiparkinsonian medications can be initiated in the ED to alleviate symptoms
- Consultation with neurology for recommended medication regimens and ongoing support and monitoring is prudent
- For patients with mild disease, no medication may be required
- For moderate disease involvement including symmetrical tremor and postural imbalance, anticholinergic medications and dopaminergic medications should be used
- Treat underlying infection if present

MEDICATIONS

- Trihexyphenidyl: 1–2 mg 4 times daily
- Benztropine: 0.5–1 mg 3 times daily
- Amantadine: 100 mg twice daily
- Levodopa/dopacarboxylase inhibitor (carbidopa) combination: 25 mg/100 mg daily
- Bromocriptine: 15 mg daily

Disposition

ADMISSION CRITERIA

- Patient with intercurrent infections, dehydration, or other medical problems
- Depression with intent to do self-harm
- Medication regimen adjustment

DISCHARGE CRITERIA

- Mild to moderate disease without medications
- Moderate to severe disease with medications and urgent neurological outpatient follow-up

Miscellaneous

ICD9: 332.0

CORE CONTENT CODE: 11.13

SUGGESTED READINGS

Fahn S, et al. Recent advances in parkinson's disease. New York: Raven, 1986.

Flint MB, Beal M, Richardson EP, Martin JB. Parkinson's disease. In: Isselbacher KJ, et al., eds. Harrison's principles of internal medicine. New York: McGraw Hill, 1994.

Lieberman, A. Managing the neuropsychiatric symptoms of Parkinson's disease. Neurology. 1998 Jun; 50 (6 Suppl 6):533–38.

Rajput A, et al. Epidemiology of parkinsonism: Incidence, classification, and mortality. Ann Neurol 1984;16:178.

Author: James M. Leaming, Gary Johnson

Paronychia

Clinical Presentation

SIGNS AND SYMPTOMS

- Begins as swelling, pain, and erythema in the dorsolateral corner of the nail fold bulging out over the nail plate, which progresses to a subcuticular abscess

MECHANISM/DESCRIPTION

- Disruption of the seal between the nail plate and the nail fold may allow entry of bacteria into the eponychial space
- Inflammation of the nail folds surrounding the nail plate

ETIOLOGY

- Acute paronychia: predominantly *Staphylococcus aureus* but also Streptococcal organisms
- Chronic paronychia: predominantly *C. albicans,* but may also be other fungi, atypical mycobacteria; commonly coexisting with Staphylococcus species

RISK FACTORS

- Acute: minor nail trauma such as hangnails, vigorous manicures, nail biting. Underlying disease such as diabetes
- Chronic: occupations with persistent moist hands such as dishwashers, bartenders. Also increased in patients with peripheral vascular disease

PEDIATRIC CONSIDERATIONS

- Frequently anaerobic mouth flora in children from nail biting

Pre-Hospital

N/A

Diagnosis

ESSENTIAL WORKUP

- History and physical exam with special attention to evaluating for concomitant infections such as felon or cellulitis
- Evaluate tetanus status

LABORATORY

- No specific tests are useful

IMAGING/SPECIAL TESTS

- Soft tissue x-rays if foreign body is suspected

DIFFERENTIAL DIAGNOSIS

- Felon
- Herpetic Whitlow
- Trauma or foreign body
- Primary squamous cell carcinoma
- Metastatic carcinoma
- Osteomyelitis

Treatment

INITIAL STABILIZATION

- No specific stabilization necessary

ED TREATMENT

Acute Paronychia

- Early paronychia without purulence present may be managed with oral antibiotics
  - —Cephalexin, dicloxacillin
  - —Clindamycin, or erythromycin if associated with nail biting or oral contact or allergy
- Early superficial subcuticular abscess
  - —Elevation of the eponychial fold by sliding the flat edge of a No. 11 blade (18-gauge needle or small clamps may be used) gently between the proximal nail fold and the nail plate near the point of maximal tenderness
  - —A digital nerve block or local anesthesia may be necessary
- Partial nail involvement
  - —If the lesion extends beneath the nail, remove a longitudinal section of the nail to allow drainage, followed by Vaseline or iodoform gauze packing for 24 hours
- Runaround abscess
  - —If the lesion extends beneath the base of the nail to the other side, remove 1/4 to 1/3 of the proximal nail with 2 small incisions at the dorsolateral edges of the nail fold, and pack eponychial fold with petroleum or iodoform gauze to prevent adherence
- Extensive subungual abscess
  - —Remove entire nail
- Antibiotics may be used as adjunct
  - —Dicloxacillin or a first-generation cephalosporin such as cephalexin for 5–10 days if there is any apparent cellulitis, abscess, or systemic signs of infection

Chronic Paronychia

- Eponychial marsupialization involving removal of a crescent-shaped piece of skin just proximal to the nail fold including all thickened tissue down to, but not including, germinal matrix
  - —Topical steroids with a topical antifungal have been used with success
  - —Antistaphylococcal treatment should also be considered

MEDICATIONS

- Cephalexin: adult: 500 g po qid for 7 d; peds: 40 mg/kg/d po div q 6 hrs
- Clindamycin: adult: 300 mg po qid for 7 d; peds: 20–40 mg/kg/d div q 6 hrs po, IV, IM
- Dicloxacillin: adult: 500 mg po qid for 7 d; peds: 12.5–50 mg/kg/d po div q 6 hrs
- Erythromycin: adult: 500 mg po qid for 7d; peds: 40 mg/kg/d div q 6 hrs po

Disposition

ADMISSION CRITERIA

- Patients with uncomplicated paronychia can be managed as outpatients

DISCHARGE CRITERIA

- Patients with uncomplicated paronychia that has been managed in the ED may be discharged with appropriate follow-up instructions
- Patients with packing must return in 24 hours for reevaluation

Miscellaneous

ICD9: 681.9

CORE CONTENT CODE: 10.6.3

SUGGESTED READINGS

Canales FL, Newmeyer WL, Kilgore ES. The treatment of felons and paronychias. Hand Clin 1989;5(4):515–523.

Hochman LG. Paronychia: More than just an abscess. Int J Dermatol 1995;34(6):385–386.

Moran GJ, Talan DA. Hand infections. Emerg Med Clin 1993;11(3):601–619.

Author: Gene Ma

Patellar Injuries

Clinical Presentation

SIGNS AND SYMPTOMS

Dislocation

- History of feeling knee "go out"; popping, ripping, or tearing sensation
- Pain
- Inability to bear weight
- Obvious lateral deformity of knee
- Knee held in slight flexion
- Mild to moderate swelling
- Occasionally hemarthrosis
- Often reduced spontaneously prior to ED evaluation
- Tenderness along patella
- Positive apprehension or Fairbanks's sign
  —Attempts to push the patella laterally elicit patient apprehension

Fracture

- Pain over anterior knee
- Difficulty ambulating
- Increased pain with movement of patella
- Tenderness and swelling over patella
- Difficulty or inability to extend knee
- Palpable defect, crepitus, or joint effusion/hemarthrosis

MECHANISM/DESCRIPTION

Dislocation

- Usually caused by sudden flexion and external rotation of tibia on femur, with simultaneous contraction of quadriceps muscles
- Lateral dislocation of patella most common, with patella displaced laterally over the lateral femoral condyle
- Uncommon dislocations include superior, medial, and rare intra-articular dislocation
- Direct trauma to patella

Fracture

- Direct trauma
  —Most common mechanism of injury
  —Secondary to direct blow or fall on patella
  —Usually results in comminuted or minimally displaced fracture
- Indirect forces
  —Avulsion injury secondary to contraction of the quadriceps tendon
  —Usually results in transverse or displaced fracture (often both)
- Types of patellar fractures
  —Transverse: 50–80% (usually middle or lower third of patella)
  —Comminuted (or stellate): 30–35%
  —Longitudinal: 25%
  —Osteochondral

ETIOLOGY

Dislocation

- Risk factors for patellar dislocation
  —Genu valgum ("knock knee")
  —Genu recurvatum (hyperextension of knee)
  —Shallow lateral femoral condyle
  —Deficient vastus medialis
  —Lateral insertion of patellar tendon
  —Shallow patellar groove
  —Patella alta (high-riding patella)
  —Deformed patella
  —Pes planus (flatfoot)
- Common injury in adolescents, especially girls
- The younger the patient at time of initial dislocation, the greater the risk of recurrent dislocation

Fracture

- Direct trauma
- Indirect forces caused by forcible quadriceps tendon contraction
- 2:1 predominance in males
- Highest incidence in 20–50-year-old age group

Pre-Hospital

- Patient should be transported in supine position with knee flexed and supported

Diagnosis

ESSENTIAL WORKUP

- Radiographs are essential, even if patella spontaneously reduced prior to ED arrival
  —Anteroposterior (AP) and lateral views of knee should be obtained
  —Postreduction radiographs should include AP, lateral, and sunrise (or skyline, axial) views to exclude osteochondral fracture
  —Bipartite patella (patella with an accessory bony fragment connected to main body by cartilage) may be mistaken for fracture; comparison view may help differentiate

DIFFERENTIAL DIAGNOSIS

- Patellar subluxation
- Femoral or tibial fracture
- Traumatic bursitis

Treatment

INITIAL STABILIZATION

- Patient placed in supine position with knee flexed and supported
- Appropriate history and physical exam to identify any associated injuries (e.g., femoral fracture, hip fracture, posterior hip dislocation)

ED TREATMENT

Dislocation

- For simple lateral patellar dislocation, reduce dislocation by extending the knee gently to 180°. Occasionally may need to apply simultaneous pressure over lateral aspect of patella in medial direction
- For other types of patellar dislocation (superior, medial, intra-articular) do not attempt reduction; obtain orthopedic consultation
- Aspiration of joint with sterile technique necessary if reduction is difficult secondary to hemarthrosis
- If osteochondral fracture present (28–50% of cases), obtain orthopedic consultation
- Although reduction is typically easy to accomplish, conscious sedation or parenteral analgesia may facilitate

Fracture

- Orthopedic consultation when patellar fracture is confirmed
- Initial treatment often consists of long leg bulky splint and subsequent operative repair

MEDICATIONS

- Fentanyl citrate: adult: 1–2 μg/kg IV; peds: 0.5–1.0 μg/kg IV
- Midazolam HCL: adult: 1–3 mg IV; peds: 0.05–0.1 mg/kg (max dose 2.5 mg) IV
- Morphine sulphate: adult: 2–5 mg/dose IV; peds: 0.1–0.2 mg/kg/dose IV
- Meperidine: adult: 50–150 mg IM; peds: 0.5–0.8 mg/lb IM
- Toradol: adults: 60 mg IM

Disposition

ADMISSION CRITERIA

- Patients with superior, medial or intra-articular dislocation, or inability to reduce lateral dislocation require orthopedic consultation in ED and possible admission
- Patellar dislocation associated with a fracture (osteochondral or lateral femoral condyle) require orthopedic consultation in ED
- Operative intervention indicated if fragments are displaced greater than 4 mm; or patient unable to raise extended leg off bed; or articular step-off greater than 3 mm
- All open fractures require debridement and irrigation and should be admitted

DISCHARGE CRITERIA

- Patients with successful reduction of lateral patellar dislocation and normal postreduction x-rays may be discharged with knee immobilization, crutches, and orthopedic follow-up
- Fracture is displaced less than 3 mm and patient has full active knee extension
- Knee immobilizer, or bulky long-leg splint, partial to full weight-bearing as tolerated with crutches, and orthopedic follow-up within a few days

Miscellaneous

ICD9: 836.3, 822.0

CORE CONTENT CODE: 18.4.13.2.5, 18.4.13.1.6

SUGGESTED READINGS

Cash JD, Hughston JC. Treatment of acute patellar dislocation. Am J Sports Med 1988;16:244–249.

Cofield RH, Bryan RS. Acute dislocation of the patella: Results of conservative treatment. J Trauma 1977;17:526–531.

Maguire JK, Canale ST. Fractures of the patella in children and adolescents. J Pediatr Orthop 1993;13:567–571.

Simon RR, Koenigsknecht SJ. The knee, fibular, and patellar dislocations. In: Simon RR, Koenigsknecht SJ, eds. Emergency orthopedics—The extremities. 3rd ed. East Norwalk, CT: Appleton & Lange, 1995:463–470.

Stewart C. Knee injuries: Diagnosis and repair. Emerg Med Reports 1997;18(1):1–12.

Authors: Kelly Anne Foley; Francis Counselman

Patent Ductus Arteriosus

Clinical Presentation

SIGNS AND SYMPTOMS

- Asymptomatic when the patent ductus arteriosus (PDA) is small
- Recurrent pulmonary infections
- Congestive heart failure
- Retardation of physical growth
- Wide pulse pressure
- Prominent apical impulse
- Thrill
  - —Maximal in the second left intercostal space
  - —Radiates toward the left clavicle, down the left sternal border or toward the apex
  - —Systolic or continuous
- Continuous murmur
  - —Humming top or rolling thunder
  - —Begins soon after onset of the first sound, reaches maximal intensity at the end of systole, and wanes in late diastole
  - —Localized to the second left intercostal space, or radiates down the left sternal border or to the left clavicle

MECHANISM/DESCRIPTION

- The ductus arteriosus
  - —Patent vessel in the fetus connecting the pulmonary trunk to the descending aorta
  - —Changes shortly after birth normally provoke contraction and closure
    - -Sudden increase in the partial pressure of oxygen
    - -Changes in the synthesis and metabolism of vasoactive eicosanoids
- In the preterm infant, patency of the ductus may be life-saving
  - —The patent ductus usually has a normal structural anatomy
  - —Patency is the result of hypoxia and immaturity
- In the full-term newborn, patency of the ductus is a true congenital malformation
  - —Deficiency of both the mucoid endothelial layer and the muscular media of the ductus
  - —As pulmonary vascular resistance falls, aortic blood is shunted into the pulmonary artery
  - —The extent of the shunt depends on the size of the ductus and on the ratio of pulmonary to systemic vascular resistances
- Up to 70% of the left ventricular output may be shunted through the ductus to the pulmonary circulation
- Risk factors
  - —Maternal rubella infection
  - —Premature birth
  - —High altitudes
  - —Coexisting cardiac anomalies
  - —Conditions resulting in hypoxia
  - —Female patients outnumber males 2:1

ETIOLOGY

- Prematurity
- Congenital
- Hypoxia
- Prostaglandins

Pre-Hospital

CAUTIONS

- Supplemental oxygen if signs of congestive heart failure

Diagnosis

ESSENTIAL WORKUP

- Establish the diagnosis with imaging studies
- Rule out complications such as heart failure and endocarditis

LABORATORY

- Unhelpful in making the diagnosis

IMAGING/SPECIAL TESTS

- Chest radiograph
  - —Usually normal in infants
  - —In children and adults
    - -Increased intrapulmonary markings
    - -Calcifications
    - -Left ventricle and left atrial enlargement
    - -Dilated ascending aorta
    - -Dilated pulmonary arteries
- Electrocardiogram
  - —Abnormal if the ductus is large
  - —Left ventricular hypertrophy
  - —Right ventricular hypertrophy is a sign of severity
- Echocardiography
  - —Normal if the ductus is small
  - —Left atrial enlargement
  - —Size of the ductus can be determined by scanning from the suprasternal notch
  - —Doppler will determine aortic to pulmonary artery flow during diastole
- Cardiac catheterization
  - —Normal or increased right-sided pressure
  - —Oxygenated blood in the pulmonary artery confirms left-to-right shunt
  - —Injection of contrast into the ascending aorta shows opacification of the pulmonary arteries

DIFFERENTIAL DIAGNOSIS

- Venous hum
  - —Common insignificant bruit
  - —Heard in the neck or anterior portion of the chest
  - —Soft humming sound in systole and diastole
  - —Decreased by light compression of the jugular venous system
- Aorticopulmonary septal defect
  - —Murmur is often only systolic
  - —Heard at the right upper sternal border
- Ruptured sinus of Valsalva
- Coronary arteriovenous fistulas
- Anomalous origin of left coronary artery from pulmonary artery
- Absence or atresia of pulmonary valve
- Aortic insufficiency with ventricular septal defect
- Peripheral pulmonary stenosis
- Truncus arteriosus

Treatment

INITIAL STABILIZATION

- Small, asymptomatic shunts may not need closure
- Pulmonary support
- Supplemental oxygen

ED TREATMENT

- Sodium and fluid restriction
- Correction of anemia
- Antibiotic prophylaxis for endocarditis
- Preterm infant
  —Usually closes spontaneously
  —Varies with the magnitude of shunting and the severity of hyaline membrane disease
  —Pharmacological inhibition of prostaglandin synthesis with indomethacin during the first 2–7 days of life
- Full term infant and children
  —Surgical closure is required, even in asymptomatic patients, as spontaneous closure is rare
  —Ligation and division
  —Transfemoral catheter technique to occlude PDA with foam plastic plug or double umbrella

MEDICATIONS

- Indomethacin: 0.2–0.25 mg/kg/dose; repeat every 12–24 hours × 3 doses

Disposition

ADMISSION CRITERIA

- Presence of a complication
  —Heart failure
  —Endocarditis
  —Pulmonary hypertension

DISCHARGE CRITERIA

- Asymptomatic
- Prophylactic antibiotics
- Close followup with plans for early surgical closure

Miscellaneous

ICD9: 747.0

CORE CONTENT CODE: 13.2.2; 13.2.2.1

SUGGESTED READINGS

Burton DA, Cabalka AK. Cardiac evaluation in infants. Pediatr Clin North Am 1994;41:991–1015.

Friedman WF. Congenital heart disease in infancy and childhood. In: Braunwald E, ed. Heart disease. 5th ed. Philadelphia: WB Saunders, 1997:877–962.

Riemenschneider TA. The cardiovascular system. In: Behrnam RE, Vaughan VC, eds. Nelson's textbook of pediatrics. 13th ed. Philadelphia: WB Saunders 1987:987–89.

Author: Richard Wolfe

Pediatric Exanthams

Clinical Presentation

SIGNS AND SYMPTOMS

- Fever
- Generalized rash
- Specific presentation depends on
  —Characteristic of the rash
  —Where it arises
  —How it progresses
  —Associated signs and symptoms
  —Age, previous exposures, and immunizations

MECHANISM/DESCRIPTION

- Exanthem is usually one manifestation of systemic illness
- Life-threat is a reflection of the underlying disease process and patient's immunologic status

ETIOLOGY

- Infection: viral, bacterial, Rickettsia
- Drug reaction
- Systemic disease

Pre-Hospital

- Identify exanthems associated with potentially life-threatening illness or that need special isolation precautions
- Petechiae or purpura with fever: meningococcemia, Rocky Mountain Spotted Fever
- Diffuse scarlatiniform rash with fever: toxic shock syndrome, Kawasaki syndrome (also hypotension, vomiting, diarrhea, intense myalgia, mucous membrane changes, arthralgia)
- Vesicles, diffuse maculopapular rash with fever: roseola, chickenpox, rubella are highly contagious and spread by respiratory pathogens; isolation needed

Diagnosis

ESSENTIAL WORKUP

- Clinical examination and history are usually adequate except for some specific entities
  —Meningococcemia: blood cultures and lumbar puncture
  —EB virus exanthem: mono spot and EB virus titer
  —Scarlet fever: rapid strep test and routine culture
  —Varicella: if uncertain, Tzanck preparation and direct immunofluorescence

LABORATORY

- CBC with differential if systemic disease suspected
- Electrolytes and renal function to evaluate patients with suspected dehydration and those with scarlatiniform rash (exclude glomerulonephritis)
- Lumbar puncture if meningeal or encephalitis process suspected (varicella, rubeola, meningococcemia, Rocky Mountain Spotted Fever)

IMAGING/SPECIAL TESTS

- Chest x-ray for systemic disease
- Specific tests to evaluate multisystem disease
- Viral cultures and specific titers to confirm diagnosis
- Bacterial cultures as indicated

DIFFERENTIAL DIAGNOSIS

- Infection
- Drug reaction
- Systemic inflammatory disease (JRA, SLE, etc.)

Treatment

INITIAL STABILIZATION

- Systemic disease with cardiovascular collapse, ARDS, DIC and sepsis
- Toxic shock syndrome, meningococcemia, Rocky Mountain Spotted Fever
- Scalded skin syndrome needs to be treated with fluid resuscitation as a burn
- Isolation if appropriate

ED TREATMENT

- Beyond life-threatening conditions, support is usually required
  —Antipyretics and nonsteroidal anti-inflammatory agents are helpful
- Each entity requires specific pharmacologic agents
- Toxic shock syndrome needs identification and removal of foreign body such as a tampon or diaphragm

MEDICATIONS

- Meningococcemia: penicillin G 2 million units q 2 hrs IV (peds: 250,000–400,000 units/kg/day q 4 hrs); alternative: ampicillin 2 g q 6 hrs IV (peds: 100–200 mg/kg/day q 6 hrs) or ceftriaxone 2 g q 12 hrs IV (peds: 100 mg/kg/day); prophylaxis will be required for close household and school contacts and health care professionals having contact with secretions
- Rocky Mountain Spotted Fever: doxycycline 100 mg po bid if >8 years of age
- Kawasaki syndrome: immune globulin 2 g/kg IV over 10–12 hrs and aspirin 25 mg/kg/dose po q 6 hrs
- Varicella: acyclovir 800 mg po qid (peds: 20 mg/kg/dose) with pulmonary or CNS involvement; give 10–12 mg/kg/dose IV q 8 hrs in the immunocompromised patient; *NO* aspirin should be used
- Toxic shock syndrome or scalded skin syndrome: nafcillin or oxacillin 2 g IV q 4 hrs (peds: 200 mg/kg/day IV q 4 hrs); alternative: cefazolin 2 g q 8 hrs (ped: 100 mg/kg/day IV q 8 hrs)
- Scarlet fever: penicillin V 500 mg po qid (peds: 250 mg po qid) for 10 days; alternative: erythromycin 250–500 mg po qid (peds: 12.5 mg/kg/dose po qid) for 10 days or azithromycin 500 mg po QD (peds: 12 mg/kg/day po QD) for 5 days

Disposition

ADMISSION CRITERIA

- Life-threatening conditions: meningococcemia, Rocky Mountain Spotted Fever, toxic shock syndrome, Kawasaki syndrome
- Other illnesses associated with systemic illness or potential deterioration; scalded skin syndrome, rubeola, and varicella, as well as others, may require inpatient care

DISCHARGE CRITERIA

- Exanthems associated with self-limited entities in stable children

Miscellaneous

ICD9: 782.1

CORE CONTENT CODE: 13.12.4, 3.2.4.6

SUGGESTED READINGS

Cherry JD. Contemporary infectious exanthems. Clin Infect Dis 1993;16:199–207.

Report of the Committee on Infectious Diseases. 24th ed. Elk Grove, IL: American Academy of Pediatrics, 1997.

Frieden HJ, Resnick SD. Childhood exanthems. Pediatr Clin North Am 1991;38:859–887.

Hogan PA. Viral exanthems in childhood. Australas J Dermatol 1996;37:S14–S16.

Author: Bruce Webster

Pediatric Trauma

Clinical Presentation

SIGNS AND SYMPTOMS

- Mechanism of injury and size of child determine nature of potential injuries
- Vital signs reflect blood loss and associated injuries
  —Hemodynamic instability
  —Respiratory distress
- Frequent thorough reassessments essential
  —Respiratory distress
  —Neurologic deficits, altered mentation
  —Bleeding, pain, deformity

MECHANISM/DESCRIPTION

- Size and shape
  —Greater force applied per unit body mass secondary to smaller size
  —Less fat, less elastic connective tissue, more pliable bones, close proximity of organs
- Pelvic organs often abdominal in location
  —Fluids and medications must be weight-specific
  —Disproportionately large head with short neck, relatively poor cervical musculature
  *flat facet joint surfaces
  result in increased risk of head, spinal cord and vertebral injuries
- Surface area
  —Higher ratio of body surface area to body volume
  -More rapid heat loss
- Physiology
  —Smaller blood volume (80 cc/kg)
  —Hemodynamic compensation excellent
  —Hypotension is a late finding preceded by tachycardia, pallor or decreased mental status
  —25–30% loss of blood volume may produce few findings
  —Decompensation may occur rapidly
- Psychologic status
  —Scared and hurting in a strange environment
  —Family anxious and scared
  —Potential of inconsistent story implying child abuse
- Motor vehicle crashes and falls account for 80% of pediatric injuries
  —Passengers, pedestrians, bicyclists
  —Alcohol often involved

ETIOLOGY

- Leading cause of death and disability in children >1 year (U.S.)
  —20,000 casualties and 2,000,000 deaths per year
- Permanent disabilities
  —30,000–150,000 per year
- Relative frequency of injuries (mortality)
  —Falls: 23.9% (0.6%)
  —Electrical injuries and burns: 23.1% (0.6%)
  —Bicyclist/pedestrian versus motor vehicle: 18.8% (2.8%)
  —Motor vehicle crash: 10.4% (4.4%)
  —Child abuse: 2.2% (13%)
  —Penetrating (stab or gunshot): 1.2% (11.6%)

Pre-Hospital

- Regionalized trauma system facilitates appropriate disposition
- Airway, breathing, and circulation
- Cervical spine and extremity immobilization, as appropriate
- Control bleeding
- Communicate and transport

Diagnosis

ESSENTIAL WORKUP

- Primary survey and trauma resuscitation (ATLS)
  —Airway, breathing, and circulation
  —Cervical spine and extremity immobilization
  —Shock
  —Mental status and pupillary response
- Secondary "head-to-toe" survey and reassessment
  —Neurologic considerations
  —Cardiac
  —Abdomen
  —Musculoskeletal
  —Facial and soft injuries
- Determine mechanism to assist in defining injuries
  —What was the speed of the vehicle and extent of damages? (Or height of fall, etc.)
  —Was a seat belt and car seat used appropriately?
  —Was the victim wearing a bicycle helmet?
  —Is the history consistent with the physical findings? (E.g., child abuse)
  —Were there any predisposing factors which may have given rise to the injury? (E.g., seizure, developmental delay, intoxication, suicide gesture, metabolic disorder)?

LABORATORY

- Individualize to nature and extent of injury and physiologic status
- Type and screen/cross match
- CBC, platelet count, coagulation studies (prothrombin time, partial thromboplastin time)
- Electrolytes, BUN, glucose, amylase, and liver transaminases (with abdominal findings)
- Urinalysis to exclude significant hematuria (>20 RBC/HPF)
- Toxicologic studies, alcohol level, pregnancy test as indicated

IMAGING/SPECIAL TESTS

- Standard radiographic trauma studies
  —Cervical spine
    -Patients with intoxication, neck pain/tenderness, abnormal neurologic findings, "distracting" injury
    -Epiphyses and anomalies present
    -Normal film does not exclude injury
  —Chest, abdomen/pelvis
- Computed tomography (CT)
  —Head CT for loss of consciousness, depressed sensorium or focal neurologic findings
    -Usually no contrast needed acutely
  —Abdominal CT in stable patients with potential intraabdominal injury
    -May need oral and IV contrast
  —Spine CT if plain films or history are suggestive of unstable injury

- Ultrasound
  - —Increasingly used to exclude intraperitoneal bleeding
- Diagnostic peritoneal lavage may be useful in evaluating the abdomen in the unstable patient needing emergent intervention and in those patients with suspected mesenteric or diaphragmatic injuries that are not defined by CT scan

DIFFERENTIAL DIAGNOSIS

- Parallel those seen in adults with some anatomical and function differences

Treatment

INITIAL STABILIZATION

- Airway, breathing, and circulation per ATLS protocols
- Spinal immobilization
- Primary and secondary surveys
- Intubate and initiate resuscitation as indicated
- Thorough examination with removal of all clothing
- Establish monitoring

ED TREATMENT

- TEAM approach is essential
  - —Approach early consultations and activation of trauma protocols
- Reassessment and completion of surveys
- Define a systematic management plan
- AMPLE history: allergy, medications, past medical history, time of last meal, and events leading up to injury
- Aggressive management
  - —Treatment based upon clinical findings; diagnosis may not always be confirmed because of time constraints
  - —Assume the most serious diagnosis based upon findings and mechanism of injury
  - —Consider the mechanisms of the injury
- Technical steps
  - —Intravenous lines, usually two
    - -Central and intraosseous lines are alternatives
  - —Nasogastric tube—may delay if facial fractures
  - —Urinary catheter if no blood at meatus
  - —Cardiac monitor and oximetry
  - —Laboratory and x-ray studies
- Avoid hypothermia because of large body surface area
- Splenic and sometimes liver injuries are often treated conservatively

MEDICATIONS

- Crystalloid: lactated ringers (LR) at 20 ml/kg repeated as needed
- Blood: indicated after 60 ml/kg of crystalloid infusion and little response or in the presence of an estimated blood loss of 40 ml/kg
- Tetanus immunization if indicated
- Antibiotics only indicated for cause

Disposition

ADMISSION CRITERIA

- Multiple trauma or significant mechanism of injury
- Hemodynamic instability
- Airway injury or respiratory distress
- Life or limb-threatening injury
- Injury requiring surgical intervention
- Neurologic or vascular injury
- Abdominal pain or tenderness that is not fully explained
- Orthopedic or other organ injury requiring inpatient observation
- Comorbid condition requiring admission or observation such as child abuse or poisoning
- Unreliable followup

DISCHARGE CRITERIA

- Absence of any of the above admission criteria
- Timely followup possible

Miscellaneous

ICD9: 959.9

CORE CONTENT CODE: 18.6

SUGGESTED READINGS

Moront ML, Williams JA, et al. The injured child—an approach to care. Pediatr Clin North Am 1994;41:1201–1226.

Peclet MH, Newman KD, et al. Patterns of injury in children. J Pediatr Surg 1990;25:85–91.

Polgheers A, Ruddy RM. An update on pediatric trauma. Emerg Med Clin North Am 1995;13:267–289.

Ross AJ III. The delicate matter of the spleen. Contemp Pediatr 1989;6:111–122.

Author: Scott D. Berns

Pediculosis

Clinical Presentation

SIGNS AND SYMPTOMS

Head Lice

- Scalp and posterior neck erythema, scaling, and excoriated papules
- Nits (egg casings) attached to hair shafts
- Excoriations may lead to pyoderma, posterior cervical lymphadenopathy and febrile episodes

Body Lice

- Linear excoriations of neck and trunk
- Pus or serum stains on clothing
- Nits found in seams of clothing

Pubic Lice

- Intense pruritus, particularly at night
- Occasional urticaria with typical flare/wheal formation
- May infest eyelashes and scalp in children
- Characteristic bluish macules (maculae ceruleae) appear infrequently on trunk and thighs

ETIOLOGY

- Infestation by *Pediculus capitus* (head louse), *Pediculus corporis* (body louse), or *Pthirus pubis* (pubic louse)
- Bites are painless
- Signs and symptoms result from host response to saliva and anticoagulant injected during feeding
- Transmitted by direct contact and fomites; pubic lice are transmitted by sexual contact

Pre-Hospital

CAUTIONS

- Maintain universal precautions

Diagnosis

ESSENTIAL WORKUP

- Examine hair for adult lice and nits
- Nits are cemented on hair shafts and are not easily removed
- Head lice and pubic lice infestation is confirmed by differentiating nits from scales, hair casts, and other easily brushed-off artifacts
- Empty nits are not diagnostic of active infection
- Body lice are observed only in very heavy infestation; infestation is confirmed by finding nits in clothing seams

LABORATORY

- Nits may be visualized under low-power microscopy along hair shafts

DIFFERENTIAL DIAGNOSIS

- Scabies
- Contact or allergic dermatitis

Treatment

INITIAL STABILIZATION

- Not applicable for routine cases

ED TREATMENT

Head Lice

- Topical pediculicidal agents: *Permethrin 1% cream rinse* (nix) is the best first line agent. It has low toxicity and is ovicidal. *Pyrethrin* (rid) also has low toxicity but is less effective. Lindane shampoo is effective but may cause CNS toxicity and seizures if applied incorrectly or overused
- All agents require reapplication in 7–10 days if further adult lice or nits noted
- Remove nits with fine tooth comb
- Examine all members of household; treat infested individuals
- Change clothing and machine wash and dry (using hot cycles) all clothing, towels, linens, and headgear. Vacuum floors and furniture. Wash combs and brushes in hot water for 10–20 minutes or coat with pediculicide for 15 minutes and wash

Pubic Lice

- Topical pediculicide applied to hairy areas of chest, axilla, and groin
- Remove nits with fine tooth comb
- Treat sexual contacts simultaneously
- Wash and dry bedding and clothing using hot cycles
- Treat eyelash involvement with topical petrolatum twice daily for 9 days

Body Lice

- Wash and dry bedding and clothing using hot cycles
- Apply topical pediculicide cream or lotions from chin to toes
- Oral antihistamines and topical steroids may help pruritic symptoms of all lice infestations

MEDICATIONS

Pediculicidals

- Lindane (γ-benzene hexachloride) 1% shampoo: lather for 4 minutes then rinse.
  —Lotion: apply chin to toes, wash off after 8 hours; avoid use in children, lactation, pregnancy, or seizure disorder
- Permethrin 1% cream rinse (NIX): apply to scalp and hair, rinse after 10 minutes; reapply in 7–10 days if needed
- Pyrethrin/piperonyl butoxide (RID): apply to scalp and hair, wash after 10 minutes; repeat in 7–10 days

Antipruritics

- Cetirizine (Zyrtec): adult (age >12): 5–10 mg po q day; peds: not recommended
- Diphenhydramine (Benadryl): adult: 25–50 mg po q 6 hrs; peds: 5 mg/kg/day div q 6 hrs
- Hydroxyzine (Atarax): adult: 25 mg po q 8 hrs; peds: 12.5 mg per dose q 6 hrs

Disposition

ADMISSION CRITERIA

- Extensive bacterial superinfection; systemic hypersensitivity reaction with cardiorespiratory compromise

DISCHARGE CRITERIA

- Mild to moderate infestation with absence of significant superinfection or hypersensitivity reaction

Miscellaneous

ICD9: 132.9

CORE CONTENT CODE: 3.2.3.1, 13.12.2.1

SUGGESTED READINGS

Brown S, Becher J, Brady W. Treatment of ectoparasitic infections: Review of the English-language literature. Clin Infect Dis 1995;20(Suppl 1):S104–S109.

Ibarra J, Hall D. Head lice in schoolchildren. Arch Dis Child 1996;75(6):471–473.

Orkin M, Maibach H. Mite infestations and pediculosis. In: Sams MW, Lynch P, eds. Principles and practice of dermatology. 2d ed. New York: Churchill Livingstone, 1996:209–213.

Author: Guy Tarleton

Pelvic Fracture

Clinical Presentation

SIGNS AND SYMPTOMS

- Localized pain, swelling, ecchymoses, tenderness over hips, groin, and lower back
- Pain on hip movement, ambulation, sitting, standing, defecation
- Tenderness on lateral compression of pelvis, palpation of symphysis pubis or sacroiliac (SI) joints
- Often presents with other traumatic injuries including neurologic, intra-abdominal, genitourinary, perineal, rectal, vaginal, and vascular injury
- Gross pelvic instability, deformity, asymmetry in lower extremity
- Evidence of hemorrhagic shock (see chapter: Hemorrhagic Shock)
- Inability to actively or passively perform range of motion of involved hip

MECHANISM/DESCRIPTION

Key-Conwell Classification System

- Type I fractures
  - —Fracture of individual pelvic bone with no break in ring continuity
  - —Isolated rami fractures: commonly seen in falls in the elderly
  - —Avulsion fractures
    - -Three types: anterior superior, inferior iliac spine, and ischial tuberosity
    - -Result of sudden forceful muscle contraction or stretch
  - —Iliac wing fractures (Duverney's fractures) due to direct trauma or lateral compression
  - —Sacral fractures
  - —Coccygeal fractures
- Type II fractures
  - —Single break in pelvic ring continuity
  - —Two ipsilateral ischiopubic rami fractures; most common Type II fracture
  - —Symphysis pubis fracture: often associated with genitourinary injury
  - —Sacroiliac joint fracture or subluxation
- Type III fractures
  - —Multiple breaks in pelvic ring continuity
  - —High risk for associated injuries and pelvic hemorrhage
  - —Malgaigne fracture (see chapter: Malgaigne Fracture)
  - —Anterior and posterior break in the ring on the same side
  - —Straddle fracture
    - -Fractures of all 4 pubic rami or ipsilateral fracture of 2 pubic rami with dislocation of symphysis pubis
    - -Due to lateral compression or straddle injury (i.e., fall on object)
  - —Open book fracture
    - -Wide separation of symphysis pubis (often >2.5 cm) associated with sacroiliac joint disruption from anterior/posterior pelvic compression
  - —Severe multiple fractures
    - -Crush injuries or falls resulting in multiple fractures and gross instability
- Type IV fractures
  - —Fractures involving the acetabulum

ETIOLOGY

- 60% of pelvic fractures occur from motor vehicle accidents, most commonly pedestrians struck by automobiles
- 30% are due to falls from heights
- Mortality rate from pelvic fractures reported is 6%–19%
- Increases to nearly 50% with hemorrhagic shock
- Significant pelvic hemorrhage can occur in unstable pelvic fractures, particularly Type III fractures
  - —Bleeding most commonly arises from the venous plexuses
  - —Significant hemorrhage results in retroperitoneal hematoma formation that may tamponade in the enclosed pelvic space

PEDIATRIC CONSIDERATIONS

- Children can have proportionately greater hemorrhage
- Nonaccidental trauma is a concern

Pre-Hospital

CAUTIONS

- Pneumatic antishock garment (PASG) is an option, particularly when faced with a prolonged transport time or hemodynamically instability
- Aggressive fluid resuscitation must occur before deflation of the PASG

Diagnosis

ESSENTIAL WORKUP

- Pelvic radiology is the most valuable initial diagnostic test
- A single AP view of the pelvis should be obtained as early as possible
  - —Most significant unstable pelvic fractures will be seen on the single AP view
  - —Other views include
    - -Inlet projection: 30° caudal view, allows visualization of posterior arch
    - -Outlet projection: 30° cephalic angulation, allows visualization of sacrum
    - -Judet oblique views (internal and external): allows evaluation of acetabulum

LABORATORY

- Type and crossmatch
- Hemoglobin/hematocrit, platelet count, and coagulation studies (PT/PTT)

IMAGING/SPECIAL TESTS

- CT scan may further delineate pelvic fracture(s) and retroperitoneal hematoma
- MRI is indicated when there is evidence of neurologic injury
- Abdominal ultrasound (US) or diagnostic peritoneal lavage (DPL) are rapid bedside evaluations for intraperitoneal hemorrhage
  - —There is a high mortality rate in victims with pelvic fractures who undergo celiotomy; caution must be exercised to avoid false positive results
  - —In the setting of pelvic fracture, the supraumbilical open approach for DPL should be used

DIFFERENTIAL DIAGNOSIS

- Normal variants (i.e., os acetabuli epiphyseal line can mimic Type I fracture on x-ray)
- Ligamentous injury
- Spinal injury
- Intra-abdominal injury and hemorrhage

Treatment

INITIAL STABILIZATION

- ABCs of trauma care
  - —Avoid using lower extremity IV sites
  - —Aggressive resuscitation with blood or crystalloid, O-negative or type-specific blood if hemodynamically unstable
  - —Immobilize the pelvis to prevent further injury and decrease bleeding
    - -PASG: use in ED is controversial but allows rapid pelvic immobilization and pelvic compression to slow bleeding
    - -External fixator requires more time to place than PASG but "splints" pelvis in a similar manner; contraindicated in severely comminuted pelvic fracture
    - -Placement of a stabilization device should not interfere with further workup and care (DPL, etc.)

ED TREATMENT

- Determine which pelvic fractures are stable and unstable
- Type I and II fractures are generally stable
- Type III fractures are unstable

Type I Fractures

- Treated conservatively with bed rest, analgesics, and comfort measures

Type II Fractures

- Treated conservatively but management decisions should be made in conjunction with orthopedics
- Insure there is no other break in the pelvic ring

Type III Fractures

- Immediate orthopedics consultation; patient should remain NPO
- May require ED pelvic stabilization measures
- Assess for pelvic hemorrhage (see below)

Type IV Fractures

- Orthopedics consultation; patient to remain NPO

Pelvic Hemorrhage

- Angiography and selective vessel embolization
- Direct operative control of pelvic bleeding

Prioritization of Studies: CT, Angiography, or Surgery

- In the hemodynamically *unstable* patient, a rapidly performed DPL or US can determine treatment course
  - —If the DPL or US is positive, the patient should go for celiotomy with external pelvic fixation followed by selective angiography
  - —If the DPL or US is negative, the patient should go to angiography
  - —In the hemodynamically stable patient, the patient can go to CT scan for evaluation of the abdomen, pelvis, and retroperitoneum

MEDICATIONS

- Crystalloid fluids: NS *or* LR, IV bolus 2 L; peds: 20 cc/kg
- Blood products: crossmatched, type-specific, or O-negative 4–6 IU; peds: 10 cc/kg

Disposition

ADMISSION CRITERIA

- Hemodynamic instability, and pelvic hemorrhage to the ICU
- Type III or IV pelvic fracture
- Other related injuries (genitourinary, intra-abdominal, neurologic, etc)
- Intractable pain

DISCHARGE CRITERIA

- Type I or II fractures; hemodynamically stable with no evidence of other injuries

Miscellaneous

ICD9: 808.8

CORE CONTENT CODE: 18.4.15

SUGGESTED READINGS

Berger JJ, Britt LD. Pelvic fracture hemorrhage: Current strategies in diagnosis and management. Surg Annu 1995;27:107–112.

Cryer H, Miller F, Evers B. Pelvic fracture classification: correlation with hemorrhage. J Trauma 1988;28:973–980.

Cwinn AA. Pelvis and hip. In: Rosen P, et al., eds. Emergency medicine: Concepts and clinical practice. 4th ed. St. Louis: CV Mosby, 1998:739–762.

Jerrard DA. Pelvic fractures. Emerg Med Clin North Am 1993;11(1):147–163.

Author: Ted Chan

Pelvic Inflammatory Disease

Clinical Presentation

SIGNS AND SYMPTOMS

- Lower abdominal pain, usually bilateral
- Vaginal discharge
- Abnormal uterine bleeding
- Dysuria
- Dyspareunia
- Nausea and vomiting
- Fever
- Lower abdominal tenderness
- Bilateral adnexal tenderness
- Cervical motion tenderness
- Adnexal mass or fullness
- Right upper quadrant pain

MECHANISM/DESCRIPTION

- Pelvic inflammatory disease is an infection of the uterus, fallopian tubes, ovaries, and adjacent structures. Progressive disease can lead to the formation of a tubo-ovarian abscess
- Fitz-Hugh-Curtis syndrome is a capsular inflammation of the liver that is associated with pelvic inflammatory disease. It frequently presents as a sharp right upper-quadrant abdominal pain that is worse with inspiration, movement, or coughing

ETIOLOGY

- Risk factors for pelvic inflammatory disease include young age, multiple sexual partners, intrauterine devices, instrumentation of the female genital tract
- Most common cause of pelvic inflammatory disease is *Neisseria gonorrhea* and *Chlamydia trachomatis*
- Other organisms include streptococci, anaerobes, and Gram-negative rods

Pre-Hospital

- No specific pre-hospital considerations
- Maintain ABCs, appropriate pain management

Diagnosis

ESSENTIAL WORKUP

- History and physical exam including pelvic examination
- Pregnancy test
- Cervical culture for *Neisseria gonorrhea* and *Chlamydia trachomatis;* swab for *Chlamydiazyme*

LABORATORY

- CBC, ESR, or C-reactive protein may be helpful
- Gram stain of endocervix
- Liver enzymes may be elevated in Fitz-Hugh-Curtis syndrome

IMAGING/SPECIAL TESTS

- Patients with adnexal fullness or an adnexal mass on exam should have immediate pelvic ultrasound to exclude a tubo-ovarian abscess (TOA)
- Consider obtaining a pelvic ultrasound in patients who use a intrauterine device, fail outpatient antibiotic therapy for pelvic inflammatory disease, or who have inadequate pelvic exams due to pain or obesity
- Minimum criteria for clinical diagnosis
  - —Lower abdominal tenderness
  - —Bilateral adnexal tenderness
  - —Cervical motion tenderness
- Supportive criteria for diagnosis
  - —Fever >38.3°C
  - —Intracellular Gram-negative diplococci on endocervical Gram stain
  - —Leukocytosis >10,000/mm^3
  - —Elevated erythrocyte sedimentation rate or C-reactive protein
  - —White blood cells or bacteria in peritoneal fluid obtained by culdocentesis or laparoscopy
  - —Cervical discharge

DIFFERENTIAL DIAGNOSIS

- Acute appendicitis
- Endometriosis
- Hemorrhagic corpus luteum cyst
- Ectopic pregnancy
- Pelvic adhesions
- Benign ovarian cyst
- Chronic salpingitis

Treatment

INITIAL STABILIZATION

- Manage ABCs and shock as indicated

ED TREATMENT

Outpatient

- Cefoxitin plus probenecid plus doxycycline; or ceftriaxone plus doxycycline

Inpatient

- Cefoxitin; or cefotetan plus doxycycline; or gentamycin plus clindamycin

MEDICATIONS

- Cefotetan: 2 g IV q 12 hrs
- Cefoxitin: 2 g IM single dose (outpatient); 1 g IV q 8 hrs (inpatient)
- Ceftriaxone: 125 mg IM single dose
- Clindamycin: 900 mg IV q 8 hrs
- Doxycycline: 100 mg po bid × 14 days (outpatient); 100 mg IV q 12 hrs (inpatient)
- Gentamicin: 2 mg/kg loading dose followed by 1.5 mg/kg q 8 hrs IV
- Probenecid: 1 g po single dose
- Tubo-ovarian abscesses may require drainage or surgical intervention in addition to antibiotics
- Laparoscopy can be used to lyse adhesions in the acute and chronic stages of Fitz-Hugh-Curtis syndrome

Disposition

ADMISSION CRITERIA

- Uncertain diagnosis and toxic appearing
- Pelvic abscess is suspected, including TOA
- Pregnancy
- Adolescent
- Severe illness (e.g., vomiting or severe pain) precludes outpatient therapy
- Noncompliance
- Consider admission if appropriate clinical follow-up cannot be arranged

DISCHARGE CRITERIA

- Most patients that do not meet admission criteria may be treated as outpatients

Miscellaneous

ICD9: 614.9

CORE CONTENT CODE: 19.1.5.3, 19.1.5.3.3, 19.1.5.3.4

SUGGESTED READINGS

Centers for Disease Control. Pelvic inflammatory disease: Guidelines for prevention and management. MMWR Recom Rep 1991;40(rr-5):1–25.

Lopez-Zeno JA, Keith LG, Berger GS. The Fitz-Hugh-Curtis syndrome revisited. J Reprod Med 1985;30:567–582.

McCormack WM. Pelvic inflammatory disease. N Engl J Med 1994;330:115–119.

Pastorek JG. Pelvic inflammatory disease and tubo-ovarian abscess. Obstet Gynecol Clin North Am 1989;16:347–361.

Author: Bing Pao

Pemphigus

Clinical Presentation

SIGNS AND SYMPTOMS

- Generalized or focal flaccid bullae (blisters) of the skin and mucosa
- Painful nonhealing oral erosions
- Painful skin erosions with shreds of detached epithelium
- Crusting, partially healing skin erosions from ruptured bullae
- Hypertrophic, hyperplastic erosive plaques with pustules in intertriginous areas (pemphigus vegetans)
- Malar distribution of erythematous, scaly, crusting skin lesions (pemphigus erythematosus)
- Nikolsky's sign (separation of the epidermis with lateral pressure) is characteristic but not diagnostic

MECHANISM/DESCRIPTION

- Pemphigus is an autoantibody-mediated blistering disease of the skin and mucous membranes
  - —If untreated mortality rates average greater than 73%
- Pemphigus is a rare disease with a worldwide incidence of 0.1–0.5 cases per 100,000
- Four major subtypes exist (vulgaris, vegetans, foliaceus, erythematosus)
- *Pemphigus vulgaris* accounts for 80% of all cases
- 70% of patients with vulgaris or vegetans present with oral lesions
- Superficial pemphigus (foliaceus, erythematosus) often lack oral lesions and have a better prognosis
- Pemphigus is most common in individuals 40–60 years old but has been reported in people with ages ranging from neonates to 89 years

ETIOLOGY

- IgG autoantibodies are directed against pemphigus antigen found in all keratinocytes
- The autoantibodies cause acantholysis (separation of the epidermis), which causes blistering
- Immunogenetic predisposition secondary to higher frequencies of specific HLA haplotypes contributes to this disease
- Drugs may induce or trigger pemphigus (penicillamine, captopril, rifampin, piroxicam, phenobarbital)
- Endemic pemphigus foliaceus (fogo selvagem) may be triggered or transmitted by bites from flying insects

PEDIATRIC CONSIDERATIONS

- Pemphigus is rare in children
- Neonates may develop the disease secondary to transplacental transfer of IgG
- Neonatal pemphigus spontaneously resolves in several weeks as the maternal antibodies are catabolized

Pre-Hospital

CAUTIONS

- Patients with severe pemphigus may require rapid transport and fluid resuscitation secondary to the loss of the skin barrier function as in a severe burn patient

Diagnosis

ESSENTIAL WORKUP

- Pemphigus is suspected by clinical findings
- Biopsy with histologic and immunofluorescence testing is essential for definitive diagnosis (arrange with a dermatologist)

LABORATORY

- Serum antibody titers, detected by indirect immunofluorescence, are often used as a marker of disease activity. The emergency physician would not routinely order this test

IMAGING/SPECIAL TESTS

- No imaging test is helpful

DIFFERENTIAL DIAGNOSIS

- Bullous pemphigoid
- Dermatitis herpetiformis
- Erythema multiforme
- Toxic epidermal necrolysis
- Epidermolysis bullosa
- Hand, foot, and mouth disease
- Systemic lupus erythematosus
- Systemic vasculitis
- Oral candidiasis
- Herpes simplex gingivostomatitis
- Erosive lichen planus
- Seborrheic dermatitis

Treatment

INITIAL STABILIZATION

- ABCs
- If severe disease, establish a safety net at presentation (IV, O_2 saturation monitor, cardiac monitor)
- Crystalloid resuscitation should be guided by the Parkland burn formula if symptoms of hypotension or sepsis are present
  —4 ml crystalloid/kg body weight/percent body surface area involvement per 24 hours
  —Give half of total calculated fluid in first 8 hours, remainder in the next 16 hours
  —Adjust fluids to keep urine output greater than 0.5 ml/kg/hour
- Stress-dose steroids if patient is steroid-dependent
- Early broad spectrum antibiotic coverage if signs or symptoms of sepsis are present

ED TREATMENT

- Systemic corticosteroids are the mainstay of therapy
- *Severe disease:* conventional high-dose corticosteroids
  —If severe symptoms are unresponsive to high-dose po corticosteroids, consider pulse intravenous corticosteroids and admission for plasmapheresis
- *Mild to moderate disease* should receive po prednisone and consider intralesional triamcinolone acetonide 20 mg/ml; inject 0.1 ml into each superficial lesion
- *Adjuvant therapy* may be added by a primary physician to decrease the symptoms of high-dose systemic corticosteroids or in patients with contraindications to steroid therapy
  —Dapsone, gold, azathioprine, cyclophosphamide, cyclosporine, methotrexate

Medications

- Hydrocortisone: 100–300 mg IV stress-dose steroids
- Methylprednisolone (pulse IV therapy): 1 g over 3 hrs q day IV (adults)
- Prednisone: 20–400 mg/day po (adults); severe disease: 200–400 mg/day po for 5–10 weeks then taper; mild to moderate disease: 20–80 mg/day po
- Triamcinolone acetonide: 20 mg/ml 0.1 ml injection into each lesion

Disposition

ADMISSION CRITERIA

- Admit to the ICU if any signs or symptoms of sepsis are present or aggressive fluid resuscitation is required secondary to massive skin involvement with third spacing into blisters
- Admit to a floor bed if pulse parenteral steroid therapy and plasmapheresis is indicated
- Most first-time presentations of disease should be admitted for definitive diagnosis and stabilization

DISCHARGE CRITERIA

- Discharge to home if mild to moderate disease
- Arrange follow-up for reevaluation of progression of disease and biopsy if not previously obtained

Miscellaneous

ICD9: 694.4

CORE CONTENT CODE: 3.6.1

SUGGESTED READINGS

Becker BA, Gagpari AA. Pemphigus vulgaris and vegetans. Dermatol Clin 1993;11(3):429–452.

Bystryn JC, Steinman NM. The adjuvant therapy of pemphigus. Arch Dermatol 1996;132:203–212.

Fine J. Bullous diseases. In: Moschella SL, Hurley HJ, eds. Dermatology. 3rd ed. Philadelphia: WB Saunders, 1992:655–692.

Korman NJ. Pemphigus. Dermatol Clin 1990;8(4):689–700.

Stanley JR. Pemphigus skin failure mediated by autoantibodies, JAMA 1990;264(13):1714–1717.

Wooldridge WE. The blistering diseases. Post Grad Med 1990;88(3):103–106.

Author: James T. Vandenberg

Penile Shaft Fracture

Clinical Presentation

SIGNS AND SYMPTOMS

- Sudden sharp painful sensation in erect penis during sexual intercourse or soon after with loss of erection. May hear cracking or crunching sound at the time of trauma
- Swelling and bluish black discoloration at base of penis, usually on one side
- Ecchymosis may also involve scrotum
- Penis flaccid and edematous with angulation away from the side of tear
- Defect in corpus cavernosum may be palpable at the site of tear in tunica albuginea
- When there is an associated urethral injury, patient may have blood at tip of penis or frank hematuria. May also have dysuria, inability to void, or an increase in size of the swelling with voiding because of extravasation of urine

MECHANISM/DESCRIPTION

- Traumatic rupture of tunica albuginea, surrounding corpus cavernosum. Usually unilateral, caused by blunt trauma to erect penis during,
  - —Sexual intercourse
  - —Manipulation
  - —Fall on erect penis
- During erection, pressure within corpus cavernosum is maximum, close to arterial pressure, increasing volume in each corpus to maximum, which thins tunica albuginea making it susceptible to rupture
- Penile erection also stretches spongiosum to the limit, which will limit movement vertically, while still allowing lateral movements. This forms a bend at base of penis making it vulnerable to lateral swing and rupture of corpus cavernosum
- About 25–30% have associated urethral injury, which may be partial or complete

ETIOLOGY

- Peyronie's disease
- Urethritis in past
- Surgical procedure on corpus cavernosum or trauma to corpus cavernosum resulting in weak scar tissue

Pre-Hospital

- Application of ice to penis and elevation to reduce swelling and hematoma

Diagnosis

ESSENTIAL WORKUP

- Urinalysis to evaluate urethral trauma. May have frank blood or microscopic hematuria
- Retrograde urethrography—recommended in all cases of suspected urethral trauma; should be done with low pressure during injection, prior to urethral catheterization
- Cavernosography and MRI of penis may be needed to confirm diagnosis and site of tear

DIFFERENTIAL DIAGNOSIS

- Contusion of penis
- Paraphimosis
- Cellulitis of penis
- Vasculature rupture especially deep dorsal vein or artery
- Trauma because of constrictive ring or other structure
- Neoplasm of penis

Treatment

INITIAL STABILIZATION

- ABCs if associated trauma present
- Needle suprapubic cystotomy in patients with urethral trauma and full bladder to relieve patient discomfort
- Local treatment: ice packs locally to penis; splinting with tongue blade

ED TREATMENT

- Combined efforts of emergency physician and urologist are aimed toward restoration of normal shape of penis and sexual and urinary functions
- ED treatment directed to reduce hemorrhage, prevent further complications
- Prophylactic antibiotic use is questionable
- Urethral catheterization in all cases after excluding urethral trauma
- Urological evaluation and early surgical treatment is essential to prevent complications such as erectile dysfunction, impotence, penile deformity, urethral stenosis
- All patients with suspected or definite diagnosis *must* have early urological evaluation

MEDICATIONS

- Diazepam: 2–5 mg IV
- Lorazepam: 0.5–1.0 mg IV
- Meperidine: 1 mg/kg IV
- Morphine sulfate: 0.1 mg/kg IV

Disposition

ADMISSION CRITERIA

- *All* patients with penile fracture must be hospitalized for prompt surgery

TRANSFER

- If immediate urological consultation and treatment unavailable, patient may be transferred to a suitable hospital after initial stabilization, following appropriate criteria for transfer

Miscellaneous

ICD9: 959.1

CORE CONTENT CODE: 19.2.2

SUGGESTED READINGS

Asgari MA, et al. Penile fractures: Evaluation therapeutic approaches and long-term results. J Urol 1996;155:148–149.

Fedel M, et al. The value of MRI in diagnosis of suspected penile fracture with atypical clinical findings. J Urol 1996;155(6):1924–1927.

Koga S, et al. Sonography in fracture of penis. Brit J Urol 1993;72:228–229.

Authors: Shyambhai Rao; Joseph LaMantia

Peptic Ulcer

Clinical Presentation

SIGNS AND SYMPTOMS

- Epigastric pain or tenderness (80–90%)
  - —Burning, gnawing, aching pain
  - —Location: midline, xiphoid, or umbilicus
- Duodenal ulcers
  - —Pain occurs 90 minutes to 3 hours after meals
  - —Usually awakens the patient at night
  - —Food and antacids relieve the pain
- Gastric ulcers
  - —Pain worsens after meals
  - —Nausea and anorexia
- Difficult to differentiate clinically between gastric and duodenal ulcers
- Relief of pain with antacids
- Heme-positive stools
- Complications of PUD
  - —Acute perforation
    - -Rigid "boardlike" abdomen
    - -Generalized rebound tenderness
    - -Pain radiation to back or shoulder
  - —Obstruction
    - -Pain with vomiting
    - -"Succussion" splash from retained gastric contents and abdominal distention
  - —Hemorrhage
    - -Hematemesis
    - -Melena
    - -Hypotension
    - -Tachycardia
    - -Skin pallor
    - -Orthostatic changes

MECHANISM/DESCRIPTION

- Produced by a breakdown in the gastric or duodenal mucosal defenses
- Imbalance between production of acid and ability of mucosa to prevent damage

ETIOLOGY

- Major causes
  - —*Helicobacter pylori*
    - -Gram-negative spiral bacteria that lives in the mucus layer
    - -Responsible for 90–95% of duodenal ulcers and 80% of gastric ulcers
    - -Increases antral gastrin production and decreases mucosal integrity
  - —NSAIDs
    - -Interfere with prostaglandin synthesis
    - -Leads to a break in the mucosa
  - —Aspirin
  - —Cigarette smoking
  - —Alcohol

Pre-Hospital

CAUTIONS

- Initial stabilization with 2 large-bore IVs of LR or 0.9%NS to fluid resuscitate for
  - —Perforation with peritonitis
  - —Massive upper gastrointestinal hemorrhage with hemodynamic compromise
  - —Hypotension

Diagnosis

ESSENTIAL WORKUP

- Careful physical examination including hemoccult testing and vital signs with orthostatics
- For stable patients oral "GI cocktail" typically relieves pain
  - —Antacid: 30 cc
  - —Viscous lidocaine: 10 cc

LABORATORY

- Normal lab values in uncomplicated ulcer disease
- CBC
  - —Low Hct with bleeding
  - —Leukocytosis with perforation/penetration
- Amylase/lipase
  - —Elevated with perforation/penetration
  - —Pancreatitis in differential diagnosis
- Electrolytes, BUN/Cr, glucose for critically ill
- Type and cross match
  - —For significant blood loss

IMAGING/SPECIAL TESTS

- ECG
  - —For elderly patients
  - —Myocardial ischemia in differential diagnosis
- CXR/abdominal series for
  - —Perforation
  - —Bowel obstruction
- Endoscopy
  - —Procedure of choice
  - —Outpatient unless significant hemorrhage
  - —Allows for biopsies of gastric/duodenal ulcers for the presence of *H. pylori*
  - —Detects malignant gastric ulcers
- UGI series
  - —Single contrast barium diagnose 70–80%
  - —Double contrast diagnose 90%
- Gastrin level is elevated in Zollinger-Ellison syndrome

DIFFERENTIAL DIAGNOSIS

- Gastroesophageal reflux
- Biliary colic
- Cholecystitis
- Pancreatitis
- Gastritis
- Abdominal aortic aneurysm
- Aortic dissection
- Myocardial infarction
- Subset with symptoms and no ulcer on endoscopy called "nonulcer dyspepsia"

Treatment

INITIAL STABILIZATION

- For ulcer complications (hemorrhage, perforation, and obstruction)
- ABCs
- Treat hypotension with LR or 0.9%NS IV fluid bolus via 2 large-bore IVs
- Nasogastric tube for gastric decompression/check for hemorrhage

ED TREATMENT

- Pain control with antacids (GI cocktail) or IV H_2 antagonists
- Avoid narcotics—may mask serious illness
- Promotion of ulcer healing
  —Antacids
  —H_2 antagonists (cimetidine, famotidine, ranitidine, nizatidine)
  —Sucralfate
  —Prostaglandin congers (misoprostol)
  —Protease pump inhibitors (omeprazole)
- Gastric outlet obstruction
  —Decompress stomach with NG tube
  —IV hydration
- Gastric hemorrhage
  —IV fluid resuscitation
  —Blood transfusion depending on loss/Hct
  —Foley to monitor volume status
- Perforation
  —IV hydration
  —Foley
  —Preoperative antibiotics
  —Emergency surgical consultation
- Treatment of *H. pylori* infection
  —Invasive or noninvasive testing to confirm infection
  —Oral (po) eradication antibiotic therapy options
    -Proton pump inhibitor (omeprazole 20 mg bid) and two antibiotics (clarithromycin 250 mg bid plus metronidazole 500 mg bid) for 7 days
    -H_2 blocker, bismuth subsalicylate (pepto bismol) plus either amoxicillin 500 mg qid or tetracycline 500 mg qid in combination with either metronidazole 250 mg tid or clarithromycin 500 mg tid for 14 days

MEDICATIONS

- Bismuth subsalicylate: 262 mg tabs 2 po qid
- Cimetidine (H_2 blocker): 800 mg po qhs for 6–8 weeks
- Famotidine (H_2 blocker): 40 mg po qhs for 6–8 weeks
- Misoprostol: 100–200 μg po qid
- Maalox plus: 2–4 tablets po qid
- Mylanta II 2–4 tablets po qid
- Nizatidine (H_2 blocker): 300 mg po qhs for 6–8 weeks
- Omeprazole: 20 mg po qd for 4 weeks
- Ranitidine (H_2 blocker): 300 mg po qhs for 6–8 weeks
- Sucralfate: 1 g po qid for 6–8 weeks

Disposition

ADMISSION CRITERIA

- Gastric obstruction
- Perforation
- Active upper GI bleed
- Melena
- Uncontrolled pain

DISCHARGE CRITERIA

- Unremarkable physical examination with normal CBC and heme-negative stools
- If heme-positive stools, discharge if stable vital signs, normal Hct, and negative NG tube aspiration for upper GI hemorrhage

Miscellaneous

ICD9: 533.9

CORE CONTENT CODE: 1.5.3

SUGGESTED READINGS

McGuirk TD, et al. Upper gastrointestinal tract bleeding. Emerg Med Clin North Am 1996;14(3):530–533.

Moss SF. Treatment of *H. pylori* infection—who, how and when. Resid Staff Physician 1996;42:11–18.

Peptic ulcer disease: Current medical diagnosis and treatment. 33rd ed. Chap. 14. 1994:490–498.

Author: Marco Cordero

Perforated Viscous

Clinical Presentation

SIGNS AND SYMPTOMS

- Sudden severe abdominal pain
  - —Initially local
  - —Rapidly becoming diffuse
- Rigidity
- Guarding
- Rebound tenderness
- Absent bowel sounds
- Hypovolemic shock
  - —Tachycardia
  - —Hypotension

MECHANISM/DESCRIPTION

- Perforation of any segment of gastrointestinal tract due to
  - —Inflammation
  - —Ulceration
  - —Shearing/crushing or bursting forces in trauma
  - —Obstruction
- Chemical peritonitis occurs as a result of spillage of gastric or intestinal contents into peritoneal cavity
- Massive outpouring of extracellular fluid into peritoneum follows shortly

ETIOLOGY

- Peptic ulcer disease
- Appendicitis
- Inflammatory bowel disease
- Diverticular disease
- Colon carcinoma
- Foreign body ingestion
- Trauma
- Radiation enteritis

PEDIATRIC CONSIDERATIONS

- Blunt trauma—more common cause of bowel rupture than penetrating trauma in children
  - —Jejunum is the most common site of rupture

Pre-Hospital

CAUTIONS

- Treat hypotension/tachycardia with 500 cc–1 L bolus (peds: 20 cc/kg) of 0.9%NS

Diagnosis

ESSENTIAL WORKUP

- Upright CXR
  - —Best demonstrates pneumoperitoneum
  - —When in upright position for 5–10 minutes may detect as little as 1–2 ml of free air under the diaphragm

LABORATORY

- CBC
- Electrolytes, BUN/Cr, glucose
- Amylase/lipase
- Urinalysis

IMAGING/SPECIAL TESTS

- Abdominal radiographs
  - —Left lateral decubitus film
  - —Supine abdomen
    - -Double-wall or "Rigler's" sign: air in intestinal lumen and peritoneal cavity allows for visualization of both serosal (not normally seen) and mucosal surfaces of intestine
- ECG

DIFFERENTIAL DIAGNOSIS

- Intra-abdominal abscess
- Pneumomediastinum with peritoneal extension
- Pancreatitis
- Peptic ulcer disease
- Inferior wall myocardial infarction
- Cholecystitis

Treatment

INITIAL STABILIZATION

- ABCs
- Correct hypovolemia
  - —Rapid fluid resuscitation with 0.9%NS 1 L in adults (20 cc/kg in children)
  - —Pressure support for persistent hypotension

ED TREATMENT

- Nasogastric tube
- Foley
- Administer broad spectrum antibiotics (second-generation cephalosporin)

MEDICATIONS

- Cefoxitin: 1–2 g q 6–8 hrs (peds: 0–7 days: 40mg/kg/24hrs q 12 hrs; >7 days: 80–160 mg/kg/24hrs q 6 hrs) IVPB
- Demerol: 25 mg increments (peds: 1 mg/kg) IV PRN
- Morphine sulfate: 2–4 mg increments (peds: 0.1 mg/kg) IV PRN

Disposition

ADMISSION CRITERIA

- Suspected or confirmed perforation requires admission and immediate surgical consultation

DISCHARGE CRITERIA

- None

Miscellaneous

ICD9: 799.8

CORE CONTENT CODE: 1.1.2.3 PERFORATION

SUGGESTED READINGS

Shaffer H. Perforation and obstruction of the gastrointestinal tract. Radiol Clin North Am 1992;30(2):405.

Sivit C. Gastrointestinal emergencies in older infants and children. Radiol Clin North Am 1997;35(4):865.

Author: Julio Silva

Peri-lunate Dislocation

Clinical Presentation

SIGNS AND SYMPTOMS

- Pain in the wrist
- Swelling or mass in the wrist

MECHANISM/DESCRIPTION

- Fall from height, violent palmar or dorsiflexion of the hand
- Dislocation of the carpal bones (usually the capitate) volar or dorsal from the lunate
- Radiocarpal ligament intact

Pre-Hospital Considerations

CAUTIONS

- Consider other more serious injuries
- Dress open wounds
- Immobilize in neutral position
- Elevation, cold to reduce swelling
- Age appropriate social management

Diagnosis

ESSENTIAL WORKUP

- Physical examination with special attention to skin integrity and neurovascular status, including two-point discrimination
- This diagnosis is often missed by the clinical exam
- Radiographic imaging that includes three views of the wrist

IMAGING/SPECIAL TESTS

- Peri-lunate dislocation is visualized best on the true lateral view with the distal carpal row dorsal or volar to the lunate and with the lunate in its normal relationship to the radius

DIFFERENTIAL DIAGNOSIS

- Lunate fracture
- Lunate dislocation
- Scapholunate dissociation
- The scaphoid is frequently fractured with this injury

Treatment

INITIAL STABILIZATION

- Immobilize, ice, elevate pending definitive evaluation
- Identify other, more serious, associated injuries

ED TREATMENT

- Reduction of dislocation
  —The patient is given appropriate conscious sedation
  —The hand is placed in finger traps and counterweights are used
  —Finger pressure is placed at the level of the dislocation and the injury is gently exaggerated, then brought to appropriate position, maintaining pressure over the dislocated segment
  —The wrist is immobilized using a thumb spica-splint in neutral position

MEDICATIONS

- Pain control
- See chapter on conscious sedation

PEDIATRIC CONSIDERATIONS

- Wrists are rarely sprained in children and the x-ray is difficult to interpret
- Although peri-lunate dislocation is unusual in pediatric patients, children with wrist pain should be splinted and referred for ongoing evaluation of possible dislocations or fractures

Disposition

ADMISSION CRITERIA

- Open fracture, presence of multiple trauma or other, more serious, injuries
- Inability to reduce the fracture or maintain reduction
- Neurovascular compromise

DISCHARGE CRITERIA

- Closed injuries, adequate reduction, no neurovascular involvement
- Next day orthopedic follow-up

Miscellaneous

ICD9: 833.00

CORE CONTENT CODE: 18.4.12.2.3.2

SUGGESTED READINGS

American Society for Surgery of the Hand. The hand: Primary care of common problems. 2d ed. New York: Churchill Livingston, 1990:637-649.

Eisenhauer MA. Forearm and wrist injuries. In: Rosen P, et al., eds. Emergency medicine: Concepts and clinical practice. 4th ed. St Louis: Mosby-Year Book 1998:669–689.

Simon RR, Slobodkin. Injuries to the wrist and hand. In: American College of Emergency Physicians. Emergency medicine: A comprehensive study guide. 4th ed. New York: McGraw Hill, 1996:1217–1226.

Uehara DT. The hand in emergency medicine. Emerg Clin North Am 1993;11(3): 781–796.

Author: Matthew Walsh

Perianal Abscess

Clinical Presentation

SIGNS AND SYMPTOMS

Local

- Perianal pain
  - —Present constantly
  - —Aggravated by defecation, sitting, and coughing or sneezing
- Perianal swelling in
  - —Perianal abscess
  - —Large ischiorectal abscess
- Intra-anal and intrarectal swelling
  - —Intersphincteric abscess
  - —Submucosal abscess
  - —Small, deep ischiorectal abscess
  - —Supralevator abscess

Systemic

- Malaise
- Pyrexia
- Advanced lesions may lead to septic shock

MECHANISM/DESCRIPTION

- Infected anal glands spread to perianal, ischiorectal, supralevator, intersphincteric, or submucosal spaces

ETIOLOGY

- Majority from infected anal glands in the anal crypts
- Foreign body
- Crohn's disease
- Abdominal infection (PID or diverticulitis)
- Trauma
- Radiation
- Carcinoma
- Leukemia

PEDIATRIC CONSIDERATIONS

- Rectal duplication may mimic perianal abscess

Pre-Hospital

CAUTIONS

- Sitz baths will reduce pain
- Antibiotics contraindicated as drainage is the treatment

Diagnosis

ESSENTIAL WORKUP

- Typical signs/symptoms in history
- Abdominal examination for abdominal or pelvic suppurative disease draining to the perineum
- Careful observation of the external anal and perianal region
  - —Any swelling with cellulitis is presumed abscess requiring incision and drainage
  - —Identify if drainage has occured spontaneously
- Gentle rectal exam
  - —To identify deep ischiorectal, supralevator, submucosal, and intersphincteric abscesses
- Vital signs for signs of systemic infection/sepsis
  - —Fever
  - —Tachycardia
  - —Hypotension

LABORATORY

- CBC if suspicious of systemic infection
  - —Leukocytosis
- Glucose for diabetes mellitus

DIFFERENTIAL DIAGNOSIS

- Anal fissure
- Sentinel pile in the posterior midline or anterior midline
- Thrombosed external hemorrhoids
- HIV anal ulcer
- Gonococcal proctitis
- Leukemic infiltrate
- Rectal duplication in children

Treatment

INITIAL STABILIZATION

- None required if no systemic signs
- With systemic signs of sepsis
  - —Treat hypotension with IV fluids/pressors
  - —Broad spectrum antibiotics
  - —Urgent abscess drainage poststabilization

ED TREATMENT

- Needle aspiration
  - —If it not clearly an abscess
  - —Use 16-gauge needle
  - —Do not aspirate all of pus
  - —Leave needle in to accurately incise and drain deeper abscesses
- Incision and drainage
  - —Visible abscesses under local anesthesia with epinephrine
  - —Perform with an eliptical incision as the pus and necrotic fat is thick and will drain for several days
  - —Large ischiorectal abscesses—caution
    - -Do not I+D if drainage already occurring inside the rectum
    - -I+D of draining abscess may result in high extrasphincteric fistulae
- Operative debridement under anesthesia and IV antibiotics for
  - —Large abscesses (≥10 cm)
  - —Large amount of necrotic tissue
  - —Deep internal abscesses
  - —Unable to drain under local anesthetic
  - —Immunosuppressed (HIV, diabetics, transplant patients, patients on chemotherapy)
- Pain medication/sedation for procedure
- Antibiotics (cefoxitin) for
  - —Systemic toxicity
  - —Large area of cellulitis
  - —Lymphangitis
  - —Immunocompromise

MEDICATIONS

- Cefoxitin: 1–2 g (peds: 100 mg/kg/24hrs) IV q 8 hrs

Disposition

ADMISSION CRITERIA

- Need for operative drainage
- Systemic toxicity/signs of sepsis

DISCHARGE CRITERIA

- Adequate incision and drainage with return of discernible pus
- Ability to ambulate and care for wound

Miscellaneous

ICD9: 566

CORE CONTENT CODE: 1.8.1.7

SUGGESTED READINGS

Abcarian H, Alexander-Williams J, Christiansen J, et al. Benign anorectal disease: Definition, characterization and analysis of treatment. Am J Gastroenterol 1994;89:S182–S193.

Ramanujam P, Prasad ML, Abcarian H. Perianal abscesses and fistulas: A study of 1023 patients. Dis Colon Rectum 1984;27:593–597.

Read DR, Abcarian H. A prospective survey of 474 patients with anorectal abscess. Dis Colon Rectum 1979:22:566–568.

Author: Charles Orsay

Pericardial Effusion/Tamponade

Clinical Presentation

SIGNS AND SYMPTOMS

- Pericardial effusion
- Majority asymptomatic
- Symptoms
  - —Dyspnea
  - —Chest pain
  - —Fatigue
  - —Malaise
- Signs
  - —Pericardial friction rub
  - —Signs of shock or right heart failure
  - —Pulsus paradoxus
  - —Fall in the systolic blood pressure >10 mm Hg with inspiration
  - —Dressler's syndrome
  - —Fever
  - —Chest pain
  - —Pericardial friction rub several weeks after an MI
  - —Beck's triad
  - —Classic presentation of cardiac tamponade
  - —Hypotension
  - —Jugular venous distention (JVD)
  - —Hypovolemic patients may not have JVD
  - —Muffled heart sounds (present in one-third of patients)

MECHANISM/DESCRIPTION

- Pericardial effusion
  - —Accumulation of fluid in the pericardial sac
  - —Occurs in 10% of cancer patients
- Pericardial tamponade
  - —Accumulation of pericardial fluid with elevation of pressure in the pericardial space that results in impairment of ventricular filling and decreased cardiac output
  - —Rapid accumulation of 200 cc of fluid in the pericardial space causes hemodynamic compromise and pericardial tamponade
  - —Occurs in 2% of patients with penetrating chest trauma

ETIOLOGY

- Medical causes
  - —Viral or bacterial pericarditis
  - —Malignancy
  - —Uremia
  - —Radiation therapy
  - —Autoimmune disorders
  - —Drug reactions
  - —Postmyocardial infarction (Dressler's syndrome)
- Surgical causes
  - —Trauma
  - —Thoracic aortic dissection
  - —Complications of central line placement

Pre-Hospital

CAUTIONS

- Insert large-bore IV lines in all cases of suspected cardiac tamponade

Diagnosis

ESSENTIAL WORKUP

- ECG
  - —Low voltage
  - —Electrical alternans
  - —Alternating beat-to-beat variation in QRS amplitude
  - —Rare in patients with traumatic pericardial effusions or tamponade
- CXR
  - —Enlarged cardiac silhouette only in cases of pericardial effusion/tamponade that develop over time
- Echocardiogram
  - —Fluid in pericardial sac
  - —Transesophageal echo is the most accurate for penetrating cardiac injury and effusion
  - —Right ventricular or atrial diastolic collapse—characteristic findings suggestive of tamponade

LABORATORY

- Complete blood count
- Electrolytes, BUN/Cr, glucose for renal failure in suspected uremic pericarditis
- Blood cultures if an infectious source suspected

IMAGING/SPECIAL TESTS

- Chest computed tomography for detecting hemopericardium
- Pericardiocentesis and fluid analysis
  - —Further workup for medical causes of pericardial effusion with determination of the etiology of the pericardial fluid
- Central venous pressure (CVP) determination
  - —Penetrating chest trauma should undergo central line placement for penetrating chest trauma
  - —CVP >15 cm H_2O suggests tamponade, but may be normal in the hypovolemic patient

DIFFERENTIAL DIAGNOSIS

- Other causes of shock
- Myocardial infarction
- Pulmonary embolus
- Sepsis
- Ruptured abdominal aortic aneurysm
- Gastrointestinal bleeding
- Congestive heart failure
- Postrauma
- Hemothorax
- Air embolism
- Tension pneumothorax

Treatment

INITIAL STABILIZATION

- IV fluid resuscitation with normal saline or blood
- Pericardiocentesis for unstable patient to decompress the tamponade
- ED thoracotomy with pericardiotomy for patients in cardiac arrest after penetrating thoracic trauma or those who remain unstable after volume replacement and pericardiocentesis

ED TREATMENT

- Bacterial pericardial effusion
  —Initiate antibiotic therapy to cover Gram-negative and anaerobic organisms and *Staphylococcus aureus*
  —May require partial surgical resection of the pericardium
- Uremic pericardial effusion
  —Arrange urgent dialysis
- Dressler's syndrome and postirradiation pericardial effusion
  —Initiate nonsteroidal anti-inflammatory drugs
- Medical causes of tamponade in patients who are unstable
  —Perform pericardiocentesis with placement of an indwelling catheter for continued drainage.
- Suspected traumatic pericardial tamponade
  —Consult trauma surgeon immediately
- Definitive treatment: subxiphoid pericardial window and thoracotomy in the operating room

MEDICATIONS

- Ibuprofen: 600–800 mg po q 8 hrs
- Indomethacin: 25–75 mg po bid

Disposition

ADMISSION CRITERIA

- ICU admission for acute, symptomatic pericardial effusion/tamponade
- New pericardial effusion

DISCHARGE CRITERIA

- Cardiac injury excluded in trauma patient
- Known effusion in asymptomatic patient

Miscellaneous

ICD9: 429.0

CORE CONTENT CODE: 2.3.2

SUGGESTED READINGS

Asensio JA, Stewart BM, Murray J, et. al. Penetrating cardiac injuries. Surg Clin North Am 1996;76:685–724.

Cox GR. Pericardial and myocardial disease. In: Rosen P, et al., eds. Emergency medicine: concepts and clinical practice. 3rd ed. St Louis: CV Mosby, 1992:1391–417.

Hals GD, Carleton SC. Pericardial disease and tamponade. Emerg Med Rep 1996;17(16):161–72.

Jordan RC. Penetrating chest trauma. Emerg Med Clin North Am 1993;11:97–106.

Stewart C. Chest injuries: emergency management of cardiovascular and other manifestations. Emerg Med Rep 1996;17(19):191–98.

Author: Carlo Rosen

Pericarditis

Clinical Presentation

SIGNS AND SYMPTOMS

- Chest pain
  - —Retrosternal or precordial
  - —Usually sharp
  - —Pleuritic
  - —Radiating to the shoulder or the trapezial ridge
  - —Worsened with cough or inspiration
  - —Increased with recumbency
  - —Improved with leaning forward
- Fever
- Mild dyspnea
- Cough
- Hoarseness
- Nausea
- Anorexia
- Tachypnea
- Tachycardia
- Odynophagia
- Friction rub
  - —Heard best at lower left sternal border
  - —Any of three components
    - -Presystolic
    - -Systolic
    - -Early diastolic
  - —Intermittent and exacerbated by leaning forward
- Beck's triad with the accumulation of pericardial fluid
- Muffled heart sounds
- Increased venous pressure (distended neck veins)
- Decreased systemic arterial pressure (hypotension)
- Worsened dyspnea
- Ewart's sign
- Dullness and bronchial breathing between the tip of the left scapula and the vertebral column
- Pulsus paradoxus
- Exaggerated decrease (>10 mm Hg) in systolic pressure with inspiration
- Constrictive pericarditis
- Signs of both right- and left-sided heart failure
- Pulmonary and peripheral edema
- Ascites
- Hepatic congestion

MECHANISM/DESCRIPTION

- Inflammation, infection, or infiltration of the pericardial sac which surrounds the heart
  - —Pericardial effusion may or may not be present
- Acute pericarditis
  - —Rapid in onset
  - —Potentially complicated by accumulation of pericardial fluid leading to cardiac tamponade
- Constrictive pericarditis
  - —Results from chronic inflammation causing thickening and adherence of the pericardium to the heart

ETIOLOGY

- Idiopathic (most common)
- Viral
  - —Echovirus
  - —Coxsackie
  - —Adenovirus
  - —Varicella
  - —Epstein-Barr
  - —Cytomegalovirus
  - —Hepatitis B
  - —AIDS
- Bacterial
  - —Staphylococcus
  - —Streptococcus
  - —Haemophilus
  - —Salmonella
  - —Legionella
  - —Tuberculosis
- Fungal
  - —Candida
  - —Aspergillus
  - —Histoplasmosis
  - —Coccidioidomycosis
  - —Blastomycosis
  - —Nocardia
- Parasitic
  - —Amebiasis
  - —Toxoplasmosis
  - —Echinococcosis
- Neoplastic
  - —Lung
  - —Breast
  - —Lymphoma
  - —Leukemia
  - —Melanoma
- Uremia
- Myxedema
- Myocardial infarction, Dressler's syndrome
- Connective tissue disease
  - —Systemic lupus erythematosus
  - —Rheumatoid arthritis
  - —Scleroderma
- Radiation
- Chest trauma
- Postpericardiotomy
- Aortic dissection
- Pancreatitis
- Inflammatory bowel disease
- Drugs
  - —Procainamide
  - —Cromolyn sodium
  - —Hydralazine
  - —Dantrolene
  - —Methysergide
  - —Mesalamine
- Amyloidosis

Pre-Hospital

CAUTIONS

- Differentiation between acute pericarditis and myocardial infarction necessitates rapid transport to the ED for evaluation with a 12-lead ECG
- Treat the hypotensive patient in cardiac tamponade with aggressive prehospital fluid resuscitation and rapid transport to point of definitive care

Diagnosis

ESSENTIAL WORKUP

- ECG
  - —Stage 1
    - -ST segment elevation diffusely except AVR and V1
    - -ST segments concave up
    - -No reciprocal ST segment depression in other leads (in contradistinction to the changes seen in acute myocardial infarction)
  - —Stage 2
    - -ST segments return to normal
    - -T waves flatten
    - -PR segments may become depressed
  - —Stage 3
    - -T-wave inversion
  - —Stage 4
    - -Eventual resolution of all changes
    - -Differentiation from myocardial infarction
    - -No Q waves formed
    - -T-wave inversion occurs after the resolution of the ST segment changes

LABORATORY

- CBC
- Leukocytosis
- ESR may be elevated
- Cardiac enzymes
  - —Helpful in distinguishing pericarditis from myocardial infarction
  - —Reported elevated with the inflammation of pericarditis

IMAGING/SPECIAL TESTS

- CXR
  - —Can be normal
  - —May show enlargement of the cardiac silhouette
  - —No change in heart size until >250 ml of fluid have accumulated in the pericardial sac
- Echocardiography
  - —Diagnostic method of choice for the detection of pericardial fluid
  - —Can detect as little as 15 ml of fluid in the pericardial sac
- Chest CT
  - —Useful for the detection of calcifications or thickening of the pericardium
- Pericardiocentesis
  - —Used to obtain fluid for protein, glucose, culture, cytology, Gram and acid-fast stains, and fungal smears

DIFFERENTIAL DIAGNOSIS

- Acute myocardial infarction
- Pulmonary embolism
- Pneumothorax
- Aortic dissection
- Pneumonia
- Empyema
- Cholecystitis
- Pancreatitis

Treatment

INITIAL STABILIZATION

- ABCs
- Pericardiocentesis for hemodynamic compromise secondary to cardiac tamponade
  - —Removal of even a small amount of fluid can lead to a dramatic improvement
- Guided ultrasound is safest

ED TREATMENT

- Treatment dependent on the underlying etiology
- Idiopathic, viral, rheumatologic, and post-traumatic
  - —Nonsteroidal antiinflammatory drug regimens effective
  - —Corticosteroids reserved for refractory cases
- Bacterial
  - —Aggressive treatment with intravenous antibiotics along with drainage of the pericardial space
  - —Search for primary focus of infection
  - —Therapy guided by determination of pathogen from pericardial fluid tests
- Neoplastic
  - —Treat underlying malignancy
- Uremia
  - —Intensive 2–6-week course of dialysis
  - —Caution should be used if using nonsteroidal medications
- Expected course/prognosis
  - —Majority of patients will respond to treatment within 2 weeks
  - —Most have complete resolution of symptoms
  - —Small number progress to recurrent bouts with eventual development of constrictive pericarditis or cardiac tamponade

MEDICATIONS

- Aspirin: 350–500 mg po q 3–4 hrs
- Ibuprofen: 400–600 mg po q6 –8 hrs
- Indomethacin: 25–50 mg po q 6 hrs

Disposition

ADMISSION CRITERIA

- ICU
  - —Hemodynamic instability
  - —Cardiac tamponade
  - —Associated malignant arrhythmia
  - —Any suspicion of myocardial infarction
  - —Severe pain unresponsive to oral medications
  - —Suspicion of bacterial etiology
  - —Patients having undergone pericardiocentesis due to the relatively high incidence of complications

DISCHARGE CRITERIA

- Mild symptoms in patients without any hemodynamic compromise
- Close follow up
- Able to tolerate a regimen of oral medication

Miscellaneous

ICD9: 423.9

CORE CONTENT CODE: 2.3.1

SUGGESTED READINGS

Jourilles NJ. Pericardial and myocardial disease. In: Rosen P, et al., eds. Emergency medicine: concepts and clinical practice. 4th ed. St. Louis: CV Mosby, 1998;1716–1726.

Maisch B. Myocarditis and pericarditis—old questions and new answers. Herz 1992;17(2):65–70.

Maisch B. Pericardial diseases, with a focus on etiology, pathogenesis, pathophysiology, new diagnostic imaging methods, and treatment. Curr Opin Cardiol 1994;9:379–88.

Sternbach GL. Pericarditis. Ann Emerg Med 1988;17(3):214–20.

Author: Andrew T. McAfee

Periodontal Abscess

Clinical Presentation

SIGNS AND SYMPTOMS

- Dental pain
- Malaise
- Regional lymphadenitis
- Fever
- Diffuse or localized swelling
- Parulis
  - —Small, inflammatory nodule that develops on the alveolar mucosa at the oral termination of a draining sinus tract
  - —Tends to occur on the buccal or labial aspect of the alveolus
  - —May also appear on the palatal aspect
- Expression of pus from the sinus opening

MECHANISM/DESCRIPTION

- Results from the progression of periodontal disease and its associated bone loss
  - —Formation of periodontal pockets where food and debris accumulate
  - —These become secondarily infected
  - —Unlike a periapical abscess, the tooth is vital
- The infection may spread to the alveolar bone and soft tissues surrounding the offending tooth
- The source of infection may be from a tooth or from the periodontal tissues
- Complications
  - —Dentocutaneous fistula
  - —Osteomyelitis
  - —Cavernous sinus thrombosis
  - —Ludwig's angina

ETIOLOGY

N/A

Pre-Hospital

N/A

Diagnosis

ESSENTIAL WORKUP

- Clinical diagnosis that does not require ancillary studies

LABORATORY

N/A

IMAGING/SPECIAL TESTS

- Electric pulp testing is used to verify that the tooth is vital
  - —Generally performed by the dental consultant

DIFFERENTIAL DIAGNOSIS

- Periapical abscess
- Tumors of the salivary glands
- Asymptomatic parulis
  - —Fibroma
  - —Pyogenic granuloma
  - —Peripheral giant cell granuloma
  - —Peripheral ossifying fibroma
  - —Kaposi's sarcoma

Treatment

INITIAL STABILIZATION

N/A

ED TREATMENT

- Systemic signs of infection should be managed with antibiotics before definitive pulpal therapy
- Fluctuant abscesses are best treated with an incision and drainage
  - —The gingiva is anesthetized superficially with 2% lidocaine with 1:100,000 epinephrine
  - —A stab incision is made toward the alveolar bone and must extend through the periosteum
  - —Blunt dissection is carried out with a mosquito hemostat
  - —The cavity is irrigated
  - —If there is sufficient space, place an iodoform drain
- Antibiotics
  - —Only indicated if the abscess is extensive and systemic signs are present
  - —Tetracycline for patients over 8 years of age
  - —Penicillin VK in patients with a contraindication to tetracycline

MEDICATIONS

- Doxycycline: 100 mg po bid
- Penicillin VK: 250 mg po qid

Disposition

ADMISSION CRITERIA

- Severe infection or complication requiring parenteral antibiotics
  - —Ludwig's angina

DISCHARGE CRITERIA

- Uncomplicated cases
- Warm saline rinses 4 times a day
- Followup with a dentist as soon as possible

Miscellaneous

ICD9: 523

CORE CONTENT CODE: 6.3.7

SUGGESTED READINGS

Amsterdam JT. Dental disorders. In: Rosen P, et al., eds. Emergency medicine: Concepts and clinical practice. 4th ed. St Louis: CV Mosby, 1998:2680–696.

Ferrera PC. Uncommon complications of odontogenic infections. Am J Emerg Med 1996;14:317–22.

Author: Richard Wolfe

Periorbital Cellulitis

Clinical Presentation

SIGNS AND SYMPTOMS

- Erythema
- Warmth
- Tenderness
- Swelling
- Unilateral location

Bacteremic Periorbital Cellulitis

- Children <2 years old
- Preceding upper respiratory infection
- Fever (>39°C)
- Erythematous or violaceous swelling of the eyelid
  - —Obscured eye from swelling within 12 hours

Complication of Sinusitis

- URI
- Low grade fever
- Gradual swelling over days
  - —Inflammatory edema in the periorbital tissue does not contain actual infection
  - —Secondary to vascular and lymphatic congestion

Orbital Cellulitis

- Proptosis
- Limitation of eye movement
- Eye pain
- Abnormal pupillary reaction
- Decreased visual acuity
- Diplopia
- Toxicity
- Fever
- Leukocytosis
- Chemosis
  - —Associated with both periorbital and orbital cellulitis

MECHANISM/DESCRIPTION

- Periorbital (preseptal) cellulitis
  - —Inflammatory process of the tissues anterior to the orbital septum
- Orbital septum
  - —Connective tissue extension of the orbital periosteum that is reflected into the upper and lower eyelids
  - —Represents a nearly impervious barrier to the spread of infection into the orbit
- Orbital cellulitis
  - —Inflammatory process in the structures posterior to the orbital septum

Three Mechanisms

- Localized infection of the eyelid or adjacent structures
  - —Blepharitis
  - —Hordeolum
  - —Chalazion
  - —Dacryoadenitis
  - —Dacryocystitis
  - —Impetigo
  - —Abscess
  - —Surrounding skin disruptions (minor trauma, insect bites, dermatologic disorders)
  - —Organisms include
    - -*S. aureus*
    - -*S. pyogenes*
    - -Less commonly *S. epidermidis,* anaerobes
- Hematogenous dissemination
  - —Pathogens migrate to the periorbital tissues
  - —Organisms include
    - -*S. pneumoniae*
    - -*S. pyogenes*
    - -*Haemophilus influenzae* type b (Hib)
- Inflammation and edema from an underlying sinusitis
  - —Organisms include
    - -*S. pneumoniae*
    - -Nontypeable *H. influenzae*
    - -*M. catarrhalis*

ETIOLOGY

- Prior to *H. influenzae* type b (Hib) immunization *H. influenzae* accounted for 80% of bacteremic periorbital cellulitis cases
- Currently *Streptococcal* infections (group A and pneumococcus) are the primary causative organisms
- Consider nonbacteremic causes

PEDIATRIC CONSIDERATIONS

- Child who has had at least the second Hib vaccination a week prior to the onset of the cellulitis is unlikely to have *H. influenzae b* infection

Pre-Hospital

CAUTIONS

- Establish IV access and administer oxygen if associated serious complications
  - —Sepsis
  - —Meningitis

Diagnosis

ESSENTIAL WORKUP

- Clinical diagnosis
  - —Typical signs/symptoms
  - —Perform thorough neurologic exam
  - —Assess for orbital involvement

LABORATORY

- CBC
  - —WBC >15,000 is usually associated with bacteremic periorbital cellulitis
- Blood culture
- Gram stain and culture of either a tissue aspirate or swab of draining purulent material
- Lumbar puncture/CSF evaluation
  - —If ill-appearing
  - —Signs of meningeal irritation
  - —Without adequate Hib vaccinations

IMAGING/SPECIAL TESTS

- Sinus x-rays
- CT scan
  - —Indicated if
    - -Concern for orbital cellulitis or traumatic penetration of the orbital septum
    - -Failure to respond to parenteral antimicrobial therapy
  - —Demonstrates
    - -Sinusitis
    - -Subperiosteal abscess
    - -Presence of a foreign body
    - -Proptosis

DIFFERENTIAL DIAGNOSIS

- Lack of fever and leukocytosis suggest noninfectious causes
  - —Trauma
  - —Insect bite
  - —Allergy
  - —Tumor
  - —Local eye/eyelid infection
- Early orbital cellulitis
  - —May have the same appearance as periorbital cellulitis

Treatment

INITIAL STABILIZATION

- 0.9%NS IV bolus (500 cc or 20 cc/kg) for dehydration, sepsis, hypotension

ED TREATMENT

- Administer IV antibiotics for toxic/ill appearing/suspected bacteremic periorbital cellulitis
  —Consider vancomycin in geographic areas with prevalent penicillin-resistant pneumococci
- Children with signs of orbital cellulitis require
  —Parenteral antibiotics
  —CT scan
  —Ophthalmologic consultation
  —Prompt surgery may be necessary

MEDICATIONS

- Augmentin: 500 mg (peds: 45 mg/kg/24hrs) po bid
- Cefazolin: 1 g (peds: 100 mg/kg/24hrs) IV q 6–8 hrs
- Cefotaxime: 1–2 g (peds: 150 mg/kg/24 hrs) q 6–8 hrs
- Ceftriaxone: 1 g (peds: 50–100 mg/kg/24 hrs) IV q 24 hrs or q 12 hrs
- Cephalexin: 500 mg (peds: 100 mg/kg/24 hrs) po qid
- Clindamycin: 600 mg (peds: 40 mg/kg/24 hrs) IV q 6 hrs; 300 mg (peds: 20 mg/kg/24hrs) po qid
- Dicloxacillin: 500 mg (peds: 100 mg/kg/24 hrs) po qid
- Nafcillin: 1–2 g (peds: 150 mg/kg/24 hrs) IV q 6 hrs
- Oxacillin: 1–2 g (peds: 150 mg/kg/24 hrs) IV q 6 hrs
- Vancomycin: 500 mg (peds: 40 mg/kg/24 hrs) q 6 hrs

Disposition

ADMISSION CRITERIA

- Toxicity
- Signs of orbital cellulitis
- Progression of infection on oral antibiotics

DISCHARGE CRITERIA

- Oral antibiotics for modest swelling, nontoxic appearance, and reliable parents
- Monitor for progressive swelling, irritability, increased fever, or vision changes

Miscellaneous

ICD9: 376.01

CORE CONTENT CODE: 6.4.4.2

SUGGESTED READINGS

Powell KR. Orbital and periorbital cellulitis. Pediatr Rev 1995;16:1163–1167.

Schwartz GR, Wright SW. Changing bacteriology of periorbital cellulitis. Ann Emerg Med 1996;28:6:617–620.

Author: J. Wathen

Peripheral Vascular Disease

Clinical Presentation

SIGNS AND SYMPTOMS

- Chronic arterial insufficiency, acute arterial insufficiency and atheroembolism have differing signs and symptoms
- Differentiation essential to correct management

Chronic Arterial Insufficiency

- Claudication
  —Most common symptom
  —Aching pain in the calves or buttocks
  —Occurs with activity and slowly relieved by rest
- Severe disease present when limb pain occurs at rest, rapidly progressive claudication or ulceration
- Disease of the aortoiliac region
  —Causes pain in the buttocks and thighs
- Disease of the femoropopliteal region
  —Causes pain in the calves
- Physical examination
  —Absent or decreased peripheral pulses
  —Muscle and skin atrophy
  —Pallor and dependent rubor of the leg
  —Thickened nails
  —Delayed capillary refill

Acute Arterial Insufficiency

- Acute limb ischemia
  —Six Ps
  -Pain (first symptom)
  -Pallor
  -Pulselessness
  -Poikilothermic
  -Paresthesias (late findings)
  -Paralysis (late findings)
- Identification of a source of a possible embolic process is crucial

Atheroembolism

- Ischemic and painful toes
- Renal insufficiency and livedo reticularis
  —Common systemic signs of atheroembolism
  —Proximal aortic emboli may be showered into distal arterial networks
- Both feet may be symptomatic
- Atheroemboli may be triggered by
  —Invasive arterial procedures such as cardiac catheterization
  —Atherosclerotic disease of proximal vessels

MECHANISM/DESCRIPTION

- Collection of vascular syndromes affecting the lower extremities
- Three distinct entities
  —Chronic arterial insufficiency (CAI)
  -Prevalent in populations at risk for atherosclerotic disease
  -Primary symptom is claudication
  —Acute arterial insufficiency (AAI)
  -Presents dramatically with a painful, pale, cool, and pulseless extremity
  -Causes limb ischemia
  -Warrants rapid diagnosis and restoration of blood flow
  -Caused by either arterial thrombosis or embolism
  —Atheroembolism
  -Syndrome of cholesterol microemboli which results in ischemia to capillary beds
  -"Blue toe" syndrome

ETIOLOGY

- Chronic arterial insufficiency
  —Most common cause is progressive atherosclerotic disease
  —Complications
  -Arterial aneurysm
  -Thrombosis
  -Ulceration
- Acute arterial insufficiency
  —Two separate processes
  -Arterial embolism
  -Thrombosis
  —Sources of acute arterial embolus
  -Cardiac arrhythmias
  -Valvular heart disease
  -Aneurysms
  -Infection
  -Tumor
  -Vasculitides or foreign body
  —80% of emboli arise in the heart
- Atheroembolism
  -Caused by rupture or partial disruption of an atherosclerotic plaque
  -Gives rise to cholesterol emboli showers and obstructing arteriolar networks

Pre-Hospital

CAUTIONS

- Maintain hemodynamic stability
- Apply cardiac monitor
- Place the ischemic limb at rest and in a dependent position
- Provide oxygen if low oxygen saturation or pulmonary symptoms

Diagnosis

ESSENTIAL WORKUP

Clinical Diagnosis

- Chronic arterial insufficiency
  —Ankle-brachial index
  —Bedside test to determine whether CAI is present
  —Ratio of the systolic blood pressure at the ankle divided by that of the arm
  —Ratio of <0.8 is abnormal and <0.5 indicates severe disease
- Acute arterial insufficiency
  —Physical diagnosis using the six Ps
  —Those with acute-on-chronic arterial insufficiency tolerate limb ischemia better than those without CAI due to well-developed collateral circulation
- Atheroembolism
  —Affected areas painful, tender, and may be either dusky or necrotic
  —Classic "blue-toe syndrome"

LABORATORY

- CBC and platelets
- Electrolytes, BUN, Cr, glucose
- Coagulation studies
- ECG
- CPK if prolonged ischemia
- Hold blood for special hematologic studies if a hypercoagulable state suspected
- Blood cultures if endocarditis possible

IMAGING/SPECIAL TESTS

- Doppler ultrasound
  —Visualizes both venous and arterial systems
  —Identifies level of arterial occlusion, as well as thrombosis and aneurysm
  —Sensitivity and specificity >80–90 percent for occlusion of vessels proximal to the popliteal vessels
- Plethysmography
  —Detects areas of arterial insufficiency
  —Uses measurements of the volume and character of blood flow in an extremity
  —Less widely available than ultrasound
  —Requires an experienced technician
  —Approximates ultrasound in sensitivity and specificity
- Angiography
  —Determines details about the intravascular environment including the level of occlusion, stenosis, and collateral flow
  —Useful where the diagnosis of AAI is uncertain, or prior to emergent bypass grafting
- CT and MRI
  —For diagnosis of occlusive aortic disease or dissection
  —MRI is being investigated as a tool to evaluate CAI

DIFFERENTIAL DIAGNOSIS

- Acute thrombosis or emboli
- Arterial dissection
- Compartment syndrome
- Acute neurologic syndrome
- Massive venous insufficiency

Treatment

INITIAL STABILIZATION

- 0.9% IV fluid bolus for hypotension
- Cardiac monitor
- Supplemental oxygen for hypoxia

ED TREATMENT

- Acute arterial insufficiency
  —Limit further clot propagation with heparin
  —Do not anticoagulate patients suspected of having an aortic dissection or symptomatic aneurysm
  —Emergent consultation with a vascular surgeon
  -To determine which diagnostic study will be employed
  -To begin arrangements for operative therapy
  —Options for operative therapy include thrombectomy, embolectomy, regional arterial thrombolysis or bypass grafting
  —Blood flow to the affected limb must be reestablished within 4–6 hours after onset of ischemic symptoms
  —Complications of AAI include
  -Compartment syndromes
  -Irreversible ischemia requiring amputation
  -Rhabdomyolysis
  -Electrolyte disturbances
- Atheroembolism
  —Treat conservatively if a limited amount of tissue is involved and renal function is not significantly compromised
  —No available therapy for the ischemic digits besides supportive wound care and analgesia
  —Amputation for irreversibly necrotic toes
  —Vascular surgeon referral within 12–24 hours of ED visit
  —Prevent further embolic events by a thorough investigation and correction of the source of atheroemboli
- Chronic arterial insufficiency
  —Initiate measures to prevent disease progression
  -Tobacco cessation
  -Aggressive management of hyperlipidemia
  -Exercise
  *Not to be restricted
  *May improve exercise tolerance and reduce symptoms of claudication
  -Antiplatelet and anticoagulant drugs have not been definitively shown to prevent progression of CAI
  -Aspirin recommended for cardioprotective effects (80–325 mg/day).
  -Pentoxifylline (400 mg tid) and ticlopidine (150–225 mg/day) have been shown in some trials to improve symptoms of claudication
  —Invasive therapy
  —Atherectomy
  —Bypass grafting
  —Balloon angioplasty

MEDICATIONS

- Heparin: 80 units/kg bolus IV followed by 18 units/hr IV

Disposition

ADMISSION CRITERIA

- Acute arterial insufficiency
- Rapidly progressive claudication or ischemic pain at rest
- To undergo heparinization and angiography to rule out an acute thrombosis

DISCHARGE CRITERIA

- Atheroembolism
- If they have small lesions, adequate pain control, no evidence of renal compromise or superinfection, and followup within 24 hours
- Chronic arterial insufficiency

Miscellaneous

ICD9: 414.0

CORE CONTENT CODE: 2.5.1.2

SUGGESTED READINGS

Barnes RW. Noninvasive diagnostic assessment of peripheral vascular disease. Circulation 1991;83(suppl I):I20–I27.

Brewster DC. Current controversies in the management of aortoiliac occlusive disease. J Vasc Sur 1997;25:365–79.

Hertzer NR. The natural history of peripheral vascular disease. Circulation 1991;83(suppl I):I12–I19.

Spittell JA Jr. Peripheral arterial disease. Dis Mon 1994;40(12):650–700.

Author: Sally Santen

Peritonsillar Abscess

Clinical Presentation

SIGNS AND SYMPTOMS

Symptoms

- Sore throat
- Fever
- Dysphagia
- Trismus
- Muffled voice
- Drooling
- Feeling of oropharyngeal fullness
- Symptoms usually develop 2–4 days after the inciting pharyngitis or upper respiratory infection

Signs

- Erythematous
- Bulging tonsil, often displacing the uvula
- Fullness of the superior tonsil and adjacent soft palate
- Tonsillar exudate or fluctuantes are not common findings

MECHANISM/DESCRIPTION

- Most commonly encountered head and neck abscess
- Two theories explain the development of peritonsillar abscess (PTA)
  —Direct bacterial invasion into deeper tissues in the patient with acute pharyngitis
  —Acute obstruction and bacterial infection of small salivary glands present in the superior tonsil
- PTA can occur despite prior antibiotic therapy
- Complications
  —Uncommon, but can be life-threatening
  —Airway obstruction
  —Sepsis
  —Spontaneous perforation
  —Aspiration
  —Extension to the lateral neck or mediastinum

ETIOLOGY

- Affects all age groups, with highest rates in teens and young adults
- Most common pathogens
  —β-Hemolytic streptococcus
  —Other streptococcal species
  —Anaerobes
  —Staphylococcal species
  —Mixed organisms

PEDIATRIC CONSIDERATIONS

- PTA occurs in children (<18 years) in 24–39% of reported cases
- Presentation and therapy are similar in older children and adults
- Young children may need sedation or general anesthesia if incision and drainage (I&D) or aspiration of the abscess is attempted

Pre-Hospital

CAUTIONS

- Rarely associated with acute airway compromise, but as the diagnosis is likely to be uncertain during transport, patients should be treated as potential airway emergencies
- Apply cardiac and pulse-oximetry monitoring
- Place patient in position of comfort
- Administer supplemental oxygen
- Have suction and equipment for bag-valve mask ventilation and intubation readily available
- Initiate intravenous access in cooperative patients

PEDIATRIC CONSIDERATIONS

- Children should be exposed to minimal stimulation and accompanied by a parent if feasible
- Do not attempt oropharyngeal exam and IV access in uncooperative children who are maintaining their airway

Diagnosis

ESSENTIAL WORKUP

- PTA is evident by physical exam in most cases, unless trismus obscures full adequate examination

LABORATORY

- Throat culture and monospot
  —Indicated in persons thought to have Streptococcal pharyngitis or EBV, because this may alter antimicrobial therapy

IMAGING/SPECIAL TESTS

- Soft tissue lateral neck x-ray
  —Useful in excluding other causes of upper airway obstruction, especially in young children at risk for epiglottitis
- Chest x-ray in patients with respiratory symptoms or draining abscesses
- CT scanning of the neck
  —Differentiates tonsillar cellulitis from abscess
  —Determines if deeper tissues of the neck are involved
  —Unnecessary in simple cases of PTA

DIFFERENTIAL DIAGNOSIS

- Peritonsillar cellulitis
- Retropharyngeal abscess
- Croup
- Epiglottitis
- Bacterial tracheitis
- Cervical adenitis
- Lateral neck abscess
- Odontogenic abscess

PEDIATRIC CONSIDERATIONS

- Obtain soft tissue lateral neck x-ray prior to oral examination in young children with symptoms of upper airway obstruction

Treatment

INITIAL STABILIZATION
- ABCs
- Administer supplemental oxygen for respiratory distress
- IV hydration with 0.9%NS 500 cc bolus (peds: 20 cc/kg) for dehydration

ED TREATMENT
- Keep NPO in anticipation of drainage procedure
- Administer analgesia
  —Topical sprays
  —Parenteral narcotics/toradol
- Perform needle aspiration or incision and drainage
  —Should be performed by person experienced in drainage procedure
  —Tonsillar aspiration
    -More readily accomplished and tolerated than I&D
    -Cure rates of >85% in children and adults with a single aspiration
    -Tonsil lies in close proximity to the internal carotid artery and special equipment may be needed
    -Aspiration may not always yield abscess fluid; in these patients, medical therapy and timely reexamination is recommended
    -Cooperative patient is essential
    -Sedation or general anesthesia may be needed for young or uncooperative persons
  —Perform in the presence of personnel adept at advanced airway techniques
- Antibiotics
- Penicillins or cephalosporins are the initial choice
- Clindamycin in patients with penicillin and cephalosporin allergy

MEDICATIONS
- Ampicillin: 2 g (peds: 100–200 mg/kg/24 hrs) IV q 6 hrs
- Amoxicillin: 500 mg (peds: 20–40 mg/kg/24 hrs) po qid
- Penicillin VK: 500 mg (peds: 25–50 mg/kg/24 hrs) po qid
- Ceftriaxone: 1 g (peds: 50 mg/kg/24 hrs) IV/IM q d
- Clindamycin
  —900 mg (peds: 25–40 mg/kg/24 hrs) IV q 8 hrs
  —300 mg (peds: 10–30 mg/kg/24 hrs) po tid

Disposition

ADMISSION CRITERIA
- Patients unable to maintain oral intake or comply with antibiotic therapy
- Signs of sepsis or complicated PTA

DISCHARGE CRITERIA
- Adequate hydration
- Ability to take antibiotics
- After I&D or aspiration
- Follow-up within 24–48 hours

Miscellaneous

ICD9: 475

CORE CONTENT CODE: 6.3.8

SUGGESTED READINGS

Herzon FS, Nicklaus P. Pediatric peritonsillar abscess: management guidelines. Curr Probl Pediatr 1996;26(8):270–278

Passy V. Pathogenesis of peritonsillar abscess. Laryngoscope 1994;104(2):185–190

Author: Keith Wrenn

Pertussis

Clinical Presentation

SIGNS AND SYMPTOMS

- Presence of a chronic cough in family members
- Catarrhal stage
  - —Approximately 1 week duration
  - —Rhinorrhea
  - —Mild cough
  - —Minimal fever
- Paroxysmal stage
  - —Classic "whooping" cough
    - -Increasingly severe cough
    - -Coughing spasm that ends with a sudden inflow of air—the "whoop"
  - —Posttussive emesis
  - —Cyanosis
  - —Apnea
    - -Infants younger than 6 months
  - —Normal physical examination between coughing spells
- Convalescent stage
  - —Waning cough
  - —Improving respiratory status
- Atypical presentations
  - —Chronic cough in adolescents and adults
  - —Asymptomatic
- Complications
  - —HEENT
    - -Epistaxis
    - -Subconjunctival hemorrhage
  - —Respiratory
    - -Acute respiratory arrest
    - -Pneumonia
    - -Bronchiectasis
  - —Gastrointestinal
    - -Umbilical hernia
    - -Inguinal hernia
    - -Rectal prolapse
  - —Neurologic
    - -Seizures
    - -Encephalitis
    - -Coma
    - -Intracranial hemorrhage
    - -Spinal epidural hemorrhage

MECHANISM/DESCRIPTION

- Acute respiratory infection spread by small respiratory droplets
- Mostly young children
- Increasing incidence in adolescents
- Adults are the primary reservoir
- Peak incidence—late summer/fall
- Preventable with vaccines
  - —Newly introduced acellular vaccines have less side effects and equal efficacy to cellular vaccines
- Uncomplicated cases last 6–10 weeks
- Complications
  - —Complete obstruction of the airway by a mucus plug
  - —Secondary bacterial infection
  - —Encephalitis
  - —Sudden increases in intrathoracic pressure
    - -Intracranial hemorrhage
    - -Rectal prolapse
    - -Diaphragmatic rupture
    - -Abdominal wall hernias
- Mortality
  - —Mortality greatest in those <1 year of age
  - —1.3% for patients younger than 1 month of age
  - —0.3% in children between 2 and 11 months
  - —90% of fatalities are due to secondary bacterial pneumonia

ETIOLOGY

- *Bordetella pertussis*
  - —A fastidious, Gram-negative, pleomorphic bacillus
- *Bordetella parapertussis*
- *Bordetella bronchiseptica*
- Adenoviruses

Pre-Hospital

CAUTIONS

- Universal precautions, notably a mask
  - —If exposed, consider chemoprophylaxis of pre-hospital personnel
- Suction in patients with respiratory arrest
  - —Complete airway obstruction from a mucus plug is a life-threatening complication

Diagnosis

ESSENTIAL WORKUP

- The ED diagnosis should be made on clinical grounds
- Attempt to establish a history of a contact
- Observe the paroxysmal cough with the characteristic whoop
- Use ancillary studies to further support the clinical diagnosis and rule out complications

LABORATORY

- White blood cell count
  - —Leukocytosis (20,000–50,000 cells/mm^3)
  - —Marked lymphocytosis is characteristic

IMAGING/SPECIAL TESTS

- Chest x-ray
  - —Most often normal
  - —Perihilar infiltrates
  - —Atelectasis
  - —Occasionally characteristic "shaggy" right heart border
  - —Secondary bacterial pneumonia
- Fluorescent staining of nasopharyngeal mucus
  - —Diagnostic of pertussis
- Fluorescent antibody to exclude respiratory syncytial virus

DIFFERENTIAL DIAGNOSIS

- Bronchiolitis
- Foreign body
- Bacterial pneumonia
- Mycoplasmal pneumonia
- Chlamydia pneumonia
- Reactive airway disease
- Cystic fibrosis
- Tuberculosis

Treatment

INITIAL STABILIZATION

—Oxygen
—Suction mucus plugs

ED TREATMENT

- Universal precautions
  - —Specifically requires droplet precautions
- Maintenance of adequate hydration
- Monitor oxygenation during paroxysms
- Airway management may be life saving in younger children
- Antibiotics
  - —Effective in the catarrhal stage
  - —Prevent further transmission in the paroxysmal stage
  - —Erythromycin is the first-line agent
  - —Alternatively clarithromycin or trimethoprim-sulfamethoxazole may be used

MEDICATIONS

- Erythromycin: 10 mg/kg po qid
- Clarithromycin: 7.5 mg/kg po bid
- Trimethoprim sulfamethoxazole: 4 / 20 mg/kg po bid

Disposition

ADMISSION CRITERIA

- Patients <1 year of age
- Apnea
- Cyanosis during paroxysms of cough
- Associated pneumonia
- Encephalitis

DISCHARGE CRITERIA

- Antibiotics for 14 days
- Antipyretics for fevers
- Warm liquids to treat coughing spasm
- Remove thick secretions with bulb suction in infants
- Drink lots of fluids
- Avoid cough triggers
  - —Cigarette smoke
  - —Pollutants
  - —Perfumes
- All exposed persons should seek chemoprophylaxis

Miscellaneous

ICD9: 033.9

CORE CONTENT CODE: 13.9.7

SUGGESTED READINGS

Behrman R, Vaughn V, eds. Nelson's textbook of pediatrics. 13th ed. Philadelphia: WB Saunders, 1987:396–398.

Cattaneo L, Edwards K. Bordetella pertussis (whooping cough). Semin Pediatr Infect Dis 1995;6(2):107–118.

Peter G, ed. 1997 Red Book: Report of the Committee on Infectious Diseases. 24th ed. Elk Grove Village, IL: American Academy of Pediatrics, 1997:394–407.

Author: Kristine Kay Rittichier

Phalangeal Injuries, Foot

Clinical Presentation

SIGNS AND SYMPTOMS

- Pain, swelling, and ecchymosis are common findings
- Subungual hematoma frequently encountered with tuft fracture

MECHANISM/DESCRIPTION

- Typically results from direct trauma (e.g., sledgehammer or falling object) or stubbed toe
- Dislocation of interphalangeal joint are common with axial load injury (kicking an immovable object)

Pre-Hospital

CAUTIONS

- It is frequently difficult to distinguish fracture from dislocation; therefore, reduction of a suspected dislocation should not be attempted in the pre-hospital setting unless there is obvious neurologic or vascular compromise

Diagnosis

ESSENTIAL WORKUP

- X-ray of involved digit

Treatment

NONDISPLACED FRACTURES

- Buddy tape nondisplaced fractures (remember to place absorptive padding between toes)
- Hard-sole shoe
- Weight-bearing as tolerated with crutches or cane
- Oral analgesics
- Pain improves over 2–3 weeks

DISPLACED INTRA-ARTICULAR FRACTURES OF INTERPHALANGEAL JOINT

- Closed reduction with longitudinal traction
- Short leg-walking cast with toe platform
- If unstable after closed reduction, then open reduction internal fixation (ORIF) is required

INTERPHALANGEAL JOINT DISLOCATIONS

- Digital block anesthesia
- Longitudinal traction with gentle downward pressure on distal phalanx to reduce dislocation
- Buddy tape to next toe for 2–3 weeks
- Rarely sesamoid bone block attempts at reduction
- Unstable reductions require operative management

DISTAL TUFT FRACTURE

- Hard soled shoe
- Oral analgesics
- Drain subungual hematoma if present
- Weight-bearing as tolerated

Disposition

ADMISSION CRITERIA

- Unstable or blocked dislocations and unstable fractures of great toe require ORIF

DISCHARGE CRITERIA

All other fractures may be discharged with follow-up in 2–3 weeks to evaluate healing

Miscellaneous

ICD9: 959.7

CORE CONTENT CODE: 18.4.13.1.1

SUGGESTED READINGS

Heckman JD. Fractures and dislocations of the foot. In: Rockwood CA, Green DP, Bucholz RW, Heckman JD, eds. Rockwood and Green's fractures in adults. 4th ed. New York: Lippincott-Raven, 1996:2267–2405.

Simon RS, Koeningsknecht SJ. Metatarsal fractures. In: Simon RS, Koeningsknecht SJ, eds. Emergency orthopedics: The extremities. 2d ed. Norwalk, CT: Appleton & Lange, 1987:288–291.

Author: Kevin Reilly

Phalangeal Injuries, Hand

Clinical Presentation

SIGNS AND SYMPTOMS

- Pain in the area of injury
- Deformity of the digit
- Loss of motion at the joint involved

MECHANISM/DESCRIPTION

- The fingers are most frequently injured in athletic or occupational accidents

PEDIATRIC CONSIDERATIONS

- Fractures may be more difficult to diagnose in children who are unable to cooperate for a full examination. Also, their radiographs may be less definitive. Careful repeated examination is necessary

Pre-Hospital

CAUTIONS

- Pre-hospital personnel should not attempt to reduce a phalangeal dislocation at the scene unless there will be an unusually long transport time or unless vascular or neurologic compromise. Reduction may be successful, but prompt the physician to miss the full diagnosis, and may result in the patient receiving inadequate overall care of the injury

Diagnosis

ESSENTIAL WORKUP

- A careful history and complete physical exam should be accompanied by a full x-ray series of the affected hand
- Special attention should be directed at assessing neurovascular status and identifying rotational deformity

IMAGING/SPECIAL TESTS

- It is imperative that views of all involved digits include complete true laterals and obliques. It is unacceptable to have one lateral with several overlapping phalanges

DIFFERENTIAL DIAGNOSIS

- Tendon rupture
- Complicated open injuries may include several injuries and the entire hand should be examined carefully

PEDIATRIC CONSIDERATIONS

- Many fractures in children are torus (buckle) fractures of the phalanges

Treatment

INITIAL STABILIZATION

- Assess for other, more serious, injuries
- Immobilize the involved digit by splinting or buddy-taping pending definitive evaluation
- Intermittent ice application, elevation
- Dislocations or severely deformed fractures producing vascular compromise should be reduced immediately to a neutral position and immobilized

ED TREATMENT

- Most phalangeal dislocations are dorsal or dorsolateral. These may be reduced under digital block by gentle distraction, hyperextension, and guiding the base of the dislocated phalanx into proper position with mild thumb pressure
- Simple transverse or small corner fractures not exceeding 25% of a joint surface and dislocations may be treated with "buddy" splinting in a functional position allowing stable motion, or with a padded splint in a neutral position for several days, with arrangements for "buddy" splinting later
- Unstable fractures (rotational deformity, oblique fractures, fractures involving larger portion of a joint or angulated fractures) should be referred for orthopedic care
- Any fracture with a subungual hematoma should have the blood released by using a heated paperclip, electric cautery, or a hole drilled with an 18-gauge needle. This injury does not have to be treated as an open injury just because of the subungual hematoma

MEDICATIONS

- Mild analgesics may be necessary, but narcotics are usually not indicated

Disposition

ADMISSION CRITERIA

- Open injuries are admitted for irrigation and debridement and early repair
- Closed injuries requiring surgical management may be admitted for early operative intervention but it is acceptable to wait for a day or two for semielective repair

DISCHARGE CRITERIA

- Patients with a stable fracture in an appropriate splint may be discharged for early orthopedic follow-up

PEDIATRIC CONSIDERATIONS

- If the child does not have significant rotational deformity, simple fractures can be treated with splinting
- Epiphyseal fractures (Salter-Harris) should be referred to an orthopedist

Miscellaneous

ICD9: 959.5

CORE CONTENT CODE: 18.4.12.1.1, 18.4.12.2.4.2

SUGGESTED READINGS

American Society for Surgery of the Hand. The Hand: Examination and diagnosis. 2d ed. New York: Churchill Livingston, 1983, 585–600.

American Society for Surgery of the Hand. The Hand: Primary care of common problems. 2d ed. New York: Churchill Livingston, 1990, 437–649.

Antosia RE, Lyn E. The hand. In: Rosen P, et al., eds. Emergency medicine: concepts and clinical practice. 4th ed. St Louis: Mosby YearBook, 1988:625–668.

Uehara DT. The hand in emergency medicine. Emerg Clin North America 1993;11 (3):781–96.

Author: Matthew Walsh

Pharyngitis

Clinical Presentation

SIGNS AND SYMPTOMS

- Sore throat
- Odynophagia
- Dysphagia
- Fever
- Cervical adenopathy
- Rash
- Diminished oral intake
- Fatigue
- Pharynx
  - —Erythematous
  - —Exudates
- Cervical adenopathy
- Fever
- Scarlatiniform rash
- Diphtheria
  - —Exuberant gray, airway-threatening pharyngeal membrane
- Mononucleosis
  - —Hepatosplenomegaly
- Gonococcal pharyngitis
  - —In children with signs of sexual abuse
  - —In adults with sexually transmitted disease

MECHANISM/DESCRIPTION

- Inflammation/infection of the pharynx
- Third most common complaint of patients seeking medical attention

ETIOLOGY

- Viral
  - —Most common cause of infectious pharyngitis
  - —Influenza
  - —Adenovirus
  - —Epstein Barr virus (mononucleosis)
- Bacterial
  - —Many bacterial pathogens cause pharyngitis
  - —Direct attention toward organisms with potentially serious sequelae
- *Group A β-hemolytic streptococcus*
  - —Strep throat
  - —Causes <10% of adult pharyngitis and <30% of childhood pharyngitis
- *Corynebacterium diphtheriae* (diphtheria)
- *Neisseria gonorrhoeae* (gonococcal pharyngitis)
- Noninfectious
  - —Chemical burns
  - —Foreign bodies
  - —Inhalants
  - —Postnasal drip

Pre-Hospital

CAUTIONS

- Direct attention to airway control for difficulty with respirations
- Initiate 0.9%NS IV fluid for hypotension or significant signs of dehydration

Diagnosis

ESSENTIAL WORKUP

- Physical exam
  - —Does not allow physician to differentiate between various etiologies of pharyngitis
  - —Ability to differentiate *Group A β-hemolytic streptococcus* from nonstreptococcal etiologies
    - -50% false-negative rate
    - -75% false-positive rate when attempting to differentiate *Group A β-hemolytic streptococcus* based solely on clinical grounds

LABORATORY

- Throat culture
  - —Gold standard
  - —Cumbersome due to 48-hour delay and difficulties with ER followup
  - —False-negative rate = 10%
  - —False-positive rate = 20%
- Rapid strep tests (RST)
  - —Convenient
  - —Results within 30 minutes
  - —Sensitivity = 85–95%
  - —Specificity = 96–99%
  - —Few false-positives and many false-negatives
  - —Treat all positive-RST
  - —Confirm all negative-RST by throat culture and treated empirically
- Monospot for suspected mononucleosis

DIFFERENTIAL DIAGNOSIS

- Epiglottitis
- Peritonsillar/retropharyngeal abscess
- Diphtheria
- Acute leukemia
- Oropharyngeal cancer
- Foreign body
- Postnasal drip

IMAGING/SPECIAL TESTS

- Lateral neck x-ray for suspected epiglottitis or foreign body

Treatment

INITIAL STABILIZATION

- ABCs
- Administer 1-L (peds: 20 cc/kg) 0.9%NS fluid bolus for signs of volume depletion or if patient is unable to tolerate oral solutions

ED TREATMENT

- Administer antipyretics
  —Acetaminophen
  —Ibuprofen

Group A β-Hemolytic Streptococcus

- Administer antibiotics for confirmed or highly suspicious
  —Objectives of treatment
    -Prevent rheumatic fever
    -Diminish symptoms
    -Prevent the suppurative complications
  —Options
    -Penicillin
    -Erythromycin
- Corticosteroids
  —Dexamethasone 10 mg IM × 1
  —Provides symptomatic relief in patients with severe streptococcal pharyngitis
- Children should not return to school until they have had at least 24 hours of antibiotics
- Complications
  —Acute rheumatic fever
    -Usually occurs 2.5 weeks following infection
    -Attack rate 0.5–3.0 % in untreated patients
    -Preventable if patients are treated within 9 days of infection
  —Poststreptococcal glomerulonephritis
    -Rarely causes permanent renal failure
    -Antibiotics do not prevent occurrence
  —Peritonsillar/retropharyngeal abscess
    -<1% of those treated
    -Retropharyngeal abscess occurs primarily in children <3 years old
    -Retropharyngeal nodes regress after age 3

Diphtheria

- Goals of therapy
  —Protect patient against the local dangers of the airway-compromising membrane
  —To treat the infection
  —Counteract the exotoxin which, unabated, causes myocarditis and neuritis
- Horse antitoxin
  —Dose dictated by illness severity
- Penicillin or erythromycin
- Complications
  —Myocarditis
    -Occurs in two-thirds
    -Clinically significant in 10%
  —Peripheral neuritis usually involves the cranial nerves

Gonococcal Pharyngitis

- Treat as per usual sexually transmitted disease protocol
  —third-generation cephalosporin/azithromycin

MEDICATIONS

- Penicillin
  —Intramuscular
    -<27 kg: Pen G benzathine (LA) 0.6 million units × 1
    ->27 kg: Pen G benzathine (LA) 1.2 million units × 1
  —Oral
    -<12 years: 250 mg bid × 10 d
    ->12 years: 500 mg bid × 10 d
- Erythromycin
  —Erythromycin base 500 mg po qid × 10 d (peds: erythroethylsuccinate 40 mg/kg/d po + tid × 10 d)

Disposition

ADMISSION CRITERIA

- Airway compromise
- Severe dehydration
- Child sexual abuse

DISCHARGE CRITERIA

- Able to tolerate oral intake

Miscellaneous

ICD9: 462

CORE CONTENT CODE: 6.3.9

SUGGESTED READINGS

Kline J. Streptococcal pharyngitis: a review of pathophysiology, diagnosis and management. J Emerg Med 1994;12:665–680.

Quayle K. Otitis and pharyngitis in children. In: Tintinalli J, et al., eds. Emergency medicine: a comprehensive study guide. 4th ed. 1996:604–610.

Shulman S. Evaluation of penicillins, cephalosporins, and macrolides for therapy of streptococcal pharyngitis. Pediatr Infect Dis J 1994;13(Suppl 1):955–959.

Slay R. Upper respiratory tract infection. In: Rosen P, et al., eds. Emergency medicine: concepts and clinical practice. 3rd ed. St. Louis: CV Mosby, 1997.

Authors: Annie Jewel Sadosty; Brian I. Browne

Phencyclidine, Poisoning

Clinical Presentation

SIGNS AND SYMPTOMS

Central Nervous System

- Altered mental status
  - —Agitation
  - —Bizarre/violent behavior
  - —Belligerence
- Coma
- Seizures
- Nystagmus (vertical, horizontal, or rotatory)

Cardiovascular

- Hypertension
- Tachycardia

Musculoskeletal

- Traumatic injury (decreased pain perception)
- Rhabdomyolysis (due to vigorous muscular contraction)

Vital Signs

- Hyperthermia

MECHANISM/DESCRIPTION

- Dissociative anesthetic structurally related to ketamine
  - —Causes decreased perception of pain, and agitation
- Half-life of 21–24 hours, but may be longer in overdose
- Enterohepatic recirculation—recirculated into the stomach

ETIOLOGY

- Drug of abuse
  - —Frequently encountered as an adulterant of marijuana
- Street names for PCP include
  - —Angel dust
  - —Wicky stick
  - —Wicky weed
  - —Wacky weed
  - —Embalming fluid
  - —Sherman

PEDIATRIC CONSIDERATIONS

- Exposure in toddlers reported via passive exposure

Pre-Hospital

CAUTIONS

- Use restraints/additional personnel to control combative patient

Diagnosis

ESSENTIAL WORKUP

- Clinical diagnosis based on presentation supported by urine toxicology screen
- Careful physical examination for occult trauma
- Exclude other causes of altered mental status

LABORATORY

- CBC
- Electrolytes, BUN/Cr, glucose
- Urinalysis
  - —Dip for myoglobin (rhabdomyolysis)
- CPK
  - —If urine dip for blood is positive
- Ethanol level
- Serum osmolality to rule out toxic alcohol ingestion

IMAGING/SPECIAL TESTS

- CXR for aspiration pneumonia
- Extremity/spine radiographs when there is associated trauma
- CT scan head when there is head trauma/altered mental status

DIFFERENTIAL DIAGNOSIS

Drugs of Abuse

- Cocaine
- Amphetamines
- Designer drugs
  - —Nethcathinone (Cat)
  - —Ecstasy
  - —ICE
- Ketamine
- Other sympathomimetics
- Alcohols

Drugs that Cause Nystagmus

- Lithium
- Carbamazepine
- Sedative Hypnotics
- Alcohols
- Phenothiazines

Treatment

INITIAL STABILIZATION

- ABCs
- IV
- Cardiac monitor
- Naloxone, thiamine, glucose (or Accucheck) if altered mental status
- Protect patient/staff from injury

ED TREATMENT

- Maintain patient in a quiet place; avoid stimulation
- Physical restraints for violent patient
- Sedation
  —Benzodiazepines
  —Butyrophenones (haloperidol) can lower the seizure threshold
- Activated charcoal/sorbitol if oral coingestants
- IV 0.9%NS hydration/mannitol/sodium bicarbonate for rhabdomyolysis

MEDICATIONS

- Activated charcoal slurry: 1–2 g/kg up to 90 g po
- Ativan (lorazepam): 2 mg IV increments
- Dextrose: D50W 1 amp (50 ml or 25 g) (peds: D25W 2–4 ml/kg) IV
- Diazepam: 5 mg IV increments
- Haloperidol: 5 mg IM/IV increments
- Mannitol: 25–50 g IV
- Naloxone (narcan): 2 mg (peds: 0.1 mg/kg) IV or IM initial dose
- Sodium bicarbonate: 2 amp diluted in 1 L of D5W, given at 125–250 cc/hr (for rhabdomyolysis) to urine pH of 7.0
- Sorbitol: 1–2 g/kg to a max of 100 g (peds: >1-year-old: 1–1.5 g/kg as a 35% solution to a max of 50 g) po mixed in the activated charcoal slurry—only use for first dose
- Thiamine (vitamin B_1): 100 mg (peds: 50 mg) IV or IM

Disposition

ADMISSION CRITERIA

- Prolonged altered mental status
- Significant traumatic injuries
- Rhabdomyolysis
- Hyperthermia

DISCHARGE CRITERIA

- Become lucid after a period of observation (6 hours)

Miscellaneous

ICD9: 968.3

CORE CONTENT CODE: 17.2.19

SUGGESTED READINGS

Ellenhorn MJ, Schoonwald S, Ordog G, Wasserberger J. Phencyclidine. In: Ellenhorn MJ, ed. Ellenhorn's medical toxicology. 2d ed. Baltimore: Williams & Wilkins, 1997:400–403.

Patel R, Connor G. A review of thirty cases of rhabdomyolysis-associated acute renal failure among phencyclidine users. Clin Toxicol 1986;23:547–556.

Silber TJ, Iosefsohn M, Hicks JM, et al. Prevalence of PCP use among adolescent marijuana users. J Pediatr 1988;112:827–829.

Author: Steven Aks

Phenothiazine, Poisoning

Clinical Presentation

SIGNS AND SYMPTOMS

- Overdose
  - —Exhibits mild symptoms
  - —Serious toxicity associated with concomitant ingestion of sympathomimetic, lithium, antihistamines, or cyclic antidepressants
- Neurologic
  - —CNS depression
  - —Agitation
  - —Seizures
  - —Coma
  - —Extrapyramidal signs
  - —Neuroleptic malignant syndrome
- Cardiovascular
  - —Hypotension
  - —Ventricular tachycardia
  - —Torsades de pointes
  - —Ventricular fibrillation
  - —Atrioventricular block
  - —Widened QRS complex
- Respiratory
  - —Respiratory depression
  - —Pulmonary edema
- Gastrointestinal
  - —Constipation
  - —Dry mouth
- Genitourinary
  - —Urinary retention
  - —Priapism
- Hyperthermia
- Ocular—mydriasis
- Hematologic—agranulocytosis, anemia
- Hepatic—cholestatic jaundice
- Neuroleptic malignant syndrome
  - —Hyperthermia
  - —Skeletal muscle rigidity
  - —Impaired consciousness
  - —Autonomic dysfunction

MECHANISM/DESCRIPTION

- Phenothiazines used for the management of
  - —Psychotic disorders
  - —Depressive neurosis
  - —Dementia in the elderly
  - —Behavioral problems in children
  - —Chemotherapy-induced emesis
  - —Alcohol withdrawal symptoms
- Toxic and potentially fatal dose between 15–150 mg/kg depending on the agent ingested
- Peak plasma levels within 2–4 hours
- Cardiovascular toxicity peak 10–15 hours postingestion
- Dystonic reactions occur from 5–18 hours up to 72 hours postingestion

PHENOTHIAZINE	*ANTICHOLINERGIC EFFECTS*	*EXTRAPYRAMIDAL EFFECTS*
Thioridazine, Serentil, Mellaril, Parsidol	High	Low-moderate
Prolixin, Trilafon, Compazine, Stelazine	Low-moderate	Moderate-high

ETIOLOGY

- Blocks
  - —Postsynaptic mesolimbic dopaminergic receptors in the brain
  - —Peripheral dopaminergic receptors
- Exhibits a strong α-adrenergic block
- Depresses the release of hypothalamic and hypophyseal hormones

Pre-Hospital

CAUTIONS

- Do not induce emesis due of risk of seizures and sedation

Diagnosis

ESSENTIAL WORKUP

- Monitor vital signs with significant exposure
- Cardiac monitor/pulse oximetry

LABORATORY

- Electrolytes, BUN, Cr, glucose
- Liver function tests for significant overdose
- Urinalysis
  —Dip for myoglobin if neuroleptic malignant syndrome (NMS) suspected
- CPK levels if NMS suspected
- Qualitative colorimetric tests are useful if positive
- Quantitative phenothiazine levels are rarely useful

IMAGING/SPECIAL TESTS

- ECG
  —QT/QRS prolongation
  —Conduction disturbances
- Abdominal radiograph
  —Unabsorbed phenothiazine radiopaque
  —Absence of visible tablets does not eliminate possibility of ingestion

DIFFERENTIAL DIAGNOSIS

- Tricyclic antidepressants overdose
- Antihistamines overdose
- Cocaine overdose
- Amphetamine overdose

Treatment

INITIAL STABILIZATION

- ABCs
  —Administer supplemental oxygen
  —Intubate if respiratory depression

ED TREATMENT

- Supportive care
- Decontamination
  —Lavage for recent large ingestion
  —Administer multidose activated charcoal and cathartic after lavage
  —Hemodialysis and hemoperfusion of limited value (large volume of distribution and high protein binding)
- Hypotension
  —0.9%NS IV fluid bolus
  —Treat resistant hypotension with norepinephrine
  —Avoid dopamine due to the potent β-adrenergic activity when α-adrenergic activity is blocked
- Ventricular dysrhythmias
  —Lidocaine or phenytoin (often ineffective)
  —Temporary pacing often required
  —Avoid class 1 antidysrhythmics—potential exacerbation of phenothiazine's quinidine-like effect
- Dystonic reactions
  —Administer diphenhydramine or benztropine mesylate
- Malignant hyperthermia
  —Administer dantrolene or bromocriptine
- Seizures
  —Treat initially with diazepam
  —Phenobarbital or phenytoin for persistent seizures

MEDICATIONS

- Activated charcoal: 1–2 g/kg
- Benztropine: 1–2 mg IV
- Bromocriptine: 5 mg q 8 hrs po
- Dantrolene: 2.5 mg/kg IV
- Diazepam: 5–10 mg IV q 10–15 min (0.2–0.5 mg/kg)
- Diphenhydramine: 25–50 mg IV (1 mg/kg)
- Lidocaine: loading dose: 1 mg/kg IV q 5–10 min (3 mg/kg max); maintenance dose: 2–4 mg/min IV
- Norepinephrine: 1–2 μg/kg/min titrate to blood pressure
- Phenobarbital: 15–20 mg/kg IV (loading dose)
- Phenytoin: 15–20 mg/kg IV (loading dose)
- Sorbitol: 0.5–1 g/kg to a max of 100 g of 70% solution (peds: >1-year-old: 0.5–1 g/kg as a 35% solution to a max of 50 g) po mixed in the activated charcoal slurry—only use for first dose

Disposition

ADMISSION CRITERIA

- Admit overdose with CNS excitation, sedation, vital sign abnormalities, or extrapyramidal effects to monitored bed

DISCHARGE CRITERIA

- Asymptomatic after 4 hours of observation

Miscellaneous

ICD9: E853.0

CORE CONTENT CODE: 17.2.10

SUGGESTED READINGS

Ellenhorn MJ, Schonwald S, Ordog G, Wasserberger J. Neuroleptic drugs. In: Ellenhorn MJ, ed. Ellenhorn's medical toxicology. 2d ed. Baltimore: Williams & Wilkins, 1997:662–683.

Knight ME, Roberts RJ. Phenothiazines and butyrophenone intoxication in children. Pediatr Clin North Am 1986;33:299–309.

Le Blaye I, Donatini B, Hall M, Krupp P. Acute overdosage with thioridazine: A review of the available clinical exposure. Vet Hum Toxicol 1993;35:147–150.

Lewin NA, Wang RY. Neuroleptic agents. In: Goldfrank LR, Weisman RS, Flomenbaum NE, Howland MA, Lewin NA, Hoffman RS, eds. Goldfrank's toxicologic emergencies. East Norwalk, CT: Appleton & Lange, 1994:739–747.

Author: Robert June

Clinical Presentation

SIGNS AND SYMPTOMS

- Levels 20–40 μg/ml
  - —Nystagmus
  - —Dizziness
  - —Ataxia
  - —Drowsiness
  - —Nausea/vomiting
  - —Diplopia
  - —Slurred speech
- Levels 40–90 μg/ml
  - —Confusion
  - —Disorientation
- Level >90 μg/ml
  - —Coma
  - —Respiratory depression
  - —Paradoxical seizures
- Hypotension/bradycardia with rapid IV administration
  - —Fosphenytoin injection does not contain propylene glycol
  - —Hypotension/dysrhythmia unlikely with fosphenytoin
- Hypersensitivity reaction following chronic use
  - —Rash
  - —Fever
  - —Neutropenia
  - —Agranulocytosis
  - —Hepatitis
  - —Cholangitis

MECHANISM/DESCRIPTION

- Follows zero order pharmacokinetics
  - —Small incremental increase in dose can result in a large increase in plasma concentration
- Half life in overdose—up to 70 hrs
- Cardiovascular toxicity from IV administration due to the diluent, propylene glycol
- Fosphenytoin, a prodrug for parenteral administration, is metabolized to its active moiety phenytoin

ETIOLOGY

- Phenytoin intoxication results from acute, chronic, or acute on chronic ingestion
- If the etiology of the intoxication is unclear in a patient on phenytoin consider
  - —Change in the brand of phenytoin
  - —Change in dosage form
  - —Drug interaction

Pre-Hospital

CAUTIONS

- Differentiate phenytoin-induced altered mental status from other potentially serious causes
  - —Head trauma common in seizure population
- Collect/transport prescription bottles and medications to aid in identification and quantification of ingestion

Diagnosis

ESSENTIAL WORKUP

- Determine the time and amount of ingestion
- Phenytoin level
  - —After oral overdose, the peak plasma concentration may not be reached until 24 hours or more postacute ingestion
  - —Repeat levels every 4 hours until levels have peaked and are declining
  - —Once levels begin declining check every 24 hours until <30 μg/ml
  - —Fosphenytoin levels are measured as phenytoin
  - —Measure fosphenytoin after conversion to phenytoin is complete (2 hours post-IV infusion/4 hours post-IM injection)
  - —Prior to complete conversion to phenytoin, immunoanalytical techniques may overestimate plasma phenytoin concentrations due to cross-reactivity with fosphenytoin

LABORATORY

- Electrolytes, BUN, Cr, glucose
  - —Check for anion gap metabolic acidosis due to coingestant
  - —Determine glucose with altered mental status
  - —Hyperglycemia often present

DIFFERENTIAL DIAGNOSIS

- Intoxication with other CNS depressants
- Guillain-Barré syndrome
- Botulism
- Posterior fossa tumor
- Acute cerebellitis

Treatment

INITIAL STABILIZATION

- ABCs
  —IV access
  —Cardiac monitor (with IV overdose)
- Treat hypotension with IV fluids and Trendelenburg position
  —Dopamine for refractory hypotension
- Treat paradoxical seizures with diazepam

ED TREATMENT

- Gastric lavage if within 1 hour of ingestion
- Activated charcoal
  —Administer single dose
  —Multiple-dose activated charcoal may increase the clearance of phenytoin; does not correlate with clinical improvement in patients with phenytoin toxicity

MEDICATIONS

- Activated charcoal slurry: 1–2 g/kg up to 90 g po
- Dextrose: D50W 1 amp (50 ml or 25 g) (peds: D25W 2–4 ml/kg) IV
- Dopamine: 2–20 μg/kg/min IV titrated to desired blood pressure
- Naloxone (narcan): 2 mg (peds: 0. 1 mg/kg) IV or IM initial dose
- Sorbitol: 1–2 g/kg to a max of 100 g (peds: >1 year old: 1–1.5 g/kg as a 35% solution to a max of 50 g) po mixed in the activated charcoal slurry—only use for first dose
- Thiamine (vitamin B_1): 100 mg (peds: 50 mg) IV or IM

Disposition

ADMISSION CRITERIA

- Altered mental status, severe ataxia, increasing phenytoin level
- Level >25 μg/ml
- ICU admission with intoxication from IV phenytoin

DISCHARGE CRITERIA

- Level <25 μg/ml
- Ambulatory without ataxia

Miscellaneous

ICD9: 966.1

CORE CONTENT CODE: 17.2.6

SUGGESTED READINGS

Browne TR. Fosphenytoin (cerebyx). Clin Neuropharmacol 1997;20:1–12.

Ellenhorn MJ. Anticonvulsants Ellenhorn's medical toxicology:Diagnosis and treatment of human poisoning. 2d ed. Baltimore: Williams and Wilkins, 1997: 605–607.

Howard CE, Roberts RS, Ely DS, et al. Use of multiple-dose activated charcoal in phenytoin toxicity. Ann Pharmacother 1994:28;201–203.

Larsen JR, Larsen LS. Clinical features and management of poisoning due to phenytoin. Med Toxicol Adverse Drug Exp 1989:4;229–245.

Author: Michele Kanter

Pheochromocytoma

Clinical Presentation

SIGNS AND SYMPTOMS

- 60% have sustained hypertension; 40% hypertensive only during attacks

Hypertensive Crisis

- *Classic presentation*—paroxysms of
  - —Hypertension
  - —Headache
  - —Tachycardia
  - —Diaphoresis/anxiety
- Moderate to malignant hypertension
- Chest pain
- Palpitations
- Tremors
- Abdominal pain
- Diarrhea
- Flushing
- Pallor

Acute Hemorrhagic Tumor Necrosis

- Acute abdomen
- Marked hypertension followed by declining BP leading to hypotensive shock

Complications

CNS Complications

- Hypertensive encephalopathy
  - —Altered mental status
  - —Focal neurologic signs
  - —Seizures
  - —CVA (infarction, hemorrhagic or embolic)

Cardiac Complications

- Tachydysrrhythmias due to catecholamine release
- Orthostatic hypotension due to
  - —Diminished plasma volume
  - —Blunted sympathetic reflexes

Respiratory Complications

- Cardiogenic or noncardiogenic pulmonary edema

Genitourinary Complications

- Renal artery stenosis (mass effect)
- Renal infarction due to severe vasospasm

Endocrine and Metabolic Complications

- Hyperglycemia
- Hypoglycemia—usually postoperative
- Lactic acidosis in the absence of shock
- Transient thyrotoxicosis
- Hypercalcemia secondary to excess parathyroid hormone (PTH) production
- Diarrhea secondary to excess VIP
- Hypokalemic alkalosis secondary to excess ACTH

MECHANISM/DESCRIPTION

- Hypertensive episode may occur
  - —Spontaneously
  - —Due to any activity that displaces abdominal contents
  - —Acute hemorrhagic necrosis of the tumor
  - —Precipitation by drugs: TCA, metoclopramide, opiates, histamine, β-blockers

ETIOLOGY

- Catecholamine-producing tumor arising from the chromaffin tissues of the sympathetic nervous system
- Incidence ranges from 0.3% to 1.9%
- 10% extraadrenal in location
- 10% malignant
- Associated with MEN IIA and IIB (multiple endocrine neoplasia), neurofibromatosis, Von-Hippel-Lindau, tuberous sclerosis, Sturge-Weber syndrome
- Alterations occur in levels of circulating catecholamines as well as the cardiovascular response to them

Pre-Hospital

N/A

Diagnosis

ESSENTIAL WORKUP

- ECG abnormalities ranging from
  - —Ischemia
  - —Dysrhythmias—tachydysrrhythmia, AFib, VFib

LABORATORY

- CBC
  - —Indicated when abdominal pain/infection
- Electrolytes, BUN, Cr, glucose
  - —Lactic acidosis
  - —Renal failure secondary to hypertension/renal damage
  - —Hyper/hypoglycemia due to impaired response to insulin and effect of catecholamines
- Calcium
  - —Hypercalcemia due to excess PTH
- Urinalysis
  - —Protein in urine due to hypertension

IMAGING/SPECIAL TESTS

- Confirmatory diagnostic studies (usually not in ED)
  - —Plasma catecholamines
  - —24-hour urine for metabolites including metanephrine, normetanephrine, and vanillylmandelic acid
  - —Clonidine suppression test
  - —Glucagon stimulation test
  - —Chromogranin A
  - —Adrenal imaging following biochemical confirmation of diagnosis via CT Scan, MRI, MIBG (^{131}I met-iodobenzylguanidine) scan
- CXR for pulmonary edema
- CT scan head if abnormal neurologic exam for CVA, intracranial bleed

DIFFERENTIAL DIAGNOSIS

- Hypertension with associated
  - —Anxiety
  - —Severe migraines
  - —Hyperthyroidism
  - —MI
  - —Drug abuse (amphetamines, crack, cocaine)
- Alcohol withdrawal
- Monoamine oxidase inhibitor and hypertensive crisis
- Septic shock (pure epinephrine-producing tumor may cause peripheral vasodilation.)
- Surgical abdomen (due to tumor necrosis)

Treatment

INITIAL STABILIZATION

- IV access
- Continuous cardiac/blood pressure monitoring

ED TREATMENT

- Hypertensive crisis
  - —α-Blockade with phentolamine—first-line agent
  - —Nitroprusside for uncontrolled hypertension
  - —Vigorous fluid resuscitation required as vasoconstriction is relieved
- β-Blockade (labetalol or esmolol)
  - —For further BP control
  - —If tachycardia develops during induction of α-blockade
  - —Caution: institution of β-blockade without prior α-adrenergic blockade may exacerbate hypertension by antagonizing β-mediated vasodilatation in smooth muscle
- Ventricular tachydysrrhythmias
  - —β-Blockade
  - —Lidocaine
  - —Amiodarone

MEDICATIONS

- Amiodarone: rapid-loading regimen: 5 mg/kg (max: 450 mg) mixed in D5W infused over 10–30 minutes (max rate 30 mg/min)
- Esmolol: load 500 μg/kg over 1 minute, followed by 50 μg/kg/min for 4 minutes. If adequate therapeutic effect not achieved within 5 minutes, repeat loading dose and increase infusion to 100 μg/kg/min. Repeat loading dose and titrate infusion rate upwards at 50 μg/kg/min q 4–5 minutes as needed. Omit further loading doses once nearing therapeutic target
- Labetalol: incremental doses beginning at 20–40 mg IV. BP should fall within 5 minutes, with maximum effect at 10 minutes. Can double IV dose q 30–60 minutes until target reached, with maximum total dose of 300 mg
- Lidocaine: 0.7–1.4 mg/kg IVP, may repeat in 5 minutes; maximum 200–300 mg over 1 hour. Follow bolus with infusion of 2–4 mg/min
- Phentolamine: 5–10 mg (peds: 0.05–0.1 mg/kg/dose max 5 mg) IV, repeat as needed to 20 mg total. Can be administered as IV drip
- Sodium nitroprusside: 0.5–10.0 μg/kg/min continuous IV infusion, max 800 μg/min. Stop infusion if adequate BP control not achieved at 10 μg/kg/min within 10 minutes

Disposition

ADMISSION CRITERIA

- Suspicion of pheochromocytoma in an ill patient mandates α-blockade and aggressive volume expansion in a closely monitored setting

DISCHARGE CRITERIA

- Stable patient with mild hypertension, suspicious for pheochromocytoma may be referred for prompt outpatient investigations

Miscellaneous

ICD9: 227.0

CORE CONTENT CODE: 4.7

SUGGESTED READINGS

Bravo E, Gifford R. Pheochromocytoma. Endocrinol Metab Clin North Am 1993;22(2):329–341.

Gifford R. Management of hypertensive crisis. JAMA 1991;266(6):829–835.

Landsberg L, Young J. Pheochromocytoma. In: Isselbacher K, et al., ed. Harrison's principles of internal medicine. 13th ed. New York: McGraw Hill, 1987:1775–1778.

Salehi A, et al. Pheochromocytoma and bowel ischemia. J Emerg Med 1997;15(1):35–38.

Werbel S, Ober K. Pheochromocytoma. Med Clin North Am 1995;79(1):131–153.

Author: Steven Friedman

Phimosis

Clinical Presentation

SIGNS AND SYMPTOMS

- Whitish, narrowed preputial opening of the foreskin
- Dysuria, hematuria
- Poor urinary stream
- Edema, erythema and tenderness of prepuce
- *Balanoposthitis* (inflammation of the glans and foreskin)
- Ballooning of foreskin on urination in severe cases

MECHANISM/DESCRIPTION

- True phimosis is the inability to retract the foreskin over the glans of the penis as a result of *scarring*. The inability to retract a normal, supple foreskin is not true phimosis
- The foreskin is rarely retractable at birth. This is due to normal adhesions between the glans and the inner prepuce. Approximately 90% are retractable by 3 years of age, and 99% are retractable by age 17, as the epithelial cells that comprise *smegma* are shed. Parents should be instructed not to forcibly retract the foreskin

ETIOLOGY

- Possible causes of true phimosis include
  —Trauma from forcible retraction of the foreskin
  —Repetitive bouts of diaper dermatitis
  —Recurrent balanoposthitis
  —Poorly performed circumcision
  —Congenital anomalies

Pre-Hospital

CAUTIONS

- Pre-hospital personnel and family members should be instructed *not* to attempt retraction of the foreskin prior to medical evaluation. Unwarranted attempts may traumatize a normal, nonretractable prepuce, or convert the situation to a more emergent *paraphimosis*

Diagnosis

ESSENTIAL WORKUP

- In the majority of cases, no workup is necessary
- In patients with severe stenosis, the complication of an *obstructive uropathy* may occur. This may result from structural compression, but should be investigated by evaluation of kidney function (BUN and creatinine) and a renal sonogram
- Phimosis secondary to recurrent balanoposthitis should prompt a workup for *diabetes mellitus* (urinalysis, serum glucose, or glucose tolerance test)

DIFFERENTIAL DIAGNOSIS

- Preputial "adhesions" are normal in young children
- Balanoposthitis without phimosis

Treatment

INITIAL STABILIZATION

- None required in most cases. Examination should include an evaluation for potential complications such as *obstruction* and *vascular compromise* to the glans. These occur only in the most extreme cases

ED TREATMENT

- Relieve obstructive uropathy, if present, with urethral catheterization or suprapubic aspiration
- If vascular flow to the glans is compromised, a dorsal slit must be made in the foreskin. This is performed with infiltration of local anesthetic without epinephrine at the base of the penile shaft and possibly sedation. This is rarely necessary in phimosis
- In uncomplicated cases, provide patients with urologic follow-up for elective dilation of the preputial opening, operative repair, or elective circumcision as necessary
- Potent topical steroids have been reported to successfully reduce phimosis but are inappropriate for emergent cases

MEDICATIONS

- Pain control as required

Disposition

ADMISSION CRITERIA

- Obstructive uropathy
- Severe balanoposthitis with ischemia or necrosis

DISCHARGE CRITERIA

- Ability to urinate
- Adequate urologic follow-up

Miscellaneous

ICD9: 605

CORE CONTENT CODE: 19.2.1.3, 13.13.2.2

SUGGESTED READINGS

Dewan PA, Tieu HC. Phimosis: Is circumcision necessary? J Ped and Child Health. 1996 Aug;32(4):285–9.

Pontari MA. Phimosis and paraphimosis. In: Seidman EJ, Hanno PM, eds. Current urologic therapy. 3rd ed. Philadelphia: WB Saunders, 1994:392–397.

Super DM. Phimosis. In: Hoekelman R, et al., eds. Primary pediatric care. St. Louis: CV Mosby, 1987:1232–1234.

Authors: Lorne Sherman; Joseph LaMantia

Pityriasis Rosea

Clinical Presentation

SIGNS AND SYMPTOMS

- *Herald patch:* solitary, erythematous, slightly raised papule 2–10 cm in diameter and seen in 50–90% of cases
- *Secondary eruption:* widespread salmon colored, elliptic, finely scaling 1 cm macular or papular lesions with longest axis along lines of skin tension (a "fir tree" distribution)
  —Generally follows the herald patch by 7–14 days. Lesions are concentrated on the trunk and proximal extremities
- Pruritus accompanies the rash in up to 75% of cases
- Prodromal symptoms may be seen in approximately 5% of cases including fever, headache, malaise, arthralgias, and gastrointestinal symptoms
- Atypical forms of individual lesions occasionally occur including papular, urticarial, pustular, and purpuric

ETIOLOGY

- Unknown. Weak evidence exists for an infectious (viral) cause
- Medications including barbiturates, captopril, clonidine, gold, isotretinoin, metronidazole, and penicillamine have been associated with a pityriasislike eruption

PEDIATRIC CONSIDERATIONS

- Atypical presentations including oral involvement and inverse pityriasis rosea are more common in children
- Oral lesions may include punctate hemorrhages, ulcerations, erythematous macules, and vesicles
- Lesions concentrated on the face and distal extremities with minimal trunk involvement characterize *inverse pityriasis*

Pre-Hospital

N/A

Diagnosis

ESSENTIAL WORKUP

- Syphilis testing: secondary syphilis can mimic pityriasis rosea, so an RPR or VDRL is required if the diagnosis is in question, especially with history of chancre or absence of herald patch
- KOH preparation may be needed to differentiate the herald patch from tinea corporis

DIFFERENTIAL DIAGNOSIS

- Herald patch
  —Nummular eczema
  —Tinea corporis
- Generalized eruption
  —Secondary syphilis
  —Drug eruption
  —Guttate psoriasis
  —Kaposi's sarcoma
  —Lichen planus
  —Occult malignancy
  —Scabies
  —Seborrheic dermatitis
  —Tinea versicolor

Treatment

INITIAL STABILIZATION
- None required

ED TREATMENT
- Pityriasis is treated symptomatically

MEDICATIONS
- Diphenhydramine: adult: 50 mg po qid; peds: 5 mg/kg/day divided qid
- Hydrocortisone: adult: 1% cream tid; peds: 1% cream tid
- Prednisone: adult: 15–40 mg qd; peds: 0.25–0.5mg/kg/qd
- Ultraviolet B (UVB): 5 daily erythemogenic doses

Disposition

ADMISSION CRITERIA
None

DISCHARGE CRITERIA
- Pityriasis rosea is a self-limited disease. Admission is not required

Miscellaneous

ICD9: 696.3

CORE CONTENT CODE: 3.3.1

SUGGESTED READINGS
Allen RA, Janniger CK, Schwartz RA. Pityriasis rosea. Cutis 1995;56(4):198–202.

Bjornborg A. Epidermal-dermal inflammatory conditions of unknown etiology. In: Fitzpatrick TB, et al., eds. Dermatology in general medicine. 4th ed. Chap. 83. New York: McGraw Hill, 1993:1117–1123.

Horn T, Kazakis A. Pityriasis rosea and the need for a serologic test for syphilis. Cutis 1987;39(1):81–82.

Parsons J. Pityriasis rosea update: 1986. J Am Acad Dermatol 1986;15(2):159–167.

Author: Nate Rudman

Placenta Previa

Clinical Presentation

SIGNS AND SYMPTOMS

- Vaginal bleeding in the second half of pregnancy may be catastrophic
- Hallmark is bright red, painless, vaginal bleeding occurring at the end of the second trimester
- Profuse hemorrhage at the onset of labor
- Uterine cramps are variably present
- First trimester vaginal bleeding may be a sentinel bleed with previa implantation

MECHANISM/DESCRIPTION

- Implantation of the placenta over the cervical os
- Spontaneous placental separation and blood vessel disruption with growth of the lower uterine segment and dilation of the cervix
- The lack of myometrium in the lower uterine segment weakens the contractile response of the uterus
- Four degrees of previa exist
  - —Low lying placenta: placenta in the lower uterine segment
  - —Marginal: edge of the placenta at margin of internal os
  - —Partial: internal os is partially covered by placenta
  - —Total: internal os is completely covered by the placenta
- Degree of previa will depend on degree of cervical dilation
- Low-lying placenta may become partial previa as dilation occurs
- Placenta accreta/increta/percreta are abnormally firm attachments of the placenta due to poorly developed decidua in the lower uterine segment

ETIOLOGY

- Unknown cause
- Approximately 6% of all pregnancies

RISK FACTORS

- Previous placenta previa
- Multiparity
- Advanced maternal age
- Smoking
- Previous cesarean section
- Previous D&C
- Previous twin gestation
- Uterine anomalies

Pre-Hospital

N/A

Diagnosis

ESSENTIAL WORKUP

- Do not perform bimanual or speculum examination in patients with third trimester bleeding
  - —May cause uncontrolled hemorrhage in placenta previa
- Rapid hemoglobin/hematocrit
- Blood type, Rh, and crossmatch

LABORATORY

- CBC, platelets
- PT/PTT
- BUN, creatinine
- Fibrinogen, fibrin-split products
- Wall clot
  - —10 cc venous blood in red top tube, tape to wall. No clot after 9 minutes should raise suspicion of clotting abnormality
- Wright stain vaginal blood may contain cord (nucleated) RBCs
- Kleihauer-Betke

IMAGING/SPECIAL TESTS

- Transabdominal ultrasound—98% sensitive
  - —Position of placenta, estimated gestational age of fetus
  - —Empty bladder preferred
  - —Do not perform vaginal probe US
- MRI is most sensitive if patient hemodynamically stable
- Examination in the operating room may be necessary
  - —"Double setup" approach involves pelvic examination in the OR/delivery suite with subsequent ability to attempt vaginal delivery or cesarean section

DIFFERENTIAL DIAGNOSIS

- Vasa Previa
- Placental abruption
- Cervical/uterine trauma
- Lacerations
- Spontaneous abortion
- Cervical lesions; polyps, hypervascularity

Treatment

INITIAL STABILIZATION

- ABCs
  - —Two large bore intravenous lines with normal saline bolus therapy
  - —Hypotensive patients >20 weeks gestation should be placed in left lateral recumbent position
  - —Intubation if altered mental status or shock
  - —Immediate obstetrical consultation
  - —Early transfusion if hypotension not responsive to 2 L NS

ED TREATMENT

- Tocolytics may benefit some preterm patients and with transfusion bleeding may stabilize
  - —Tocolytics: β-agonists, $MgSO_4$ may precipitate worsened hypotension
- Consumptive coagulopathy; restore with platelets, FFP
- Foley drainage may improve lower uterine segment contractility
- "Delivery" may be necessary for continued hemorrhage, or fetal compromise
- Hemodynamically unstable patients should be taken directly to the OR for delivery and management of hemorrhage

MEDICATIONS

Tocolytic

- Magnesium sulfate: 4–6 g IV over 30 min, followed by 2–4 g/hr
- Terbutaline: 0.25 mg subcutaneously, may repeat same dose in 30 min

Disposition

ADMISSION CRITERIA

- All patients with bleeding from placenta previa must be admitted to a monitored setting and frequently need urgent operative intervention

DISCHARGE CRITERIA

- Preterm patients found to have placenta previa with no active bleeding may on occasion be considered for outpatient management if arrangement can be made for rapid transport to the ED if bleeding occurs
  - —Pelvic rest and bleeding precautions must be stressed
  - —Decision made in conjunction with OBGyn and with close follow-up
  - —Most studies have shown outcome benefit to admission and monitoring
- First trimester, stable bleeding with previa may undergo outpatient management and further evaluation after OBGyn consultation and evaluation with ultrasound

Miscellaneous

ICD9: 641.10

CORE CONTENT CODE: 12.3.5

SUGGESTED READINGS

Charles D, Hurry D, eds. Obstetrics and gynecology. 6th ed. New York: Elsevier Science, 1986.

Cunningham FG, MacDonald PC, Grant NF, eds. Williams' Obstetrics. 19th ed. Norwalk, CT: Appleton & Lange, 1993.

Reid A, Duncan G, Christian C, eds. Controversy in obstetrics and gynecology II. 2nd ed. Philadelphia: WB Saunders, 1974.

Rosen P, et al., eds. Emergency medicine. 3rd ed. St. Louis: CV Mosby, 1992.

Scott CJ, et al. Emergencies in pregnancy. Patient Care 1991;15:132–151.

Author: Shawn D. Evans

Clinical Presentation

SIGNS AND SYMPTOMS

Herbs

- Shave grass and horsetail
  - —CNS stimulant
  - —Confusion
  - —Ataxia
- Pokeweed, juniper berries, senna
  - —Fulminant gastroenteritis
  - —Abdominal pain/colic
- Pennyroyal oil, sassafras root
  - —Hepatorenal syndrome
- Chamomile, chrysanthemums: histamine-releasing/anaphylactic reactions
  - —Angioedema
  - —Bronchospasm
  - —Hypotension
  - —Shock
  - —Death
- Tonka beans, sweet woodruff (natural coumarin): hemorrhage
- Nutmeg
  - —Nausea, vomiting
  - —Chest pain
  - —Abdominal pain
  - —Agitation, "feelings of doom"
- Ginseng
  - —Tachycardia
  - —Hypertension
  - —Hypoglycemia
  - —Increased GI motility
- *Jimson weed* (locoweed, datura)
  - —Anticholinergic toxidrome
  - —Dry mouth, skin, eyes
  - —Dilated pupil
  - —Tachycardia
  - —Altered mental status

Indoor/Outdoor Plants

- Lectins group (castor bean and rosary pea)
  - —CNS depression
  - —Seizures
  - —Severe gastroenteritis
- Colchicine group (autumn crocus and glory lily)
  - —3 phases
    - -Gastrointestinal (24 hours): severe abdominal pain, nausea, vomiting, diarrhea
    - -Multisystem failure (2–7 days): ascending paralysis, ARDS, DIC, pancytopenia, cardiac arrhythmias, hepatic insufficiency, delirium
    - -Recovery (>7 days): resolution of organ systems failure, rebound of leukocytosis, alopecia
  - —Requires large amount of plant (>0.8 mg/kg is lethal)
- Solanine group (deadly nightshade)
  - —Nausea, vomiting, diarrhea
  - —Headaches, muscle weakness
  - —Begin 2–24 hours after ingestion

Nicotine-Containing Plants (Tobacco Plants)

- Rapid onset
- Abdominal pain/nausea/vomiting
- Initially tachycardia/hypertension followed by bradycardia/hypotension
- CNS stimulation initially: tremor/seizures/confusion/restlessness
- CNS depression later: decreased mental state/coma
- Hypotonia/decreased reflexes/motor paralysis occur sequentially

Grayanotoxin-Containing Plants (Rhododendrons and Azaleas)

- Dose-dependent bradycardia
- Hypotension
- CNS depression
- Most ingestions asymptomatic

Cyanogenic Plants (Seeds of Apples, Pear, and Crab Apple; Lima Beans, Cassava, and Bamboo)

- Headache
- Dyspnea
- Cyanosis
- Convulsions
- Coma, cardiovascular collapse
- Identical to cyanide poisoning due to inhibition of oxidative phosphorylation

Cardiac Glycosides-Containing Plants (Foxglove, Oleander, Yellow Oleander, Lily of the Valley)

- Resembles digoxin toxicity
- Nausea/vomiting
- Alteration in vision
- Cardiac effect
  - —Bradyarrhythmias
  - —Tachyarrhythmias

Hallucinogenics (Marijuana, Morning Glory, Catnip, Peyote, Juniper)

- Mood alteration—euphoria or depression
- Dry mouth/thirst
- Tachycardia
- Toxic psychosis/panic reactions

Gastrointestinal Symptoms

- Irritation of oral mucosa from calcium oxalate crystallization (philodendron)
- Irritation of gastric mucosa (daffodil, narcissus)
- Irritation of intestinal mucosa (pokeweed, horse, chestnut)

PEDIATRIC CONSIDERATIONS

- Often present with lip, tongue, and oropharyngeal irritation and swelling from oxalate crystal-containing plants
  - —Potential for airway compromise
- Usually consume the leaves and seeds—most concentrated forms
- Nicotine group: 1–2 cigarettes potentially lethal
- Jimson weed: seeds highly concentrated; 4–5 g of the leaf lethal
- Yellow oleander: 2 leaves lethal in 12.5-kg child

Pre-Hospital

CAUTIONS

- Nontoxic houseplants
  - —African violet
  - —Aluminum plant
  - —Baby's tears
  - —Bird's nest fern
  - —Corn plant
  - —Creeping Charlie
  - —Creeping Jenny
  - —Gardenia
  - —Grape ivy
  - —Jade plant
  - —Parlor palm
  - —Peacock plant
  - —Piggyback begonia
  - —Prayer plant
  - —Rubber tree
  - —Snake plant
  - —Spider plant
  - —Swedish ivy
  - —Velvet plant
  - —Wandering Jew
  - —Wax plant
  - —Zebra plant
- Collect seeds, leaves, spores in paper bag
- Contact local botanist

CONTROVERSIES

- Syrup of ipecac not recommended in setting of severe GI distress, altered mental status

Diagnosis

ESSENTIAL WORKUP

- Identification of ingested material
- Exact work-up depends on plant ingested

LABORATORY

- Electrolytes, BUN, Cr, glucose
- ABG
  —Check pH
  —Methemoglobinemia
  —Oxygen saturation
- Digoxin level for cardioglycoside plants
- Cyanide level for cyanogenic plants

IMAGING/SPECIAL TESTS

- EKG: arrhythmias/bradycardia

DIFFERENTIAL DIAGNOSIS

- Altered mental status
  —Drug use/alcohol
  —Seizures
  —Trauma
  —CVA
- Digoxin toxicity
- Gastroenteritis
- Agents causing metabolic acidosis (MUD-PILES)-see Acidosis chapter

Treatment

INITIAL STABILIZATION

- ABCs
- 0.9%NS IV
  —Aggressive volume replacement for dehydration/hypotension
  —Initiate pressors (dopamine) for hypotension unresponsive to fluids
- Cardiac monitoring
- Supportive care for most ingestants

ED TREATMENT

- Gastric decontamination
  —Lavage with Ewald tube for recent (<1 hour) ingestion of plant with serious potential toxicity
  —Charcoal
- Oxalate crystal irritation from philodendron
  —Ice
  —Local wound care
  —Close follow-up
- Gastric decontamination, fluid therapy, and supportive care for
  —Solanine group
  —Lectins Group
- Jimson weed poisoning
  —Physostigmine in severe cases; consult toxicologist
- Cyanogenic group poisoning
  —Lilly cyanide antidote kit
  —In Europe, hydroxocobalamin and DMAP followed by sodium thiosulfate
- Grayanotoxin group poisoning
  —Atropine if significant bradycardia
- Colchicine group
  —Multidose activated charcoal
- Cardiac glycosides group
  —Digibind may be useful, initial dose 10 vials
  —Correct hypokalemia
  —Magnesium
- Nicotine group
  —Airway control (due to neuromuscular paralysis)
  —Atropine for symptomatic bradycardia

MEDICATIONS

- Atropine: 0.5 mg (peds: 0.02 mg/kg) IV repeat 0.5–1.0 mg IV (peds: 0.04 mg/kg)
- DMAP: 3.25 mg/kg IV
- Hydroxocobalamin: 50x cyanide dose or 50 mg/kg IV
- Magnesium: 2–4 g IV
- Physostigmine: 0.5–2 mg IV
- Sodium thiosulfate: 150–250 mg/kg

Disposition

ADMISSION CRITERIA

- Cardiac monitoring/dysrhythmias
- Intractable vomiting
- Refractory hypotension
- Evidence of end organ damage
- Altered mental status

DISCHARGE CRITERIA

- Baseline mental status
- Tolerating fluids
- Normal cardiac activity
- No delayed sequelae

PEDIATRIC CONSIDERATIONS

- Lower threshold to admit children
  —Tend to eat the more concentrated parts
  —Lower doses are lethal
  —Symptoms more nonspecific

Miscellaneous

ICD9: NEC 988.1

CORE CONTENT CODE: 5.7

SUGGESTED READINGS

Braithberg G, Kunkel DB, et al. Toxic plant ingestions. In: Auerbach P, et al., eds. Wilderness medicine: Management of wilderness and environmental emergencies. 3rd ed. St. Louis: CV Mosby, 1995: 862–890.

Koppel C. Clinical symptomatology and management of mushroom poisoning. Toxicon 1993;31(12):1513–1540.

Langford SD, Boor PJ. Oleander toxicity: An examination of human and animal toxic exposures. Toxicology 1996;109:1–13.

Author: Chris Ervin

Pleural Effusion

Clinical Presentation

SIGNS AND SYMPTOMS

- Dyspnea on exertion or at rest
- Decreased breath sounds
- Increased egophony
- Dullness to chest percussion
- Pleural rub
- Primary pathologic process (pneumonia, pulmonary embolus, pancreatitis) not the pleural effusion is often the source of symptoms

MECHANISM/DESCRIPTION

- Normal conditions
  —Pleural space contains about 30 ml of clear, protein-free fluid that helps facilitate movement of the pulmonary parenchyma within the thoracic space
  —Fluid formation and reabsorption is governed by the hydrostatic and colloid forces acting at the parietal and visceral surfaces
  —Normally, the sum of these forces results in movement of fluid into the pleural space from the parietal surface and reabsorption at the visceral surface
  —Lymphatics help remove any excess fluid
  —Alteration of any of the above factors will result in excess accumulation and pleural effusion
- Transudative effusion
  —Results from alteration of systemic hydrostatic and colloid factors
  —Pleural surface is not involved in the primary pathologic process
- Exudative effusion
  —Results from pathologic disease of the pleural surface or disruption of lymphatic reabsorption

ETIOLOGY

- Transudative effusions
  —Hydrostatic factors
    -Congestive heart failure (right or left ventricular)
    -Peritoneal dialysis
    -Cirrhosis
  —Colloid factors
    -Acute glomerulonephritis
    -Myxedema
    -Hypoproteinemia
    -Meigs' syndrome
    -Sarcoidosis
    -Trauma: hemothorax, chylothorax
    -Medication: nitrofurantoin, methysergide
- Exudative effusions
  —Infection
    -Pneumonia (viral, bacterial, tuberculosis)
    -Parasitic
    -Fungal
    -Neoplasm, metastasis, mesothelioma
  —Pulmonary embolization or infarction
  —Gastrointestinal disorders
  —Pancreatitis
  —Subdiaphragmatic abscess (hepatic)
  —Esophageal rupture

Pre-Hospital

CAUTIONS

- Place high-flow oxygen
- Apply cardiac monitor and pulse oximeter
- Initiate IV line access

Diagnosis

ESSENTIAL WORKUP

- CXR
  —Blunting of the costophrenic angle
  —Most sensitive radiographic sign
  —Requires at lease 250 ml of fluid
    -Lateral decubitus films may reveal a lateral layer of fluid
    -Presence of subpulmonic effusions may be indicated by loss of supradiaphragmatic vascular markings or an increased space between the gastric bubble and pulmonary parenchyma
    -Provide hints to the primary source (malignancy, pneumonia)

LABORATORY

- CBC
- Electrolytes, BUN/Cr, glucose
- Pulse oximetry/arterial blood gas
- Coagulation profile
- Pleural fluid analysis
  —Protein, LDH, and specific gravity
  —Differentiates between transudative and exudative effusions
  —Criteria for exudate
    -Pleural fluid protein/serum protein >0.5
    -Pleural fluid LDH/serum protein >0.6
- Culture and Gram's stain
- Red cell count
  —5000–100,000/mm^3 nonspecific
  —>100,000/mm^3 suggestive of malignancy, infarction
- White cell count
  —1000–10,000/ mm^3 nonspecific
  —>10,000/ mm^3 suggestive of parapneumonic effusion, pancreatitis, collagen vascular disease, malignancy, or tuberculosis
- Wright stain identifies presence of mesothelial cells, macrophages, plasma cells, lymphocytes, PMNs, eosinophils, and malignant cells
- Cytology identifies malignant cells
- Glucose
  —Levels <50% of serum glucose suggestive of rheumatoid/lupus induced effusion, bacterial
- Empyema, malignancy, or esophageal rupture
- Triglyceride/cholesterol
  —Triglycerides >110 mg/dl suggestive of chylous effusion from disruption of thoracic duct
- Amylase
  —Elevated levels suggestive of pancreatitis or esophageal rupture

IMAGING/SPECIAL TESTS

- Diagnostic/therapeutic thoracentesis
- Examination of pleural fluid to identify and treat underlying disease
- Method
  —Position patient upright with arms crossed in front in order to elevate scapula
  —Identify superior border of effusion via percussion, ultrasound, or egophony
  —Mark area one interspace below this at the posterior axillary space
  —Cleanse area with iodophor, dry, and drape for sterile field
  —Anesthetize with 2% lidocaine
  —Enter superior border of rib with needle bevel down using 14-gauge syringe/catheter gently aspirating while advancing
  —Advance catheter through needle once pleural space accessed
    -Minimum of 100 cc required for basic studies (protein, LDH, cell count, and culture)—more required for cytology and additional studies
  —After obtaining fluid, withdraw needle, apply pressure, dress, and obtain postprocedural CXR for pneumothorax

Treatment

INITIAL STABILIZATION

- ABCs
- High-flow oxygen for shortness of breath
- Emergency thoracentesis for significant respiratory compromise

ED TREATMENT

- Identify and treat underlying primary pathologic process (CHF, pneumonia, pancreatitis)
- Surgical consult if empyema found for surgical drainage

Disposition

ADMISSION CRITERIA

- Respiratory compromise
- Unknown cause of the effusion
- Primary process requires hospitalization
- Presence of a parapneumonic effusion or empyema
- ICU admission for severe hemodynamic and respiratory compromise

DISCHARGE CRITERIA

- Source of the pleural effusion is known
- No evidence of respiratory compromise exists
- Majority of effusions will resolve if the primary process is treated appropriately

Miscellaneous

ICD9: 511.9

CORE CONTENT CODE: 16.3.5

SUGGESTED READINGS

Grogan DR, Irwin RS, Corwin RW. Thoracentesis. In: Rippe JM. Intensive care medicine. 2nd ed. Boston: Little, Brown and Co., 1991.

McEwen JI. Pleural disease. In: Rosen P, Barken RM, et al. Emergency medicine: Concepts and clinical practice. 4th ed. St. Louis: CV Mosby, 1998:1511–528.

Vukich DJ. Diseases of the pleural space. Emerg Med Clin North Am 1989;7(2):309–24.

Author: Walter G. Belleza

Pneumocystis Carinii Pneumonia

Clinical Presentation

SIGNS AND SYMPTOMS

- Subacute presentation
- Dyspnea on exertion or at rest
  —Progressive over days (most common in non-HIV immunocompromised hosts)
  —Indolent, developing over weeks to months (more frequently in HIV-positive hosts)
- Cough with none or minimal amount of white sputum
- Fever
- Weight loss
- Chest pain
- Night sweats
- Chills
- Fatigue
- Hemoptysis
- Tachypnea
- Tachycardia

MECHANISM/DESCRIPTION

- Organism has a tropism for human lungs
- Unknown life cycle
- Unknown environmental reservoir
- Some studies have suggested person-to-person transmission

ETIOLOGY

- Controversy surrounds the classification of pneumocystis as a parasite or fungus
- Pneumocystis occurs in hosts with altered cellular immunity
  —HIV infection (most common)
  —Cancer
  —Chemotherapy
  —Corticosteroid treatment
  —Organ transplantation
  —Malnutrition

PEDIATRIC CONSIDERATIONS

- Pneumocystis carinii pneumonia (PCP) in children is more severe

Pre-Hospital

CAUTIONS

- Provide adequate oxygenation via 100% non-rebreather for symptomatic patients

Diagnosis

ESSENTIAL WORKUP

- Chest x-ray
  —Classically reveals diffuse interstitial or alveolar infiltrates, more prominent in the bases and midlung zone
  —Atypical presentations include
    -Lobar infiltrates
    -Cysts
    -Pneumothoraces
    -Pleural effusions
    -Nodular infiltrates
    -Mass lesions
    -Cavitations
    -Hilar adenopathy
    -Bronchiectasis
    -Normal chest x-rays
- Prophylaxis with aerosolized pentamidine is a risk factor for developing predominantly upper lobe infiltrates

LABORATORY

- Arterial blood gas
  —Obtain in all cases of PCP
  —Calculate the A-a gradient—usually increased
  —Adjunctive corticosteroid therapy for A-a gradient greater than 35 or PaO_2 less than 70
- Pulse oximetry
  —Useful to titrate the oxygen to a saturation level of 92–95%
- CBC
- Electrolytes, BUN/Cr, glucose
- LDH
  —Elevated in AIDS patients with PCP compared with non-PCP pneumonias
- Blood cultures

IMAGING/SPECIAL TESTS

- Diagnosis is established by demonstrating the presence of pneumocystis organisms in an appropriately stained respiratory specimen
- Stains include Gomori's, toluidine blue, modified Gram, and silver
  —All stains of comparable accuracy
  —Choice of stains is by laboratory preference
- The initial respiratory specimen obtained is an induced sputum
  —Sensitivity of 60–80% in HIV-infected patients is higher than in non-HIV-infected patients
- Bronchoalveolar lavage
  —Next step to perform if the induced sputum is negative, and the suspicion for PCP is still high
  —Sensitivity of 80–90%
- Transbronchial biopsy
  —Has demonstrated the organism in cases with a negative bronchoalveolar lavage

DIFFERENTIAL DIAGNOSIS

- Constellation of dyspnea, fever, diffuse radiographic infiltrates, and minimal or nonproductive cough suggests atypical causes of the pneumonia
  —Legionella
  —Mycoplasma
  —*Coxiella burnetii*
  —Chlamydia pneumoniae
  —Psittaci
  —Tuberculosis

Treatment

INITIAL STABILIZATION

- ABCs
- Provide adequate oxygenation with nasal cannula up to nonrebreather 100% oxygen
- Perform oral tracheal intubation in those with refractory hypoxemia (pO_2 <100 mm Hg on 100% nonrebreather) despite maximal oxygenation or hypercarbic respiratory failure
- 500 cc–1 L 0.9%NS IV bolus for hypotension, sepsis, or dehydration

ED TREATMENT

- Initiate antibiotics
  —Moderate-severe disease
    - Bactrim is the first-line agent
    -IV pentamidine for those who cannot tolerate bactrim
  —Mild to moderate disease (A-a gradient less than 35 or PaO_2 >70)
    -Oral therapy is an option
    -Bactrim preferred agent
    -Alternative regimens include trimethoprim-dapsone, clindamycin-primaquine, atovaquone
  —Continue antibiotics for 21 days
- Adjunctive corticosteroids
  —Initiate within the first 72 hours of treatment with an A-a gradient of greater than 35 or PaO_2 <70
- Isolate suspected PCP from others who are immunocompromised
  —Organism can be aerosolized

MEDICATIONS

- Atovaquone: 750 mg po tid
- Clindamycin-primaquine: clindamycin 300–450 mg orally q 6 hrs and primaquine 15–30 mg po q day (rule out G6PD deficiency before dosing)
- Pentamidine: 4 mg/kg/24hrs IV over 1 hour
- Prednisone: 40 mg po bid for 5 days, 40 mg po q day for 5 days, then 20 mg q day for 11 days (IV methylprednisolone at 80% of the prednisone dose may be substituted)
- Trimethoprim/dapsone: 15–20 mg/kg/24hrs of trimethoprim po q 6–8 hrs plus dapsone 100 mg po as q day (rule out G6PD deficiency before dosing)
- Trimethoprim/sulfamethoxazole: 15–20 mg/kg/24hrs of trimethoprim and 75–100 mg/kg/24hrs of sulfamethoxazole IV or po q 6–8 hrs

PEDIATRIC CONSIDERATIONS

- Treatment of choice is IV bactrim, followed by IV pentamidine
- Doses are the same as for adults
- Consult pediatrician for doses of corticosteroids

Disposition

ADMISSION CRITERIA

- Moderate to severe disease (PaO_2 <70, or Alveolar-arterial gradient >35)
- Inability to ingest medications
- Inability to return for careful follow-up (in 2–3 days)

DISCHARGE CRITERIA

- Mild disease
- Ability to tolerate medications
- Close follow-up arranged
- If results of induced sputum not available, add a macrolide to the empirical regimen

Miscellaneous

ICD9: 136.3

CORE CONTENT CODE: 13.10

SUGGESTED READINGS

Levine, SJ. Pneumocystis carinii. Clin Chest Med 1997;17:665–696.

Petersen C, Mills J. Parasitic infections. In: Murray JF, Nadel JA, eds. Textbook of respiratory medicine. 2d ed. Philadelphia: WB Saunders, 1994:1201–1244.

Santamauro JT, Stover DE. Pneumocystis carinii pneumonia. Med Clin North Am 1997;81:299–318.

Author: Richard Lenhardt

Pneumomediastinum

Clinical Presentation

SIGNS AND SYMPTOMS

- Chest pain
  - —Sharp
  - —Pleuritic
  - —Often positional
- Dyspnea
- Neck pain
  - —Occurs in association with dissection of air into the soft tissues of the neck
  - —Often described as "neck swelling," "neck pain," "throat pain," or "difficulty swallowing"
  - —Subcutaneous emphysema
- Hamman's crunch
  - —Presence of a crinkling or crepitant sound that varies with the heart beat

MECHANISM/DESCRIPTION

- Presence of air or gas within the mediastinum
- Secondary pneumomediastinum occurs
  - —Secondary to thoracic barotrauma
  - —As a complication of positive pressure ventilation
  - —In association with esophageal rupture
  - —In association with a mediastinal infection caused by gas-forming organisms
- Primary or spontaneous pneumomediastinum
  - —Occurs secondary to alveolar rupture
  - —Often in the setting of a Valsalva maneuver or in association with inhalational drug use
- Occasionally unclear triggering etiology

ETIOLOGY

- Relatively rare entity that may occur spontaneously or as a result of trauma or other pathologic processes

Pre-Hospital

CAUTION

- Initiate treatment with an IV, oxygen, cardiac monitoring, and pulse oximetry

Diagnosis

ESSENTIAL WORKUP

- CXR
  - —Most valuable initial test
  - —Important to include a lateral view because mediastinal air is often missed on the PA view
  - —Excludes pneumothorax
  - —Identification of a pleural effusion or parenchymal infiltrate should heighten the suspicion for an esophageal rupture

LABORATORY

- CBC if suspicious of mediastinitis

IMAGING/SPECIAL TESTS

- Esophagram with gastrografin
  - —Study of choice to exclude the diagnosis of esophageal rupture

DIFFERENTIAL DIAGNOSIS

- Pericarditis
- Pulmonary embolus
- Pneumonia
- Coronary ischemia
- Aortic dissection

Treatment

INITIAL STABILIZATION

- ABCs

ED TREATMENT

- Spontaneous pneumomediastinum
  - —Does not require specific treatment
  - —Efforts should focus on pain relief and reassurance once the diagnosis is confirmed
  - —Condition is self-limiting and can be expected to resolve over 2–5 days
- Secondary pneumomediastinum
  - —Direct therapy toward underlying cause

Disposition

ADMISSION CRITERIA

- Secondary pneumomediastinum
- Associated pneumothorax
- Possibility of esophageal rupture has not been excluded
- Abnormal vital signs

DISCHARGE CRITERIA

- Spontaneous pneumomediastinum with normal vital signs and no pneumothorax may be discharged
- Close outpatient follow up
- Caution against use of inhalational drugs or any activities associated with Valsalva-type or breath-holding maneuvers

Miscellaneous

ICD9: 518.1

CORE CONTENT CODE: 16.3.7

SUGGESTED READINGS

Brody S, Anderson G, Gutman J. Pneumomediastinum as a complication of "crack" smoking. Am J Emerg Med 1988;6: 241–43.

Panacek E, Singer A, Sherman B, et al. Spontaneous pneumomediastinum: clinical and natural history. Ann Emerg Med 1992;21:1222–27.

Sands D, Ledgerwood A, Lucas C. Pneumomediastinum on a surgical service. Am Surg 1988;54:434–37.

Author: R. Dart

Pneumonia, Adult

Clinical Presentation

SIGNS AND SYMPTOMS

- Cough
- Sputum production
- Shortness of breath
- Pleuritic chest pain
- Chills
- Sweats
- Fever
- Tachypnea
- Lung exam
  - —Dullness to percussion
  - —Egophony
  - —Rales
  - —Rhonchi
  - —However, pneumonia may be present in the setting of an unremarkable exam

MECHANISM/DESCRIPTION

- Inflammation of the lung parenchyma with consolidation of the infected area due to accumulation of exudate in alveolar air spaces
- An estimated 4 million cases of pneumonia occur annually in the United States
  - —Sixth leading cause of death
- Comorbid conditions impact the etiology and outcome
  - —Chronic obstructive pulmonary disease
  - —Diabetes mellitus
  - —Renal insufficiency
  - —Congestive heart failure
  - —Chronic lung disease
  - —Ethanol abuse
  - —Immunosuppression

ETIOLOGY

- Age ≤60 years
  - —*Streptococcus pneumoniae*
  - —*Mycoplasma pneumoniae*
  - —Respiratory viruses
  - —*Chlamydia pneumoniae*
  - —*Haemophilus influenzae*
- Age >60 years *or* comorbid conditions
  - —*Streptococcus pneumoniae*
  - —Respiratory viruses
  - —*Haemophilus influenzae*
  - —Aerobic Gram-negative bacilli
    - -Enterobacter
    - -Klebsiella
    - -Pseudomonas species
    - -Staphylococcus aureus
- Severely ill despite age or comorbid conditions in addition to the aforementioned organisms
  - —*Moraxella catarrhalis*
  - —*Mycobacterium tuberculosis*
  - —Endemic fungi
  - —Legionella species
  - —Polymicrobial infections to include anaerobic bacteria

Pre-Hospital

- Supplemental oxygen
- Consider endotracheal intubation in patients with severe respiratory distress
- Intravenous access

Diagnosis

ESSENTIAL WORKUP

- Patients should first be classified
  - —Age greater than or less than 60 years old
  - —The presence of one or more comorbid conditions listed above
  - —Immunocompetent versus possibly immunosuppressed
    - -Asplenic
    - -Oncology/chemotherapy patient
    - -Chronic corticosteroid use
    - -Human immunodeficiency virus (HIV) infection
  - —Community-acquired versus possibly a nosocomial pathogen
    - -Patients discharged from an inpatient facility within 10–14 days

LABORATORY

- Pulse oximetry to evaluate for hypoxemia
- White blood cell counts, arterial blood gases
  - —Unlikely to change the management of younger patients without comorbid illnesses who do not appear toxic
- Gram stain of sputum
  - —Not reliable method to identify organisms
  - —This should not be used to narrow the spectrum of empirical antibiotic coverage
- Blood cultures and sputum gram stain and culture
  - —For patients deemed sufficiently ill that hospitalization is required

IMAGING/SPECIAL TESTS

- Chest radiography
  - —Most useful study in the elderly, patients with comorbid conditions, and those that appear toxic
  - —Not needed in young, otherwise healthy persons when antibiotic treatment for bronchitis is planned
    - -However, reasonable screening test because antibiotic treatment for bronchitis is not beneficial
- Diagnostic thoracentesis
  - —When parapneumonic effusions are detected to determine the etiologic organism
  - —If chest tube drainage is indicated

DIFFERENTIAL DIAGNOSIS

- Pulmonary edema
- Pulmonary embolus
- Occupational or environmental exposures
- Tumor
- Immunologic disease
  - —Sarcoidosis
  - —Goodpasture's syndrome
- Bronchitis

Treatment

INITIAL STABILIZATION

- Supplemental oxygen
  —Guided by the pulse oximeter
- Endotracheal intubation if worsening respiratory distress

ED TREATMENT

- Empirical approach to initial antimicrobial therapy
  —Clinical features of pneumonia (symptoms, signs, and radiographic findings) have insufficient sensitivity and specificity to predict an etiologic organism
  —A pathogen is not identified in up to 50% of patients
- Age ≤60 years without comorbid illness
  —Macrolide or tetracycline
- Age >60 years or with comorbid condition(s)
  —Second generation cephalosporin
    -Cefuroxime
    -Cefoxitin
  —Other options include trimethoprim-sulfamethoxazole or β-lactam plus β-lactamase inhibitor with erythromycin or other macrolide
- Duration of treatment
  —Usually 7–10 days
- Severely ill, toxic appearing patients
  —Third-generation cephalosporin with antipseudomonal activity
    -Cefotaxime
    -Ceftazidime
  —Other agent with antipseudomonal activity as well as a macrolide as empirical therapy on admission

MEDICATIONS

- Azithromycin: 500 mg po then 250 mg po qid × 4 days
- Cefotaxime: 2 g q 8 hrs IV
- Cefoxitin: 2 g q 8 hrs IV
- Ceftazidime: 2 g q 8 hrs IV
- Cefuroxime: 0.75–1.5 g q 8 hrs IV
- Clindamycin: 0.15–0.45 g q 6 hrs po; 150–900 mg q 8 hrs IV
- Doxycycline 100 mg po bid
- Erythromycin: 500 mg qid po; 1 g q 6 hrs IV
- Imipenem: 0.5 g q 6 hrs IV

Disposition

ADMISSION CRITERIA

- Immunosuppression
- Nosocomial pathogen
- Risk factors for a complicated course of pneumonia
  —Age >60 years
  —1 comorbid condition
  —Severe alteration in vital signs
    -Respiratory rate >30 per minute
    -Systolic blood pressure <90 mm Hg
    -Temperature >101°F
    -1 lobe involvement
  —Pleural effusion
  —Leukopenia or leukocytosis
  —Hypoxia
- Patients who appear ill even without one of the above risk factors
- Patients who return to the emergency department after a trial of outpatient therapy

DISCHARGE CRITERIA

- Patients <60 years
- No comorbid risk factors
- Nontoxic appearing
- Most young patients without comorbid conditions should have improvement in their symptoms and signs within several days of initiating antimicrobial therapy
- The majority return to their usual activities by the end of their course of antibiotics
- Persistent or worsening symptoms or signs should prompt a more aggressive evaluation
- Primary care or telephone follow up after 72 hours of outpatient therapy is advised

Miscellaneous

ICD9: 480; 481; 482

CORE CONTENT CODE: 13.9.6

SUGGESTED READINGS

American Thoracic Society. Guidelines for the initial management of adults with community-acquired pneumonia: Diagnosis, assessment of severity, and initial antimicrobial therapy. Am Rev Respir Dis 1993;148:1418–426.

Bartlett JG. Community-acquired pneumonia. N Engl J Med 1995;333(24):1618–624.

Author: Michael F. Minogue

Pneumonia, Pediatric

Clinical Presentation

SIGNS AND SYMPTOMS

- Tachypnea
- Tachycardia
- Retractions
- Fever
- Cough
- Rales
- Vocal fremitus
- Bronchiolar breath sounds
- Decreased breath sounds
- Dullness to percussion
- Severe pneumonia
  - —Dyspnea
  - —Grunting
  - —Nasal flaring
  - —Cyanosis
  - —Poor perfusion
  - —Decreased muscle tone
  - —Lethargy
  - —Hypoxic agitation
- Infants under 6 months
  - —Nonspecific symptoms
  - —Poor feeding
  - —Vomiting
  - —Decreased activity
  - —Irritability
  - —Apnea
  - —Infants under 3 months may be afebrile or even hypothermic depending on the agent and severity of illness
  - —Difficult to appreciate fremitus, change in breath sounds
- Children over 5 years old
  - —Pleuritic chest pain
  - —Rigors
  - —Productive cough with bacterial pneumonia
- Bacterial pneumonia
  - —More severe and rapid onset of signs and symptoms
  - —Toxic appearance
- Viral pneumonia
  - —Slower onset than with bacterial
  - —Lower fever than with bacterial
  - —Wheezing

MECHANISM/DESCRIPTION

Neonates

- Organisms causing pneumonia typically reflect those aspirated on passage through the birth canal or from infected amniotic fluid
  - —Most commonly
    - -Group B streptococci
    - -*E. coli*
    - -*Klebsiella pneumoniae*
    - -*Chlamydia trachomatis*
  - —Less commonly
    - -*Listeria monocytogenes*
    - -Cytomegalovirus
    - -Herpes simplex
- Postnatal-acquired organisms include
  - —Gram-negative enteric
  - —Staphylococcal species from nurseries
  - —Respiratory viruses from community and family contacts

Infants 1–3 Months

- Organisms causing pneumonia in this age group include those infecting neonates (see above) and older infants (see below)
- *Bordetella pertussis* is another possible agent

Older Infants–5 Years

- Viruses predominate
  - —Especially respiratory syncytial virus (RSV)
  - —Parainfluenza
  - —Influenza
  - —Adenovirus
- Bacterial infection is less prominent
  - —*Streptococcal pneumoniae* is the most frequent cause
  - —*Haemophilus influenzae type B* (*HiB*) in unimmunized children
  - —Group A Streptococci
  - —*Staphylococcal aureus* in ill children

6–18 Years

- *Mycoplasma pneumoniae* most frequent
- *Streptococcal pneumoniae* second most common
- Viruses much less frequent

Recent Immigrants from Developing Countries

- *M. tuberculosis*

Immunocompromised Children

- *Pneumocystis carinii*
- *M. tuberculosis*

Pre-Hospital

- Administer high-flow oxygen for respiratory difficulties
- IV 0.9%NS 20 cc/kg bolus for volume depleted, hypotensive children

Diagnosis

ESSENTIAL WORKUP

- Chest radiograph
  - —Gold Standard for diagnosis
  - —Much overlap between viral and bacterial findings
  - —Viral and mycoplasma pneumonias tend to show interstitial infiltrates, often perihilar and peribronchial
  - —Bacterial pneumonias may show focal lobar consolidation, focal alveolar infiltrates, and possibly effusion
  - —Lateral decubitus films may aid in demonstrating effusion

LABORATORY

- CBC with differential
  - —May help distinguish bacterial (higher WBC with left shift) from viral pneumonia (variable WBC with lymphocytosis)
- Blood culture
  - —If suspicious of bacterial etiology
  - —Low yield (2–30%)
  - —Immensely helpful if positive
- Sputum for Gram stain and culture may be obtained in older children
- ABG is helpful in determining degree of respiratory insufficiency or failure

IMAGING/SPECIAL TESTS

- Mycoplasma IgM or cold agglutinin titers
  - —Useful if suspecting this organism
  - —More likely positive with severe illness
- Nasopharyngeal washes for direct fluorescent antibody and culture
  - —Identify RSV, chlamydia trachomatis, and bordetella pertussis infections
- Pleural fluid (if present) for culture, Gram stain, protein, glucose, and cell counts

DIFFERENTIAL DIAGNOSIS

- Asthma
- Bronchiolitis (age <2 years)
- Foreign body aspiration
- Aspiration of gastric contents
- Congestive heart failure
- Cystic fibrosis
- Neoplasm
- Sequestered lobe
- Hydrocarbon aspiration

Treatment

INITIAL STABILIZATION

- If moderate or severely ill
  - —Secure airway
  - —High-flow oxygen
  - —Intubate for clinical respiratory failure
  - —IV hydration with 0.9%NS 20 cc/kg bolus if in shock or dehydration
- Monitor
- Apply pulse oximetry
- Check bedside glucose in severely ill-appearing infants and toddlers
  - —Administer glucose D_{25} at 2 cc/kg IV for toddlers or D_{10} at 5 cc/kg IV for neonates if hypoglycemic

ED TREATMENT

- Perform thoracentesis if pleural effusion compromising respiratory function and for diagnostic tests

Antibiotics

- Initiate IV antibiotic therapy for moderate to severely ill children who require admission
- IV antibiotic options by age
  - —Neonatal (weight >2 kg)
    - -Ampicillin and cefotaxime or gentamicin
    - -Erythromycin ethylsuccinate for suspected chlamydia trachomatis or bordetella pertussis pneumonia
  - —Infants 1–3 months of age
    - -Ampicillin and cefotaxime
    - -Erythromycin for suspected chlamydia trachomatis or bordetella pertussis
  - —Children 3 months and older
    - -Cefotaxime or cefuroxime or ceftriaxone
    - -Vancomycin for suspected or confirmed penicillin resistant *Streptococcal pneumoniae*
    - -Erythromycin or clarithromycin for suspected *Mycoplasma pneumoniae*
- Outpatient empiric antibiotic therapy by age
  - —Infants <3 months old
    - -Outpatient treatment generally not recommended
  - —Children 3 months–5 years acceptable regimens
    - -Amoxicillin
    - -Amoxicillin-clavulanate
    - -Trimethoprim-sulfamethoxazole
    - -Erythromycin-sulfisoxazole
    - -Clarithromycin
  - —Children 5–18 years acceptable regimens
    - -Erythromycin
    - -Clarithromycin

MEDICATIONS

- Amoxicillin: 30–50 mg/kg/24hrs divided q 8 hrs po
- Amoxicillin-clavulanate: 25–40 mg/kg/24hrs divided q 8 hrs po
- Ampicillin: 100–150 mg/kg/24hrs divided q 6–8 hrs IV
- Cefotaxime: 150 mg/kg/24hrs divided q 8 hrs IV, max 2 g q 8 hrs
- Ceftriaxone: 75 mg/kg/24hrs divided q 12–24hrs IV, max 2 g q 12 hrs
- Cefuroxime: 150 mg/kg/24hrs divided q 8 hrs IV, max 2 g q 8 hrs
- Clarithromycin: 15 mg/kg/24hrs divided q 12 hrs po, max 500 g q 12 hrs
- Erythromycin: 40 mg/kg/24hrs divided q 6 hrs po or IV max 2 g/day
- Erythromycin ethylsuccinate: 30 mg/kg/24hrs divided q 8 hrs po
- Erythromycin-sulfisoxazole: 40 mg/kg/24hrs as erythromycin divided q 8 hrs po
- Gentamicin: 5–7.5 mg/kg/24hrs divided q 8–12hrs IV
- Trimethoprim-sulfamethoxazole: 6–10 mg/kg/24hrs as TMP divided q 12 hrs po
- Vancomycin: 40 mg/kg/24hrs divided q 6 hrs IV, max 500 mg q 6 hrs

Disposition

ADMISSION CRITERIA

- Infants <3 months old
- Moderate or severe distress
- Toxic appearance
- Hypoxia
- Apnea
- Pleural effusion
- Dehydration/vomiting
- Poor response to outpatient oral therapy
- Immunocompromised children
- Noncompliant parents

DISCHARGE CRITERIA

- Most cases are mild and can be discharged home if no evidence of hypoxia, significant work-of-breathing, dehydration, or vomiting
- Assured follow-up within 1–2 days

Miscellaneous

ICD9: 482.9, 480.9, 483.1

CORE CONTENT CODE: 13.10

SUGGESTED READINGS

Campbell PW, Hazinski TA. Acute pneumonia. In: Hoekelman RA, ed. Primary pediatric care. 3rd ed. St. Louis: CV Mosby, 1997:521–523.

Jadavji T, Law B, Lebel MH, et al. A practical guide for the diagnosis and treatment of pediatric pneumonia. Can Med Assoc J 1997:156 (Suppl):S703–S711.

Letourneau MA, Schuh S, Gausche M. Pneumonia. In: Barkin RM, ed. Pediatric emergency medicine: Concepts and clinical practice, 2d ed. St. Louis: CV Mosby, 1997:1102–1108.

Author: Guy Upshaw

Pneumothorax

Clinical Presentation

SIGNS AND SYMPTOMS

- Chest pain on the ipsilateral side of the pneumothorax (PTX)
  —Sharp, pleuritic pain and dyspnea with sudden onset
  —Dull chest ache in delayed presentations
- Shortness of breath, tachypnea
- Severity of symptoms are generally proportional to size of PTX
- Heart rate <140 generally seen in simple spontaneous PTX
- Hypotension, diaphoresis, cyanosis, cardiovascular collapse, and tracheal deviation are indications of more severe PTX, i.e., tension PTX
- Rarely cough, asymptomatic, or generalized malaise

MECHANISM/DESCRIPTION

- Presence of free air in the intrapleural space
- Spontaneous PTX are due to atraumatic rupture of alveolus, bronchiole, or bleb
- Tension PTX
  —Air continues to enter pleural space through bronchoalveolar disruption and becomes trapped via "ball-valve mechanism"
  —Intrapleural pressure increases
  —Venous return to right heart decreases resulting in decrease in cardiac output
  —Mediastinum shifts towards uninvolved side mechanically interfering with right atrial filling
  —Ventilation compromised and v/q mismatch resulting in hypoxemia

ETIOLOGY

- Trauma: blunt (i.e., rib fracture) or penetrating
- Iatrogenic—most commonly during central line placement
- Primary spontaneous PTX (two-thirds of incidences)
  —No underlying pulmonary pathology present
  —Rupture of small subpleural cyst or bleb
  —Primarily young healthy 20–40-years old, tall and thin body habitus
- Secondary spontaneous PTX from underlying pulmonary pathology
  —Airway disease: COPD, asthma, cystic fibrosis
  —Infections: bacteria, tuberculosis, fungal
    -AIDS: associated with *Pneumocystis carinii*
  —Neoplasm
  —Interstitial lung disease

Pre-Hospital

CAUTIONS

- Suspected tension PTX requires immediate needle thoracostomy by a qualified provider

Diagnosis

ESSENTIAL WORKUP

- Tension PTX is a clinical diagnosis based on the above signs and symptoms; initiate intervention for suspected tension PTX immediately, do not wait for CXR confirmation
- Upright chest radiograph (CXR) is the definitive diagnostic test for other than tension PTX
- Patients unable to tolerate upright CXR can be taken in decubitance position with the suspected side up
- Expiratory CXR will improve detection
- A rough estimate of PTX size is sufficient to make clinical decisions

IMAGING/SPECIAL TESTS

- Electrocardiograms (ECG)
  —Often necessary to rule out cardiac etiologies of chest pain
  —Nonspecific changes include T-wave inversion, left axis deviation and decreased R-wave amplitude
- Chest CT is very sensitive for small PTX but little practical advantage over CXR

DIFFERENTIAL DIAGNOSIS

- Exacerbation of COPD, asthma, or pulmonary embolus
- Myocardial infarction, pericarditis
- Pneumomediastinum, dissection of aortic aneurysm
- Chest wall pain, pleuritis
- Acute abdominal processes

Treatment

INITIAL STABILIZATION

- ABCs of trauma care if appropriate
- Patients with chest pain or dyspnea of unconfirmed etiology need to be placed on continuous cardiac monitor and pulse oximetry, provided oxygen by nasal cannula or face mask and have an IV placed.
- Suspected *tension PTX require immediate needle thoracostomy* by placing a 14–18-gauge angiocatheter in the second intercostal space at midclavicular line or 4th or 5th intercostal space at anterior axillary line
- Tube thoracostomy is the definitive treatment for tension PTX
- Patients should receive 100% O_2 via nonrebreather face mask while workup occurs

ED TREATMENT

- Tube thoracostomy for all suspected tension PTX
- Chest procedures should be performed with adequate analgesia or conscious sedation
- PTX estimated at <15% collapse and no cardiovascular or respiratory compromise
  —Observe with 100% oxygen support for 4–6 hours
  —Repeat CXR and discharge if unchanged
  —Sequential approach to management of >15% collapse
  —15–30% collapse or increase in size during observation, go to step 1
  —>30% collapse, go to step 4
  —(−)PTX means <10% remaining collapse
  —Step 1: simple aspiration
    -Placement of aspiration catheter (typically 8 Fr) with three-way stopcock
    -Aspirate air until resistance or 3 L air aspirated
    -Repeat CXR, (−)PTX = continue; otherwise repeat aspiration once then go to step 2
    -Observe in department for 4 hours
    -Repeat CXR, (−)PTX = remove catheter and continue; otherwise go to step 2
    -Observe in department for 2 hours
    -Repeat CXR, (−)PTX = stop; otherwise go to step 2
  —Step 2—Heimlich valve
    -Attach Heimlich valve to aspiration catheter or use Tru-Close kit
    -Observe in department for 1 hour
    -Repeat CXR, (−)PTX = stop; otherwise go to step 3
  —Step 3—suction
    -Attach aspiration catheter/ Tru-Close to suction at 20 cm H_2O
    -Observe in department for 1 hour
    -Repeat CXR, (−)PTX = stop; otherwise go to step 4
  —Step 4—Chest tube insertion with suction
  —Reexpansion edema is a rare complication requiring supportive care
  —Tru-Close thoracic vent is a commercially available kit for these procedures with a 13 Fr catheter, insertion is as follows
    -Sterile preparation of the chest region over the second intercostal space at the midclavicular line on the side of the PTX
    -Infiltrate region with local anesthetic
    -Prepare the instrument by inserting the trocar into the catheter with tip extending slightly beyond end of catheter
    -With scalpel, make an incision through the skin over sight of insertion
    -Introduce trocar/catheter into the pleural space immediately superior to rib border
    -Remove trocar immediately once the pleural space is entered to avoid laceration of lung tissue and feed remaining catheter until it is completely within the chest wall
    -Attach device to chest wall with adhesive pads and suture
    -Follow the above sequential approach starting at step 1, simple aspiration
    -Leave in place with built in Heimlich valve if simple aspiration successful

Disposition

ADMISSION CRITERIA

- Tension PTX, or chest tube and suction required

DISCHARGE CRITERIA

- <15% collapse, no expansion while in the ED or successful aspiration with catheter removed
  —Discharge with follow-up in 24 hours and 1 week for CXR to assure reexpansion
- Reliable patients with the thoracic vent and successful aspiration or secured catheter and Heimlich valve
  —Discharge with 24- and 48-hour follow-up
  —At 48-hour follow-up
    -Clamp catheter, observe for 2 hours, and repeat CXR
    -Remove Thoracic Vent or catheter if no re-expansion
    -Observe for 2 hours and repeat CXR
    -If no reexpansion, discharge with 24-hour and 1-week follow-up
- Discharge instruction include prompt return for new onset of chest pain or dyspnea
- Patients without reexpansion at 1 week require a cardiothoracic surgery consult

Miscellaneous

ICD9: 512.8

CORE CONTENT CODE: 18.4.10.12, 16.3.7

SUGGESTED READINGS

Jantz MA, Pierson DJ. PTX and barotrauma. Clin Chest Med 1994;15(1):75–91.

McEwen JI. Pleural disease. In: Rosen P, et al., eds. Emergency medicine: Concepts and clinical practice. 4th ed. St. Louis: CV Mosby, 1997:1511–1521.

Paape K, Fry, WA. Spontaneous PTX. Chest Surg Clin N Am 1994;4(3):517–538.

Vallee P, Sullivan H, et al. Sequential treatment of a simple PTX. Ann Emerg Med 1988;17(9):119–125.

Author: Allen Marino

Clinical Presentation

SIGNS AND SYMPTOMS

- Neurologic
  - —Lethargy
  - —Agitation
  - —Coma
  - —Hallucinations
  - —Seizures
- Respiratory
  - —Inadequate ventilation
  - —Inability to protect airway
- Cardiovascular
  - —Tachydysrhythmias
  - —Torsades de Pointes
  - —Hypo/hypertension
- Vital signs
  - —Wide variety depending on toxic substance
  - —Hyper/hypothermia
  - —Bradycardia/tachycardia
  - —Hypertension/hypotension
- Selected toxidromes (see chapter: Poisoning, Toxidromes)
  - —Anticholinergic
    - -Altered mental status (confusion, delirium, lethargy)
    - -Dry skin and mucous membranes
    - -Fixed dilated pupils
    - -Tachycardia
    - -Hyperthermia/flushing
    - -Urinary retention
  - —Cholinergic
    - -Salivation
    - -Constricted pupils
    - -Sweating
    - -Wheezing
  - —Narcotic
    - -CNS and respiratory depression
    - -Pinpoint pupils
  - —Sympathomimetic
    - -CNS excitation
    - -Seizures
    - -Tachycardia
    - -Hypertension

MECHANISM/DESCRIPTION

- Pharmacologic mechanism specific to agent

ETIOLOGY

- Intentional
  - —Depression
  - —Suicide
  - —Recreational drug abuse
- Accidental
  - —Common cause in children

PEDIATRIC CONSIDERATIONS

- Accidental ingestions—typically young children (ages 1–5)
- Consider child abuse, especially if >5 years old

Pre-Hospital

CAUTIONS

- Search for clues from scene
  - —Pills
  - —Drug paraphernalia
  - —Witnesses
- Transport all drugs and pill bottles for identification
- Restrain uncooperative patients
- Consider comorbid conditions
  - —Trauma
  - —Medical illness
  - —Environmental exposure
- Ipecac *contraindicated* in ambulance setting

CONTROVERSIES

- Decreased time to activated charcoal (AC) administration when given in the pre-hospital setting
- Decreased drug absorption in a simulated ingestion while volunteers were lying in the left lateral versus the right lateral decubitus position
- Home use of ipecac for
  - —Ingestion of substance known *not* to cause neurological or cardiovascular deterioration
  - —Patient >1 hour to healthcare facility
  - —Consider administration after consultation with the regional poison center

Diagnosis

ESSENTIAL WORKUP

- Electrolytes, BUN/Cr, glucose
  - —Calculate anion gap
  - —Anion gap acidosis associated with pneumonic *ACAT MUDPILES*
    - -*A*lcoholic ketoacidosis
    - -*C*yanide, CO, H_2S, others
    - -*A*SA, other salicylates
    - -*T*oluene
    - -*M*ethanol, metformin
    - -*U*remia
    - -*D*iabetic ketoacidosis
    - -*P*araldehyde, phenformin
    - -*I*ron, INH
    - -*L*actic acidosis from other causes
    - -*E*thylene glycol
    - -*S*tarvation ketosis

LABORATORY

- Serum osmolality
  - —Obtain if elevated anion gap acidosis from unknown etiology
  - —Determine osmol gap
    - -Osmol gap = measured osmolality − calculated osmolarity
    - -Calculated osmolarity = 2(Na^+) + glucose/18 + BUN/2.8 + ethanol (in mg/dl)/4.6
    - ->10 increased
  - —Osmal gap
    - -Screens for toxic alcohols
    - -Most sensitive early in poisoning
    - -Normal osmol gap does *not* rule out toxic alcohol ingestion
  - —Substances that increase osmol gap—pneumonic: *ME DIE A*
    - -*M*ethanol
    - -*E*thanol
    - -*D*iuretics (mannitol, glycerin, sorbitol)
    - -*I*sopropyl alcohol
    - -*E*thylene glycol
    - -*A*cetone, ammonia
- Pregnancy test
- Acetaminophen level for all suicide ingestions
- Toxicology screen

IMAGING/SPECIAL TESTS

- ECG for tachycardia/widened QRS
- CT of head for altered mental status not clearly due to toxin

DIFFERENTIAL DIAGNOSIS

- Causes of altered mental status
  - —Intracranial mass, infection, bleeding
  - —Sepsis
  - —Hypoglycemia
  - —Hypothermia
  - —Hypoxia
  - —Uremia
  - —Endocrine/electrolyte abnormalities

Treatment

INITIAL STABILIZATION

- ABCs
  - —Endotracheal intubation as needed for airway protection, oxygenation/ventilation, and orogastric lavage
  - —Oxygen for hypoxia
  - —Cardiac monitor
  - —Pulse oximetry
  - —0.9%NS IV access
- For hypotension
  - —Administer 500 cc–1 L (peds: 20 cc/kg) 0.9%NS fluid bolus
  - —Initiate vasopressors for hypotension unresponsive to fluid bolus
- For bradycardia
  - —Atropine
  - —Cardiac pacing
  - —Glucagon
- If altered mental status, administer coma cocktail: thiamine, D50W (or Accucheck), naloxone

ED TREATMENT

Decontamination

- See chapter: Poisoning, Gastric Decontamination
- Ipecac
  - —Delays administration of activated charcoal
  - —Offers no advantage over activated charcoal alone when both treatments potentially effective
  - —Orogastric lavage
  - —Effectiveness dependent on the time interval since ingestion, timing of the last meal, and toxin ingested
  - —Protected airway essential prior to any attempts at orogastric lavage
  - —Indications
    - -Present within 1 hour of taking a potentially lethal ingestion with no known antidote
    - -Poisoned intubated patients
- Activated charcoal
  - —Administer in every toxic ingestion (for exceptions see below)
  - —Optimal for toxic ingestions presenting within 1 hour of ingestion
  - —Contraindications
    - -Caustic ingestions
    - -Unprotected airway
    - -Bowel obstruction or ileus
  - —Drugs not effectively bound to charcoal
    - -Metals (borates, bromide, iron, lithium)
    - -Alcohols
    - -Potassium
    - -Potassium cyanide (poorly absorbed)
- Multiple-dose activated charcoal
  - —Use in toxic ingestions that are well absorbed by charcoal and undergo enterohepatic circulation
  - —Never use cathartics in conjunction with multiple-dose activated charcoal
  - —Indications
    - -Theophylline
    - -Salicylates
- Cathartics
  - —Used in combination with activated charcoal to prevent constipation and to enhance gastrointestinal transit time
- Whole-bowel irrigation
  - —Cleansing of the bowel with polyethylene glycol (colyte, golytely)
  - —Indications
    - -Toxins not well absorbed by charcoal; toxic iron and lithium ingestions
    - -Toxins in sealed containers (body packers) without signs of gastrointestinal perforation
    - -Toxic sustained-release product ingestions

Antidotes

- See chapter: Poisoning, Antidotes
- Acetaminophen: n-acetylcysteine
- Arsenic: BAL (British anti-Lewisite)
- Atropine: physostigmine
- Benzodiazepines: flumazenil
- Beta blockers: glucagon
- Calcium channel blockers: calcium chloride
- Carbon monoxide: oxygen, hyperbaric oxygen
- Coumadin: vitamin K
- Cyanide: cyanide antidote kit
- Digoxin: digibind
- Ethylene glycol: ethanol/hemodialysis/4-methylpyrazole
- Iron: deferoxamine
- Lead: calcium disodium edetate *or* dimercaptosuccinic acid
- Mercury: BAL (British anti-Lewisite)
- Methanol: ethanol/hemodialysis/4-methylpyrazole
- Nitrites: methylene blue
- Opiates: naloxone
- Organophosphates: atropine, pralidoxime
- Tricyclic antidepressants: $NaHCO_3$

Consultation

- Poison control center
- Psychiatry
- Social services (especially pediatric patients)

MEDICATIONS

- Activated charcoal slurry: 1–2 g/kg up to 90 g po
- Sorbitol: 1–2 g/kg to a max of 150 g (peds: >1 year old: 1–1.5 g/kg as a 35% solution to a max of 50 g) po mixed in the activated charcoal slurry
- Dextrose: D50W 1 amp (50 ml or 25 g) (peds: D25W 2–4 ml/kg) IV
- Naloxone (narcan): 2 mg (peds: 0.1 mg/kg) IV or IM initial dose
- Thiamine (vitamin B_1): 100 mg (peds: 50 mg) IV or IM
- See chapters: Poisoning, Antidotes; Poisoning, Gastric Decontamination; and specific chapters for other medications

Disposition

ADMISSION CRITERIA

- Altered mental status
- Cardiopulmonary instability
- Suicidal
- Laboratory abnormalities
- Potential for decompensation from delayed acting substance

DISCHARGE CRITERIA

- Psychiatrically clear
- Detoxified

Miscellaneous

ICD9: N/A

CORE CONTENT CODE: 17.1

SUGGESTED READINGS

Flomenbaum NE, Goldfrante LR, Weisman RS, et al. General management of the poisoned or overdosed patient. In: Goldfrank LR, et al. Goldfrank's toxicologic emergencies. 5th ed. 25–41. Prentice Hall Press Year: 1994.

Hoffman RS, Goldfrank LR. The poisoned patient with altered consciousness. JAMA 1995;274:562–569.

Author: Martin Horak

Poisoning, Antidotes

ANTIDOTE	INDICATIONS	WARNINGS	DOSE
n-Acetyl cysteine (NAC)	Acetaminophen overdose	Unpleasant odor, nausea, vomiting; most effective within 12 hrs	po: 140 mg/kg then 70 mg/kg q 4 hrs × 17; IV: 140 mg/kg then 70 mg/kg q 4 hrs × 12
Antibody, digoxin (Digibind)	Digoxin, digitoxin toxicity	False-elevated digoxin levels after use; development of CHF or rapid Afib in patients requiring digoxin	1 vial (40 mg) binds 0.6 mg digoxin; Dose estimate: acute overdose 10–20 vials; chronic overdose 4–6 vials, Dose calculaion: # vials = digoxin level (ng/ml) × wt (kg)/100
Antitoxin, botulin trivalent A, B, E	Clinical botulism (prior to onset of paralysis)	Only binds free toxins; not for infant botulism; horse serum precautions—immediate hypersensitivity; serum sickness in 10–14 days	1–2 vials IV q 4 hrs for 4–5 doses
Antivenin, black widow spider	Severe hypertension, muscle spasms, age <5 or >60 years old	Horse serum-derived—immediate hypersensitivity; serum sickness in 10–14 days	1 vial = 6000 IU; reconstitute with supplied diluent; further dilute to 50 ml with NaCl; administer IV over 30 min; before administering skin test for horse serum sensitivity
Antivenin, coral snake (*Micrurus fulvius*)	Eastern or Texas coral snake	Horse serum-derived—immediate hypersensitivity; serum sickness in 10–14 days	4–10 vials, each vial reconstituted with 10 ml diluent; then dilute to 100–200 ml with NaCl; administer IV over 15–30 min
Antivenin, rattle snake (*Crotalidae*)	Eastern, western diamondback; Mojave rattlesnake	Horse serum-derived—immediate hypersensitivity; serum sickness in 10–14 days	mild: 5 vials; moderate: 10 vials; Severe: 15 vials
Atropine	Bradycardia due to drugs, organophosphate insecticides	Carbamates, myasthenia gravis, narrow angle glaucoma, hypertension, coronary ischemia, urinary obstruction	0.5–1.0 mg (peds: 0.02 mg/kg min) 0.1 mg IV; large repeated doses in organophosphates
Benztropine (Cogentin)	Acute dystonic reactions	See atropine	1–2 mg (peds: 0.02 mg/kg) IV for acute reaction or po to prevent reaction
Benzodiazepine	Agitation, stimulant drugs, seizures; for sedation	Respiratory/CNS depression	Midazolam: 1 mg IV q 2–3 min PRN (peds: age 1–5: 0.05–0.1 mg/kg; age 6–12: 0.10–0.2 mg/kg) Diazepam: 2–5 mg IV/IM, repeat in 10–15 min (peds: 0.2–0.5 mg/kg)
β-Blocker	SVT, hypertension	Bradycardia, bronchospasm, increased BP in cocaine excess	Esmolol: 500 μg/kg IV load then 50 μg/kg/min titrate up Metoprolol: 5 mg IV, repeat q 5–10 min Propranolol: 0.5–1.0 mg IV, repeat q 10 min
Bicarbonate, sodium	Cyclic antidepressant poisoning, metabolic acidosis, urinary alkalinization	May cause CHF; excessive alkalosis hypokalemia	0.5–1.0 mEq/kg IVP; 100–150 mEq in 1 L D5W, titrated
Calcium	Hyperkalemia with cardiac toxicity; hydrofloric acid, calcium channel blocker; citrate, oxalate, phosphate poisoning	Avoid in digoxin toxicity, hypercalcemia; CaCl corrosive to skin, SC tissue; incompatible with certain IV solutions	Ca gluconate SC or IA for topical HF acid burns; $CaCO_3$ 2–3 g po for oral fluoride or oxalate toxicity
Cyanide antidote kit	Cyanide poisoning	Hypotension, methemoglobinemia	Amyl nitrite 1–2 amp crushed, inhaled; then sodium nitrite 300 mg in 10 ml IV over 5 min (peds: 0.3 ml/kg of 3% solution); then Sodium thiosulfate 12.5 g IV (peds: 50 mg/kg), may repeat in 1 hr
Dantrolene	Malignant hyperthermia, drug-induced rhabdomyolysis, muscle rigidity	Muscle weakness, respiratory depression	1–2 mg/kg IV bolus, repeat q 5–10 min PRN to max 10 mg/kg

ANTIDOTE	INDICATIONS	WARNINGS	DOSE
Deferoxamine (Desferal)	Iron toxicity	Hypotension if >15 mg/kg/hr, flushing, urticaria	10–15 mg/kg/hr IV until serum Fe <350 or 6 g total
Dimercaprol (BAL)	Arsenic, gold, mercury lead-induced encephalopathy	Renal toxicity, fever, nausea, vomiting, urticaria, cholinergic symptoms	3 mg/kg deep IM q 4 hrs × 2 days; then q 12 hrs × 7 days; follow metal levels. In Pb level >100 μg/dl: 4–5 mg/kg IM q 4 hrs until Pb <50 μg/dl
Diphenhydramine (Benadryl)	Antihistamine, acute dystonic reactions	Sedation, excitation in children, anticholinergic symptoms	25–50 mg (peds: 0.5–1.0 mg/kg) IV, IM or po q 4–6 hrs
DMSA (chemet)	Lead poisoning (only peds approved)	Caution in renal impairment—urinary eliminated; nausea, vomiting, diarrhea,	10 mg/kg po q 8 hrs × 5 days, then q 12 hrs × 14 days; then reassess blood levels
EDTA (edetate disodium), calcium	Lead, chromium, nickel, manganese, zinc toxicity	Nausea, vomiting, chills, nephrotoxicity, hypercalcemia	20–30 mg/kg over 24 hrs based on Pb level as 6 divided doses q 4 hrs or as continuous IV (concentration = 2 mg/ml); follow Pb level
Epinephrine	Angioedema, anaphylaxis, acute asthma, spinal shock, β-blocker overdose	Dysrhythmias, hypertension, tremor, anxiety	Mild to moderate: 0.3–0.5 mg SC (peds: 0.01 mg/kg); adult severe: 0.05–0.1 μg/kg IV q 5 min or 1–4 μg/min; adult endotracheal: 1 mg in 10 cc NS; adult hypotension: 1 μg/min titrate up q 3–5 min
Ethanol	Methanol or ethylene glycol toxicity	Disulfiram reaction, CNS sedation	IV: 750 mg/kg load as 5% or 10% solution in D5W; po: 1.5 ml/kg of 100-proof dose to level of 100 mg/dl
Flumazenil (Romazicon)	Benzodiazepine overdose	Contraindicated in TCA overdose; lower seizure threshold; induce withdrawal	Adult: 0.2 mg IV slow, repeat q 2–3 min to 1 mg max; (peds: 0.01–0.05 mg/kg over 30 min–1 hr)
Fomepizole 4-MP (Antizol)	Ethylene glycol or methanol toxicity (no FDA approval for methanol)	Nausea, dizziness, headache	15 mg/kg load then 10 mg/kg q 12 hrs × 4, then 15 mg/kg q 12 hrs
Glucagon	Hypoglycemia with no IV access; β-blocker overdose with hypotension or bradycardia	Nausea, vomiting, hyperglycemia; hypotension from diluent	Hypoglycemia: 1.0 mg IM or SC; β-blocker: 50 μg/kg IV repeat in 3–5 min PRN
Methylene blue	Methemoglobinemia with dyspnea or level >25%	G-6-PD deficiency	1–2 mg/kg slow IV as 1% solution, repeat in 1 hr
Narcotic antagonists (naloxone, nalmefene) 0.5–2.0 mg	Opiate poisoning, empiric treatment of coma	Acute opiate withdrawal, severe agitation	Naloxone: 0.4–2.0 mg IV or IM, repeat to 8 mg; nalmefene: IV, IM, or SC
Oxygen, hyperbaric	CO poisoning	TM perforation, seizures due to oxygen toxicity	At 2–3 ATM 100% oxygen
Penicillamine	Arsenic, copper, lead mercury with or following BAL or EDTA	Contraindicated in penicillin allergy, renal insufficiency	Lead: 25–50 mg/kg/day po on empty stomach divided in 4 doses; arsenic: 100 mg/kg/day po divided in 4 doses (peds max: 1 g)
Phentolamine	Hypertensive crisis; stimulants, sympathomimetic, MAO-tyramine reaction, extravasated pressers	Hypotension, tachycardia, dysrhythmias	HTN: 1–5 mg IV (peds: 0.02–0.1 mg/kg) bolus, repeat q 5–10 min; extravasation: 2× above dose diluted in 10–15 ml saline SC
Physostigmine	Severe anticholinergic syndrome	Contraindicated in TCA overdose, cholinergic crisis with succinylcholine seizures	0.5–1.0 mg (ped: 0.02 mg/kg) IV repeat in 10 min PRN
Pralidoxime (2-PAM)	Organophosphate toxicity: reversal of nicotinic effects; reactivates enzyme; atropine for muscarinic symptoms	Myasthenic crisis if myasthenia gravis; nausea, headache dizziness, laryngospasm, muscle rigidity	1–2 g (peds: 25–50 mg/kg) in 100 ml NaCl over 15 min,repeat in 1 hr PRN; repeat in 6–12 hrs if nicotinic symptoms return

Poisoning, Antidotes

ANTIDOTE	*INDICATIONS*	*WARNINGS*	*DOSE*
Protamine	Heparin anticoagulation reversal	Avoid benzyl alcohol diluent in neonates	1–1.5 mg for each 100 IU heparin, 1/2 dose if 30–60 min and 1/4 dose if 2 hrs after heparin bolus or for heparin infusion
Pyridoxine (Vitamin B_6)	Isoniazid-induced seizures; gyromitra mushroom	Nontoxic	INH: 5 g IV over 30–60 min or dose = INH overdose dose; gyromitra: 25 mg/kg IV over 30 min–1 hr
Vitamin K (Aqua mephyton)	coumarin anticoagulation reversal	Hypersensitivity from IV	2–10 mg slow IV or IM q 8 hrs based on PT times

Author: Ed Michelson

Clinical Presentation

N/A

Pre-Hospital

CAUTIONS

- Ipecac *contraindicated* in ambulance setting

CONTROVERSIES

- Decreased time to activated charcoal (AC) administration when given in the pre-hospital setting
- Decreased drug absorption in a simulated ingestion while volunteers were lying in the left lateral versus the right lateral decubitus position
- Home use of ipecac if all of the following criteria is met:
  —Ingestion of substance known *not* to cause neurological or cardiovascular deterioration
  —Patient >1 hour to healthcare facility
  —Consider administration after consultation with the regional poison center

Diagnosis

N/A

Treatment

INITIAL STABILIZATION

- ABCs
  —Secure airway for decreased mental status/inability to protect airway
  —IV access/cardiac monitor
- Naloxone, thiamine, dextrose (or Accucheck) with altered mental status from overdose

ED TREATMENT

Ipecac

- Derived from the roots of the plant *Cephaelis acuminata*
- Exerts emetic action by direct gastric irritation and centrally mediated chemoreceptive trigger zone stimulation
- Delays administration of activated charcoal
- Offers no advantage over activated charcoal alone when both treatments potentially effective

Dosage

- >12 years old: 30 ml
- Ages 1 through 12 years old: 15 ml
- Ages 6 months through 1 year: 5–10 ml plus 15 ml clear fluid

Indications

- No utility in ED

Adverse effects

- Vomiting may complicate and worsen the clinical presentation
- Delay to administration of activated charcoal or oral antidotes

Contraindications

- Caustics (acids & alkali)
- Hydrocarbons
- Agents that rapidly depress mental status
- Patients actively vomiting

Orogastric Lavage

- Placement of a large-bore tube (32–36 French) in the stomach for removal of ingested toxins
- Effectiveness of orogastric lavage dependent on the time interval since ingestion, timing of the last meal, and toxin ingested
- Protected airway essential prior to any attempts at orogastric lavage

Indications

- Present within 1 hour of taking a potentially lethal ingestion with no known antidote
- Poisoned intubated patients

Adverse Effects

- Inadvertent intubation of the respiratory tree
- Esophageal or gastric perforation
- Charcoal aspiration
- Patient discomfort

Contraindications

- Large pills (limited by lavage tube port size)

- Caustics (acids and alkali)
- Hydrocarbons
- Agents that rapidly depress mental status
- Unprotected airway

Pediatric Considerations

- Avoid in children
- Unlikely to result in any clinically significant pill extraction secondary to the smaller bore orogastric tube (i.e., 18 French)
- Risk of aspiration increased in children

Controversies

- Several randomized controlled trials have documented *no benefit* when lavage plus activated charcoal is compared to activated charcoal alone

Activated Charcoal

- Prepared by treating heated wood pulp, which creates a large surface area to bind toxins
- Mainstay of gastric decontamination
- Effective when contents have reached the small intestines

Dose

- 1–2 g/kg of body weight or an activated charcoal-to-drug ratio of 10:1; often mixed with sorbitol (see below)
- Oral or nasogastric tube administration

Indications

- Administer in every toxic ingestion (for exceptions see below)
- Optimal for toxic ingestions presenting within one hour of ingestion

Adverse Effects

- Vomiting and constipation
- Charcoal aspiration and subsequent charcoal pneumonitis

Contraindications

- Caustic ingestions
- Unprotected airway
- Bowel obstruction or ileus

Drugs not Effectively Bound to Charcoal

- Metals (borates, bromide, iron, lithium)
- Alcohols
- Potassium
- Potassium cyanide (poorly absorbed)

Pediatric Considerations

- Mix with a palatable substance (cola or juice) to facilitate intake or administer via gastric tube

Controversies

- Randomized controlled trials have shown a slightly worse outcome and higher complication rate when *asymptomatic* patients received charcoal versus nothing

Multiple-Dose Activated Charcoal

- Used in toxic ingestions that are well absorbed by charcoal and undergo enterohepatic circulation

Dose

- 1 g/kg followed by 0.5 g/kg every 2–6 hours
- *Never* use cathartics in conjunction with multiple-dose activated charcoal

Indications

- Theophylline
- Salicylates

Cathartics

- Used in combination with activated charcoal to prevent constipation and to enhance gastrointestinal transit time
- Limited data available to demonstrate any decreased absorption when a cathartic (sorbitol) is added to activated charcoal

Dose

- Magnesium citrate 10% solution: 250 ml (peds: 4 ml/kg)
- Magnesium sulfate: 15–20 g (peds: 250 mg/kg)
- Sorbitol: 0.5–1 g/kg to a max of 100 g of 70% solution (peds: >1-year-old: 0.5–1 g/kg as a 35% solution to a max of 50 g) po mixed in the activated charcoal slurry—only use in 1st dose

Adverse Effects

- Dehydration
- Hypermagnesemia
- Diarrhea
- Abdominal discomfort

Contraindications

- Preexisting dehydration
- Children
- Renal disease (cathartics containing magnesium)

Whole-Bowel Irrigation

- Cleansing of the bowel

Indications

- Toxins not well absorbed by charcoal—toxic iron and lithium ingestions
- Toxins in sealed containers (body packers) without signs of gastrointestinal perforation
- Toxic sustained-release product ingestions

Dose

- Polyethylene glycol (colyte, Go-Lytely)
- Solution at 2 L/hr in adults (0.5 L/hr in children) until rectal excretions clear
- Administer via a nasogastric tube with activated charcoal as indicated via a continuous or bolus method

Adverse Effects

- Bloating
- Rectal irritation
- Frequent bowel movements

Contraindications

- Mechanical or pharmacological ileus
- Bowel obstruction
- Intestinal perforation
- Unprotected airway

Disposition

N/A

Miscellaneous

ICD9: 977.9

CORE CONTENT CODE: 17.3.2

SUGGESTED READINGS

American College of Emergency Physicians. Clinical policy for the initial approach to patients with acute toxic ingestions or dermal or inhalation exposure. Ann Emerg Med 1995;25:570–585.

Ellenhorn MJ, Schoonwald S, Ordog G, Wasserberger J. Gut decontamination. In: Ellenhorn MJ, ed. Ellenhorn's medical toxicology. 2d ed. Baltimore: Williams & Wilkins, 1997:66–78.

Perrone J, Hoffman RS, Goldfrank LR. Special considerations in gastric decontamination. Emerg Med Clin 1994;12:285–299.

Pond SM, Lewis-Driver DJ, Williams GM, et al. Gastric emptying in acute overdose: A prospective randomized controlled trial. Med J Aust 1995;163:345–349.

Author: Frank LoVecchio

Poisoning, Toxidromes

Clinical Presentation

SIGNS AND SYMPTOMS

TOXICOLOGIC PNEUMONICS

Anion Gap Acidosis: ACAT MUD PILES

- AKA
- CO/cyanide
- ASA
- Toluene
- Methanol
- Uremia
- DKA
- Paraldehyde
- Iron/INH
- Lactic acidosis
- Ethylene glycol
- Starvation

Increased Osmolar Gap: ME DIE

- Methanol
- Ethylene glycol
- Diuretics (mannitol)
- Isopropyl alcohol
- Ethanol

Seizures: OTIS CAMPBELL

- Organophosphates
- Tricyclic antidepressants
- INH/insulin
- Sympathomimetics, salicylates
- Camphor/cocaine
- Amphetamines, anticholinergic agents
- Methylxanthines, mushrooms (monomethyl hydrazine group)
- PCP, pethidine (demerol), propoxyphene, plants (nicotine, water hemlock)
- β-Blockers
- Ethanol withdrawal
- Lithium, local anesthetics
- Lead, lindane

Mydriasis: AAAS

- Antihistamines
- Antidepressants
- Anticholinergics/atropine
- Sympathomimetics

Miosis: COPS

- Cholinergic/clonidine
- Opiates/organophosphates
- Phenothiazines/pilocarpine/pontine bleed
- Sedative hypnotics

Hypertension: CT SCAN

- Cocaine
- Theophylline
- Sympathomimetics
- Caffeine
- Anticholinergics/amphetamines
- Nicotine

Bradycardia: PACED

- Propranolol (β-blockers)
- Anticholinesterase drugs
- Clonidine/calcium channel blockers
- Ethanol/alcohols
- Digoxin/darvon (opiates)

Tachycardia: FAST

- Free base (cocaine)
- Anticholinergic/antihistamines/amphetamines
- Sympathomimetics
- Theophylline

MECHANISM OF TOXICITY

- Anticholinergic
  —Adrenergic imbalance results from inhibition of acetylcholine
- Cholinergic
  —Excess parasympathetic stimulation and *cholinergic crisis* result from inhibition of acetylcholinesterase or increased activity at the acetylcholine receptor
- Narcotic
  —Differ in their agonist and antagonist properties at various opioid receptor sites
  —μ-Receptor stimulation-full agonist
  —κ and Δ receptors share partial agonist and antagonist properties
- Sympathomimetic
  —Stimulation of sympathetic effector organs (particularly the CNS)
- Withdrawal
  —Hyperactivity of sympathetic nervous system predominates

Pre-Hospital

CONTROVERSIES

- Ipecac
  —Generally not indicated in the home or ambulance
  —Ipecac administration may be justified if
    -Arrival to the ED will be delayed $>$1 hour
    -Recent ingestion
    -No contraindications

CAUTIONS

- Ipecac contraindicated
  —Strong alkali or acid ingestion
  —Patients not able to protect their airway
  —In infants $<$6 months of age

Diagnosis

ESSENTIAL WORKUP

- Acquire essential historical features
  —Specific agent
  —Quantity consumed
  —Time of poisoning
- Focus PE on
  —Vital signs
  —Cardiopulmonary and neurologic function
  —Abdominal and dermatologic findings
  —Physical findings specific for toxidromes
- Base diagnosis on history and physical findings with laboratory studies serving to guide definitive care and confirm the diagnosis

LABORATORY

- Depends on agent and presentation
- ABG/pulse oximetry
- CBC
- Electrolytes, BUN/Cr, glucose
- Ketones
- Serum osmolality
- Liver function
- Urinalysis

IMAGING/SPECIAL TESTS

- EKG
- Levels
  —Acetaminophen: obtain routinely because toxicity can occur without signs or symptoms
  —Salicylate
  —Methanol/ethylene glycol
  —Iron
  —Lithium
  —Theophylline
  —Digoxin
  —Carbon monoxide
- Abdominal radiograph for common radiopaque ingestions
  —Chloral hydrate
  —Cocaine/opiate packets
  —Calcium, heavy metals (arsenic and lead), iron, iodides
  —Phenothiazines, potassium, enteric-coated and slow-release preparations

Common Toxidromes

SYNDROME	CLASSIC SIGNS AND SYMPTOMS	CAUSATIVE AGENTS
Anticholinergic	Unreactive mydriasis Hypertension Absent bowel sounds Tachycardia Flushed skin Urinary retention Hyperthermia Dry skin/mucus membranes Toxic delirium Auditory/visual hallucinations Seizures Coma Cardiogenic pulmonary edema	Antihistamines, antiparkinsonian drugs, antipsychotics, antispasmodics, cyclic antidepressants, belladonna alkaloids *Ophthalmic products:* cyclopentolate hydrochloride (cyclogel), tropicamide (Mydriacyl) *Skeletal muscle relaxants:* orphenadrine citrate (norflex), cyclobenzaprine hydrochloride (flexeril) *Plants:* deadly nightshade, mandrake, and jimson weed *Mushrooms: Amanita muscaria, Amanitapantherina.*
Cholinergic	*Muscarinic effects:* Hypotension Bradycardia Miosis Abdominal cramps Vomiting Diarrhea Sweating Salivation Urinary incontinence Wheezing Respiratory failure or arrest *Nicotinic effects:* Hypertension Tachycardia Muscle fasciculations and cramps *CNS effects:* Anxiety Respiratory/circulatory depression Absent reflexes Seizure Coma	Organophosphate insecticides Carbamate insecticides *Medications:* acetylcholine, bethanechol, carbachol, methacholine, muscarine, pilocarpine *Plant: Areca catechu* *Mushroom: Clitocybe, Pilocarpus* species
Narcotic	CNS depression Miosis Depressed respirations Hypotension Response to naloxone CNS excitation and mydriasis (with meperidine and lomotil) Seizures and arrhythmias (with meperidine and propoxyphene metabolites)	Opiate-related medications/products
Sympathomimetic	CNS excitation Tachycardia Hyperthermia Hypertension Mydriasis Seizures Hypotension (with end stage toxicity)	Aminophylline, amphetamines, caffeine, cocaine, dopamine, ephedrine, epinephrine, levarterenol, LSD, methylphenidate (ritalin), pemoline, phencyclidine, phenmetrazine, phentermine, phenylpropanolamine
Withdrawal	Hypertension Tachycardia Mydriasis Piloerection Insomnia Lacrimation Muscle cramps Diarrhea	Alcohol, barbiturates, benzodiazepines, chloral hydrate, glutethimide, meprobamate, methaqualone, opioids, paraldehyde

Common Toxidromes

SYNDROME	CLASSIC SIGNS AND SYMPTOMS	CAUSATIVE AGENTS
Withdrawal (continued)		
	Restlessness Yawning Hallucinosis Seizure	

Treatment

INITIAL STABILIZATION

- ABCs
- Naloxone, thiamine, D50W (or Accucheck) for altered mental status

ED TREATMENT

- Treat hypotension initially with fluid bolus and, if unresponsive, with vasopressors
- Treat cardiac dysrhythmias with standard agents or agents chosen based on the pharmacology of the ingested agent
- Initiate IV bicarbonate if hypotension refractory to fluid boluses and dysrhythmias refractory to standard agents especially with poisioning due to
  —Cyclic antidepressants
  —Anticholinergic agents
  —Type Ia antidysrhythmic agents
  —Sotalol
  —Cocaine
- Decontaminate skin with dermal exposure
- Gastric lavage most effective when performed within the first hour of ingestion
- Administer activated charcoal
- Treatment with specific antidotes without delay (see Poisioning, Antidote chapter)
- Consult with a regional poison control center

MEDICATIONS

- Dextrose: D50W 1 amp (50 ml or 25 g) (peds: D25W 2–4 ml/kg) IV
- Naloxone: 2–4 mg (peds: 0.1 mg/kg) IV or IM
- Thiamine: 100 mg (peds: 50 mg) IV or IM

Disposition

ADMISSION CRITERIA

- Development of symptoms related to ingested toxin
- Overdose of oral hypoglycemic agents, lomotil, and long-acting or sustained-release preparations

DISCHARGE CRITERIA

- Asymptomatic and normal laboratory values after 6 hours of observation
- Intentional overdose must be evaluated psychiatrically prior to discharge

Miscellaneous

ICD9: N/A

CORE CONTENT CODE: 17.0

SUGGESTED READINGS

Ellenhorn MJ, Schoonwald S, Ordog G, Wasserberger J. The clinical approach. In: Ellenhorn MJ, ed. Ellenhorn's medical toxicology. 2d ed. Baltimore: Williams & Wilkins, 1997:3–46.

Erickson TB. Dealing with the unknown overdose. Emerg Med 1996;6:74, 79–88.

Goldfrank LR, et al., eds. Vital signs and toxic syndromes. Chap. 9. In: Goldfrank's toxicologic emergencies. 5th ed. Norwalk, CT: Appleton & Lange, 1994:143.

Graves HB, et al. Clinical policy for the initial approach to patients with acute toxic ingestion or dermal or inhalation exposure. Ann Emerg Med 1995;25(4):570.

Smilkstein MJ. A rational approach to the unknown ingestion. Emerg Med 1993;25(2):73.

Authors: Donald Duke; Leslie R. Wolf

Polio

Clinical Presentation

SIGNS AND SYMPTOMS

- Fever (37–39°C)
- Malaise
- Anorexia/nausea/vomiting
- Upper respiratory tract symptoms
- Headache, photophobia
- Nuchal rigidity

Neurologic changes

- Muscle soreness that becomes severe muscle spasm, progressing rapidly to spotty flaccid weakness and paralysis
- Asymmetric paralysis more prominent in the lower than the upper extremities
- Urinary retention (50% of paralytic cases)
- Reflexes
  —Initially hyperactive then absent
- Apprehensive and irritable, occasionally drowsy
- No sensory loss associated with the motor deficit

MECHANISM/DESCRIPTION

- Incubation period 9–12 days
- Duration <1 week
- Clinical manifestations are defined as
  —Subclinical (i.e., not apparent) 90–95%
  —*Abortive poliomyelitis* 4–8%
    -Clinically indistinct from many other viral infections (fever, myalgias, malaise)
    -Only suspected to be polio during an epidemic
  —*Nonparalytic poliomyelitis* 1–2%
    -Differs from abortive poliomyelitis by the presence of meningeal irritation
    -Course similar to any aseptic meningitis
  —Paralytic poliomyelitis 0.1%, which is further subdivided
    -*Spinal paralytic poliomyelitis* (frank polio)
    -*Bulbar paralytic poliomyelitis* (10% of paralytic polio): paralysis of muscle groups innervated by cranial nerves; involves the circulatory and respiratory centers of the medulla with high mortality
    -*Mixed bulbospinal poliomyelitis*
- *Postpoliomyelitis syndrome*
  —New onset of muscle weakness, pain and atrophy
  —Occurs many years after the active illness, usually in the previously affected limb
  —Gradual progression

ETIOLOGY

- Polioviruses
  —Picornoviruses
  —Small, nonenveloped, RNA viruses of the enterovirus genera
- Fecal-oral route transmission
- Humans are the only natural host and reservoir
- Poliovirus selectively destroys motor and autonomic neurons
- Natural (wild) virus is completely eliminated in North and Latin America
- Oral poliovirus vaccine (OPV)
  —Accounts for only poliomyelitis seen in the U.S. (8–10 cases per year of vaccine-associated paralysis (VAP))
  —Incidence of VAP: 1 in 700,000
  —Confers immunity to unvaccinated contacts by fecal-oral spread
  —Inexpensive
- Inactivated polio virus (IPV)
  —Costly
  —Painful
  —No conferred immunity
  —No VAP

PEDIATRIC CONSIDERATIONS

- More likely to have a biphasic acute course
  —Viral-type syndrome for 1–2 days
  —Symptom-free period of 2–5 days
  —Then an abrupt onset of the major illness

Pre-Hospital

CAUTIONS

- Rare fatal case comes from respiratory insufficiency, which requires prompt ventilatory support

Diagnosis

ESSENTIAL WORKUP

- Clinical diagnosis
- Differentiate from other causes of acute paralysis
- Notify public health officials when diagnosis suspected

LABORATORY

- CBC
  —WBC normal or mildly elevated
- CSF analysis
  —Abnormalities typical of aseptic meningitis (increased lymphocytes and elevated protein)
  —Poliovirus rarely isolated from the CSF
- Diagnosis confirmed by
  —Comparing acute to convalescent sera for antigen titers
  —Isolation of virus from blood or CSF

DIFFERENTIAL DIAGNOSIS

- Abortive poliomyelitis is similar to many viral illnesses
- Nonparalytic poliomyelitis is indistinguishable from any viral, aseptic meningitis
- Paralytic poliomyelitis
  —Guillain-Barré (not febrile, symmetrical, not ill appearing)
  —Acute transverse myelitis
  —Diphtheria
  —Botulism
  —Tick paralysis
  —Encephalitis

Treatment

INITIAL STABILIZATION

- Aggressive pulmonary toilet and early intubation mandated for respiratory insufficiency

ED TREATMENT

- Supportive and symptomatic management
- Analgesics for severe muscle pain and spasm
- Bed rest to prevent augmentation or extension of paralysis
- Paralytic poliomyelitis tends to localize to a limb that has been the site of intramuscular injection or injury within 2–4 weeks prior to the onset of infection
  - —Avoid any unnecessary tissue damage in suspected cases

Prevention

- Live, attenuated, or killed polio vaccine
- No antiviral agents available

Disposition

ADMISSION CRITERIA

- All acute phase paralytic poliomyelitis for strict bed rest and observation for respiratory symptoms
  - —Isolate from nonvaccinated personnel

DISCHARGE CRITERIA

- No evidence of nervous system involvement and no danger of contact with nonvaccinated population
  - —Deterioration of muscle strength usually ends after 3–5 days

Miscellaneous

ICD9: 045.1

CORE CONTENT CODE: 9.5.5

SUGGESTED READINGS

Modlin JF, Poliovirus. In: Mandell GL, Bennett JE, Dolin R, eds. Mandell, Douglas, and Bennett's principles and practice of infectious diseases. 4th ed. New York: Churchill Livingstone, 1995:1613–1620.

Mulder DW. Clinical observations on acute poliomyelitis. Ann N Y Acad Sci 1995;753:1–10.

Pascuzzi RM. Poliomyelitis and the postpolio syndrome. Semin Neurol 1992;12(3):193–199.

Patriarca PA, Foege WH, Swartz TA. Progress in polio eradication. Lancet 1993;342(8885):1461–1464.

Plotkin SA. Inactivated polio vaccine for the United States: A missed vaccination opportunity. Pediatr Infectious Dis 1995;14(10):835–839.

Racaniello VR, Ren R. Poliovirus biology and pathogenesis. Curr Top Microbiol Immunol 1996;206:305–325.

Author: Philip Shayne

Polycythemia

Clinical Presentation

SIGNS AND SYMPTOMS

General

- Dyspnea
- Weakness
- Sweating
- Weight loss
- Epistaxis
- Pruritus
- Gout
- Erythromelalgia
  - Burning pain in the feet or hands associated with warmth and erythema of the affected areas

Neurologic

- Headache
- Vertigo/dizziness
- Paresthesias
- Scotoma, blurred vision
- Tinnitus
- CVA/TIA

Cardiovascular

- Congestive heart failure/angina
- Hypertension
- Digital artery occlusion
- DVT

Abdominal

- Epigastric discomfort
- Peptic ulcer disease/GI bleed
- Hepatomegaly/splenomegaly

MECHANISM/DESCRIPTION

- Excessive erythropoiesis leading to proliferation of erythroid, myeloid, and megakaryocyte elements in the bone marrow
- Hematocrit >52% = exponential rise in blood viscosity

Classification of polycythemia

- Relative and stress polycythemia
  - Resulting from decrease in plasma volume
- Primary polycythemia vera
  - Three stages
    - Proliferative stage: increase in RBCs, megakaryocytes, platelets
    - Stable phase: return of blood counts to normal values due to replacement of marrow by fibrosis
    - Spent phase: extensive marrow fibrosis—peripheral cytopenia
  - Occurs age >60
  - Increase incidence of leukemia later
- Secondary polycythemia
  - Appropriately increased erythropoietin caused by tissue hypoxia
  - Inappropriate autonomous erythropoietin production

Bleeding and Thrombosis

- Increased blood viscosity due to elevated hematocrit
- Platelet abnormalities in 80%
- Decreased factor XII, prekallikrein, and kallikrein inhibitors

Pre-Hospital

N/A

Diagnosis

ESSENTIAL WORKUP

- CBC
  - Elevated RBC mass
  - Low MCV due to decreased iron stores
  - Thrombocytosis with large, hypogranular platelets

LABORATORY

- Bleeding time prolonged in 11% of patients

Diagnostic Criteria

- Category A
  - A1: increased RBC mass
    - Male: >36 ml/kg
    - Female: >32 ml/kg
  - A2: oxygen saturation >92%
  - A3: splenomegaly
- Category B
  - B1: platelets >400,000/mm^3
  - B2: WBC >12,000/mm^3
  - B3: B_{12} >900 pg/ml; unbound vitamin B_{12} binding capacity >2200 pg/ml
- Diagnosis established by either of these combinations
  - Presence of all 3 category A criteria
  - A1 + A2 + any two category B criteria

IMAGING/SPECIAL TESTS

- CT scan if CVA or AMS

DIFFERENTIAL DIAGNOSIS

- Secondary polycythemia
  - Right-to-left shunt congenital heart disease
  - Pulmonary disease
  - Carboxyhemoglobinemia
  - High altitude
  - Decreased tissue oxygen release from high oxygen-affinity hemoglobinopathies
- Inappropriate autonomous erythropoietin production
  - Renal origin: carcinoma, hydronephrosis cyst
  - Other lesions: uterine fibroids, hepatoma of adrenal origin, cerebellar hemangioma
  - Congenital overproduction

Treatment

INITIAL STABILIZATION

- ABCs

ED TREATMENT

- IV rehydration for relative polycythemia (dehydration)
- Pruritis
  - —H_1 blockers: cyproheptadine 4 mg po tid
  - —H_2 blockers: cimetidine 300 mg po tid
- Hyperuricemia: allopurinol 100–400 mg po QD

Primary Polycythemia Vera

- Antithrombotic therapy
  - —Low-dose aspirin
- Phlebotomy
  - —For Hct >60%
  - —To bring hematocrit to 45%
  - —500 cc blood withdrawn followed by infusion of 500 cc 0.9%NS
  - —May need to remove 1–1.5 L over 24 hours
- Myelosuppressive therapy
  - —^{32}P (radioactive phosphorus)
  - —Hydroxyurea
  - —Interferon
- Thrombocytosis
  - —Plateletpheresis for platelet count >1,000,000 mm^3 or with thrombosis or hemorrhage
- Splenectomy
  - —If severe thrombocytopenia
  - —Contraindicated if DIC due to uncontrolled hemorrhage
- Surgery with polycythemia
  - —Increased morbidity and mortality
  - —Elective procedures until polycythemia is under control;
  - —For emergency surgery need
    - -Emergent phlebotomy to lower hematocrit to <45%
    - -Control thrombocytosis with therapeutic plateletpheresis

Cautions

- No studies have shown that lowering the Hct improves survival or reduces rate of thrombotic complications
- Difficult to decrease Hct while maintaining adequate oxygenation (right-to-left shunt or COPD)
- If reduced plasma volume, phlebotomy may worsen hypovolemia and produce shock

Disposition

ADMISSION CRITERIA

- New diagnosis of polycythemia
- Unstable vital signs/underlying medical problems
- Inability to comply with outpatient treatment or follow-up

DISCHARGE CRITERIA

- Previous diagnosis of polycythemia and requiring outpatient phlebotomy
- Stable vital signs

Miscellaneous

ICD9: 238.4

CORE CONTENT CODE: 7.5.2

SUGGESTED READINGS

Berk PD, Goldberg JD, Fruchtman SM, Berlin NI, Wasserman LR. Therapeutic recommendations in polycythemia vera based on polycythemia vera study group protocols. Semin Hematol 1986;23(2):132–143.

Bilgrami S, Greenberg BR. Polycythemia rubra vera. Semin Oncol 1995:22(4):307–326.

Braunwald E, Isselbacher K, et al., eds. Harrison's principles of internal medicine. 13th ed. New York: McGraw Hill, 1994.

Hoffman R, Benz E, Shattil S, et al., eds. Hematology: Basic principles and practice. New York: Churchill Livingstone, 1991.

Landaw S, Williams W. Deciphering polycythemia. Hosp Pract 1996;3:155–166.

Rosen P, Barkin R, eds. Emergency medicine: Concepts and clinical practice. 4th ed. St. Louis: CV Mosby, 1998.

Author: Marc Gelman

Postpartum Hemorrhage

Clinical Presentation

SIGNS AND SYMPTOMS

- Ongoing blood loss, usually painless
- Significant hypovolemia: tachycardia, tachypnea, narrow pulse pressure, decreased urine output, cool clammy skin, poor capillary refill, altered mental status
- Due to relative hypervolemia, maternal tachycardia and hypotension may not manifest until blood loss exceeds 1500 ml
- Bleeding at other sites—consider coagulopathy

MECHANISM/DESCRIPTION

- *Immediate postpartum hemorrhage(PPH):* hemorrhage occurring within 24 hours of delivery
- *Delayed PPH:* hemorrhage occurring over 24 hours after delivery, often 1–2 weeks postpartum

ETIOLOGY

- *Immediate PPH:* uterine atony, lower genital lacerations, retained placental tissue, placenta accreta, uterine rupture, uterine inversion, puerperal hematoma, coagulopathies
- *Delayed PPH:* retained products of conception, postpartum endometritis, withdrawal of exogenous estrogen, puerperal hematoma
- Coagulopathies: preexisting ITP, TTP, von Willebrand's disease, DIC

Pre-Hospital

CAUTIONS

- Patients with postpartum hemorrhage may be hemodynamically unstable and require intravenous access and fluid resuscitation

Diagnosis

ESSENTIAL WORKUP

- Abdomen and pelvic examination to access for uterine atony, retained products, or other anatomic abnormality
- Type and crossmatch for packed red blood cells (PRBCs)
- Rapid hemoglobin determination

LABORATORY

- CBC
- PT, PTT, platelets, fibrinogen
- Type and crossmatch

IMAGING/SPECIAL TESTS

- Ultrasound may be helpful to evaluate for retained products in delayed PPH

DIFFERENTIAL DIAGNOSIS

- Consider puerperal hematomas if perineal, rectal, or lower abdominal pain in conjunction with tachycardia and hypotension

Treatment

INITIAL STABILIZATION

- Attempts to control bleeding and stabilize hemodynamic status proceed simultaneously
- ABC
  —Supplemental oxygen
  —Cardiac monitor
- Large-bore peripheral IV (preferably 2)
- IV Fluid resuscitation with normal saline (NS) or lactated ringers (LR)
- Foley catheter

ED TREATMENT

- Management of uterine atony
  —Bimanual message
  —Oxytocin (pitocin) administered IV/IM
  —Methylergonovine (methergine) or ergonovine (ergotrate) IM if oxytocin fail; avoid if known hypertensive; onset in minutes
  —15-methyl PGF_{2a} (hemabate) IM if above fails; relatively contraindicated in asthma
  —Surgery if medical intervention fails
- Inspect closely for genital tract laceration
  —2 cm or greater require repair
  —00 or 000 absorbable suture; continuous, locked recommended
- Management of uterine inversion (acute)
  —Reposition uterus using Johnson maneuver or Harris method
  -Use left hand on abdominal wall to stabilize fundus of uterus. Place right hand with fingers spread into vagina and push steadily on inverted part to reduce
  —If unsuccessful, give terbutaline IV or $MgSO_4$ to produce cervical relaxation and reposition
  —Surgery if unsuccessful or if subacute or chronic inversion
- Management of coagulopathies
  —FFP, platelets, cryoprecipitate as indicated. See appropriate chapter on blood products
  —Careful attention to volume status
  —Continuous reassessment

MEDICATIONS

Uterotonics: Stimulate Uterine Contraction to Control Bleeding

- Ergonovine (ergotrate): 0.2 mg IM, avoid if known hypertensive
- Methylergonovine (methergine): 0.2 mg IM; 0.2 mg po q 6 hrs; avoid if known hypertensive
- Oxytocin (pitocin): 20–40 IU in 1 L NS at 200 ml/hr; do not use for resuscitation
- 15-methyl PGF_{2a} (hemabate): 0.25 mg IM; may repeat in 15–60 min

Cervical Relaxation: Facilitate Uterine Inversion Reduction

- Magnesium sulfate 20%: 2 g IV bolus over 10 min
- Terbutaline: 0.25 mg IV; avoid if hypotensive

Disposition

ADMISSION CRITERIA

- All patients with immediate PPH require admission to a closely monitored setting
- Early obstetrics consultation recommended
- Early surgical intervention dependent upon etiology
- ICU setting if DIC or evidence of hemodynamic compromise
- Patients with endometritis should be admitted for parenteral antibiotics

DISCHARGE CRITERIA

- Delayed PPH without excessive bleeding which is easily controlled
- Outpatient management with methylergonovine 0.2 mg orally every 6 hours may be considered in consultation and close follow-up with obstetrician

Miscellaneous

ICD9: 666.10

CORE CONTENT CODE: 12.8.2

SUGGESTED READINGS

Druelinger L. Postpartum emergencies. Emerg Med Clin North Am 1994;12(1):219–237.

Gilstrap LC, Ramin SM. Postpartum hemorrhage. Clin Obstet Gynecol 1994;37(4):824–830.

Roberts WE. Emergent obstetric management of postpartum hemorrhage. Obstet Gynecol Clin North Am 1995;22(2): 283–302

Author: Clyde Turner, Marco Coppola

Postpartum Infection

Clinical Presentation

SIGNS AND SYMPTOMS

- Fever and chills
- Localized pain and swelling
- Lower abdominal pain
- Foul-smelling lochia, cervical motion tenderness, uterine tenderness
- Absence of other sources of infection
- "Picket fence" shaped fever curve, tachycardia and normal examination consider septic pelvic thrombophlebitis

MECHANISM/DESCRIPTION

- *Early postpartum endometritis (PPE):* develops within 48 hours; most often complicating cesarean section
- *Late postpartum endometritis:* develops after 3 days to 6 weeks, usually following vaginal delivery
- *Septic pelvic thrombophlebitis:* diagnosis of exclusion; two distinct clinical presentations
  —Acute thrombosis: most common right ovarian vein, usually occurring in first 48 hours as acute, progressive lower abdominal pain
  —Enigmatic fever: spiking fever and persistent tachycardia

ETIOLOGY

- Polymicrobial infection result of ascending spread from lower genital tract
- Anaerobic (up to 80%) and aerobic (~70%)
  —Gram-positive aerobes: Group A, B streptococcus, enterococcus and *Gardnerella vaginalis*
  —Gram-negative aerobes: *Escherichia coli,* enterobacter
  —Anaerobes: bacteroides, peptostreptococcus
  —Other genital mycoplasmas (ureaplasma urealyticum and mycoplasma hominis), *Chlamydia trachomatis*—common in late PPE

Pre-Hospital

N/A

Diagnosis

ESSENTIAL WORKUP

- Abdominal and pelvic examination
- Cervical cultures for chlamydia
- Transcervical endometrial cultures

LABORATORY

- CBC
- Urinalysis and culture
- Blood Cultures

IMAGING/SPECIAL TESTS

- CT or MRI for ovarian vein thrombosis—nonurgent
- Ultrasound—sensitive for abscess

DIFFERENTIAL DIAGNOSIS

- Fever from other sources—see Table below

Fever Differential by Timing of Occurrence

<6 hours	Early streptococcal infection Transfusion reaction Thyroid crisis
<48 hours	Atelectasis
<72 hours	Urinary tract infection Pneumonia
3–5 days	Wound infection Breast engorgement Necrotizing fasciitis
3–7 days	Mastitis Septic thrombophlebitis
7–14 days	Abscess
>2 weeks	Mastitis Pulmonary embolism

Treatment

INITIAL STABILIZATION

- ABC
  - —Prompt evaluation of respiratory and hemodynamic status
  - —Supplemental oxygen, cardiac monitor as needed
  - —Venous access

ED TREATMENT

- IV antibiotics and close observation
  - —Clindamycin (cleocin) plus gentamycin (garamycin)—standard
  - —Add ampicillin if severe; metronidazole (flagyl) may replace clindamycin when ampicillin added
  - —β-Lactamase-stable antibiotic, i.e., ticarcillin/clavulanate (timentin), mezlocillin (mezlin), ampicillin/sulbactam (unasyn)—effective alternative
  - —Cefoxitin (mefoxin)—also shown quite effective
- Heparin if suspicion or evidence of thrombophlebitis
- Infected wound should be opened to establish drainage
- Necrotizing fasciitis requires wide surgical debridement, parenteral antibiotics, and adjunctive hyperbaric oxygen therapy
- Peritonitis requires imaging to evaluate cause

MEDICATIONS

- Ampicillin: 2 g q 4 hrs IV
- Ampicillin/sulbactam: 3 g q 6 hrs IV
- Cefoxitin: 2 g q 6 hrs IV
- Clindamycin: 900-mg load, then 600 mg q 6–8 hrs IV
- Gentamycin: 2 mg/kg load, then 1–1.5 mg/kg q 8 hrs IV
- Metronidazole: 1-g load, then 500 mg q 6 hrs IV
- Mezlocillin: 4 g q 6 hrs IV
- Ticarcillin/clavulanate: 3.1 g q 4 hrs IV
- Heparin: 80 IU/kg loading dose, then 18 IU/kg/hr IV

Disposition

ADMISSION CRITERIA

- Patients with endometritis or suspicion for septic pelvic thrombophlebitis should be admitted

DISCHARGE CRITERIA

- Nontoxic, mildly symptomatic patient with late PPE may be considered for outpatient management with erythromycin (500 mg orally qid) in consultation and close follow-up with obstetrics

Miscellaneous

ICD9: 615.9

CORE CONTENT CODE: 12.8.3

SUGGESTED READINGS

Calhoun BC, Brost B. Emergency management of sudden puerperal fever. Obstet Gynecol Clin North Am 1995;22(2):357–367.

Druelinger L. Postpartum emergencies. Emerg Med Clin North Am 1994;12(1):219–237.

Authors: Clyde Turner; Marco Coppola

Preexcitation Syndromes

Clinical Presentation

SIGNS AND SYMPTOMS

- Asymptomatic
- Palpitations
- Dyspnea
- Dizziness
- Nausea
- Abnormal heart rate
  - —Rapid and regular (SVT)
  - —Irregular (atrial fibrillation)
- Signs of instability
  - —Chest pain
  - —Hypotension
  - —Change in mental status
  - —Rales
  - —Cyanosis

MECHANISM/DESCRIPTION

- A group of conditions characterized by an accessory pathway
  - —Connects the atria and the ventricles outside of the SA node
  - —Conduction is faster and the refractory period is shorter
  - —Prototypical pathways are the bundle of Kent and the Mahaim fibers
  - —Allows for early depolarization of the ventricles generating rapid supraventricular tachycardias
- Wolff-Parkinson-White syndrome
  - —Type A, or orthodromic, is the most common (70%)
    - -Impulse travels down the A-V node and then up the retrograde pathway
    - -A circuit is created that potentiates reentrant tachycardia
  - —Type B or antidromic
    - -Less common than Type A
    - -The circuit operates in the opposite direction
- Lown-Ganong-Levine syndrome
  - —Rare preexcitation syndrome with an accessory pathway in the A-V node
- The majority of patients with accessory pathways never become symptomatic
- Risk of death is very low
  - —Preexcitation with wide complex tachycardia is most at risk for ventricular dysrhythmias
- Prevalence is estimated at 0.1–0.3% of the population
- Males are affected twice as often as females

PEDIATRIC CONSIDERATIONS

- Most supraventricular tachycardias in children are the result of AV nodal reentry
- 10% are the result of an identified preexcitation syndrome

ETIOLOGY

- Idiopathic
- In association with structural heart disease
  - —Cardiomyopathy
  - —Transposition of he great vessels
  - —Mitral valve prolapse
  - —Ebstein's anomaly

Pre-Hospital

CAUTIONS

- Supplemental oxygen
- Monitor
- Synchronized cardioversion if signs of instability

CONTROVERSIES

- Pre-hospital use of adenosine
  - —Stable patients do not require emergent conversion
  - —Unstable patients should undergo cardioversion not adenosine

Diagnosis

ESSENTIAL WORKUP

- The diagnosis is made on the 12-lead EKG
- Stable patients much be carefully monitored and reassessed for signs of instability

LABORATORY

- Cardiac enzymes only if signs of ischemia

IMAGING/SPECIAL TESTS

- EKG
  - —Wolff-Parkinson-White syndrome
  - —Short PR $<$0.12s
  - —Prolonged QRS $>$0.10s
  - —Delta wave: Small slurred upstroke at the beginning of the QRS

DIFFERENTIAL DIAGNOSIS

- AV nodal reentry SVT
- Ventricular tachycardia

Treatment

INITIAL STABILIZATION

- Unstable patients
  - —Synchronized cardioversion starting with 50 J-min
  - —Increase incrementally until sinus rhythm is restored
- Stable patients with wide complex tachycardia
  - —Procainamide

ED TREATMENT

- Stable patients with narrow complex, regular tachycardia
  - —Vagal maneuvers such as a Valsalva
  - —Right carotid artery massage for no more than 10 seconds
    - -Auscultate the artery first for a bruit that would contraindicate this procedure
  - —Fluid replacement and Trendelenburg if the patient has mild hypotension
  - —Pharmacologic conversion if carotid massage fails
    - -Adenosine
    - -Verapamil
- Irregular wide complex tachycardia
  - —Procainamide or magnesium is effective
  - —Never use calcium channel blockers, β-blockers, or digoxin
    - -These medications block the AV node
    - -Conduction occurs exclusively down the faster accessory pathway
    - -Precipitation of ventricular dysrhythmias

PEDIATRIC CONSIDERATIONS

- Children may develop ventricular rates up to 320 bpm that are poorly tolerated
- Cardiovert unstable children with 0.5–2 J/kg
- Vagal maneuvers and adenosine are safe in stable children

MEDICATIONS

- Adenosine: 6 mg rapid IV push; if ineffective repeat with 12 mg; peds: 0.1 mg/kg rapid IV push
- Diltiazem: 0.25 mg/kg IV over 2 min followed in 15 min by 0.35 mg/kg IV over 2 min
- Esmolol: 0.5 mg/kg over 1 min; maintenance infusion at 0.05 mg/kg/min over 4 min, then 0.1–0.2 mg/kg/min continuously
- Lidocaine: 1 mg/kg IV bolus followed in 10 min by 0.5 mg/kg bolus; infusion at 2–4 mg/min
- Magnesium: 2 g IV bolus
- Procainamide: 6–13 mg/kg IV at 0.2–0.5 mg/kg/min until arrhythmia controlled; up to a total dose of 1,000 mg, then 2–6 mg/min
- Verapamil: 2.5–5 mg IV bolus over 2 min; may repeat with 5–10 mg every 15–30 min to max of 20 mg

Disposition

ADMISSION CRITERIA

- Patients with signs of instability require admission to a monitored bed
- Failure of outpatient therapy for continuous pharmacologic control or ablation

DISCHARGE CRITERIA

- The majority of patients will be stable and can be discharged once converted to sinus rhythm
- Follow up should be arranged
- Electrophysiologic studies can be determined during the outpatient workup
- Consider low-dose verapamil prophylaxis

Miscellaneous

ICD9: 426.7

CORE CONTENT CODE: 2.4.1.3

SUGGESTED READINGS

Gonzales RP, Schrinman MM, et al. Clinical and electrophysiologic spectrum of fascicular tachycardias. Am Heart J 1994;128(1):147–156.

Medeiros CM, Zimmerman LI, et al. Atrioventricular junctional and orthodromic atrioventricular reentrant tachycardia in Wolff-Parkinson-White syndrome. J Electrocardiol 1993;26(1):83–89.

Nattel S. Comparative mechanisms of actions of antiarrhythmic drugs. Am J Cardiol 1993;72(16):13F–17F.

Oren JW, Beckman KJ, et al. A functional approach to preexcitation syndromes. Cardiol Clin 1993;11(1);121–149.

Author: Eric Glasser

Preeclampsia/Eclampsia

Clinical Presentation

SIGNS AND SYMPTOMS

Preeclampsia

- Most common in late third trimester
- Sudden weight gain may precede other symptoms (>2 lb/wk)
- Hypertension BP 140/90 if unknown baseline, SBP >30 or DBP >15 on two occasions
- Dependent edema progressing to constant edema
- Proteinuria develops later than edema, hypertension, and weight gain
- Epigastric pain/RUQ pain mimicking cholelithiasis
  - —Edema/hemorrhage and stretch of hepatic capsule
- Abdominal pain
- Hematologic abnormalities
- Thrombocytopenia
- Hyperreflexia

Severe Preeclampsia

- Visual disturbances, headache, edema, abdominal pain
- Hematologic abnormalities, oliguria, proteinuria >3+ dipstick, and BP >160/110

Eclampsia

- Tonic-clonic seizure activity is the hallmark,
- Seizures may occur after delivery, usually within 48 hours. Case reports exist 10 days after delivery
- Premonitory facial twitching, headache, blurred vision

MECHANISM/DESCRIPTION

Preeclampsia

- Relative or absolute hypertension associated with proteinuria and edema during pregnancy
- Syndrome accompanied by progressive weight gain and diffuse symptoms

Risk Factors

- Multiparity, advanced maternal age
- Young and nulliparous
- Lower socioeconomic status
- Diabetes, collagen vascular disturbances
- Hydrops fetalis, molar pregnancy
- Preexisting renal disease or hypertension

Eclampsia

- Eclampsia is the presence of tonic-clonic convulsions that develop in pregnancy-induced hypertension or pregnancy aggravated hypertension
- Clinical end point of severe pregnancy-induced hypertension
- Preeclampsia transitions to severe eclampsia which may develop eclampsia
  - —Up to 2% of preeclamptic women will progress to eclampsia

ETIOLOGY

- Diffuse arteriolar vasospasm
- Abnormal fluid retention with fluctuating renal vasospasm
- Heightened vascular permeability
- Hypertension
- Microthrombi

Pre-Hospital

- Patients should be transported in left lateral recumbent position
- Manage seizures as described in treatment section
- Patients should be transported to the nearest facility with high-risk obstetric capability

Diagnosis

ESSENTIAL WORKUP

- History and physical examination with special attention to mental status, neuro exam, abdominal exam
- Vital signs (blood pressure)
- Stat blood sugar
- Urinalysis for protein

LABORATORY

- Proteinuria on dipstick >1, send urine for 24 hours
- Urine sediment for RBC, WBC Casts
- PT/PTT, Platelets (<150 k)
- BUN, Creatinine
- Liver function tests
- Urine toxicology-sympathomimetics
- Fetal monitoring/stress test

IMAGING/SPECIAL TESTS

- Emergent ultrasound for EGA, fetal viability
- Head CT after airway stabilization if concern for intracranial masses, bleeding
- Lumbar puncture to assess intracranial hemorrhage, meningitis

PATHOLOGIC FINDINGS

- Widespread fibrin deposits in small vessels especially the kidney and liver
- Microvascular changes in placental flow may effect fetal well being

DIFFERENTIAL DIAGNOSIS

Preeclampsia

- Pregnancy induced hypertension (PIH), chronic with superimposed PIH, worsened chronic HTN
- Flare in underlying renal or collagen vascular diseases
- Hydatidiform mole
- Hydrops fetalis
- Concomitant drug abuse

Eclampsia

- Epilepsy
- Encephalitis
- Meningitis
- Encephalopathy
- Brain tumor
- Intracranial hemorrhage
- Hysteria

Treatment

INITIAL STABILIZATION

- ABCs
- Left lateral decubitus position
- 100% O_2, maternal cardiac and tocographic monitoring, and fetal monitoring
- $MgSO_4$ is first line agent for severe preeclampsia with seizure prophylaxis and treatment of seizures
- Valium, and phenytoin are considered second- and third-line treatments for seizures
- Manage hypertension with hydralazine

ED TREATMENT

- Immediate obstetrical consult
- Emergent delivery if symptoms severe
- Possible Cesarean delivery

MEDICATIONS

- $MgSO_4$: 2–4 g IVP; followed by 2 g/hr IV drip *or* 10 mg IM; $MgSO_4$ infusion should not exceed 1 g/min; monitor blood pressure, respiratory rate, and DTRs carefully
- Valium: 5–10 g IV if no analeptic response to $MgSO_4$
- Phenytoin: 15–18 mg/kg, 25–50 mg/min IV
- Hydralazine: 5–20 mg IV, may use diazoxide 30 mg IV if no response to 20 mg hydralazine

Disposition

ADMISSION CRITERIA

- All patients with preeclampsia should be admitted
- Eclampsia should be admitted to ICU or delivery room/OR

DISCHARGE CRITERIA

- Patients that are completely asymptomatic and felt not to have preeclampsia may be considered for outpatient management with close OBGyn follow-up

Miscellaneous

PROGNOSIS

- Improved mortality with aggressive seizure prophylaxis and termination/delivery
- Determined by gestational age of fetus if preeclampsia is not severe
- Improved with early delivery
- Neonatal loss largely due to preterm delivery
- Perinatal mortality increased if preexisting hypertension or PIH

ASSOCIATED CONDITIONS

- Renal failure
- Collagen vascular diseases
- Slight increased incidence of abruption

ICD9: 642.40, 780.39

CORE CONTENT CODE: 12.3.6.1, 12.3.6.2

SUGGESTED READINGS

Charles D, Hurry D, eds. Obstetrics and gynecology. 6th ed. New York: Elsevier Science, 1986.

Cunningham FG, MacDonald PC, Grant NF, eds. Williams' obstetrics. 19th ed. Norwalk, CT: Appleton & Lange, 1993.

Dambro M, et al. Griffith's 5 minute clinical consult. Baltimore: Williams & Wilkins, 1997.

Reid A, Duncan G, Christian C, eds. Controversy in obstetrics and gynecology II. 2nd ed. Philadelphia: WB Saunders, 1974.

Rosen P, et al., eds. Emergency medicine. 3rd ed. St. Louis: CV Mosby, 1992.

Scott CJ, et al. Emergencies in pregnancy. Patient Care 1991;15:132–151.

Author: Shawn D. Evans

Pregnancy, Trauma in

Clinical Presentation

SIGNS AND SYMPTOMS

- Abdominal pain
- Uterine contraction
- Vaginal bleeding, leakage of fluid
- Contusion, lap belt marks

MECHANISM/DESCRIPTION

- Fetal and maternal injury specific to pregnancy is evident after the first trimester
  - —There is an increased rate of fetal loss, but not maternal mortality
- The likelihood of fetal injury increases with the severity of maternal insult
- The hypervolemic gestational state frequently leads to an underestimation of blood loss
  - —Clinical shock may be apparent only after a 30% maternal blood loss
- Abdominal findings are less evident in the gravid patient
- Less frequent bowel injury
- More frequent retroperitoneal hemorrhage due to the engorgement of pelvic organs and veins
- Increased morbidity and mortality with pelvic fractures due to pelvic and uterine engorgement
- Fetal or uterine trauma includes placental abruption, fetal maternal hemorrhage, premature labor, uterine rupture or contusion, fetal demise, premature membrane rupture, and hypoxemic or anatomic fetal injury (skull fracture)
- Abruption occurs in up to 38–50% of severe trauma and >2% of minor injuries
  - —Hallmark is uterine contractions
- Fetal/maternal hemorrhage (FMH) occurs in more than 30% of severe trauma
  - —Isoimmunization of Rh-negative mothers
- Penetrating trauma results in direct injury to fetus, maternal shock, and premature delivery

ETIOLOGY

- Trauma occurs in about 7% of all pregnancies
- Motor vehicle (54–70 %)
- Falls
- Direct abdominal trauma
- Penetrating (stab or gunshot)
- Electrical or burn
- Domestic violence (reported at over 17% of all pregnant women)

Pre-Hospital

CAUTIONS

- Patients in late second and third trimester should be transported to a trauma center
- Advise trauma center early of pregnancy and estimated gestational age to facilitate early mobilization of fetal monitors, sonography, and of neonatal and obstetric consultants and equipment
- Place patient (while on backboard) in the left lateral recumbent position to avoid supine hypotension
- Mast suit inflation over the abdomen is contraindicated

Diagnosis

ESSENTIAL WORKUP

- Identify maternal condition first
- Follow ATLS guidelines
- Determine the gestational age (EGA) to assess viability
  - —Estimate LMP
  - —Fundal height (FH) − EGA = FH (cm) × 8/7 after week 16
  - —Doppler fetal heart tones
  - —Sonography
- Fetal/maternal monitoring for a minimum of 4 hours
  - —Abruption does not occur in patients that have no contractions during the first 4 hours of monitoring
  - —With >1 contraction/10 min, a 20% abruption incidence is reported
  - —The occurrence of bradycardia, poor variability or Type II "late" deceleration (after the peak of uterine contraction) indicates fetal distress

LABORATORY

- CBC, urinalysis
- Blood gas and electrolyte panel
- Type, Rh, and screening of blood
- The Kleihauer-Betke (KB) stain: a citric acid elution that identifies fetal maternal hemoglobin (FMH) in vaginal fluid or blood

IMAGING/SPECIAL TESTS

- Shield the uterus if possible but *do not avoid necessary maternal x-rays*
- Fetal radiation injury is less than 1 event/1000/rad exposure
- The rad exposure is estimated at the following
  - —C-spine and chest x-rays: <0.005 rad
  - —Femur: <0.012 rad
  - —AP pelvis, spine, KUB: 0.14–0.5 rad each
  - —IVP: 0.2–0.8 rad
  - —CT head: <0.05 rad; thorax: <1 rad; upper abdomen: <3 rad; lower abdomen/pelvis: 3–9 rad
- Ultrasonography
  - —Evaluate for solid organ injury or hemoperitoneum, fetal heart activity, gestational age, abruptions, and amount of amniotic fluid
  - —Test vaginal fluid with nitrazine paper (turns blue), and for ferning
  - —Patients with stable penetrating trauma, triple-contrast CT is advocated, particularly with stab wounds

PEDIATRIC CONSIDERATIONS

- Fetal survival begins at the 24th week (9.9%); it becomes significant after the 26th week (54.7%)

Treatment

INITIAL STABILIZATION

- Direct therapy at the mother with no delays due to pregnancy
- ABCs of trauma care
- Cardiac, pulse-oximetry and cardiotocographic monitoring
- Tilt the patient or board 15–30° to the left to relieve vena caval compression

ED TREATMENT

- Use LR for IV fluids, NS may induce a hyperchloremic acidosis
- Replace estimated blood loss in a 3:1 ratio
- Resort to transfusions after 1 L of estimated blood loss or if hypovolemia persists after 2 L of crystalloid
- Nasogastric tube decompression due to higher risk of aspiration in pregnancy
- Foley catheterization to assess urinary output
- If DPL is necessary, use supraumbilical open technique
- Use tocolytic therapy only for hemodynamically stable patients
  - —Contraindicated if cervix dilated >4 cm and FMH and abruption have been reasonably ruled out
  - —Use tocolytics only when over 8 contractions per hour have lasted more than 4 hours
- See chapter: Cesarean Section, Emergency
- In minor trauma after the 20th week, fetal and maternal monitoring is best done in the labor and delivery area

MEDICATIONS

- RhoGAM in Rh-negative women: 50 μg IM in women <12 weeks pregnant; 300 μg IM in women >12 weeks pregnant
- Tocolytics: magnesium sulfate 4 g IV
- Avoid: aspirin; hypnotics; nonsteroidals; vasopressors
- Contraindicated: chloramphenicol; dilantin; gentamycin; sulfonamides; tetracyclines

Disposition

ADMISSION CRITERIA

- Vaginal bleeding or amniotic fluid leakage
- Feto-maternal hemorrhage
- Abdominal Pain
- Uterine contractions
- Evidence of fetal distress
- Abruption placenta
- Hemoperitoneum or visceral or solid organ injury

DISCHARGE CRITERIA

- All following criteria must be met
- No uterine contractions for over 4 hours of tocodynamometry
  - —Some authors however recommend 24 hours of monitoring
- No evidence of fetal distress
- No vaginal bleeding or amniotic fluid leakage
- No abdominal pain or tenderness
- Timely obstetric follow-up
- Specific instructions to return if any of the above symptoms occur

Miscellaneous

ICD9: 760.5

CORE CONTENT CODE: 18.5

SUGGESTED READINGS

Kuhlman RS, Cruikshank DP. Maternal trauma during pregnancy. Clin Obstet Gynecol 1994;37(2):274–293.

Lavery JP, Staten-McCormick M. Management of moderate to severe trauma in pregnancy. Obstet Gynecol Clin North Am 1995;22(1):69–90.

Morris AM, et al. Infant survival after cesarean section for trauma. Ann Surg 1996;223(5):481–488.

Pearlman MD, Tintinalli JE, Lorenz RP. A prospective controlled study of outcome after trauma during pregnancy. Am J Obstet Gynecol 1990;162:102–110.

Author: A. Antoine Kazzi

Pregnancy, Uncomplicated

Pregnancy is not a disease process but rather a physiologic state in which a female provides gestational support to an unborn offspring. The changes associated with pregnancy are mediated by alterations in maternal endocrine function, fetal metabolic and physical requirements, and the interaction of fetal and placental function. All women of reproductive age with abdominal pain are considered pregnant until proven otherwise!

Clinical Presentation

SIGNS AND SYMPTOMS

- Amenorrhea
  - —The most common cause of secondary amenorrhea in a woman of reproductive age is pregnancy
- Nausea and vomiting (morning sickness), heartburn/pyrosis
- Breast tenderness (mastodynia)
- Urinary frequency
- Headache, backache
- Pica
- Edema, fatigue, weight gain

ETIOLOGY

- All of the preceding signs and symptoms can be explained by elevations in various hormones levels secreted by the mother as well as the placenta, or changes in anatomy which is a function of the progression of the pregnancy
- Placental human chorionic gonadotropin (HCG)
  - —Prevents the normal involution of the corpus luteum at the end of the menstrual cycle
  - —Causes the corpus luteum to secrete even larger quantities of estrogen and progesterone
  - —Elevated HCG levels are responsible for the nausea and vomiting
- Placental progesterone
  - —Causes decidual cells in the endometrium to develop and provide nutrition for the early embryo
  - —Decreases contractility of the gravid uterus and risk of spontaneous abortion
  - —Helps estrogen prepare the breasts for lactation
- Placental estrogen
  - —Responsible for enlargement of uterus, breasts, and mammary ducts
  - —Enlargement of female external genitalia, relaxation of pelvic ligaments, symphysis pubis, and sacroiliac joints

MECHANISM/DESCRIPTION

- The changes associated with pregnancy are accounted for by the production of large amounts of placental hormones, in particular placental estrogen and progesterone
- Feedback mechanisms occur between maternal and fetal endocrine systems

PEDIATRIC CONSIDERATIONS

- In the United States, the range for menarche is 11–15 years with the average age 12.7 years
- Pregnant adolescents who present to the ED may be either unaware of the pregnancy or be reluctant to admit it. Assume pregnancy in adolescents regardless of the chief complaint

Pre-Hospital

- Assume that the patient is pregnant
- Administer medications only when necessary to avoid teratogenetic side affects or placental-fetal compromise, i.e., epinephrine
- ACLS or ATLS Protocols as indicated
- If greater than 24 weeks gestation, transport in left lateral recumbent position

Diagnosis

ESSENTIAL WORKUP

- Determine first day of last menstrual period (LMP)
  - —40% of women cannot accurately remember their LMP
  - —The single most important part of the initial assessment is the pelvic examination. Estimate expected date of delivery by determining uterine fundal height

LABORATORY

- Pregnancy tests: various techniques that detect HCG include agglutination-inhibition, radioimmunoassay, enzyme-linked immunosorbent assay, and immunochromatography. These tests may be performed on urine or serum. Qualitative urine tests are sensitive to 50 IU HCG

IMAGING/SPECIAL TESTS

- Ultrasonography can estimate gestational age, confirm intrauterine or ectopic pregnancy, evaluate fetal viability, as well as evaluate for a number of fetal abnormalities. It does not replace a complete history and physical examination
- Vaginal probe ultrasound is contraindicated in premature rupture of membranes and third trimester vaginal bleeding

DIFFERENTIAL DIAGNOSIS

- The most common cause of secondary amenorrhea is pregnancy. Any woman who is of the age to be sexually active who presents to the ED should be assumed to be pregnant until proven otherwise. There are a multitude of other etiologies (medications, endocrine, psychiatric) responsible for secondary amenorrhea but these can be evaluated in the clinic

PEDIATRIC CONSIDERATIONS

- The recognition of pregnancy in an adolescent is difficult because of vague and misleading complaints. This can result in delay of prenatal care. Assume pregnancy in the adolescent regardless of the chief complaint

Treatment

INITIAL STABILIZATION

- ACLS, ATLS measures as needed: oxygen, cardiac monitor, IV access, and fluids
- If greater than 24 weeks gestation, place in left lateral recumbent position

ED TREATMENT

- The goal is to optimize maternal condition to improve fetal condition

MEDICATIONS

- Avoidance of certain medications and exposure to noxious agents is particularly important during the first trimester when organogenesis is occurring. The risk of fetal malformation continues beyond the first trimester. *Before using any drug,* it is prudent to refer to its FDA safety classification in pregnancy. This classification system categorizes drugs as Category A, B, C, D, and X with category A being the safest and category X being the most toxic
- Analgesics: acetaminophen is the preferred OTC analgesic. Aspirin and NSAIDs are not teratogenic but are best utilized in consultation with an obstetrician. Propoxyphene, codeine, synthetic codeine, meperidine, and morphine have no known teratogenic affect and can be used for the control of severe pain in pregnancy for short periods of time (3–4 days)
- Antibiotics: selecting the right antibiotic in a gravid female is dependent upon three factors
  1. Maternal drug allergies
  2. Type of infection and associated pathogens
  3. Gestational age
- For antibiotic usage, it is particularly helpful to review their respective FDA safety classifications. Consultation with an obstetrician is prudent.

Disposition

ADMISSION CRITERIA

- Pregnant women with the following diagnoses should be admitted to the hospital
  - —Hyperemesis gravidarum with inability to tolerate oral fluids
  - —Complicated urinary tract infection
  - —Ectopic or molar pregnancy
  - —Placenta previa or abruptio placenta
  - —Septic abortion
  - —Preeclampsia
  - —Preterm labor
  - —Premature rupture of membranes
  - —Other medical conditions which would warrant admission in a non-gravid female

DISCHARGE CRITERIA

- Women without the above conditions may be discharged from the ED

Miscellaneous

ICD9: V22.2

CORE CONTENT CODE: 12.2

SUGGESTED READINGS

American College of Obstetrics and Gynecology. Antepartum care. In: PRECIS V: An update in obstetrics and gynecology. Washington, DC: American College of Obstetrics and Gynecology, 1994:124–142.

Benson MD. Obstetrical pearls: A practical guide for the efficient resident. 2d ed. Philadelphia: FA Davis, 1989.

Causey AL, Seago K, Wahl NG, Voelker CL. Pregnant adolescents in the emergency department: Diagnosed and not diagnosed. Am J Emerg Med 1997;15:125–130.

Author: James S. Walker

Priapism

Clinical Presentation

SIGNS AND SYMPTOMS

- Penile erection in the absence of sexual arousal that is prolonged and frequently painful
- Urinary retention is possible

MECHANISM/DESCRIPTION

- Engorgement of corpora cavernosa
- *Low-flow priapism* is most common, and is caused by *poor venous outflow*. Pain is characteristic. The presence of stagnant, hypoxic blood can lead to ischemia and thrombosis after a few hours. Fibrosis and impotence are late sequelae
- *High-flow priapism* is rare and is usually associated with penile arterial laceration with *uncontrolled inflow* of arterial blood. It is usually painless. Presentation may be later than in low-flow priapism, and ischemia and impotence are uncommon sequelae

ETIOLOGY

- Idiopathic
- Pharmacological agents
  - —Intracavernosal injectables for the treatment of impotence: PGE-1, papaverine, phentolamine. These agents are an increasingly prevalent cause of priapism in adults
  - —Psychotropics: phenothiazines, butyrophenones, trazodone, sedative-hypnotics, selective serotonin uptake inhibitors (SSRIs)
  - —Antihypertensives: prazosin, hydralazine, phenoxybenzamine, guanethidine
  - —Rarely implicated agents include anticoagulants, cocaine, marijuana and ethanol
- Sickle cell anemia, leukemia, and other hematologic disorders predisposing to sludging of blood may cause low-flow priapism
- Penile trauma can result in arterial laceration and high-flow priapism
- Spinal trauma may cause priapism from loss of inhibitory adrenergic tone
- Rare causes include pelvic neoplasms and infections, dialysis, and parenteral nutrition solutions containing a fat emulsion

PEDIATRIC CONSIDERATIONS

- Sickle cell anemia is the cause of the majority of priapism in children

Pre-Hospital

- IV Flush
- O_2 administration
- Pain Medication

Diagnosis

ESSENTIAL WORKUP

- The cause of priapism can frequently be determined by history
- High-flow priapism may be suspected in a patient with painless priapism and a history of trauma
- Low-flow priapism should be suspected in patients presenting with painful priapism

LABORATORY

- Complete blood count and coagulation profile may be helpful
- Intracavernosal blood gas analysis can help differentiate high-flow from low-flow priapism. Near-normal values are found in high-flow priapism, whereas acidosis and hypoxia (O_2 <30 torr) are found in low flow priapism. Because of the possibility for penile arterial injury, a urologist best performs this procedure

IMAGING/SPECIAL TESTS

- Duplex Doppler ultrasound can verify and localize the arterial laceration in high-flow priapism
- Angiography enables localization and embolectomy of the arterial laceration in high-flow priapism

DIFFERENTIAL DIAGNOSIS

- Penile erection from sexual arousal is usually painless and transient
- Penile implants are discovered by history and physical examination

PEDIATRIC CONSIDERATIONS

- Sickle cell anemia evaluation may be undertaken in pediatric patients

Treatment

INITIAL STABILIZATION

- Supplemental oxygen
- Analgesia and sedation
- Intravenous hydration
- Urgent urological consultation

ED TREATMENT

- Management for specific etiologies should be undertaken
  - —Sickle cell anemia: RBC transfusion, exchange transfusion, hyperbaric oxygen if other measures fail
  - —Leukemia: chemotherapy
- Terbutaline is a β-agonist that may be administered in consultation with a urologist to initiate the treatment of low-flow priapism
- Intracavernosal injection/aspiration is an invasive technique that should be performed by an urologist if medical therapy for low-flow priapism fails. If specialty care is unavailable for several hours, the procedure may be performed by the ED physician as follows
  1. Administer local anesthesia to the glans or perform a pudendal nerve block
  2. Prep the penis in a sterile fashion
  3. Positioning yourself to the right of the patient, grasp the penile shaft with the left hand
  4. Enter the corpus cavernosum with a 19-gauge butterfly needle inserted through the glans
  5. Aspirate blood while "milking" the penile shaft. Aspirating both corpora cavernosa is unnecessary as they are connected by shunts. Aspirate until arterial blood is obtained. Irrigation with saline may be necessary
  6. Epinephrine, phenylephrine, or pseudoephedrine may be injected through the butterfly needle if tumescence recurs. Monitor heart rate and blood pressure if these agents are utilized, and do not administer them to patients with cardiovascular or cerebrovascular disease or patients taking monoamine-oxidase inhibitors (MAOIs) because of the risk of hypertensive crisis
- Embolectomy following angiographic localization of the arterial injury is effective in high-flow priapism
- Surgical shunt (i.e., corpus cavernosum to spongiosum) may be necessary if the above measures fail

MEDICATIONS

- Terbutaline: 0.25–0.5 mg SQ or 5 mg po q 4–6 hrs
- Epinephrine: dilute 1 mg in 100 ml saline; inject 1–3 ml boluses in the corpus cavernosum, up to 10 ml
- Phenylephrine: dilute 1 mg in 100 ml saline; inject 10 ml boluses in the corpus cavernosum
- Pseudoephedrine: 60–100 mg in the corpus cavernosum

Disposition

ADMISSION CRITERIA

- Persistent priapism despite noninvasive treatments
- Serious underlying disease (sickle cell anemia, leukemia)

DISCHARGE CRITERIA

- Detumescence is complete and has not recurred after several hours of observation
- Urological consultation has been obtained
- Short-term follow-up has been arranged
- The patient has been advised to return to the ED if tumescence recurs, and the ED physician and the consulting urologist have discussed the possibility of impotence with the patient

Miscellaneous

ICD9: 607.3

CORE CONTENT CODE: 19.2.2.3

SUGGESTED READINGS

Hakim LS, Kulaksizoglu H, Mulligan R, Greenfield A, Goldstein I. Evolving concepts in the diagnosis and treatment of arterial high flow priapism. J Urol 1996;155:541–548.

Mulhall JP, Honig SC. Priapism: Diagnosis and management. Acad Emerg Med 1996;3:810–816.

Shantha TR, Finnerty DP, Rodriquez AP. Treatment of persistent priapism using terbutaline. J Urol 1990;144:1483–1484.

Winter CC, McDowell G. Experience with 105 patients with priapism: Update and review of all aspects. J Urol 1988;140:980–983.

Authors: David Barlas; Joseph LaMantia

Prostatitis

Clinical Presentation

SIGNS AND SYMPTOMS

- Irritative voiding symptoms (frequency, urgency, dysuria)
- Acute prostatitis presents with fever and chills, malaise, arthralgias, and myalgias
- The hallmark of chronic prostatitis is relapsing dysuria
- Low-back pain
- Perineal, suprapubic, or testicular pain
- Bladder outlet obstruction and urinary retention
- Ejaculatory symptoms such as hematospermia
- Examination may reveal exquisitely tender, warm, swollen, and firm or boggy prostate in acute prostatitis. *The acutely inflamed prostate should not be massaged because of the possibility of precipitating hematogenous spread of organisms*
- Examination is usually normal in chronic prostatitis

MECHANISM/DESCRIPTION

- Can be subdivided into 5 categories
- Prostatic abscess
  - —Once common after acute prostatitis, now rare except in immunocompromised patients
  - —The presence of continuing fevers, rectal symptoms, and leukocytosis despite treatment, along with a fluctuant mass on rectal exam, suggest abscess
- Acute (bacterial) prostatitis
  - —The easiest entity to diagnose and treat
  - —Acute febrile illness in which systemic symptoms may appear days before localizing urinary symptoms appear
  - —Patients often appear toxic and usually have a concurrent cystitis
- Chronic bacterial prostatitis
  - —About 10% of cases of prostatitis, but probably the most common cause of recurrent urinary tract infection in men
  - —White blood cells and bacteria may be present in expressed prostatic secretions (EPS), and bacteria may be cultured from the urine or EPS
- Chronic nonbacterial prostatitis (also called prostatosis)
  - —Same symptoms as chronic bacterial prostatitis but unable to culture organisms from urine or EPS
- Prostatodynia
  - —Symptoms referable to the prostate but no inflammatory cells are found and no bacteria can be cultured from the urine or prostatic secretions

ETIOLOGY

- Usually a single organism bacterial infection of the prostate
- Exact mechanism by which bacteria infect the prostate isn't known. Various routes have been proposed but none have been firmly substantiated
- Acute prostatitis
  - —Age <35 years: *Neisseria gonorrhoeae* and *Chlamydia trachomatis* are usual etiologies
  - —Age >35 years: Enterobacteriaceae or *E. coli* (usual), *Klebsiella, Pseudomonas, Enterococcus,* and *Proteus* also seen
  - —Rarely may be caused by *Salmonella, Clostridia,* tuberculosis, or fungi (*Cryptococcus neoformans* in AIDS patients.)
- Chronic bacterial prostatitis
  - —Enterobacteriaceae (80%), Enterococcus (15%), and *Pseudomonas aeruginosa*
- Chronic nonbacterial prostatitis:
  - —Possible role for *Chlamydia, Ureaplasma urealyticum, Trichomonas vaginalis,* and *Mycoplasma hominis*
  - —Inconclusive evidence implicating Gram-positive commensals such as Micrococci, Streptococci, diphtheroids, and coagulase-positive Staphylococci

Pre-Hospital

N/A

Diagnosis

ESSENTIAL WORKUP

- Urinalysis (with microscopy) and culture
- Rectal and prostatic examination, do not massage prostate in acute prostatitis

LABORATORY

- *Acute prostatitis:* complete blood count, electrolytes, blood cultures, and arterial blood gas analysis may be helpful in the acutely ill patient. If <35 years old or suspected sexual transmission, testing for syphilis (VDRL or RPR) is recommended
- *Chronic prostatitis/prostatodynia:* prostatic massage between voiding may be used to capture EPS for Gram stain and culture if organism or white cells not present in the urine

IMAGING/SPECIAL TESTS

- Not indicated in acute prostatitis
- If prostatic abscess suspected, pelvic computed tomography (CT) scan with intravenous (IV) and rectal contrast are necessary to confirm diagnosis
- Pelvic radiographs may reveal prostatic calculi (common in men), which may serve as a nidus for infection in chronic prostatitis

DIFFERENTIAL DIAGNOSIS

- Cystitis
- Pyelonephritis
- Urolithiasis
- Vesicular calculi
- Seminal vesiculitis
- Proctitis
- Perirectal/perianal abscess
- Urethritis
- Epididymitis
- Orchitis
- Prostatic infarction
- Benign prostatic hyperplasia
- Prostatic carcinoma
- Other causes of lower back pain (strain, disk disease, sacroiliac joint disease, etc.)

Treatment

INITIAL STABILIZATION

- Initial resuscitative measures (ABCs) on all patients who are acutely ill, toxic-appearing, or septic

ED TREATMENT

- Prostatic abscess requires urgent urologic consultation and operative management
- Antibiotic therapy should be initiated in ED (see Medications below)
- Urinary tract instrumentation should be avoided
  —If patient has painful urinary retention in acute prostatitis, suprapubic needle aspiration, or suprapubic catheter placement should be performed
- Patients will benefit from adequate IV fluid
- Pain control with NSAIDs and narcotic analgesics as needed
- Stool softeners
- Bed rest
- Irritative voiding systems may persist for months after antibiotic therapy and may be treated with NSAIDs

MEDICATIONS

- Oral antibiotics for outpatient treatment of acute (>35 years old) or chronic prostatitis
  —Ciprofloxacin: 500 mg po bid 14–28 days acute, 14 days–4 weeks chronic
  —Ofloxacin: 300 mg po bid 14–28 days acute, 6 weeks chronic
  —Trimethoprim/sulfamethoxazole: 1 DS tab or 2 regular-strength tablets po bid 1–3 months
- Parenteral antibiotic therapy for acute prostatitis
  —Ampicillin: 2 g IV q 6 hrs *plus* gentamicin: 3–5 mg/kg/day IV *or* tobramycin: 3 mg/kg/day IV
  —Ciprofloxacin: 400 mg IV bid
  —Ofloxacin: 200 mg IV bid
- Empiric antibiotic therapy for acute prostatitis in patients <35 years old
  —Ofloxacin: 300 mg po bid × 2 weeks
  —Ceftriaxone: 125 mg IM *or* cefixime: 400 mg po (single dose); *plus* doxycycline: 100 mg po bid × 14 days *or* azithromycin: 1 g po single dose
- Chronic nonbacterial prostatitis (prostatosis)
  —Doxycycline: 100 mg po bid × 14 days
  —Erythromycin: 500 mg po qid × 14 days
- Prostatodynia
  —Peripheral α-adrenergic blocking agents have been used with some success. Consult a urologist
  —Terazosin: 1 mg po qhs
  —Prazosin: 1 mg po bid/tid
  —Doxazosin: 1 mg po qd

Disposition

ADMISSION CRITERIA

- Acute prostatitis: patients who appear ill or toxic with fever, chills, and urinary retention should be admitted for parenteral antibiotics and close observation
- Chronic prostatitis: admission generally not warranted unless patient has signs or symptoms of acute prostatitis

DISCHARGE CRITERIA

- Acute prostatitis: patient must be nontoxic, able to take fluids and oral medications (analgesia and antibiotics), urinate without difficulty, immunocompetent, relatively free of concurrent underlying disease, and have appropriate follow-up care
- Chronic prostatitis: appropriate follow-up care should be available

Miscellaneous

ICD9: 601.9

CORE CONTENT CODE: 19.2.3.4

SUGGESTED READINGS

Harwood-Nuss AL, Etheredge W, McKenna I. Urologic Emergency. In: Rosen P, et al., eds. Emergency medicine: Concepts and clinical practice. 4th ed. St. Louis: CV Mosby, 1998:2227–2260.

Robert RO, Lieber MM, Bostwick DG, Jacobsen SJ. A review of clinical and pathological prostatitis syndromes. Urology 1997;49:809–821.

Stewart C. Prostatitis. Emerg Med Clin North Am 1988;6:391–402.

Author: Robert S. Hamilton

Pruritus

Clinical Presentation

SIGNS AND SYMPTOMS

- Onset
  - —Shortly after fresh water bathing in swimmer's itch
  - —More intense at night with scabies
  - —Paroxysmal with multiple sclerosis
  - —Sudden changes in temperature with polycythemia vera
- Dermatologic
  - —Absence of rash
  - —Hives
  - —Urticaria
  - —Grouped papules
  - —Interdigital, pubic, axillary, or nipple lesions
  - —Generalized morbilliform eruptions
  - —Discrete weeping patches with vesicles
  - —Dry skin
  - —Jaundice
  - —Excoriations
  - —Prurigo papules
    - -Thickened papular areas of skin from constant rubbing
- Psychogenic
  - —The patient believes that itching is caused by invisible parasites in the skin
  - —Constant rubbing in areas that the patient can readily reach
    - -Extremities, scalp, upper back

MECHANISM/DESCRIPTION

- Mediated by unmyelinated C fibers found in the upper portion of the dermis
  - —The afferent C fibers enter the dorsal horn of the spinal cord, synapse, cross the midline, and ascend the spinothalamic tracts to the thalamus and then to the sensory area of the postcentral gyrus
- Peripheral mediators stimulate the C fibers and induce itching
  - —Histamine
  - —Trypsin
  - —Proteases
  - —Peptides that release histamine
    - -Bradykinin
    - -Vasoactive intestine peptide
    - -Substance P
  - —Bile salts
- Prostaglandins lower the threshold to pruritus
- Opiates cause pruritus by acting on central receptors
- No single pharmacologic agent effectively treats all kinds of pruritus
- "Itch-scratch-itch" cycle
  - —Itching triggers scratching, which damages the skin and stimulates nerve endings, thereby producing even greater itching
  - —Pathogenic basis for lichen simplex chronicus and prurigo nodularis that may complicate a primary cause of pruritus
  - —This cycle in chronic pruritus often causes anxiety adding a psychogenic component

ETIOLOGY

- Allergy
- Iron deficiency
- Kidney disease
- Liver disease
- Aquagenic
- Malignancies
- Atopy
- Polycythemia vera
- Collagen vascular disease
- Infections
  - —Parasitic
  - —Bacterial
  - —Fungal
  - —Viral including HIV
- Lymphomas
- Carcinoid
- Thyroid disease

Pre-Hospital

N/A

Diagnosis

ESSENTIAL WORKUP

- A detailed history and physical is the most important component of the ED workup
  - —Onset
  - —Medications
  - —Use of new topical products
    - -Soap
    - -Hair spray
    - -Lotions
    - -Cosmetics
    - -Perfume
  - —Family history of atopic dermatitis
  - —Personal history of allergies or asthma
  - —History of HIV or AIDS
- Characterization of skin lesions
  - —Follicular
    - -Around the hair
    - -Folliculitis
  - —Nonfollicular
    - -Insect bites, scabies
  - —Primary lesions
    - -Papular, pustular, urticarial, or polymorphic

LABORATORY

- CBC with differential
  - —Suspicion of iron deficiency or polycythemia
- Serum chemistry
  - —Including liver and kidney screens in selected patients
- Thyroid function tests
- Stool examination for ova and parasites

IMAGING/SPECIAL TESTS

- Skin biopsy
  - —May be required to determine the underlying diagnosis
  - —Performed by the dermatologist during the followup visit

DIFFERENTIAL DIAGNOSIS

Dermatologic

- Xerosis (dry skin)
- Insect infestations
  - —Scabies
    - -Vesicles and burrows on intertriginous areas
  - —Pediculosis
  - —Insect bites
    - -Localized clusters of papules
- Dermatitis
  - —Atopic
  - —Contact dermatitis
    - -Includes poison ivy contact
  - —Nummular dermatitis
    - -Round eczematous or vesicular eruption
- Drug induced
  - —Opiates, aspirin, quinidine
  - —Suspect when pruritus occurs without a rash

- Lichen planus
  - —Lichenification, hyperpigmentation, skin thickening
- Urticaria
- Eosinophilic folliculitis
- Dermatitis herpetiformis
  - —Burning itch
- Sunburn
- Fiberglass dermatitis
- Seborrheic dermatitis
  - —Scaly plaques on scalp, hairline, eyebrows, central face and other sebaceous gland-bearing areas like axillae and chest
- Swimmer's itch
  - —Schistosome cercarial dermatitis
  - —Repeated fresh water exposure
  - —Itching starts as water evaporates
  - —Highly pruritic papules develop hours later

Infectious

- HIV
  - —Pruritus may be a manifestation of HIV infection
  - —Other etiologies may occur as with non-HIV patients but often these are more difficult to treat
- Chronic phase of intestinal helminthic infections

Cholestatic

- Obstructive biliary disease
- Primary biliary cirrhosis
  - —Early sign usually starting on hands and soles
- Cholestatic hepatitis secondary to drugs (chlorpropamide)
- Intrahepatic cholestasis of pregnancy
- Extrahepatic biliary obstruction

Hematologic-Oncologic

- Lymphoma including Hodgkin's disease
- Mycosis fungoides
- Polycythemia vera
- Iron deficiency anemia
- Carcinoid
- Visceral malignancies
  - —Breast, stomach, lung

Metabolic-Endocrine

- Uremia
- Thyrotoxicosis
- Hypothyroidism
- Diabetes

Neurologic

- Multiple sclerosis
  - —Paroxysmal itching
- Notalgia paraesthetic
  - —Local itch of back, medial shaft scapula
- Brain abscess
- CNS infarct

Psychiatric

- Stress
- Delusions of parasitosis

Treatment

INITIAL STABILIZATION

N/A

ED TREATMENT

- Antihistamines are the initial agents of choice for pruritus of undetermined etiology
  - —Nonsedative agents are of use in urticaria, but not with atopic dermatitis
- Topical glucocorticoids are the agents of choice for contact dermatitis
- Emollients are indicated for pruritus secondary to dry skin
- Treatment for scabies and lice should be treated when the rash is suggestive with permethrin cream
- Discontinue medications that may cause an allergic reaction
- Swimmer's itch
  - —Itching is controlled with antihistamines, cool compresses, and calamine lotion
  - —Intense inflammation may be suppressed with topical steroids
  - —Towel drying immediately after leaving the water is an effective preventative measure

MEDICATIONS

- Sedative antihistamines
  - —Chlorpheniramine: 4 mg po qid
  - —Diphenhydramine: 25–50 mg po qid
  - —Hydroxyzine: 10–25 mg po qid
- Nonsedative antihistamines
  - —Terfenadine: 60 mg po bid
  - —Astemizole: 10 mg po qd
- White petroleum emollients: apply after a short bath in warm (not hot) water
- Permethrin 5% cream: apply from the neck down after a bath
  - —Shower thoroughly to remove the medication in 8–12 hours

Disposition

ADMISSION CRITERIA

- Anaphylaxis
- Generalized exfoliating lesions

DISCHARGE CRITERIA

- Refer patients with skin lesions to the primary care physician or dermatologist
- Patients with pruritus without skin lesions should be discharged on antipruritic medication and referred a physician for an underlying systemic illness
- Recommend bicarbonate or oatmeal baths in patients with dry skin

Miscellaneous

ICD9: 698

CORE CONTENT CODE: N/A

SUGGESTED READINGS

Greco PJ, Ende J. Pruritus: A practical approach. J Gen Intern Med 1992;7:340–49.

Kantor GR. Evaluation and treatment of generalized pruritus. Cleve Clin J Med 1990;57:521–26.

Klecz RJ, Schwartz RA. Pruritus. Am Fam Physician 1992;45:2681–686.

Author: Richard Wolfe

Pruritus Ani

Clinical Presentation

SIGNS AND SYMPTOMS

- Itching
  - —Generally worse at night in this very sensitive and richly innervated area
- Relief provided by scratching is very short-lived
- Perirectal appearance
  - —Area may be entirely normal or showing only slight moisture
  - —Erythema and edema common with more chronic symptoms
  - —Maceration, lichenification, and excoriation with more severe symptoms

MECHANISM/DESCRIPTION

- Pruritus ani is not a specific diagnosis, but a symptom, the causes of which are many and diverse

ETIOLOGY

- Hygiene—either poor or overly zealous hygienic practices can result in itching
  - —Most soaps are alkaline and therefore irritating, and too much friction from scrubbing may cause symptoms
- Warm climate, tight and occlusive clothing, obesity, and exercise contribute to perianal moisture and sweating
- Dermatologic causes include
  - —Seborrhea
  - —Psoriasis
  - —Atopic eczema
  - —Urticaria
  - —Lichen planus
  - —Contact dermatitis (consider soaps, powders, deodorants, ointments)
- Over the counter (OTC) remedies including topical anesthetics can make pruritus ani worse
- Parasitic and infectious dermatoses include
  - —Pinworm (Enterobius vermicularis)
  - —Scabies
  - —Lice
  - —Trichomonads
  - —Tinea
  - —Candida—often present but not necessarily the cause of pruritus
- Most anorectal diseases can cause pruritus either primarily or by promoting leakage of irritating stool through the anal sphincter
  - —Skin tags
  - —Hemorrhoids
  - —Fissures
  - —Fistulae
  - —Condylomata
  - —Tumors
  - —Prolapse
  - —Anal sphincter dysfunction
- Loose, irritating loose stools that are more alkaline and that may contain more active digestive enzymes than normal stools
- Psychogenic

Pre-Hospital

N/A

Diagnosis

ESSENTIAL WORKUP

- History
  - —Relationship of pruritus to foods (especially coffee, tea, cola, chocolate, citrus fruit, peppers, milk, alcohol) and activities
  - —Important factors include bowel habits, hygiene, type of clothing, antibiotics, topical compounds, and generalized symptoms including pruritus elsewhere
- Physical examination
  - —Inspection of the anus and perianal skin
  - —Any of the specific diseases listed in differential diagnosis (below) should be apparent

LABORATORY

- Scrapings of the perianal skin mixed with 10% KOH and examined microscopically to diagnose candidiasis
- Cellophane tape pressed onto the perianal skin then placed on a glass slide for microscopy
  - —For suspected pinworm
  - —Best on awakening in the morning

IMAGING/SPECIAL TESTS

- Biopsy
  - —If there is any question about the diagnosis of a lesion
  - —Refer to a colon and rectal surgeon or a dermatologist for examination and procedure

Treatment

INITIAL STABILIZATION

N/A

ED TREATMENT

- Treat specific entity causing symptoms (e.g., pinworm or rectal fissure)
- When no specific lesion is found, the general approach below should be followed
- Avoid all foods which can result in alkaline or irritating stools
  - —Restart one at a time to identify which are problematic
  - —Malt soup extract and foods containing Lactobacillus acidophilus (e.g., yogurt) promote acidic colon flora
- Stop all topical preparations, antibiotics and any other medication which would cause loose stools
- Avoid tight and occlusive clothing
- Practice good hygiene after defecation such as cleansing with moist cotton or soft tissue; possibly a pad such as Tuck's should be used
- Topical preparations
  - —Small amount of plain talcum powder to promote dryness in moist lesions
  - —Petroleum jelly to protect fragile irritated skin
  - —Hydrocortisone cream
  - —Antihistamine (hydroxyzine or diphenhydramine) to stop pruritus

MEDICATIONS

- Diphenhydramine: 25–50 mg (peds: 5 mg/kg/24 hrs) q 4–6 hrs PRN itching
- Hydrocortisone cream 1%: applied sparingly to skin up to 4 times a day to help get over the acute episode (most helpful at night on a PRN basis)
- Hydroxyzine (atarax): 25–50 mg up to every 4 hours PRN itching (may cause drowsiness)

Disposition

ADMISSION CRITERIA

None

DISCHARGE CRITERIA

- Virtually all patients with pruritus ani can be sent home safely with appropriate follow-up

Miscellaneous

ICD9: 698.0

CORE CONTENT CODE: 22.4.24

SUGGESTED READINGS

Daniel GL, Longo WE. Vernava AM 3rd. Pruritus ani: causes and concerns. Dis Colon Rectum 1994;37(7):670–674.

Hoexter B, Labow SB, Moseson M. Common diseases of the anus and rectum. Hosp Med 1985;(Sep):119–144.

Lieberman DA. A basic approach to anorectal ailments. Acute Care Med 1985;(Jun):339–341.

Schrock TR. Diseases of the anorectum. In: Sleisenger MH, Fordtran JS, eds: Gastrointestinal disease. 4th ed. Philadelphia: W.B. Saunders, 1989:1582–1583.

Author: Charles Pattavina

Psoriasis

Clinical Presentation

SIGNS AND SYMPTOMS

- The classic skin lesion is a round red patch with an adhered central plaque of silvery white scale that appears on extensor surfaces (psoriasis vulgaris). The lesions are not usually intensely pruritic, but do itch
- The plaques display a positive Auspitz sign. New lesions may appear in an area of recent skin trauma (Koebner's phenomenon). Pustules may or may not be present. Mucous membranes may be affected. Because areas of disease may coalesce and portions of the lesions may heal, the pattern may be gyrate, nummular, annular, arcuate or circinate
- Scalp lesions may be confused with seborrhea. Lesions that extend beyond the hair borders indicate psoriasis
- Nails may exhibit stippling and pitting and oncolysis. A yellow or brown band across the nail will help differentiate psoriasis (+ band) from onychomycosis (− band)
- The classic arthritis (<5% of cases) is found in the DIP joints of the hands and feet. Asymmetric oligoarticular arthritis is present in the majority of cases (70%) with swelling of the juxtarticular tissue giving a classic "sausage-shape" appearance to the affected digits. There are five arthritis variants

MECHANISM/DESCRIPTION

- The disease displays an autosomal dominant inheritance pattern with incomplete penetration
- Caucasians and atopics are most affected. Cases occur from infancy to adulthood with the majority of cases occurring between 10 and 30 years of age. Equal number of adult male and female cases. In the United States, there are 1000–2000 cases per 100,000 population
- The pathophysiology involves defective inhibition of epidermal proliferation with shortening of the cell cycle and marked increase in cell proliferation and turnover
- The disease is chronic and unpredictable. It has several clinical presentations
  - —Chronic plaque psoriasis: most common form with classic lesions on the scalp, limbs and trunk
  - —Guttate psoriasis: occurs more commonly in children with most lesions found on the trunk
  - —Pustular psoriasis: collections of pustules on one area of the body, usually palms or soles
  - —Erythrodermic psoriasis: the patient may exhibit pustules (von Zumbusch psoriasis) or simple confluent erythroderma
  - —Light-sensitive psoriasis: a Koebner phenomenon response to sunburning
  - —Inverse flexural psoriasis: a variant that causes lesions in flexural areas that don't exhibit scaling due to moisture in these areas
  - —HIV-induced psoriasis: may be a first manifestation of AIDS with an explosive onset of the disease of the erythroderma or pustular variety
  - —Keratoderma blennorrhagicum: psoriasis of the penis seen with Reiter's syndrome with a distinctive winding pattern to the lesion (balanitis circinata)
- In addition to the morphological variants noted above, there are variations in location, presentation, and severity of each of the clinical forms

ETIOLOGY

- The disease has numerous triggers but precise pathogenesis is unknown. Triggers include
  - —Drugs: lithium, β-blockers, antimalarials, steroids, NSAIDs, alcohol, tetracycline, penicillin, amiodarone, morphine, procaine, potassium iodide, sulfapyridine, and sulfonamides
  - —Infections: streptococcal pharyngitis, HIV, viral URI
  - —Local trauma: frostbite, sunburn, routine skin breaks
  - —Stress: emotional and physical
  - —Winter (low light exposure)

PEDIATRIC CONSIDERATIONS

- There are congenital forms of psoriasis and statistical analysis shows that 37% of all cases occur before 20 years of age. In childhood forms, the female cases outnumber male cases 2:1. A child presenting for the first time should have a throat culture and possible antistreptolysin O titer as streptococcal infection is a common precipitant. The younger the patient at onset of disease the worse the course

Pre-Hospital

N/A

Diagnosis

ESSENTIAL WORKUP

- The diagnosis is clinical and rarely is biopsy necessary. History should address
  - —Age at first appearance of eruption
  - —Specific location of eruptions
  - —New lesions in sites of recent trauma (Koebner phenomenon)
  - —Drug history
  - —Family history of the disease
  - —Recent illnesses
  - —History of improvement with sun exposure, or if recurrent, success of prior regimens
  - —Systemic symptoms like fevers and chills or joint pain
- Physical examination should concentrate on diagnostic clues the lesions may exhibit. These clues include
  - —Scalp lesions that extend beyond the hairline
  - —Nails with pits, staining, and hyperkeratosis
  - —Auspitz sign when plaques are removed
  - —Koebner's phenomenon along the lines of recent trauma
  - —"Sausage-shaped" digits from arthritis

LABORATORY

- Elevated sedimentation rate and uric acid
- Decreased serum albumin
- Anemia with B_{12}, folate, and iron deficiency
- Positive streptococcal cultures and titers
- Hypocalcemia and leukocytosis in pustular disease
- Negative rheumatoid factor
- Key biopsy traits include dilated tortuous capillaries (Auspitz sign), hyperkeratosis, epidermal hyperplasia, and Munro microabscesses

IMAGING/SPECIAL TESTS

- Plain radiographs of the hands or feet may show osteoporosis and bone loss at the distal phalanx causing the pencil-in-cup deformation at the MTP or MCP joints. Sacroiliitis and ankylosing spondylitis may also be seen on radiographs

DIFFERENTIAL DIAGNOSIS

- Best thought of by region
  - —Scalp: seborrhea
  - —Flexure creases: candidiasis, intertrigo
  - —Nails: onychomycosis
  - —Trunk and extremities: nummular eczema, pityriasis rosea or rubra pilaris, tinea, SLE, syphilis, drug eruption, atopy, mycosis fungoides, squamous cell carcinoma

PEDIATRIC CONSIDERATIONS

- Do not let young age eliminate the diagnosis
- Order streptococcal tests if the history supports the testing

Treatment

INITIAL STABILIZATION

- Patients are rarely systemically ill except in the generalized erythroderma and pustular forms. These rare patients require general resuscitation efforts aimed at correcting fluid and electrolyte abnormalities and treating sepsis if present. Cultures of skin, blood, and urine should be obtained. Soothing moist compresses are appropriate but occlusive dressings and ointments are contraindicated
- Systemic steroids should not be used as they may predispose to severe complications

ED TREATMENT

- Depending on the severity of the disease therapy may be topical and/or systemic with or without phototherapy
- Phototherapy is not an ED treatment modality
- Systemic therapy should be reserved for the acute erythroderma variant with or without pustulosis as above noted
- Dermatology consult should be obtained in all severe cases

MEDICATIONS

- Localized disease is treated with topical therapy alone. More diffuse disease is treated with topicals and phototherapy. Systemic medication is used in resistant or severe cases
  —Mild to moderate disease: topical treatment is usually reserved for patients with only 10–20% skin involvement. Topical agents include:
    -Emollients: hydrates and softens plaques. Greasier choices work best, but are poorly tolerated by patients for cosmetic reasons
    -Keratolytics: help to remove plaques. Salicylic acid (2–10%) is the mainstay of treatment. Caution must be used near the eyes
    -Tar preparations: usually used alternatively with steroids, with ultraviolet light, or alone. Ointments and shampoos are available. Tar is malodorous, an irritant may be acneiform and rarely induces skin cancer
    -Anthralin: may be used in complex treatment regimens with other topical agents and ultraviolet light. It oxidizes to colored products that stain skin and clothes. It irritates normal skin
    -Corticosteroids: the mainstay of treatment in the U.S. The patients tolerate them well. In doses needed to control the disease, there may be skin thinning, striae, hypopigmentation, and adrenal-pituitary suppression, and tolerance may develop. Best results are obtained by rotating drugs and using occlusive dressings. Fluorinated compounds should be avoided on the face. Small lesions may be treated with intralesional Kenalog as may psoriatic nails. Steroids have been implicated in serious relapses and pustular psoriasis
    -Vitamin D derivatives: calcipotriene is applied to the lesions twice daily. It is well tolerated. It is as effective as medium potency steroids. Hypercalcemia has been reported with excessive use
  —Moderate to severe disease: the above named agents may be employed along with phototherapy and systemic medications
  —Phototherapy
    -The original phototherapy is of course sunlight exposure; however, patients must be warned not sunburn to avoid Koebner phenomenon
    -Ultraviolet B irradiation is combined with coal tar and has reports of 80% remission. It is poorly tolerated, expensive, and time-consuming. Ultraviolet B may be used alone in guttate psoriasis
    -Ultraviolet A irradiation (PUVA) is used with topical agents and systemic agents to gain remission in over 85% of patients using it. Immediate side effects are few and it is well-tolerated
    -Skin damage does occur with intensive therapy and squamous cell carcinoma is a real possibility with cumulative doses
  —Systemic agents: these may be used in various combinations with the above modalities
    -Methotrexate: folic acid antagonist blocks DNA synthesis and cell proliferation. Useful in selected patients. The patient needs renal, liver, and hematological function assessed prior to therapy. Cirrhosis is the most common side effect
    -Etretinate: a retinoid that has several putative actions to treat psoriasis. It causes dryness, scaling, redness, and tenderness of the skin. Patients cannot get pregnant while on this drug. It may be used with PUVA
    -Systemic corticosteroids: not in favor due to iatrogenic Cushing's syndrome. It may worsen the disease when stopped. It may have a role in acute erythrodermic psoriasis where the patient is extremely ill
    -Cyclosporine: the drug blocks steps in the formation of interleukin-2 thereby preventing clinical expression of the disease. Side effects include hypertension and possible irreversible renal disease. It should not be used with phototherapy

PEDIATRIC CONSIDERATIONS

- The emotional side of this chronic disease may be paramount in children whose body image is being formed. In general, the topical agents are well tolerated but PUVA and the systemic agents are generally avoided in children

Disposition

ADMISSION CRITERIA

- Acute erythroderma and acute pustular psoriasis warrant admission for supportive therapy and systemic treatment as above noted

DISCHARGE CRITERIA

- Patients without the above mentioned forms may be safely sent home. Advise patients the disease is not contagious. Warn the patients against excessive scrubbing to loosen scale as it may worsen the disease. Educate the patient on avoiding medications that trigger relapses. Refer patients to the National Psoriasis Foundation (503-244-7404) to help them learn about their diagnosis

PEDIATRIC CONSIDERATIONS

- Except as noted above, no special criteria exist

Miscellaneous

ICD9: 696.1

CORE CONTENT CODE: 3.1.7

SUGGESTED READINGS

Dambro M. Griffith's 5 minute clinical consult. Baltimore: Williams & Wilkins, 1996

Habif T. Psoriasis In: Habif T, ed. Clinical dermatology. 3rd ed. St. Louis: CV Mosby, 1996. pp 190–212.

Schwartz M. Guzzo, C. ed. Psoriasis in 5 Minute pediatric consult. Baltimore: Williams & Wilkins, 1997. pp 622–30.

Wood J. Treatment of psoriasis. N Engl J Med 1995;332:581–588.

Author: Michael G. LaMar

Psychiatric Commitment

Clinical Presentation

SIGNS AND SYMPTOMS

- Psychotic patient
  —Hallucinations
  —Delusions
  —Difficulty concentrating
  —Idiosyncratic speech
- Manic patient
  —Agitated
  —Hyperkinetic
  —Pressured speech
  —Perseveration
  —Delusions of grandeur
  —Hallucinations
  —Acutely manic patient may be indistinguishable from the schizophrenic patient
- Depressed patient
  —Psychomotor retardation
  —Dysphoric mood or affect
  —Suicidal ideation
  —Alteration in eating or sleeping habits
  —Hopelessness
  —Inability to take pleasure in any activities
- Most important signs and symptoms
  —Gross cognitive deficits
  —Suicidal and homicidal ideation

MECHANISM/DESCRIPTION

- Technically, psychiatric commitment refers to an order by a judge for continued hospitalization of an inpatient in a mental health facility for treatment of psychiatric disease against the patient's wishes
- In common usage, the term refers to involuntary admission of an outpatient to a psychiatric hospital by any individual, most commonly a physician

Pre-Hospital

N/A

Diagnosis

ESSENTIAL WORKUP

- Clinical diagnosis through history/mental status exam
  —Areas to focus on
    -Prior diagnosis of psychiatric disease
    -Recent change in behavior or thinking
    -Potentially dangerous behaviors such as violence or those that interfere with activities of daily living
    -Disabling thought patterns such as hallucinations, delusions, and severe deficits in judgment
  —Complete history of medications/substances, including
    -Over-the-counter medications
    -Drugs of abuse
    -Dosages at which the patient has been taking their medications
  —Include tests of thought content and process in mental status exam with attention to the signs and symptoms noted above
  —Rule out organic pathology through
    -A complete and thorough physical exam with attention to the neurologic exam
    -Appropriate use of the lab and radiology

LABORATORY

- Initiate as indicated through history and physical
  —Laboratory investigation not necessary part of every workup
- Electrolytes, BUN, creatinine, glucose
- CBC
  —Attention to the WBC for evidence of infection
- Toxicology screen

IMAGING/SPECIAL TESTS

- CT head if there is evidence of structural CNS pathology

DIFFERENTIAL DIAGNOSIS

- Organic causes of mental status change must be excluded
- Delirium is most important item to rule out
  —Acute alteration of consciousness with an organic etiology characterized by
    -Fluctuating level of consciousness
    -Clouding of sensorium
    -Difficulty focusing attention appropriately
  —Etiology of delirium includes
    -Toxic/metabolic
    -CNS structural
    -Infectious causes

Treatment

INITIAL STABILIZATION

- Assure patient and staff safety

ED TREATMENT

- Restrain dangerous psychiatric patients; options include
  - —Nurse or security guard standing outside the room
  - —Physical restraints
  - —Chemical restraint options
    - -Haldol
    - -Droperidol
    - -Navane
    - -Valium
    - -Ativan
  - —Closely observe patients when using physical or chemical restraints
- Determine if patient is a danger to self or to others or is gravely disabled
  - —Features which indicate danger to self or others include
    - -Suicidal ideation (especially with a plan)
    - -Any desire to harm self
    - -Intention to cause harm to another individual
    - -Grave disability
    - -Any lack of judgment or impairment of cognition so severe as to render the patient unable to care for themselves
  - —Involuntary psychiatric commitment if it is determined that patient is a danger to self or to others, or is gravely disabled
    - -Legal procedures required for involuntary commitment vary from state to state and the physician should be aware of the laws in his or her area
    - -Usually there is a form the physician must sign attesting that the patient meets one of the above mentioned criteria and explaining why
    - -Often leads to 72-hour mandatory hospitalization
  - —Voluntary psychiatric admission for psychiatric patients whose condition is causing them great emotional distress, but do not meet the above criteria

MEDICATIONS

- Ativan: 1–3 mg IV/IM/PO
- Droperidol: 1.25–5 mg IV/IM
- Haldol: 2.5–10 mg IM
- Navane: 10 mg IM
- Valium: 5–10 mg IV/IM/PO

Disposition

ADMISSION CRITERIA

- Danger to self or to others or gravely disabled

DISCHARGE CRITERIA

- Even if a patient's ideas are vastly different from one's own *it is only if the ideas place patient's health or the health of others in danger* that the patient may be involuntarily committed
- Patients who can care for themselves adequately and have no intentions of harm may be discharged, if they wish

Miscellaneous

ICD9: N/A

CORE CONTENT CODE: 14.10

SUGGESTED READINGS

Burzan RD, Weissberg MP. Suicide: risk factors and therapeutic considerations in the emergency department. J Emerg Med 1992;10:335.

Folstein MF, Folstein FE, McHugh PR. The "mini-mental state": a practical method for grading the cognitive state of patients for the clinician. J Psychiatr Res 1975;12:189.

Nickens HW. Assessment and management of the violent patient. In: Dubin WR, Homke N, Nichory H, eds. Clinics in emergency medicine: psychiatric emergencies. Vol. 4. Churchill Livingstone: Edinburgh. 1984:101–11.

Author: Nicholas A. Schwartz

Psychosis, Acute

Clinical Presentation

SIGNS AND SYMPTOMS

- Delusions
  - —Erroneous beliefs that involve a misinterpretation of perceptions
  - —Beliefs are clearly implausible, are not derived from normal life experiences
  - —These beliefs are often persecutory, religious or somatic in nature
- Hallucinations
  - —A sensory experience that does not exist except in the mind of the person experiencing it
  - —Hallucinations can involve any sense but auditory or visual are most common
- Disorganized speech
  - —Loose associations
  - —Neologisms
  - —Perseverations
  - —Poverty of content
  - —Word salad
- Disorganized or catatonic behavior
  - —Difficulty in performing goal-directed behavior
  - —Lack of awareness of the environment
- Negative symptoms
  - —Flattened affect
  - —Poverty of speech
  - —Avolition
    - -An inability to initiate and persist in goal-directed activities
- Features suggesting an organic etiology
  - —Sudden onset
  - —>40 years old
  - —Fluctuating course
  - —Confusion
  - —Headaches
  - —Loss of consciousness
  - —Focal neurologic symptoms
  - —Speech difficulties
  - —Abnormal vital signs
  - —Disorientation
  - —Psychomotor retardation
  - —Visual hallucinations
  - —Global impairment of attention and cognitive function
  - —Delusions are disorganized
  - —Labile affect
  - —Incoherent speech
  - —Social immodesty

MECHANISM/DESCRIPTION

- A description of behavior that does not imply a specific cause or diagnosis in general
- The psychosis may be secondary to functional (psychiatric) or organic (medical) causes
- Medical psychoses are generally secondary to systemic or neurologic diseases, or neuroactive medications
- Neurodevelopmental abnormalities in the dopaminergic and serotonergic systems are implicated in functional psychosis

ETIOLOGY

Organic

- Central nervous system
- Encephalopathy
- Seizure
- Head injury
- Neoplasms
- Migraine
- Huntington's chorea
- CVA
- Metabolic
  - —Intoxication or withdrawal
  - —Hypercarbia
  - —Hypoglycemia
  - —Hypoxia
  - —Poisoning
  - —Electrolyte imbalance
- Endocrine
  - —Addison's disease
  - —Thyroid dysfunction
  - —Parathyroid dysfunction
- Other
  - —Autoimmune disorders
  - —Hepatic encephalopathy
  - —Renal failure

Pharmacologic

- Psychoactive agents
- Benzodiazepines
- Chlordiazepoxide
- Antidepressants
- Antiepileptics
- Antibiotics
  - —Isoniazid
  - —Rifampin
- Cardiovascular agents
- Captopril
- Digoxin
- Methyldopa
- Procainamide
- Propranolol
- Reserpine
- Drugs of abuse
  - —Alcohol
  - —Amphetamines
  - —Cocaine
  - —Opioids
  - —Hallucinogens
- Other
  - —Steroids
  - —Heavy metals
  - —Antihistamines
  - —Cimetidine
  - —Disulfiram

Functional

- Brief psychotic disorder
  - —Usually secondary to acute emotional stress
- Schizophreniform disorder
  - —Symptoms present 1–6 months
- Schizophrenia
- Mood disorder with psychotic features or schizoaffective disorder

Pre-Hospital

CAUTIONS

- Prevention of violent behavior must be established before transport
- If the patient is violent, threatening, or an immediate perceived danger, involve police backup to reduce risk of violence and to place restraints

CONTROVERSIES

- Chemical restraints are rarely included in field protocols, but may be a useful adjunct to physical restraints

Diagnosis

ESSENTIAL WORKUP

- The workup is case-specific and is primarily based upon the suspected etiology
- Functional and organic etiologies are generally distinguished by features of the history and physical examination described below
- Collateral history is important as the patient history is often unreliable
- Complete physical exam with particular attention to the neurological exam, vital signs, and mental status exam
- Mental status exam
  - —Orientation
  - —Memory (short and long)
  - —Attention (or calculation)
  - —Recall
  - —Language
  - —Thoughts
  - —Perception
  - —Mood/affect
  - —Judgement

LABORATORY

- Laboratory evaluation is needed in patients at risk for an organic etiology
  - —Specific studies should be guided by the suspected underlying etiologies
  - —Serum glucose
  - —Toxicological screen
  - —Serum electrolytes
  - —Urinalysis

IMAGING/SPECIAL TESTS

- Head CT Scan indicated in patients at risk for a neurologic etiology
- Lumbar puncture indicated if signs and symptoms suggest delirium

DIFFERENTIAL DIAGNOSIS

- See etiology

Treatment

INITIAL STABILIZATION

- Prevention of violence
  - —Psychotic patients are irrational, unpredictable, and potentially violent in their behavior
  - —Patient and staff safety must be immediately assessed
  - —If the patient is violent, threatening, or there is an immediate perceived danger, call security and employ physical or chemical restraint

ED TREATMENT

- Antipsychotic agents are symptom-specific, not disease-specific, and therefore are useful in psychoses of both organic or functional etiology
- High potency, intravenous antipsychotics, such as haloperidol and droperidol, are most commonly utilized in the ED setting
- Rapid tranquilization may be achieved with the addition of a benzodiazepine
- If a specific organic etiology is identified, therapy should be directed towards the treatment of the medical condition
- Treatment of adverse effects from antipsychotic medications
  - —Extrapyramidal symptoms
    - -Dystonia, akathisia, pseudoparkinsonism and tardive dyskinesia
    - -Treat with diphenhydramine or benztropine
  - —Neuroleptic malignant syndrome
    - -Life-threatening complication
    - -Characterized by hyperthermia, muscle rigidity, autonomic instability and altered consciousness
    - -Treat with supportive measures and dantrolene

MEDICATIONS

- Antipsychotics
  - —Droperidol: 2.5–5.0 mg IV or IM
  - —Haloperidol: 2–5 mg IV or IM; 0.5–2.0 mg for elderly
  - —Risperidone: 1–2 mg po
- Treatment of medication side-effects
  - —Benztropine: 2 mg IM or IV
  - —Diphenhydramine: 50 mg IV, IM, or po
  - —Dantrolene: 1 mg/kg IV repeated to symptom resolution or total of 10 mg/kg

Disposition

ADMISSION CRITERIA

- If the cause is determined to be medical in origin, admission to the appropriate medical service is indicated
- Acute psychosis of psychiatric etiology requires admission to a psychiatric service
- Safety of staff and patient must be maintained in the hospital after disposition from the ED, including possible chemical and physical restraint or a one-on-one sitter
- If the patient is felt to be a danger to either self or others, the patient *cannot* be discharged
- Involuntary commitment is required if patient is uncooperative and a threat to self or others

DISCHARGE CRITERIA

- If the psychotic behavior was caused by a temporary, reversible organic cause (e.g., drug intoxication) and the patient is now deemed to be in control, competent, and not a danger to self or others the patient may be discharged
- Psychiatric consultation prior to discharge is recommended

Miscellaneous

ICD9: 297, 298, 299

CORE CONTENT CODE: 13.8.4

SUGGESTED READINGS

Anderson WH, Kuehanle JC. Diagnosis and early management of acute psychosis. N Engl J Med 1989;305:1128.

Frame DS, Kercher EE. Acute psychosis: Functional vs. organic. Emerg Med Clin North Am 1991;9:123–36.

Hutzler JC, Rund DA. Behavioral disorders: Emergency assessment and stabilization. In: Tintinalli JE, Ruiz E, Krome RL, eds. Emergency medicine: A comprehensive study guide. 4th ed. New York: McGraw-Hill, 1996.

Author: Robert J. Vissers

Psychosis, Medical vs. Psychiatric

Clinical Presentation

SIGNS AND SYMPTOMS

- Psychosis characterized by
  - —Impaired reality testing
  - —Inappropriate affect
  - —Poor impulse control
  - —Regressive or inappropriate behavior
- Hallucinations
  - —Auditory
  - —Visual
  - —Olfactory
  - —Tactile
- Delusions
  - —False beliefs held strongly by the patient even in the face of reasonable evidence to the contrary
- Affective symptoms include mania and catatonic states
- Focal and diffuse central nervous system (CNS) impairment result in derangements of
  - —Thinking
  - —Communicating
  - —Perceiving
- Responding appropriately

MECHANISM/DESCRIPTION

- Wide variety of medical and neurological illnesses have psychosis as one of their presenting manifestations or which emerge during the course of the illness
- Difficult to determine whether medical or psychiatric illness is the cause of psychotic behavior
- Nature of impairment determines whether a primarily psychiatric disorder or a secondary psychosis based on a medical, neurological, or toxic etiology
- Evaluation for underlying medical or neurologic condition essential for patients with psychotic presentation without previous history of psychosis

ETIOLOGY

- Age factor
  - —Late adolescence/early adulthood presentation more likely to be schizophrenia
  - —Middle to late life presentation more likely to be medical cause
- Etiology of the CNS impairment that results in a psychotic presentation include
  - —Neurological disorders
  - —Metabolic conditions
  - —Toxic or drug effects
  - —Nonorganic or psychiatric

Pre-Hospital

N/A

Diagnosis

ESSENTIAL WORKUP

- Careful history and physical examination
- Laboratory investigation for new or previously undiagnosed psychosis
- Use history and physical to guide direction

LABORATORY

- CBC
- Electrolytes, BUN/Cr, glucose
- Toxicology screen
- Ammonium level
- Urinalysis
- Thyroid function tests

IMAGING/SPECIAL TESTS

- CT head
- Lumbar puncture/CSF analysis

DIFFERENTIAL DIAGNOSIS

- Neurologic
  - —Head trauma
  - —Space-occupying lesions
  - —Cerebrovascular disease
  - —Postanoxic encephalopathy
  - —Seizure disorders
- Degenerative diseases
  - —Alzheimer's
  - —Pick's
  - —Huntington's
  - —Parkinsonism
  - —Hydrocephalus
- CNS infections
- Viral
- Herpetic
- Nonherpetic (e.g., rabies, mumps, influenza)
- Slow virus diseases
  - —Cerebral malaria
  - —Syphilis
  - —Toxoplasmosis
  - —Trypanosomiasis
  - —Schistosomiasis
- Myelin diseases
- Multiple sclerosis
- Leukodystrophies
- Marchiafava-Bignami disease
- Narcolepsy
- Endocrine
- Thyroid disorders
- Parathyroid disorders
- Diabetes mellitus
- Pituitary abnormalities
- Adrenal abnormalities
- Postpartum psychosis
- Metabolic
  - —Electrolyte imbalance
- End-organ failure
  - —Respiratory cardiac
  - —Renal
  - —Hepatic
  - —Pancreatic

- Ketoacidosis
- Porphyria
- Wilson's disease
- Deficiency diseases
  —Pernicious anemia
  —Beriberi, Wernicke-Korsakoff syndrome
  —Pellagra
  —Pyridoxine deficiency
- Systemic illnesses
  —Carcinomatosis
  —Infections, sepsis
- Viral syndromes
  —Hepatitis
  —Mononucleosis
- Collagen and autoimmune disorders
- Postoperative states
  —Delirium
  —Psychosis
  —Depression
- Intoxicants
  —Alcohol
  —Barbiturates
- Stimulants
- Hallucinogens
- Opiates
- Heavy metals
- Bromide
- Organic phosphates
- Anticholinergic compounds
- Carbon monoxide
- Industrial agents
- Withdrawal states
  —Alcohol withdrawal (delirium tremens)
  —Barbiturate withdrawal
- Medication side effects
  —Antipsychotics
  —Steroids
  —Sedative-hypnotics
  —Antidepressants
  —Lithium carbonate
  —Cimetidine
  —Disulfiram
  —Belladonna alkaloids
  —Levodopa
  —Anticonvulsants
  —Antituberculous drugs
  —Anti-inflammatory drugs
  —Antihypertensive agents
  —Cardiac drugs digitalis lidocaine propranolol procainamide
  —Idiosyncratic drug reaction of any medication
- Psychiatric
  —Schizophrenia
  —Manic-depressive illness
  —Stress reactions including posttraumatic stress disorder (PTSD)
  —Intermittent explosive disorder
  —Impulse control disorder

Treatment

INITIAL STABILIZATION

- ABCs
- If uncooperative and dangerous, control behavior with neuroleptics or benzodiazepines

ED TREATMENT

- Determine if a medical cause for psychosis
- Treat underlying illness
- Psychiatric evaluation for true psychosis
- Control psychotic behavior with psychotropic medications
  —Treatment approach based on the severity of the psychotic features of the medical or psychiatric illness
  —Severe behavioral disturbance of medical psychosis requires sedating the patient to adequately attend to the medical work up and treatment
  —The more behaviorally unstable the patient, the more difficult it is to stabilize medical derangements
- Haloperidol or droperidol in combination with lorazepam
  —Safest, fastest, and least disruptive of the ongoing mental examination of the patient
  —Calms and sedates the behaviorally agitated, psychotic, medical patient effectively

MEDICATIONS

- Neuroleptics
  —Droperidol: 2.5–5 mg IV
  —Haloperidol: 2.5–10 mg IM/IV
- Benzodiazepines
  —Lorazepam: 0.5–2 mg IV/IM
  —Diazepam: 5–10 mg IV
  —Midazolam: 1–5 mg IV

Disposition

ADMISSION CRITERIA

- Psychosis primarily psychiatric (i.e., schizophrenia/manic depressive)
- Admission same as for involuntary commitment
  —Suicidal/homicidal behavior
  —Inability to care for self
  —Deranged thought pattern that can be threat to self or others
- Psychosis primarily medical etiology
- Admission dictated by specific medical condition and behavior

DISCHARGE CRITERIA

- Stable medical condition
- Not suicidal/homicidal
- Able to care for self
- Decisionally capacitated

Miscellaneous

ICD9: 289.9

CORE CONTENT CODE: N/A

SUGGESTED READINGS

Cummings JL. Secondary psychoses, delusions, and schizophrenia. In: Cummings, JL, ed. Clinical neuropsychiatry. Orlando, FL: Grune & Stratton, 1985:163–82.

Goff D, Manschreck TC, Groves JE. Psychotic patients. In: Cassem NH, ed. Handbook of general hospital psychiatry. St Louis: Mosby Yearbook, 1991:217–36.

Author: K. Sanders

Pulmonary Contusion

Clinical Presentation

SIGNS AND SYMPTOMS

- Dyspnea, tachypnea; onset may be insidious, increasing over time
- Ecchymosis, bony crepitus and tenderness associated with rib fractures
- Hemoptysis
- Cyanosis, tachycardia, hypotension
- Assume all patients with flail chest have a pulmonary contusion
- Auscultation: initially normal breath sounds progressing to wet rales or absent breath sounds

MECHANISM/DESCRIPTION

- Direct chest wall trauma or sudden deceleration, fall from height, motor vehicle accident, missile wounds
- Direct injury from the transfer of kinetic energy to the lung parenchyma results in disruption of the alveolocapillary membrane
- Microhemorrhage, localized pulmonary edema, and extravasation of blood into the interstitial and alveolar spaces produce arteriovenous shunting, ventilation-perfusion mismatch, decreased lung compliance, hypoxemia, and potential respiratory failure
- The major problem with pulmonary contusion is the ensuing hypoxemia

PEDIATRIC CONSIDERATIONS

- Relatively more elastic chest wall may transmit greater force to the thoracic contents in children

Pre-Hospital

CAUTIONS

- Patients with chest trauma associated with a motor vehicle accident, significant fall, or preexisting lung disease should be routed to the nearest trauma facility
- Patients with significant respiratory distress from pulmonary contusion benefit from early intubation to correct hypoxemia and decrease the work of breathing

Diagnosis

ESSENTIAL WORKUP

- Chest radiograph
  - —Radiographic findings may not appear until 6–12 hours postinjury
  - —Patchy alveolar infiltrates to frank consolidation
  - —Associated intrathoracic injury such as rib fractures, pneumothorax, hemothorax, and widened mediastinal silhouette

LABORATORY

- Arterial blood gas may be helpful in assessing the degree of hypoxemia and demonstrate an elevated A-a gradient

IMAGING/SPECIAL TESTS

- Thoracic computed tomography (CT) may be a useful adjunct in defining associated thoracic injuries

DIFFERENTIAL DIAGNOSIS

- Adult respiratory distress syndrome (ARDS)
- Pulmonary laceration
- Congestive heart failure
- Pneumonia or other infectious process
- Noncardiogenic causes of pulmonary edema

Treatment

INITIAL STABILIZATION

- ABCs
- *Control airway as needed,* endotracheal intubation made be indicated for patients with severe hypoxemia (PaO_2 <60 mm Hg on room air, <80 mm Hg on O_2), significant underlying lung disease or impending respiratory failure
- Early intubation and institution of positive end expiratory pressure (PEEP) is beneficial to correct hypoxemia and acidosis, as well as decrease the work of breathing

ED TREATMENT

- Maintain adequate oxygenation, monitor O_2 saturation and respiratory rate
- In the conscious and alert patient, passive O_2 administration via facemask is first-line therapy. If the patient cannot maintain a PaO_2 >80 mm Hg on high flow oxygen then continuous positive airway pressure (CPAP) via mask or nasal BiPAP can be attempted
- *Avoid overhydration.* Intravenous crystalloid administration needed for resuscitation must be balanced with the risk of increasing interstitial pulmonary edema. Frequent reexamination and serial chest radiographs are required to monitor alveolar fluid accumulation

MEDICATIONS

- The benefits of *steroids* are controversial and remain unproven
- *Prophylactic antibiotics are not indicated*

Disposition

ADMISSION CRITERIA

- Patients with pulmonary contusion must be admitted to the hospital for observation in anticipation of delayed onset respiratory compromise

DISCHARGE CRITERIA

- Patients with minimal chest trauma, no evidence of respiratory distress, or hypoxemia, and clear chest x-ray may be discharged
- Strict instructions should be given to return for shortness of breath, chest pain, or development of any of the above signs of pulmonary contusion

Miscellaneous

ICD9: 861.21

CORE CONTENT CODE: 18.4.10.8

SUGGESTED READINGS

Committee on Trauma, American College of Surgeons. Advanced trauma life support instructor manual. 5th ed. Chicago: American College of Surgeons, 1993.

Vukich D, Markovchick V. Thoracic trauma. In: Rosen P, et al., eds. Emergency medicine: Concepts and clinical practice. 4th ed. St. Louis: CV Mosby, 1998:514.

Wilson R. Thoracic trauma. In: Tintinalli J, et al., eds. Emergency medicine: A comprehensive study guide. 4th ed. New York: McGraw Hill, 1996:1156.

Author: Greg Lampe

Pulmonary Edema

Clinical Presentation

SIGNS AND SYMPTOMS

- General
  - —Weakness
  - —Fatigue
  - —Anxiety
  - —Diaphoresis
  - —Cold, ashen, or cyanotic skin
- Respiratory
  - —Shortness of breath
  - —Dyspnea with exertion
  - —Orthopnea, paroxysmal nocturnal dyspnea
  - —Cough,
    - -Pink, frothy sputum
  - —Noisy respirations
  - —Tachypnea
  - —Wheezing, rhonchi, gurgles
  - —Moist, crepitant rales noted initially at bases and progressing to apices
  - —Dilated alae nasi
  - —Inspiratory retraction of the intercostal spaces or supraventricular fossae
  - —Cheyne-Stokes respirations
- Cardiovascular
  - —Tachycardia
  - —Jugular venous hypertension
  - —Abnormal heart sounds
    - -Increased P2
    - -S3
    - -S4
  - —Nocturnal angina
  - —Pulsus alternans or presence of valvular heart disease

MECHANISM/DESCRIPTION

- A pathological increase in the net flux of liquid, colloid, and solutes from the pulmonary vasculature into the interstitial space
- Four possible mechanisms may lead to pulmonary edema
  - —Hydrostatic edema
    - -Determined by the Starling equation

$$Q_{(iv\text{-}int)} = K_f\,[(P_{iv}-P_{int}) - \Sigma_f\,(II_{iv}-II_{int})]$$

Q = net rate of transudation

P_{int} = interstitial hydrostatic pressures

P_{iv} = intravascular hydrostatic pressures

II_{int} = interstitial colloid osmotic pressure

II_{iv} = intravascular colloid osmotic pressure

S_f = reflection coefficient for proteins

K_f = hydraulic conductance

  - —Acute respiratory distress syndrome
    - -Permeability edema caused by diffuse alveolar damage
  - —Permeability edema without alveolar damage
  - —Mixed hydrostatic and permeability edema
- Mortality approximately 50–60% for noncardiogenic pulmonary edema and up to 80% for cardiogenic shock

ETIOLOGY

Hydrostatic

- Cardiogenic
  - —Left heart failure
  - —Ischemic heart disease
  - —Acute myocardial infarction
  - —Aortic and mitral valvular disease
  - —Hypertensive heart disease
  - —Cardiomyopathy
  - —Volume overload
  - —Arrhythmias
  - —Endocarditis
  - —Myocarditis
  - —Congenital heart disease
  - —Acute rheumatic fever and rheumatic heart disease
  - —Septal defects
  - —High cardiac output states
    - -Thyrotoxicosis
    - -Beriberi
- Hypoalbuminemia
  - —Renal failure
  - —Hepatic failure
  - —Protein-losing enteropathic
  - —Severe dermatological disease with high protein losses
  - —Starvation
- Increased negativity of interstitial pressure
  - —Rapid decompression of a pneumothorax
  - —Asthma
- Lymphatic obstruction
  - —Postlung transplant
  - —Lymphangitic carcinomatosis
  - —Fibrosing lymphangitis

Adult Respiratory Distress Syndrome

- Pneumonia
- Inhaled toxins
- Circulating foreign substances
  - —Snake venom
  - —Endotoxins
- Aspiration
- Acute radiation pneumonitis
- Disseminated intravascular coagulation
- Hypersensitivity pneumonitis
- Shock lung in association with nonthoracic trauma
- Acute hemorrhagic pancreatitis

Unknown Mechanism

- High-altitude pulmonary edema
- Neurogenic pulmonary edema
- Narcotic overdose
- Pulmonary embolism
- Eclampsia
- Postcardioversion
- Postanesthesia
- Postcardiopulmonary bypass

Pre-Hospital

- Intravenous access
- Supplemental oxygen
  - —100% non rebreather mask
- Cardiac monitor
- Pulse oximetry
- Sublingual nitrates
- Furosemide
- Endotracheal intubation may be required in severe cases

CAUTIONS

- Administration of morphine
  - —Pulmonary edema may be difficult to distinguish from an acute exacerbation of COPD

Diagnosis

ESSENTIAL WORKUP

- A careful history and physical should determine if the underlying etiology is cardiogenic

LABORATORY

- Studies are nonspecific for pulmonary edema but may be helpful in determining the underlying etiology
- Serum electrolytes
  - —Generally normal before treatment
  - —Hyperkalemia with severe low output states
- BUN and creatinine
  - —Elevation in severe CHF
- Cardiac enzymes may be useful if ischemia or infarction is presumed to be the underlying cause
- Serum lipase if pancreatitis is suspected as the underlying cause
- Arterial blood gas
  - —Clinical assessment and pulse oximetry are more cost-effective in determining ED management

IMAGING/SPECIAL TESTS

Chest radiograph

- 3 phases of pulmonary findings
  - —Pulmonary redistribution
    - -Cephalization of vessels
  - —Interstitial edema
    - -Effusions
    - -Kerley B lines
    - -Classic butterfly infiltrate
  - —Frank alveolar infiltrates
    - -May be asymmetric and mistaken for pneumonia
    - -Especially common in patients with COPD

EKG

- Assess for underlying cardiac disorders

Echocardiography

- Excludes acute valvular pathology
- Assessment for focal or global LV dysfunction
- Measurement of cardiac output

DIFFERENTIAL DIAGNOSIS

- Pneumonia
- Asthma
- COPD exacerbation
- Pulmonary embolism
- Hyperventilation syndrome
- Pericardial tamponade

Treatment

INITIAL STABILIZATION

- Intravenous access
- Supplemental oxygen
- Place patient in an upright position
- Cardiac monitor
- Pulse oximetry
- Control airway as needed
  - —Continuous positive airway pressure
    - -CPAP
    - -Nasal Bi-PAP
    - -May decrease the need for intubation
- Endotracheal intubation for impending respiratory failure

ED TREATMENT

- Normotensive or hypertensive patients with cardiogenic pulmonary edema
  - —Rapid-acting nitrates
  - —IV nitroglycerin
  - —Morphine sulfate
  - —Intravenous diuretics
    - -Lasix or bumex
  - —Sodium nitroprusside for afterload reduction may be required for severe persistent hypertension
- Hypotensive patients
  - —Avoid nitrates, morphine and diuretics
  - —Use agents that increase myocardial contractility
    - -Dopamine
    - -Dobutamine
    - -Amrinone
    - -Milrinone
- Renal dialysis patients
  - —Emergent renal dialysis is the treatment of choice
  - —If rapid dialysis cannot be rapidly achieved
    - -IV nitroglycerin
    - -Phlebotomy of 1 unit of blood
      - *If collected properly, can then be autotransfused postdialysis

MEDICATIONS

- Furosemide: 20–80 mg IV
- Morphine sulfate: 2–5 mg IV
- Nitroglycerin paste: 1–2 inches; begin drip at 5 μg/min and increase by 5–10 μg/min every few minutes; titrate to blood pressure
- Isosorbide: 60 mg po tid-qid
- Nitroprusside: begin drip at 10 μg/min and increasing by 5–10 μg/min every few minutes
- Dobutamine: begin at 2 μg/kg/min IV; titrate to blood pressure, cardiac output, and pulmonary capillary wedge pressure
- Captopril: 25–25 mg po tid
- Digoxin: 0.125–0.25 mg po qd
- Enalapril: 5–15 mg po qd-bid
- Furosemide: 400 mg daily
- Hydralazine: 100 mg po qid
- Hydrochlorothiazide: 5–50 mg po qd
- Lisinopril: 5–20 mg po qd

Disposition

ADMISSION CRITERIA

- Intensive care unit
  - —Intubated patients
  - —Patients on Bi-PAP
  - —Adult respiratory distress syndrome
- Monitored unit
  - —New onset pulmonary edema
  - —Electrocardiographic changes
- Observation
  - —Known congestive heart failure with mild to moderate disease

DISCHARGE CRITERIA

- Patients with known congestive heart failure presenting with mild pulmonary edema
  - —Complete resolution of symptoms after ED management
  - —Normal oxygenation on room air at the time of discharge
  - —No new electrocardiographic changes
- Followup arranged within the next 48 hours
- Low-salt diet
- Serial weights to assess fluid accumulation

Miscellaneous

ICD9: 518.4

CORE CONTENT CODE: 2.2.1; 2.2.1.1; 2.2.1.2; 5.4.3; 16.5

SUGGESTED READINGS

Braunwald E. Pulmonary edema. In: Braunwald E. Heart disease: A textbook of cardiovascular medicine. 5th ed. Philadelphia: WB Saunders, 1997:464–467.

Ketai LH, Godwin JD. A new view of pulmonary edema and acute respiratory distress syndrome. J Thorac Imaging 1998;13:147–71.

Pang D, Keenan SP, Cook DJ, et al. The Effect of positive pressure airway support on mortality and the need for intubation in cardiogenic pulmonary edema. A systematic review. Chest 1998;114:1186–192.

Authors: Jonathan Edlow; Richard Wolfe

Pulmonary Embolism

Clinical Presentation

SIGNS AND SYMPTOMS

- Most common
  - —Dyspnea
  - —Pleuritic chest pain
  - —Tachycardia
- General
  - —Apprehension
  - —Diaphoresis
- Pulmonary
  - —Cough
  - —Hemoptysis
  - —Rales
  - —Wheezing
- Cardiovascular
  - —Syncope
  - —Loud P2
  - —S3 or S4 gallop
  - —Diaphoresis
  - —Cardiac murmurs
- Cyanosis
  - —Extremities
  - —Evidence of thrombophlebitis
  - —Lower extremity edema

MECHANISM/DESCRIPTION

- Vast majority arise from thrombi in the deep veins of the femur and pelvis
- Thrombi in the lower extremities occasionally propagate to the popliteal veins from where they embolize

ETIOLOGY

- Most patients with pulmonary embolus (PE) have an identifiable risk factor
- Risk factors
  - —Recent surgery
  - —Pregnancy
  - —Cardiac disease
  - —Stroke or recent paraplegia
  - —Malignancy
  - —Age past the fifth decade
  - —Previous DVT
  - —Immobilization
  - —Oral contraceptives
  - —Major trauma
  - —Factor deficiency state
    - -Mutations in factor 5 resulting in activated protein C resistance
    - -Protein C and S
    - -Plasminogen and antithrombin 3 deficiency
  - —Antiphospholipid antibody syndrome

PEDIATRIC CONSIDERATIONS

- Risk factors for children in decreasing order of prevalence
  - —Presence of central venous catheter
  - —Immobility
  - —Heart disease
  - —Ventriculoatrial shunt
  - —Trauma
  - —Neoplasm
  - —Surgery
  - —Infection
  - —Medical illness
  - —Dehydration
  - —Shock

Pre-Hospital

CAUTIONS

- Initiate supplemental oxygen
- Establish IV access
- Cardiac monitor

Diagnosis

ESSENTIAL WORKUP

- CXR
  - —To rule out other causes
  - —Most common findings with PE
    - -Normal
    - -Nonspecific pulmonary infiltrates
    - -Atelectasis
  - —Other findings with PE
    - -Pleural effusions
    - -Pleural based opacities (when wedged shaped called Hampton hump)
    - -Elevated hemidiaphragms
    - -Local oligemia (Westermark's sign)
    - -Enlarged right descending pulmonary artery (Palla's sign)
- ECG
  - —To rule out a cardiac etiology
  - —Findings in PE
    - -Nonspecific ST-T wave changes
    - -T-wave inversion in anterior leads
    - -Sinus tachycardia
- Normal ECG
  - —Left axis deviation
  - —RBBB pattern
  - —Atrial fibrillation
  - —S1Q3T3 pattern—uncommon and not specific enough to rule-in diagnosis of PE
- Assess oxygenation
  - —Pulse oximetry
    - -Rapidly attained
  - —Arterial blood gases
    - -Assesses pO_2 and pCO_2
    - -Do not aid in the diagnosis
    - -PE possible with normal Alveolar-arterial gradient

LABORATORY

- CBC
  - —Anemia may be a contributing factor to dyspnea
  - —Very high WBC might suggest infectious etiology
- d-dimer enzyme-linked immunosorbent assay (ELISA)
  - —High sensitivity with low specificity for PE
  - —High negative predictive value (>90%)
  - —Requires 3–4 hours to perform

IMAGING/SPECIAL TESTS

- Ventilation perfusion (V/Q) scan
  - —Results reported in probabilities: normal, low, intermediate, or high probability
  - —Probability of PE with V/Q results
    - -Normal or near normal V/Q scan: 4% probability for PE
    - -Low probability V/Q scan with low clinical suspicion: 4% probability for a PE
    - -Low probability V/Q scan with high clinical suspicion: 16–40% probability for a PE

- –Intermediate V/Q scan: 16–66% probability of PE
- –High probability V/Q scan with low clinical suspicion: 56% probability of PE
- –High probability V/Q scan with high clinical suspicion: 96% probability of PE

- Spiral chest CT with IV contrast
  - —Accurate for identifying PE in proximal pulmonary vascular tree
  - —May be normal with small distal PE
  - —Pulmonary angiography
  - —Gold standard
  - —Use when diagnosis not excluded or confirmed
  - —Intermediate probability (10–80%) VQ scan
  - —Normal CT when distal PE suspected
  - —Higher complication rate than other modalities
  - —Lower extremity duplex ultrasound
  - —Used in patients who would otherwise require pulmonary angiography
  - —Presence of deep vein thrombosis requires same anticoagulation as PE

DIFFERENTIAL DIAGNOSIS

- Pneumonia
- Cardiac dysrhythmias (due to syncope)
- Asthma
- Pneumothorax
- Pleural effusion
- Pericarditis
- Myocardial infarction
- Rib fracture
- Musculoskeletal pain
- Pulmonary edema

Treatment

INITIAL STABILIZATION

- ABCs
- Provide supplemental oxygen to maintain adequate oxygen saturation with nasal cannula or face mask
- Intubation for if unable to provide adequate oxygen
- Administer IV fluid carefully for hypotensive patients
- Excessive fluid expansion may worsen right heart failure

ED TREATMENT

- —Initiate heparin
  - –Prevents additional thrombus from forming
  - –Goal is to maintain the PTT between 1.5 and 2.5 times the control value (60–80 seconds)
- Warfarin
  - —Begin once a therapeutic PTT is achieved
  - —Continue for 5 days with concurrent heparin administration
  - —Goal is INR of 2–3
- Thrombolysis
  - —Initiate in hemodynamically unstable patients with massive PE
  - —Stop heparin while infusing TPA
  - —Restart heparin when PTT falls in therapeutic range (1.5–2.5 times control)
- Inferior vena cava (IVC) filter
  - —Indicated in patients who cannot tolerate anticoagulation and who have been on therapeutic anticoagulation but failed
- Norepinephrine
  - —Initiate with massive PE and hypotension

MEDICATIONS

- Heparin options
  - —Initial bolus of 80 units/kg IV followed by continuous infusion of 18 units/kg/hr
  - —Initial bolus of 5,000 units IV followed by 1,280 units/hr
  - —TPA 100 mg IV over 2 hrs
- Norepinephrine: 2–20 μg/min IV
- Coumadin: 5 mg loading dose orally each day, titrate PT to an INR of 2–3

PEDIATRIC CONSIDERATIONS

- Heparin dosing: 50 IU/kg bolus IV followed by 10–25 IU/kg/hr continuously
- Thrombolytic dosing
  - —TPA: 0.1–0.5 mg/kg body weight per hour (use for as long as 3 days)
    - –TPA is not approved by the FDA for use in children
  - —Streptokinase: 3,500–4,000 IU/kg loading dose over 30 min followed by 1,000–1,500 IU/kg/hr
  - —Urokinase: 4,400 IU/kg loading dose over 10 min followed by 4,400 IU/kg/hr

Disposition

ADMISSION CRITERIA

- Admit all patients with PE for heparin therapy
- Cases with a high suspicion for PE, no contraindication to anticoagulation, and a lack of V/Q scanning or angiographic availability may be anticoagulated and studied when resources are available in the morning or upon transfer

DISCHARGE CRITERIA

N/A

Miscellaneous

ICD9: 415.1

CORE CONTENT CODE: 16.9

SUGGESTED READINGS

ACCP Consensus Committee on Pulmonary Embolism. Opinions regarding the diagnosis and management of venous thromboembolic disease. Chest 1996;109:233–37.

Becker DM, Philbrick JT, Bachhuber TL, Humphries JE. d-dimer testing and acute venous thromboembolism. Arch Intern Med 1996;156:939–46.

Evans DA, Wilmott RW. Pulmonary embolism in children. Pediatr Clin North Am 1994;41:569–84.

Ginsburg JS. Management of venous thromboembolism. N Engl J Med 1996;335:1816–28

Goldhaber SZ. Pulmonary embolism. N Engl J Med 1999:339;93–104.

PIOPED Investigators. Value of the ventilation/perfusion scan in acute pulmonary embolism. JAMA 1990;263:2753–59.

Turkstra F, Kuijer PM, Van Beek EJ, et al. Diagnostic utility of ultrasonography of leg veins in patients suspected of having pulmonary embolism. Ann Intern Med 1997;126:775–81.

Author: Richard Lenhardt

Purpura

Clinical Presentation

SIGNS AND SYMPTOMS

- Lesions that do not blanch with pressure
  - Purpura
    - Circumscribed deposit of blood from 0.2 cm to 1 cm in diameter
  - Petechiae
    - Circumscribed deposits of blood smaller than 0.2 cm in diameter
    - Generally caused by platelet disorders
    - Typically present in areas subjected to increased hydrostatic force
  - Ecchymosis
    - Circumscribed deposit of blood from greater than 1 cm in diameter
    - Generally caused by coagulation disorders
- Palpable purpura
  - Indicative of a vascular disorder
  - Infectious emboli
    - Irregular in outline
  - Leukocytoclastic vasculitis
    - Circular in outline
- Purpura fulminans
  - Rapidly progressive hemorrhagic necrosis of the skin with hematologic features of DIC
- Ecthyma gangrenosum
  - Begin as edematous, erythematous papules or plaques and then develop central purpura and necrosis
  - Bullae formation also occurs in these lesions, and they are frequently found in the girdle region
- Henoch Schönlein Purpura
  - The majority of lesions are found on the lower extremities and buttocks
  - Systemic manifestations include fever, arthralgias (primarily of the knees and ankles), abdominal pain, gastrointestinal bleeding, and nephritis
- Rocky Mountain Spotted Fever
  - Rash appears within 1 week of the onset of the fever chills, severe headache, and photophobia
  - Located initially on the wrists and ankles
  - Spreads to the palms and soles and then centripetally to the trunk and face
  - Erythematous macules, which rapidly become palpable and a few hours later purpuric
- Disseminated gonococcal infection
  - Small number of papules and vesicopustules
  - Central purpura or hemorrhagic necrosis are found over the joints of the distal extremities
  - Arthralgias, tenosynovitis, and fever
- Meningococcemia
  - Small, stellate, gray-purple, occasionally with raised borders and slightly depressed centers
  - Found primarily on the trunk, lower extremities, and sites of pressure
  - Size varies from 1 mm to several centimeters, and the organisms can be cultured from the lesions
  - Associated findings
  - History of a preceding upper respiratory tract infection, fever, headache, altered mental status, hypotension
- Underlying bleeding disorder
  - Spontaneous mucous membrane bleeding
  - Hematomas
  - Hemarthroses
  - Delayed bleeding after trauma or surgery

MECHANISM/DESCRIPTION

- Extravasation of red blood cells from the vasculature into the skin
- Results from abnormalities in any of the three components of hemostasis
  - Platelets
  - Coagulation factors
  - Blood vessels
- Infection may cause purpura by several mechanisms
  - Direct vessel wall invasion
  - Thrombocytopenia
  - DIC
  - Purpura fulminans
  - Immunologically mediated vasculitis
  - Septic emboli
  - Direct effect of toxins released by the infecting organism

ETIOLOGY

Palpable Purpura

- Vasculitic
  - Leukocytoclastic vasculitis
    - Also known as allergic vasculitis
    - One most commonly associated with palpable purpura
  - Henoch-Schönlein purpura
    - Subtype of acute leukocytoclastic vasculitis
  - Polyarteritis nodosa
    - Specific cutaneous lesions result from a vasculitis of arterial vessels rather than postcapillary venules
    - Leads to ischemia of the skin
- Infectious emboli
  - Gram-negative cocci
  - Meningococcus
  - Gonococcus
  - Gram-negative rods
    - Enterobacteriaceae
  - Gram-positive cocci
    - Staphylococcus
  - Rickettsia
  - Candida
  - Aspergillus
- Cholesterol emboli
  - Usually on the lower extremities of patients
  - History of anticoagulant therapy or an invasive vascular procedure
  - Associated findings include livedo reticularis, gangrene, cyanosis, subcutaneous nodules, and ischemic ulcerations
  - Petechiae are also an important sign of fat embolism and occur primarily on the upper body 2–3 days after a major injury

Ecthyma Gangrenosum

- Pseudomonas aeruginosa
- Other Gram-negative rods
- In immunocompromised hosts, candida and aspergillus

Platelet Disorders

- Underproduction
  - Drug-induced
  - Viral suppression
  - Marrow infiltration (myelophthisis)
- Increased destruction
  - Immune thrombocytopenic purpura
  - Posttransfusion purpura
  - HIV-associated thrombocytopenia
    - Thrombotic thrombocytopenic purpura
    - Thrombocytopenia during pregnancy
  - Hypersplenism

Vasculitis

- Large vessel disease
  - ArteritisTemporal (giant cell) arteritis
  - Takayasu's arteritis
  - Primary (idiopathic)
  - Hepatitis B or C spondylitis
- Medium and small vessel disease
  - CMV
  - Herpes zoster
  - HIV
  - Associated with malignancy
  - Hairy cell leukemia
  - Familial Mediterranean fever
  - Granulomatous vasculitis
  - Wegener's granulomatosis
  - Lymphomatoid granulomatosis
  - Behçet's disease
  - Kawasaki disease (mucocutaneous lymph node syndrome)
- Predominantly small vessel disease
  - Hypersensitivity vasculitis
  - Mixed cryoglobulinemia
  - Serum sickness
  - Systemic lupus erythematosus
  - Sjögren's syndrome
  - Primary biliary cirrhosis
  - Lyme disease
  - Chronic active hepatitis
  - Drug-induced vasculitis
  - Churg-Strauss syndrome
  - Goodpasture's syndrome
  - Erythema nodosum
  - Panniculitis
  - Buerger's disease (thrombophlebitis obliterans)

Purpura Fulminans

- Protein C and S deficiencies in neonates
- Severe bacterial infections
- "Classic" during the convalescence of an otherwise benign "preparatory" infectious disease

—Varicella
—Streptococcal infections
—Febrile exanthems
—Urticaria
—Drug hypersensitivity
—Smallpox and diphtheria vaccinations

Neonatal Purpura

- Extramedullary erythropoiesis (blueberry muffin baby)
- Coagulation defects
  —Protein C and S deficiency (neonatal purpura fulminans)
  —Hemorrhagic disease of the newborn
  —Hereditary clotting factor deficiencies
- Platelet abnormalities
  —Immune platelet destruction
  —Alloimmune neonatal thrombocytopenia
  —Maternal autoimmune thrombocytopenia (ITP, lupus)
  —Drug-related immune thrombocytopenia
  —Primary platelet production/function defects
  —Thrombocytopenia with absent radii syndrome
  —Wiskott-Aldrich syndrome
  —Fanconi anemia
  —Congenital megakaryocytic thrombocytopenia
  —X-linked recessive thrombocytopenia
  —Other hereditary thrombocytopenias
  —Giant platelet syndromes
  —Trisomy 13 or 18
  —Alport syndrome variants
  —Gray platelet syndrome
  —Glanzmann thrombasthenia
  —Hermansky-Pudlak syndrome
  —Kasabach-Merritt syndrome
- Infections
  —Congenital (TORCH)
  —Sepsis
  —HIV
  —Parvovirus B19
- Trauma

Pre-Hospital

- Intravenous access and monitor if patient appears septic

CAUTION

- Safety precautions
  —Mask and gloves
  —Antibiotic prophylaxis is required if unprotected exposure to respiratory secretions in patients with meningococcemia

Diagnosis

ESSENTIAL WORKUP

- Obtain a complete medical history
  —Prolonged bleeding following procedures and injury
  —Pertinent medical history
  —Liver disease
  —Malabsorption
  —HIV infection
- Family history
  —Inherited disorders of coagulation or platelet function
- Use of medications
  —Aspirin
  —Nonsteroidal anti-inflammatory drugs
  —Anticoagulants
  —Oral contraceptives
  —Antibiotics
- Alcohol use

LABORATORY

- Platelet count
  —Abnormal counts must be verified by manual examination of a peripheral blood smear
- Bleeding time
- Von Willebrand's disease screen
- Platelet function studies
- PTT
- PT
- Disseminated intravascular coagulation screen

IMAGING/SPECIAL TESTS

N/A

DIFFERENTIAL DIAGNOSIS

See etiology

Treatment

INITIAL STABILIZATION

- Not required in the majority of cases
- Aggressive ED resuscitation if purpura appears to be secondary to a bacterial infection
  —Airway support
  —Intravenous access
  —Intravenous antibiotics should be administered as possible
    -Penicillin, cefotaxime, or ceftriaxone

ED TREATMENT

- Treat underlying etiology

MEDICATIONS

- Penicillin: 40,000 U/kg IV q 4 hrs; max dose: 20 million U/24 hrs
- Cefotaxime: 50 mg/kg IV q 6 hrs; max dose: 12 g/24 hrs
- Ceftriaxone: 50 mg/kg IV q 12 hrs; max dose: 4 g/24 hrs
- Rifampin: 600 mg PO bid for 2 days

Disposition

ADMISSION CRITERIA

- Determined by the underlying etiology

DISCHARGE CRITERIA

- After exclusion of life-threatening etiologies
  —Bacterial infection
  —Critical thrombocytopenia
- Appropriate follow up arranged

Miscellaneous

ICD9: 287

CORE CONTENT CODE: 3.3.2

SUGGESTED READINGS

Baselga E. Purpura in infants and children. J Am Acad Dermatol 1997;37:673–705.

Schneiderman P. The vascular purpuras. In: Beuler E, Lichtman MA, Coller BS, Kipps TJ, eds. Williams' hematology. 5th ed. New York: McGraw-Hill; 1995:1401–412.

Author: Richard Wolfe

Pyelonephritis

Clinical Presentation

SIGNS AND SYMPTOMS

- Dysuria/urgency/frequency
- Back, flank or abdominal pain
- Body aches, fever, chills, malaise
- Nausea, vomiting
- Costovertebral angle tenderness or suprapubic tenderness
- Ill/toxic appearing
- Dehydration
- Occult pyelonephritis
  —Invasion of the upper urinary tract without clinical symptoms
  —Suspect in lower UTI which doesn't resolve with standard treatment

MECHANISM/DESCRIPTION

- Ascension of bacteria from a lower urinary tract infection into the renal parenchyma
- Male:female ratio
  —1:5 in first year of life
  —1:10 children
  —1:50 reproductive years
  —1:1 fifth decade and older

ETIOLOGY

- Bacteriology
  —*E. coli* 80–95%
  —*S. saprophyticus* 5–15%
  —*Proteus mirabilis*
  —*Klebsiella* species
  —*Citrobacter freundii*
  —*Serratia*
  —*Enterobacter*
  —*Pseudomonas*
- Predisposing factors
  —Recent instrumentation: catheterization, cystoscopy, indwelling urinary catheter
  —Urinary obstruction: stricture, stone, prostatic enlargement, tumor, other foreign body,
  —Anatomic abnormalities: hypospadius, ureteral ectopia, bifid ureter, renal scarring
  —Neurologic conditions: neurogenic bladder, spinal cord injury
  —Previous UTIs (in childhood, more than 3 in past year)
  —Recent pyelonephritis within one year
  —Diabetes mellitus
  —Immunosuppression
  —Pregnancy

PEDIATRIC CONSIDERATIONS

- Fever, irritability, lethargy, poor feeding or jaundice may be the only symptoms in infants
- Enuresis in the previously toilet-trained child
- UTIs
  —Spread hematogenously in neonates and immunocompromised children
- Renal scarring
  —More common sequelae in young children than adults
- Group B streptococci
  —Etiologic agents in neonates

Pre-Hospital

CAUTIONS

- Treat shock secondary to urosepsis

Diagnosis

ESSENTIAL WORKUP

- Urinalysis
  —Clean catch or catheterized urine specimen
  —Pyuria
  —Hematuria
- Urine culture and sensitivity
  —>100,000 CFU/ml
  —10^2–10^4 CFU considered positive in
    -Early infection
    -Clinical scenario consistent with UTI
    -Catheter or suprapubic specimen
  —Identifies bacteria in the event that infection does not respond to empiric therapy
- Assess for dehydration

LABORATORY

- CBC
  —Optional
  —Does not rule in or out upper tract infection
- Blood cultures
  —Not needed
  —Bacteria identified more readily on urine culture

IMAGING/SPECIAL TESTS

- Helical CT, IVP or renal ultrasound if concomitant stone or obstruction suspected
- Consider elective evaluation of the genitourinary tract in males with pyelonephritis

DIFFERENTIAL DIAGNOSIS

- Lower tract UTI
- Pelvic inflammatory disease
- Prostatitis
- Epididymitis
- Urethritis
- Nephrolithiasis
- Renal abscess
- Appendicitis
- Diverticulitis
- Cholecystitis
- Lower lobe pneumonia

PEDIATRIC CONSIDERATIONS

- "Bag" urine specimen
  —Vast majority of positive cultures are contaminants
  —Helpful only in ruling out disease if culture is negative
- Catheterized or suprapubic specimens >1000 CFU is positive
- Blood cultures usually performed for children <1 year of age
- Renal cortical scan using dimecaptosuccinic acid (DMSA)
  —Sensitive and specific test for diagnosis of pyelonephritis
  —Decreased cortical uptake without volume loss indicates acute pyelonephritis
- All children with first episode of pyelonephritis should have urinary tract imaging performed later
  —Renal ultrasound
    -Within 48 hours if no clinical improvement
    -Within 3–6 weeks if clinical improvement
  —Girls 4–10 years old
    -Radionuclide isocystogram for vesicoureteral reflux
  —Boys 4–10 years old
  —Voiding cystourethrogram after urine is sterile and bladder spasm has subsided

Treatment

INITIAL STABILIZATION

- Bolus with 0.9%NS 500 cc–1 L for shock/dehydration

ED TREATMENT

- Parenteral antibiotics for
  —Inability to comply with oral therapy
  —Extremes of age
  —Failure of oral therapy
  —Urinary obstruction
  —Toxic patients
  —Immunosuppressed patients
  —Pregnancy
  —Suspected antibiotic resistant organisms
- Preferred empiric intravenous antibiotics
  —Aminoglycoside (gentamicin) plus ampicillin
  —Third-generation cephalosporin (ceftriaxone)
  —Quinolones (ciprofloxacin)—not approved for children
  —Bactrim (TMP-SMZ)
  —In pregnancy, use third-generation cephalosporin or aminoglycoside/ampicillin
- Outpatient oral antibiotics
  —For nontoxic otherwise healthy patient
  —10–14 day course
  —Bactrim (TMP-SMZ) or quinolones preferred agents
- Administer one dose of parenteral antibiotics prior to oral antibiotics
  —Assures a prompt cessation of bacterial proliferation
  —Avoids delays in oral antibiotic administration
- Antiemetics for vomiting
- Analgesia for pain

MEDICATIONS

- Oral antibiotics
  —Bactrim (TMP-SMZ): 160 mg/800 mg bid
  —Cephalexin: 500 mg qid
  —Ciprofloxacin: 250 mg bid
  —Ofloxacin: 200 mg bid
  —Norfloxacin: 400 mg bid
- IV antibiotics
  —Ampicillin: 1 g q 6 hrs
  —Bactrim (TMP-SMZ): 160 mg/800 mg q 12 hrs
  —Cefazolin: 1–1.5 g q 8 hrs
  —Ceftriaxone: 2 g q 24 hrs
  —Ciprofloxacin: 500 mg q 12hrs
  —Gentamicin: 2–5 mg/kg load
  —Imipenem-cilastatin: 0.5–1 g q 8 hrs
  —Ticarcillin-clavulanate: 3.1 g q 6 hrs

PEDIATRIC CONSIDERATIONS

- Oral antibiotic liquid preparations for children
  —Amoxicillin: 30–50 mg/kg/24hrs tid
  —Amoxicillin/clavulanic acid: 45 mg/kg/24hrs tid
  —Cephalexin: 50–75 mg/kg/24hrs qid
  —Cefixime: 8 mg/kg/24hrs q day
  —Cefpodoxime: 10 mg/kg/24hrs bid
  —Erythromycin/sulfisoxazole: 50 mg EM/kg/24hrs qid
  —Loracarbef 15–30 mg/kg/24hrs bid
  —TMP-SMZ: 6–12 mg TMP, 30–60 mg SMZ per kg/24hrs bid
- Parenteral antibiotics for admitted children
  —Age 0–3 months
    -Cefotaxime (50–180 mg/kg/day tid) plus ampicillin (50–100 mg/kg/day qid)
    -Gentamicin (1–2.5 mg/kg/day tid) plus ampicillin
  —Age >3 months
    -May substitute ceftriaxone (50–100 mg/kg/day bid to qd) for cefotaxime

Disposition

ADMISSION CRITERIA

- Inability to comply with oral therapy
  —Nausea/vomiting
  —Social situation prevents compliance
- Pregnancy
- Indwelling urinary catheter
- Urinary obstruction/anatomic abnormalities
  —Proximal obstruction (such as a kidney stone) places the patient at high risk for development of a renal abscess or sepsis and so requires emergent urologic consultation
  —Immunosuppression/diabetes mellitus
  —Extremes of age (all children <6 months)
  —Failure of outpatient therapy/recent antibiotics
- Short-term observation unit
  —Ideal setting in which to hydrate a patient, control pain and begin IV antibiotics, allowing for early discharge
- Unstable vital signs/toxic appearance

DISCHARGE CRITERIA

- Ability to maintain oral hydration
- Pain controlled with oral analgesic
- 48–72-hour follow-up

Miscellaneous

ICD9: 590.80

CORE CONTENT CODE: 15.2.1.1

SUGGESTED READINGS

Gibly R. Infections of the urinary tract and male genitalia. In: Brillman JC, Quenzer RW, eds. Infectious disease in emergency medicine. 2d ed. Philadelphia: Lippincott 1998:602–629.

Hellerstein S. Urinary tract infections: Old and new concepts. Pediatr Clin North Am 1993;42(6):1433–57.

Stamm WE, Hooton TM. Management of urinary tract infection in adults. N Engl J Med 1993;329:1328–1334.

Author: Judith Brillman

Pyloric Stenosis

Clinical Presentation

SIGNS AND SYMPTOMS

- Vomiting
  - —Nonbilious
  - —May be blood tinged
  - —Progressively worsening
  - —Postprandial
  - —Often projectile vomiting
- "Lean and hungry" infant
- Constipation or small green stools
- Variable dehydration and wasting depending on duration of symptoms
- Peristaltic waves moving from left to right in the left upper quadrant
- 1.5–2-cm olive-shaped mass at the lateral margin of the right rectus abdominis muscle in the right upper quadrant
  - —Represents the hypertrophied pylorus
  - —Confirms diagnosis
  - —Requires a relaxed abdomen
  - —Best felt immediately after vomiting or after the stomach is emptied via gastric suction as the dilated body of the stomach overlies the pylorus

MECHANISM/DESCRIPTION

- Most common cause of gastrointestinal obstruction in infants with an incidence of 1 in 3000
- Males affected 5 times more commonly than females
- Familial
  - —Recurrence risk in subsequent male children is 10%; 2% in females
  - —20% of sons and 7% of daughters of female patients develop pyloric stenosis
  - —5% of sons and 2.5% of daughters of male patients develop pyloric stenosis
- Most commonly presents between 2–6 weeks of life (range: 1 week to 3 months)

ETIOLOGY

- Neuronal nitric oxide synthase (NOS 1) may be a genetic susceptibility locus
- Postnatal hypertrophy and hyperplasia of smooth muscle cells causing a thickened pylorus and antrum leads to worsening gastric outlet obstruction

Pre-Hospital

N/A

Diagnosis

ESSENTIAL WORKUP

- If "olive" palpable, further diagnostic evaluation is unnecessary and surgical consultation should be sought
- Abdominal ultrasound
  - —Study of choice
  - —Ultrasonic diagnosis hinges on identification and measurement of pyloric muscle mass and observation of fluid movement through the pylorus
  - —Positive predictive value approaches 100%
  - —Serial ultrasounds for equivocal or negative exams

LABORATORY

- Electrolytes, BUN/Cr, glucose
  - —Hypokalemic, hypochloremic metabolic alkalosis
  - —Normal electrolytes do not exclude the diagnosis
- CBC
- Urinalysis

IMAGING/SPECIAL TESTS

- Flat plate abdominal film
  - —If ultrasound is not available
  - —Dilated stomach and no air distal to the pylorus
  - —Most useful to rule out other serious abdominal pathology, such as malrotation or volvulus
- Upper GI series
  - —"String sign" representing contrast passing through a narrowed gastric outlet
  - —95% accurate
  - —Remove contrast from the stomach after the study to prevent aspiration

DIFFERENTIAL DIAGNOSIS

- Esophageal reflux
- Gastroenteritis
- Urinary tract infection
- Gastric or duodenal web
- Adrenal insufficiency
- Formula intolerance
- Increased intracranial pressure
- Drug withdrawal
- Psychosocial entities
- Poor maternal interaction
  - —Overzealous feeding

Treatment

INITIAL STABILIZATION

- IV access
- Rapid bedside glucose test to exclude hypoglycemia
- Correct volume deficit with 20 cc/kg bolus of 0.9%NS

ED TREATMENT

- Correct electrolyte abnormalities
- Hydrate with dextrose-containing solution after fluid resuscitation at 1–1.5 times maintenance rate
  —Add potassium after ensuring adequate urine output
- Insert nasogastric tube to decompress the stomach
- Restrict oral intake
- Consult pediatric surgeon for pyloromyotomy

Disposition

ADMISSION CRITERIA

- All patients should be admitted to the hospital for surgical correction

DISCHARGE CRITERIA

- None

Miscellaneous

ICD9: 537.0

CORE CONTENT CODE: 13.1.15

SUGGESTED READINGS

Bishop HC. Diagnosis of pyloric stenosis by palpation. Clin Pediatr 1973;12(4):226–227.

Garcia VF, Randolph JG. Pyloric stenosis: diagnosis and management. Pediatr Rev 1990;11:292–296.

Touloukian RJ, Higgins E. The spectrum of serum electrolytes in hypertrophic pyloric stenosis. J Pediatr Surg 1983;18(4):394–397.

Authors: Mara Stankovich; Dale Steele

Rabies

Clinical Presentation

SIGNS AND SYMPTOMS

Prodrome

- Malaise
- Fever
- Headache
- URI
- Nonspecific GI complaints
- At site of bite
  - —Pain
  - —Itching
  - —Paresthesia
  - —Spreads to entire limb
  - —Due to virus multiplication in dorsal root ganglion of sensory nerve

Classic (Encephalitic–Furious) Rabies (80%)

- Hydrophobia
  - —Violent reflexive intense contractions of the diaphragm with
    - -Attempts to swallow
    - -Sight of liquid
    - -Blowing air on face (aerophobia)
  - —Possibly exaggerated airway protective reflex
- Fever
- Terror
- Excitement
- Agitation
- Cluster breathing with long periods of apnea
- Respiratory failure
- Cardiac dysrhythmia
- Autonomic instability
- Seizures
- Coma

Paralytic Rabies (20%)

- Ascending paralysis
  - —Symmetric or asymmetric
- Myoedema
- Piloerection
- Fever
- May progress to classic rabies

MECHANISM/DESCRIPTION

- Fatal central nervous system infection transmitted to humans from animal reservoirs
- Incubation period 4–8 weeks on average (range of days to a year)
  - —Shorter incubation period with bites of the face and neck, with a large inoculum of virus or more virulent strains
- Delay in onset of disease related to multiplication of virus in peripheral tissues (skeletal muscle) prior to entering nervous system
  - —Virus may be eliminated during this period by host immune mechanisms/prophylactic postexposure immunization
- Virus enters a peripheral nerve and travels centrally by axoplasmic transport
  - —Immune systems unable to suppress once virus enters nervous system

ETIOLOGY

- Small number of human cases in the U.S.
  - —Half of these are acquired outside of the U.S.
- Neurotropic RNA virus of Rhabdovirus family
- Exposure through bite or contact with saliva or neural tissue of natural carrier animal on mucous membrane or nonintact skin
  - —Wildlife (account for 90% of confirmed rabies in the U.S.)—treat as rabid unless negative by laboratory tests
    - -Bats (most common)
    - -Raccoons
    - -Skunks
    - -Foxes
    - -Coyotes
    - -Bobcats
  - —Domestic sources—treat exposure if rabid or suspected rabid
    - -Cats
    - -Dogs
    - -Livestock
  - —Rodents not natural carriers
    - -Squirrels
    - -Hamsters
    - -Guinea pigs
    - -Gerbils
    - -Chipmunks
    - -Rats
    - -Mice
    - -Rabbits
    - -Hares
- Human/human transmission through corneal transplants

PEDIATRIC CONSIDERATIONS

- Children at greater risk for unrecognized exposure
- Shorter incubation period

Pre-Hospital

Controversies

- Rabies seldom recognized

CAUTIONS

- Theoretical risk to personnel via human-human transmission (except for corneal transplants)
  - —One reported case from human bite

Diagnosis

ESSENTIAL WORKUP

- Virus isolation from (positive in the first 2 weeks, but confirmation takes 3 weeks)
  - —Saliva
  - —CSF
- Rabies antibody titers
  - —Serum
    - -Any titre confirms diagnosis if patient never vaccinated
    - -Not useful if ever vaccinated
    - -Day 6—earliest positive
    - -Day 13—most positive
  - —CSF is always diagnostic, but probably not positive until day 9 or later
- Rabies Flourescent Antibody (RFA) for antigen
  - —Hair follicle nerve ending biopsy from nape of neck (50–60% positive)
  - —Brain biopsy
- CSF analysis
  - —Nondiagnostic by usual tests

LABORATORY

- CBC
- Electrolytes, BUN/Cr, glucose
- Blood cultures

IMAGING/SPECIAL TESTS

- CXR for aspiration pneumonia
- Head CT scan for altered mental status

DIFFERENTIAL DIAGNOSIS

- Classic rabies
  - —Tetanus
  - —Delirium tremens
  - —Encephalitis
  - —Psychosis
  - —Hysteria
- Paralytic
  - —Guillain-Barré
  - —Polio
  - —Immune mediated polyneuritis
  - —Tick bite paralysis

Treatment

INITIAL STABILIZATION

- ABCs
  - —Intubation for altered mental status/respiratory depression

ED TREATMENT

Prophylaxis

- Local wound cleansing with soap (virucidal) or iodine
- Tetanus prophylaxis if indicated
- Bite of natural rabies carrier (wild) or domestic with aberrant behavior
  - —Rabies immune globulin 20 IU/kg on day 0
    - -Half-dose injected locally into wound
    - -Half-dose IM (deltoid in adults, anterolateral thigh in children)
  - —Human diploid cell vaccine (HDCV)
    - -1 ml on days 0, 3, 7, 14, and 28
  - —Same therapy in pregnancy
  - —Begin, if indicated, up to 6 months after exposure occurred
  - —If anaphylaxis before full vaccine series
    - -Consult Centers for Disease Control (CDC)
    - -Send titers, if further dose is needed
    - -Pretreat with steroids and diphenhydramine
    - -Before administering dose, establish IV, prepare epinephrine for administration and set up for possible intubation
    - -Must achieve adequate titers
- Preexposure prophylaxis
  - —Virus laboratory workers, veterinarians, forest rangers, zookeepers
  - —HDCV 0.1 ml IM or intradermal

Classic/Paralytic Rabies Therapy

- Supportive care
- Sedation for agitation
- Analgesics
- Almost 100% fatal despite intensive care

Disposition

ADMISSION CRITERIA

- ICU admission for all suspected rabies

DISCHARGE CRITERIA

- Rabies exposure only—discharge after
  - —Appropriate wound management
  - —Prophylaxis

Miscellaneous

ICD9: 71.0

CORE CONTENT CODE: 9.5.6

SUGGESTED READINGS

Centers for Disease Control and Prevention. Human rabies. Florida. JAMA 1996;276(11):865–866.

Vodopija I. Current issues in human rabies immunization. Rev Infect Dis 1988;10(4):S758–S762.

Warrell DA, Warrell MJ. Human rabies and its prevention: An overview. Rev Infect Dis 1988;10(2):S726–S731.

Author: Constance Greene

Radiation Injury

Clinical Presentation

SIGNS AND SYMPTOMS

- Tissues with greater rates of cellular division more radiosensitive
- GI and heme systems most vulnerable

Skin

- With increasing radiation exposure develop
  - —Epilation
  - —Erythema
  - —Dry desquamation
  - —Wet desquamation
- Erythema that develops within 48 hours usually progresses to ulceration or chronic radiodermatitis
- Treat as thermal burn

Gastrointestinal

- Anorexia/nausea/vomiting/diarrhea
- Dehydration due to transudation of plasma into the GI tract
- Major source of septicemia when combined with bone marrow suppression
- Higher doses result in an earlier onset and more protracted course
  - —<0.5 Gy: onset >6 hours
  - —<2 Gy: onset 2–6 hours
  - —>4 Gy: onset < 2 hours
  - —>10 Gy: onset <30 minutes

Hematopoetic

- Pancytopenia due to bone marrow suppression
  - —Anemia
  - —Thrombocytopenia with doses exceeding 2–4 Gy after about 4 weeks
  - —Lymphopenia/neutropenia causing fever and increased risk of infection
- Bone marrow depression develops after a latent phase

Central Nervous System

- Headache
- Altered mental status
- Vertigo
- Occurs after massive exposure—associated with near 100% mortality within 48 hours
- Survivable if exposure is limited to the head

MECHANISM/DESCRIPTION

- Acute radiation syndrome results after a major portion of the body is irradiated by deeply penetrating radiation with a dose usually >1 Gy
- Measuring radiation
  - —Rad (radiation absorbed dose) is a measure of energy imparted to matter
    - -1 rad = 100 ergs/g
  - —1 Gray (Gy) (the SI (International System of Units) Measure) = 100 rad

Types of exposure

- External
  - —Follows irradiation from an external source (e.g., radiation therapy)
  - —No contamination hazard
- Internal contamination
  - —Inhalation or ingestion of radioactive material
  - —Treat as heavy metal ingestion
- External contamination
  - —Radioactive material in contact with a patients clothing or skin
  - —Must remove radioactive material
  - —Contain radioactive material to prevent further contamination

ETIOLOGY

- α, β, x, and γ rays emitted during the decay of unstable isotopes
  - —Responsible for acute radiation syndrome
- α particles
  - —Penetration limited to the epidermis
  - —Contamination treated by skin cleaning
- β particles
  - —Skin penetration of 8 mm causes thermal-like burns
  - —Clothing blocks penetration
  - —Measured by radiation meters
  - —Removed by skin cleaning
- Gamma (γ) rays
  - —Primary cause of radiation injury
  - —Deeply penetrating high energy wave

Pre-Hospital

CAUTIONS

- Activate disaster plan when predefined criteria met
- Early notification of type of incident to receiving hospital
- Transport after decontamination if medically stable
- Site decontamination
  - —Remove/bag clothing and leave at scene for disposal
  - —Clean skin with soap and water
- Protective clothing including respirators, rubber gloves, and shoe covers for rescue personnel

Diagnosis

ESSENTIAL WORKUP

- Radiation monitoring to ensure decontamination

LABORATORY

- CBC/platelet count
  - —Baseline important
  - —Absolute lymphocyte count (ALC) at 48 hours correlates with prognosis
    - ->1200/mm^3, good prognosis
    - -300–1200/mm^3, fair prognosis
    - -<300 mm^3, poor/critical prognosis

DIFFERENTIAL DIAGNOSIS

- Suspect radiation illness in unknown burns with GI symptoms and bone marrow suppression
- Thermal burns
- Gastroenteritis
- Carbon monoxide poisoning

Illness Categorization

DEGREE	GY	CLINICAL SCENARIO	TREATMENT/DISPOSITION
Mild	<2	Mild GI for 24 hrs ALC (48 hrs) >2000	Discharge if asymptomatic Follow daily CBC and platelets
Moderate	2–4	Moderate GI for 4 days ALC (48h)>1200	Admit for supportive care and observation
Severe	4–10	Severe GI for 7 days ALC (48 hrs) <1200 Symptomatic anemia Infections common	Admit for reverse isolation, antibiotics, transfusions, consider bone marrow transplant About 50% mortality
Fatal	>10	GI and CNS within 30 min ALC (48 hrs) <300	Admit for palliative measures Death expected within 1 week

Treatment

INITIAL STABILIZATION

- Field decontamination except for patients in extremis
- ABCs
  —0.9%NS IV fluid bolus for extensive thermal burns/hypotension

ED TREATMENT

- Protect all hospital personal
  —Cover skin with gown
  —Use radiation survey monitors to prevent contamination
  —Set up containment and decontamination areas with running water and drainage
  —Cover floors with disposable paper/plastic
- Irrigate open wounds with saline followed by 3% hydrogen peroxide if contamination persists
- Irrigate contaminated eyes and ears
- Gently scrub skin with soap and water 3 minutes (do not abrade)
- GI decontamination for ingestions
  —Whole-bowel irrigation and activated charcoal within 2 hours of exposure
- Pulmonary decontamination
  —Consider bronchoalveolar lavage
- Supportive treatment
  —IV fluids to replace GI losses
  —Antiemetics and analgesics
  —Monitor for need of reverse isolation
  —Cover severe burns with sterile dressing
  —Early and broad spectrum antibiotics for fevers or other signs of infection
  —Early surgery for associated trauma to reduce risk of infection and bleeding
- Potassium iodine to prevent thyroid uptake of radioactive ^{131}I ingestion
  —Indications: >100 rad for adult/>50 rad for child
  —Blocks 90% ^{131}I if given within 1 hour; 50% if given within 5 hours
- Chelating agents for radioactive heavy metals
  —Aluminum reduces absorption of strontium
  —Barium precipitates radium
  —EDTA precipitates lead
  —Penicillamine for lead, copper, cobalt
  —Prussian blue for thallium, cesium, rubidium
  —DTPA for transuranic, heavy metals
  —Deferoxamine for plutonium, iron
  —Water diuresis for tritium, Na^+, K^+
  —Dimercaprol for mercury, arsenic, bismuth, chromium, nickel, lead
- For expert assistance contact Radiation Emergency Assistance Center in Tennessee (615) 481-1000 (24 hrs/day)

MEDICATIONS

- Potassium iodide: 100 mg po

Disposition

ADMISSION CRITERIA

- Exposure to a dose of radiation >1Gy

DISCHARGE CRITERIA

- Asymptomatic patients with dose of radiation less than 1 Gy with close laboratory follow-up

Miscellaneous

ICD9: NEC 990

CORE CONTENT CODE: 5.5

SUGGESTED READINGS

Heifetz IN. Radiation Accidents. In: Harwood-Nuss A, et al. The clinical practice of emergency medicine. Philadelphia: Lippincott-Raven, 1996:1493–1497.

Markovchick V. Radiation injuries. In: Rosen P, et al., eds. Emergency medicine: Concepts and clinical practice. 4th ed. St. Louis: CV Mosby, 1998:1066–1074.

Author: Kirk Dufty

Clinical Presentation

SIGNS AND SYMPTOMS

Lesion Morphology

- Macule
  - —Localized nonpalpable changes in skin color
  - —Purpura or petechiae if nonblanching when pressure is applied
- Maculopapule
  - —Slightly elevated lesions with localized changes in skin
- Papule
  - —Solid, elevated lesions smaller than 5 mm in diameter
  - —Keratotic (rough-surfaced lesion)
  - —Nonkeratotic (smooth lesion)
  - —Palpable purpura if nonblanching when pressure is applied
- Plaque
  - —Solid, elevated lesions larger than 5 mm in diameter
  - —Often results from a confluence of papules
- Nodule
  - —Solid, elevated lesions extending deep into the dermis or subcutaneous tissue larger than 5 mm in diameter
- Wheal
  - —Circular, irregular lesions varying from red to pale
- Vesicle
  - —Clear fluid filled lesions less than 5 mm in diameter
- Bullae
  - —Clear fluid filled lesions larger than 5 mm in diameter
- Pustules
  - —Pus-filled lesions

Secondary Lesions

- Scales
  - —Thin plates of dried cornified epithelium partially separated from the epidermis
- Lichenification
  - —Dried plaques resulting in furrowing of the skin
- Erosion
  - —Moist surface uncovered by rupture of vesicles or bullae
- Excoriation
  - —Linear loss of the skin secondary to trauma
- Ulcer
  - —Deep loss of the skin involving the epidermis and a variable amount of the dermis and subcutaneous tissue

Configuration

- Circles or arcs
- Serpiginous (creeping or wormlike)
- Iris grouping (Bull's eye appearance)
- Irregular grouping
- Zosteriform grouping
- Linear grouping
- Retiform grouping

Associated Signs and Symptoms

- Fever
- Pruritus
- Joint pain
- Abdominal pain

MECHANISM/DESCRIPTION

- Most dermatologic emergencies in children are due to an underlying infection
- In children with fever and a rash, viruses account for 72% and bacteria for 20%
- The color of a particular lesion or the entire skin may be due to a number of substances
  - —Red or red-brown lesions result from oxyhemoglobin found in red blood cells
  - —The macular erythematous lesions seen in viral exanthema usually represent dilated superficial cutaneous vessels
  - —Purpura and petechiae result from leakage of red blood cells out of the vasculature space
  - —Hypopigmentation or hyperpigmentation represent postinflammatory change from either increases or decreases in melanin production
  - —Depigmentation refers to the total loss of pigment secondary to an autoimmune effect (vitiligo) or in congenital disorders from a genetic inability to produce melanin (albinism)
- Scales represent a proliferative disorder of epidermal cell turnover

ETIOLOGY

Papulosquamous

- Infections
  - —Viral
  - —Bacterial
  - —Rickettsial
  - —Fungal
- Allergic Reactions
- Autoimmune disorders

Purpura and Petechiae

- Clotting disorder
- Platelet disorder
- Vascular fragility disease
- Vasculitis
- Overwhelming infection

Vesicobullous

- Infection
- Drug reaction
- Autoimmune disorder

Ulcer

- Infection
- Vascular insufficiency

Pre-Hospital

- Field management is indicated when there are signs of systemic instability
  - —Airway management using precautions to avoid exposure to respiratory secretions
  - —Intravenous access

CAUTIONS

- Mask and gloves should be worn to prevent contagion

Diagnosis

ESSENTIAL WORKUP

- Obtain a detailed history
  - —Age group
    - -Many conditions occur more commonly at specific ages
    - -Distribution and appearance vary with age
  - —Development, progression, and duration of the rash
  - —Associated symptoms
    - -Fever
    - -Pruritus
  - —Family history
    - -Generic dermatoses
    - -Atopic dermatitis
    - -Psoriasis
- Classify the rash based on the primary lesions
  - —Papulosquamous
  - —Vesicobullous
  - —Purpuric

LABORATORY

- Indicated if the rash is purpuric
  - —Platelet count
  - —Bleeding time
  - —PTT
  - —PT
  - —Disseminated intravascular coagulation screen

IMAGING/SPECIAL TESTS

- Potassium hydroxide preparations
  - —Indicated with scaling lesions to differentiate dermatophytosis from nummular eczema and pityriasis rosea
  - —Superficial scale should be removed from the skin with a scalpel or the edge of a glass slide
  - —The sample should be obtained from the active border of the lesion
    - -Place on a slide and add 1 drop of 10% KOH
    - -Place a cover slip and heat slowly without boiling
    - -Allow the slide to set for a few minutes
    - -Scan for hyphae

- Scabies preparations
  - —The majority of the mite population resides on the hands and feet in young children
  - —A drop of mineral oil should be placed on the lesion and then scraped with a #15 blade
  - —The scraping should be deep enough to produce just a speck of blood
  - —Examine under low power for the mite, ova, larva, or fecal matter

DIFFERENTIAL DIAGNOSIS

Maculopapular Rash

- Solid, skin colored or yellow
  - —Keratotic
    - -Wart
    - -Corn
    - -Callus
  - —Nonkeratotic
    - -Wart
    - -Molluscum contagiosum
    - -Sebaceous cyst
    - -Basal and squamous cell carcinoma
    - -Nevi
    - -Jaundice
- Solid, brown
  - —Café au lait patch
  - —Nevi
  - —Freckle
  - —Melanoma
  - —Photoallergic drug eruption
  - —Phototoxic drug eruption
  - —Tinea nigra palmarisHypopigmentation
- Solid, red, nonscaling
  - —Nonpurpuric
    - -Exanthems
      - *Rubeola
      - *Scarlet fever
      - *Toxin-producing staphylococcal or streptococcal disease
      - *Erythema infectiosum (fifth disease)
      - *Roseola
      - *Rubella
      - *Rubella like rash (echoviruses, Coxsackie A viruses)
    - -Varicella (early manifestations)
    - -Epstein-Barr virus
    - -Enterovirus
    - -Adenovirus
    - -Mycoplasma
    - -Kawasaki disease
    - -Erythema multiforme
  - —Localized, pruriginous
    - -Insect bites
    - -Scabies
    - -Allergic contact dermatitis
    - -Irritant contact dermatitis
  - —Purpuric
    - -Bacteremia-Sepsis
      - *Meningococcemia
      - **Haemophilus influenzae*
      - *Pneumococcemia
      - *Gonococcemia
      - *Endocarditis
      - *Plague
    - -Disseminated intravascular coagulation
    - -Rocky Mountain spotted fever
    - -Henoch-Schönlein purpura
    - -Idiopathic thrombocytopenic purpura
    - -Leukemia
    - -Underlying bleeding disorder
    - -Ecthyma gangrenosum
    - -Rarely pityriasis rosea
- Solid, red, scaling
  - —Without epithelial disruption
    - -Tinea corporis, capitus, pedis, or cruris
    - -Pityriasis rosea
    - -Secondary syphilis
    - -Lupus erythematosis
  - —With epithelial disruption
    - -Papular urticaria
    - -Eczema
    - -Seborrheic, diaper, contact, or stasis dermatitis
    - -Impetigo
    - -Candidiasis
    - -Tinea corporis, capitus, pedis, or cruris

Vesicular-Bullous Rash

- Varicella
- Herpes simplex
- Herpes zoster
- Hand-foot-and-mouth syndrome
- Scabies
- Drug hypersensitivity toxic epidermal necrolysis
- Staphylococcal scalded-skin syndrome
- Bullous impetigo
- Cat-scratch disease
- Dermatitis herpetiformis
- Eczema
- Erythema multiforme
- Impetigo
- Lichen planus

Pustular

- Acne
- Folliculitis
- Candidiasis
- Gonococcemia
- Meningococcemia

Treatment

INITIAL STABILIZATION

- Aggressive, empiric management of children with a purpuric rash associated with fever or unstable vital signs
  - —Airway support, intravenous access
  - —Intravenous antibiotics should be administered as possible
    - -Penicillin, cefotaxime, or ceftriaxone

ED TREATMENT

- Specific ED treatment should be directed to the underlying etiology
- Acetaminophen is indicated in children with fever
- Diphenhydramine should be used when an allergic reaction is suspected

MEDICATIONS

- Acetaminophen: 10–15 mg/kg PO/PR q 4–6 hrs
- Diphenhydramine: 1.25 mg/kg PO/IM/IV q 6 hrs
- Penicillin: 40,000 U/kg IV q 4 hrs; max dose: 20 million U/24 hrs
- Cefotaxime: 50 mg/kg IV q 6 hrs; max dose: 12 g/24 hrs
- Ceftriaxone: 50 mg/kg IV q 12 hrs; max dose: 4 g/24 hrs

Disposition

ADMISSION CRITERIA

- Hospital admission is determined by the underlying disorder

DISCHARGE CRITERIA

- —Discharge instructions should be based on the underlying disorder
- —Followup with a primary care physician or a dermatologist should be arranged

Miscellaneous

ICD9: N/A

CORE CONTENT CODE: 13.12.4; 13.12.4.1; 13.12.4.2; 13.12.4.3; 13.12.4.4; 13.12.4.5

SUGGESTED READINGS

Barkin RM. Rash. In: Barkin RM, ed. Emergency pediatrics. A guide to ambulatory care. St Louis: CV Mosby, 1999:285–290.

Pomeranz AJ. The systematic evaluation of the skin in children. Pediatr Clin North Am 1998;45:49–63.

Resnick SD. New aspects of exanthematous diseases of childhood. Dermatol Clin 1997;15:257–266.

Authors: Bruce Webster; Richard Wolfe

Rectal Prolapse

Clinical Presentation

SIGNS AND SYMPTOMS

- Protruding rectum
- Bleeding
- Mucous discharge
- Sensation of rectal mass
- Tenesmus
- Constipation and incontinence

MECHANISM/DESCRIPTION

- Full thickness rectum intussuscepts through the rectum to the outside

ETIOLOGY

- Unknown—possibilities include
  —Chronic constipation
  —Outlet obstruction
  —Sphincters with decreased tone
    -Birth trauma
    -Neurologic disease

PEDIATRIC CONSIDERATIONS

- True rectal prolapse unusual in children—more likely intussusception

Pre-Hospital

CAUTIONS

- Reduce pressure on rectum
  —Avoid straining
  —Avoid prolonged sitting

Diagnosis

ESSENTIAL WORKUP

- History with emphasis on bowel obstruction and duration of prolapse
- Rectal examination—must differentiate rectal prolapse, internal hemorrhoids, or intussusception
  —Intussusception identified by placing the examining finger between the protruding rectum and the anus
  —Internal hemorrhoids identified by identifying the folds of mucosa radiating out like spokes in a wheel
  —Folds of mucosa in rectal prolapse are circular

LABORATORY

- No laboratory test necessary for uncomplicated prolapse
- Preoperative tests for acutely incarcerated prolapse with necrosis preoperative
  —CBC
  —Urinalysis
  —Electrolytes, BUN/Cr, glucose

DIFFERENTIAL DIAGNOSIS

- Prolapsed internal hemorrhoids
- Intussusception from above

Treatment

INITIAL STABILIZATION

- No stabilization needed for elective rectal prolapse
- Incarcerated nonreducible prolapse
  —NPO
  —IV fluids rehydration
  —Prepared for surgery

ED TREATMENT

- Reduce prolapse gently
  —If reduction accomplished without difficulty—correct prolapse electively
  —If prolapse incarcerated—admission for reduction and surgical correction before the swelling creates a full thickness necrosis
- If the reduction is easy—recurrence is likely
  —Elective surgical correction

Disposition

ADMISSION CRITERIA

- Necrotic or anoxic mucosa on the prolapse
- Inability to easily reduce the prolapse

DISCHARGE CRITERIA

- Chronic, easily reduced rectal prolapse
- Refer to an appropriate surgeon

Miscellaneous

ICD9: 569.1

CORE CONTENT CODE: 1.8.1.4

SUGGESTED READINGS

Heine JA., Wong WD. Rectal prolapse. In: Mazier PW, et al. Surgery of the colon, rectum, and anus. Philadelphia: WB Saunders, 1995:515–537.

Author: Charles Orsay

Rectal Trauma

Clinical Presentation

SIGNS AND SYMPTOMS

- Perineal, anal, or lower abdominal pain
- Signs of peritonitis with guarding, rebound tenderness, or fever
- Signs of perforation
- Pelvic fracture
- Rectal bleeding
- Obstipation
- History of anal manipulation, foreign body insertion, sexual abuse

ETIOLOGY

- Penetrating trauma
  - —Gunshot wound: accounts for 80%
  - —Knife wound
  - —Impalement injuries
- Blunt trauma: accounts for 10%
  - —Motor vehicle collision
  - —Motor cycle accident
  - —Falls
  - —Sharp bony edges from pelvic fractures may penetrate the rectum
- Iatrogenic trauma
  - —Diagnostic and therapeutic procedures
  - —Colonoscopy
  - —Barium enema
  - —Urologic and OB/Gyn procedure
  - —Episiotomy
- Foreign body
  - —Autoeroticism
  - —Assault
  - —Anal intercourse
  - —Ingestion of sharp objects

MECHANISM/DESCRIPTION

- Some anatomical differences between the rectum and the colon
- 2/3 of the rectum is extraperitoneal
- Rectum is surrounded by the rigid bony pelvis
- The rectum is accessible via the anus

PEDIATRIC CONSIDERATIONS

- Thermometer insertion can give rise to rectal injury
- Child abuse

Pre-Hospital

CAUTIONS

- Do not attempt to remove foreign body from rectum.

Diagnosis

ESSENTIAL WORKUP

- History
  - —Type of injury
  - —Time of the injury
  - —All patients with GSW, stab wound, or impalement injury to trunk, buttocks, perineum, or upper thigh should be suspected as having a rectal injury
  - —Any patient with anal manipulation who complains of lower abdominal or pelvic pain should also be evaluated for a rectal injury
- Physical Examination
  - —Inspect and palpate thoroughly the buttocks, anus, and perineum
  - —In penetrating wound, find the entrance and exit wound
  - —Digital anal examination should always be performed to evaluate for blood or guaiac positive stool. Also note the position of the prostate
  - —Obtain retrograde urethrogram prior to Foley insertion if there is blood at the urethral meatus or prostate is high riding to prevent exacerbating urethral injury
  - —Exclude injury to genitourinary system by doing a through vaginal examination in all female patients
- Anoscopy and sigmoidoscopy
  - —Must be performed if rectal injury is suspected by history, the rectum is in the pathway of a penetrating object or blood is found in the rectum
  - —Irrigate and suction feces and blood
  - —Avoid insufflating large amount of air during sigmoidoscopic exam because stool can be forced into the peritoneal cavity if proximal bowel perforation exists
- Sexual assault
  - —If history suggests sexual assault, an evidentiary examination should be undertaken looking for anal bruising, mucosal laceration, and sperm sampling

LABORATORY

- CBC
- Type and Screen
- Urinalysis

IMAGING/SPECIAL TESTS

- Supine/Upright abdominal films, pelvis x-ray
  - —Allow the identification of the location, size, and shape of object, or to look for pneumoperitoneum
- Look for extraperitoneal or extrarectal tissue densities or gas suggesting perforation
- Diastasis of symphysis pubis or pelvic fracture often accompanies rectal injury

DIFFERENTIAL DIAGNOSIS

- Colonic injuries
- Genitourinary injuries

Treatment

INITIAL STABILIZATION

- In penetrating or blunt abdominal trauma, follow ATLS protocol, which includes primary survey, resuscitation, secondary survey, and treatment

ED TREATMENT

- Rectal injuries are usually evaluated during the secondary survey
- If skin abrasion is present administer antibiotic. Also administer tetanus as prophylaxis against *Clostridial* infections
- If perforation or peritonitis is suspected immediate trauma surgical consultation is mandatory
- Place a Foley catheter
  - —Foley catheter is contraindicated with high riding prostate or blood in the urethral meatus
- If peritonitis is present, a multiple antibiotic regimen may be required. Must cover both Gram-negative aerobic and anaerobic organisms. See medication list below
  - —Antibiotics active against anaerobic Gram-negative bacilli: clindamycin, or metronidazole
  - —Antibiotics active against aerobic Gram-negative bacilli: aminoglycosides, cephalosporins 2nd/3rd/4th-generation, antipseudomonal penicillin, aztreonam
  - —Antibiotics active against both aerobic/anaerobic Gram-negative bacteria: cefoxitin, cefotetan, cefmetazole, ticarcillin/clavulanate, piperacillin/tazobactam, and ampicillin/sulbactam

Rectal Foreign Body Removal in ED

- Treatment is determined by the location and type of foreign object
- Extraction in emergency department is successful in 60% of the cases and should be attempted only after adequate IV sedation and gentle digital sphincter dilatation
- Local anesthesia may be used to get maximal anal sphincter dilation
- Removal of foreign body may be assisted with obstetric forceps, ring forceps, tenaculum, biopsy forceps, or suctioning devices
- For some smooth objects try passing a Foley catheter above the object and then inflating the balloon to permit retraction while preventing the suction
- May use plaster of Paris placed in hollow objects and a gauze or instrument inserted into the plaster can act as a handle when plaster hardens
- High riding or sharp objects should be removed under general anesthesia
- After the extraction rigid sigmoidoscopy should be done to look for mucosal tear

MEDICATIONS

GENERIC NAME	TRADE NAME	ADULT DOSE	PEDIATRIC DOSE
Ampicillin/sulbac tam	Unasyn	3.0 g IV	50 mg/kg IV
Cefazolin	Ancef	1 g IV	30 mg/kg IV
Cefotetan	Cefotan	2 g IV	40 mg/kg IV
Cefoxitin	Mefoxin	2 g IV	40 mg/kg IV
Clindamycin	Cleocin	450–900 mg IV	10 mg/kg IV
Ciprofloxacin	Cipro	400 mg IV	
Metronidazole	Flagyl	1 g IV	15 mg/kg IV
Piperacillin/tazobactam	Zosyn	3.375 g IV	75 mg/kg IV
Ticarcillin/clavulanate	Timentin	3.1 g IV	75 mg/kg IV

Disposition

ADMISSION CRITERIA

- Perforation
- Significant bleeding
- Unstable vital signs
- Abdominal pain
- Torn anal sphincter
- Foreign body that cannot be extracted
- Broken glass or other sharp object in rectum requiring surgical removal

DISCHARGE CRITERIA

- Stable vital signs
- No abdominal pain
- Normal sigmoidoscopy/anoscopy exam

Miscellaneous

ICD9: 863.45

CORE CONTENT CODE: 1.8

SUGGESTED READINGS

Carrillo EH, Somberg LB, Ceballos CE, et al. Blunt traumatic injuries to the colon and rectum. J Am Coll Surg 1996;183:548–552.

Cohen JS, Sackier JM. Management of colorectal foreign bodies J R Coll Surg Edinb 1996;41:312–315.

Fry RD. Anorectal trauma and foreign bodies. Surg Clin North Am 1994;74(6) 1491–505.

Coates WC. Disorders of the anorectum. In: Rosen P, et al eds. Emergency Medicine. 4th ed. St. Louis, Mosby, 1998:2037–2052.

Author: Carlyn Ko

Red Eye

Clinical Presentation

SIGNS AND SYMPTOMS

- Discharge
- Pruritus
- Pain
  —Foreign body sensation
- Ectropion
- Entropion
  —Eyelash against globe (trichiasis)
  —Conjunctival injection
  —Corneal abrasion, ulcer or opacity
  —Anterior chamber cells or flare
  —Photophobia (from movement of an inflamed iris)
  —Proptosis
  —Preauricular or submandibular lymphadenopathy
  —Rosacea (may cause blepharitis)
  —Facial skin lesions (herpes)
- Associated
  —Sinusitis
  —Otitis
  —Pharyngitis

MECHANISM/DESCRIPTION

- Red eye
  —May be caused by almost any eye disorder
  —Often benign
  —May represent systemic disease
- Pathophysiology—conjunctival vascular engorgement (common to all nontraumatic red eyes) which may be associated with
  —Inflammatory diseases
    -Uveitis (anterior and posterior)
    -Episcleritis (70% idiopathic)
    -Scleritis (50% associated with systemic disease)
  —Inflammation/allergy
    -Histamine release and increased vascular permeability, which results in swelling of the conjunctiva (chemosis), sometimes with watery discharge and pruritus
  —Infection
    -Bacterial—purulent mucous discharge
    -Viral—watery or no discharge, pruritus
  —Trauma
    -Corneal abrasion
    -Conjunctival hemorrhage
    -Foreign bodies

ETIOLOGY

- Categorize by location of conjunctival injection
  —Perilimbal
    -Anterior uveitis (iritis)
  —Sectorial
    -Pinguecula
    -Pterygium
    -Hemorrhage
    -Episcleritis
    -Scleritis
      *Occult perforation
  —Diffuse
    -Bacterial or viral conjunctivitis
    -Blepharitis
    -Dry eye syndrome
    -Acute angle closure glaucoma
    -Endophthalmitis
- Categorize red eyes by the presence of discharge or pain
  —With discharge
    -More common
      *Conjunctivitis
      *Ophthalmia neonatorum
      *Blepharitis
    -Less common
      *Allergic reaction
      *Dacryocystitis
      *Caniculitis
  —Without discharge
    -No pain
      *Subconjunctival hemorrhage
      *Conjunctival tumor
    -Mild to moderate pain
      *Inflamed pinguecula/pterygium
      *Blepharitis
      *Dry eye syndrome conjunctivitis
      *Foreign body
      *Corneal disorder
      *Episcleritis
      *Posterior uveitis
      *Orbital cellulitis
    -Moderate to severe pain
      *Corneal ulcer/abrasion/erosion
      *Anterior uveitis
      *Scleritis
      *Acute angle-closure glaucoma
      *Endophthalmitis

Pre-Hospital

N/A

Diagnosis

ESSENTIAL WORKUP

- Visual acuity
  —Pupil exam
  —Confrontational visual field exam
  —Extraocular muscle function
  —Slit-lamp examination with fluorescein
  —Lid eversion
- Funduscopy and tonometry when applicable

IMAGING/SPECIAL TESTS

- Direct towards the suspected etiology of the red eye
  —Dacryocystitis: culture discharge
  —Corneal ulcers: ophthalmologist should scrape the cornea for cultures
  —Bacterial conjunctivitis: obtain conjunctival swab
  —Moderate discharge: routine culture and sensitivity (usually *S. aureus, Streptococcus,* and *H. influenzae* [children])
  —Severe discharge: Neisseria gonorrhea and Chlamydia
    -Treat systemic infection and sexual partners
  —Foreign body or orbital disease: Plain films or CT scan of the orbits
  —Uveitis
    -If unilateral, nongranulomatous, and history and physical are unremarkable: no systemic workup is necessary
    -If bilateral, recurrent, or granulomatous: CBC, ESR, ANA, VDRL, FTA Ab. PPD, ACE level, CXR (sarcoidosis and TB), Lyme titer and HLA B-27, Toxoplasma and CMV titers

DIFFERENTIAL DIAGNOSIS

- Trauma
- Uveitis
- Arthritic disease
- Ankylosing Spondylosis
- Ulcerative colitis
- Reiter's syndrome
- TB
- Herpes
- Syphilis
- Sarcoidosis
- Toxoplasma
- CMV
- Lyme

Treatment

INITIAL STABILIZATION

N/A

ED TREATMENT

- Direct therapy toward specific etiology
  - —Differentiate between a corneal abrasion and a corneal ulcer
    - -Most abrasions will heal with or without patching
    - -Ulcers will get worse and may perforate if patched
  - —Never patch an eye with significant infection risk
    - -Contact lens wearers
    - -Abrasions from tree branch
    - -Fingernails
  - —Do not spread infection from the affected eye to the unaffected eye
- Trauma or uveitis
  - —Rule out intraocular foreign body
- Antibiotic drops
  - —Polytrim
  - —Gentamycin 0.3%
  - —Ciprofloxacin 0.35%
  - —Sulfacetamide10%
  - —Trifluridine 1%
- Antibiotic ointments
  - —Bacitracin
  - —Erythromycin
  - —Gentamycin
  - —Neosporin
  - —Polysporin
  - —Sulfacetamide
  - —Vidarabine
- Mydriatics and Cycloplegics
  - —Atropine
  - —Cyclopentolate
  - —Homatropine
  - —Phenylephrine
  - —Tropicamide
- Corticosteroid drops (always with ophthalmology consultation)
  - —Cortisporin
  - —Maxitrol
  - —Metimyd
  - —Neo-decadron
  - —Prednisolone
  - —TobraDex
- Glaucoma agents (always with ophthalmology consultation)
  - —Acetazolamide
  - —Betaxolol
  - —Carteolol
  - —Dipivefrin
  - —Pilocarpine
  - —Timolol
  - —Mannitol
  - —Pilocarpine (only if mechanical closure is ruled out)
- Consult ophthalmologist for
  - —Dacryocystitis
  - —Corneal ulcer
  - —Scleritis
  - —Angle-closure glaucoma
  - —Uveitis
  - —Proptosis
  - —Orbital cellulitis
  - —Vision loss
  - —Uncertain diagnosis

Disposition

ADMISSION CRITERIA

- Endophthalmitis
- Perforated corneal ulcers
- Orbital cellulitis

DISCHARGE CRITERIA

- Depends on the diagnosis
  - —If the diagnosis is certain and visual loss will not result, the patient may be discharged without consultation

Miscellaneous

ICD9: N/A

CORE CONTENT CODE: 22.2.18

SUGGESTED READINGS

Bertolini J, Pelicio M. The red eye. Emerg Med Clin North Am 1995;13(3):561–79

Cullom R, Chang B. The Wills eye manual: office and emergency room diagnosis and treatment of eye disease. 2ns ed. Philadelphia: JB Lippincott, 1994.

Juang P, Ahn D, Rosen P. Ocular examination techniques for the emergency department. J Emerg Med 1997;15:793–810.

Author: Pascal S.C. Juang

Reiter's Disease

Clinical Presentation

SIGNS AND SYMPTOMS

- This syndrome is typically characterized by lower extremity asymmetric polyarticular arthritis, urethritis, and uveitis
- Constitutional symptoms are common early including joint stiffness, low back pain worsening with rest, and myalgias. Knees, ankles, metatarsophalangeal, and heel joints are the most commonly involved, though the wrist may be an early target
- Extra-articular symptoms may include
  —Noninfectious conjunctivitis
  —Urethritis/Cervicitis
  —Mild dysentery
  —Balanitis circinata, crusty (circumcised) or moist (uncircumcised) penile lesions
  —Keratoderma blennorrhagica, clear vesicles on an erythematous base progressing to macules, papules, and then keratotic lesions. Common on soles, palms, penis, and trunk
  —Uveitis, iritis
  —Carditis and aortic regurgitation have been described in chronic disease
- There may be a prior history of dysentery or urethritis/cervicitis, commonly occurring 2–6 weeks before the disease presentation

MECHANISM/DESCRIPTION

- Reactive arthritis, occurring after infectious process, most commonly dysentery or genital tract infection often with *Chlamydia trachomatis.* Defined as a triad of urethritis/cervicitis/dysentery followed by conjunctivitis then arthritis
  —Incomplete forms exist and all three need not be present for diagnosis
- The characteristic joint finding is a local enthesopathy: inflammation of tendinous insertions into bone. This may manifest in the digits as "sausage finger"
  —This finding suggests Reiter's syndrome or psoriatic arthritis
- Males are affected more commonly than females by a ratio of 5–10:1 in the posturogenital infection group
  —There is an equal sex distribution in the postdysentery group
- Predominantly a disease of the young with peak onset between ages 15 and 35

ETIOLOGY

- This syndrome develops in a genetically susceptible host following a bacterial infectious process, usually urethritis, cervicitis or dysentery. The suspect pathogens are *Salmonella, Shigella, Yersinia, Campylobacter,* and *Chlamydia*
- Bacterial antigens may be present in synovial fluid, but organisms have not been found
- A strong correlation with HLA-B27 exists; 70–80% of patients have this marker. The disease is uncommon in persons of African dissent
- There is an association with HIV infection

PEDIATRIC CONSIDERATIONS

- This disease is rare in the pediatric population. However, the diagnosis can be made using adult criteria

Pre-Hospital

N/A

Diagnosis

ESSENTIAL WORKUP

- Includes a search for the bacterial infection by history and exam, especially in females where cervicitis is often asymptomatic
- Urethral or cervical swab for *Chlamydia* infection is mandatory and best tested for by direct fluorescent antibody or DNA-probes for *Chlamydial* ribosomal RNA

LABORATORY

- Arthrocentesis and fluid analysis is often necessary to rule out an infectious process, especially in the presence of monoarticular arthritis with constitutional symptoms
  —Synovial fluid may reveal mild to severe inflammation, but culture will be negative
- CBC with differential may show a moderate neutrophilic leukocytosis and ESR may be mildly elevated
- C-reactive protein and C3/C4 levels will be mildly elevated (not specific)
- Rheumatoid factor and HLA-B27 may be useful adjuncts
- HIV testing should be considered, especially if use of immunosuppressive therapy is contemplated
- Electrocardiogram may show a prolonged P-R interval in chronic disease

IMAGING/SPECIAL TESTS

- Plain radiography of affected joint. Soft tissue swelling is common, but bone density is preserved. Periosteal spurs with indistinct margins and fluffy periostitis can be seen at sites of tendinous insertions (enthesitis) especially of lower extremity. Joint space narrowing is common in the small joints of the hand
- Plain radiography of lumbar spine, sacroiliac joints and heel(s). Sacroiliitis occurs in 10% of patients early in disease and tends to be unilateral
  —Eventually 70% will have SI involvement

DIFFERENTIAL DIAGNOSIS

- Gonococcal arthritis
- Ankylosing spondylitis
- Psoriatic arthritis
- Arthritis related to inflammatory bowel disease
- Undifferentiated spondyloarthropathy
- Lyme disease
- Gonococcal arthritis
- Rheumatoid arthritis
- Gout/pseudogout
- Viral arthritis

Treatment

INITIAL STABILIZATION

- Hypovolemia may be present from GI bleeding secondary to NSAID use or dysentery
  - —IV fluid and blood products may be necessary

ED TREATMENT

- NSAIDs are the mainstay of therapy
- Sulfasalazine is useful for NSAID failure or contraindications
- Treatment for urethritis/cervicitis is mandatory if present
  - —This may ameliorate the arthropathy and extraarticular symptoms
- Antibiotic therapy for post-dysenteric disease is not indicated
- Systemic or intra-articular corticosteroids may be useful in patients failing NSAID therapy

MEDICATIONS

- Indomethacin: 100–250 mg/day po divided q 6 hrs
- Ibuprofen: 600 mg po q 6 hrs
  - —A minimum of 1 month of NSAID treatment at maximum dosage is mandatory before evaluating effectiveness
- Sulfasalazine: 2000 mg/day for NSAID failure or contraindication
- Doxycycline: 100 mg bid × 10 days for chlamydia-induced disease
- In difficult cases, further therapy listed below may be initiated in consult with rheumatologist
  - —Systemic corticosteroids
  - —Intra-articular corticosteroids
  - —Methotrexate: 15–25 mg po per week may be necessary for aggressive unremitting disease

PEDIATRIC CONSIDERATIONS

- Doxycycline: 5 mg/kg/day bid; max dose 200 mg/day
- Methotrexate: 0.5–1 mg/kg/week; max 15–25 mg/week (may be indicated for ANA-positive patients with polyarticular disease or NSAID failures)
- NSAIDs are the mainstay of treatment
  - —Ibuprofen: 20–40 mg/kg/day in 3 doses
  - —Sulfasalazine: 30–60 mg/kg/day in 4 doses; max dose is 2 g/day

Disposition

ADMISSION CRITERIA

- Concomitant disease(s) that require admission
- Unremitting pain or inability to ambulate

DISCHARGE CRITERIA

- Most patients can be discharged. Close follow-up with a rheumatologist or a primary care physician is required. Physiotherapy may be useful

Miscellaneous

ICD9: 099.3

CORE CONTENT CODE: 8.5.2.3

SUGGESTED READINGS

Ansell BA. Juvenile rheumatoid arthritis, juvenile chronic arthritis, and juvenile spondyloarthropathies. Curr Opin Rheumatol 1992;4:706–712.

Buxbaum J. Therapy for the seronegative spondyloarthropathies. Curr Opin Rheumatol 1992;4:500–506.

Cuellar ML, Espinoza LR. Management of spondyloarthropathies. Curr Opin Rheumatol 1996;8:288–295.

El-Khoury GY, et al. Seronegative spondyloarthropathies. Radiol Clin North Am 1996;34(2):343–357.

Espinoza LR, et al. There is an association between human immunodeficiency virus infection and spondyloarthropathies. Rheum Dis Clin North Am 1992;18(1):257–266.

Author: Robert Hitchcock

Renal Calculus

Clinical Presentation

SIGNS AND SYMPTOMS

- Sudden onset of severe pain in the costovertebral angle, flank and lateral abdomen
- Colicky or constant pain
  —Patient cannot find a comfortable position
- Hematuria
- Nausea/vomiting
- Restlessness
- Diaphoresis
- History of prior stone formation
- Abdominal tenderness is not present

MECHANISM/DESCRIPTION

- Urinary tract obstruction
- Intermittent distention of the renal pelvis of proximal ureter produces pain
- Kidney stones
  —Most common cause of renal colic
- Theories of stone formation
  —Urinary supersaturation of solute followed by crystal precipitation
  —Decrease in the normal urinary proteins inhibiting crystal growth
  —Urinary stasis from a physical anomaly, catheter placement, neurogenic bladder, or the presence of a foreign body
- Stone composition
  —75%: calcium in conjunction with phosphate and/or oxalate
  —15%: magnesium-phosphate (struvite)
    -Associated with infections caused by urea-splitting organisms (e.g., *Pseudomonas, Proteus, Klebsiella*) along with an alkalotic urine
  —5% uric acid
- 90% of urinary calculi radiopaque

ETIOLOGY

- 1% of the population
- 3 times more common in males than females

PEDIATRIC CONSIDERATIONS

- Rare in children
  —When present—indication of an overt metabolic or genetic disorder
- Painless hematuria common presentation (up to 30%)
- Pediatric patients under the age of 16 comprise approximately 7% of all cases of renal stones
- 1:1 sex distribution
- Metabolic abnormalities
  —Most common etiologies of stone formation in the pediatric population (50%)
- Urological abnormalities present in 20%
- Infection comprises 15%

Pre-Hospital

CAUTIONS

- Parenteral opiates may be required for pain control with long transport times

Diagnosis

ESSENTIAL WORKUP

Physical Examination

- Obtain vital signs
  —Fever suggests an occult infection
  —Hypotension, along with an altered mental status is suggestive of urosepsis
- Abdominal examination
  —Pain on palpation, rebound tenderness and or guarding suggests a more serious intra-abdominal process
  —Palpate the abdominal aorta for tenderness or pulsatile enlargement suggestive of an aneurysm
- Examine the genitalia for evidence of epididymitis, torsion, or testicular masses

LABORATORY STUDIES

- Urinalysis
  —Microscopic hematuria present in >80%
  —Gross hematuria
  —Absent urinary blood in 10%
  —No correlation between the amount of hematuria and the degree of urinary obstruction
  —WBC/bacteria suggestive of infection
- CBC
  —WBC >15,000 suggestive of concomitant infection
- Urine culture
- Electrolytes, glucose, BUN, and Cr
- Pregnancy test when suggestive

IMAGING/SPECIAL TESTS

Kidney—Ureter-Bladder Radiograph

- Indicated when allergy to IVP dye and when renal scanning and ultrasound not available
- Assists in locating radiopaque stones and the exclusion of other pathologies in nonpregnant patients
- Difficult to distinguish radiopaque body
  —Phlebolith
  —Bowel contents
  —Obstruction within the urinary tract on the KUB
- Oblique films assist in localizing suspicious calcifications

Intravenous Pyelogram (IVP)

- Establishes diagnosis in 95%
- Demonstrates the severity of obstruction
- Scout film prior may localize stones that would otherwise be obscured by the dye
- Postvoiding film
  —Useful to identify stones at the ureteral vesicular junction or distal ureter that are obscured by a full bladder

Ultrasound

- For patients who are not candidates for IV contrast
- Useful in the detection of larger stones and hydronephrosis
- Provides anatomical information only
- Helpful in diagnosing obstruction and localizing stones in the proximal and distal portions of the ureter
- Limitations
  - —May miss stones <5 mm in size
  - —May miss an obstruction in the early phase of renal colic
    - -Time delay until the onset of pyelocaliectasis even after total obstruction

Renal Scan

- Useful in patients with a known allergy to contrast media
- Excellent functional test
- Does not provide the anatomical detail of the IVP, US, or computed tomography

Computed Tomography

- Helical CT has replaced IVP as test of choice
- Indications:
  - —1st time diagnosis
  - —Persistent pain
  - —Clinical confusion with pyelonephritis

DIFFERENTIAL DIAGNOSIS

- Do not miss a catastrophe mimicking renal colic
- Dissecting or rupturing abdominal aortic aneurysm (AAA)
- Pyelonephritis
- Papillary necrosis (sickle cell disease, NSAID analgesic abuse, diabetes, or infection)
- Renal infarction (vascular dissection or arterial embolus)
- Ectopic pregnancy
- Ovarian cyst/torsion
- Appendicitis (subacute prodrome differentiates)
- Biliary tract disease (RUQ tenderness makes renal calculi unlikely)
- Musculoskeletal strain (worsening of discomfort during physical exam maneuvers)
- Lower lobe pneumonia (quscultate the lungs)

Treatment

INITIAL STABILIZATION

- Rapid dipstick urine test for blood
  - —Positive test in conjunction with clinical findings sufficient to begin analgesic therapy

ED TREATMENT

- Hydration
  - —Initiate IV crystalloid infusion with 1 L NS infused over 30–60 minutes followed by 200–500 cc/hr
  - —Bolus volume compromised patients with 500 cc increments until urine output adequate
- Analgesics (demerol, morphine, ketorolac)
- Antiemetics (prochlorperazine, droperidol, vistaril)

MEDICATIONS

- Droperidol (inapsine): 2.5 mg IV or IM q 3–6 hrs
- Hydroxyzine hydrochloride (vistaril): 25–50 mg IM (*Not IV*) q 4–6 hrs
- Ketorolac (toradol): 30–60 mg IM or 30 mg IV (alone or with opiates)
- Meperidine (demerol): 50–100 mg (peds:1–2 mg/kg/dose) q 3–4 hrs IV/IM
- Morphine sulfate: 1–3 mg IV may be administered q 15 min as needed to control pain (peds: 0.1–0.2 mg/kg/dose q 2–4 hrs)
- Prochlorperazine (compazine): 5–10 mg IV/IM q 4–6 hrs; 25 mg suppository PR

Disposition

ADMISSION CRITERIA

- Obstruction in the presence of infection mandates immediate urologic intervention
- Intractable pain with refractory nausea and vomiting
- Severe volume depletion
- Urinary extravasation
- Hypercalcemic crisis
- Solitary kidney and complete obstruction
- Relative admission indications (discuss with urologist)
  - —High grade obstruction
  - —Renal insufficiency
  - —Intrinsic renal disease
  - —Stone size <5 mm usually pass spontaneously; those >8 mm rarely do

DISCHARGE CRITERIA

- Normal vital signs
- No evidence of concomitant urinary tract infection
- Adequate analgesia
- Able to tolerate po fluids to maintain hydration status
- Reliable patient with an adequate home situation
- Appropriate outpatient followup arranged
- Normal renal function
- Provide a urine strainer to collect the stone for possible future stone analysis
- Arrange urologic follow-up

Miscellaneous

ICD9: 592.0

CORE CONTENT CODE: 15.1.1

SUGGESTED READINGS

Callaham ML, Barton CW, Schumaker HM. Decision making in emergency medicine. Philadelphia: BC Decker, 1990.

Harwood-Nuss A, Luten RC. Handbook of emergency medicine. Philadelphia: JB Lippincott, 1995.

May HL, Aghababian RV, Fleisher GR. Emergency medicine. 2d ed. Boston: Little, Brown and Company, 1992.

Tintinalli JE, Ruiz E, Krome RL. Emergency medicine: A comprehensive study guide. 4th ed. New York: McGraw Hill, 1996.

Author: Lawrence Heiskell

Renal Failure

Clinical Presentation

SIGNS AND SYMPTOMS

Acute Renal Failure (ARF)

- Typically asymptomatic
  - —Diagnosed incidentally from routine BUN/Cr
- Oliguria
  - —<400 ml per day
- Fluid overload
  - —Dyspnea
  - —Hypertension
  - —Jugular venous distension
  - —Pulmonary edema
  - —Peripheral edema
  - —Ascites
  - —Pericardial effusion
  - —Pulmonary effusion
- Nausea/vomiting

Prerenal Failure

- Absolute or relative volume deficit
- Dry mucous membranes
- Hypotension
- Tachycardia
- Low cardiac output
  - —CHF
- Systemic vasodilation
  - —Sepsis
  - —Anaphylaxis

Intrarenal (Intrinsic) Failure

- Renal artery thrombosis
  - —Flank or abdominal pain
  - —Atrial fibrillation
  - —Recent myocardial infarction
- Renal vein thrombosis
  - —Nephrotic syndrome (see chapter: Nephrotic Syndrome)
  - —Pulmonary embolus (see chapter: Pulmonary Embolism)
  - —Flank pain
- Glomerulonephritis/vasculitis
  - —Recent infection
    - -Sinusitis
    - -Rash (palpable purpura)
    - -Pulmonary hemorrhage
- Hemolytic uremic syndrome (HUS)
  - —Preceded by a viral or bacterial infection
  - —Upper respiratory infection or diarrhea
- Thrombotic thrombocytopenic purpura (TTP)
  - —Headache
  - —Confusion
  - —Seizures
  - —Cranial nerve palsies
  - —Coma
- Allergic interstitial nephritis following drug ingestion
  - —Fever
  - —Rash
  - —Arthralgias

Postrenal Failure

- Abdominal or flank pain
- Distended bladder
- Oliguria or anuria

Complications of ARF

Uremic syndrome

- Pericarditis
- Pericardial effusion
- Cardiac tamponade
- Ileus
- Altered mental status
- Asterixis
- Hyperreflexia
- Restless leg syndrome
- Focal neurologic abnormality
- Seizures

Hematological Disorders

- Anemia
- Increased bleeding time
- Leukocytosis

MECHANISM/DESCRIPTION

- Decline in glomerular filtration
- Disrupts the extracellular fluid volume, electrolyte, and acid-base status
- Results in accumulation of nitrogenous waste

ETIOLOGY

- Prerenal failure
  - —Caused by renal hypoperfusion
  - —Renal tissue remains normal unless severe/prolonged hypertension
- Intrarenal failure
  - —Caused by diseases of the renal parenchyma
- Postrenal failure
  - —Due to acute obstruction of the urinary tract
- Iatrogenic causes include
  - —Aminoglycoside antibiotics
  - —Radiocontrast material administration

Pre-Hospital

CAUTIONS

- Avoid rapid administration of IV fluid
- Administer calcium/sodium bicarbonate for suspected hyperkalemic cardiac arrest

Diagnosis

ESSENTIAL WORKUP

- Electrolytes
  - —Hyperkalemia
  - —Hyponatremia
  - —Hyperphosphatemia
  - —Hypocalcemia
  - —Hypermagnesemia
  - —Metabolic acidosis
  - —Elevated anion gap
- BUN/Cr
  - —Elevated
- Urinalysis
  - —Centrifuged specimen helps to distinguish between different etiologies of ARF
  - —Examined for casts, blood, white blood cells, and crystals
- CBC
  - —Anemia with chronic renal failure

LABORATORY

Prerenal

- UA
  - —Specific gravity >1.018
  - —Osmolality >500 mmol/kg
  - —Sodium <10 mmol/L
  - —Hyaline casts
- BUN/Cr ratio >20
- Rapid recovery renal function when renal perfusion normalized

Intrarenal

- BUN/Cr ratio <10–15
- Glomerulonephritis/vasculitis
  - —UA with red cell or granular casts
  - —Complement and autoimmune antibodies
- Hemolytic uremic syndrome (HUS) or thrombotic thrombocytopenic purpura (TTP)
  - —UA normal
  - —Anemia
  - —Thrombocytopenia
  - —Schistocytes on blood smear
  - —Elevated LDH
- Nephrotoxic acute tubular necrosis (ATN)
  - —UA
    - -Brown granular or epithelial cell casts
    - -SG 1.010
    - -Urine osmolality <350 mmol/kg
    - -Urine Na >20 mmol/L
  - —Ethylene glycol ingestion
    - -UA: calcium oxalate crystals
    - -Anion gap metabolic acidosis
    - -Osmolal gap
- Rhabdomyolysis
  - —UA: heme+ without red cells
  - —Elevated serum K^+, $PO_4^{=}$, myoglobin, CPK–MM, uric acid
  - —Decreased serum Ca^{++}

- Tubulointerstitial disease
- Allergic interstitial nephritis
  - -UA with white cell casts, white cells, red cells, and proteinuria
  - -Systemic eosinophilia

Postrenal

- UA
  - —Usually normal
  - —May have some hematuria but no casts or protein

IMAGING/SPECIAL TESTS

- Intravenous pyelography
  - —Avoid contrast with renal insufficiency
  - —Predisposes to further renal decompensation
- Ultrasound
  - —98% sensitive for excluding obstruction
- Helical CT scan without contrast detects for obstruction
- Duplex scan for
  - —Renal artery or vein thrombosis
- Renal arteriogram
  - —Definitive diagnosis or renal artery thrombosis
- Inferior vena cava and renal vessels venogram for
  - —Renal vein thrombosis
- ECG
  - —Severe hypertension
  - —CHF
  - —Hyperkalemia

Treatment

INITIAL STABILIZATION

- ABCs
  - —Supplemental oxygen for hypoxia
- Correct electrolyte disturbances
- Indications for emergent dialysis
  - —Life-threatening hyperkalemia
  - —Intractable hypertension or pulmonary edema
  - —Fluid overload unresponsive to other treatments
  - —BUN >100 mg/dl
  - —Cr >10 mg/dl
  - —Metabolic acidosis (pH <7.2)
  - —Severe uremia—pericarditis
- Avoid nephrotoxins
- Monitor urine output

ED TREATMENT

Prerenal

- Treat hypoperfusion
  - —Consider PRBC for blood loss
- Invasive cardiac monitoring if unable to assess cardiac failure versus hypovolemia
- Administer 0.9%NS fluid challenge cautiously to avoid fluid overload in liver failure with ascites
  - —Response: good indicator of the degree to which hypovolemia is a factor

Intrarenal

- Glomerulonephritis
  - —Immunosuppressive agents (glucocorticoids) or plasma exchange
- ATN—therapeutic options
  - —Low-dose dopamine
  - —Mannitol
  - —Furosemide
  - —Calcium channel blockers
- Acute interstitial nephritis
  - —Withdrawal of causative agent
  - —Treat underlying disease process
- Euvolemic patients with acute oliguric renal failure
  - —Trial of dopamine 0.5–2.5 μg/kg/min

Complications of ATN

- Volume overload
  - —Furosemide (up to 400 mg)
  - —Low dose dopamine
  - —Dialysis
- Hyponatremia
  - —Fluid restriction
- Hyperkalemia
  - —Sodium polystyrene sulfonate for asymptomatic with K^+>5.5 mEq/L
  - —For K^+ >6.5 mEq/L or ECG abnormalities consistent with hyperkalemia
    - -Calcium gluconate: for cardiac and neuromuscular protection
    - -Glucose and insulin: onset 30–60 minutes, duration several hours
    - -Sodium bicarbonate: onset <15 minutes, duration 1–2 hours
    - -Dialysis for intractable hyperkalemia
- Metabolic acidosis
  - —Consider sodium bicarbonate for pH <7.2 or HCO_3 <15 mEq/L
  - —Dialysis
- Hyperphosphatemia
  - —Calcium carbonate
  - —Aluminum hydroxide
- Myoglobinuria
  - —Mannitol
  - —Sodium bicarbonate to alkalinize the urine
  - —Aggressive fluid resuscitation with 0.9%NS

MEDICATIONS

- Aluminum hydroxide (amphojel): 500–1500 mg po
- Calcium carbonate (os-cal): 250–3000 mg po
- Calcium gluconate: 10 ml of 10% solution over 5 min
- Dextrose: D50W 1 amp (50 ml or 25 g) (peds: D25W 2–4 ml/kg) IV
- Furosemide: 20–400 mg IVP
- Insulin: 10 IU regular IV with dextrose
- Mannitol: 12.5–25 g IVP
- Sodium bicarbonate: 1–2 mEq/kg IV
- Sodium polystyrene sulfonate (kayexalate): 1 g/kg up to 15–60 g po or 30–50 g retention enema in sorbitol q 6 hrs

Disposition

ADMISSION CRITERIA

- New onset acute renal failure
- Hyperkalemia/significant electrolyte abnormalities
- Fluid overload with hypoxia/CHF

DISCHARGE CRITERIA

- Stable
- Normal electrolytes

Miscellaneous

ICD9: 586

CORE CONTENT CODE: 15.4

SUGGESTED READINGS

Brady HR, Brenner BM. Acute renal failure. In: Isselbacher KJ, Braunwald E, Wilson JD, Martin JB, Fauci AS, Kasper DL, eds. Harrison's principles of internal medicine. 13th ed. New York: McGraw Hill, 1996:1265–1274.

Brady HR, Singer GG. Acute renal failure. Lancet 1995;346:1533–1540.

Thadhani R, Pascual M, Bonventre JV. Acute renal failure. N Engl J Med 1996;334(22):1448–1460.

Author: Lauren Grossman

Renal Injury

Clinical Presentation

SIGNS AND SYMPTOMS

- Gross hematuria is a common presentation even with minor renal trauma
  - —Severity of renal trauma does not correlate with the amount of blood in the urine
- Flank mass or ecchymosis
- Tenderness in the flank, abdomen, or back
- Fracture of the inferior ribs or spinal transverse processes
- Coexisting injuries are frequent with both blunt and penetrating injuries, particularly hepatic and splenic injuries

MECHANISM/DESCRIPTION

- Occurs in approximately 8–10% of all abdominal trauma
  - —Majority resulting from blunt trauma including motor vehicle accidents, falls, and contact sports
- Mechanism of injury and kinematics are important factors in evaluating patients for possible renal injury
- Obtain details from pre-hospital providers
  - —Blunt trauma: the forces and direction (horizontal or vertical) of any deceleration or compressive forces
  - —Penetrating trauma: the characteristic of the weapon (type and caliber), distance from the weapon or the type and length of knife or impaling object
- Renal injuries are classified according to type and severity of the injury
  - —Grade I: renal contusion
  - —Grade II: cortical laceration
  - —Grade III: caliceal laceration with urinary extravasation
  - —Grade IV: complete renal tear or fracture
  - —Grade V: vascular pedicle injury or shattered kidney

PEDIATRIC CONSIDERATIONS

- The kidney is the organ most commonly damaged by blunt trauma in the pediatric population
- Contributing factors include relatively larger size of children's kidneys compared with adults and the fact that the tenth and eleventh ribs are not completely ossified until the third decade of life

Pre-Hospital

CAUTIONS

- Penetrating wounds or evisceration should be covered with sterile dressings

Diagnosis

ESSENTIAL WORKUP

- Adults with blunt trauma, microscopic hematuria (<50 RBC/HPF) and no evidence of shock have an extremely low incidence of major renal injuries and do not need radiographic imaging of the kidneys
- All adults with blunt renal trauma and gross hematuria, or microhematuria and shock, require renal imaging for further evaluation of renal injury
- Important to rule out coexisting injuries

LABORATORY

- Urinalysis: gross hematuria or >50 RBCs per HPF adult (>20 RBC/HPF peds is suggestive of renal injury
- Baseline laboratory values including hematocrit and creatinine/BUN should be obtained

IMAGING/SPECIAL TESTS

- Plain abdominal films may show fractured inferior ribs or transverse processes, a unilateral enlarged kidney shadow secondary to edema or hemorrhage, or absence of the psoas margin
- Excretory urography (IVP)
  - —Allows evaluation for renal viability and function
  - —Extravasation reflects injury to the collecting system
  - —Nonvisualization of a kidney may indicate renal pedicle injury or parenchymal shattering
- Abdominal computed tomography (preferred)
  - —Superior anatomic detail and diagnostic accuracy of 98% for renal injury
  - —Sensitive indicator of minor extravasation, parenchymal laceration, vascular injury as well as nonrenal injuries

PEDIATRIC CONSIDERATIONS

- Major blunt renal trauma can occur in the absence of gross hematuria or shock in the pediatric population thus requiring complete radiographic evaluation for the proper diagnosis and staging of renal injuries after blunt trauma with hematuria
- CT scan is the imaging modality of choice

DIFFERENTIAL DIAGNOSIS

- Renal parenchymal injury
- Renal vascular injury
- Ureteral injury
- Bladder or urethral injury

Treatment

INITIAL STABILIZATION

- ABCs
- Rule out potential life threatening injuries first

ED TREATMENT

- Immediate laparotomy may be appropriate in the acutely injured patient who is hemodynamically unstable with presumed hemoperitoneum and renal injury
- All penetrating renal trauma requires renal exploration unless complete radiographic staging reveals an injury which can be managed nonoperatively in a hemodynamically stable patient
- Management of renal injuries
  - —Classes I and II: contusions and minor lacerations with stable vital signs and urographically demonstrated normal renal function can be managed nonoperatively
  - —Class III: renal lacerations with urinary extravasation
    - -Controversy between operative versus nonoperative management
    - -Management should be based on complete radiologic definition of the degree of injury using CT scanning
  - —Classes IV and V: shattered kidney or renal pedicle injuries and hemodynamically unstable patients require emergent laparotomy

Disposition

ADMISSION CRITERIA

- Patients with significant renal injury require hospitalization for definitive laparotomy or observation

DISCHARGE CRITERIA

- Microscopic hematuria only, hemodynamically stable with no other traumatic injuries may be discharged with instructions for immediate return if gross hematuria develops

Miscellaneous

ICD9: 866.00

CORE CONTENT CODE: 18.4.11.10

SUGGESTED READINGS

Peterson N. Genitourinary trauma. In: Felicano D, et al., eds. Trauma. 3rd ed. Stamford, CT: Appleton & Lange, 1996:661–694.

Stein J, Kaji D, Eastham J, et al. Blunt renal trauma in the pediatric population: Indications for radiographic evaluation. Urology 1994;(44):406–410.

Wessells H, McAninich J. Update on upper urinary tract trauma. AUA Update Series 1996;(15):110–115.

Zoller G. Genitourinary trauma. In: Rosen P, et al., eds. Emergency medicine: Concepts and clinical practice. 4th ed. St. Louis: CV Mosby, 1998.

Author: Tom Moats

Respiratory Distress

Clinical Presentation

SIGNS AND SYMPTOMS

- Tachypnea
- Dyspnea
- Tachycardia
- Anxiety
- Diaphoresis
- Cough ("barking," productive)
- Stridor
- Hoarse voice
- Difficulty swallowing or handling oral secretions
- Upper airway rhonchi (wheezes)
- Lower airway crackles (rales)
- Increased work of breathing
- Accessory and intercostal muscle use
- Hypoxemia
- Hypocapnia or hypercapnia if severe
- Respiratory acidosis
- Cyanosis
- Lethargy, then obtundation

ETIOLOGY

- Upper airway obstruction
  —Epiglottitis
  —Croup Syndromes
  —Laryngotracheobronchitis
  —Foreign Body
  —Angioedema
  —Retropharyngeal abscess
- Cardiovascular
  —Pulmonary edema/CHF
  —Dysrhythmias
  —Cardiac ischemia
  —Pulmonary embolus
  —Pericarditis
  —Tamponade
- Pulmonary
  —Asthma
  —COPD/Emphysema
  —Pneumonia
  —Bronchiolitis
  —Aspiration
  —Adult respiratory distress syndrome (ARDS)
  —Pulmonary edema
  —Pneumothorax
  —Pleural effusion
  —Toxic inhalation injury
- Neuromuscular
  —Guillain-Barré syndrome
  —Myasthenia gravis
- Metabolic/systemic/toxic
- Anaphylaxis
- Anemia
- Acidosis
- Hyperthyroidism
- Sepsis
- Salicylate intoxication
- Drug overdose
- Amphetamines
- Cocaine
- Sympathomimetic
- Obesity
- Psychogenic
  —Anxiety disorder
  —Hyperventilation syndrome

PEDIATRIC CONSIDERATIONS

- Respiratory failure is most common cause of cardiac arrest in infants
- Croup syndromes include
  —Viral
  —Spasmodic
  —Bacterial
  —Congenital defects
  —Noninflammatory causes (foreign body, gastroesophageal reflux, trauma, tumors)
- Most common cause of upper airway obstruction
  —Under 6 months: congenital laryngomalacia
  —Over 6 months: viral croup
- Epiglottitis
  —Highest incidence ages 2–4
  —Abrupt onset
  —Fever
  —Respiratory distress and stridor
  —Difficulty swallowing oral secretions
  —Restlessness and anxiety

Pre-Hospital

CAUTION

- Assume a position of comfort for patient
- 100% oxygen
  —Assisted ventilation if obtunded
- Airway adjunct devices (oral or nasal) to maintain patency if tolerated
- Intubation for severe respiratory distress
- Needle aspiration of suspected tension pneumothorax

Diagnosis

ESSENTIAL WORKUP

- Pulse oximetry
- Cardiac and blood pressure monitoring
- Thorough history
  - —Previous history of asthma, COPD, cardiac disease or dysrhythmia, CHF; foreign body aspiration
  - —Recent fever or URI, cough, sputum production, sore throat, systemic disease, anxiety disorder
- Physical examination
  - —Observe: mental status, level of distress, work of breathing, JVP, skin color
  - —Feel/palpate: distal pulses, heart PMI, chest wall, peripheral edema
  - —Percuss: lungs for dullness or resonance, abdominal distention or hepatomegaly
  - —Auscultate: heart sounds, lung wheezes or crackles, neck for upper airway stridor, abdomen bowel sounds
- EKG if suspected cardiac etiology

LABORATORY

- Arterial blood gas for severity and acid-base determination
- CBC
- Electrolytes, BUN/Cr, glucose
- Blood, sputum, urine cultures for fever or sepsis
- Urinary output monitoring for CHF
- Toxicology screen or salicylate level if suspected

IMAGING/SPECIAL TESTS

- CXR for
  - —Pneumonia
  - —Pneumothorax
  - —Hyperinflation
  - —Atelectasis
  - —CHF/pulmonary edema
- Spirometry (peak expiratory flow rates) for asthma, COPD
- Neck radiographs to assess epiglottis and soft tissue spaces, foreign body
- Fiberoptic laryngoscopy to assess epiglottis, vocal cords, and pharyngeal space
- Ventilation/perfusion scan for pulmonary embolus
- Bronchoscopy for foreign body in trachea or bronchus
- Pulmonary artery (Swan-Ganz) catheter for severe CHF, ARDS, pulmonary edema

PEDIATRIC CONSIDERATIONS

- Evaluate retractions, behavior, respiratory rate, breath sounds, and color
  - —Weak cry, expiratory grunting, nasal flaring, tachypnea, and tachycardia, retractions and cyanosis in neonates
- Chest/neck radiograph may show "steeple sign" in croup syndromes
- Chest fluoroscopy may be used to assess inspiratory and expiratory excursions if foreign body is suspected

Treatment

INITIAL STABILIZATION

- ABCs
- Insure patent airway; BVM assist or intubate for severe distress or arrest
- IV fluids if hypotensive
- 100% oxygen by face mask
  - —Use cautiously in patients with severe COPD or chronic C02 retention
- Monitor blood pressure, heart rate, respirations, pulse oximetry
- ACLS for dysrhythmias or arrest

ED TREATMENT

- Treat underlying etiology as appropriate
- CHF or pulmonary edema
  - —Furosemide
  - —Nitroglycerin
  - —Nitroprusside if hypertensive
  - —Pulmonary artery catheter if severe
- Asthma, bronchiolitis, COPD
  - —Bronchodilators
  - —Steroids
  - —Antibiotics for infection
- ARDS, aspiration, toxic lung injury
  - —Mechanical ventilation as needed
  - —Steroids controversial
- Pneumonia
  - —Antibiotics
- Pneumothorax
  - —Needle thoracostomy if suspected tension pneumothorax
  - —Thoracostomy (see Pneumothorax)
- Pleural effusion
  - —Determine etiology
  - —Diagnostic and symptomatic thoracentesis
- Croup
  - —Cool, misted air or oxygen
  - —Steroids
  - —Racemic epinephrine
  - —Antibiotics for bacterial infection
- Epiglottitis
  - —Immediate airway stabilization with intubation or tracheostomy in operating room if possible
  - —Antibiotics for *Haemophilus influenzae*
- Anaphylaxis, angioedema
  - —IV steroids
  - —H_1/H_2 blockers
- Retropharyngeal abscess
  - —Drainage
  - —IV antibiotics
  - —ENT consult
- Cardiac
  - —Treat dysrhythmias or ischemia
  - —Pericardiocentesis for tamponade
  - —NSAIDs or aspirin for pericarditis
- Neuromuscular
  - —Support ventilation
  - —Pyridostigmine bromide or neostigmine for myasthenia gravis
- Metabolic/toxic
  - —Treat underlying cause
- Psychogenic
  - —Anxiolytics

PEDIATRIC CONSIDERATIONS

- Transtracheal jet ventilation if unable to intubate (cricothyrotomy not recommended in children <10 years old)
- Bronchiolitis
  - —Bronchodilators
  - —Inhaled ribavirin for RSV
  - —Antibiotics for infection
- Spasmodic croup
  - —Very sensitive to misted air
- Bacterial croup (membranous laryngotracheobronchitis)
  - —Treat *Staphylococcus aureus*

Disposition

ADMISSION CRITERIA

- Continued supplemental oxygen requirement
- Cardiac or hemodynamic instability
  - —Requiring IV therapy or hydration
  - —Requiring close airway observation or repeated treatments
- As required by underlying cause or significant comorbid disease

DISCHARGE CRITERIA

- Correction of underlying disease
- Stable airway
- Acute supplemental oxygen not required

Miscellaneous

ICD9: 786.09

CORE CONTENT CODE: 22.3.3

SUGGESTED READINGS

Williams SA, Hutson HR, Speals HL: Dyspnea. In Emergency medicine: Concepts and clinical practice. 4th ed. St Louis: Mosby 1998, pp 1460–1469.

Author: Erik D. Barton

Restraints, Physical

Clinical Presentation

SIGNS AND SYMPTOMS

- Physical restraints should be considered
  - —When a patient is a potential danger to self or others
  - —When the patient, by virtue of a medical or psychiatric condition, is unable to be reasoned with or control themselves
  - —To facilitate control, prevent harm, and allow appropriate evaluations
  - —When requested by the patient
- Physical restraints should *not* be used
  - —As a threat
  - —As punitive therapy
  - —To facilitate medical treatment in a competent, cooperative patient

MECHANISM/DESCRIPTION

- Used to prevent harm, allow for examination of the violent patient
- Up to 25% of emergency departments restrain at least one patient daily
- 13% of hospitals reported injuring patients during restraint, including some deaths
- In one survey, 15% of hospitals had a lawsuit pending against them for restraining patients
- When used appropriately restraints are considered more humane than allowing self-harm or harm others

ETIOLOGY

N/A

Pre-Hospital

- Physical restraints in the field requires authorization from
  - —Police
  - —Base station physician

Diagnosis

N/A

Treatment

INITIAL STABILIZATION

ED TREATMENT

- Approach to the unrestrained patient
  - —When the decision is made to restrain a patient, follow a prearranged restraint procedure
  - —Do not attempt restraint without adequate resources
  - —Do not underestimate the potential for violence
- Principles of patient restraint
  - —Should be individualized and afford as much dignity as possible
  - —Should be humanely and professionally administered
  - —Protocols to ensure patient safety should be developed
  - —Carefully document reasons for and means of restraint and periodic assessment
  - —Should be the least-restrictive necessary
  - —Should conform to applicable laws, rules, regulations, and accreditation standards
- Guidelines for the use of restraints
  - —At least four persons should assist with restraining the patient, while a fifth person controls the head and prevents biting
  - —One or two persons should never attempt to restrain a patient
  - —One person should be the "team leader"
  - —Explain why to the patient but do not negotiate once the decision is made
  - —Emphasize the therapeutic reasons, not to be used punitively or as a threat
  - —Allow the opportunity for cooperation
  - —At a signal, the team brings the patient to the floor in a backward motion, avoiding injury
  - —Start with 4-point restraint, one arm above and one below the shoulders
  - —Leather restraints are the safest and most secure

ED TREATMENT

- After the patient is safely restrained
  - —Undress and remove all personal objects
  - —Begin verbal intervention or rapid tranquilization
  - —Perform a physical examination
  - —Never leave only one limb in restraint
  - —Stabilize associated or etiologic medical conditions
  - —Consult psychiatry if the behavior is secondary to a psychiatric condition

Restraint Record

- There should be a standardized physical restraint record that contains the following
  - —Indications for restraint
  - —Type of restraint
  - —Mental status exam
  - —Frequent patient rechecks of mental status and extremity neurovascular exams (may be performed by nursing staff)
  - —Physician to reassess need for restraints at least every 2 hours

MEDICATIONS

- Benztropine: 2 mg IM or IV
- Diphenhydramine: 50 mg IV, IM, or po
- Droperidol: 5–10 mg IV or IM
- Haloperidol: 5–10 mg IV or IM, 0.5–2.0 mg for elderly
- Lorazepam: 1–2 mg IV, IM, or po

Disposition

ADMISSION CRITERIA

N/A

DISCHARGE CRITERIA

- Patient demonstrates a level of control and cooperation to ensure the safety of the patient and others
- Chemical control has been achieved
- Reversal of the precipitating etiology has occurred
  - —No longer intoxicated
- Restraints are causing harm to the patient
  - —Neurovascular compromise
- The restraints can be removed in a stepwise fashion until one arm and leg remain restrained
- Never leave a patient in one restraint

Miscellaneous

ICD9: N/A

CORE CONTENT CODE: 14.11.13

SUGGESTED READINGS

American Council of Emergency Physicians. Use of patient restraint. *ACEP policy statement,* approved January, 1996.

Lavoie FW. Consent, involuntary treatment, and the use of force in an urban emergency department. Ann Emerg Med 1992;21(1):25–32.

Moore GP, Jackimczyk KC. The violent patient. In: Rosen P, et al., eds. Emergency medicine: Concepts and clinical practice. 4th ed. St. Louis: CV Mosby, 1997:2871–878.

Author: Robert J. Vissers

Resuscitation, Termination

Clinical Presentation

SIGNS AND SYMPTOMS

- A combination of signs and symptoms in which the patient has lost the ability to maintain a normal physiologic state
- Unwitnessed cardiac arrest suggests a bad prognosis in nearly all situations

MECHANISM/DESCRIPTION

- Resuscitation is any series of clinical interventions designed to restore a patient to a normal physiologic state

ETIOLOGY

- Illnesses
- Injuries
- Pharmacological agents
- Environmental factors
- Anatomical or physiological abnormalities

Pre-Hospital

- Resuscitative efforts should *not* be withdrawn or withheld on the basis of DNR tattoos or other nonstandard requests that do not involve discussions with patients or their legal surrogate decision-makers
- Decisions to implement or to terminate resuscitative efforts should *not* be based on the patient's age, socioeconomic status, insurance coverage, cultural background, or relationship to the criminal justice system
- Resuscitative efforts may be terminated (or withheld) if attempting resuscitation would clearly jeopardize the health care workers' safety
- Decisions to terminate or withhold resuscitation attempts in the field should be made in conjunction with base hospital physicians
  - —Communicate such information as response to efforts thus far
  - —If cardiac rhythm absent (i.e., asystole in the contiguous leads)
  - —Discussions with patient or family if appropriate
- It is becoming more common to terminate resuscitative efforts in the field if patient maintains asystole in 3 leads and fails to respond to usual ACLS measures
- Emergency physicians should pronounce dead in the field (and stop any resuscitative efforts on) patients who EMS personnel find have any one of the following
  - —Rigor mortis
  - —Livor mortis
  - —Evidence of decomposition
  - —Burned beyond recognition
  - —Injuries clearly incompatible with life (such as decapitation)
- Rescuers may stop resuscitative efforts if they cannot physically continue or when signs of death (e.g., livor mortis) become evident

Diagnosis

- Patients are dead when a physician pronounces them dead

ESSENTIAL WORKUP

- Criteria for death
  - —Patient unresponsive to all stimuli
  - —No spontaneous respiration or cardiac activity
  - —No pulse
  - —Blood pressure unobtainable
    - -Check vital signs more than once
  - —Isoelectric cardiac activity in at least 3 ECG leads
  - —Anatomical injuries (such as decapitation) that are incompatible with life

LABORATORY

N/A

IMAGING/SPECIAL TESTS

- Emergency echocardiography
  - —Absence of organized cardiac activity

Treatment

Withholding or Not Instituting

- Base termination (or noninstitution) of resuscitative efforts on
  - —Patient (or legal surrogate) wishes, if known
    - -Advance directives, living will, etc., and the patient can be identified using the clinician's "good-faith efforts."
  - —Evidence (i.e., patient history, lack of success with current resuscitative efforts, and anatomical or physiological abnormalities incompatible with life) that resuscitative efforts will not succeed
- If patient has capacity to make decisions
  - —The patient will be given appropriate information and be allowed to decide whether resuscitative efforts will be instituted (e.g., massive burns)
  - —If resuscitative efforts are not instituted, patient should receive appropriate comfort care
- Inadequate resources exist to treat all patients (e.g., disasters)
  - —Resources (i.e., time, personnel, equipment) should be devoted to those patients with the greatest chance of benefitting
  - —Patients not receiving resuscitative efforts should receive pain relief and comfort care
- Arrest from blunt trauma is nearly uniformly fatal
- Deciding not to resuscitate equates to terminating resuscitative efforts
- Patient without capacity to make decisions
  - —If inadequate information is available about patient wishes usual clinical indications must guide resuscitation attempts
  - —If validated information is obtained, after resuscitation has begun, demonstrating a patient (or their legal decision-maker) does not want the resuscitation to continue, it can be halted at that point
- Do not continue resuscitation to practice or teach procedures, or to complete research protocols
- Cardiac arrest in cases of acute hypothermia or lightning strike often have good clinical outcomes after prolonged resuscitation attempts
- Decisions to withhold or withdraw resuscitative efforts are ultimately clinical determinations based on the patient's condition, potential reversibility of altered physiologic state, history, and desires, in the context of currently available information
- The most senior physician present (or on-line with EMS personnel) is responsible for deciding to withhold or withdraw resuscitative efforts

PEDIATRIC CONSIDERATIONS

- Terminate or withhold resuscitation efforts for neonates who exhibit anatomical and physiological evidence of in utero development inadequate for survival using currently (and regionally) available resources
  - —These criteria should be predetermined
  - —Developed in conjunction with neonatologists
- Cardiac arrest in a child suggests at least as bad a prognosis as it does in adults, and resuscitations need not be continued any longer than would be justified continuing in adults

Disposition

- Neurological evaluations during and immediately after cardiac resuscitations cannot be used as a predictor of final neurological status
- "Success" in resuscitative efforts is defined by the patient's (or legal surrogate's) desired outcomes

Miscellaneous

ICD9: N/A

CORE CONTENT CODE: N/A

SUGGESTED READINGS

Ardagh M. Preventing harm in resuscitation medicine. N Z Med J 1997;110 (1041):113–15.

Handley AJ, Becker LB, Allen M, van Drenth A, Kramer E, Montgomery WH. Single-rescuer adult basic life support: an advisory statement from the basic life support working group of the international liaison committee on resuscitation. Circulation 1997;95:(8):2174–179.

Iserson KV. The "no code" tattoo—an ethical dilemma. West J Med 1992;156:3:309–12.

Iserson KV. Withholding and withdrawing medical treatment: an emergency medicine perspective. Ann Emerg Med 1996;28:(1):51–55.

Kloeck W, Cummins RO, Chamberlain D, et al. Special resuscitation situations: an advisory statement from the international liaison committee on resuscitation. Circulation 1997;95:(8):2196–210.

Author: Kenneth V. Iserson

Resuscitation, Neonatal

Clinical Presentation

SIGNS AND SYMPTOMS

- Apnea
- Hypoventilation
- Decreased tone
- Lack of response to stimuli
- Temperature instability
- Signs of shock
  - —Altered mental status
  - —Respiratory distress
    - -Tachypnea
    - -Grunting
    - -Ineffective respirations
  - —Tachycardia
  - —Pallor
  - —Cyanosis
  - —Cool extremities
  - —Weak peripheral pulses
  - —Hypotension
  - —Bradycardia
- Maternal risk factors for neonatal distress
  - —Premature delivery or miscarriage
  - —Perinatal loss
  - —Previous baby with fetal growth retardation or malformation
  - —Toxemia of pregnancy
  - —Gestational diabetes
  - —Prolonged rupture of membranes
  - —Clinical chorioamnionitis
  - —Prolonged labor
  - —Breech or face delivery
  - —Abruptio placentae
  - —Placenta previa
- Fetal risk factors for neonatal distress
  - —Multiple births
  - —Meconium stained fluid
  - —Abnormal presentation
  - —Prematurity
  - —Congenital anomalies
- Apgar Score
  - —Does not replace the primary survey in neonatal resuscitation
  - —Measured at 1 and 5 minutes
  - —Muscle Tone (*A*ctivity))
  - —*P*ulse
  - —Reflex irritability (*G*rimace)
  - —Color (*A*ppearence)
  - —*R*espirations

MECHANISM/DESCRIPTION

- Aggressive life support
  - —Rarely required in the ED
  - —6% of all newborns
  - —80% of in premature infants weighing less than 1500 g
- High-risk pregnancy and likely ED delivery
  - —Lack of prenatal care
  - —Teenage pregnancy
  - —Placental abruption
  - —Trauma-induced labor
  - —Substance abuse
- Meconium aspiration
  - —Meconium is a sign of intrauterine distress
    - -Occurs in 10–20% of all deliveries
    - -Meconium aspiration syndrome occurs in about 2–5% of these cases
  - —Mortality rate of 40%

ETIOLOGY

- Immediately following delivery
  - —Perinatal aspiration
  - —Hypoxia
  - —Hypoglycemia
  - —Hypothermia
  - —Hypovolemia
  - —Acidosis
  - —Anemia
  - —Sepsis
  - —Meconium aspiration
  - —Prematurity
  - —Congenital anomalies
- First two weeks of life
  - —Infection
  - —Anemia
  - —Trauma
  - —Dehydration
  - —Metabolic disease
  - —CNS abnormalities
  - —Electrolyte abnormalities
  - —Congenital heart disease

Pre-Hospital

- Keep equipment in a separate neonatal kit
- Problems during transport
  - —Hypothermia
  - —Hypoglycemia
  - —Maintaining the airway
    - -Dislodged endotracheal tubes are a major cause of morbidity during transport
    - -Frequent reassessment of tube position
    - -Bagging should not be overly zealous to avoid barotrauma and pneumothorax
  - —Maintaining intravenous access

CAUTIONS

- Bradycardia is an oxygenation problem

Diagnosis

ESSENTIAL WORKUP

- Detailed physical examination
- Cardiac assessment
  - —Heart sounds
  - —Murmurs
  - —Liver size
  - —Peripheral pulses
  - —Lower-extremity blood pressures
  - —Skin perfusion

LABORATORY

- Bedside serum blood glucose
- If vigorous resuscitation
  - —Arterial blood gases
  - —Complete blood count
- Blood cultures if sepsis is a concern

IMAGING/SPECIAL TESTS

- Chest radiography
  - —Significant respiratory distress
  - —Congenital heart disease
- Other workup is based on clinical suspicion
  - —Echocardiography
  - —Computed tomography
  - —Lumbar puncture

DIFFERENTIAL DIAGNOSIS

See etiology

Treatment

INITIAL STABILIZATION

- Most infants will respond to simple maneuvers
  - —Maintain body temperature
    - -Warm environment
    - -Dry the infant
    - -Remove wet towels
    - -Place the infant under a radiant warmer
  - —Positioning
    - -Supine with the neck mildly hyperextended (sniffing position)
    - -A 2.5-cm roll under the shoulders
  - —Suctioning
    - -Use a wall suction device or a bulb syringe
    - -Suction the mouth first then the nose
    - -Avoid deep suctioning to prevent vagally mediated bradycardia or apnea
  - —Tactile stimulation
    - -Absence of adequate spontaneous respirations
    - -Flick the soles of the feet or rub the back
- Oxygen
  - —100% oxygen is always used
  - —Oxygen toxicity is not a concern during resuscitation
- Positive pressure ventilation (PPV)
  - —Indications
    - -Apnea
    - -Inadequate respirations to maintain oxygenation
    - -Persistent central cyanosis despite delivery of 100% oxygen
    - -Heart rate less than 100 beats per minute
  - —Ventilations are delivered at a rate of 40–60 breaths per minute
  - —The initial breath may require up to 70 cm H_2O pressure, and the pop-off valve may need to be bypassed
  - —If available, pressure manometers should be used
  - —After 15–30 seconds reevaluate
    - -Heart rate greater than 100 and spontaneous respirations, discontinue PPV
    - -If the heart rate is between 60 and 100 and increasing, continue PPV
    - -If the heart rate is between 60 and 100 and not increasing, check the adequacy of the ventilation
    - -If the heart rate remains below 60, begin chest compressions
  - —Insertion of an orogastric tube is needed with prolonged ventilation
- Tension pneumothorax due to barotrauma
  - —Insertion of a 23–25-gauge catheter or butterfly
  - —Second intercostal space at the midclavicular line
  - —Connect via a three-way stopcock to a 50 cc syringe
- Endotracheal intubation
  - —Indications
    - -Ineffective bag-valve-mask ventilation
    - -Need for prolonged ventilation
    - -Meconium aspiration
    - -Known diaphragmatic hernia
  - —Miller 0 (premature infants) or Miller 1 straight blades may be used
  - —Suggested tube size by weight and gestational age
    - -2.5 mm: below 1000 g; below 28 weeks
    - -3.0 mm: 1000–2000 g; 28–34 weeks
    - -3.5 mm: 2000–3000 g; 34–38 weeks
    - -3.5–4.0 mm: above 3000 g; above 38 weeks
- Chest Compressions
  - —Indications
    - -Heart rate of less than 60 or a heart rate of 60–80 that is not rapidly increasing
    - -Compressions are delivered at a rate of 120 times per minute
- Access
  - —Umbilical venous catheter is the route of choice
  - —Endotracheal route
    - -Instill medications via a feeding tube
    - -Flush the tube with 0.5–1 cc of normal saline

ED TREATMENT

- Epinephrine
  - —Heart rate less than 80 beats per minute
  - —Adequate ventilation with 100% oxygen
  - —Chest compressions for a minimum of 30 seconds
- Naloxone
  - —Indicated for respiratory depression related to narcotic administration to the mother
  - —May precipitate withdrawal seizures in an infant of a chronically addicted mother
- Sodium bicarbonate
  - —Prolonged resuscitation or documented metabolic acidosis
- Glucose
  - —Serum glucose less than 35 mg/dl in a term infant or less than 25 mg/dl in a premature infant
- Hypovolemia
  - —Volume expanders
    - -Normal saline
    - -Ringer's lactate
    - -5% albumin
    - -O-negative blood crossmatched with the mother's blood
- Dopamine
  - —Prolonged resuscitation with continued evidence of shock
- Prematurity
  - —Avoid hypothermia, rapid infusion of fluid boluses, and all hypertonic solutions
- Meconium aspiration
  - —Suctioning of the mouth, oropharynx, and then the nose after delivery of the head
  - —Intubate immediately with thick or particulate meconium prior to any stimulation
  - —Suction the trachea via the ETT until clear
  - —Reintubation followed by repeat suctioning as needed

MEDICATIONS

- Epinephrine: 0.1–0.3 ml/kg IV, ET 1:10,000 solution
- Sodium bicarbonate: 1–2 mEq/kg IV 4.2% solution; give slowly over at least 2 min
- Dextrose: 2–4 ml/kg IV 10% solution; give slowly over 10 min
- Naloxone: 0.1 mg/kg IV, ET
- Dopamine: begin at 5 μg/kg/min, up to 20 μg/kg/min; IV
- Volume expanders: 10 cc/kg bolus

Disposition

ADMISSION CRITERIA

- All neonates requiring resuscitation should be admitted for observation
- Neonatal intensive care unit
  - —If more than simple maneuvers
  - —Premature infants for surfactant therapy

DISCHARGE CRITERIA

N/A

Miscellaneous

ICD9: N/A

CORE CONTENT CODE: 13.17

SUGGESTED READINGS

Jain L, Vidyasagar D. Controversies in neonatal resuscitation. Pediatr Ann 1995;25:540–545.

Khan NS, Luten RC. Neonatal resuscitation. Emerg Med Clin North Am 1994;12:239–256.

Leuther SR, Jansen RD, Hageman JR. Cardiopulmonary resuscitation of the newborn, an update. Pediatr Clin North Am 1994;41:893–907.

Sims DG, Heal CA, Bartle SM. Use of adrenaline and atropine in neonatal resuscitation. Arch Dis Child 1994;70:F3–F10.

Author: Joan Bothner

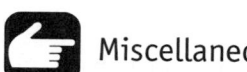

Resuscitation, Pediatric

Clinical Presentation

SIGNS AND SYMPTOMS

- Cardiopulmonary arrest
  - —Progressive deterioration of respiration function and circulatory shock
- Vital signs initially compensated, deteriorating to decompensated findings
  - —Orthostatic vital signs helpful
- Respiratory failure
  - —Tachypnea, followed preterminally by slow irregular breathing
  - —Cyanosis
  - —Grunting, flaring, stridor
  - —Retractions, diminished breath sounds
  - —Decreased level of consciousness, poor skeletal muscle tone
- Shock
  - —Tachycardia, followed by bradycardia
  - —Hypotension, although early in shock BP may be normal or high
  - —Weak, thready pulse
  - —Mottled, pale skin
  - —Increased capillary refill time >2 seconds
  - —Altered or decreased level of consciousness
  - —Decreased urine output

MECHANISM/DESCRIPTION

- Primary respiratory or circulatory failure leads to hypoxia and acidosis
- Multiple organ failure subsequently develops

ETIOLOGY

- Primary respiratory or circulatory failure
- Respiratory
  - —Upper airway: croup, epiglottitis, foreign body, tracheitis
  - —Lower airway: asthma, bronchiolitis, pneumonia, foreign body
- Shock: hypovolemia secondary to fluid loss (vomiting and diarrhea, trauma, burn), distributive, sepsis
- Vascular: congenital heart disease, dysrhythmia, myocarditis, pericarditis
- Hypoventilation: coma, status epilepticus
- Trauma: hypovolemia, subdural/epidural
- Infection: meningitis, sepsis
- Metabolic: hypoglycemia, hypercalcemia, hypo/hyperkalemia
- Sudden infant death syndrome (SIDS)/apparent life-threatening event (ALTE)

Pre-Hospital

- Early recognition of impending arrest
- EMS personnel must recognize and stabilize child
- Priorities of airway, breathing, and circulation
- Requires experienced personnel, equipment, and protocols
- Communication with receiving institution is essential

Diagnosis

ESSENTIAL WORKUP

- Assess patient's airway, breathing and circulation
- History of preceding events from pre-hospital personnel and parents
- Airway patency: observe respirations, listen to patient talk/cry, observe for signs of obstruction
- Respiratory rate: tachypnea initial response to stress; slow or irregular respiratory pattern is sign of impending respiratory failure
- Work of breathing: assess for grunting, nasal flaring, chest retractions, and head bobbing with respiration
- Air movement: chest wall should normally expand smoothly and symmetrically with equal breath sounds
- Skin: look for mottled, pale, gray, or cyanotic skin; feel skin for its temperature and consistency (i.e., tenting in severe dehydration)
- Pulse and blood pressure: look for tachycardia or bradycardia (more ominous) while assessing pulse pressure (wide pulse pressure in early septic shock)
- Capillary refill: normally >2 seconds; delayed with poor perfusion or cold ambient temperature
- Mental status: inadequate oxygen delivery can result in confusion, agitation, and lethargy
- Pulse oximetry: reflects hemoglobin oxygen saturation, not necessarily oxygen delivery

LABORATORY

- Initial studies should reflect assessment needs and potential etiologic considerations
- Arterial blood gas to assess ventilation, oxygenation, and acid-base status
- Electrolytes and serum glucose; metabolic studies as indicated
- Trauma studies if indicated
- Toxicology studies as indicated

IMAGING/SPECIAL TESTS

- Chest radiograph to evaluate for pulmonary and cardiac status; look for potential etiologies
- Cervical spine film and other trauma studies if preexisting injury

DIFFERENTIAL DIAGNOSIS

- Potential endpoint of all untreated or unresponsive critical illness
- Child abuse should be considered when the history is inconsistent with nature of the illness

Treatment

INITIAL STABILIZATION

- Focus on resuscitation
- ABCDE
  - —Airway: check for signs of obstruction; talk to patient
  - —Breathing: observe chest excursion; auscultate chest
  - —Circulation: evaluate heart rate, blood pressure, pulse pressure, level of consciousness, capillary refill
  - —Disability: determine level of consciousness and assess for neurological deficit
  - —Exposure/environment: undress child for full exposure while keeping ambient temperature adequate to prevent hypothermia

ED TREATMENT

- Continuous monitoring for response to therapy and changes in conditions
- Airway: must be secured for resuscitative efforts to succeed
  - —Correct tongue obstruction using jaw thrust and chin lift
  - —Clear airway by suctioning blood, secretions, foreign body
  - —Airway adjuncts: nasopharyngeal and oropharyngeal airways, bag-valve mask ventilation, endotracheal intubation
- Breathing: assure ventilation and oxygenation
- Circulation
  - —Control hemorrhage: pressure/elevation for external hemorrhage, surgical intervention for internal injuries
  - —Intravascular access: peripheral, intraosseous, cut down, central venous
  - —Fluid therapy: initial bolus of 20 ml/kg crystalloid, repeat as necessary; if inadequate response, consider red cell transfusion
- Cardiopulmonary resuscitation (CPR)
  - —Formal algorithms are available from the American Heart Association
  - —Provide blood flow to vital organs while restoring spontaneous circulation
  - —Infant <1 year: Check for pulse at the brachial or femoral artery. Compressions are on the lower half of the sternum using two fingers placed just below the nipple line. Alternatively, the lower chest and abdomen are gripped by both hands and lower sternum compressed by both thumbs. Compression rate at least 100 per minute; 5 compressions to 1 ventilation; compress 0.5–1.0 inches (⅓ chest)
  - —Children 1–8 years: Check for pulse at carotid artery. Compressions are applied with one hand midway between the xiphoid notch and nipple line. Compression rate of 100 per minute. Compress 1.0–1.5 inches (⅓ chest)
- Cardiac rhythm disturbances
  - —Usually secondary to respiratory insufficiency or metabolic disturbances
  - —Absent pulse: ventricular fibrillation, pulseless ventricular tachycardia, asystole, and electromechanical dissociation (EMD)
  - —Slow pulse: sinus bradycardia, atrioventricular nodal block, escape rhythms
  - —Fast pulse: sinus tachycardia, supraventricular tachycardia, ventricular tachycardia

MEDICATIONS (FIRST OR LOADING DOSE)

- Adenosine: 0.1 mg/kg IV
- Atropine: 0.01 mg/kg IV (min dose: 0.1 mg)
- Bretylium: 5 mg/kg IV
- Calcium chloride: 20 mg/kg IV slowly
- Cardioversion: 0.5 joules/kg
- Defibrillation: 2 joules/kg
- Epirephrine: 0.01 mg/kg IV (second or ET dose: 0.1 mg/kg IV)
- Glucagon: 0.03–0.1 mg/kg IV
- Lidocaine: 1 mg/kg IV
- Naloxone: 0.1 mg/kg IV
- Procainamide: 2–6 mg/kg IV slowly
- Sodium bicarbonate: 0.5–1.0 mEq/kg IV
- Verapamil: 0.1–0.15 mg/kg IV (> 1 year olds)

Disposition

ADMISSION CRITERIA

- All survivors should be admitted to an intensive care unit with personnel, equipment, and expertise in the management of children
- Patients require aggressive management of hypoxemia, hypercapnia, hemodynamic instability, altered sensorium
- Consultation often required, which reflects the specific pathophysiology

DISCHARGE CRITERIA

N/A

Miscellaneous

ICD9: 427.5

CORE CONTENT CODE: 13.17, 18.6.1.3, 18.1.3

SUGGESTED READINGS

Chameides L, Hazinski MF, eds. Textbook of pediatric advanced life support. Dallas: American Heart Association, 1994.

Jaffe D, Wesson D. Emergency management of blunt trauma in children. N Engl J Med 1991;324:1477.

Rockney RM, Alario AJ, Lewander WJ. Pediatric advanced life support: Part 1 and 2. Am Fam Physician 1991;43:1712.

Authors: Scott D. Berns; Stuart J. Spitalnic

Retinal Detachment

Clinical Presentation

SIGNS AND SYMPTOMS

- Flashes of light
- Floaters
- "Curtain" or shadow over visual field
- Peripheral or central vision loss
- Visual field defects
- May be asymptomatic, especially in tractional retinal detachments

MECHANISM/DESCRIPTION

- Three distinct classifications of retinal detachments—treatments for each are different and exclusive
  —Rhegmatogenous retinal detachments (RRD)
  —Tractional retinal detachments (TRD)
  —Exudative retinal detachments (ERD)
- RRD
  —Most common
  —Occur when a break in the sensory retina allows fluid from the vitreous to separate the rods and cones from the villi of the pigment epithelium
  —Occur as an acute event, with symptoms of flashes due to the separation of the nerve fibers, and spots due to bleeding from the rupturing of retinal blood vessels
- TRD
  —Occur because of contraction of fibrous vitreous bands pulling the sensory retina off of the pigment epithelium
  —Chronic progressive disorder
  —May remain without symptoms unless hemorrhage or retinal tear occurs
- ERD
  —Abnormal collections of fluid are produced, separating the layer of the retina
  —Usually asymptomatic until involvement of the macula occurs, with impairment of the central vision
  —Occasionally, the retina can become so elevated and anteriorly displaced by underlying fluid as to be visible with a penlight just behind the lens

ETIOLOGY

- RRD occurs as a result of either structural/developmental abnormalities of the eye
  —High myopia
  —Marfan's syndrome
  —Structural degeneration of the underlying anatomy of the eye (including the pigment epithelium, the sensory retina, and the vitreous body, or occasionally as a result of trauma)
- TRD occur in association with
  —Diabetes
  —Vasculopathy
  —Perforating injury
  —Severe chorioretinitis
  —Retinopathy of prematurity, sickle cell retinopathy, or toxocariasis
- ERD arise from
  —Tumors of the choroid (e.g., melanoma) or retina (e.g., retinoblastoma)
  —Inflammatory disorders as Coats' or Harada's diseases

Pre-Hospital

N/A

Diagnosis

ESSENTIAL WORKUP

- History, especially
  —Age
  —Speed of onset of symptoms
  —Associated symptoms
  —Previous episodes
- Complete ophthalmologic examination, especially
  —Assessment of pupillary function
  —Evaluation of the vitreous for cells
  —Dilated retinal exam

LABORATORY

- As indicated for underlying disease

IMAGING/SPECIAL TESTS

- Visual field testing

DIFFERENTIAL DIAGNOSIS

- Senile retinoschisis (retinoschisis—a splitting of the retina)
- Juvenile retinoschisis
- Choroidal detachment

Treatment

INITIAL STABILIZATION

N/A

ED TREATMENT

- Bedrest
- Urgent ophthalmologic consultation

Disposition

ADMISSION CRITERIA

- Admit acute RRDs that threaten the macula for bedrest pending urgent repair of the detachment
- Admit TRDs involving the macula for bedrest and urgent repair

DISCHARGE CRITERIA

- RRDs that do not threaten the macula may be repaired at the earliest convenience, ideally within 1–2 days
- Chronic retinal detachments may be repaired or treated within 1 week
- Exudative retinal detachments will generally resolve with successful treatment of the underlying condition

Miscellaneous

ICD9: 361.9

CORE CONTENT CODE: 6.4.3.4

SUGGESTED READINGS

LaVene D, Halpern J, Jagoda A. Loss of vision. Emergency treatment of the eye. Emerg Med Clin North Am 1995;13(3):539–560.

Lincoff H, Kreissig I. Retinal detachment. In: Fraunfelder, FT. Current Ocular Therapy. 4th ed. Philadelphia: WB Saunders, 1995:474–476.

Author: Evan Liu

Retropharyngeal Abscess

Clinical Presentation

SIGNS AND SYMPTOMS

- Often preceded by nasopharyngitis or otitis media
- Fever (100%)
- Torticollis or refusal to move the neck (75%)
  - —Aggravated by swallowing
- Dysphagia
- Stridor/drooling (20–40%)
- Cervical adenopathy (100%)
- Pharyngitis (60%)
- Bulging of the posterior pharynx (25%)
- Trismus
- Meningismus
- Difficult diagnosis in infants
  - —Fever
  - —Irritability
  - —Poor feeding
  - —Pain with neck movement
  - —Stridor
  - —Do not palpate the posterior pharynx
    - -Spontaneous perforation and aspiration may occur

MECHANISM/DESCRIPTION

- An infection lying between the middle cervical and alar fascia
  - —Anterior to the prevertebral space
- Wide spectrum of pathogens
  - —Primarily Gram-positive and anaerobic bacteria
  - —Gram-negative
  - —Acid-fast bacilli
  - —Broad spectrum antibiotic coverage should be used initially
- Primarily a disease of preschool children
  - —The posterior pharyngeal nodes regress well before puberty
  - —Reported in all age groups
  - —Resurgence of cases in later adulthood
- Complications
  - —Sepsis
  - —Airway obstruction
  - —Mediastinitis
  - —Spontaneous perforation
  - —Aspiration pneumonia
  - —Thrombosis of the internal jugular vein
  - —Erosion into the carotid artery
- Prognosis with prompt therapy and diagnosis is very good

ETIOLOGY

- Suppurative adenitis of the posterior pharyngeal nodes
- Otitis media
- Pharyngitis
- Recent upper airway instrumentation
- Upper airway trauma
- Foreign body
- Pharyngotonsillitis
- Cervical osteomyelitis

Pre-Hospital

CAUTIONS

- The child should be kept calm
- A parent may hold or comfort the child in transport if this is feasible
- Place on pulse oximetry and cardiac monitors
- Provide with supplemental oxygen as needed
- Transport with suction and intubation equipment
- Airway control
  - —Prior to lengthy transports
  - —Airway compromise

Diagnosis

ESSENTIAL WORKUP

- Evaluation should occur after the airway is controlled in patients with respiratory compromise
- Determine presence of a fluid collection
- Determine the need for surgical intervention

LABORATORY

- Blood cultures
- CBC
- Throat culture patients with pharyngitis

IMAGING/SPECIAL TESTS

- Soft tissue lateral neck radiographs
  - —Taken in inspiration with partial neck extension
  - —Crucial in establishing the diagnosis
  - —Widening of the retropharyngeal space anterior to C2
    - ->7 mm
    - -less than one-half the width of the vertebral body
  - —The retrotracheal space anterior to C6
    - ->14 mm in preschool aged children
    - ->22 mm in adults
- Chest radiograph is used to evaluate for aspiration or mediastinal widening
- Contrasted CT of the neck
  - —Delineates the extent of deep space involvement
  - —Differentiate abscess formation from cellulitis
  - —Detection of abnormalities of adjacent vertebra and vasculature

DIFFERENTIAL DIAGNOSIS

- Tonsillopharyngitis
- Epiglottitis
- Tracheitis
- Croup
- Foreign body
- Cervical osteomyelitis
- Epidural abscess
- Retropharyngeal hemorrhage
- Meningitis
- Dystonic reactions
- Other deep space neck infections

Treatment

INITIAL STABILIZATION

- Patients with significant airway obstruction
- Supplemental oxygen
- Controlled oral intubation or tracheotomy, preferably in an operating suite
- Intravenous access but delay to avoid upsetting children when the airway is compromised

ED TREATMENT

- Antibiotics
  —Primarily directed toward Gram-positive organisms
  —Other second- or third-generation cephalosporins may also be used initially *in lieu* of ceftriaxone
- Patients are made NPO in anticipation of diagnostic or therapeutic intervention
- Surgical consultation

MEDICATIONS

- Ceftriaxone: 50 mg/kg IV (peds) or 1 g IV (adult); *plus*
- Clindamycin: 10 mg/kg IV (peds) or 600–900 mg IV (adult) *or*
- Ampicillin/sulbactam: 50 mg/kg IV (peds) or 1.5–3.0 g IV (adult)

Disposition

ADMISSION CRITERIA

- All patients with RPA should be admitted to a hospital with readily available otolaryngologists and anesthesiologists
- ICU admission
  —Infants and toxic-appearing children
  —Patients with airway compromise
  —Altered mental status
  —Hemodynamic instability
  —Those with evidence of other complications

DISCHARGE CRITERIA

- None

Miscellaneous

ICD9: 478.24

CORE CONTENT CODE: 6.3.10; 13.7.15

SUGGESTED READINGS

Bank DE, Krug SE. New approaches to upper airway disease. Emerg Med Clin North Am 1995;13(2):473–487.

Marra S, Hotaling AJ. Deep neck infections. Am J Otolaryngol 1996;17(5):287–298.

Pontell J, Har-El G, Lucente FE. Retropharyngeal abscess: clinical review. Ear Nose Throat J 1995;74(10):701–704.

Author: Keith Wrenn

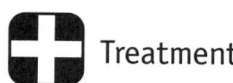

Reye's Syndrome

Clinical Presentation

SIGNS AND SYMPTOMS

- History of a viral illness or prodrome
- Profuse and repeated vomiting
  —Typically 4–5 days after the start of the viral illness
- Infants
  —Tachypnea
  —Apnea
  —Irritability
  —Seizures
  —Hypoglycemia
- Usually the patient is afebrile
- Tachycardia
- Hyperventilation
- No focal neurological signs
- No meningismus
- Hepatomegaly in 40% of cases
- Clinical staging of Reye's syndrome with Lovejoy's Classification
  —Stage I
    -Vomiting
    -Lethargy
    -Sleepiness
  —Stage II
    -Disorientation
    -Delirium
    -Combativeness
    -Hyperventilation
    -Hyperreflexia
    -Appropriate response to noxious stimuli
  —Stage III
    -Obtunded
    -Coma
    -Hyperventilation
    -Inappropriate response to noxious stimuli
    -Decorticate posturing
    -Preservation of pupillary light reflexes
    -Preservation of oculovestibular light reflexes
  —Stage IV
    -Deeper coma
    -Decerebrate rigidity
    -Loss of oculovestibular reflexes
    -Dilated, fixed pupils
    -Dysconjugate eye movements in response to caloric stimulation
  —Stage V
    -Seizures
    -Absent deep tendon reflexes
    -Respiratory Arrest
    -Flaccid paralysis

MECHANISM/DESCRIPTION

- Reversible clinicopathologic syndrome of unknown etiology
- Primary mitochondrial injury
- Decrease enzyme activity
  —Krebs cycle
  —Gluconeogenesis
  —Urea biosynthesis
- Fatty infiltration
  —Liver
    -Hyperammonemia due to decreased conversion from ammonia to urea
    -Hepatorenal syndrome may be the end result
    -Rapid recovery of liver function in survivors
  —Brain
    -Encephalopathy of unclear etiology
    -Cytotoxic edema
    -Herniation is the most common cause of death
    -Normal recovery of neurologic function in survivors
  —Skeletal and myocardial muscle
    -Fatty infiltration and distorted mitochondria
- Fewer than 10% of cases occurs before the age of 1 year
  —Average age is 7 years
  —Peak age is 4–11 years
- Regional differences
  —Highest incidence in the Midwestern states
  —Lower incidence in the states of the Southeast and far West
- More common in whites than in blacks
- Peak incidence is in winter and early spring

ETIOLOGY

- Not known with certainty
- Multifactorial causes have been epidemiologically implicated
  —Antecedent viral syndrome
    -Influenza B and A
    -Varicella
    -Diarrhea illness
  —Genetic predisposition
  —Exposure to salicylates
  —Other undefined factors

Pre-Hospital

CAUTIONS

- Decreased mental status
  —Glucose
  —Narcan
- Coma
  —Assist respirations with bag-valve-mask

Diagnosis

ESSENTIAL WORKUP

- Establish the presence of encephalopathy and liver abnormalities
- Laboratory testing to assess for characteristic biochemical abnormalities
- Liver biopsy confirms the diagnosis

LABORATORY

- Liver function tests
  - —A three-fold or greater rise in AST, ALT
  - —Serum ammonia level at least 1.5 times greater than normal
  - —Serum bilirubin should be normal or slightly elevated
- The prothrombin time may be prolonged
- Hypoglycemia may be present, especially in infants
- Elevated BUN
- Ketonuria
- Normal platelet count and blood smear
- Negative toxic screen
- Bleeding screen
  - —Liver dependent clotting factors decreased

IMAGING/SPECIAL TESTS

- Head CT scan
  - —May show diffuse cerebral edema
- Lumbar puncture
  - —Perform after head CT
  - —Edema is diffuse and LP is not contraindicated
  - —Measure opening pressure
  - —Less than 8 leukocytes per mm^3

DIFFERENTIAL DIAGNOSIS

- Inborn errors of metabolism
  - —Consider in children <1 year of age
  - —Disorders of the urea cycle
  - —Disorders of fatty acid oxidation
  - —Systemic carnitine deficiency
  - —Organic acidemias
  - —Disorders of the electron transport chain
- Sepsis with dehydration
- Toxin exposure
  - —Toxic encephalopathy without liver dysfunction (Gall's syndrome)
  - —Lead
  - —Hydrocarbons
- Drug intoxication
  - —Acetaminophen
  - —Salicylates
- CNS infection
  - —Meningitis
  - —Encephalitis
- Varicella hepatitis

Treatment

INITIAL STABILIZATION

- Place on a cardiorespiratory monitor
- Supplemental oxygen
- Rapid sequence intubation is airway management required
- Glucose if there is altered mental status
  - —10% glucose solution intravenously
    - -rate of two-thirds maintenance requirement after dehydration corrected
  - —Follow serum glucose hourly
- Avoid early overhydration

ED TREATMENT

- Institute treatment before the liver biopsy
- Vitamin K
  - —Indicated if there is an elevated prothrombin time
- Fresh frozen plasma
  - —To control bleeding
  - —To correct a severe coagulopathy
- Interventions aimed at lowering intracranial pressure
  - —Stage III or greater
  - —Stage II with serum ammonia >300 μg/L
  - —Intubation using rapid sequence intubation
  - —Hyperventilation
  - —Fluid restriction
  - —Barbiturate coma
  - —Osmotically active agents
    - -Mannitol
    - -Furosemide
  - —Monitor Intracranial pressure
    - -Subarachnoid bolt
    - -Intraventricular cannula

MEDICATIONS

- D50W: 1–2 cc/kg/dose (0.5–1.0 g/kg) IV over the age of 3 years
- D25W: 2–4 cc/kg/dose (0.5–1.0 mg/kg) IV under the age of 3 years; maintenance infusion 10% dextrose solution at a rate of 2/3
- Lasix: 1 mg/kg IV
- Mannitol: 0.25–1.0 g/kg IV q 4–6 hrs
- Vitamin K: 1–2 mg/dose (Infants and children) 2–10 mg/dose (Adolescents)
- Pentobarbital: 3–20 mg/kg IV slowly while monitoring blood pressure; maintenance infusion 1–2 mg/kg/h; maintain level at 25–40 μg/dl

Disposition

ADMISSION CRITERIA

- All children with suspected Reye's syndrome should be admitted to the intensive care unit
- Hospital capable of ICP monitoring

DISCHARGE CRITERIA

N/A

Miscellaneous

ICD9: 331.81

CORE CONTENT CODE: 13.5.1.1

SUGGESTED READINGS

Hails KA. Reye's syndrome. In: Reisdorff EJ, Roberts MR, Wiegenstein JG, eds. Pediatric emergencies. Philadelphia: WB Saunders, 1993:371–377.

National Institutes of Health Consensus Conference. Diagnosis and treatment of Reye's syndrome. JAMA 1981;246:2441–2444.

Quam DA. Recognizing a case of Reye's syndrome. Am Fam Physician 1994;50:1491–1496.

Author: Brian Everle

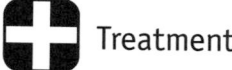

Rhabdomyolysis

Clinical Presentation

SIGNS AND SYMPTOMS

- Can vary dramatically, reflect underlying disease process
- Obvious crushing injury
- Hypothermia/hyperthermia
- Alert/obtunded
- Muscle pain (only 50%), tenderness, swelling
- Hypovolemic state, dry mucous membrane, poor skin turgor, tachycardia, hypotension
- Decreased urine output
- Change in urine color

MECHANISM/DESCRIPTION

- Syndrome associated with muscle injury and systemic release of its content (CPK)
- Combination of myoglobinuria, hypovolemia, and aciduria lead to acute renal failure
- Direct release of potassium from damaged muscle tissue may lead to dysrhythmias and sudden death

ETIOLOGY

- Muscle injury due to trauma, exercise, seizure, burn, electrical shock
- Hypothermia, hyperthermia
- Prolonged immobile state
- Drugs/toxins (alcohols, cocaine, amphetamines, opiates, antihistamines, barbiturates, PCP, caffeine, carbon monoxide, cholesterol lowering agents, succinylcholine, snake venom, bee/hornet venom, etc.)
- Neuroleptic malignant syndrome
- Metabolic disorder (hypokalemia, hypophosphatemia, hyperthyroid state, DKA, hyperosmolar state, hypoxia)
- Infections (viral, bacterial, parasitic, protozoan, rickettsial)
- Genetic disorders (McArdle's disease, Tarui's disease)
- Immunological disorders (dermatomyositis, polymyositis)
- Idiopathic

Pre-Hospital

- Need for rapid extrication in case of crush injury
- *Early IV fluids* to prevent complications of restored blood flow to injured limb (hypovolemia, acute renal failure (ARF), hyperkalemia, etc.)

Diagnosis

ESSENTIAL WORKUP

- History and physical are insensitive in making the diagnosis
- *Serum CPK level is criterion standard and must be sent if any clinical suspicion exists*
- Urine dipstick which is positive for heme but absent for RBCs suggests rhabdomyolysis
  - —Becasue of rapid urinary excretion of myoglobin, up to 26% of patients with rhabdomyolysis have negative urine dipstick
- Serum electrolytes (potassium, calcium, magnesium, phosphorus, bun, creatinine, uric acid)

LABORATORY

- Arterial blood gas
- Urine/serum myoglobin is too transient to be useful
- Serum glucose, LDH, SGOT, albumin, toxicology screen in absence of physical injury
- PT/PTT, platelet count, fibrinogen, fibrin-split products if DIC is suspected

IMAGING/SPECIAL TESTS

- MRI is 90–95% sensitive in visualizing muscle injury, but does not change initial ED treatment

DIFFERENTIAL DIAGNOSIS

- The following conditions may present with elevated serum CPK but may not lead to complications of rhabdomyolysis
  - —Nontraumatic myopathies
  - —Renal failure
  - —Intramuscular injections
  - —Myocardial injury
  - —Hypothyroidism
  - —Hyperthyroidism
  - —Stroke
  - —Surgery

Treatment

INITIAL STABILIZATION

- ABCs
- Immobilization of trauma/crush injuries
- IV fluids for hypotension and hypovolemia

ED TREATMENT

- Directed toward treating or reversing the cause of rhabdomyolysis
- *Prevent ARF:* IV fluid, mannitol, furosemide (keep urine output >30 cc/hr)
- *Hyperkalemia:* IV fluid, dextrose, insulin, kayexalate, calcium gluconate, monitor/EKG
- *Acidosis:* bicarbonate IV (keep urine PH >6.5)
- *Overdose:* activated charcoal, lavage, antidote
- *Infection:* broad spectrum antibiotics
- *Compartment syndrome:* fasciotomy (compartment pressure >35 mmHg)
- *Neuroleptic malignant syndrome:* dantrolene, bromocriptine
- *Need for hemodialysis:* refractory to treatment, hyperkalemia, hyperphosphatemia, hyperuricemia, volume overload, overdose

MEDICATIONS

- Bicarbonate: 50–100 cc of 8.4% solution IV; peds: 1 mEq/kg up to 50–100 mEq
- Furosemide: 20 mg IV bolus; peds: 1 mg/kg/dose IV

Disposition

ADMISSION CRITERIA

- *Because it is impossible to predict which patients will develop complications all patients with significant elevated CPK or suspicion for rhabdomyolysis must be admitted*
- Admit to monitored bed for patients with electrolyte abnormalities
- Admit to ICU bed for patients who might require hemodialysis or closer fluid and electrolyte monitoring

DISCHARGE CRITERIA

- No patients suspected of having rhabdomyolysis should be discharged from the ED

Miscellaneous

ICD9: 728.89

CORE CONTENT CODE: 10.5.2

SUGGESTED READINGS

Cheney P. Early management and physiologic changes in crush syndrome. Crit Care Nurs Q 1994;17(2):62–73.

Pina EM, Mehlman CT. Rhabdomyolysis—A primer for the orthopaedist. Orthop Rev 1994;23(1):28–32.

Prendergast BD, George CF. Drug-induced rhabdomyolysis—Mechanisms and management. Postgrad Med J 1993;69(811):333–336.

Sinert R, Kohl L, Rainone T, Scalea T. Exercise-induced rhabdomyolysis. Ann Emerg Med 1994;23(6):1301–1306.

Zager RA. Rhabdomyolysis and myohemoglobinuric acute renal failure [Editorial Review]. Kidney Int 1996;49(2):314–326.

Authors: Marcelo Sandoval; Nicholas K. Han

Rheumatic Fever

Clinical Presentation

SIGNS AND SYMPTOMS

- Acute rheumatic fever (ARF) presents with fever and malaise
- Symptoms begin within 2–6 weeks following a streptococcal pharyngitis
  - —One-third of patients are unaware of preceding pharyngitis
- In adults, ARF may present with joint symptoms alone
- In children, the full spectrum of disease, including fever, rash, chorea, arthritis, and carditis, is more likely
- Spontaneous resolution of ARF within 3 months is the rule, though carditis/valvulitis may persist

Major Manifestations

- *Polyarthritis* in 60–75% of initial attacks
  - —Often migratory, involves the knees, ankles, elbows, and wrists
  - —Lower extremities joints are more commonly involved
  - —Rheumatic arthritis generally responds to salicylates
- *Carditis* occurs in one-third of new cases
  - —Pericardium, myocardium, and endocardium may be affected (pancarditis)
  - —Myocarditis may lead to heart failure, but is frequently asymptomatic
  - —Valvular disease and endocarditis are the most serious sequela of ARF
  - —Carditis is heralded by a new murmur, tachycardia, gallop rhythm, pericardial friction rub, or congestive heart failure
- *Chorea* occurs in 10% of cases
  - —Syndenham's chorea predominantly affects teenage females
  - —Purposeless uncoordinated movements of the extremities characterize chorea
  - —The movements are more apparent during periods of anxiety and disappear with sleep
  - —Chorea may be the sole manifestation of ARF
- *Erythema marginatum* occurs in less than 5% of cases
  - —Nonpruritic pink eruptions with central clearing and well-demarcated irregular borders
  - —Usually seen on the trunk and the extremities
- *Subcutaneous nodules* in 20% of patients
  - —Crops of small subcutaneous painless nodules located most commonly on extensor surfaces

Minor Manifestations

- Clinical
  - —Fever (>38°C)
  - —Arthralgia
  - —Previous rheumatic fever or rheumatic heart disease
  - —History of positive throat culture
- Laboratory
  - —Prolong PR interval
  - —Increased antistreptolysin O (>250)
  - —Elevated erythrocyte sedimentation rate or C-reactive protein
  - —Leukocytosis

PEDIATRIC CONSIDERATIONS

- In children, cardiac involvement is usually a dominant feature and occurs early
- Chorea is a late finding, and is not seen in conjunction with carditis

ETIOLOGY

- Genetic predisposition
- Patients with prior ARF are at greater risk for recurrence
- Group A streptococcus contain antigens that are thought to be immunologically cross-reactive with antigens in human tissue
  - —The magnitude of the immune response is strongly correlated with the attack rate of rheumatic fever following streptococcal pharyngitis
- Risk factors associated with ARF are the same for streptococcal pharyngitis, including overcrowding, age, dampness, and socioeconomic status
- ARF is relatively rare in the United States, and remains more prevalent in the developing world where in some places it is the leading cause of mortality in people between the ages of 5 and 24

Pre-Hospital

- Patients with significant congestive heart failure may require early airway management

Diagnosis

- *Jones' criteria* for diagnosis of ARF requires the presence of two of the major manifestations listed above, or one major and two minor; in addition, there must be evidence of an antecedent streptococcal infection

ESSENTIAL WORKUP

- CXR
- EKG
- Throat culture
- Antistreptolysin O
- Erythrocyte sedimentation rate, C-reactive protein
- CBC

LABORATORY

- Throat culture is helpful if previous Group A Streptococcal infection is demonstrated
  - —In 90% of patients, throat culture is negative by the time symptoms of ARF are seen
- Antistreptolysin O greater than 250 Todd units, though may normally be found up to 300 in healthy school-age children in crowded urban environments
- Increased P-R interval on ECG is useful for diagnosis
- Approximately 50% of patients will have mild proteinuria or casts in their urine

IMAGING/SPECIAL TESTS

- Echocardiogram may reveal pericardial effusion, valvular disease, or cardiomyopathy

DIFFERENTIAL DIAGNOSIS

- Rheumatoid arthritis
- Infective endocarditis
- Lyme disease
- Reiter's syndrome and other reactive arthritis
- SLE
- Postgonococcal arthritis
- Other infectious causes of arthritis and carditis included are Coxsackie B and parvovirus

Treatment

INITIAL STABILIZATION

- In the presence of heart failure, diuretics and digitalis are indicated
- Drainage of malignant pericardial effusion
- In severe carditis, steroids are recommended
- In the case of chorea, haloperidol or other tranquilizers, including phenobarbital, are useful

ED TREATMENT

- Antibiotic treatment for Streptococcal pharyngitis should be given when the diagnosis of ARF is made
  - —IM or po penicillin, or erythromycin for penicillin allergic
  - —All patients should receive aspirin or NSAIDs for the inflammatory state associated with ARF
    - -ASA/NSAIDs should be continued for 2–3 weeks after ESR approaches near normal levels
- For *carditis*
  - —Aspirin
  - —Digoxin
  - —Diuretics
  - —Prednisone
- For *chorea*
  - —Haloperidol; chlorpromazine, diazepam, or phenobarbital may also be used
- Prophylactic regimens for streptococcus include benzathine penicillin G, 1.2 million IU IM every month, or penicillin V 250 mg orally twice daily
  - —For children without cardiac involvement 5 years of prophylaxis from the time of the last episode of ARF is generally recommended
  - —Patients with cardiac involvement are placed on life-long prophylactic antibiotics

MEDICATIONS

- Aspirin: adult: 6–8 g q 4–6 hrs; peds: 100 mg/kg/day q 4–6 hrs po
- Digoxin: adult: 0.25–0.5 mg IV; peds: 0.04 mg/kg IV
- Erythromycin: adult: 250 mg po q 6 hrs × 10 days; peds: 30–50 mg/kg/day divided q 6 hrs po × 10 days
- Furosemide: adult: 20–80 mg IV; peds: 1 mg/kg/dose IV
- Haloperidol: adult: 2–10 mg q 8 hrs IM/PO; peds: 0.01–0.03 mg/kg/day q 6 hrs po
- Prednisone: 1–2 mg/kg/day for 14 days; taper steroids for an additional 2 weeks

Disposition

ADMISSION CRITERIA

- Patients with significant carditis or newly diagnosed cases with suspicion of carditis should be admitted to the hospital for stabilization and initiation of treatment

DISCHARGE CRITERIA

- A well-appearing patient who has responded to initial treatment and whose compliance can be assured
- Chorea is controlled with haloperidol or sedatives. Even severe chorea will disappear during sleep

Miscellaneous

ICD9: 390

CORE CONTENT CODE: 8.5.1

SUGGESTED READINGS

Amigo MC, Martinez-Lavin M, Reyes PA. Acute rheumatic fever. Rheum Dis Clin North Am 1993;19(2):333–350.

Bisno AL. Rheumatic fever. In: Kelley WN, et al., eds. Textbook of rheumatology. 5th ed. Philadelphia: WB Saunders, 1997:1225–1239.

Pinals RS. Polyarthritis and fever. N Engl J Med 1994;330(11):769–774.

Stollerman GH. Rheumatic fever. Lancet 1997;349:935–942.

Authors: Norvin Perez; John Lafleur

Rib Fracture

Clinical Presentation

SIGNS AND SYMPTOMS

- Localized chest pain
- *Point tenderness,* pain referred to fracture site with palpation of the involved rib elsewhere
- Bony crepitus, ecchymosis
- Intercostal muscle spasm
- Localized pain increased with deep inspiration or coughing
- Splinting respirations

MECHANISM/DESCRIPTION

- Direct chest wall trauma, fall from height, motor vehicle accident, assault
- Ribs usually break at the point of impact or the posterior angle, which is the structurally weakest region
- Pathologic fractures associated with mild trauma and significant underlying disease
- The first three ribs are relatively protected and require significant impact to fracture, indicating possible intrathoracic injury
- Ribs 9 through 12 are relatively mobile and their fracture suggests possible intra-abdominal injury

PEDIATRIC CONSIDERATIONS

- A relatively more elastic chest wall make rib fractures less common in children

Pre-Hospital

CAUTIONS

- Patients with multiple rib fractures (particularly 1–3 or 9–12) associated with a motor vehicle accident, significant fall, or preexisting lung disease should be routed to the nearest available trauma center
- Patients with a flail chest should be assumed to have a pulmonary contusion

Diagnosis

ESSENTIAL WORKUP

- Diagnosis is initially made on clinical grounds
- Chest radiography is indicated to rule out associated intrathoracic injury but misses up to 50% of rib fractures
  —Look for pneumothorax, hemothorax, pneumomediastinum, pulmonary contusion, and widened mediastinal silhouette

IMAGING/SPECIAL TESTS

- Indications for rib x-ray series
  —Suspected fractures of ribs 1–3 or 9–12
  —Multiple rib fractures
  —Elderly patients with preexisting pulmonary disease or suspected pathologic fractures

DIFFERENTIAL DIAGNOSIS

- Rib contusion or intercostal muscle strain
- Costochondral separation
- Sternal fracture and dislocation

Nontraumatic Causes of Chest Pain

- Cardiovascular: myocardial ischemia or infarction, pericarditis, aortic dissection, pulmonary embolus, valvular heart disease
- Pulmonary: infections, inflammation, barotrauma
- Musculoskeletal: costochondritis, cervical or thoracic spine disease
- Gastrointestinal: esophageal reflux or spasm, Mallory-Weiss tear, biliary or renal colic, peptic ulcer disease, gastritis, pancreatitis, hepatitis
- Other: herpes zoster, chest wall tumor

Treatment

INITIAL STABILIZATION

- For simple fractures generally no significant stabilization is required
- Multiple fractures, elderly patients or significant underlying lung disease
  - —ABCs
  - —Control airway as needed, endotracheal intubation may be indicated for patients with significant underlying lung disease and impending respiratory failure

ED TREATMENT

Simple Fractures

- *Pain control.* Adequate pain control is the key to maintaining adequate pulmonary function, avoiding atelectasis and subsequent pneumonia
- *Intercostal nerve blocks* with 0.5% bupivacaine are safe and effective when performed properly, providing 6–12 hours of pain relief
  - —Intercostal nerve block should be performed posteriorly a couple of fingerbreadths from the vertebrae
  - —Inject 0.5–1 cc just under the inferior surface of the rib where the neurovascular bundle runs
  - —Be careful to avoid the intercostal vessels
- Deep breathing or incentive spirometry should be encouraged once adequate pain control is achieved
- *Avoid* binders or banding of the chest wall as these restrict ventilation and promote atelectasis

Multiple Fractures, Elderly Patients, or Significant Underlying Lung Disease

- *Pain control*
- Search for associated injuries, treat exacerbation of underlying lung disease
- *Intercostal nerve blocks* at the involved sites as described above with 0.5% bupivacaine for multiple fractures are safe and effective when performed properly, providing 6–12 hours of pain relief

MEDICATIONS

- Combinations of oral NSAIDs and narcotic analgesics are usually effective
- Acetaminophen/codeine (tylenol #3): 1–2 tabs po q 4–6 hrs
- Acetaminophen/hydrocodone (vicodin): 1–2 tabs po q 4–6 hrs
- Acetaminophen/oxycodone (percocet): 1–2 tabs po q 6 hrs
- Bupivacaine 0.5% for intercostal nerve blocks
- Codeine: 30–60 mg po q 4–6 hrs
- Hydromorphone (dilaudid): 1–2 mg IV/IM/SC q 4–6 hrs
- Ibuprofen (motrin): 600–800 mg po q 6–8 hrs
- Meperidine (demerol): 0.75–2.0 mg/kg IV/IM q 3–4 hrs
- Morphine sulfate: 0.05–0.1 mg/kg IV/IM/SC q 4–6 hrs
- Naproxen (naprosyn): 500 mg po bid
- For the admitted patient epidural or patient-controlled analgesia (PCA) is an effective alternative to traditional parenteral narcotics. Consider these for patients with refractory pain, oversedation, or hypoventilation secondary to narcotic analgesics

Disposition

ADMISSION CRITERIA

- Patients with multiple fractures, fractures of the first three ribs, pneumothoraces, or pneumomediastinum associated with rib fracture, pulmonary contusion, elderly patients, or patients with significant underlying lung disease (COPD, CHF, exacerbated asthma) should be admitted
- Patients whose pain control is inadequate on oral analgesics

DISCHARGE CRITERIA

- Patients with normal pulmonary function, no underlying pulmonary injury and adequate pain control on oral analgesics

Miscellaneous

ICD9: 807.0

CORE CONTENT CODE: 18.4.10.2

SUGGESTED READINGS

Committee on Trauma, American College of Surgeons. Advanced trauma life support instructor manual. 5th ed. Chicago: American College of Surgeons, 1993.

Vukich D, Markovchick V. Thoracic trauma. In: Rosen P, et al., eds. Emergency medicine: Concepts and clinical practice. 4th ed. St. Louis: CV Mosby, 1998:514.

Wilson R. Thoracic trauma. In: Tintinalli J, et al., eds. Emergency medicine: A comprehensive study guide. 4th ed. New York: McGraw Hill, 1996:1156.

Author: Greg Lampe

Ring/Constricting Band Removal

Clinical Presentation

SIGNS AND SYMPTOMS

- A constricting band with swollen tissue and skin most commonly on a finger
- Other locations: wrist, ankle, toe, umbilicus, ear lobe, nipple, septum or nares of nose, penis, scrotum, vagina, labia, or tongue
- Pain on manipulation of the appendage or constricting band

MECHANISM/DESCRIPTION

- Untreated, the constricting band may become *embedded* with interruption of skin integrity
- *Primary constricting band:* the band tightened around an appendage causes the swelling and pain, e.g., a hair knotted around a toddler's toe
- *Secondary constricting band:* An injury or disease process that causes the swelling and edema which tightens against the band, e.g., an impacted ring with an underlying fracture of the finger

ETIOLOGY

- Tourniquet syndrome may result from allergic, dermatologic, iatrogenic, endocrinologic, infectious, malignant, metabolic, physiologic, traumatic conditions, or may be pregnancy related

Pre-Hospital

- Remove rings and other potential constricting bands in the pre-hospital setting before the development of the tourniquet syndrome

Diagnosis

ESSENTIAL WORKUP

- Primary constricting band: diagnosis made by history and physical examination with special attention to neurovascular status
- Secondary constricting band: diagnosis of underlying pathology may be dependent on imaging and laboratory tests

LABORATORY

- Electrolytes, BUN and creatinine, thyroid function tests and Tzanck smear of vesicular lesions may be useful in the diagnosis of secondary constricting band

IMAGING/SPECIAL TESTS

- Plain films for evaluation of underlying fracture or foreign body *after* band removal

DIFFERENTIAL DIAGNOSIS

- *Any* condition causing marked swelling and edema predisposing to the tourniquet syndrome

Treatment

INITIAL STABILIZATION

- Pain management or conscious sedation as needed

ED TREATMENT

- Removal of the constricting band either by advancing the band distally or by division
- The most benign methods should be attempted first
- These adjuvant methods may be used alone or in combination
  —Elevation of the affected extremity may help decrease vascular congestion
  —*Cooling* the extremity with ice or cold water to reduce edema and erythema
  —*Lubrication* with soap or mineral oil to allow slippage over an inflamed or edematous area
  —*Vascular flow reduction* by the placement of a proximal arterial blood pressure cuff 10–20 mm Hg above systolic or a proximal rubber band tourniquet around an injured finger to reduce blood flow
  —*Digital block* with 1–2% lidocaine (without epinephrine) decreases the discomfort of removal and manipulation of an underlying injury
    -A digital block may increase local swelling
  —*Gauze or a needle* holder may be used to manipulate the band

Distal Edema Reduction by Sequential Compression

- The distal swollen finger, especially the proximal interphalangeal joint (PIP) presents an important obstacle in constricting band removal. Distal to proximal edema reduction by sequential compression is achieved by
  —*Self-adherent tape* wrapped from distal to proximal forms a smooth and decompressed area over which the band is advanced
  —A *Penrose surgical drain* or a finger cut from a small glove is stretched to fit over the distal swelling before the attempted removal
    -With lubrication, the proximal end of the drain is pulled under the ring to form a cuff around the ring. The cuff with distal traction applied advances the band over the decompressed area
  —*Suture material* (number 0 silk or dental floss) is wrapped under tension in a tight layer advancing over the edema in a distal to proximal direction. The proximal tail of the suture material (or floss) is tucked under the ring. With lubrication, the tail under tension is pulled distally and unwound forcing the ring over the layered suture material and decompressed area

Constricting Band Removal by Division

- A *scissor* may be used to lift then cut the offending fibrous band constricting a toddler's toe or penis
- A *number 11-scalpel* blade with cutting edge up may be sufficient to cut constricting bands formed by hair, fibers, or plastic ties
- A *hand-held wire cutter/stripper* may readily divide small girth metallic rings with minimum discomfort to the underlying injury. This type of removal may impart a crush defect to the ring making repair difficult
- A *long handled bolt cutter* available in most operating rooms or hospital engineering department may be used to divide large girth or broad sized rings
  - —Long handles provide significant mechanical advantage needed to cut large rings
  - —The reinforced cutting blades may not easily fit through a constricting band with adjacent swollen tissue and skin
- A *standard hand-powered medically approved ring cutter* may be used to divide small girth metallic constricting bands
  - —This method has the advantage of a cleaner cut for subsequent repair of the ring
  - —The disadvantage is that the handheld ring cutter is labor intensive and may aggravate the pain of an underlying injury with each turn of the handle
- A *motorized high revolution per minute (RPM) cutting device* (a "drill-like" precision cutting tool) may be used to rapidly divide constricting bands irrespective of girth and size of the ring

Cutting Procedure

- The initial cut is made on band on the volar aspect of the extremity
- A tenacula may be used to further spread the band in softer metals (14–24 karat gold)
- For a second cut, the band should be rotated 180° on the extremity allowing for the second cut on the band over the volar aspect of the extremity

Motorized Cutting

- *Flammable solvents* removed from the work area
- *Protective eyewear* worn by all persons present including the patient
- A thin *aluminum splint* should be placed between the patients skin and the ring as a shield
- *Cutting* with the tungsten-carbide cutting disc should be limited to less than 60-second intervals to avoid excessive heat
  - —*Ice water irrigations* dissipate heat; dry before cutting

Postdivision Care

- Underlying injuries should be irrigated thoroughly to remove metallic dust to avoid foreign body reaction and granuloma formation
- Tetanus prophylaxis

Disposition

ADMISSION CRITERIA

- Neurovascular compromise or injury requiring surgical repair
- Concomitant infection or necrosis

DISCHARGE CRITERIA

- Successful band removal with restoration of circulation

Miscellaneous

ICD9: 443.9

CORE CONTENT CODE: 18.4.14.4

SUGGESTED READINGS

Fasano FJ, et al. Foreign body granuloma and synovitis of the finger: A hazard of ring removal by the sawing technique. J Hand Surg 1987:12A:621–623.

Hsu CK, Antonio E, Sturmann K. Removal of a penile scrotal ring with a policy statement on the use of a non-medically approved device in the emergency department. Unpublished report. New York: Beth Israel Medical Center, 1996.

Roberts JR, Hedges JR. Clinical procedures in emergency medicine. 3rd ed. Philadelphia: WB Saunders, 1997.

Authors: Carl K. Hsu; Bradley Peckler

Rocky Mountain Spotted Fever

Clinical Presentation

SIGNS AND SYMPTOMS

- Fever in nearly all cases
- Triad of fever, headache, and rash in 50%
- Tick bite reported within 14 days of rash in 60–70%
- Rash
  - —Initial rash (3–5 days)
    - -Macular, red, and flat
    - -Blanches under pressure
    - -1–4 mm diameter
  - —In hours to days
    - -Becomes darker, papular, dusky, and palpable
  - —In 2–3 days
    - -Petechial or purpuric
    - -Positive Rumpel-Leede test
    - -May coalesce or ulcerate
  - —In severe disease, necrosis of dependent peripheral parts may occur
  - —Location
    - -Begins in flexor surfaces of wrist and ankles
    - -Spreads centripetal spread
    - -15% with centrifugal spread to palms and soles
- Pulmonary
  - —Nonproductive cough
  - —Chest pain
  - —Dyspnea
  - —Rales
- Gastrointestinal
  - —Associated with fatal RMSF
  - —Secondary to vasculitis
  - —Nausea/vomiting
  - —Abdominal pain/distension
  - —Ileus
  - —Hepatosplenomegaly
- Neurologic
  - —Focal or generalized neurologic manifestation in two-thirds
  - —Meningismus
  - —Severe, unremitting headache
  - —Encephalitis
- Other
  - —Generalized edema
  - —Dehydration
  - —Malaise
  - —Myalgia
  - —Retinal hemorrhage and conjunctivitis
- Complications
  - —Disseminated intravascular coagulation (DIC)
  - —Noncardiogenic pulmonary edema
  - —Acute renal failure

MECHANISM/DESCRIPTION

- Rickettsial invasion of small blood vessels
  - —Causes direct vascular damage
  - —Superimposed vascular damage due to immunologic phenomena

ETIOLOGY

- Acute infection by *Rickettsia rickettsii* via tick vector
  - —*Dermacentor andersonii* (wood tick) in the western states
  - —*Dermacentor variabilis* (dog tick) in the eastern states
- Reported in every state with majority in south Atlantic and south-central states
- 90% occur between April and September
- Incubation 2–14 days
- Fatal in 10%
  - —Lower fatality rate in patients reporting a tick bite
- Transmission
  - —Blood meal of an infected female tick (most common)
  - —Tick feces and tick-infected pets (less common)

PEDIATRIC CONSIDERATIONS

- Highest incidence in the 5–9 years old age group

Diagnosis

ESSENTIAL WORKUP

- Clinical diagnosis

LABORATORY

- Serology
  - —Diagnose by single titer >1:64 or 4-fold increase
  - —Methods
    - -Immunofluorescent antibody
    - -Complement fixation
    - -Indirect hemagglutination test
- CBC
  - —Normal WBC
  - —Thrombocytopenia
  - —Anemia
- Electrolytes, BUN/Cr, glucose
  - —Hyponatremia <130 mEq/L
- Liver profile
  - —Elevated AST
  - —LDH
- ABG for
  - —Hypoxia
  - —Respiratory alkalosis
- Coagulation profile if disseminated intravascular coagulation suspected
- Microbiology
  - —Immunohistologic antibody stain of skin biopsy
  - —Isolation of *R. rickettsii* (time consuming/expensive)
  - —PCR Assay
- CSF
  - —Pleocytosis and increased protein

IMAGING/SPECIAL TESTS

- CXR for pulmonary edema
- Echocardiography
  - —Decreased LV contractility

DIFFERENTIAL DIAGNOSIS

- Other tick-borne diseases
  - —Ehrlichiosis: older adults
  - —Relapsing fever
  - —Lyme Disease: erythema chronicum migrans (ECM)
  - —Tularemia
  - —Babesiosis
  - —Colorado tick fever
- Infectious diseases
  - —Meningococcemia—late winter, early spring; maculopapular or petechial rash
  - —Measles—late winter, early spring, severe prodrome
  - —Rubella—palms and soles spared
  - —Varicella—does not have rash in the extremities
  - —Infectious mononucleosis—palms and soles spared
  - —Disseminated gonococcal infection—pustular lesions

- —Typhus—rash starts at the trunk with centrifugal spread
- —Secondary syphilis
- —Scarlet fever
- —Kawasaki disease—red cracked lips
- —Toxic shock syndrome
- —Gastroenteritis
- —Staphylococcal sepsis
- Inflammatory causes
  - —Allergic vasculitis
  - —Thrombotic thrombocytic purpura
  - —Collagen vascular disease
  - —Juvenile rheumatoid arthritis
- Heat illness

Treatment

INITIAL STABILIZATION

- ABCs
- 0.9%NS IV fluid bolus for dehydration
- Oxygen for hypoxia

ED TREATMENT

- Correct fluid and electrolyte deficits
- Initiate antibiotic therapy
  - —Doxycycline—drug of choice
  - —Chloramphenicol in pregnant and allergic patients
  - —Sulfonamides make the infection worse
- Administer acetaminophen for fever
- Administer high-dose steroids for severe cases complicated by extensive vasculitis, encephalitis, or cerebral edema
- Treat complications
  - —DIC
  - —ARDS
  - —Congestive heart failure

MEDICATIONS

- Acetaminophen: 1 g (peds: 15 mg/kg) po q 4 hrs
- Chloramphenicol: 75 mg/kg/24 hrs po or IV q 6 hrs for 5–7 days and 48 hrs after defervescence
- Doxycycline: 100 mg (peds: 1.5 mg/kg) po or IV bid for 5–7 days and 48 hrs after defervescence
- Solumedrol: 125 mg (peds: 1–2 mg/kg) IVP

PEDIATRIC CONSIDERATIONS

- Doxycycline is used in children due to potential for fatal cases

Disposition

ADMISSION CRITERIA

- Moderate to severe symptoms

DISCHARGE CRITERIA

- Mild, early disease
- Notify family due to clustering

Miscellaneous

ICD9: 82.0

CORE CONTENT CODE: 9.4.1

SUGGESTED READINGS

Bolgiano EB, Sexton J. Tick-borne illness. In: Rosen P, Barkin R, et al., eds. Emergency medicine. 4th ed. St. Louis: CV Mosby, 1998:2598–2629.

Fischer JJ. Rocky mountain spotted fever: When and why to consider the diagnosis. Postgrad Med 1990;87:109–118.

Author: Moses Lee

Roseola

Clinical Presentation

SIGNS AND SYMPTOMS

- Sudden, high fever 39.4–41.2°C (103–106°F)
- Febrile seizures in 5–35%
- Absence of physical findings
  - —Child looks well
- Temperature normalizes in 3–4 days
- Maculopapular eruption from trunk to arms and neck after temperature normalization
  - —Rash fades within 3 days
- Enlarged lymph nodes
- Diarrhea
- Irritability
- Erythematous papules in pharynx (Nakayama's spots)
- Rarely causes severe or fatal disseminating diseases
  - —Infectious mononucleosis syndrome of hepatitis
- Reactivation in immunocompromised individuals

MECHANISM/DESCRIPTION

- Incubation period of 5–15 days
- Mode of acquisition unknown
  - —Horizontal spread by oral shedding suggested
- Pathophysiology
  - —Complex immune response (cytokines, antibody responses, T-cell reactivity)

ETIOLOGY

- Exanthem subitum
- Human herpesvirus 6 (HHV-6)
  - —Large, double-stranded DNA
  - —Closely related to human cytomegalovirus
- Peak incidence at 6–12 months; 90% occurrence within the first year
- Highest incidence in the late spring and early summer

PEDIATRIC CONSIDERATIONS

- Most newborns are seropositive for HHV-6 due to transplacental antibodies
- By age 1–2 years >90% of infants seropositive

Pre-Hospital

N/A

Diagnosis

ESSENTIAL WORKUP

- Clinical diagnosis
  - —High fever in well-appearing child

LABORATORY

- CBC
  - —Initial increase in WBC, then normalization with lymphocytosis
- HHV-6 DNA
  - —Detected by polymerase chain reaction (PCR)
  - —Available at research level
- IgM appears early, and declines as IgG is produced

DIFFERENTIAL DIAGNOSIS

- Fever of unknown origin
- Scarlet fever
  - —"Sandpaper" rash, "Pastia's" lines, and strawberry tongue
- Measles (rubeola)
  - —Koplik's spots, cough, coryza, conjunctivitis, and fever
- RMSF
  - —Rash begins at ankles and wrists
- Rubella
  - —Fever after rash
- Fifth disease (erythema infectiosum)
- Dengue fever
- Pneumococcal bacteremia
- Meningitis

Treatment

INITIAL STABILIZATION

- ABCs

ED TREATMENT

- Supportive
- Antipyretics
  —Acetaminophen
  —Ibuprofen

MEDICATIONS

- Acetaminophen: 650 mg (peds: 15 mg/kg) po q 4 hrs
- Ibuprofen: 200–600 mg (peds: 5–10 mg/kg; suspension 100 mg/5 ml; oral drops 40 mg/ml) po q 6 hrs

Disposition

ADMISSION CRITERIA

- Fever in child who is toxic and does not respond to initial supportive care

DISCHARGE CRITERIA

- Usually, all patients may be discharged

Miscellaneous

ICD9: 57.8

CORE CONTENT CODE: 13.12.4.3

SUGGESTED READINGS

Asano Y, Yoshikawa T, Suga S, et al. Clinical features of infants with primary human herpesvirus 6 infection (exanthem subitum, roseola infantum). Pediatrics 1994;93:104–108.

Hall CB, Long CE, Schnabel KC, et al. Human herpesvirus-6 infection in children: a prospective study of complications and reactivation. N Engl J Med 1994;331:482–438.

Nelson WE, ed. Textbook of pediatrics. Philadelphia: WB Saunders, 1996:890–892.

Author: Moses Lee

Rubella

Clinical Presentation

SIGNS AND SYMPTOMS

- Acute viral disease
- Low-grade fever
- Malaise
- Headache
- Upper respiratory symptoms
- Rash
  - —Red macular rash evolving to pink-red maculopapules, with occasional pruritus
  - —Begins in the face with rapid caudal spread
  - —Completed in first day and disappears in 3 days
  - —May have hemorrhagic manifestations
- Lymphadenopathy
  - —Postauricular
  - —Occipital
  - —Posterior cervical
- Complications
  - —Congenital Rubella syndrome (CRS)—infected women in first trimester
  - —Arthritis
    - -More common in women
    - -Begins after 2–3 days of illness
    - -Knees, wrists, fingers affected
  - —Hemorrhagic manifestations
    - -Secondary to thrombocytopenia
    - -More common in children
  - —Neurologic sequelae
    - -Encephalitis most common in children

MECHANISM/DESCRIPTION

- Transmission via droplets from respiratory secretions
- Infants with congenital rubella shed large quantities of virus for several months
- Infectious period 7 days before to 5 days after appearance of rash
- Incubation period: 14–21 days

ETIOLOGY

- Also known as German Measles or Three-Day Measles
- Rubella virus (family: Togaviridae, genus: rubivirus)
- Live, attenuated virus vaccine indications
  - —All children >12 months and entering school
  - —All women of child bearing age

Pre-Hospital

N/A

Diagnosis

ESSENTIAL WORKUP

- Clinical diagnosis

LABORATORY

- CBC
  - —Decreased WBC, platelets (more common in children)
- UA
  - —Hematuria
- ELISA to detect rubella IgM
- Rubella antibody titer
  - —Hemagglutination-inhibition test most common
  - —Definitive diagnosis in acute infection
  - —Compare infant with maternal sera for CRS
- CSF
  - —Few WBCs (monocytes) in encephalitis

DIFFERENTIAL DIAGNOSIS

- Scarlet fever
  - —"Sandpaper" rash, "Pastia's" lines, and strawberry tongue
- Measles (rubeola)
  - —Koplik's spots, cough, coryza, conjunctivitis, and fever
- Roseola infantum
  - —Spring and fall
- RMSF
  - —Rash begins at ankles and wrists
- Rheumatoid arthritis

Treatment

INITIAL STABILIZATION

- ABCs

ED TREATMENT

- Symptomatic therapy
- Antipyretics and anti-inflammatory agents
  - —Acetaminophen
  - —Ibuprofen
- Isolate rubella patients from susceptible persons (e.g., pregnancy)
- Vaccine
  - —Measles-Mumps-Rubella (MMR)
  - —Indications
    - ->12 months old and entry to school
    - -Susceptible postpubertal females
    - -High-risk groups (colleges, military, places of employment)
    - -Unimmunized contacts
  - —Contraindicated in pregnant women
  - —Avoid pregnancy for 3 months postvaccination
- Immune globulin
  - —Will not prevent viremia but may modify symptoms

MEDICATIONS

- Acetaminophen: 650 mg (peds: 15 mg/kg) po q 4 hrs
- Ibuprofen: 200–600 mg (peds: 5–10 mg/kg; suspension 100 mg/5ml; oral drops 40 mg/ml) po q 6 hrs
- Immune globulin: 0.5 cc reconstituted vial SQ (0.25–0.50 ml/kg)

Disposition

ADMISSION CRITERIA

- Congenital Rubella syndrome
- Encephalitis

DISCHARGE CRITERIA

- Most cases may go home
- Inquire regarding vaccination status of family members

PEDIATRIC CONSIDERATIONS

- Issues of parental education should be considered in nonimmunized child

Miscellaneous

ICD9: 56.9

CORE CONTENT CODE: 13.12.4.4

SUGGESTED READINGS

Centers for Disease Control. Rubella and congenital rubella—United States, 1984–1986. MMWR Morb Mortal Wkly Rep 1987(b);36:664–675.

Maldonado Y. Rubella virus (German or three-day measles). In: Nelson WE, ed. Textbook of pediatrics. 15th ed. 1996:871–873.

Author: Moses Lee

Sacral Fracture

Clinical Presentation

SIGNS AND SYMPTOMS

- Pain in buttocks, perirectal area, and posterior thigh
- Swelling and ecchymosis over the sacral prominence
- Possible sacral nerve dysfunction
  - —Absence or diminished anal sphincter tone is an important finding
  - —Bowel or bladder incontinence

MECHANISM/DESCRIPTION

- Sacral fractures are rarely isolated injuries (<5%)
- They are frequently associated with pelvic fractures
- They are defined by the orientation of the fracture line
- Axial compression
- Direct posterior trauma
- Massive crush injury

Pre-Hospital

- Sacral fractures are frequently associated with other spine and intra-abdominal injuries
- Immobilize with backboard and C-spine collar

Diagnosis

ESSENTIAL WORKUP

- History and examination with attention to loss of anal sphincter tone, sensation in the perineum, and bowel and bladder sphincter control
- Sacral fractures rarely occur in isolation, look for associated injuries
- Rectal exam will elicit pain in the sacrum
- Displacement can be assessed with bimanual rectal exam

IMAGING/SPECIAL TESTS

- Only 30% of sacral fractures detected on x-ray
- Rostrally and caudally angulated AP views and coned down views of the lumbosacral junction may help
- CT scan may better delineate the fracture and associated injuries

DIFFERENTIAL DIAGNOSIS

- Contusion

Fracture Classification

DIRECTION	SUBTYPE	ASSOCIATED FINDINGS	NEUROLOGIC EXAM
Transverse	*High Sacral:* fall from height	Transverse process fracture, alar fracture, (+) kyphosis	Rare motor weakness, (+) cauda equina syndrome
	Low Sacral: direct blow	Rectal tears, CSF leaks	Rare motor weakness, (+) cauda equina syndrome
Vertical	*Alar* (Zone I)	Sciatica, L5 root injury	Neurologic deficit *infrequent*
	Foraminal (Zone II)	Bowel/bladder dysfunction, L5, S1, S2 root injury, sciatica, foot drop	Neurologic deficit *frequent*
	Canal (Zone III)	Bowel/bladder dysfunction, sexual dysfunction, sciatica, L5,S1 root injury	Neurologic deficit *very frequent*

Treatment

INITIAL STABILIZATION

- ABCs of trauma care
- Early immobilization in unstable pelvis or spine fractures
- Pain control with NSAIDs or narcotic analgesics

ED TREATMENT

- Vertical unstable fractures require a rapid and thorough assessment for life-threatening injuries, and orthopedic consultation (see chapter: Pelvic Fracture)
- Nondisplaced isolated sacral fractures are treated symptomatically with bedrest
- Surgery may be required for fractures associated with neurological injury
- Early orthopedic referral

Disposition

ADMISSION CRITERIA

- Critically injured trauma patient with unstable pelvic fracture
- Neurologic impairment

DISCHARGE CRITERIA

- All other types of isolated sacral fractures
- Consider intermediate care for elderly patients

Miscellaneous

ICD9: 805.6

CORE CONTENT CODE: 18.4.3.1.4

SUGGESTED READINGS

Cwinn AA. Pelvis and hip. In: Rosen P, et al., eds. Emergency medicine: Concepts and clinical practice. 4th ed. St. Louis: CV Mosby, 1998:739–762.

Pollack C. Pelvic trauma. In: Harwood-Nuss A, et al., eds. The clinical practice of emergency medicine. 2d ed. Philadelphia: Lippincott-Raven, 1996.

Simon R, Koenigsknecht S. Traumatic conditions of the hip. In: Simon R, et al., eds. Emergency Orthopedics: The extremities. 3rd ed. Norwalk CT, Appleton & Lange, 1993:425–427.

Authors: Jaime B. Rivas; Teresa Carlin

Salicylate, Poisoning

Clinical Presentation

SIGNS AND SYMPTOMS

Gastrointestinal

- Nausea
- Vomiting
- Epigastric pain
- Hematemesis

Pulmonary

- Tachypnea
- Noncardiogenic pulmonary edema

CNS

- Tinnitus
- Deafness
- Delirium
- Seizures
- Coma

MECHANISM/DESCRIPTION

- Respiratory alkalosis and metabolic acidosis
  —Secondary to inhibition of Krebs cycle and uncoupling of oxidative phosphorylation
- Dehydration, hyponatremia or hypernatremia, hypokalemia, hypocalcemia
  —Due to increased sweating, vomiting, tachypnea
- Noncardiogenic pulmonary edema
  —Because of a toxic effect of salicylate on the pulmonary endothelium resulting in extravasation of fluids
- Pharmacokinetics of salicylate change from First Order to Zero Order in the overdose setting

PEDIATRIC CONSIDERATIONS

- Children exhibit a faster onset and more severe signs and symptoms than adults
  —Results from the salicylate being distributed more quickly into the target organs such as the brain, kidney, and liver
- Respiratory alkalosis (hallmark of salicylate poisoning in adults) may not occur in children
- Metabolic acidosis occurs quicker in children than adults
- Hypoglycemia more common than hyperglycemia

Pre-Hospital

CAUTIONS

- Morbidity and mortality from chronic salicylate poisoning is much greater than from acute poisoning
  —Manage chronic intoxication more aggressively
- Elderly patients
  —Greater morbidity
  —Respiratory distress/altered mental status indicative of severe toxicity
  —Diagnosis of salicylate intoxication delayed because the signs and symptoms are masked by underlying disease states

Diagnosis

ESSENTIAL WORKUP

- Guidelines for assessing poisoning severity
  —Acute ingestion of
    -<150 mg/kg—considered nontoxic
    -150–300 mg/kg—mild to moderately toxic
    ->300 mg/kg—potentially lethal
- Salicylate level
  —At presentation and then every 2 hours until the level begins to decline
  —Manage patient on clinical findings and not level alone
  —In the chronic overdose setting
    -Clinical findings a better indication of severity than plasma salicylate levels
    -Done nomogram not valid
  —Salicylate levels needed to achieve antiinflammatory effect (20–25 mg/dl) approach toxic levels

LABORATORY

- ABG
  —Respiratory alkalosis
  —Metabolic acidosis
- CBC
- Electrolytes, BUN/Cr, glucose
  —Anion gap metabolic acidosis
  —Hypokalemia
  —Baseline renal function
- Urinalysis
  —Urine pH
- PT/PTT with significant ingestions
- Ferric chloride test
  —Purple color if salicylate present
  —Positive 30 minutes postingestion
- In the presence of salicylate, Phenistix will turn brown-purple and may detect concentrations as low as 20 mg/dl

IMAGING/SPECIAL TESTS

- Abdominal flatplate radiograph for concretions
- CXR for pulmonary edema

DIFFERENTIAL DIAGNOSIS

Acute Salicylate Poisoning

- Considered with change in mental status, unexplained noncardiogenic pulmonary edema, mixed acid-base disorder
  —Methanol
  —Ethylene glycol
  —Conditions causing noncardiogenic pulmonary edema

Chronic Salicylism

- Impending myocardial infarction
- Alcohol withdrawal
- Organic psychoses
- Sepsis
- Dementia

Treatment

INITIAL STABILIZATION

- ABCs
- Naloxone, thiamine, glucose (or Accucheck) for altered mental status
- IV rehydration with 0.9%NS for hypotension

ED TREATMENT

Gastric Decontamination

- Perform gastric lavage for ingestion >150 mg/kg and
  —Patient comatose (after airway control) or at risk of having seizures
  —If patient presents within 1-hour postingestion and has an intact gag reflex
    -If no gag reflex is presented, intubate with a cuffed endotracheal tube prior to performing gastric lavage
- Administer activated charcoal plus sorbitol immediately or post lavage
- Whole-bowel irrigation
  —For concretions on the KUB
  —For ingestion of a sustained-release preparation
  —If the salicylate levels continue to increase despite appropriate management

Enhanced Elimination

- Alkalinization
  —Enhances elimination of ionized salicylate
  —Indications
    -Acidosis
    -Presence of symptoms
    -Elevated salicylate levels
  —1–2 ampules of sodium bicarbinate followed by IV D5W with 3 ampules sodium bicarbonate
    -Goal: urine pH of 7.5–8 at 3–6 ml/kg/hr rate
    -Add 20–40 mEq KCl per L to avoid hypokalemia
    -Avoid fluid overload with CHF, coronary artery disease
  —Closely monitor serum potassium
- Indications for hemodialysis include
  —CHF
  —Noncardiogenic pulmonary edema
  —CNS depression
  —Seizures
  —Unstable vital signs
  —Severe acid-base disorder
  —Hepatic compromise
  —Coagulopathy
  —Underlying disease state compromising the elimination of salicylate
  —Absolute salicylate level should not be used as a sole criteria for making a decision to dialyze without considering the patient's clinical status unless the level exceeds 80–100 mg/dl in an acute ingestion
- Lower threshold to dialyze patients with chronic overdose

MEDICATIONS

- Activated charcoal slurry: 1–2 g/kg up to 90 g po
- Dextrose: D50W 1 amp (50 ml or 25 g) (peds: D25W 2–4 ml/kg) IV
- Naloxone (narcan): 2 mg (peds: 0.1 mg/kg) IV or IM initial dose
- Sorbitol: 1–2 g/kg to a max of 100 g (peds: >1 year old: 1–1.5 g/kg as a 35% solution to a max of 50 g) po mixed in the activated charcoal slurry—use only with 1st dose
- Thiamine (vitamin B_1): 100 mg (peds: 50 mg) IV or IM

Disposition

ADMISSION CRITERIA

- Monitor patients with salicylate levels >25 mg/dl until level drops below 25 mg/dl and symptoms abate
- ICU admission for altered mental status, metabolic acidosis, pulmonary edema

DISCHARGE CRITERIA

- Salicylate level <25 mg/dl and symptoms have resolved

Miscellaneous

ICD9: 965.1

CORE CONTENT CODE: 17.2.41

SUGGESTED READINGS

Ellenhorn MJ, Schonwald S, Ordog G, Wasserberger J. Salicylate. In: Ellenhorn MJ, ed. Ellenhorn's medical toxicology. 2d ed. Baltimore: Williams & Wilkins, 1997:210–223.

Leatherman JW, Schmitz RG. Fever, hyperdynamic shock and multiple system organ failure: A pseudo-sepsis syndrome associated with chronic salicylate intoxication. Chest 1991;100:1391–1397.

Mayer AL, Sitar DS, Tenenbein M. Multiple-dose charcoal and whole-bowel irrigation do not increase clearance of absorbed salicylate. Arch Intern Med 1992;152:393–396.

Notarianni L. A reassessment of the treatment of salicylate poisoning. Drug Saf 1992;7:292–303.

Author: Michele Kanter

Sarcoidosis

Clinical Presentation

SIGNS AND SYMPTOMS

- Respiratory
  - —Dyspnea on exertion or at rest
  - —Wheezing
  - —Cough
  - —Hemoptysis
- Skin
  - —Erythema nodosum
  - —Nodules
  - —Maculopapular eruptions
  - —Plaques
  - —Lupus pernio
- Ocular
  - —Anterior uveitis
- Neurological
  - —Aseptic meningitis
  - —Cerebral vasculitis
  - —Mass lesions
  - —Myelopathy
  - —Hydrocephalus
  - —Peripheral neuropathy
  - —Cranial nerve palsy
- Cardiac
  - —Ventricular dysrhythmias
  - —Congestive heart failure
  - —Pericarditis
  - —Mitral regurgitation
  - —Acute myocarditis
  - —Conduction disturbances including third-degree heart block
- Gastrointestinal
  - —Asymptomatic liver granulomas with an increased alkaline phosphatase
- Constitutional
  - —Fatigue
  - —Anorexia
  - —Weight loss
  - —Fevers
- Lofgren's syndrome
  - —Bilateral hilar adenopathy
  - —Erythema nodosum
  - —Arthralgias

MECHANISM/DESCRIPTION

- Symptoms generally arise due to a local inflammatory reaction associated with noncaseating granulomas

ETIOLOGY

- Has not been elucidated

Pre-Hospital

- 100% nonrebreather face mask for patients with respiratory symptoms

Diagnosis

ESSENTIAL WORKUP

- Chest x-ray
  - —Stage 0: no pulmonary involvement
  - —Stage 1: bilateral hilar adenopathy only
  - —Stage 2: adenopathy and interstitial lung involvement
  - —Stage 3: interstitial lung involvement only
  - —Stage 4: diffuse scarring reflecting end-stage lung disease
- Pulse oximetry
- Electrocardiogram
- Pulmonary function testing

LABORATORY

- Serum angiotensin-converting enzyme inhibitor (ACE) level
  - —Not accurate enough to establish the diagnosis
- Serum sodium: hyponatremia due to involvement of the hypothalamus
- Serum calcium: hypercalcemia due to oversynthesis of vitamin D
- BUN and creatinine: urinary tract disease, which may be intrarenal or postrenal

IMAGING/SPECIAL TESTS

- Biopsy
  - —Establishes the diagnosis
  - —Demonstrates noncaseating granulomas and is negative for special stains for fungi and tuberculosis
  - —May involve skin, lymph node, transbronchial, or mediastinal biopsy
- Slitlamp examination by an ophthalmologist if ocular sarcoidosis is suspected

DIFFERENTIAL DIAGNOSIS

- Idiopathic pulmonary fibrosis
- Wegener's granulomatosis
- Alveolar proteinosis
- Bronchiolitis obliterans with organizing pneumonia
- Coal worker's pneumoconiosis
- Berylliosis

Treatment

INITIAL STABILIZATION

- Provide adequate oxygenation with nasal cannula or face mask
- Intubate patients with refractory hypoxemia

ED TREATMENT

- Oral corticosteroids
  —Severe ocular, neurologic or cardiac sarcoidosis, malignant hypercalcemia, or symptomatic respiratory disease
  —Respiratory involvement with significant pulmonary function abnormalities or deterioration
- Topical corticosteroids for mild uveitis
- Nonsteroidal anti-inflammatory agents for arthralgias

MEDICATIONS

- Prednisone: 30–40 mg daily for patients with mild to moderate disease; 60–80 mg daily for patients with severe involvement of the cardiac, ocular, or neurological systems
- Oxygen: maintain oxygen saturation of 92–95%

Disposition

ADMISSION CRITERIA

- Any patient who is hypoxemic
- Patients with moderate to severe symptoms without a diagnosis and thought to represent sarcoidosis

DISCHARGE CRITERIA

- Outpatient evaluation for suspected sarcoidosis
- Minimal to mild symptoms
- The patient does not potentially have a life-threatening condition
- Follow up is established

Miscellaneous

ICD9: 135

CORE CONTENT CODE: 8.5.2.5

SUGGESTED READINGS

Chesnutt A. Enigmas in sarcoidosis. West J Med 1995;162:519–526.

Fanberg B, Lazarus D. Sarcoidosis. In: Murray JF, Nadel JA, eds. Textbook of respiratory medicine. 2nd ed. Philadelphia: WB Saunders, 1994:1873–1888.

Newman L, Rose C, Maier L. Sarcoidosis. N Engl J Med 1997;336:1224–1234.

Sharma O. Pulmonary sarcoidosis and corticosteroids. Am Rev Respir Dis 1993;147:1598–1600.

Author: Richard Lenhardt

Scabies

Clinical Presentation

SIGNS AND SYMPTOMS

- Intensely pruritic eruption 10–30 days after the onset of infestation
- Pruritus begins immediately if patient is infected a second time
- Primary lesion is a linear papule to 1 cm with a small vesicle containing a black dot at the end
- Found in the web spaces of fingers, flexor surfaces of elbows and wrist, penis, vulva, areola, and in infants and young children may affect the face
- Secondary lesions: crusted papules, nodules, excoriations, and secondary impetigo or folliculitis seen on back, shoulders, axilla, waist, buttocks, and flexor aspects of the elbows. Children may be infested from head to toe
- Secondary lesions may be few if patient using topical steroids
- *Norwegian scabies* (crusted scabies) is an atypical form of scabies seen in handicapped, immunocompromised, and institutionalized patients
  - —*Norwegian scabies* produces gross scaling with hyperkeratotic plaques on hands, feet, scalp, and pressure bearing areas

ETIOLOGY

- Scabies is produced by the human scabies mite *Sarcoptes scabiei var. hominis* or from animal scabies mites
- Transmitted by direct personal contact or rarely by infected bedding and clothing

MECHANISM/DESCRIPTION

- Mites mate on skin and gravid female burrows into the stratum corneum to lay eggs. Animal scabies burrow but cannot reproduce
- Symptoms result from host sensitization to the mite and its products

Pre-Hospital

- No specific considerations in routine cases, maintain universal precautions

Diagnosis

ESSENTIAL WORKUP

- Careful history and skin exam for characteristic lesions
- Obtain skin scraping with mineral oil and a No. 15 blade, observe under low power microscope for mites, eggs, or fecal material

DIFFERENTIAL DIAGNOSIS

- Atopic dermatitis, dermatitis herpetiformis, papular urticaria folliculitis
- Pruritic urticarial papules and plaques of pregnancy (PUPPP)
- Adult linear IgA bullous dermatosis
- Syphilis, pityriasis rosea, impetigo, seborrheic dermatitis, and lymphoma

PEDIATRIC CONSIDERATIONS

- Lesions may also effect the face (rare in children over 3 years old)
- Distribution typically involves the proximal half of the foot and heel
- Neonatal scabies is associated with poor feeding, weight gain, and frequent superinfection

Treatment

INITIAL STABILIZATION

- No specific stabilization necessary in routine cases

ED TREATMENT

- Treat patient and all persons in immediate contact with topical scabicide
- Permethrin cream is 89–92% effective and best tolerated
- Lindane is slightly less effective and associated with rare nausea, vomiting and seizures, especially in infants
- Crotamiton is 50–60% effective and used when other scabicides are not tolerated
- Crusted scabies first requires removal of hyperkeratotic scale with 6% salicylic acid in petroleum jelly to facilitate entry of scabicide
- Machine wash and dry in hot cycles or dry clean all clothes worn within 2 days of treatment
- Vacuum household floors, carpets, mattresses, and furniture
- Emphasize that itching may continue 1–4 weeks after mites are killed due to skin inflammatory reaction
- Topical steroids and oral antihistamines reduce pruritic symptoms
- Reevaluate after 2 weeks for recurrence; retreat if live mites found

MEDICATIONS

Scabicides

- Crotamiton 10% lotion or cream: apply topically from neck down in adults and entire skin surface in children qhs for 2 nights then rinse 48 hours after last application
- Lindane (γ-benzene hexachloride) 1% lotion or cream: apply topically from neck down and rinse after 8–12 hours, contraindicated in infants, pregnancy, lactation, excessive excoriations, or seizure disorder
- Permethrin 5% cream (elimite): apply topically from neck down in adults and entire skin in children qhs, rinse off after 8–14 hours

Antipruritics

- Cetirizine (Zyrtec): adult (age>12): 5–10 mg po q day; peds: not recommended
- Diphenhydramine (Benadryl): adult: 25–50 mg po q 6 hrs; peds: 5 mg/kg/24hrs divided q 6 hrs
- Hydroxyzine HCl (Atarax): adult: 25 mg po q 8 hrs; peds: 50 mg po daily divided q 6 hrs

Disposition

ADMISSION CRITERIA

- Patients with severe topical or systemic superinfection

DISCHARGE CRITERIA

- Nontoxic-appearing patients with routine symptoms

Miscellaneous

ICD9: 133.0

CORE CONTENT CODE: 3.2.3.2, 13.12.2.2

SUGGESTED READINGS

Brown S, Becher J, Brady W. Treatment of ectoparasitic infections: Review of the English-language literature, 1982–1992. Clin Infect Dis 1995;20(Suppl 1):S104–S109.

Fischer T. Lindane toxicity in a 24-year-old woman. Ann Emerg Med 1994;24(5):972–974.

Molinaro M, Schwartz R, Janniger C. Scabies. Cutis 1995;(56):317–321.

Author: Guy Tarleton

Scaphoid Fracture

Clinical Presentation

SIGNS AND SYMPTOMS

- Pain and tenderness in the anatomic snuffbox
- Pain at the anatomic snuffbox on axial loading of the thumb
- Occasionally, there may be incidental damage to the superficial branches of the radial nerve

MECHANISM/DESCRIPTION

- Generally, from a fall on an outstretched or dorsiflexed hand (FOOSH injury)
- The scaphoid is the most commonly fractured carpal bone (60–70% of all traumatic wrist injuries)
- Scaphoid fractures occur more frequently in the middle third, or waist of the bone
- The blood supply to the scaphoid enters distally, therefore, proximal fractures of the bone may result in avascular necrosis
- Carpal fractures are unusual in children, and it is very uncommon for avascular necrosis to occur
- Fractures are missed on initial x-rays up to 10% of the time
- The scaphoid is the stabilizer between the distal and proximal carpal rows. Injury to this bone may result in instability of the wrist and significant disability

Pre-Hospital

CAUTIONS

- Consider other injuries
- Dress open wounds
- Immobilize in neutral position
- Elevation; cold to reduce swelling
- Age-appropriate social management

Diagnosis

ESSENTIAL WORKUP

- Examination with special attention to skin integrity and neurovascular status including two-point discrimination
- Radiographic imaging that includes three views of the wrist

IMAGING/SPECIAL TESTS

- Some authorities recommend specialized views of the scaphoid or full wrist films with gentle radial and ulnar deviation
- Avoid stress-testing of thumb metacarpal-phalangeal joint until radiography is completed
- Approximately 10% of fractures are not visible on x-ray at time of the injury

DIFFERENTIAL DIAGNOSIS

- Bennett's fracture
- Rolando's fracture
- Extra-articular fracture at the base of the thumb metacarpal
- Gamekeeper's thumb
- Perilunate dislocation
- Scapholunate dissociation
- Lunate fracture or dislocation

PEDIATRIC CONSIDERATIONS

- Wrists are rarely sprained in children and the x-ray is difficult to interpret
- Children with wrist injury should be splinted and referred for appropriate follow-up

Treatment

INITIAL STABILIZATION

- Immobilize thumb in neutral position, ice, elevate pending definitive evaluation

ED TREATMENT

- Thumb spica-splint with the thumb in neutral position
  —Some authorities recommend a long arm splint to prevent rotation at the wrist
  —Splinting is recommended *any time snuffbox tenderness is present,* whether initial x-rays reveal an obvious fracture or not
- Splint instructions provided to patient
- 72-hour orthopedic referral
- Counsel patient regarding the risk of malunion and avascular necrosis

MEDICATIONS

- Pain control with NSAIDs, acetaminophen, or oral narcotic preparations

PEDIATRIC CONSIDERATIONS

- No specific considerations

Disposition

ADMISSION CRITERIA

- Open fracture, presence of other more serious injuries

DISCHARGE CRITERIA

- Closed injuries, with 72-hour orthopedic follow-up

Miscellaneous

ICD9: 814.01

CORE CONTENT CODE: 18.4.12.1.3

SUGGESTED READINGS

American Society for Surgery of the Hand. The hand: Examination and diagnosis. 2d ed. New York: Churchill Livingston, 1983: 585–600.

American Society for Surgery of the Hand. The hand: Primary care of common problems. 2d ed. New York: Churchill Livingston, 1990:637–649.

Eisenhauer MA. Forearm & Wrist. In: Rosen P, et al., eds. Emergency medicine: Concepts and clinical practice. 4th ed. St. Louis: Mosby-Year Book, 1998:669–689.

Uehara DT. The hand in emergency medicine. Emerg Clin North Am 1993;11(3): 781–96.

Author: John MacKay, MD

Schizophrenia

Clinical Presentation

SIGNS AND SYMPTOMS

- Psychotic Symptoms
  - —Delusions (fixed, false beliefs)
    - -Bizarre, paranoid, or grandiose
    - -Often involve the conviction that others are tampering with one's mind or body
  - —Hallucinations
    - -Typically hearing voices
    - -May involve any sensory modality
  - —Thought disorder
    - -Disorganized speech ranging from odd idiosyncratic logic to incoherence
- Negative symptoms
  - —Apathy
  - —Flat affect
  - —Social isolation
  - —Anhedonia
  - —Inattention

MECHANISM/DESCRIPTION

- Genetic component (concordance rate of 50% in monozygotic twins)
- Stressors during second trimester of pregnancy may increase risk
  - —Influenza
  - —Famine
  - —Birth complications
- Onset typically early in adult life
- Substance abuse (alcohol and stimulants) is common
- Approximately 15% of patients commit suicide
- Violence may result from impaired judgment, paranoia, and command hallucinations
- Patients with schizophrenia can have abnormally high pain thresholds that can complicate the detection of medical illness

Pre-Hospital

CAUTIONS

- Pre-hospital personnel must protect themselves from harm
- Patients can display unpredictable, and violent behavior
- Patients may require restraint to protect themselves or EMS crew
  - —Know local laws as they apply to involuntary restraint

Diagnosis

ESSENTIAL WORKUP

- Obtain history from additional sources
  - —Friends or family
  - —Assists in establishing the diagnosis
  - —Evaluate potential dangerousness to self or others
- Medical and neurological screening
  - —Assessment for drug-induced psychosis (see "Psychosis, Medical vs. Psychiatric")
  - —The content of delusions and the nature of auditory hallucinations should be explored to assess safety
  - —Evaluate for acute delirium
    - -Schizophrenia does not affect orientation nor memory

LABORATORY

- Toxicology screen
- Electrolytes, BUN, creatinine, glucose, calcium
- Thyroid panel (see "Psychosis, Medical vs. Psychiatric")

IMAGING/SPECIAL TESTS

- None are helpful in the ED

DIFFERENTIAL DIAGNOSIS

- Delirium
- Drug-induced psychosis
- Huntington's chorea
- Temporal lobe epilepsy
- Bipolar (manic depressive) disorder
- Psychotic depression
- Delusional disorder
- Schizotypal personality

Treatment

INITIAL STABILIZATION

- Safety of health care workers and patient is paramount
- Patient may require a quiet room
- Presence of security staff
- Physical or chemical restraints as appropriate
  - —Agitation may be treated with a high-potency antipsychotic and benzodiazepine
    - -Haloperidol or Droperidol combined with Lorazepam is synergistic
  - —Negative symptoms tend to be less responsive to pharmacotherapy than psychotic symptoms

ED TREATMENT

- Psychiatric consultation after medical evaluation is completed
- High-potency conventional antipsychotic agents (haloperidol, fluphenazine)
  - —Minimal cardiovascular effects
  - —Produce extrapyramidal symptoms
    - -Dystonia
    - -Parkinsonism
    - -Akathisia (restlessness of lower extremities)
- Low-potency conventional agents (chlorpromazine, thioridazine)
  - —Fewer extrapyramidal symptoms
  - —More sedating
  - —Orthostatic hypotension
  - —Anticholinergic side effects
- Atypical antipsychotic agents (risperidone, olanzapine, sertindole, quetiapine)
  - —Better tolerated with fewer extrapyramidal symptoms
  - —Risperidone and sertindole can cause orthostatic hypotension
  - —Sertindole delays cardiac conduction
  - —Clozapine is the only agent that is clearly more effective for psychotic symptoms
    - -Requires weekly monitoring of WBC due to agranulocytosis
    - -Highly sedating, anticholinergic, hypotensive
  - —Haloperidol decanoate and fluphenazine decanoate are long acting depot preparations

MEDICATIONS

- Chlorpromazine (thorazine): 300–800 mg/day
- Clozapine (clozaril): 200–900 mg/day
- Droperidol: acute agitation; 2.5–10 mg IV/IM repeat q 15–60 min
- Fluphenazine (prolixin): 5–20 mg/day
- Haloperidol (haldol): 5–20 mg/day, acute agitation; 5–20 mg IV/IM repeat q 30–60 min
- Lorazepam: acute agitation; 2–4 mg IV/IM repeat q 30–60 min
- Olanzapine (zyprexa): 10–20 mg/day
- Quetiapine (seroquel): 250–750 mg/day
- Risperidone (risperdal): 4–12 mg/day
- Sertindole (serlect): 16–24 mg/day
- Thioridazine (mellaril): 5–30 mg/day
- If a conventional antipsychotic agent is administered, patients younger than age 40 should be started on benztropine (cogentin) 2 mg bid for 10 days to reduce the risk of dystonic reactions

Disposition

ADMISSION CRITERIA

- Admit if patient is a danger to self or others, or gravely disabled
- Criteria for involuntary hospitalization vary by state
- Patients with new onset psychosis should also be admitted for evaluation and stabilization

DISCHARGE CRITERIA

- Patients not a danger to self or others and able to perform activities of daily living
- Psychiatric followup is arranged
- Psychotic symptoms may persist at time of discharge

Miscellaneous

ICD9: 295.90

CORE CONTENT CODE: 14.1.1

SUGGESTED READINGS

Carpenter WT, Buchanan RW. Schizophrenia. N Engl J Med 1994;330:681–90.

Goff DC, Manschreck T, Groves J. Psychotic patients. In: Hackett TP, Cassem NH, eds. Massachusetts General Hospital handbook of general hospital psychiatry. St. Louis: Mosby-Year Book, 1991.

Author: D. Goff

Sciatica/Herniated Disc

Clinical Presentation

SIGNS AND SYMPTOMS

- Low back pain (LBP) precedes onset of leg pain, but with time, leg pain predominates
  - —Sharp, well localized, *radiates distal to knee*
  - —Exacerbated by trunk flexion/rotation, Valsalva, cough, prolonged sitting/standing
  - —Constellation of pain, dermatomal paraesthesias/sensory loss, motor and reflex deficits
- 98% involve L5 or S1 nerve root
- Paravertebral muscle spasm, loss of lumbar lordosis
- +/− spinous process point tenderness
- Muscle atrophy (long-standing)
- *Waddell Signs* are five categories of signs/symptoms that suggest "nonorganic" disease/malingering if at least 3/5 positive
  - —Nonspecific tenderness-superficial or nonanatomical
  - —Simulation tests-axial loading or passive rotation of pelvis and shoulders causes LBP
  - —Distraction-inconsistent performance, e.g., between supine and sitting straight leg raise
  - —Regional disturbances-nonanatomical changes in strength/sensation
  - —Overreaction-verbalization, grimacing, collapse

MECHANISM/DESCRIPTION

- *Sciatica* = *radicular* pain in the distribution of lumbar nerve root, often accompanied by sensory and motor deficits, usually secondary to mechanical compression and inflammation
  - —Peaks at the 4th to 5th decade of life
  - —2–10% of LBP
  - —50–80% improve with conservative management; 1–10% require surgery
- *Disc* = colloidal gel (*nucleus pulposis*) surrounded by fibrous capsule (*annulus fibrosis*), functions as hydraulic shock absorber between vertebrae
- *Herniated nucleus pulposis* (*herniated disc*) = protrusion of nucleus pulposis through weakened annulus fibrosis
  - —Long-standing degenerative changes predispose to herniation

ETIOLOGY

- Risk factors for developing sciatica from herniated disc include
  - —Smoking
  - —Repetitive lifting in forward bend and twist position
  - —Vehicular/machinery vibration
  - —Sedentary lifestyle
  - —Obesity

PEDIATRIC CONSIDERATIONS

- Usually secondary to trauma as degenerative changes do not occur in healthy children

Pre-Hospital

CAUTIONS

- C-collar and backboard for all trauma victims
- Elderly patients may need immobilization with padded backboard if suspicious for pathological fracture

DISC (NERVE)	LEG PAIN	SENSORY LOSS	MOTOR WEAKNESS	REFLEX
L3-4 (L4)	Front	Anteromedial leg, knee, medial malleolus	Knee extension (quadriceps), hip adduction	Knee
L4-5(L5)	Side	Lateral lower leg, dorsal aspect foot medially including great toe	Foot dorsiflexion, great toe extension	None
L5-S1(S1)	Back	Back of lower leg, dorsum of foot laterally including lateral malleolus	Foot plantarflexion	Ankle

Diagnosis

ESSENTIAL WORKUP

- Complete history and physical/neurologic exam including rectal tone and anal sensation
- *Straight leg raise* (*SLR*) = elevate involved leg by heel between 30° and 60°; reproduces radicular pain, *not just LBP;* variants
  - —*Sitting knee extension*
  - —Bowstring sign = compress midline popliteal fossa
  - —*Lasègue sign* = elevate leg; dorsiflex foot before SLR pain threshold
- *Crossed straight leg raise* (pathognomonic) = elevate uninvolved leg; pain in involved leg

LABORATORY

- Based upon clinical suspicion for differential diagnosis (especially elderly/pediatrics), not limited to
  - —CBC, ESR if suspect discitis/osteo/cancer
  - —Urinalysis

IMAGING/SPECIAL TESTS

- PA/lateral of lumbar spine
  - —Not diagnostic for disc disease
  - —Indications
    - -Neurologic deficits
    - -Extremes of age (<18, >50 years)
    - -Trauma
    - -Unresolved back pain >4–6 weeks
    - -Back pain + risk factors for ddx; e.g., temperature >38°C, unexplained weight loss, known cancer, IVDA
- MRI or CT myelography
  - —Indications
    - -Suspected cauda equina syndrome
    - -After 6 weeks failed conservative therapy for sciatica
  - —CT best to identify trauma, bony disease
  - —MRI best to identify neoplasm, disc infection, disc herniation

DIFFERENTIAL DIAGNOSIS

- Hematoma, extrinsic nerve compression (wallet, etc.)
- Neoplasm (primary/met)
- Peripheral nerve entrapment
- Infection (osteomyelitis, epidural abscess, discitis)
- Spondylosis/spondylolisthesis
- Subarachnoid hemorrhage
- Aneurysm (iliac/hypogastric a.)
- Spinal stenosis (pseudoclaudication)
- Paget's disease
- Synovial cyst
- Hip arthritis
- Herpes zoster
- Psychogenic

PEDIATRIC CONSIDERATIONS

- <10 years old, ddx: infection, tumor, AVM
- >10 years old, ddx: spondylolisthesis,

Scheuermann's disease, disc herniation (trauma), overuse syndrome, tumor
- Back pain or radicular symptoms in a child often indicate serious underlying disease and should prompt a complete work-up

Treatment

INITIAL STABILIZATION

- Evaluate for neurosurgical emergency, e.g., cauda equina syndrome
- Pain relief

ED TREATMENT

- Appropriate analgesia and muscle relaxants
- Conservative treatment is the rule initially
- Bedrest 3–7 days (flex hip and knee with pillows)
- Gradual physical activity tailored to increase movement without symptoms
- Abstain from activity that exacerbates pain; no lifting more than 5–10 lbs until symptoms resolve
- Unproven therapies: transcutaneous electrical nerve stimulation (TENS), traction, back brace/corset, ultrasound, diathermy, spinal manipulation

MEDICATIONS

- Ativan (lorazepam): 0.5–2 mg po tid qid
- Cyclobenzaprine (Flexeril): 10–30 mg po tid
- Ibuprofen (Motrin, Advil, Nuprin, Rufen): adult: 800 mg po tid; peds: 5–10 mg/kg/dose
- Methocarbamol (Robaxin): 1000–1500 mg po qid
- Morphine sulfate: adult: 2–4 mg IV, may repeat; peds: 0.1 mg/kg/dose titrate to effect
- Naproxen (Naprosyn, Aleve): 500 mg po bid
- Tylenol #3: 1–2 po q 4–6 hrs PRN pain
- Ketorolac (Toradol): 30 mg IV/IM ×1
- Valium (diazepam): adult: 2–10 mg po tid qid; peds: 0.1 mg/kg/dose titrate to effect
- Vicodin: 1–2 po q 6–8 hrs PRN pain

PEDIATRIC CONSIDERATIONS

- Children require surgery more than adults and have a higher success rate

Disposition

ADMISSION CRITERIA

- Cauda equina syndrome
- Severe neurological deficit
- Progressive neurological deficit
- Multiple nerve root involvement
- Social situation/pain suggest an inability to manage as outpatient

DISCHARGE CRITERIA

- Patient is able to ambulate, follow instructions, reliable home situation, and has planned follow-up

Miscellaneous

ICD9: 722.10

CORE CONTENT CODE: 10.3.3.1

SUGGESTED READINGS

Deyo RA, et al. Herniated lumbar intervertebral disk. Ann Intern Med 1990;112:598–603.

Frymoyer JW. Back pain and sciatica. N Engl J Med 1988;318(5):291–300.

McCowin PR, et al. The current approach to the medical diagnosis of low back pain. Orthop Clin North Am 1991;22(2):315–325.

Campana BA. Soft tissue spine injuries and back pain. In: Rosen P, et al., eds. Emergency medicine: Concepts and clinical practice. 4th ed. St. Louis: CV Mosby, 1998:878–905.

Author: Ruth M. Wold

Scorpion Bite

Clinical Presentation

SIGNS AND SYMPTOMS

- Onset within minutes and progresses to maximum severity in about 5 hours
- Scorpion species determines symptoms
- Local effects
  - —Wheal
  - —Flare
  - —Erythema
  - —Induration
  - —Muscle pain
- Allergic reactions
  - —Urticaria
  - —Pruritus
  - —Angioedema
  - —Dyspnea
  - —Hypotension
- Sympathetic stimulation
  - —Tachycardia
  - —Hypertension
  - —Noncardiogenic pulmonary edema
  - —Seizures
  - —Perspiration
  - —Apprehension
- Parasympathetic stimulation
  - —SLUDG (salivation, lacrimation, urination, defecation, gastric hyperdistention)
  - —Bradycardia
  - —Hypotension
  - —Miosis
  - —Bronchoconstriction
- Skeletal muscle stimulation
  - —Fasciculations
  - —Severe muscle contractions
  - —Poor control of pharyngeal, ocular, respiratory, and extremity muscles
- Respiratory failure
  - —Secondary to excessive secretions, fatigue, anaphylaxis, prolonged apnea
- Grading severity of envenomation
  - —Grade I: local pain or paresthesias at site of envenomation
  - —Grade II: local pain and pain or paresthesias distant from site
  - —Grade III: either cranial nerve or somatic skeletal muscle dysfunction
    - -Cranial nerve: blurred vision, wandering eye movements, hypersalivation, trouble swallowing, tongue fasciculations, slurred speech
    - -Somatic skeletal muscle dysfunction: jerking of extremities, restlessness, severe involuntary shaking and jerking
  - —Grade IV: both cranial nerve and somatic skeletal muscle dysfunction

MECHANISM/DESCRIPTION

- Neurotoxic venom—causes the stabilization of sodium channels in the open position leading to repetitive and unsynchronized firing of neuronal axons of somatic motor, sympathetic, and parasympathetic neurons

ETIOLOGY

- *Centruroides sculpturatus* found in southwestern U.S.
- India, Africa, Brazil, and Mexico have other venomous species that may require therapy with distinct antivenin

PEDIATRIC CONSIDERATIONS

- More rapid progression and increased severity of symptoms
- Bradycardia found in infants and children

Pre-Hospital

- Compression band
  - —Wide band (>0.5-inch) placed above level of bite on extremity
  - —Advance to keep above level of swelling
  - —Delays circulation of venom by constricting lymphatics and superficial venous return
  - —Do not place tourniquet
- Immobilize envenomated limb in position of function and hold below level of heart
- Calm and reassure patient to lower heart rate and blood pressure to minimize transport of venom

CONTROVERSIES

- Manually extracting the venom ("The Extractor")
  - —Designed to create up to 1 ATM of negative pressure
  - —Apply to the bite site after incision made at the site
  - —No animal studies on scorpion envenomation
  - —Use if delay in transport
- Oral extraction contraindicated

Diagnosis

ESSENTIAL WORKUP

- Identify species
- Suspect envenomation in endemic areas with characteristic clinical findings

LABORATORY EVALUATION

- Routine laboratory evaluation unnecessary in mild envenomations
- Baseline screening labs in severe envenomations that require significant supportive care
  - —CBC
  - —Electrolytes, BUN, Cr, glucose
  - —Urinalysis
- ABG when respiratory symptoms

IMAGING/SPECIAL TESTS

- ECG for elderly patients with cardiac risk factors who have tachycardia/hypertension

DIFFERENTIAL DIAGNOSIS

- Other envenomations
  - —Snakes/lizards
  - —Biting marine animals
  - —Spiders (brown recluse, black widow spider)
- Organophosphate poisoning
- Sympathomimetic overdose
- Tetanus

Treatment

INITIAL STABILIZATION

Severe Envenomations (Grade III or IV)

- ABCs
  - —Oxygen
  - —Airway management with endotracheal intubation for obstruction, secretions, impending respiratory failure
  - —Cardiac monitor
  - —IV access with 0.9%NS
- ED treatment

Mild Envenomations (Grade I and II)

- Cool compresses
- Oral/parental analgesics
- Antihistamines/steroids for allergic reactions (diphenhydramine, cimetidine)
- Tetanus prophylaxis

Severe Envenomations (Grade III and IV)

- IV fluids/pressors (dopamine) for hypotension
- Epinephrine/steroids for anaphylaxis
- Treat sympathomimetic effects (tachycardia/hypertension) with β-blockers or calcium channel blockers
- Treat dysrhythmias in standard fashion
- *Antivenin:* Not FDA approved; obtained by special approval through the Arizona State Board of Pharmacy. Available through the Antivenin Production Laboratory at Arizona State University Microbiology Department
  - —1–2 vials diluted in 50 cc of crystalloid (normal saline or lactated ringers) per vial given IV over 20–30 minutes
  - —Rarely need >2 vials per envenomation
  - —Type I (anaphylactic) and type III (serum sickness) reactions occur
  - —Skin test with 0.1 cc of antivenin diluted 1:10 with normal saline—place 0.02 cc of this solution as a wheal under the skin; if no reaction in 10 minutes may use antivenin
  - —Resolution of symptoms begins within minutes to 1.5 hours after administration
- Central Arizona Regional Poison Management (602) 253-3334
  - —Excellent resource for information regarding evaluation and management of scorpion envenomations

MEDICATIONS

- Cimetidine: 300 mg (peds: 20 mg/kg/24hrs q 6 hrs) IV/PO
- Diltiazem: 20 mg (peds: 0.25 mg/kg) IV, followed by drip 5–15 mg/hr
- Diphenhydramine: 50 mg (peds: 1.0 mg/kg) IV/IM
- Dopamine: 2–20 μg/kg/min IV
- Epinephrine: 0.3cc 1:1000 solution (peds: 0.01 cc/kg) SQ; infuse drip at 0.1 μg/kg/min for severe anaphylaxis
- Esmolol: 100–500 μg/kg IV over 1 min followed by infusion of 25–100 μg/kg/min; increase infusion rate by 25–50 μg/kg/min q 5–10 min PRN
- Hydralazine: 10–40 mg (peds: 0.1–0.2 mg/kg/dose) IV/IM q 4-6 hrs
- Labetalol: 20 mg (peds: 0.3–1 mg/kg/dose) IV q 10 min up to 300 mg PRN; start infusion 2 mg/min (peds: 0.4–1 mg/kg/hr to a max of 3 mg/kg/hr) as needed
- Methylprednisolone: 125 mg (peds: 1–2 mg/kg) IV/IM
- Propranolol: 1 mg (peds: 0.01–0.1 mg/kg) IV
- Verapamil: 5–10 mg (peds: 0.1–0.3 mg to a max of 5 mg) IV

PEDIATRIC CONSIDERATIONS

- Antivenin treatment is based on venom burden, not patient's size so equal doses are given to adults and children (1–2 vials in 50 cc crystalloid)

Disposition

ADMISSION CRITERIA

- Serious (grade III and IV) envenomations requiring significant supportive care (airway support, blood pressure support) to ICU
- Serious envenomations without need for airway or circulatory support to a less intensive monitored setting

DISCHARGE CRITERIA

- Mild (grade I and II) envenomations after 3–6 hours of observation without progression of symptoms
- Patients who received antivenin who have good resolution of symptoms and no recurrence of symptoms after 3–6 hours of observation
  - —Advise regarding the risks of developing serum sickness (1–3 weeks after antivenin, arthralgia, malaise, low-grade temperature, rash) and to return if serum sickness develops
  - —Inform patients as to the possibility of persistent pain or paresthesias at bite site and to follow-up if there is a progression of symptoms

Miscellaneous

ICD9: 989.5 VENOMOUS BITE

CORE CONTENT CODE: 5.10.5

SUGGESTED READINGS

Allen C. Arachnid envenomations. Emerg Med Clin North Am 1992;10(2):269–297.

Connor DA, Seldon BS. Scorpion envenomation. In Auerbach PS, ed. Wilderness medicine. 3rd ed. St. Louis: CV Mosby, 1995:831–841.

Sofer S. Scorpion envenomation [Review]. Intensive Care Med 1995;21(8):626–628.

Author: Christy Coerver

Seborrheic Dermatitis

Clinical Presentation

SIGNS AND SYMPTOMS

- Common, chronic eruptive skin disorder
- Erythematous, greasy, yellow, scaly, and crusting lesions
- Effect areas of high sebaceous gland concentration
- Periods of remission and exacerbation are frequent in adults

Infants

- Onset typically at 1 month of age and usually resolves by 12 months
- Flexural fold involvement may appear as diaper dermatitis, which frequently develops a bacterial or fungal superinfection
- Cradle cap is a thick, greasy, adherent scale on the vertex of the scalp, which may be accompanied by inflammation or secondary infection

Young Children

- Blepharitis is a white scale adherent to eyelashes and eyelid margins with characteristic erythema
  - —Resistant to treatment and may persist for years

Adolescents and Adults

- Classic seborrheic dermatitis is characterized by a greasy, fine, dry, white scaling with inflammation, erythema, and minor itching
  - —Often exacerbated by avoidance of washing
  - —Usually bilateral and symmetrical, affecting the scalp, eyebrows, eyelids, external ear canals, posterior auricular folds, and presternal region

ETIOLOGY

- Etiology is uncertain and most likely multifactorial with genetic, environmental, and hormonal influences
- Cutaneous *Pityrosporum ovale* yeast has been suggested
- Disease flares are common with stress or illness

PEDIATRIC CONSIDERATIONS

- Generalized seborrheic dermatitis may develop in infants with HIV

Pre-Hospital

N/A

Diagnosis

ESSENTIAL WORKUP

- Diagnosis is made clinically with thorough history and physical examination

LABORATORY

- Potassium hydroxide preparations of skin scrapings may suggest yeast involvement

IMAGING/SPECIAL TESTS

- None required

DIFFERENTIAL DIAGNOSIS

- Atopic dermatitis: characteristically affects antecubital and popliteal fossa in adults—axillary involvement favors the diagnosis of seborrheic dermatitis. Pruritus, oozing, and weeping support the diagnosis of atopic dermatitis. A strong family history of atopy may suggest the diagnosis. Atopic dermatitis is frequently recurrent
- Candidiasis: presence of pseudohypha on cytologic examination with potassium hydroxide is suggestive of candida, but does not exclude the diagnosis of seborrheic dermatitis
- Dermatophytosis: may occur in the groin area. Can be difficult to distinguish from seborrheic dermatitis but is generally distributed asymmetrically
- Histiocytosis X: infants affected with acute disseminated histiocytosis X, or Letterer-Siwe disease (Langerhans cell histiocytosis), may display scaling erythematous scalp eruptions clinically similar to seborrheic dermatitis but with associated splenomegaly, reddish-brown papules or vesicles, purpuric lesions, and systemic signs such as fever and adenopathy. The condition fortunately is quite rare
- Leiner's disease: caused by complement dysfunction and characterized by severe generalized erythematous and exfoliative seborrheic dermatitis with associated severe diarrhea and failure to thrive
- Lupus: a classic erythematous malar rash of the nose and malar eminences that may be difficult to distinguish from seborrheic dermatitis characterizes acute cutaneous lupus erythematosus. Chronic, or discoid, lupus erythematosus is characterized by discrete erythematous papules or plaques with a thick adherent scale which when removed reveals a "carpet tack" appearance
- Psoriasis vulgaris: difficult to distinguish from seborrheic dermatitis—may be termed Sebopsoriasis. Less likely confined to scalp. Lacks the reddish color of seborrhea. Psoriasis elsewhere is supportive of this diagnosis
- Rosacea: patients usually present with central facial erythema, or forehead involvement
- Tinea capitis: presence of hyphae on cytologic examination with potassium hydroxide

is suggestive of tinea but does not exclude the diagnosis of seborrheic dermatitis
- Tinea versicolor: presence of short hyphae with spores (spaghetti and meatball pattern) on cytologic examination with potassium hydroxide is suggestive of tinea but does not exclude the diagnosis of seborrheic dermatitis

PEDIATRIC CONSIDERATIONS

- Infants with seborrheic dermatitis and cradle cap may present with concurrent atopic dermatitis

Treatment

INITIAL STABILIZATION

- None necessary

ED TREATMENT

- Seborrheic dermatitis is a chronic condition, treatment is not emergent unless secondarily infected
- Many medications can be utilized
- Demonstrating proper cleansing of scaly lesions may be of educational benefit
- Moderate exposure to sunlight may be beneficial
- Increase frequency of showering and wash all affected areas

MEDICATIONS

- Scales may be softened with mineral oil, or petrolatum before washing
- For thick scalp scale the patient may apply 10% liquor carbonis detergens (LCD) in nivea oil (prescription required) at bedtime, then shampoo with Dawn detergent each morning until scale resolves; up to 3 weeks
- Antiseborrheic shampoos containing sulfur, coal tar or salicylic acid are the most commonly prescribed
  —Sebulex 1–3 times per day
- Zinc pyrithione based shampoos for more stubborn cases
  —Head and Shoulders, DHS Zinc, Zincon, or X Seb shampoo used daily
- Selenium sulfide shampoos are equally effective
  —Exsel or Selsun
- Low- to midpotency topical glucocorticoids
  —Hydrocortisone 1% lotion: 2–4 times/day—may be applied to scalp as well
- When fungal infection is suspected ketoconazole (nizoral)
  —Topical cream applied 1 time each day or 2% shampoo
- In blepharitis, sodium sulfacetamide ophthalmic ointment or solution, and gentle cleansing with baby shampoo may be beneficial

Disposition

ADMISSION CRITERIA

- Seborrheic dermatitis is unlikely to require admission unless severe secondary infection is present

DISCHARGE CRITERIA

- Patients can be discharged home with the recommended medications and an appropriate follow-up appointment
- Improvement should be seen within 7–10 days but may take months to resolve completely
- The adolescent and adult forms may persist as a chronic dermatitis
- Return precautions for signs of secondary bacterial or fungal infections such as fever, erythema, tenderness, or ulceration should be explained

PEDIATRIC CONSIDERATIONS

- The prognosis in infants is excellent
- Most infants are free of seborrhea by their first birthday

Miscellaneous

ICD9: 690.10

CORE CONTENT CODE: 3.1.8

SUGGESTED READINGS

Fleisher GR, Ludwig S, eds. Textbook of pediatric emergency medicine. 3rd ed. Baltimore: Williams & Wilkins, 1993.

Habif TP. Clinical dermatology. 3rd ed. St. Louis: CV Mosby, 1996.

Hurwitz S. Clinical pediatric dermatology. 2d ed. Philadelphia: WB Saunders, 1993.

Janninger CK, Schwartz, RA. Seborrheic dermatitis. Am Family Physician 1995;52:1.

Ruiz-Maldonado R, et al., eds. Pediatric dermatology. Philadelphia: Grune & Stratton, 1989.

Author: Ian Glen Ferguson

Seizure, Adult

Clinical Presentation

SIGNS AND SYMPTOMS

- Altered level of consciousness
- Involuntary, repetitive muscle movements (i.e., tonic posturing or clonic jerking)
- Seizures have abrupt onset; aura may precede a focal seizure
  —Duration is usually 90–120 seconds
  —Impaired memory of the event
  —Postictal state is a brief period of confusion and somnolence following a seizure
- Evidence of recent seizure activity
  —Confusion or somnolence
  —Acute intraoral injury
  —Urinary incontinence
  —Posterior shoulder dislocation
  —Temporary paralysis (Todd's paralysis)
- Other findings may suggest etiology of the seizure
  —Fever and nuchal rigidity (CNS infection)
  —Needle tracks; stigmata of liver disease (drugs and alcohol)
  —Head trauma
  —Papilledema (increased intracranial pressure)
  —Lateralized weakness, sensory loss, or asymmetric reflexes

MECHANISM/DESCRIPTION

Generalized Seizures

- Classically a tonic-clonic (grand mal) which begins as myoclonic jerks followed by loss of consciousness and sustained generalized skeletal muscle contractions
- Nonconvulsive generalized seizures include absence seizures (petit mal) which are brief episodes of sudden immobility and blank stare

Partial Seizures

- Simple: brief sensory, or motor manifestations without loss of consciousness (i.e. Jacksonian)
- Complex: patients manifest mental and psychological symptoms including affect changes, confusion, automatisms, or hallucinations associated with impairment of consciousness

Status epilepticus

- Seizure greater than 1 hour or serial seizures that produce an enduring epileptic condition for greater than 1 hour
- Life threatening emergency with mortality rate of 10%–12%

ETIOLOGY

- CNS infections (meningitis, abscess, encephalitis)
- Vascular disease (ischemic or hemorrhagic stroke)
- Neoplasm (primary or metastatic)
- Metabolic abnormalities
- Electrolytes (hypernatremia, hyponatremia, hypocalcemia)
- Hypo/hyperglycemia
- Hypoxia
- Uremia
- Toxins/drugs (lidocaine, TCAs, cocaine, alcohol withdrawal, etc.)
- Eclampsia
- Hypertensive encephalopathy
- Trauma
- Congenital abnormalities
- Idiopathic

PEDIATRIC CONSIDERATIONS

- Febrile seizure is a generalized seizure occurring between 3 months and 5 years of age typically lasting less than 15 minutes in duration
- Associated with a rapid rise in temperature without evidence of CNS infection or other definitive cause

Pre-Hospital

CAUTIONS

- Placing something in the mouth of a seizing patient is contraindicated because it can result in injury to the patient and the bystander
- Anticonvulsant as per local protocol

Diagnosis

ESSENTIAL WORKUP

- A thorough history is the most valuable part of the workup
  —Witness accounts, prior seizures, presence of acute illnesses, past medical problems, and substance abuse
  —Patients with chronic seizure disorder and typical seizure pattern may only need to have serum glucose and anticonvulsant levels checked
  —New onset seizure mandates work up including electrolytes, head CT, and search for specific underlying cause
  —The patient's condition and resources for follow-up determines whether all these tests need to be done in the emergency department
- Children with first febrile seizure should receive fever workup as dictated by clinical condition
  —Frequently there is a family history of febrile seizure
  —CBC, blood culture, urinalysis, CXR if any signs of respiratory distress
  —Lumbar puncture for first febrile seizure if age <1 year, any concern about mental status or reliability of exam, or unreliable follow-up

LABORATORY

- Serum anticonvulsant levels
- Other labs as indicated by concomitant disease

IMAGING/SPECIAL TESTS

- Noncontrast head CT for patients with persistent or progressive alteration of mental status, focal deficits, or seizure associated with trauma
- CT scan with contrast should be obtained in HIV positive patients to rule out toxoplasmosis
- MRI is sensitive for low grade tumors, small vascular lesions, early inflammation, and early cerebral infarcts, and should be considered as an elective study in new onset seizures
- EEG may be arranged as an outpatient with neurology

DIFFERENTIAL DIAGNOSIS

- Syncope (may also have incontinence, twitching, and jerking)
- Hyperventilation syndrome
- Psychogenic seizures
- Transient ischemic attacks
- Sleep disorders

PEDIATRIC CONSIDERATIONS

- Children with complicated febrile, or new onset seizures without fever need similar seizure workup as adults
- Toxicology screening should be done if there is any suspicion of ingestion, or overdose

Treatment

INITIAL STABILIZATION

- ABCs, pulse oximetry, and oxygen; suction available
  - —C-spine precautions
  - —Rapid sequence intubation if patient cannot control airway, hypoxic, or head trauma
  - —IV access, rapid glucose, and if hypoglycemic give IV dextrose 1 amp
  - —Lorazepam or diazepam for actively seizing patients

ED TREATMENT

- Phenytoin or phenobarbital as second-line drugs
- Rectal paraldehyde, or pentobarbital coma for refractory patients
- Treat the underlying cause if identifiable (hypoglycemia, infection, etc.)
- Load with anticonvulsants if levels are low (e.g., phenytoin)
- Fosphenytoin is an option in patients that IV dilantin is considered unsafe
- If no cause is identifiable in new onset seizure patient, begin single agent anticonvulsant therapy: e.g., phenytoin
- Notify appropriate department of motor vehicles

PEDIATRIC CONSIDERATIONS

- Fever control with acetaminophen and ibuprofen
- Anticonvulsants are not necessary for febrile seizures
- Anticonvulsants should be prescribed in conjunction with neurologist

MEDICATIONS

- Acetaminophen: 10–15 mg/kg po or PR
- Diazepam: 0.2 mg/kg IV per dose (max 20 mg), 0.5 mg/kg PR
- Fosphenytoin: 15–20 mg/kg at rate of 100–150 mg/min IV
- Ibuprofen: 5–10 mg/kg po
- Lorazepam: 0.1 mg/kg IV per dose (max 10 mg)
- Paraldehyde: 0.3–0.5 ml/kg PR 1:1 in mineral oil; peds: 0.3 ml/kg PR 1:2 in mineral oil
- Phenobarbital: 15–20 mg/kg IV at rate of 1 mg/kg/min
- Phenytoin: 15–20 mg/kg IV at rate of 40–50 mg/min; peds: use rate of 0.5–1.0 mg/kg/min

Disposition

ADMISSION CRITERIA

- Status epilepticus should be admitted to the ICU
- Seizures secondary to underlying disease (e.g., meningitis, intracranial lesion) must be admitted for appropriate treatment and monitoring
- Poorly controlled repetitive seizures should be admitted for monitoring
- Delirium tremens

DISCHARGE CRITERIA

- Patient with normal workup and appropriate neurology follow-up
- Uncomplicated seizure in patient with chronic seizure disorder
- Seizure secondary to reversible cause (e.g., hypoglycemia, alcohol withdrawal)
- Simple febrile seizure

Miscellaneous

ICD9: 780.39

CORE CONTENT CODE: 11.9, 13.5.3

SUGGESTED READINGS

Gilad R, Lampl Y, Gabby U, Eshol Y, Sarova-Pinhas I. Early treatment of a single generalized tonic-clonic seizure to prevent recurrence. Arch Neurol 1996;53(11):1149–1152.

Pelligrino TR. An emergency department approach to first-time seizure. Emerg Med Clin North Am 1994;12(4):925–939.

Shepherd SM. Management of status epilepticus. Emerg Med Clin North Am 1994;12(4):941–961.

Stenklyft PH, Carmona M. Febrile seizure. Emerg Med Clin North Am 1994;12(4):989–999.

Authors: Paul David; Rebecca Smith-Coggins

Clinical Presentation

SIGNS AND SYMPTOMS

Neonates

- Subtle abnormal motor activity
  - —Facial movements
  - —Eye deviations
  - —Eyelid fluttering
  - —Lip smacking/sucking
- Respiratory alterations
- Apnea
- Seizure activity
  - —Focal or generalized tonic seizures
  - —Focal or multifocal clonic seizure
  - —Myoclonic movements

Older Infants and Children

- Generalized seizures
  - —Tonic-clonic
  - —Tonic
  - —Clonic
  - —Myoclonic
  - —Atonic ("drop")
  - —Absence
- Partial or focal seizures
  - —Simple
    - -Consciousness is maintained
    - -Simple partial seizures
      - *May include motor, sensory and/or cognitive symptoms
      - *Motor activity is localized to one part or side of the body
      - *Paresthesias, metallic tastes, and visual or auditory hallucinations
  - —Complex
    - -Consciousness is impaired
    - -Complex partial seizure
      - *Often a simple partial seizure which progresses to include impaired consciousness
      - *Often an aura precedes altered consciousness; auditory, olfactory, or visual hallucination
      - *May generalize making these difficult to distinguish from a primary generalized seizure
- Status epilepticus
  - —Generalized and convulsive are most common
  - —Sustained partial seizures
  - —Absence seizures
    - -Persistent confusion

MECHANISM/DESCRIPTION

- Seizures are caused by sudden, abnormal discharges of neurons resulting in a change in behavior or function

ETIOLOGY

Neonates/Young Infants

- Perinatal hypoxia
- Intracranial hemorrhage
- Drug actions
- Drug withdrawal
- Hypoglycemia
- Hypocalcemia
- Brain malformations
- Infection
- Inborn errors of metabolism
- Hypernatremia
- Hyponatremia

Infants Over 6 months, Toddlers

- Febrile seizures
- Infection
- Trauma
- Toxic ingestion
- Inborn errors of metabolism
- CNS structural anomalies or degenerative diseases

Children Over 3 years old

- Idiopathic (most common)
- Trauma
- Meningitis
- Encephalitis
- CNS structural anomalies or degenerative disease

Pre-Hospital

CAUTIONS

- Avoid empiric treatment as many events are mistaken by parents as seizures
  - —Breath-holding spells
  - —Night terrors
  - —Syncope
  - —Pseudoseizures
- Immobilize the cervical spine if trauma is suspected
- Check fingerstick glucose or administer dextrose

Diagnosis

ESSENTIAL WORKUP

- Obtain a detailed history of the seizure
  - —Movements
  - —Duration
  - —State of consciousness
- A careful neurologic exam should be performed once the seizure resolves
- Rapid glucose testing for those in status epilepticus

LABORATORY

- Bedside glucose test
- Routine laboratory studies should only be performed in a subset of children presenting with seizure
  - —Young infants
  - —Patients in status epilepticus
  - —New onset seizure without a fever
- Otherwise select studies based on the presentation
  - —Electrolytes
  - —BUN
  - —Creatinine
  - —Glucose
  - —Calcium
  - —Magnesium
  - —CBC
  - —Toxicologic screen
- Patients on anticonvulsant therapy
  - —Obtain drug levels only
- Febrile seizure
  - —Laboratory studies are only indicated when a serious underlying bacterial infection is suspected
- ABG
  - —Status epilepticus
  - —Ill-appearing children

IMAGING/SPECIAL TESTS

- Head CT
  - —Focal seizure
  - —New focal neurologic abnormality
  - —Suspected intracranial hemorrhage or mass lesion
  - —New onset status epilepticus without identifiable cause
  - —Patients with recent new, generalized, single seizure who are currently alert with a nonfocal neurologic exam
- Lumbar puncture
  - —Suspicion of meningitis or encephalitis
  - —No indication of increased ICP
- MRI
  - —Rarely urgently indicated for seizures
- EEG
  - —Rarely needed emergently

DIFFERENTIAL DIAGNOSIS

Neonates

- Apnea due to other causes
- Jitters or tremors
  —Will stop with passive flexion of the limb
  —Shivering with micturition

Infants and Toddlers

- Breath-holding spells
- Night terrors

Children and Adolescents

- Migraine headache
- Vasomotor syncope
- Tics
- Toxins/drugs
- Pseudoseizures
- Hysteria

Treatment

INITIAL STABILIZATION

- Meticulous support of airway, breathing, and circulation if actively seizing
- Airway
  —Oxygen
  —Nasopharyngeal airway preferred over oral airway
  —Bag-valve mask support or intubation, if persistently hypoxic in spite of O_2 placement
  —Intubation only if seizures are refractory or the airway is persistently compromised
- IV access
- If hypoglycemic
  —D_{25} for children
  —D_{10} for neonates
- Maintain spine precautions if trauma suspected

ED TREATMENT

Status epilepticus

- Children
  —Benzodiazepine
    -Lorazepam is preferred due to its longer duration of action
    -Valium is acceptable
    -Repeat every 10 minutes for 2–3 doses
    -If IV access is not available
      *Diazepam may be given per rectum; use a T.B. syringe or 14-gauge angiocatheter
      *Midazolam IM is also effective if IV access is not available
  —Phenytoin
    -If benzodiazepines fail
    -For longer term control
  —Phenobarbital
    -Use if benzodiazepines and phenytoin fail to break the seizure
    -Risk of respiratory depression greatly increases if a benzodiazepine has also been given
  —Second-line drug therapy in the event of refractory status epilepticus
    -Lidocaine
    -Paraldehyde (per rectum)
    -Barbiturate coma
      *Pentobarbital
      *Thiopental
      *High-dose phenobarbital
      *Barbiturate coma requires intubation and EEG monitoring to be sure the seizure is suppressed
    -General anesthesia
      *A final resort
      *Halothane or isoflurane and neuromuscular blockade to facilitate mechanical ventilation
      *Continuous EEG is needed to be sure the seizure is abolished
- Neonates
  —Phenobarbital if acceptable first-line therapy
  —Preferred maintenance drug

MEDICATIONS

- Calcium gluconate: 0.5 cc/kg IV of a 10% solution over 5 min
- D_{10}: 5 cc/kg IV
- D_{25}: 2 cc/kg IV for children
- Diazepam: 0.3 mg/kg IV; 0.5 mg/kg PR
- Lidocaine: 2 mg/kg IV; maintenance: 4 mg/kg/hr IV
- Lorazepam: 0.1 mg/kg IV
- $MgSO_4$: 25–50 mg/kg/dose over 20 min IV; may be given every 4–6 hours × 3 doses if necessary
- Midazolam: 0.2 mg/kg IM
- Paraldehyde: 0.4 ml/kg PR mixed 1:1 with vegetable oil given with a glass syringe
- Pentobarbital: 10–20 mg/kg IV; maintenance: 0.5–5.0 mg/kg/hr IV
- Phenobarbital: 15–20 mg/kg IV; should not be given faster than 1–2 mg/kg/min; maintenance: 3–8 mg/kg/24hrs po; high-dose phenobarbital 10 mg/kg doses every 30 min until seizure abates for up to 120 mg/kg in 24 hours
- Phenytoin: 15–20 mg/kg IV; must be given in saline as it will precipitate in dextrose solutions; it should not be given faster than 1 mg/kg/min; maintenance: 5–10 mg/kg/24hrs po
- Thiopental: 30 mg/kg IV; maintenance: 5 mg/kg/hr IV

Disposition

ADMISSION CRITERIA

- Intensive Care Unit
  —Active status epilepticus, intubated, or with persistent mental status changes
- Wards
  —Status epilepticus resolved in the ED
  —Underlying cause of seizure not resolved or controlled
    -Intracranial hemorrhage
    -Mass lesion
    -Meningitis/encephalitis
    -Drug
    -Toxin ingestions

DISCHARGE CRITERIA

- The child is completely alert
- Normal neurologic exam
- No evidence of an underlying cause requiring hospitalization
- Reliable parent
- Home telephone
- Provide "seizure precautions" after care instructions
- Follow-up with a primary care physician or pediatric neurologist
  —Consult, prior to discharge
- Prophylactic anticonvulsant
  —Indicated for certain seizure types with high recurrence rates
    -Myoclonic, absence, atonic seizures, and infantile spasms

Miscellaneous

ICD9: 780.3, 780.31

CORE CONTENT CODE: 13.5.3; 13.16.4

SUGGESTED READINGS

Roberts MR, Eng-Bourguin J: Status epilepticus in children. Emerg Med Clin North Am 1995;13:489–507.

Roddy SM, McBride MC. Seizure disorders. In: Hoekelman RA, ed. Primary pediatric care. 3rd ed. St. Louis: CV Mosby, 1997:1564–574.

Vining EPG. Pediatric seizures. Emerg Med Clin North Am 1994;12:973–88.

Author: Guy L. Upshaw

Seizures, Febrile

Clinical Presentation

SIGNS AND SYMPTOMS

Fever

- Seizure is often the first sign of the febrile illness

Seizure

- Generalized tonic-clonic seizure activity is most common
  —Occurs during an acute fever spike
  —Initially a cry, followed by loss of consciousness
  —Tonic phase
    -Muscular rigidity
    -May be associated with apnea and incontinence
    -Seizures are usually self-limited and last only a few minutes
  —Other seizure types
    -Staring with stiffness
    -Limpness
    -Jerking movements without prior stiffening

MECHANISM/DESCRIPTION

- Seizure occurring between the ages of 3 months and 5 years in association with a fever
  —No evidence of intracranial infection or another defined cause
  —The average age of onset is 18–22 months
  —Children with previous nonfebrile seizures are excluded
- Most common pediatric convulsive disorder
  —2–4% of young children in the United States
- Most occur in normal children
- Higher incidence
  —Neurologically impaired children
  —Males
- Subgroups
  —Simple febrile seizures
    -Brief, self-limited lasting <10–15 minutes, resolve spontaneously
    -Generalized without any features suggesting focal CNS onset
  —Complex febrile seizures
    -Duration of more than 15 minutes
    -Focal features may be evident
    -Occurrence of more than a single seizure within a 24-hour period
- Risk factors for a first febrile seizure
  —Higher temperature
  —Family history of febrile seizures
  —Parental report of slow development
  —Low serum sodium levels
- Risk of recurrence
  —Occurs in about 30% of cases
  —Early age of onset
  —Positive family history of febrile seizure
  —Decreased frequency of recurrence with therapeutic levels of phenobarbital and valproic acid
    -These drugs are not initiated in the acute setting
  —No alterations in school performance, intelligence testing or behavior
  —Less than 5% of children will develop a seizure disorder

ETIOLOGY

- Common childhood infections
  —Upper respiratory illnesses
  —Otitis media
  —Roseola
  —Gastrointestinal infections
    -*Shigella* gastroenteritis

Pre-Hospital

- Protect the airway
- Oxygen
- Support breathing as needed

CAUTIONS

- Keep the child from incurring injury while actively convulsing
- Respiratory insufficiency and apnea occur secondary to overaggressive treatment with benzodiazepines
- Simple febrile seizures are self-limited and require no anticonvulsant therapy

Diagnosis

ESSENTIAL WORKUP

- The only essential components of the workup is the clinical examination
- A careful history and physical examination will help confirm the diagnosis and rule out other etiologies
  —Symptoms of infectious illness
  —Medication exposure
  —Trauma
  —Developmental level
  —Family history of febrile or afebrile seizures
  —A complete description of the seizure
  —The presence of meningismus or a tense or bulging fontanelle
  —Abnormalities or focal differences in muscle strength or tone

LABORATORY

- Routine laboratory studies are not indicated
- Evaluate for a source of fever if a serious bacterial infections is suspected
  —White blood cell count
  —Urine analysis
  —Blood and urine cultures
- Electrolytes and bedside glucose in infants or in children with vomiting or diarrhea

IMAGING/SPECIAL TESTS

- Chest radiograph only in patients with significant respiratory symptoms
- Head computed tomography
  —Should not be performed routinely
  —Indicated with traumatic injuries or focal neurologic findings
- Lumbar puncture
  —Patients with meningismus
  —Febrile or "toxic"-appearing infants
- Electroencephalogram
  —Not helpful in the evaluation of febrile seizure
  —May show an abnormality, usually consisting of occipital slowing up to 1 week after the event
  —The EEG does not help predict recurrences or risk for later epilepsy

DIFFERENTIAL DIAGNOSIS

- Febrile delirium
- Febrile shivering with pallor and perioral cyanosis
- Breath-holding spell during fever event
- Acute life-threatening event
- Other causes of seizure
  —Afebrile seizure occurring during fever event
  —Sudden discontinuance of anticonvulsants
  —Meningitis
  —Encephalitis
  —Dehydration and electrolyte imbalance
  —Head trauma
  —Toxic ingestions

- -Diphenhydramine
- -Tricyclic antidepressants
- -Amphetamines
- -Cocaine
- —Hypoxia
- —Metabolic disease
- —Intracranial masses
- —CNS vascular lesions

Treatment

INITIAL STABILIZATION

- Benzodiazepines
  - —Prolonged seizures or compromised patients
  - —Lorazepam or diazepam
- Support the airway and breathing

ED TREATMENT

- Seizures refractory to benzodiazepines
  - —Phenytoin
  - —Phenobarbital
  - —Aggressive workup to exclude other etiologies
- Administer antipyretics acutely and schedule for at least the next 24 hours
  - —Acetaminophen or ibuprofen
- If a bacterial source of fever is diagnosed, appropriate antibiotic treatment is indicated

MEDICATIONS

- Acetaminophen: 15 mg/kg po, PR
- Ibuprofen: 10 mg/kg po
- Lorazepam: 0.05–1.0 mg/kg IV
- Diazepam: 0.1–0.3 mg/kg IV; 0.3–0.5 mg/kg PR
- Phenytoin: 10–20 mg/kg IV
- Phenobarbital: 10–20 mg/kg IV or IM

Disposition

ADMISSION CRITERIA

- Patients with persistent fever
- Recurrent or prolonged seizures

DISCHARGE CRITERIA

- Simple febrile seizures
  - —Normal neurologic examination
  - —Source of their fever has been determined to be responsive to outpatient treatment
    - -Otitis media
    - -Gastroenteritis
- Reassurance to parents
- Antipyretic therapy for 24 hours

Miscellaneous

ICD9: 780.3

CORE CONTENT CODE: 13.5.3.1

SUGGESTED READINGS

American Academy of Pediatrics, Provisional Committee on Quality Improvement, Subcommittee on Febrile Seizures. Practice parameter: The neurodiagnostic evaluation of the child with a first simple febrile seizure. Pediatr 1996;97:769–771.

Camfield PR, Camfield CS. Management and treatment of febrile seizures. Curr Probl Pediatr 1997;27:6–14.

Green SM, Rothrock SG, Clem KJ. Can seizures be the sole manifestation of meningitis in febrile children? Pediatr 1993;92:527–34.

Gonzalez Del Rey JA. Febrile seizures. In: Barkin RM, ed. Pediatric emergency medicine: Concepts and clinical practice. 2nd ed. St. Louis: CV Mosby, 1997:1017–1019.

Author: Joan Bothner

Sepsis

Clinical Presentation

SIGNS AND SYMPTOMS

- Fever
- Tachycardia
- Tachypnea
- Hypothermia (poor prognosis)
- Hypoxemia

Cardiovascular

- Blood pressure
  - —Normal early in sepsis
  - —Hypotension when septic shock occurs
- Poor perfusion with septic shock
  - —Prolonged capillary refill
  - —Cool and clammy extremities
  - —Oliguria

Gastrointestinal/Genitourinary

- Abdominal pain
- Nausea, vomiting
- Diarrhea
- Dysuria/frequency
- Reduced urine output
- Abdominal tenderness
  - —Diffuse
  - —Localized to right upper-quadrant (liver or gallbladder source)
  - —Right lower-quadrant (appendicitis with or without abscess)
  - —Suprapubic area or lower quadrants (urinary tract or pelvic source or diverticulitis)
- Flank pain
  - —With pyelonephritis or retroperitoneal abscess

Pulmonary

- Shortness of breath
- Cough (productive or nonproductive)
- Localized wheeze or rales
  - —With pneumonia
- Tachypnea
  - —Present even when the lungs are not the source of sepsis

Dermatologic

- Any rash is important
- Localized erythema with lymphangitis (streptococcal or staphylococcal cellulitis)
- Rash involving palms of hands and soles of feet (Rickettsial infection)
- Petechiae scattered on the torso and extremities (meningococcemia)
- Ecthyma gangrenosum (pseudomonas septicemia)
  - —Round, indurated, painless lesion with surrounding erythema and central necrotic black eschar
- Decubitus ulcers
- Indwelling catheter
  - —Surrounding skin erythematous with or without purulent drainage

CNS

- Change in mental status
  - —Confusion
  - —Delirium
  - —Coma
- Neck stiffness (meningitis)

MECHANISM/DESCRIPTION

- Systemic inflammatory response syndrome (SIRS)
  - —Systemic response to an unspecified stimulus manifested by two or more of the following
    - -Temperature >38°C or <36°C
    - -Heart rate >90 beats/minute
    - -Respiratory rate >20/minute or $PaCO_2$ <32 mm Hg
    - -WBC $>12{,}000/mm^3$, $<4000/mm^3$, or $>10\%$ band forms
  - —Sepsis is the most common cause of SIRS
- Sepsis
  - —two or more of the SIRS manifestations present
  - —Infectious cause is documented or strongly suspected
- Septic shock
  - —Sepsis-induced hypotension despite fluid resuscitation
    - -Systolic BP <90 mm Hg or
    - -Reduction of >40 mm Hg from baseline
  - —Perfusion abnormalities
    - -Change in mental status
    - -Lactic acidosis
    - -Oliguria
    - -Poor capillary refill

ETIOLOGY

- Gram-negative bacteria most common
  - —*Escherichia coli*
  - —*Pseudomonas aeruginosa*
- Gram-positive bacteria
  - —Enterococcus species
  - —*Staphylococcus aureus*
  - —*Streptococcus pneumoniae*
- Fungi (Candida species)
- Viruses
- *Legionella* species
- Response to sepsis
  - —Decreased peripheral vascular resistance due to various mediators of the inflammatory response causing vasodilation
  - —Elevated cardiac output
    - -Early appropriate response to afterload reduction (vasodilation)
    - -Volume resuscitation
    - -Later in sepsis, myocardial depression and reduced cardiac output (due to injury at the cellular level or mediators acting on the heart)
  - —Narrow arteriovenous oxygen difference
- Elevated lactate levels
  - -Anaerobic glycolysis
- Multiple organ dysfunction syndrome (MODS) develops if sepsis either untreated or ineffectively treated
  - —Pulmonary injury: adult respiratory distress syndrome
  - —Renal injury: acute tubular necrosis and kidney failure
  - —Hepatic injury and failure
  - —Disseminated intravascular coagulation

PEDIATRIC CONSIDERATIONS

- Major causes of bacterial sepsis
  - —*Neisseria meningitis*
  - —*Streptococcal pneumoniae*
  - —*Hemophilus influenzae*
- Meningitis—most frequent site of infection

Pre-Hospital

CAUTION

- Aggressive fluid resuscitation for hypotension

Diagnosis

ESSENTIAL WORKUP
- Careful history and physical examination
  - —Guides further evaluation and initiation of appropriate antibiotic therapy

LABORATORY
- CBC with differential
- Electrolytes, BUN, Cr, glucose
- Liver function tests
- ABG
  - —Mixed acid-base abnormalities: respiratory alkalosis with metabolic acidosis
- Blood cultures
  - —From 2 different sites
  - —One may be drawn through an indwelling central line (i.e., Broviac)
- UA and culture

IMAGING/SPECIAL TESTS
- CXR
- CSF analysis
- Cultures
  - —Sputum
  - —Wound/abscess
  - —CSF
- Lactic acid level
- Amylase/lipase
- X-rays of bone and soft tissue underlying any wound for osteomyelitis or gas gangrene
- Abdominal abscess identification
  - —Abdominal ultrasound
  - —CT of abdomen

DIFFERENTIAL DIAGNOSIS
- Causes of SIRS
  - —Sepsis (most common)
  - —Pancreatitis
  - —Burns
  - —Multiple trauma

Treatment

INITIAL STABILIZATION
- ABCs
- Supplemental oxygen to maintain $PaO_2 > 60$ mm Hg
  - —If FIO_2 requirement >0.5, then intubate and provide mechanical ventilation
- Administer 0.9%NS IV fluid to restore circulating blood volume

ED TREATMENT
- Administer antibiotics early based on the most likely organisms or site of infection
  - —No source identified after initial assessment
    - -Normal immune function
      - *Second or third generation cephalosporin and gentamicin
      - *Nafcillin and gentamicin
    - -Immunocompromised host
      - *Pipercillin and gentamicin
      - *Ceftazidime and either nafcillin or vancomycin
  - —If source identified, or highly suspected, treat the most likely organisms
    - -Pulmonary source
      - *Second- or third-generation cephalosporin and gentamicin, and possibly erythromycin
    - -Intra-abdominal source
      - *Ampicillin and metronidazole and gentamicin
      - *Cefoxitin and gentamicin
      - *Urinary tract source
      - *Ampicillin or pipercillin and gentamicin
- Vasopressors
  - —Indicated for persistent hypotension despite fluid administration
    - -Add dopamine if the patient remains hypotensive after 2 L of fluid
  - —Useful to improve renal, mesenteric, cerebral, and coronary flow
    - -Dopamine: useful to maintain renal perfusion while continuing fluid resuscitation
    - -Norepinephrine adversely affects renal perfusion; initiate if dopamine not effective

MEDICATIONS
- Ampicillin: 1–2 g (peds: 50–200 mg/kg/24hrs) IV q 4–6 hrs
- Cefoxitin: 1–2 g (peds: 100–160 mg/kg/24hrs) IV q 6–8 hrs
- Ceftazidime: 1–2 g (peds: 100–150 mg/kg/24hrs) IV q 8–12 hrs
- Dopamine: 1–5μg/kg/min (renal dose); 5–10 μg/kg/min (pressor dose)
- Gentamicin: 1–1.5 mg/kg (peds: 2–2.5 mg/kg q 8 hrs) IV q 8 hrs
- Metronidazole: load with 1 g (peds: 15 mg/kg) IV, then 500 mg (peds: 7.5 mg/kg) q 6 hrs
- Nafcillin: 1–2 g IV q 4 hrs (peds: 50 mg/kg/24 hrs divided q 4–6 hrs)
- Norepinephrine: 2–8 μg/min
- Piperacillin: 3–4 g IV q 4–6 hrs
- Vancomycin: 500 mg (peds: 10 mg/kg) IV q 6 hrs

PEDIATRIC CONSIDERATIONS
- Antibiotic therapy based on age
  - —<3 months (2 drugs): ampicillin and gentamicin or cefotaxime (50–180 mg/kg/day divided q 4–6 hrs)
  - —>3 months: cefotaxime or ceftriaxone (50–100 mg/kg/day divided q 12–24 hrs)
- Initiate vasopressors after no response to 60 ml/kg IV fluid
- Avoid hyponatremia and hypoglycemia
- Dexamethasone for children with bacterial meningitis
  - —0.15 mg/kg q 6 hrs for 4 days
  - —Potentially may reduce sensorineural hearing loss

Disposition

ADMISSION CRITERIA
- Suspected sepsis
- ICU if hypotensive, requires vasopressors or airway management

DISCHARGE CRITERIA
- No patient with sepsis should be discharged

Miscellaneous

ICD9: 38.9

CORE CONTENT CODE: 9.0

SUGGESTED READINGS

Bone RC. Diagnosing sepsis: What we need to consider today. J Crit Ill 1996;11:658–665.

Carcillo JA, Cunnion RE. Septic shock. Crit Care Clinics 1997;13:553–574.

Cunha BA. Antibiotic treatment of sepsis. Med Clinic North Am 1995;79:351–558.

Jacobs RF, Sowell MK, Moss MM, Fiser DH. Septic shock in children: Bacterial etiologies and temporal relationships. Pediatr Infect Dis J 1990;9:196–200.

Lipton JD, Schafermeyer RW. Evolving concepts in pediatric bacterial meningitis—Part II: Current management and therapeutic research. Ann Emerg Med 1993;22:1616–1629.

Author: Janet Poponick

Sexual Assault

Clinical Presentation

SIGNS AND SYMPTOMS

- May not reveal they are a victim
  - —67% of rape victims do not tell their doctors
  - —Most will reveal history only in response to direct questions
- Tachycardia or pounding heart beat
- Headaches
- Nausea
- Back pain
- Skin problems
- Menstrual symptoms
- Sudden weight change
- Sleeping disorders
- Abdominal pain
- Gagging
- Trouble breathing
- Associated injuries
  - —Of those with injuries, 70% report no injury at presentation
  - —Lacerations of perineum
  - —Vulvar trauma
  - —Laceration of vaginal wall (more common in younger patients near introitus)
  - —Multiple contusions
  - —Abrasions
  - —Human bite
  - —Lacerations or puncture wound to extremity
  - —Burns
  - —Depressed skull fracture

MECHANISM/DESCRIPTION

- Specific legal definition varies state to state
- Defined as forced sexual contact without consent
  - —Continuum from unwanted touching and fondling to forced penetration of vagina, anus, oral cavity

ETIOLOGY

- 78–82% of women are raped by someone they know
- 50% of rape victims over 30 years old are assaulted by intimate partner
- Among women suffering physical abuse by a partner, 33–46% report being sexually assaulted
- Age distribution of female rape victims
  - —11–17 years old: 32%
  - —18–24 years old: 22%
  - —>50 years old: 22%

PEDIATRIC CONSIDERATIONS

- Must follow local laws regarding child abuse
- Patient most likely never had a pelvic exam previously
  - —If possible involve specialist
- Use smallest speculum possible
- Use toys, dolls to have child explain what happened
- Early psychiatric intervention necessary

Pre-Hospital

CAUTIONS

- Assure patient of safety
- Discourage patient from
  - —Changing clothes
  - —Eating
  - —Drinking
  - —Taking any medication
  - —Gargling
  - —Brushing teeth
  - —Urinating
  - —Defecating
  - —Douching
  - —Showering
- Keep history of assault to a minimum
  - —Repeated histories may retraumatize the patient
- Do not disturb evidence at rape site or on patient
- Do not examine genitalia
- If patient consents, contact local police per local protocol
  - —Including the patient in decision-making will help the patient to regain sense of control and start healing

Diagnosis

ESSENTIAL WORKUP

- Obtain written consent prior to any exam, test, or treatment
- Allow patient to pause and proceed at comfortable pace
- Allow advocate to stay with patient during exam with patient's consent

History

- Obtain complete history even if patient does not wish to file charges including
  - —Time and place of assault
  - —Race of assailants
  - —Number of assailants
  - —Types of penetration: vaginal, oral, rectal
  - —Assailant ejaculation
  - —Use of force
  - —Victims activity since assault
    - -Changed clothes
    - -Douched
    - -Bathed
    - -Urinated
    - -Defecated
    - -Ate
    - -Tampon use
  - —Full gynecological history
  - —Last voluntary intercourse
    - -Sperm maybe mobile up to 5 days in cervix and 12 hours in vagina
- Address all physical complaints

Physical Exam

- Use evidence kit even if victim unsure if reporting to police
- Female chaperone required if male physician
- If clothes soiled, photograph prior to undressing with patient's consent
  - —Note general appearance of clothes
    - -Staining
    - -Tears
    - -Mud
    - -Leaves
    - -Wood's lamp for seminal stains
  - —Have patient disrobe while standing on a sheet and place all clothes in a *paper* bag
    - -Plastic causes mold and increases bacteria counts
  - —Have only patient handle clothing
  - —Arrange for a change of clothes
- Complete physical should be done with emphasis on
  - —Abrasions
  - —Lacerations
  - —Bites
  - —Scratches
  - —Foreign bodies
  - —Ecchymoses
  - —Dried semen on skin
- Forensic collection
  - —Fingernail scrapings
  - —Head hair specimens

—Swab between teeth if oral penetration for acid phosphatase and sperm
—Throat culture for gonorrhea if oral sex
- Gynecological exam
  —Explain all steps and allow patient to pace exam
  —Comb and collect pubic hair per local protocol
  —Lubricate speculum with water
  —Look for genital trauma even in asymptomatic patients
  —May use toluidine blue to identify small pelvic lacerations from traumatic intercourse
    -Best applied to vaginal mucous at introitus
  —Special attention to hymen as one of most common places for trauma
  —Lacerations to vaginal wall near introitus more common in younger patients
  —Aspirate secretions pooled in posterior fornix and place in sterile container to be examined for sperm and acid phosphates
    -If no secretions in posterior fornix, wipe with a cotton tip
    -Swab and microscopically examine for sperm and acid phosphates
  —Swabs for gonorrhea and chlamydia
- Rectal exam if penetration or attempted penetration
  —Lacerations
  —Fissures
  —Bleeding
  —Gonorrhea and chlamydia cultures

LABORATORY

- Syphilis serology
- Hepatitis band C panel
- Blood type
- Pregnancy test
- Gonorrhea culture
- Chlamydia culture
- Other labs as needed based on injuries

Treatment

INITIAL STABILIZATION

- Treat life-threatening injuries

ED TREATMENT

- Place patient in quiet, private room
- Assure patient confidentiality to name and reason for visit
- Regularly assure patient of safety
- Enforce nonjudgmental behavior by staff
- Designate nursing and medical provider for entire stay who are familiar with evidence collection kit
- Contact community or in-hospital advocate to stay with patient while in ED
- Alert hospital security to possibility of assailant presenting to ED
- Contact police if patient consents or local law requires
- Collect evidence as outlined above and according to local law
- Administer pregnancy prophylaxis if not currently pregnant
  —Hormonal therapy if within 72 hours
    -100 μg ethinyl estradiol stat and repeat in 12 hours
    -Decreases risk of pregnancy 60–90%
  —72 hours to 7 days postassault
    -Consult Ob/Gyn consult for possible IUD placement
    -Estimated risk of pregnancy is 2–4% if woman not using contraceptives
- Administer prophylactic therapy for gonococcus and chlamydia
  —Suprex 400 mg po
  —Doxycycline 100 mg po bid for 7–10 days

Disposition

ADMISSION CRITERIA

- Serious traumatic injury

DISCHARGE CRITERIA

- Medical follow-up to check culture results and future HIV testing
- Safe place for patient to go

Miscellaneous

ICD9: N/A

CORE CONTENT CODE: 19.3

SUGGESTED READINGS

Dunn SFM, Gilchrist VJ. Sexual assault. Prim Care 1993;20:359–373.

Dupre AR, Hampton HL, Morrison H, Meeks GR. Sexual assault. Obstet Gynecol Surv 1993;45:640–648.

Levine DL, Kaufman LE. Rape and sexual violence: The adult and adolescent female victim. In: Bernstein E, Bernstein J, eds. Case studies in emergency medicine and the health of the public. Jones & Bartlett, Boston, 1996:100–112.

Author: David Levine

Shock

Clinical Presentation

SIGNS AND SYMPTOMS

- Anxiety
- Obtundation
- Hypotension
- Decreased urine output
- Hypovolemic shock
  - —Cool, clammy, or mottled extremities
  - —Tachycardia
  - —Tachypnea
  - —Poor capillary refill
  - —Pallor
  - —Decreased peripheral pulses
  - —Flattened neck veins
- Obstructive Shock
  - —Narrowed pulse pressure
  - —Diaphoresis
  - —Jugular venous distention
  - —Cool, clammy, sweaty extremities
  - —Rales
- Vasogenic Shock
  - —Flushing
  - —Widened pulse pressure
  - —Septic shock
    - -Hyperthermia
    - -Hypothermia
    - -Flushing
    - -Strong pulses
    - -Purpura or petechial rash
  - —Anaphylactic shock
    - -Urticaria
    - -Flushing
    - -Tachypnea
    - -Throat tightness
    - -Hoarseness
  - —Neurogenic shock
    - -Flaccid paralysis
    - -Hypotension with bradycardia

MECHANISM/DESCRIPTION

- Supply of blood flow to tissues inadequate to meet the demands of the tissues
- Nutrient requirements are not fulfilled
- Toxic metabolites are not removed
- When an insult or injury occurs, physiologic responses attempt to increase the perfusion pressures and supply of nutrients to meet the tissues' demands
- Shock occurs when the body's physiologic responses to increase organ perfusion are inadequate in meeting the tissue demands
- Main components of blood flow
  - —Cardiac output (CO)
  - —Blood volume (central venous pressure) (CVP)
  - —Peripheral resistance of arteriolar and venous system (Systemic Vascular Resistance—SVR)

Major Categories of Shock

- Hypovolemic shock
  - —↓ Blood volume (↓ CVP) causes ↓ CO, leads to ↑SVR in an attempt to normalize perfusion pressure
- Cardiogenic shock
  - —↓ Cardiac output causes venous congestion (↑CVP), reflexive ↑SVR
  - —Decreased cardiac output due to
    - -Reduction in contractility
    - -An obstruction to inflow of blood to the heart
    - -An obstruction to outflow
- Vasogenic shock
  - —↓ SVR causes a reflexive ↑CO, ↓ CVP
  - —Septic
    - -An initial infectious insult overwhelms the immune system
    - -Biochemical messengers (leukotrienes, histamines, prostaglandins) cause vessel dilatation
    - -Capillary endothelium becomes disrupted and the vessels leak
    - -Drop in total vascular resistance leads to inadequate tissue perfusion
  - —Anaphylactic
    - -An antigen stimulates the allergic reaction
    - -Mast cells degranulate
    - -Histamine release along with autocoids stimulate an anaphylaxis cascade
    - -Vascular smooth muscle relaxes
    - -Capillary endothelium leaks
    - -Drop in total vascular resistance leads to inadequate tissue perfusion
  - —Pharmacologic
    - -Any pharmacologic agent can cause hypotension through smooth muscle dilatation or myocardial depression
  - —Neurogenic shock
    - -Spinal chord insults disrupts sympathetic stimulation to vessels
    - -Loss of sympathetic tone causes arteriodilitation and vasodilitation
    - -Cardiac and thoracic vessel sympathetic innervation is from T1-T8
    - -Lesions proximal to T4 disrupt sympathetic, spares vagal innervation causing bradycardia

ETIOLOGY

- Hypovolemic shock
  - —Hemorrhage
  - —Dehydration
  - —Decreased fluid intake
  - —Excessive fluid losses
- Cardiogenic shock
  - —Myocardial infarction (↓ contractility)
  - —Cardiomyopathy (↓ contractility)
  - —Pulmonary embolism (↓ outflow)
  - —Pericardial tamponade (↓ inflow)
  - —Tension pneumothorax (↓ inflow)
- Vasogenic shock
  - —Sepsis
  - —Anaphylaxis
  - —Pharmacologic overdose
- Neurogenic shock
  - —Spinal cord injury

PEDIATRIC CONSIDERATIONS

- Hypovolemic shock
  - —Diarrhea causing volume depletion is the most common cause of pediatric shock worldwide
- Cardiogenic shock
  - —Viral myocarditis
  - —Drug ingestions
  - —Postoperative cardiac surgery
  - —Congenital heart disease
  - —Pericardial tamponade
- Vasogenic shock
- Septic shock
  - —Haemophilus influenza
  - —Neisseria meningitidis
  - —Streptococcal pneumonia

Pre-Hospital

- Focus on supportive care and stabilization of ABCs
- Intubation for airway protection, hypoxia, or extreme tachypnea
- Adequate IV access
- Fluid resuscitation for hypotension when cardiogenic shock *is not* suspected

Diagnosis

ESSENTIAL WORKUP

- History and physical exam
- Identify type or types of shock present
- Identify underlying cause of shock
- Rule out other life-threats in differential

LABORATORY TESTS

- Hemoglobin/hematocrit
  - —Low hemoglobin and hematocrit—hemorrhage
    - -A normal hematocrit does not rule out hemorrhage
  - —Very high hematocrit—dehydration
- White blood cell count
  - —High—nonspecific marker of infection
  - —Low—neutropenic infections
- Electrolytes
  - —Low CO_2—Acidosis
  - —Increased BUN—GI hemorrhage
  - —Increased Na, K, Cl, BUN/CR—dehydration
- Blood Glucose
  - —Very high—DKA—septic shock
  - —Very low—sepsis
- Arterial blood gas
  - —Acidosis as marker of shock state
- PT/PTT
  - —Increased coagulation times—DIC—septic shock
  - —Liver disease with coagulopathy and hemorrhage
- CPK, CPK-MB, Troponin I, T
  - —Elevated cardiac enzymes for myocardial infarction, cardiogenic shock
- Urinalysis
  - —High WBC/bacteria—urosepsis
  - —High glucose/ketones—DKA—septic shock
- β-HCG—women of childbearing age—ectopic—hemorrhagic
- Lactic Acid level
  - —Anaerobic metabolism of lactic acids when organ demands exceed nutrient supply
  - —Good surrogate marker of shock state

IMAGING/SPECIAL TESTS

- EKG
  - —Ischemia
  - —Electrical alternans is pathognomic for a large pericardial effusion
  - —Dysrhythmias
- Echocardiography
  - —Indicated when obstructive shock is suspected
  - —Assessment of cardiac output to classify type of shock
  - —Diagnosis of tamponade
  - —Wall motion abnormalities in cardiac ischemia, myocarditis, and cardiomyopathy
  - —Diagnosis of valvular disruption
  - —Distended right ventricle
- Abdominal Ultrasound
  - —Intraperitoneal hemorrhage
  - —Abdominal aneurysms
- CT scan of the abdomen
  - —Abscesses or infection
  - —Ruptured spleen
  - —Liver lacerations
  - —Severe pancreatitis

DIFFERENTIAL DIAGNOSIS

- Hypovolemic shock
  - —Abdominal trauma, blunt or penetrating
  - —Abortion—complete, partial, or inevitable
  - —Anemia—chronic or acute
  - —Aneurysms—abdominal, thoracic, dissecting
  - —Ectopic pregnancy
  - —Postpartum hemorrhage
  - —Diuretics
  - —Diarrhea
  - —Vomiting
  - —Diabetes
  - —Hemoptysis
  - —Epistaxis
  - —Upper GI bleed
  - —Lower GI bleed
  - —Anorexia
  - —Bulimia
  - —Burns
  - —Toxic epidermal necrolysis
  - —Severe ascites
  - —Penetrating trauma
  - —Blunt trauma
  - —Splenic rupture
  - —Aortogastric fistula
  - —Vascular injuries
  - —Retroperitoneal bleeds
  - —Fractures (especially long bones)
  - —Mallory-Weiss tear
  - —Malignancies
  - —Arteriovenous malformations
  - —Placenta Previa
- Cardiogenic shock
  - —Myocardial infarction
  - —Myocarditis
  - —Cardiomyopathy
  - —Myocardial contusion
  - —Pericardial tamponade
  - —Tension pneumothorax
  - —Valvular insufficiency
  - —Pulmonary embolus
  - —Ventricular septal defect
  - —Conduction abnormalities and arrhythmias
- Vasogenic shock
  - —Septic
  - —Acute respiratory distress syndrome
  - —Abscess
  - —Bacterial infection
  - —Bowel perforation
  - —Cellulitis
  - —Cholangitis
  - —Cholecystitis
  - —Endocarditis
  - —Endometritis
  - —Fungemia
  - —Infected indwelling prosthetic device
  - —Intra-abdominal infection or abscess
  - —Mediastinitis
  - —Meningitis
  - —Myometritis
  - —Pelvic inflammatory disease
  - —Peritonitis
  - —Pyelonephritis
  - —Pharyngitis
  - —Pneumonia
  - —Septic arthritis
  - —Thrombophlebitis
  - —Tubo-ovarian
  - —Urinary tract infection
- Anaphylactic
  - —Drug reaction
  - —Food allergy
  - —Insect sting
  - —Radiographic contrast materials
  - —Synthetic products
- Pharmacologic
  - —Antihypertensives
  - —Digoxin
  - —Narcotics
  - —Antidepressants
  - —Cholinergics
  - —Benzodiazepines
  - —Nitrates
- Neurogenic
  - —Spinal chord injury

Treatment

INITIAL STABILIZATION

- Optimize perfusion and oxygen delivery to vital organs
- Endotracheal intubation
  - —For airway protection
  - —For hypoxia and to optimize oxygenation
  - —To reduce the work of breathing
- Large-bore IV access
- Consider central venous access
- Fluid resuscitation in noncardiogenic shock patients
- Control bleeding with temporary measures
  - —Direct pressure
  - —Long-bone traction
  - —External fixation of pelvis

ED TREATMENT

Hypovolemic Shock

- Identify source of volume depletion
- Aggressive fluid resuscitation keeping SBP >100 mm Hg until definitive treatment
  - —2–3 L crystalloid initially
  - —If 2–3 crystalloids does not correct pressure transfuse packed red blood cells
    - -O-negative if type specific unavailable in women of child bearing age
    - -O-positive in males
    - -Type-specific blood if the patient is not grossly unstable
    - -Type and cross-match blood if the patient is stable
- In hemorrhage, identify source of bleeding and rapidly move towards definitive treatment
- Consider thoracotomy and aortic cross-clamping in refractory shock with torso trauma

Cardiogenic Shock

- Low threshold to ease work of breathing with intubation
- Insult-specific therapy
  - —Thrombolytics or angioplasty for MI
  - —Pericardiocentesis for pericardial tamponade
- Treat dysrhythmias
- Inotropic support as needed
  - —Dopamine
  - —Dobutamine
  - —Phenylephrine

Vasogenic Shock

- Sepsis
  - —Aggressive crystalloid fluid resuscitation
  - —Titrate fluid to urine output >30 cc/hr
  - —Blood product transfusion to maintain hct 30–35%
  - —Early antimicrobial therapy
  - —Surgical drainage of abscess
  - —Operative intervention as needed
  - —Attempt to rapidly identify and treat source of infection
  - —Ionotropic support as needed

  - -Dopamine infusion
  - -Norepinephrine infusion
- Anaphylactic
  - —Intubation for airway compromise
  - —H_1-blockers—diphenhydramine
  - —H_2-blockers—cimetidine
  - —Corticosteroids—hydrocortisone or methylprednisolone
  - —Nebulized β_2-antagonists for bronchospasm
  - —Epinephrine 1:1000 subcutaneous or IM doses—quick and usually definitive
  - —Epinephrine IV 1:10000 bolus—severe manifestations
  - —Epinephrine IV drip for refractory hypotension
- Pharmacologic
  - —Supportive therapy
  - —Decontamination of overdoses with Charcoal
  - —Inotropic agents as needed
    - -Dopamine
    - -Epinephrine
    - -Norepinephrine
    - -Dobutamine support metabolic derangements
  - —Drug-specific antidotes
    - -Opiates: narcan
    - -Calcium channel blockers and β blockers: calcium infusions; glucagon
    - -Digoxin: digoxin immune fab
    - -Neurogenic—supportive therapy; traction and fracture stabilization; corticosteroids

MEDICATIONS

- Albuterol: 2.5 mg/2.5 cc nebulizer PRN
- Calcium Gluconate: 100–1,000 mg IV
- Cimetidine: 300 mg IV
- Digoxin immune fab: 2–20 vials IV
- Diphenhydramine: 50–100 mg IV over 3 min
- Dobutamine: 5–40 μg/kg/min IV
- Dopamine: dopaminergic 1–3 μg/kg/min IV; β effects: 3–10 μg/kg/min IV; α/β effects: 10–20 μg/kg/min IV; α effects: 20 μg/kg/min IV
- Epinephrine: 1–4 μg/min IV infusion
- Epinephrine 1:1000: 0.1–0.3 mg SQ/IM repeat q 5–20 min × 3 PRN
- Epinephrine 1:100,000: 10 ml over 10 min IV
- Glucagon: 1–5 mg IV bolus initial; 1–20 mg/hr infusion
- Hydrocortisone: 5–10 mg/kg IV
- Methylprednisolone: 1–2 mg/kg IV
- Naloxone: 0.01 mg/kg initial, titrate to effect
- Norepinephrine: start 2–4 μg/min IV, titrate up to 1–2 μg/kg/min IV
- Phenylephrine: 40–180 μg/kg/min IV

Disposition

ADMISSION CRITERIA

- All patients in shock need to be admitted
- All patients with persisting shock need intensive care monitoring
  - —Patients with shock definitively reversed may be admitted to non-ICU setting

DISCHARGE CRITERIA

- Patients who present to the ED in shock should not be discharged

Miscellaneous

ICD9: 785.5, 785.51

CORE CONTENT CODE: 2.2.3.3, 9.1.8, 18.1.3.1, 18.1.3.2

SUGGESTED READINGS

Carcillo JA: Septic shock Crit Care Clin 1997;13:553–74.

Asensio JA: Invasive and noninvasive monitoring for early recognition and treatment of shock in high-risk trauma and surgical patients. Surg Clin North Am 1996;76: 985–97.

Author: Nathan Shapiro

Shoulder Dislocation

Clinical Presentation

SIGNS AND SYMPTOMS

- Severe pain in the affected shoulder is common in all types of shoulder dislocations

Anterior Dislocation

- *Over 90% of shoulder dislocations are anterior dislocations* of the humeral head in relation to the glenoid fossa
- The shoulder will be squared off with a prominent acromion process and often a palpable anterior fullness
- Arm is held in slight abduction and external rotation

Posterior Dislocation

- Often missed
- The coracoid process is prominent with a palpable posterior bulge
- Arm is held in slight adduction and internal rotation

Inferior Dislocation (Luxatio Erecta)

- Rare but easy to identify
- Arm is shortened and fixed above head. The patient's hand looks as if it were raised to ask a question
- Head of humerus may be palpable on the lateral chest wall

MECHANISM/DESCRIPTION

Anterior Dislocation

- The injury is from direct or indirect forces on the abducted and externally rotated arm, which result in anterior dislocation of the humeral head in relation to glenoid fossa
- Also may result from direct blow to posterior lateral aspect of shoulder

Posterior Dislocation

- The injury is from forces on the adducted and internally rotated arm, which result in posterior dislocation of humeral head in relation to glenoid fossa
- The most common mechanism is a seizure and sudden contraction of all the posterior muscle groups
- Other mechanisms of injury include electrocution and direct blow to anterior shoulder

Inferior Dislocation (Luxatio Erecta)

- The injury results from hyperabduction of arm, tear of rotator cuff, and rotation of arm 180° above head
- Commonly seen after a fall from a height where an arm strikes an object on descent and is thrust above the head

PEDIATRIC CONSIDERATIONS

- Dislocation is rare in children; epiphyseal fractures must be ruled out

Pre-Hospital

CAUTIONS

- Neurovascular injury should be identified and the arm splinted in the position of most comfort

Diagnosis

ESSENTIAL WORKUP

- Evaluate neurovascular status of the arm
  - —Sensory distribution of the *axillary nerve* corresponds to the lateral aspect of the shoulder
- Retest neurovascular status after any manipulation
- Dislocation requires prompt treatment, plain films of the shoulder should be obtained immediately
  - —The incidence of posttraumatic arthritis increases with length of time dislocated
  - —*Even in clinically obvious cases, films should be obtained before manipulation unless there will be a significant delay*
  - —An impacted humeral head fracture may be converted to a displaced humeral head fracture if manipulated
  - —Displaced fracture requires surgical repair and possible prosthesis

IMAGING/SPECIAL TESTS

- Two views should be obtained
  - —Anterior-posterior view
  - —Transcapular Y or axillary view

Anterior Dislocation

- A posterior, lateral compression fracture of the humeral head (Hills-Sachs deformity) may be seen. Corresponding lesion on glenoid fossa is the Bankart lesion
  - —These do not require treatment
  - —Reduction is not contraindicated
- Fractures of the greater tuberosity of the humeral head are seen in 15–35%
  - —If there is >1 cm displacement after reduction surgical intervention may be necessary

Posterior Dislocation

- Often missed on AP film
  - —Degree of overlap on x-ray is smaller and displaced superiorly producing the "meniscus sign"
  - —Rotated humerus yields "light bulb on a stick" finding on AP view from lining up lesser and greater tuberosity
- Also may see a "reverse Hill-Sachs deformity" from compression fracture of the anterior medial humeral head

DIFFERENTIAL DIAGNOSIS

- Fracture of the humeral head
- Fracture of the humeral shaft
- Acromioclavicular injury
- Septic shoulder joint
- Hemarthrosis in shoulder joint

Treatment

INITIAL STABILIZATION

- Exclude more serious injuries
- Ensure no injury to axillary vessels

ED TREATMENT

- *The key to successful reduction is adequate analgesia and muscle relaxation*
  —Conscious sedation with a short-acting opioid and a benzodiazepine
  —Recent success has also been reported utilizing intra-articular lidocaine (20 mg of 1% lidocaine) injected into shoulder joint

Anterior Dislocation Reduction Techniques

- Scapular manipulation
  —Patient seated, traction to arm in horizontal plane, counter traction with other hand against clavicle
  —Second person adducts tip of scapula towards spine, opening up shoulder joint
- Stimson
  —Patient placed in prone position on stretcher with arm dangling over side, hang 10–15 lbs around wrist; fatigue muscle over 20–30 minutes
  —Gently manipulate humeral head into place or use scapular manipulation
  —Only one person required
- Traction/counter traction
  —Patient in supine position, hold continuous longitudinal traction to arm
  —Gentle countertraction from sheet wrapped through axilla and across chest
  —Arm slightly internally or externally rotated if unsuccessful after several minutes
- Hennipen
  —Patient supine, elbow at 90°, gentle, slow external rotation of arm, and finally slow elevation arm above head. Must be done slowly with cooperative patient
- Leverage techniques such as the Kocher method are to be avoided as further injury can occur

Posterior Dislocation Reduction Techniques

- May use Stimson or traction/counter traction techniques with manipulation of humeral head anteriorly after muscles are sufficiently fatigued

Inferior Dislocation (Luxatio Erecta) Reduction Techniques

- Patient in supine position, gentle longitudinal traction to distract humeral head, gentle countertraction with sheet draped over trapezius and chest, and arm is slowly rotated from 180° to 0°

Postreduction Care

- Plain films should be repeated after manipulation to confirm successful reduction
- Place in sling and swath or shoulder immobilizer immediately after reduction
- Shoulder should remain immobilized for 3 weeks in young patients. Immobilization time should be less in older patients because they are at-risk for frozen shoulder

MEDICATIONS

- Diazepam: 5–10 mg IV
- Fentanyl: 2–5 μg/kg IV
- Midazolam: 2–5 mg IV
- Morphine: 2–8 mg IV
- Meperidine: 50–100 mg IV

Disposition

ADMISSION CRITERIA

- Failure to reduce shoulder may require admission for reduction under general anesthesia or open reduction
- Patients with neurovascular compromise

DISCHARGE CRITERIA

- Successful reductions, confirmed by plain films, may be discharged with shoulder in appropriate immobilizer and with orthopedic follow-up
- Recurrent dislocation may require elective surgery
- Patients with residual neuropraxia from injury or manipulation may be safely discharged with instructions that most symptoms will resolve but should have neurology follow-up

Miscellaneous

ICD9: 831.00

CORE CONTENT CODE: 18.4.12.2.1

SUGGESTED READINGS

Matthews DE, Roberts T. Intraarticular lidocaine versus intravenous analgesic for reduction of acute anterior shoulder dislocations. Am J Sports Med 1995;23:54–58.

McNamara RM. Reduction of anterior shoulder dislocations by scapular manipulation. Ann Emerg Med 1993;22:1140–1144.

Riebel GD, McCabe JB. Anterior shoulder dislocation: A review of reduction techniques. Am J Emerg Med 1991;9:180–188.

Authors: G. Richard Bruno; Wallace Carter

Sick Sinus Syndrome

Clinical Presentation

SIGNS AND SYMPTOMS

- Asymptomatic
- Palpitations
- Fatigue
- Confusion
- Lightheadedness
- Syncope/presyncope
- Chest pain
- Sudden death
- Bradycardia
- Tachycardia
- Altered mental status
- Transient ischemic attack
- Stroke

MECHANISM/DESCRIPTION

- Caused by progressive degeneration of the cardiac conduction system
  - —Frequently idiopathic
- Characterized by periods of unexplained sinus node dysfunction leading to bradyarrhythmias
- In a subset of patients, bradyarrhythmias may alternate with supraventricular tachydysrhythmias
  - —Atrial fibrillation is most common tachydysrhythmia
  - —Tachycardia-bradycardia syndrome is an alternative name for this syndrome
- Primarily a disease of the elderly

ETIOLOGY

- Idiopathic
- Coronary artery disease
- Longstanding hypertension
- Idiopathic cardiomyopathy
- Amyloidosis
- Collagen vascular disease
- Hemochromatosis
- Metastatic malignancy
- Myocarditis
- Rheumatic heart disease

Pre-Hospital

CAUTIONS

- ALS transport
- Cardiac monitoring
- Transcutaneous pacing for patients in shock

Diagnosis

ESSENTIAL WORKUP

- Essential workup should be focused on excluding other causes of sinus node dysfunction
- 12-lead electrocardiography (ECG) should be performed

LABORATORY

- Serum electrolytes
- Cardiac enzymes
- Digoxin levels if relevant

IMAGING/SPECIAL TESTS

- EKG
  - —Inappropriate sinus bradycardia
  - —Sinus pauses
  - —Sinus arrest or exit block
  - —Atrial fibrillation with slow ventricular response
  - —Prolonged pauses after carotid massage or cardioversion
  - —Alternating tachycardia-bradycardia syndrome

DIFFERENTIAL DIAGNOSIS

- Bradyarrhythmias
- Acute coronary syndromes
- Electrolyte disturbances
  - —Especially hyperkalemia
- Medication toxicity
  - —Digoxin
  - —β-Blockers
  - —Calcium channel blockers
- Hypothyroidism

Treatment

INITIAL STABILIZATION

- Atropine
  - —Indicated if a bradyarrhythmia is compromising circulatory function
  - —Frequently lacks efficacy in sick sinus syndrome (SSS)
- Temporary transcutaneous pacing in symptomatic patients
  - —If this fails, emergent transvenous pacing can be performed

ED TREATMENT

- Unstable supraventricular tachydysrhythmias
  - —Cardiovert
  - —Anticipate subsequent profound bradycardia
- Stable patients
  - —Rate control should be cautiously attempted
    - -Digoxin is the most common choice
    - -Diltiazem
    - -Caution: any pharmacotherapy may result in profound bradycardia
- Identification and discontinuation of medications that alter sinus node function
- Anticoagulation in patients who present with atrial fibrillation

MEDICATIONS

- Atropine: adult: 0.5 mg IV repeat every 5 min as necessary, max dose of 0.04 mg/kg; peds: 0.02 mg/kg, minimum 0.1 mg
- Epinephrine: adult: 2 μg/min, max 10 μg/min; peds: 0.01 mg/kg bolus; 0.2–2 μg/kg/min infusion
- Diltiazem: 0.25 mg/kg IV over 2 min followed in 15 min by 0.35 mg/kg IV over 2 min
- Verapamil: 2.5–5 mg IV bolus over 2 min; may repeat with 5–10 mg every 15–30 min to max of 20 mg
- Digoxin: 0.5 mg IV initially then 0.25 mg IV q 4 hrs until desired effect
- Heparin: load 80 IU/kg IV; infusion at 18 IU/kg/hr

Disposition

ADMISSION CRITERIA

- New onset
- Symptomatic
- Persistent bradyarrhythmia or tachydysrhythmia
- Syncope
- Chest pain suggestive of acute coronary syndrome
- Advanced age >60 years
- Patients should be admitted to a telemetry floor with cardiology consultation
- Most will require permanent pacing

DISCHARGE CRITERIA

- Asymptomatic otherwise healthy patients can be evaluated as outpatients
  - —Holter monitoring
  - —Exercise testing

Miscellaneous

ICD9: 427.81

CORE CONTENT CODE: 2.4.2.1

SUGGESTED READINGS

Alagona P. Advances in pacing for the patient with sick sinus syndrome. Curr Opin Cardiol 1997;12:3–11.

Cosin J, Hernandiz A, Solaz J, et al. Sick sinus syndrome: Strategies for reducing mortality. Cor et Vasa 1992;34:135–148.

Rodriguez RD, Schocken DD. Update on sick sinus syndrome, a cardiac disease of aging. Geriatrics 1990;45:26–30.

Rubenstein JJ, Schulman CL, Yurchak PM, et al. Clinical spectrum of the sick sinus syndrome. Circulation 1972;46:5–13.

Author: David F.M. Brown

Sickle Cell Disease

Clinical Presentation

SIGNS AND SYMPTOMS

- May present with either
  - —Painful episode
  - —Complications of the disease
  - —Combination of above
- Acute painful episodes
  - —Bone/joint crisis
    - -Pain in extremities, back, sternum, or joints
    - -Variable swelling, warmth
    - -Variable joint effusion
    - -"Hand-foot syndrome" in infants
  - —Abdominal crisis
    - -Abdominal pain without peritonitis
    - -Variable nausea, vomiting, diarrhea
  - —Priapism—prolonged painful erection
- Complications/progression of disease
  - —Chest crisis (or syndrome)
    - -Pleuritic chest pain
    - -Cough with variable hemoptysis
    - -Dyspnea
    - -Tachypnea
    - -Rales
  - —Splenic sequestration crisis
    - -Abdominal pain
    - -Splenomegaly
    - -Variable nausea, vomiting
    - -Fatigue, lethargy
    - -Pallor
    - -Tachycardia
    - -Hypotension, syncope, shock
  - —Aplastic crisis
    - -Variable fever, headache, nausea, vomiting
    - -Fatigue
    - -Pallor
    - -Tachycardia
  - —Cerebrovascular accident/TIA
    - -Focal neurologic deficit
    - -Mental status changes
  - —Infections
    - -Fever
    - -Localizing signs

MECHANISM/DESCRIPTION

- Affects multiple organ systems
- Inherited autosomal recessive disorder caused by a single amino acid substitution in hemoglobin gene
- Abnormal hemoglobin (hemoglobin S) polymerizes under stress, deforms RBC, resulting in hemolysis, vaso-occlusion, tissue ischemia, and infarction
- Occurs in people of African, Mediterranean, Middle Eastern, and Indian descent
- Severity is variable, even among the same phenotype
- Vaso-occlusion, ischemia, and infarction crises occur in essentially all organ systems
  - —Bone/joint crises
    - -Vaso-occlusion of bone microvasculature causes infarction
    - -Dactylitis "hand-foot syndrome" occurs ages 6–24 months
  - —Chest crisis or syndrome
    - -Vaso-occlusion of pulmonary vasculature with infarcts
    - -Fat embolism, viral and bacterial infections may contribute
    - -High mortality (2–14%)
    - -More common in children
    - -Difficult to distinguish from pneumonia
  - —Splenic sequestration
    - -Splenic sinusoids become congested with sickled red blood cells and obstruct outflow
    - -High mortality (12–20%)
    - -May be rapidly fatal
    - -More common in children under 5, rare in adults
  - —Aplastic crisis
    - -Bone marrow suppression usually occurs secondary to viral infection
    - -Increased baseline hemolysis in sickle cell patients requires maximum erythropoiesis
    - -Decrease in hematocrit may be severe
    - -Generally self-limited
    - -More common in children
  - —Cerebrovascular accident/TIA
    - -Secondary to infarction in children; hemorrhage in adults
    - -Peak incidence between ages 9 and 15; prevalence 5–20%
    - -Often preceded by TIAs
  - —Bacterial infection
    - -Sepsis is the leading cause of death in sickle cell patients
    - -Ability to fight encapsulated organisms is impaired secondary to decreased splenic function
    - -Children under 5 years have 400-fold increase in pneumococcal infections
    - -*S. pneumoniae, H. influenzae, S. aureus, E. coli,* and salmonella are leading organisms
    - -Sites: lung, central nervous system, bone, kidney

GENOTYPE	*PHENOTYPE*	*CLINICAL SEVERITY*	*INCIDENCE IN AFRICAN-AMERICANS*
SS	*Sickle cell disease*	*Marked*	0.3% (70,000)
SC	(SC) disease	Mild to moderate	0.1%
Sβthal	βThalessemia	Mild to moderate	<0.1%
AS	*Sickle cell trait*	*No manifestation of disease*	8% (1.76 million)

ETIOLOGY

- Common crisis precipitants
  - —Infection (bacterial and viral)
  - —Dehydration
  - —Hypoxemia
  - —Acidosis
  - —Surgery/trauma
  - —Weather changes
  - —Pregnancy
  - —Toxins

PEDIATRIC CONSIDERATIONS

- Infections commonly precipitate crisis
- Patients immunization history (pnemococcal and *H. influenzae*) must be confirmed
- Acute sickle cell complications in children carry high morbidity and should be screened for aggressively

Pre-Hospital

N/A

Diagnosis

ESSENTIAL WORKUP

- Thorough physical examination

LABORATORY

- CBC
  - —Anemia may be profound
  - —Compare with prior values if available
  - —Leukocytosis is common, does not necessarily indicate infection
- Reticulocyte count
  - —Generally elevated >5.0% in SS individuals
  - —A low count may indicate an aplastic crisis
- Consider the following if indicated
  - —Urinalysis
    - -Asymptomatic hematuria is a common finding
    - -Urinary tract infection may precipitate pain crisis and requires aggressive treatment
  - —Electrolytes, BUN/Cr, glucose
  - —Blood cultures
  - —Type and screen (or cross)

IMAGING/SPECIAL TESTS

- X-rays should be directed to confirm suspected diagnoses
  - —CXR if pneumonia or chest syndrome suspected
  - —Extremities if osteomyelitis suspected
  - —*Intravenous contrast may exacerbate or precipitate a crisis*
- Head CT/MRI to evaluate stroke

DIFFERENTIAL DIAGNOSIS

- Sickle cell crises may mimic or obscure more serious underlying pathology (e.g., acute abdomen, myocardial infarction, nephrolithiasis)
  - —Suspect other diagnoses if pain is more severe or atypical

Treatment

INITIAL STABILIZATION

- Identify and treat high morbidity complications
  - —Sepsis
  - —Splenic sequestration
  - —Chest crisis
  - —CVA
- Assess pain and initiate therapy

ED TREATMENT

- Analgesia
  - —Choice of analgesic agent depends on patient, severity of episode, and prior agents
  - —Evaluate patient frequently and titrate medications accordingly for relief of pain
  - —See table below for recommended agents
- Hydration
  - —1.5–2 times maintenance after correction of deficits
  - —Oral hydration if patient can tolerate fluids by mouth
  - —Parenteral IV solution .45NS for adults and children, or DSW.25NS for infants
  - —Monitor fluids closely
- Complication-specific therapy
  - —Oxygen: chest syndrome, pneumonia
  - —Antibiotics: sepsis, pneumonia, osteomyelitis
  - —Acute simple transfusion: sequestration crisis, blood loss, accelerated hemolysis
  - —Exchange transfusion may be required for more severe complications: cerebrovascular accident

Disposition

ADMISSION CRITERIA

- Refractory pain crisis
- Signs of bacterial infection or fever of undetermined etiology
- Chest syndrome
- Sequestration crisis
- Aplastic crisis
- Cerebrovascular accident or TIA
- Refractory priapism

DISCHARGE CRITERIA

- Resolution of pain crisis
- No indications for admission

Miscellaneous

ICD9: 282.60

CORE CONTENT CODE: 7.1.1

SUGGESTED READINGS

Brokoff D, Polomano R. Treating sickle cell pain like cancer pain. Ann Intern Med 1992;116:364.

Pollack CV. Emergencies in sickle cell disease. Emerg Med Clin North Am 1993;11:365.

Reid C, Carache S, Lubin B, eds. Management and therapy of sickle cell disease. Pub. No. 95–2117. Washington, DC: NIH, 1995.

Steingart R. Management of patients with sickle cell disease. Med Clin North Am 1992;76(3):669.

Author: Steven Bowman

MEDICATIONS

Suggested analgesic agents

AGENT	DOSAGE/ROUTE
Severe/Moderate Pain	
Hydrocodone	Oral: 0.15 mg/kg/dose po q 4 hrs
Hydromorphone	Parenteral: 0.01–0.02 mg/kg/dose IV q 3–4 hrs Oral: 0.04–0.06 mg/kg/dose po q 4 hrs
Ketorolac	Parenteral: 30–60 mg initial, 15–30mg IV q 6–8 hrs
Meperidine	Parenteral: 0.75–1.5 mg/kg/dose IV q 2–4 hrs
Morphine	Parenteral: 0.1–0.15 mg/kg/dose IV q 3–4 hrs Oral: 0.3–0.6 mg/kg/dose po q 4 hrs
MILD PAIN	
Acetaminophen	Oral: 1 g po q 4 hrs Peds: 15 mg/kg/dose po q 4 hrs
Codeine	Oral: 0.5–1 mg/kg/dose po; maximum dose 60 mg
Ibuprofen	Oral: 800 mg po q 8 hrs Peds: 5–10mg/kg/dose po q 6–8 hrs

Sinusitis

Clinical Presentation

SIGNS AND SYMPTOMS

- Facial pain
- Headache
- Cough
- Purulent nasal discharge
- Fever
- Edema of the nasal mucous membranes
- Pus in the nares or posterior pharynx
- Warmth, tenderness and possibly cellulitis over the affected sinus
- Frontal sinusitis
  —Pain of the lower forehead
- Maxillary sinusitis
  —Malar facial pain
  —Maxillary dental pain
  —Referred ear pain
- Ethmoid sinusitis
  —Retro-orbital pain
- Sphenoid sinusitis (very uncommon)
  —Pain over the occiput or mastoid
- Recent history of nasotracheal intubation suggests nosocomial sinusitis
  —Involves atypical pathogens such as Pseudomonas and gram negative organisms
- Rhinocerebral mucormycosis
  —Rare but rapidly progressive fungal infection
  —Occurs in diabetic and other immunocompromised patients
  —Orbital and facial pain out of proportion to physical signs
  —Lethargy, headache in a systemically ill appearing patient
  —Black eschar or pale area on the palate or nasal mucosa

MECHANISM/DESCRIPTION

- Sinusitis is inflammation of the mucous membranes lining the paranasal sinuses
- Acute bacterial sinusitis is diagnosed when signs and symptoms last less than 3 weeks
- Chronic sinusitis occurs when signs and symptoms last longer than three weeks
- Nosocomial sinusitis is associated with nasogastric and nasotracheal tubes

ETIOLOGY

- Complication of simple viral upper respiratory tract infection or allergic rhinitis
- As mucous membranes become inflamed, sinus ostia narrow and block drainage
- Air is absorbed and negative pressure develops, resulting in transudate formation
- Bacteria are trapped and multiply resulting in suppuration
- Foreign bodies, nasal polyps, tumors, or traumatic fractures can lead to obstruction of ostia
- Immunocompromised patients and patients with impaired mucociliary movement are also predisposed to sinusitis
- Pathogens
  —Acute sinusitis: *H. influenza, Strep pneumoniae, Moraxella catarrhalis, S. aureus*
  —Chronic sinusitis: *Peptostreptococcus, Fusobacterium, Bacteroides, Aspergillus*
  —Nosocomial sinusitis: *S. aureus, Pseudomonas, klebsiella*

COMPLICATIONS

- Osteomyelitis
- Extension into the CNS
  —Seizures
  —Focal neurologic signs
  —Cranial nerve palsies
  —Altered level of consciousness
  —Meningitis, subdural empyema, epidural abscess
  —Cavernous sinus thrombosis
  —Brain abscess
- Periorbital cellulitis
- Orbital cellulitis
  —Periorbital swelling, fever, ptosis, proptosis, and painful or decreased extraocular movements
  —Most frequently a complication or ethmoid sinusitis in children
- Pott's puffy tumor
  —A focal, doughy mass localized to the forehead
  —Indicative of osteomyelitis of the frontal bone

SPECIAL PEDIATRIC CONSIDERATIONS

- Ethmoid and maxillary sinuses are present at birth
- Frontal and sphenoid sinuses do not emerge until age 6–7
- Periorbital/orbital cellulitis is a common complication of ethmoid sinusitis in children
  —Periorbital swelling, fever, ptosis, proptosis, and painful or decreased extraocular movements

Diagnosis

ESSENTIAL WORKUP

- Clinical diagnosis based on history and physical exam
- Transillumination is not a reliable indicator of sinus disease
- Imaging is unnecessary in uncomplicated cases (see below)

LABORATORY

- White blood cell count if the patient appears toxic

IMAGING/SPECIAL TESTS

- Plain film radiography
  —Normal plain films do not rule out bacterial involvement
  —A water's view may help in the diagnosis of maxillary sinusitis
  —Opacification or air fluid level in involved sinus
- Computed tomography
  —Preferred to plain films if imaging is necessary
  —May assist in diagnosing complications of sinusitis

DIFFERENTIAL DIAGNOSIS

- Migraine and cluster headache
- Dental pain
- Trigeminal neuralgia
- TMJ disorders
- Temporal arteritis
- Uncomplicated viral or allergic rhinitis
- Nasal polyp, tumor, or foreign body
- CNS infection

Treatment

INITIAL STABILIZATION

- Toxic-appearing patients may require airway intervention and fluid resuscitation
  - —First dose of antibiotics in ED

ED TREATMENT

- Cost-effective approach favors appropriate antibiotic therapy and no testing
- Establishing good drainage with topical or oral decongestants and mucoevacuants
- Reducing edema with topical corticosteroids in chronic sinusitis
- Humidification and saline spray are beneficial adjunct to pharmacologic therapy

MEDICATIONS

Antibiotics

- Antibiotics listed are considered first-line drugs, except for amoxicillin where there is known drug resistance
  - —Acute sinusitis
    - -Amoxicillin: adults: 500 mg po tid; peds: 40mg/kg/day po divided tid for 10–14 days
    - -Amoxicillin-clavulanate: adults: 500 mg po tid; peds: 40 mg/kg/day po divided tid for 10–14 days
    - -Azithromycin: adults: 500 mg po day 1, 250 mg po days 2–5; peds: 10 mg/kg po day 1, 5 mg/kg po qd days 2–5
    - -Trimethoprim-sulfa DS: adults: 1 tab po bid; peds: 5 cc/10 kg (40/200 per 5 cc) po bid 10–14 days
    - -Cefuroxime: adults: 500 mg po bid; peds: 20–30 mg/kg/day po divided bid for 10–14 days
  - —Chronic
    - -Amoxicillin-clavulanate: adults: 500 mg po bid; peds: 40 mg/kg/day po divided tid for 21 days
    - -Cefaclor: adults: 500 mg po tid; peds: 20–40 mg/kg/day po divided tid for 21 days

Decongestants

- Topical: not to be used for more than 3 days
- Oxymetazoline hydrochloride 0.05%: 2–3 drops/sprays per nostril bid
- Phenylephrine hydrochloride 0.5%: 2–3 sprays per nostril q 3–4 hrs; oral: if longer than 3 days of treatment
- Phenylpropanolamine: 25 mg po q 4 hrs
- Pseudoephedrine: 60 mg po q 4–6 hrs

Mucoevacuants

- Guaifenesin: adults: 5–20 ml po q 4 hrs; peds: 5–10 ml/dose if 6–12 years old, 2.5–5ml if 2–6 years old

Corticosteroids for Chronic Sinusitis

- Beclomethasone dipropionate: 1 spray/nostril bid/tid
- Dexamethasone sodium phosphate: 2 sprays/nostril bid/tid

Disposition

ADMISSION CRITERIA

- Evidence of spread of infection beyond the sinus cavity
- Toxic-appearing patients
- Immunocompromised/diabetic patients with extensive infection
- ENT evaluation and aspiration if patient is severely ill, immunocompromised, or pansinusitis and ill-appearing

DISCHARGE CRITERIA

- Most cases of uncomplicated sinusitis may be managed as outpatients
- Followup with primary care physician or ENT if symptoms persist greater than 7 days despite antibiotic therapy

Miscellaneous

ICD9: 473.9

CORE CONTENT CODE: 6.2.5.1

SUGGESTED READINGS

Brook I. Microbiology and management of sinusitis. J Otolaryngol 1996:25(4):249–56.

Gershwin ME, Incaudo GA, eds. Diseases of the sinuses. Totowa, NJ: Humana Press, 1996. pp215–233.

Reuler JB, Lucas LM, Kumar KL. West J Med 1995:163(1):40–48.

Authors: Cara Deckelman; Michael Rolnick

Sleep Apnea

Clinical Presentation

SIGNS AND SYMPTOMS

Symptoms

- Snoring in combination with observed apnea
- Daytime drowsiness
- Sleep disturbance
  —Inadequate sleep due to repetitive apneas during sleep
- Irritability

Signs

- Predisposing physical features
  —Obesity
  —Craniofacial anomalies
  —Enlarged tonsils
- Signs of chronic disease
  —Hypertension
  —Elevated jugular veins (secondary to pulmonary hypertension)

Associated Emergencies

- Dysrhythmias
- Right and left heart failure
- Hypertension poorly controlled by medical therapies
- Myocardial infarction
- Stroke
- Motor vehicle accidents

MECHANISM/DESCRIPTION

- Sleep apnea—cessation of airflow during sleep
- Narrowing of the upper airway especially with decreased tone during REM sleep
- Airway closing at the level of nasopharynx or oropharynx during sleep produces sleep apnea

ETIOLOGY

- Risk groups
  —Obese
  —Male
  —Age over 40
  —Upper airway anomalies hypertrophy
  —Myxedema (hypothyroidism)
  —Alcohol/sedative abuse

Pre-Hospital

CAUTIONS

- Provide supplemental oxygen for shortness of breath
- Active airway management for acute respiratory insufficiency

Diagnosis

ESSENTIAL WORKUP

- ECG
- CXR

LABORATORY

- Arterial blood gas
  —Hypoxia with elevated pCO_2
  —Respiratory acidosis indicative of acute deterioration
- CBC
  —Elevated Hct in chronically hypoxic patients
- Electrolytes, BUN/Cr, glucose
- Thyroid function tests
  —Exclude hypothyroidism as etiology

IMAGING/SPECIAL TESTS

- Lateral neck soft tissue radiograph to rule out other etiologies of upper airway obstruction
- Sleep study (polysomnogram)
  —Required for diagnosis
  —Never indicated in the ED

DIFFERENTIAL DIAGNOSIS

- Central sleep apnea
  —Neurologic, rather than obstructive, cause of apnea during sleep
- Other etiologies of obstructive lung disease
  —COPD
  —Asthma
- Other etiologies of pulmonary hypertension
- Left heart failure
- Primary pulmonary hypertension
- Other sleep disorders
  —Narcolepsy
  —Idiopathic hypersomnia

Treatment

INITIAL STABILIZATION

- For acute apnea in ED
  - —Chin lift/jaw thrust maneuver for acute apnea
  - —Oral or nasal airway
- Endotracheal intubation for acute respiratory decompensation
  - —Anticipate difficult oral intubation
  - —Blind nasotracheal or fiberoptic-guided nasotracheal intubation in lieu of oral rapid sequence intubation preferable if oral pharyngeal anatomy will make oral intubation difficult
  - —Positive end-expiratory pressure (PEEP) for ventilated patients

ED TREATMENT

- Insure that patient has access to home respiratory adjunctive therapy
- Mask ventilation with continuous positive airway pressure (CPAP)
  - —Titrate pressure to individual patient needs by pulmonologist
- Oxygen therapy (0.5–3.0 L/min)
  - —Must be titrated for resting, walking, and nocturnal needs by pulmonologist
- Medical therapy
  - —Weight loss
  - —Nasal decongestants
  - —Drugs to reduce upper airway inflammation (nasal steroids)
- Avoid sedating antihypertensive medications

Disposition

ADMISSION CRITERIA

- Ventilatory failure
- Hemodynamic instability
- Severe hypoxia
- Respiratory distress

DISCHARGE CRITERIA

- Maintenance of oxygen saturation at established baseline above 85% for several hours using oxygenation or ventilation equipment available to the patient at patient's home
- Absence of respiratory distress
- Normal mental status
- No associated medical condition precluding discharge

Miscellaneous

ICD9: 780.57

CORE CONTENT CODE: 16.14

SUGGESTED READINGS

Hudgel DW. Treatment of obstructive sleep apnea. Chest 1996;109:1346–1358.

Man GCW. Obstructive sleep apnea: diagnosis and treatment. Med Clin North Am 1996;80(4):804–820.

Strollo PJ, Rogers RM. Obstructive sleep apnea. N Engl J Med 1996;334(2):99–101.

Author: Mark J. Sagarin

Slipped Capital Femoral Epiphysis

Clinical Presentation

- Slipped Capital Femoral Epiphysis (SCFE) is an urgent orthopedic condition; delay in diagnosis may lead to chronic irreversible hip joint disability

SIGNS AND SYMPTOMS

- Older child or adolescent
- Presents with limp, or limping on exertion
- Pain in the knee, thigh, groin, or hip
  - —Vague and dull for weeks in chronic SCFE
  - —Severe and sudden onset in an acute SCFE
  - —Referral of pain along the obturator nerve
- Typically hold affected leg in slight external rotation
- Often a history of minor trauma

MECHANISM/DESCRIPTION

- Femoral epiphysis translates or "slips" relative to the femoral head/neck
- Peak age of onset 13–15 years for boys and 11–13 years for girls
- Majority of patients are obese
- Males predominate
- Bilateral involvement is present in approximately 25% of cases

Pre-Hospital

- Patient should be immobilized for transport, as with suspected hip fracture or dislocation

Diagnosis

ESSENTIAL WORKUP

- Anterior-posterior and frog lateral leg X-ray of both hips should be obtained
  - —Widened or irregular physis
  - —Bird's beak appearance of the actual slipping of the epiphysis off of the femoral head

LABORATORY

N/A

DIFFERENTIAL DIAGNOSIS

- Legg-Calve-Perthes
  - —Typically seen in 4–9 years old age range
- Septic arthritis of hip
- Osteomyelitis
- Femur or pelvic fractures

Treatment

INITIAL STABILIZATION

- Immobilize hip
- Keep nonweight-bearing

ED TREATMENT

- Refer immediately to orthopedics for definitive immobilization and operative intervention

Disposition

ADMISSION CRITERIA

- Patients with SCFE require orthopedic admission

DISCHARGE CRITERIA

- None
  —It is too difficult to achieve complete nonweight-bearing status
  —Patients should be operated on urgently to prevent subsequent aseptic necrosis of femoral head

Miscellaneous

ICD9: 732.9

CORE CONTENT CODE: 13.6.4

SUGGESTED READINGS

Busch MT, Morrissy RT. Slipped capital femoral epiphysis. Orthop Clin North Am 1987;18:637–47.

Ledwith CA, Fleisher GR. Slipped capital femoral epiphysis without hip pain leads to missed diagnosis. Pediatrics 1992;89(4):660–62.

Author: Carol Ledwith

Small Bowel Injury

Clinical Presentation

SIGNS AND SYMPTOMS

- Awake, alert patients: abdominal tenderness (87–98%), abdominal pain (85%), peritoneal signs (67%)
- Abdominal wall bruising (54%), hypotension (38%), guaiac (+) rectal exam (5%)
- Inability to tolerate food or fluids, vomiting and abdominal pain in duodenal hematoma
- Small bowel injury (SBI) may initially be obscured by abnormal mental status, severe associated injuries
- Progressive abdominal pain, intestinal obstruction, decreased urine output, tachycardia indicate SBI not initially apparent

MECHANISM/DESCRIPTION

Penetrating

- Visceral injury (96% GSW, 50% stabbing)
  - —Serosal tear, bowel wall hematoma, perforation, bowel transection, mesenteric hematoma/vascular injury

Blunt

- Perforation is twice as common as mesenteric injuries
- Deceleration injury at fixed points like the ligament of Treitz
- Shearing mechanisms near fixed points like the ileocecal junction, adhesions
- Compressive force against anterior spine
- Bursting or "blowout" at antimesenteric margin from sudden closed loop intraluminal pressure rise
- Mesenteric tears may initially be asymptomatic
- Associated injuries
  - —Liver and splenic lacerations, thoracic and pelvic fractures
  - —Seatbelt syndrome: abdominal wall ecchymosis, small bowel injury, chance fracture of L1 , L2

ETIOLOGY

Penetrating

- Small bowel is the second most common injured organ (32%) in anterior abdominal stabbing
- Small bowel injury most common in gunshot wounds (49%)
- 80% of small bowel injuries are caused by gunshot wounds, 60% by stab wounds

Blunt

- Third most commonly injured organ (5–10% of all blunt trauma victims)
- Lap belts
- Motor vehicle accidents
- Nonvehicular trauma: abuse/assault, bicycle handlebars, large animal kick

PEDIATRIC CONSIDERATIONS

Penetrating

- Air gun accidents at close range (<10 feet)

Blunt

- Less common in children (1–8% of all blunt pediatric trauma)
- Wearing both shoulder and lap belts less likely to have intestinal injury

Pre-Hospital

CAUTIONS

- Do not attempt to replace eviscerated abdominal contents, cover with moist gauze, blanket and transport
- Do not remove impaled objects in the abdomen, stabilize the object with gauze and tape and transport
- Patients should be transported to the nearest trauma center

Diagnosis

ESSENTIAL WORKUP

- Physical exam noting all wounds and areas of tenderness
- Serial abdominal exams and vital signs
- For stable patients; abdominal CT
- For unstable injury; diagnostic peritoneal lavage (DPL) is superior to US in suggesting hollow viscus injuries

LABORATORY

- Baseline CBC, lytes, BUN, creatinine, ABG, type and screen, and UA
- Serum amylase, lipase and LFTs have little sensitivity for acute injury

IMAGING/SPECIAL TESTS

Plain Radiography (Chest/Abdomen)

- Not useful for SBI
- Poor sensitivity for free air (10–30%); <50% of perforations show free air

Computed Tomography

- Blunt
  - —Indications in blunt trauma (≥3 present)
    - -Abdominal distention, absent bowel sounds, blood in the NG tube
    - -Abdominal abrasions or contusions, gross hematuria, lap belt injury
    - -Assault/abuse as mechanism, abdominal tenderness, trauma score <12
  - —Used in stable patients
  - —CT is the diagnostic standard for solid organ injury, and head trauma, but is less sensitive in hollow viscus (up to 20% false-negative CT rate), pancreas, and diaphragmatic trauma
  - —Specific signs for SBI are pneumoperitoneum, extravasation of contrast
  - —Suggestive signs for SBI include unexplained free intraperitoneal fluid (most sensitive 73%), thickened bowel wall >3 mm (35% sensitive), intramural hematomas (75–88% sensitive), interloop fluid, and mesenteric streaking
- Penetrating
  - —CT not recommended (sensitivity only 14%, false-negative rate of 18%)

DPL

- Invasive but helpful in unstable patients or clinically suspicious but nondiagnostic abdominal CT
  - —Sensitive for hemoperitoneum but not source specific
  - —Positive if >100,000 RBC
  - —Lavage amylase (>20 IU/L) and WBC count (>500/mm^3) helpful but late markers of SBI
  - —Lavage microscopy for succus/vegetable matter is specific for SBI but not sensitive
  - —Lavage alkaline phosphatase (>3 IU/L) is reported to be a useful immediate marker of SBI

Ultrasonography

- Little clinical US experience, operator-dependent, not sensitive in hollow viscus injury

Laparoscopy

- Limited use in specialized centers; may play a role in diagnosing SBI in stable patients

DIFFERENTIAL DIAGNOSIS

- Hemoperitoneum due to vascular insult
- Solid visceral organ injury or gastric/colon/rectum perforation
- Vertebral injury and associated ileus

PEDIATRIC CONSIDERATIONS

- Delay in diagnosis 1–2 days is common and may increase morbidity

Treatment

INITIAL STABILIZATION

- Standard ATLS protocols including ABCs of multiple trauma care
- Aggressive fluid resuscitation, central line suggested with pressure infusion of warmed IVF (LR of NS)
- Nasogastric tube decompression, then administration of CT contrast as indicated
- Eviscerated small bowel should be covered with moist gauze; impaled foreign body should not be removed in ED

ED TREATMENT

- Immediate transfer to operating suite for patients with an indication for celiotomy
  —Evisceration, abdominal pain with hypotension, positive DPL or abdominal CT, thoracic abdominal herniation (seen on chest x-ray), impaled foreign body, gunshot wound to the abdomen
  —Tetanus and antibiotic prophylaxis for penetrating abdominal wounds and blunt injury requiring surgical exploration
- Local wound exploration is safe for abdominal stab wounds
- Serial abdominal examinations and observation
- Judicious analgesia as blood pressure permits once diagnosis established

MEDICATIONS

- Cefoxitin (mefoxin): adult: 1–2 g; peds: 40 mg/kg IV *or*
- Cefotetan (cefotan): adult: 1–2 g; peds: 20 mg/kg IV *or*
- Ceftizoxime (cefizox): adult: 1–2 g; peds: 50 mg/kg IV *plus*
- Flagyl: adult: 500 mg; peds: 7.5 mg/kg, IV

Disposition

ADMISSION CRITERIA

- Abnormal mental status/intoxication with abdominal injury
- Indication for celiotomy
- Presence of abdominal pain, tenderness or the "seat belt sign" requires admission for observation
- Stab wounds that violate the abdominal fascia, positive DPL or worsening clinical exams, and all gunshot wounds

DISCHARGE CRITERIA

- Minimal mechanism blunt trauma in a nonintoxicated patient with normal exam who has no abdominal pain and adequate follow-up
- Penetrating wounds that do not violate abdominal fascia

Miscellaneous

ICD9: 863.20

CORE CONTENT CODE: 18.4.11.4

SUGGESTED READINGS

Hagawara A, Yukioka T, Satou M, et al. Early diagnosis of small intestine rupture from blunt abdominal trauma using computed tomography: Significance of the streaky density within the mesentery. J Trauma 1995;38(4):630–633.

Marx JA. Penetrating abdominal trauma. Emerg Med Clin North Am 1993;11(1): 125–135.

Sivit CJ, Eichelberger MR, Taylor GA. CT in children with rupture of the bowel caused by blunt trauma: Diagnostic efficacy and comparison with hypoperfusion complex. AJR Am J Roentgenol 1994;163: 1195–1198.

Wisner DH, Chun Y, Blaisdell W. Blunt intestinal injury. Arch Surg 1990;125: 1319–1323.

Authors: Irene Tien; Tamas Peredy

Smoke Inhalation

Clinical Presentation

SIGNS AND SYMPTOMS

- Initially often asymptomatic, with presentation over the next 24 hours after injury
- Pulmonary
  - —Cough
  - —Hoarseness
  - —Dyspnea
  - —Wheezing
  - —Rales
- Associated signs (alert to the possibility of significant inhalation injury)
  - —Major burns
  - —Facial burns
  - —Singed nasal hairs
  - —Carbonaceous sputum
- Associated with significant carbon monoxide exposure and to a lesser extent, cyanide exposure

CO Toxicity

CO LEVEL	SYMPTOMS AND SIGNS (GUIDELINES)
10%	No symptoms
20%	Headache, nausea, vomiting, dyspnea on exertion
30%	Confusion, lethargy, ECG changes
40–60%	Coma
>60%	Death

Cyanide Toxicity

- Seizures
- Coma
- Apnea
- Severe, persistent metabolic acidosis

MECHANISM/DESCRIPTION

- *Upper airway injury:* results in stridor, respiratory arrest
- *Lower airway injury:* results in bronchospasm and noncardiogenic pulmonary edema (ARDS)
- *Cellular asphyxiation:* Interference with oxidative phosphorylation by CO and cyanide results in obtundation, seizures, myocardial ischemia

ETIOLOGY

- Thermal injury
- Chemical insult
- Chemical asphyxiation on a cellular level (e.g., carbon monoxide, cyanide)

PEDIATRIC CONSIDERATIONS

- Pediatric airway narrower than adult's and more prone to airway compromise from edema
- Fetal hemoglobin especially sensitive to CO toxicity

Pre-Hospital

CAUTIONS

- Intubation for agonal breathing
- 100% oxygen by face mask
  - —Therapeutic maneuver for CO and CN toxicity
- Transport awake, stridorous patients to the nearest ED
  - —Advanced airway management best left to the emergency physician unless prolonged transport time
  - —β-Agonist nebulization for bronchospasm
  - —IV LR or 0.9%NS at high flow rates with major burns
  - —Cover the patient with major burns with a clean sheet
  - —Cervical spine and backboard immobilization for traumatized patients

Diagnosis

ESSENTIAL WORKUP

- ABG with carboxyhemoglobin level
  - —Hypoxia
  - —Metabolic acidosis
- EKG
  - —>35 years old for associated myocardial ischemia
  - —For CO-induced myocardial ischemia
- CXR
  - —Baseline initially normal
  - —Becomes abnormal over 8–24 hours with significant lower airway injury

LABORATORY

- Pulse oximetry erroneously normal with significant carboxyhemoglobinemia
- Pregnancy testing
  - —Management of CO toxicity more aggressive in pregnancy
- Any critically burned patient
  - —Electrolytes, BUN/Cr, glucose
  - —CBC
  - —PT/PTT
  - —Cardiac enzymes
- Cyanide levels
  - —Not clinically useful
  - —Results come back hours after therapeutic decisions have been made
- Lactate levels as a marker of cyanide toxicity controversial

IMAGING/SPECIAL TESTS

- Bedside peak expiratory flow
- Bronchoscopy
  - —Visualization of upper and lower airway injuries: erythema, edema, ulcerations, desquamation
  - —Used therapeutically to suction out desquamated epithelial debris
- ^{133}Xenon lung scan
  - —Lung uptake of ^{133}Xe interfered by smoke inhalation injury
  - —Difficult test in children
  - —False-positives in adults with obstructive airway disease
  - —Minimal diagnostic value

DIFFERENTIAL DIAGNOSIS

- COPD or asthma exacerbation
- Cardiogenic pulmonary edema
- Toxic gas exposure
- In the setting of trauma: pneumothorax or hemothorax

Treatment

INITIAL STABILIZATION

- 100% oxygen by face mask
- Intubation for
  - —CNS depression
  - —Respiratory distress (stridor/drooling)
  - —Hypoxia
  - —Significant upper airway/facial burns
  - —Unable to protect airway
- IV fluids LR or 0.9%NS according to Parkland or similar formula for major burns
- Naloxone, thiamine, dextrose (or Accucheck) for altered mental status

ED TREATMENT

- Aggressive airway suctioning
- Positive end-expiratory pressure ventilation despite intubation and 100% oxygen
- Bronchospasm
  - —β-Agonist nebulization
  - —Anticholinergic nebulization
  - —IV steroids for asthma or COPD (otherwise the role of steroids is unknown)
  - —IV aminophylline: role unknown
- Carbon monoxide toxicity (see chapter: Carbon Monoxide, Poisoning)
  - —100% oxygen decreases the half-life of CO from 4–6 hours to 1 hour
  - —Hyperbaric oxygen (HBO) reduces CO half-life to 20 minutes
  - —HBO therapy for
    - -CO level >40%
    - -Loss of conciousness/seizures/significant neurologic findings
    - -Altered mental status
    - -Myocardial ischemia
    - -Pregnancy with CO level >10, fetal distress
- Cyanide toxicity (see chapter: Cyanide, Poisoning)
  - —100% oxygen
  - —Sodium thiosulfate portion of the Lilly kit
  - —Amyl nitrite and sodium nitrite portion of Lilly kit
    - -Contraindicated with significant carboxyhemoglobinemia
    - -Inducement of methylhemoglobinemia further reduces hemoglobin oxygen-carrying capacity
  - —Hydroxocobalamin (probably safe and effective, not yet available in the U.S.)
- No role for prophylactic antibiotics
- No role for steroids in the absence of bronchospasm

MEDICATIONS

- Albuterol nebulization: 2.5–5.0 mg in 2.5 cc NS q 20 min, or continuous neb 5 mg/hr (peds: 0.1–0.3 mg/kg diluted in 2.5 cc NS q 20 min, maximum 2.5 mg, or continuous neb 0.5 mg/kg/hr)
- Dextrose: D50W 1 amp (50 ml or 25 g) (peds: D25W 2–4 ml/kg) IV
- Ipratropium bromide: 0.5 mg added to 1st neb (peds: 0.25 mg/dose for children >5 years old)
- Methylprednisolone: 125 mg IV push (peds: 1–2 mg/kg)
- Naloxone (narcan): 2 mg (peds: 0.1 mg/kg) IV or IM initial dose
- Sodium thiosulfate: 50 ml slow IV push: 50 ml ampule, 25% sodium thiosulfate = 12.5 g (peds: 1.65 ml/kg of 25% sodium thiosulfate = 0.41 g/kg)
- Thiamine (vitamin B_1): 100 mg (peds: 50 mg) IV or I

Disposition

ADMISSION CRITERIA

- ICU or Burn Unit
  - —Intubated
  - —Major burn
  - —Continued dyspnea
  - —Hoarseness
  - —Cough with carbonaceous sputum
- General medical admission for 24-hour observation
  - —Persistent cough in otherwise asymptomatic patients
  - —Asthma or COPD patients with bronchospasm that has resolved with standard medical therapy in the ED
  - —Otherwise asymptomatic with carbonaceous sputum
  - —Underlying illnesses (COPD, CHF, and CAD)
  - —Singed nasal hair
  - —Facial burns
- Transfer severe CO toxicity for hyperbaric oxygen therapy (HBT)

DISCHARGE CRITERIA

- Asymptomatic with normal arterial saturation after 4–6-hour observation period
- Long-term follow-up important

Miscellaneous

ICD9: 987.9

CORE CONTENT CODE: 17.2.26

SUGGESTED READINGS

Ellenhorn MJ, Schoonwald S, Ordog G, Wasserberger J. Respiratory toxicology. In: Ellenhorn MJ, ed. Ellenhorn's medical toxicology. 2d ed. Baltimore: Williams & Wilkins, 1997:1448–1531.

Harrigan R. Smoke inhalation injury and fire toxicology: Evaluation and management. Emerg Med Rep 1994;15(21):203–210.

Nelson L, Hoffman RS. Toxic inhalations. In: Rosen P, et al., eds. Emergency medicine: Concepts and clinical practice. 4th ed. St. Louis: CV Mosby, 1998:1443–1451.

Ruddy RM. Smoke inhalation injury. Pediatr Clin North Am 1994;41(2):317–337.

Weiss SM, Lakshminarayan S. Acute inhalation injury. Clin Chest Med 1994;15(1):103–116.

Author: Ross Tannenbaum

Snake Envenomation

Clinical Presentation

SIGNS AND SYMPTOMS

Local

- Classic skin changes
  - —One or two puncture wounds
  - —Pain and swelling at the site
- Swelling and edema of the involved extremity
  - —Within an hour in severe envenomations
- Ecchymosis, petechiae, and hemorrhagic vesicles develop within several hours

Systemic

- Weakness
- Diaphoresis
- Dizziness
- Nausea
- Scalp paresthesias
- Periorbital fasciculations
- Metallic taste
- Severe bites can lead to
  - —Coagulopathies and DIC
  - —Hypotension
  - —Shock
  - —Pulmonary edema
  - —Hematuria
  - —Renal failure
  - —Cardiac dysfunction
- Compartment syndrome in the involved extremity
- Coral snake venom
  - —Primarily neurotoxic
    - -Weakness
    - -Diplopia
    - -Confusion
    - -Respiratory depression
  - —Local effects may be deceivingly minimal

MECHANISM/DESCRIPTION

- Pit viper venom
  - —Mixture of proteolytic enzymes and thrombinlike esterases
    - -Enzymes cause local muscle and subcutaneous tissue necrosis
    - -Esterases have an anticoagulant effect, leading to DIC in severe envenomations
- Bite location
  - —Head or trunk bite—more severe than on the extremities
  - —Lower extremity bites may have a delayed presentation
- Severe envenomation
  - —Direct bite into an artery or vein
  - —All coral snake venom (primarily neurotoxic)
- Bite mark significance
  - —Venomous snake: classically includes one or two puncture marks
  - —Nonvenomous snake: horseshoe-shaped row of multiple teeth marks

ETIOLOGY

- Venomous snakes indigenous to the U.S.
  - —Pit vipers
    - -Account for 95% of all envenomations
    - -Rattlesnakes, cottonmouths, and copperheads
  - —Coral snakes
    - -More severe envenomations
    - -Western coral snakes are found in Arizona and New Mexico
    - -More venomous eastern coral snakes found in the Carolinas and the Gulf states

PEDIATRIC CONSIDERATIONS

- Small children are most likely target for snake envenomations
- Those who freeze with fear in response to the snake are also more susceptible to multiple envenomations.
- Due to their low body weight, smaller children and infants are more vulnerable to severe envenomation

Pre-Hospital

CAUTIONS

- Retreat well-beyond striking range of snake
- Immobilize extremity
- Keep physical activity minimal

CONTROVERSIES

- Incision and suction of the bite wound is not recommended
  - —Can lead to further wound contamination with human mouth flora
  - —Incision attempts by the inexperienced can lead to severe tendon, nerve, and vascular damage
- Tourniquets, cryotherapy, and electrocautery
  - —Contraindicated due to tissue damage
- While mechanical suction devices do exist, no clinical human trials support their use

PEDIATRIC CONSIDERATIONS

- Increased urgency in transport to the hospital setting is indicated
  - —Envenomation more likely to be severe
  - —Due to the relatively low body weight of a small child

Diagnosis

ESSENTIAL WORKUP

- History
  - —Description of the snake
  - —Geographic location of the bite
- Physical examination
  - —Careful examination of the wound site and involved extremity
    - -Essential in judging the severity of the envenomation
  - —Careful assessment for anaphylactic reactions

LABORATORY

- CBC
- PT/PTT
- DIC panel
- Electrolytes, BUN/Cr, glucose
- CPK
- Urinalysis
- Type and crossmatch with moderate to severe envenomation

DIFFERENTIAL DIAGNOSIS

- Nonpoisonous snakes
  - —Smooth, tapered body
  - —Narrow head
  - —Round pupils
  - —No rattles
- Pit vipers
  - —Triangular or arrow-shaped head
  - —Vertical or elliptical pupils
  - —Rattles
- Coral snakes
  - —"Red on yellow—kill a fellow"
  - —"Red on black—venom lack"

Treatment

INITIAL STABILIZATION

- ABCs
- Vigorous hydration with 0.9%NS to maintain intravascular volume and renal blood flow
- Monitor
- Immobilize the bitten extremity

ED TREATMENT

- Supportive care
- Observe for compartment syndrome
- Wound severity
  - —Minimal
    - -Local swelling and tenderness
  - —Moderate
    - -Extremity swelling
    - -Evidence of systemic toxicity
  - —Severe
    - -Obvious toxicity
    - -Unstable vitals
    - -Coagulopathy
    - -Coral snake
    - -Lab abnormalities
- Tetanus prophylaxis if needed
- Broad-spectrum antibiotics for moderate to severe envenomations

Antivenin

Crotalidae Antivenin

- Fundamental treatment for pit viper envenomation
- Effective for rattlesnakes, cottonmouths, and copperheads
- Most effective if given within 4–6 hours of the bite
- Skin test with diluted horse serum (in the antivenin kit) prior to antivenin administration
- Treatment complications include anaphylaxis and serum sickness
- Dosage (each vial contains 10 ml of antivenin) by wound severity
  - —Minimal: 5 vials
  - —Moderate: 10 vials
  - —Severe: 15 vials
- Victims of severe envenomations who develop a positive skin test with horse serum
  - —May still receive the antivenin
  - —Pretreat with diphenhydramine and corticosteroids
  - —Monitor closely for anaphylaxis with epinephrine at the bedside

Coral Snake Antivenin

- Effective against the more toxic eastern coral snake, but not against the western coral snakes
- After proper skin testing, 3–5 vials of antivenin are recommended
- Treatment complications are the same as with Crotalidae antivenin

Treatment Assistance

- Contact local poison control center, local zoo, or herpetologist
- Call the Antivenom Index at (602) 626-6016 in Tucson, AZ for assistance in treatment of exotic snakes not indigenous to the United States

PEDIATRIC CONSIDERATIONS

- Proportionally more antivenin per body weight
- Children often require standard adult doses

Disposition

ADMISSION CRITERIA

- 24-Hour observation for patients requiring antivenin administration
- ICU admission for
  - —Evidence of moderate to severe envenomation, especially in children
  - —All victims of coral snake bites

DISCHARGE CRITERIA

- Suspicious bite that shows no signs or symptoms of envenomation for 6–8 hours and has a normal lab panel
  - —Discharge with follow-up in 24 hours
  - —Observe lower extremity bites for 12 hours due to delayed toxicity
  - —"Dry" bites occur in up to 25% of pit viper bites

Miscellaneous

ICD9: 989.5

CORE CONTENT CODE: 5.10.4

SUGGESTED READINGS

Cruz NS, Alvarez RG. Rattlesnake bite complications in 19 children. Pediatr Emerg Care 1994;10:30.

Erickson T, Herman BE, Bowman, MA. Snake envenomations. In: Strange G, Ahrens WR, et al. eds. Pediatric emergency medicine. Chap. 109. McGraw Hill, New York 1996:590–592.

Lawrence WT, Giannopoulos A, Hansen A. Pit viper bites: Rational management in locales in which copperheads and cottonmouths predominate. Ann Plast Surg 1996;36(3):276–285.

Sing K, Erickson T, Aks S, Rothenberg H, Lipscomb J. Eastern massasauga rattlesnake envenomations in an urban wilderness. J Wilderness Med 1994;5:77–87.

Wuster W, Golay P, Warrell DA. Synopsis of recent developments in venomous snake systematics. Toxicon 1997;35(3):319–340.

Authors: Adam Black; Timothy Erickson

Spinal Cord Injury

Clinical Presentation

SIGNS AND SYMPTOMS

- Localized back or neck pain in the region of the midline
- Tenderness over spinous processes
- Radiation of pain into one or more extremities
- Hypesthesia, hyperesthesia, paresthesia, or analgesia
- Hypoalgesia or hyperalgesia
- Paresis or plegia

MECHANISM/DESCRIPTION

- Vertebral subluxation secondary to hyperflexion or hyperextension with ligamentous rupture
- Fracture or dislocation of one or both facets
- Axial loading with burst type fractures
- Distraction of vertebral components as by hanging
- Fractures of vertebral arches
- Fractures in the vicinity of vertebral foramina with associated arterial injury
- Acute disc rupture with herniation and injury to the spinal cord or nerve root
- Most spinal injuries are caused by falls, motor vehicle accidents, and sports-related accidents

ETIOLOGY

- Spinal column and spinal cord injuries are caused by direct trauma, high-speed deceleration, electrical injury, or penetrating trauma

PEDIATRIC CONSIDERATIONS

- Always consider the possibility of child abuse in the infant or young child with an apparent spinal injury
- The cervical spine, especially the upper portion, is much more vulnerable in young children: larger head size, poorly developed muscles and ligaments

Pre-Hospital

- Maintain the patient in a neutral position and avoid any movement of the head and neck while full spinal immobilization is being performed

Diagnosis

ESSENTIAL WORKUP

- Examine the whole spinal column from top to bottom. Look for areas of tenderness, ecchymosis, hematoma, crepitus, deformity, and muscle spasm
- Perform a detailed neurologic examination
  - —Mental status
  - —Sensory: evaluate light touch, pain, and joint position senses
    - -Sensory levels of deficit
    - -C2—occiput
    - -C4—clavicular region
    - -C6—thumb
    - -C8—little finger
    - -T4—nipple line
    - -T10—umbilicus
    - -L1—inguinal region
    - -L3—knee
    - -S1—heel
    - -S5—perianal area
  - —Motor: muscle strength in all muscle groups (on a 5-point scale)
    - -Motor levels of deficit
    - -C5—elbow flexion
    - -C7—elbow extension
    - -C8—finger flexion
    - -T1—finger abduction
    - -L2—hip flexion
    - -L3—knee extension
    - -L4—ankle dorsiflexion
    - -L5—Great toe dorsiflexion
    - -S1—ankle plantar flexion
  - —Always evaluate *rectal sphincter tone* and the amount of *residual urine* after catheterization (postvoid residual)
  - —Check deep tendon reflexes and Babinski's sign
- Absence of bulbocavernous, and cremasteric reflex indicate *spinal shock* and some degree of reversal of symptoms may occur
- When performing a neurologic exam, look for symmetry and, when deficits are apparent, try to establish sensory and motor levels
- Radiographs as outlined below

IMAGING/SPECIAL TESTS

- Initial radiologic examination is always a 3-view trauma series of the cervical spine (AP, cross-table lateral, and odontoid views)
  - —All 7 cervical vertebrae must be visualized along with the top of T1
- These are followed with plain radiographs of tender areas of the spinal column (thoracic, lumbosacral)
- If suspicion is high for a spinal injury and initial x-rays are normal, perform flexion-extension views (these must be done under the direct supervision of the physician and the alert patient instructed to immediately stop all movement if pain increases)
- Further studies should also be obtained when the initial x-rays are normal, equivocal, or suspicious if severe pain is present, when neurologic deficits are found, or when obvious abnormalities are present on plain x-rays
- When defining fractures through the posterior elements (spinous processes, laminae, pedicles, and facets), CT is the test of choice
- MRI examination is the best modality to evaluate the spinal cord for compression. This includes the intervertebral disc for herniation or the presence of an epidural clot which can cause cord compression
- Also consider the use of three-dimensional (3D) CT scanning to improve the yield (not universally available and quite costly)

PEDIATRIC CONSIDERATIONS

- Abnormal radiographic findings on plain films in infants and small children may be normal anatomic variants (pseudosubluxation)
- Crying can alter the normal appearance on screening x-rays of the cervical spine
- Spinal cord injury without radiographic abnormality (SCIWORA) occurs because of the elasticity of bony structures

DIFFERENTIAL DIAGNOSIS

- It is imperative to discern whether the severe pain or motor deficits are the result of neurologic injury or trauma to other areas of the musculoskeletal system
- Vascular (arteriovenous malformation, angioma)
- Infectious (tuberculosis, osteomyelitis)
- Neoplastic (metastatic carcinoma, lymphoma)
- Demyelinating diseases (multiple sclerosis)
- Degenerative diseases (osteoporosis, ankylosing spondylitis)
- Coagulopathy, or congenital abnormalities (osteogenesis imperfecta, achondroplasia)

Treatment

INITIAL STABILIZATION

- ABCs
- If the patient arrives on their own and may have a spinal injury, immobilize the patient at once with a rigid cervical collar and a long spine board
- Until the possibility of spinal injury has been completely eliminated, maintain spinal immobilization

ED TREATMENT

- Fully evaluate the patient for associated injuries
- Obtain appropriate imaging studies
- Obtain early consultation with an orthopedic surgeon or a neurosurgeon
- Perform repeat neurologic examinations and *document them*
- If subspecialty care is not available, arrange for transfer of the patient to the nearest spine or trauma center
- Prepare for the application of skeletal traction if indicated (such as Creutzfeldt tongs or Halo device) in consult with neurosurgeon or spine specialist
- High-dose steroid protocol for neurologic deficits, administer within 8 hours post injury

MEDICATIONS

- Methylprednisolone: 30 mg/kg IV over 15 min; then 5.4 mg/kg/hr over the next 23 hrs

Disposition

ADMISSION CRITERIA

- All patients with proven or suspected spinal injuries must be admitted to the ICU
- If neurosurgical or orthopedic consultation is not available, the patient should be transferred

DISCHARGE CRITERIA

- Only those patients with negative spinal evaluations and absence of neurologic symptoms may be released from the hospital

Miscellaneous

ICD9: 952.9

CORE CONTENT CODE: 18.4.2

SUGGESTED READINGS

Meldon SW, Moettus LN. Thoracolumbar spine fractures: Clinical presentation and the effect of altered sensorium and major injury. J Trauma 1995;39(6):1110.

Neumann P, Nordwall A, Osvalder A-L. Traumatic instability of the lumbar spine. Spine 1995;20(10):1111.

Petersilge CA, Pathria MN, Emery SE, et al. Thoracolumbar burst fractures: Evaluation with MR imaging. Radiology 1995;194(1):49.

Velmahos GC, Theodorou D, Tatevossian R, et al. Radiographic cervical spine evaluation in the alert asymptomatic blunt trauma victim: Much ado about nothing? J Trauma 1996;40(5):768.

Author: Bernard Beckerman

Spinal Cord Syndromes

Clinical Presentation

SIGNS AND SYMPTOMS

- Spinal cord syndromes result from incomplete spinal cord lesions and as a result exhibit mixed motor and sensory sparing
- *Anterior cord syndrome*
  —Bilateral loss of motor function and sensation of pain and temperature below the level of the lesion
  —Preservation of dorsal column function (proprioception, and position sense)
- *Brown-Sequard syndrome (lateral cord syndrome)*
  —Ipsilateral loss of motor function and dorsal column function (proprioception and position sense)
  —Contralateral loss of pain and temperature sensation
  —Deficits usually begin two levels below the injury
- *Central cord syndrome*
  —Loss of motor function affects upper extremities more severely than lower extremities
  —Sensory loss is more variable
  —Most profound deficits occur in the distal upper extremities
- *Dorsal cord syndrome*
  —Loss of proprioception, and position sensation below the level of the lesion
- Sacral sparing is present with incomplete lesions
- Sensory deficit levels
  —C2—occiput
  —C4—clavicular region
  —C6—thumb
  —C8—little finger
  —T4—nipple line
  —T10—umbilicus
  —L1—inguinal region
  —L3—knee
  —S1—heel
  —S5—perianal area
- Motor deficit levels
  —C5—elbow flexion
  —C7—elbow extension
  —C8—finger flexion
  —T1—finger abduction
  —L2—hip flexion
  —L3—knee extension
  —L4—ankle dorsiflexion
  —S1—ankle plantar flexion

MECHANISM/DESCRIPTION

- Patients with arthritis, osteoporosis, metastatic disease, or other chronic spinal disorders are at risk for developing spinal injuries as the result of even minor trauma
- Anterior cord syndrome
  —Results from a flexion or axial loading mechanism, vertebral fractures or dislocations, and disc herniation
  —Rarely caused by a laceration or thrombosis to the anterior spinal artery
- Brown-Sequard syndrome
  —Hemisection of the spinal cord classically as a result of a penetrating wound
- Central cord syndrome
  —Most commonly occurs in elderly patients who have preexisting cervical spondylosis and stenosis
  —Forced hyperextension causes buckling of the ligamentum flavum creating a shearing injury to the central portion of the spinal cord
- Dorsal cord syndrome
  —Associated with hyperextension injuries

Pre-Hospital

- Strict spinal precautions
- Patients should be transported to the nearest trauma center

PEDIATRIC CONSIDERATIONS

- Cervical collars must be the appropriate size for the child
- If the correct cervical collar is not available, splinting the head and torso with tape and sandbags to a short backboard is adequate

Diagnosis

ESSENTIAL WORKUP

- Plain films of the cervical spine
- Thoracic and lumbosacral films as determined by level of pain or neurologic deficit
- CT of the spine when plain films are normal or to better delineate pathology
  —The CT allows assessment of the spinal canal and any impingement by bone fragments
- MRI is the study of choice in detecting spinal cord injury related to trauma
  —In acute settings, it is indicated for patients with
    -Neurologic deficits not explained by plain films or CT
    -Fractures or dislocations that may be causing direct cord injury
    -Clinical progression of a spinal cord lesion
  —Disadvantages of MRI include the inability to adequately monitor the patient while undergoing the study

IMAGING/SPECIAL TESTS

- Myelography is used in combination with CT when MRI is not available or cannot be performed

DIFFERENTIAL DIAGNOSIS

- Complete cord syndrome with or without spinal shock
- Dorsal root injury

Treatment

INITIAL STABILIZATION

- ABCs of trauma care
- Spinal immobilization must be maintained at all times
- Intubation must proceed with in-line spinal immobilization
- IV fluids should be administered at maintenance levels unless shock is present
  - —Spinal trauma may cause hypotension due to loss of sympathetic tone
  - —Other causes of hypotension (i.e., hemorrhage) should be sought before being attributed to spinal cord injury
  - —Generally hypovolemic shock causes tachycardia while neurogenic shock results in bradycardia
  - —If the blood pressure does not improve after a fluid challenge, and no other cause for hypotension can be found, vasopressor use may be necessary

ED TREATMENT

- Other injuries must be treated as indicated
- Level of spinal cord injury should be determined as a baseline to follow for improvement or deterioration
- A neurosurgeon must be consulted once a spinal cord injury is suspected even when plain films are normal
- The patient with a spinal cord injury should be managed at an appropriate regional trauma center or spinal center
  - —If necessary, transfer should occur as soon as management of other injuries allow
- High-dose methylprednisolone is started as soon as possible in the patient with spinal cord injury
  - —The greatest benefit is reported when infusion is begun within 8 hours of injury
  - —To prevent GI bleeding with steroid use, concurrently start the patient on IV pepcid
- IV antibiotics and tetanus prophylaxis are given to patients with a penetrating injury to the neck

MEDICATIONS

- Dopamine: 2–20 μg/kg/min IV (adult and peds)
- Methylprednisolone: 30 mg/kg IV loading dose given over 15 min in the 1st hr followed by a 5.4 mg/kg/hr continuous infusion for the next 23 hrs (adult and peds)
- Pepcid: adult: 20 mg IV; peds: 0.6–0.8 mg/kg/24hrs q 8–12 hrs

Disposition

ADMISSION CRITERIA

- All patients with spinal cord syndrome must be admitted to an ICU setting

DISCHARGE CRITERIA

- No patient with suspicion of spinal cord injury should be discharged

Miscellaneous

ICD9: 952.9

CORE CONTENT CODE: 18.4.3

SUGGESTED READINGS

American College of Surgeons, Committee on Trauma. Advanced trauma life support course for physicians. 1993:193–203 Chicago, IL. About College of Surgeons.

Bracken MB, et al. A randomized controlled trial of methylprednisolone or naloxone in the treatment of acute spinal cord injury. N Engl J Med 1990;322(20):1405–1411.

Hockberger RS, et al. Spinal trauma. In: Rosen, P, et al., eds. Emergency medicine: Concepts and clinical practice. 4th ed. St. Louis: CV Mosby, 1998:462–504.

Pang D, Wilberger J. Spinal cord injury without radiographic abnormalities in children. J Neurosurg 1982;57:114.

Rhee KJ, et al. Oral intubation in the multiply injured patient: The risk of exacerbating spinal cord damage. Ann Emerg Med 1990;19(5):511–514.

Author: Eileen M. Duffy

Spinal Dislocations/Subluxations

Clinical Presentation

SIGNS AND SYMPTOMS

- Symptoms will vary depending on the level of the injury
- Cervical spine injuries are the most common
  - —Greater than one-third of cervical spine fractures or dislocations will have evidence of neurologic injury
- Because of the stabilizing influence of the rib cage, a tremendous amount of force is required to cause dislocations of the thoracic spine
  - —Concomitant internal injury should be suspected
  - —Thoracic spine fracture-dislocation is less common than thoracolumbar fracture-dislocation but is associated with a higher incidence of neurologic impairment

Common Signs and Symptoms

- Localized soft tissue defect
- Pain and tenderness over spinous process, or referred to trapezium or deltoid
- Paraspinal muscle spasm
- Paresthesia or dysesthesia; often elicited only during flexion or extension
- Weakness (focal or global)
- Distal areflexia
- Flaccid plegia
- Bowel/bladder incontinence
- Priapism
- Loss of temperature control
- Spinal shock

MECHANISM/DESCRIPTION

- Baseball bat to the occiput
- Sudden deceleration in an MVA or a fall from a significant height
- The vectors of the movement of the spine will have a significant impact on the resultant injury. For example
  - —Flexion
    - -Anterior subluxation
    - -Bilateral interfacetal dislocation
  - —Flexion-rotation
    - -Unilateral interfacetal dislocation of C-spine
    - -Posterior ligament or joint capsule rupture of T/L-spine
  - —Flexion-distraction (seat belt injury)
    - -Avulsion of bone, disks and ligaments (T12–L2)
  - —Extension rotation
    - -Unilateral facet dislocation
  - —Hyperextension
    - -Hyperextension dislocation
    - -Hyperextension fracture/dislocation
  - —Hyperextension distraction
    - -Occipitocervical dislocation

ETIOLOGY

- Blunt trauma causes the majority of injuries
- Preexisting disease that increases the incidence of injury
  - —Degenerative and rheumatoid arthritis
  - —Ankylosing spondylitis
  - —Spina bifida
  - —Congenital malformation of vertebrae

Pre-Hospital

CAUTIONS

- Maintain strict C-spine precautions
- Transport to the nearest trauma center
- Do not apply traction to the C-spine, apply in-line immobilization

Diagnosis

ESSENTIAL WORKUP

- Rapid evaluation of airway, breathing, and circulation
- Detailed neurologic exam with specific attention to evidence of spinal cord injury
  - —Motor function, pain perception, reflexes, and proprioception
  - —Rectal tone, perianal sensation, post void residual
  - —Assess for bulbocavernous reflex in spinal shock
- Thorough spine exam noting any deformity or tenderness
- Radiography
  - —Midline tenderness or a nontender exam in the setting of distracting injury or intoxication mandates spine radiography

IMAGING/SPECIAL TESTS

- Ligamentous spinal disruption or occult fracture will be represented on plain films by changes in soft tissue markings or alignment
- It should be assumed that there is existing ligamentous injury with bony fractures
- Ligamentous injury without fracture may be suspected with the following findings on plain films
  - —Lateral C-spine (C1 to the top of T1)
    - -Measure prevertebral soft tissue; 5 mm or greater anterior to C3 or C4 suggests injury
    - -Evaluate the alignment of the four lordotic curves
      - *Anterior margin of the vertebral bodies
      - *Posterior margin of the vertebral bodies
      - *Spinolaminar line
      - *Tips of the spinous processes
    - -Check for abrupt change in angulation of the cervical column. Greater than 11° at a single interspace suggests injury
    - -Fanning of the spinous processes suggests posterior ligamentous disruption
    - -Widening of the predental space at C1–C2 suggests disruption of the cruciform ligament. (Normal: 3 mm or less for adults and 4 mm or less for children.)
    - -Check the atlantooccipital relation
  - —Open mouth odontoid view
    - -Check for malposition, and fracture of the odontoid
    - -Check the alignment of the lateral masses of C1 with C2
    - -Examine for symmetry of the C1–C2 interspace.
  - —AP C-spine
    - -Check alignment of the facets and pedicles
    - -Check spacing between the transverse processes
    - -Ensure that the spinous processes line up vertically

—AP T- and L-spine
 -Check for lateral subluxation
—Lateral T- and L-spine
 -Check for anterior or posterior listhesis or subluxation
- Flexion and extension lateral C-spine views should be done for patients with normal plain films and persistent tenderness
- Plain film evidence of fracture or ligamentous disruption mandates thin cut CT scan to document the presence or absence of spinal cord impingement
- A CT scan is also indicated for severe, persistent pain without plain film abnormality
- MRI is the study of choice to document soft tissue or ligamentous disruption

DIFFERENTIAL DIAGNOSIS

- Arthritis (degenerative and rheumatoid)
- Ankylosing spondylitis
- Spina bifida
- Congenital malformation
- Neoplasm

PEDIATRIC CONSIDERATIONS

- Between ages 3 and 6 the pediatric spine gradually approaches adult dimensions
- Soft tissue projection on plain film can be variable in children
  —Retropharyngeal space up to 7 mm may be normal
  —Retrotracheal space up to 14 mm may be normal
  —Prevertebral soft tissues are variable in children and can be affected by crying, position, and adenoid tissue
   -This can lead to a false impression of widened prevertebral soft tissue space
  —Anterior translation ("pseudosubluxation") of up to 4 mm (commonly C2 on C3) can be normal
   -Posterior elements will be in normal alignment with pseudosubluxation
  —Reversal of the normal smooth anterior curve can be seen in very young patients

Treatment

INITIAL STABILIZATION

- Follow the ABCs of trauma care
  —Rapid sequence orotracheal intubation with in-line immobilization has been shown to be safe
  —Preserve residual spinal cord function and prevent further injury by stabilizing the spine
  —Initiate therapy to ensure the greatest possible spinal recovery

ED TREATMENT

- Perform all needed resuscitation and diagnostic tests with the patient in full spinal immobilization
- If spinal cord injury is suspected administer high dose steroids and consult neurosurgery
- If spinal fracture or ligamentous injury is suspected without neurologic impairment arrange CT or MRI scanning
- Pain control with NSAIDs, opiates, and benzodiazepines

MEDICATIONS

- High-dose steroid protocol
  —Methylprednisolone: 30 mg/kg IV bolus then 5.4 mg/kg/hr over the next 23 hrs; begin within 8 hrs of injury

Disposition

- Patients with significant spinal cord damage, ligamentous injury, or dislocation should be transferred to a regional trauma center

ADMISSION CRITERIA

- Unstable spinal column injury
- Cord or root injury should be admitted to the ICU
- Ileus
- Pain control

DISCHARGE CRITERIA

- Patients with normal neurologic exam, and no evidence of radiologic injury may be discharged with orthopedic spine service follow-up
  —If significant neck pain persists, discharge in a hard cervical collar

Miscellaneous

ICD9: 839.40

CORE CONTENT CODE: 18.4.3.2

SUGGESTED READINGS

Chiles BW 3rd, Cooper PR. Acute spinal injury. New Engl J Med 1996;334(8):514–520.

el-Khoury GY, Whitten CG. Trauma to the upper thoracic spine: Anatomy, biomechanics, and unique imaging features. AJR Am J Roentgenol 1993;160:95–102.

Skeletal trauma. In: Browner, Jupiter, Levine, Trafton, eds. Thoracic and upper lumber spine injuries. Philadelphia: WB Saunders, 1992:729–805.

Author: Richard D. Zane

Splenic Injury

Clinical Presentation

- The spleen is the most commonly injured intra-abdominal organ

SIGNS AND SYMPTOMS

- Systemic signs from acute blood loss
  - —May present with syncope, dizziness, or weakness
  - —May progress to profound hypotension or shock
- Local signs
  - —Left upper-quadrant tenderness
  - —Referred pain to the left shoulder (Kehr's sign)
  - —Abdominal distension, rigidity, rebound tenderness
- Contusions, abrasions, or penetrating wounds to the chest, flank, or abdomen may indicate underlying spleen injury
- Fractures of lower left ribs are commonly seen in association with splenic injuries
- Physical exam is neither sensitive nor specific for splenic injury; adjunctive studies are required

MECHANISM/DESCRIPTION

- Motor vehicle accidents are the major cause of blunt abdominal trauma
- Mechanism of injury and kinematics are important factors in evaluating patients for possible splenic injury
- Obtain details from pre-hospital providers
  - —Blunt trauma: the forces and direction (horizontal or vertical) of any deceleration or compressive forces
  - —Penetrating trauma: the characteristic of the weapon (type and caliber), distance from the weapon, or the type and length of knife or impaling object
- Injuries to the spleen from blunt trauma are caused by forces to the anterior abdominal wall compressing the spleen between the posterior thoracic cage or vertebral column
- Injuries to the spleen from penetrating trauma may result in simple lacerations or complete disruption of the splenic parenchyma
- Splenic injuries are graded by severity of injury, ranging from subcapsular hematoma, mild and major lacerations to severe splenic fragmentation

PEDIATRIC CONSIDERATIONS

- Poorly developed musculature and relatively smaller anterior-posterior diameter increase the vulnerability of abdominal contents to compressive forces

Pre-Hospital

CAUTIONS

- Initiate IV access as hemorrhage is major life threat
- Penetrating wounds or evisceration should be covered with sterile dressings

Diagnosis

ESSENTIAL WORKUP

- Physical exam is neither specific nor sensitive for splenic injury
- Adjunctive imaging studies are required

LABORATORY

- No hematologic laboratory studies are specific for diagnosis of injury to the spleen
- Obtain baseline hemoglobin determination, type, and crossmatch

IMAGING/SPECIAL TESTS

- Plain abdominal x-rays are too nonspecific to be of value
- CXR findings suggestive for splenic injury include left lower rib fracture, elevation of left hemidiaphragm, or left pleural effusion
- Bedside ultrasound detects intra-abdominal fluid that may suggest splenic injury
- Diagnostic peritoneal lavage is extremely sensitive for the presence of hemoperitoneum although nonspecific for source of bleeding
- Abdominal CT scan depicts the presence and extent of splenic injury as well as injuries to adjacent organs
  - —This modality will provide the most specific information in patients stable enough to go to the CT scanner

DIFFERENTIAL DIAGNOSIS

- Intraperitoneal organ injury, especially liver
- Injury to retroperitoneal structures
- Thoracic injury

Treatment

INITIAL STABILIZATION

- ABCs (including C-spine immobilization)
  - —Adequate IV access, including central lines and cutdowns as dictated by the patient's hemodynamic status
  - —Fluid resuscitation, initially with 2 L of crystalloid (NS or LR), followed by blood products as needed

ED TREATMENT

- Immediate laparotomy may be appropriate in the acutely injured patient who is hemodynamically unstable with presumed hemoperitoneum and splenic injury
- Majority of patients with acute splenic injury are either hemodynamically stable or stabilize rapidly with relatively small amounts of fluid resuscitation
- Adjunctive diagnostic procedures supplementing the physical exam should be performed early in the evaluation, followed by laparotomy when indicated by positive diagnostic findings
- Gun shot wounds to the anterior abdomen are routinely explored
- Stab wounds can be managed by local wound exploration, followed by US or DPL when intraperitoneal penetration is demonstrated or equivocal
- Operative versus nonoperative management
  - —Patients with signs and symptoms of intraperitoneal hemorrhage, those with operative indications based on imaging/diagnostic procedures, and those who fail nonoperative management should undergo laparotomy
  - —Splenectomy versus splenic salvage procedures depends on the grade of splenic injury
  - —Patient selection for nonoperative management includes hemodynamic stability, no evidence of other intra-abdominal injury, isolated splenic injury confirmed by imaging study, most commonly CT scan
  - —Patients over 55 should be considered for operative management due to decreased physical tolerance to traumatic insult and reduced physiologic reserve
  - —In the pediatric population, nonoperative management of splenic injuries is considered safe

Disposition

ADMISSION CRITERIA

- All patients with splenic injury require hospitalization for definitive laparotomy or observation with serial abdominal examinations and hematocrit determinations

DISCHARGE CRITERIA

- Only asymptomatic patients objectively demonstrated not to have splenic or other traumatic injury may be discharged

Miscellaneous

ICD9: 865.00

CORE CONTENT CODE: 18.4.11.3

SUGGESTED READINGS

Dupuy DE, Raptopoulos V, Fink MP. Current concepts in splenic trauma. J Intensive Care Med 1995;10:76–90.

Esposito T, Gamelli R. Injury to the spleen. In: Felicano D, et al., eds. Trauma. 3rd ed. Norwalk, CT: Appleton & Lange, 1996:525–550.

Marx J. Abdominal trauma. In: Rosen P, et al., eds. Emergency medicine: Concepts and clinical practice. 4th ed. St. Louis: CV Mosby, 1998.

Author: Tom Moats

Spondylolysis/Spondylolisthesis

Clinical Presentation

SIGNS AND SYMPTOMS

- Often associated with feeling of stiffness or spasm in paravertebral muscles
- Pain occurs after varying amounts of exercise, with standing, or with coughing
- Relief of pain with rest is variable and slow, and usually requires sitting or stooping
- Pain in the back and legs that is aggravated by standing and walking
- Sitting or forward bending relieves pain
- Pain and sensory loss is in a dermatomal distribution
- May have flattening of normal lumbar lordosis
- Hamstring tightness is common
- Neurological exam usually normal

MECHANISM/DESCRIPTION

Spondylolysis

- Bony defect at the pars interarticularis (the isthmus of bone between the superior and inferior facets), which can be unilateral or bilateral
- Dysplastic: congenital defect of the neural arch or intra-articular facets
- Lytic: stress fracture from repetitive microtrauma through the neural arch

Spondylolisthesis

- The slipping forward of one vertebra upon another
- Spondylolysis is not a clinical problem but can contribute to spondylolisthesis, which is noted in approximately 5% of the population
- Of those with spondylolysis, 50% will have some degree of spondylolisthesis develop during their lifetime, and 50% of those will be symptomatic
- Spondylolisthesis predisposes to sciatica
- Spondylolisthesis is divided into four grades based on degree of slippage (Meyerding's grading system)
  - —Grade I: up to 25% of the vertebral body width
  - —Grade II: 26–50% of the vertebral body width
  - —Grade III: 51–75% of the vertebral body width
  - —Grade IV: 76–100% of the vertebral body width
- The most common location for spondylolisthesis is L5 displaced on the sacrum in 85% of cases, followed by L4 on L5

ETIOLOGY

- Unknown
- Theories include congenital anomaly, or environmental

PEDIATRIC CONSIDERATIONS

- Symptoms most often present during adolescent growth spurt between ages 10 and 15
- Athletes in sports resulting in hyperextension of the back, e.g., gymnastics, wrestling, or football
- Acute symptoms are related to trauma
- Spondylolysis in a child under 10 years of age should be monitored closely for
  - —Constant pain that lasts for several weeks
  - —Pain that occurs spontaneously at night
  - —Pain that interferes repeatedly with school, play, or sports
  - —Pain that is associated with marked stiffness and limitation of motion, fever, or neurological signs
  - —Pain at the lumbosacral junction
- Spondylolysis is one of the most common causes of serious low back pain in children

Pre-Hospital

- Spinal precautions are not needed unless there is a history of recent trauma

Diagnosis

ESSENTIAL WORKUP

- History
  - —Onset of symptoms
  - —Location of pain
  - —Aggravating/alleviating factors
  - —Systemic/neurologic symptoms
- Physical examination
  - —Neurological exam is usually normal
  - —Tight hamstrings, knees flexed to allow patient to stand upright
  - —Palpation may reveal step-off with a prominent spinous process of L5
  - —Trunk may appear shortened
  - —Rib cage approaches iliac crests

LABORATORY

- Not helpful except for identifying alternative causes of symptoms

IMAGING/SPECIAL TESTS

- Lumbosacral spine x-rays
  - —Lateral and oblique x-rays of spine most helpful
  - —Spondylolysis will manifest as a radiolucent defect in the pars interarticularis, visible as a "collar" or "broken neck" on the oblique view "Scottie dog"
  - —This is most common at lumbosacral junction
  - —Spondylolisthesis will manifest as forward slipping of the body of one vertebra on another
- CT scan
  - —Demonstrates pathology more clearly than plain films
  - —May be scheduled outpatient unless history of recent trauma
  - —Can play an important role for orthopedist in short-term and long-term management decisions through identification of new stress fractures and healing stage of old stress fractures
- MRI
  - —Useful for defining root impingement and foraminal narrowing
  - —Less valuable than CT in defining bone detail

DIFFERENTIAL DIAGNOSIS

- Tuberculosis
- Discitis
- Bone or spinal cord tumor
- Pyelonephritis
- Retroperitoneal infection
- Injury to muscles or joints of back
- Congenital hip dislocation
- Rickets
- Ruptured intervertebral disk
- Vascular claudication

PEDIATRIC CONSIDERATIONS

- Lower threshold for ordering imaging studies
- Progressive slipping more likely to occur than in adults

Treatment

INITIAL STABILIZATION

- Maintain spinal precautions if traumatic spondylolisthesis
- Vigorous attempts at traction should not be pursued

ED TREATMENT

- Pain control
- Supportive therapy if symptoms are mild
  - —Restrict activities if repetitive trauma is likely aggravating cause (e.g., sports), followed by reintroduction of activity when asymptomatic
  - —Analgesics and muscle relaxants
  - —Consider antilordotic braces or physical therapy
- Orthopedic consult or referral if symptoms are moderate to severe or unresponsive to supportive care
  - —Surgical intervention typically consists of spinal fusion in the flexed position
  - —50% of symptomatic patients with spondylolisthesis may require surgery
  - —All symptomatic grade III or IV spondylolisthesis should probably undergo surgery
- Patient education
- Exercises are not of proven benefit

MEDICATIONS

- NSAIDs
  - —Example: ibuprofen: adult: 200–800 mg po qid; peds: 5–10 mg/kg po q 6 hrs
- Opioids
  - —Example: morphine sulfate: 0.1 mg/kg up to 2–4 mg increments IV
- Muscle relaxants
  - —Example: methocarbamol: adult: 1000–1500 mg po qid; peds: safety and effectiveness for children under 12 not established

PEDIATRIC CONSIDERATIONS

- Activity restriction is not necessary if minimal or no symptoms

Disposition

ADMISSION CRITERIA

- Inability to walk
- Inability to cope at home due to pain or social situation
- Progressive neurologic deficit

DISCHARGE CRITERIA

- Most patients can be treated on outpatient basis
- Orthopedic follow-up arranged
- Social support system in place
- Pain control
- Patient education

PEDIATRIC CONSIDERATIONS

- Close follow-up is mandatory

Miscellaneous

ICD9: 721.90, 756.12

CORE CONTENT CODE: 10.3.2

SUGGESTED READINGS

Congeni J, McCulloch J, Swanson K. Lumbar spondylolysis. A study of natural progression in athletes. Am J Sports Med 1997;25(2):248–253.

Nachemson A. Newest knowledge of low back pain. Clin Orthop 1992;279:8.

Skinner H. Disorders, diseases and injuries of the spine. In: Current diagnosis and treatment in orthopedics. Norwalk, CT: Appleton & Lange, 1995:206–211.

Vitek G. Spine conference—Spondylolysis and spondylolisthesis. OrthoNews Magazine May 1995; http://www.nmis.com/onm/html/sponconf_spon.htm.

Authors: Kathleen J. Clem; Steven M. Green

Spontaneous Bacterial Peritonitis

Clinical Presentation

SIGNS AND SYMPTOMS

- *Often asymptomatic*
- Abdominal pain, usually mild
- Direct or rebound tenderness
- Fever, chills
- Hypothermia
- Onset or worsening of ascites
- Development or worsening hepatic encephalopathy
- Nausea and vomiting
- Hypoactive bowel sounds
- Hypotension
- Worsening liver or renal function

MECHANISM/DESCRIPTION

- Translocation of bacteria through edematous gut mucosa, caused by portal hypertension, into lymph nodes to the peritoneal cavity
- Transient bacteremia, along with low serum complement
- Impaired reticuloendothelial system phagocytic activity and *low ascitic fluid protein* (<1 g/dl), opsonin, and bactericidal activity

ETIOLOGY

- Usually seen in setting of liver cirrhosis, especially in decompensated jaundiced patients
- Rare in other conditions causing ascites (e.g., nephrotic syndrome, and CHF)
- Predominant organisms
  —*E. coli* (45%)
  —Pneumococcus (20%)
  —*Klebsiella* (10%)
  —Enterobacter
  —Proteus
  —*Citrobacter freundii*
  —Enterococcus (5%)
- Polymicrobial is rare (<5%)

Pre-Hospital

CAUTIONS

- IV fluid bolus for unstable vital signs or shock or hypothermia

Diagnosis

ESSENTIAL WORKUP

- Paracentesis
  —Polymorphonuclear (PMN) cell count >250/μL diagnostic
  —Inject 10 ml of ascitic fluid in each blood culture bottle to maximize the yield
  —Gram stain—infrequently positive
  —Repeat paracentesis after 48 hours of treatment to monitor response

LABORATORY

- CBC
  —Anemia
  —Leukocytosis
- Liver profile/liver enzymes
- PT/PTT
  —Elevated PT
- Blood cultures are infrequently positive
- Spot urine for sodium and creatinine
- Other tests as noted in ascites section
- Serum albumin-ascitic gradient (SAAG) remains wide (i.e., >1.1 g/dl)

IMAGING/SPECIAL TESTS

- Abdominal US
  —Confirms presence of ascites (if volume small)
  —Helps guide paracentesis
- CXR for pneumonia, CHF, effusion
- Abdominal radiograph for obstruction/perforation

DIFFERENTIAL DIAGNOSIS

- Culture-negative neutrocytic ascites
  —Ascitic PMN >250 μL but the culture is negative
  —May progress to spontaneous bacterial peritonitis (SBP)—treated similarly
  —Consider secondary cause TB or malignancy if PMN count does not drop with treatment
- Secondary bacterial peritonitis
  —Due to perforation or abscess
  —Multiple organisms, especially anaerobes
  —Ascitic glucose <50 mg/dl
  —Ascitic protein >1 g/dl
  —Ascitic PMN >10,000/μL
- Monomicrobial bacterial ascites
  —PMN <250 μL but the culture is positive
  —If contamination cannot be ruled out, treat as SBP
- Polymicrobial bacterial ascites
  —PMN <250 μL but the culture is positive for multiple organisms
  —Suspicious of accidental gut perforation by the paracentesis needle (rare)
- High acites WBC (>500/ul) with lymphocyte prominence favor TB, malignancy or chylous acites

Treatment

INITIAL STABILIZATION

- ABCs
- Aggressive IV fluid resuscitation and prompt antibiotic treatment for septic shock

ED TREATMENT

- Correct coagulopathy prior to large volume paracentesis with large-bore needle
  - —Administer 2 units FFP if PT >16
  - —Administer 10 IU platelets if platelet count <50,000
- Initiate antibiotic for ascitic fluid PMN >250 µL—*do not* wait for culture result
  - —First choice: third generation cephalosporin (cefotaxime or ceftriaxone)
  - —Second-generation cephalosporin, ampicillin and sulbactam combination, or aztreonam provides lesser cure rate
  - —*Avoid* aminoglycosides—cirrhotic patients at high risk for nephrotoxicity
- Subsequent antibiotic choice depends on culture and sensitivity result
- Administer antibiotics for 10 days
  - —May use 5-day course if the ascitic PMN drops by 50% after 48 hours of treatment
- Higher mortality rate and poor infection resolution seen with
  - —Hospital-acquired SBP
  - —High BUN
  - —High band count in the blood
  - —High AST
  - —Presence of ileus
- Oral quinolones (ofloxacin or ciprofloxacin) for patients refusing IV antibiotics
  - —Not tested in patients who have severe HE, GI bleed, ileus, septic shock, creatinine level >3 mg/dl
- Predictors of high recurrence rate (up to 69% in 1 year)
  - —Ascitic protein <1 g/dl
  - —Serum bilirubin >4 mg/dl
  - —Prolonged prothrombin time
  - —Benefit from prophylactic norfloxacin 400 mg/day, or trimethoprim-sulfamethizole 1 D.S. tablet 5 days/week

MEDICATIONS

- Bactrim DS: 1 tablet 5 days/week
- Cefotaxime: 2 g (peds: 50–180 mg/kg/24hrs) IV q 8 hrs
- Ceftriaxone: 2 g (peds: 50–75 mg/kg/24hrs) IV q 24 hrs
- Ciprofloxacin: 500 mg po bid
- Ofloxacin: 400 mg po bid
- Norfloxacin: 400 mg/day

PEDIATRIC CONSIDERATIONS

- Quinolones: not tested in children with SBP

Disposition

ADMISSION CRITERIA

- Admit all patients with SBP with a gastroenterologist consult
- ICU admission if in septic shock or hepatic encephalopathy

DISCHARGE CRITERIA

- Patients refusing inpatient care
  - —Administer dose of ceftriaxone followed by oral quinolones for 10 days

Miscellaneous

ICD9: 567.2

CORE CONTENT CODE: 1.9.3

SUGGESTED READINGS

Garcia-Tsoa G. Treatment of spontaneous bacterial peritonitis with oral ofloxacin: Inpatient or outpatient therapy? Gastroenterol 1996;11:1147.

Gilbert JA, Kamath PS. Spontaneous bacterial peritonitis. Mayo Clin Proc 1995;70:365.

Guarner C, Soriano G. Spontaneous bacterial peritonitis. Sem Liver Dis. 1997:17;203–217.

Author: Abbas Zagnoon

Sporotrichosis

Clinical Presentation

SIGNS AND SYMPTOMS

- Varies with the form of the disease
- Three forms
  - —Cutaneous
  - —Extracutaneous
  - —Multifocal extracutaneous

Cutaneous

- Distal extremities most commonly involved
- Initial lesions appear 1 week to several months following inoculation
  - —Erythematous papule
  - —Either smooth or verrucous
  - —Size: millimeters to 2–4 cm
- Multiple secondary lesions usually develop along lymphatics draining original site (lymphocutaneous)
- May ulcerate late
- Painless
- No constitutional symptoms unless lesions are secondarily infected
- May wax and wane over years if untreated

Extracutaneous

Osteoarticular

- Most common
- Single or multijoint involvement of extremities
- Indolent onset
- Joint inflammation with few systemic symptoms
- Multiple joints (become involved hematogenously)
- Tenosynovitis, osteomyelitis, and bursitis

Pulmonary

- Clinical syndrome and CXR resemble mycobacterial infection
- Low-grade fever
- Productive cough
- Weight loss

Meningitis

- Least common
- Chronic lymphocytic meningitis
- Indolent course

Multifocal Extracutaneous

- Low-grade fever
- Weight loss
- Diffuse cutaneous lesions
- Arthritis/osteolytic lesions/parenchymal involvement
- Can be fatal if untreated

MECHANISM/DESCRIPTION

Cutaneous

- Most common (75%)
- Greatest risk: farmers, gardeners, and forestry workers

Pulmonary

- From inhalation of conidia
- 66% are either alcoholics or otherwise immunosuppressed

Multifocal Extracutaneous

- Affects HIV/immunosuppressed patients

ETIOLOGY

- Fungal infection caused by *Sporothrix schenckii*
- Dimorphic fungus occurs as a mold on plants in temperate and tropical environments
- Cats and armadillos vectors
- Infection occurs by direct inoculation into the skin or through inhalation of sporelike conidia

Pre-Hospital

N/A

Diagnosis

ESSENTIAL WORKUP

- Diagnosis dependent on culture or demonstration of organism in tissue or fluid
  - —Biopsy from skin lesions or synovial tissue
  - —Blood, sputum, and CSF cultures

LABORATORY

- Blood tests not indicated with cutaneous disease

IMAGING/SPECIAL TESTS

- Tissue examination
  - —Granulomas
  - —Microabscesses
  - —Occasional cigar-shaped yeasts
- With lung involvement
  - —CXR mimics reactivation TB
  - —Sputum Gram stain—yeast
  - —Cultures usually positive
- Bone scan for multifocal disease and immunosuppressed with isolated cutaneous involvement

DIFFERENTIAL DIAGNOSIS

- Cutaneous infection
  - —Bacterial pyoderma
  - —Foreign body granuloma
  - —Inflammatory dermatophyte infections (Majocchi's granuloma)
  - —Blastomycosis
  - —Chromoblastomycosis
  - —Cutaneous tuberculosis
- Osteoarticular disease
  - —Rheumatoid arthritis
  - —Gout
  - —TB
  - —Pigmented villonodular synovitis
  - —Bacterial arthritis
- Pneumonia and meningitis
  - —Histoplasmosis
  - —Coccidioidomycosis
  - —Cryptococcal disease
  - —Mycobacterial infections

Treatment

INITIAL STABILIZATION

- ABCs for severely ill patients with extracutaneous manifestations

ED TREATMENT

Cutaneous Form

- Systemic azole antifungals (itraconazole) better than classic saturated solution potassium iodide (SSKI.)
  - —SSKI less expensive but compliance and side effects (anorexia, nausea, metallic taste, etc.) limit acceptability
- Itraconazole more effective than ketoconazole or fluconazole
- Therapy may take months

Extracutaneous Form

- Itraconazole for stable patients with disseminated and isolated osteoarticular disease
- Amphotericin B for
  - —Acutely ill
  - —Meningitis
  - —Disseminated
  - —Immunosuppressed host
- Pulmonary form
  - —Combined drug and surgical resection may be necessary

Adjunctive Measures

- Local heat kills fungus
- Especially useful in pregnancy and drug intolerance

MEDICATIONS

- Amphotericin B: start 0.25 mg/kg IV q day, advance to 0.5–1.5 mg/kg IV q day
- Itraconazole: 300 mg po bid for up to 6 months then 200 mg po bid long-term if needed
- Saturated solution of potassium iodide (SSKI): 5 drops in water or juice tid; increase by 5 drops each week up to a maximum of 40–50 drops tid as tolerated, for 6–12 weeks or until the lesions resolve

Disposition

ADMISSION CRITERIA

- Pulmonary, CNS, multifocal disease

DISCHARGE CRITERIA

Cutaneous Form

- With immunosuppressed host discharge if no evidence of occult disseminated disease

Miscellaneous

ICD9: 117.1

CORE CONTENT CODE: 9.2

SUGGESTED READINGS

Kauffman CA. Old and new therapies for sporotrichosis. Clin Infect Dis 1995;21(4):981–985.

Winn RE. A contemporary view of sporotrichosis. Curr Top Med Mycol 1995;6:73–94.

Authors: Maurice De Fina; Robert Powers

Staphylococcal Scalded Skin Syndrome

Clinical Presentation

SIGNS AND SYMPTOMS

- Prior to rash
  - —Malaise
  - —Irritability
  - —Fever
  - —Tender Skin
- Diffuse erythematous rash
- Scarlatiniform erythroderma
- Resembles a diffuse sunburn
- Abrupt onset
- Sandpaper-like appearance
- Painful
- Increased erythema in skin creases
- Cracks in the mouth and eyes
- Skin desquamation
- Absence of bullae
- Initial common locations
  - -Neck
  - -Intertriginous areas
  - -Around the eyes and mouth
- Flaccid bullae
  - —Within 1–3 days after onset of erythematous rash
  - —Initially over flexures
  - —Bullae migrate through epidermis with light lateral pressure (Nikolsky's sign)
  - —Rupture within a few hours
  - —Epidermis is then shed in sheets of tender moist red skin
  - —Complete healing within 2 weeks
- Pharyngitis
- Superficial erosions of oral mucosa
- Conjunctivitis
  - —Purulent discharge without conjunctival injection

MECHANISM/DESCRIPTION

- Rash resulting from an exotoxin produced by *Staphylococcal aureus*
- Water-soluble epidermolytic toxin
  - —Produced at a remote location of the infection
  - —Disseminates and lyses desmosomes of granular cells in the superficial epidermis
  - —Results in desquamation
- Coagulase positive phage Group II staph
  - —Rarely Group I or Group III
- Multiple presentations based on the age and rash
  - —Classic staphylococcal scalded skin syndrome (Ritter's disease)
  - —Pemphigus neonatorum
- Disease of children less than 10 years of age
- Complications are rare
  - —Electrolyte imbalance
  - —Septicemia
  - —Pneumonia
  - —Cellulitis

ETIOLOGY

- Infection of circumcision site in male infants
- Conjunctivitis
- Minor skin wounds
- Preceding impetigo skin eruptions
- Pharyngitis
- Gastroenteritis

Pre-Hospital

N/A

Diagnosis

ESSENTIAL WORKUP

- Clinical presentation is diagnostic
- Determine source of staph infection

LABORATORY

- CBC and urinalysis
  - —Assess for sepsis if the diagnosis is not absolutely clear
- Electrolytes
  - —Indicated is signs of dehydration or widespread rash
- Blood cultures
  - —Rarely positive

IMAGING/SPECIAL TESTS

- Fluid aspirated from bullae
  - —Sterile in staph scalded skin syndrome
  - —Purulent fluid is more consistent with bullous impetigo
- Skin biopsy
  - —Children on medication preceding the rash
  - —Children >6 years of age
  - —Mixed rash

DIFFERENTIAL DIAGNOSIS

- Neonates
  - —Bullous impetigo
  - —Epidermolysis bullosa
  - —Epidermolytic hyperkeratosis
  - —Boric acid poisoning
- Drug hypersensitivity toxic epidermal necrolysis
  - —Much more common in adults
- Scarlet fever
  - —Involves the mucous membranes
  - —Painful desquamation does not occur
  - —Strawberry tongue
- Bullous impetigo
  - —Turbid or cloudy bullae fluid
- Bullous varicella
  - —5 days after the onset of varicella
  - —Tzank prep of viral base reveals giant cells
- Toxic shock syndrome
- Secondary rash of an underlying disorder
  - —Lymphoma
  - —Aspergillosis
  - —Irradiation
  - —Graft vs. host reaction
  - —Kawasaki's disease
  - —Leptospirosis

Treatment

INITIAL STABILIZATION

- Management is similar to that for burns
  - —Large percentage of involved skin surface requires intravenous fluids
- Undress and place on sterile linen
- Handle child as little as possible
- Apply cool saline compresses
- Parenteral fluids if signs of dehydration

ED TREATMENT

- Intravenous antibiotics effective against penicillinase resistant staph
  - —Cefazolin
  - —Oxacillin
  - —Nafcillin
- Oral antibiotics for mild involvement
  - —Dicloxacillin
  - —Erythromycin

MEDICATIONS

- Cefazolin: 5–50 mg/kg IV divided qid
- Nafcillin: 50–100 mg/kg/day IV divided q 6 hrs in the newborn; 100–200 mg/kg/day IV divided q 6 hrs in children; 1–2 g IV q 6 hrs in adults
- Dicloxacillin: 12–25 mg/kg po divided qid
- Erythromycin: 30–50 mg/kg po divided qid

Disposition

ADMISSION CRITERIA

- Children <1 year of age
- All toxic appearing children
- Widespread skin involvement
- Dehydration
- Electrolyte imbalance

DISCHARGE CRITERIA

- Older children
- Mild involvement
- Oral antibiotics for 7 days
- Follow-up within 48 hours

Miscellaneous

ICD9: 695.1

CORE CONTENT CODE: 3.6.2

SUGGESTED READINGS

Cribier B, Piemont Y, Grosshans E. Staphylococcal scalded skin syndrome in adults. A clinical review illustrated with a new case. J Am Acad Derm 1994;30(2):319–324.

Feigin RD, Cherry JD, eds. Textbook of pediatric infectious diseases. Philadelphia: WB Saunders, 1992:1254–1257.

Gemell CG. Staphylococcal scalded skin syndrome. J Med Microbiol 1995;43(5):318–327.

Mandell GL, Douglass RG, Benett JE. Principles and practice of infectious diseases. 4th ed. New York: Churchill Livingstone, 1994:1759–1761.

Author: J. Brian Liddy; Timothy J. Mader

Sternoclavicular Joint Injury

Clinical Presentation

SIGNS AND SYMPTOMS

- Patient presents with the affected arm foreshortened and supported across the chest by opposite hand
- Inability to abduct or externally rotate the affected arm because of severe pain over sternoclavicular junction
- In *anterior dislocation,* medial end of the clavicle is visibly prominent, palpable, and may be fixed or mobile
- In *posterior dislocation,* loss of normal inner prominence of the clavicular head may be masked by significant local swelling
  - —Head tilted toward injured side because of spasm of the sternocleidomastoid muscle
  - —Venous congestion in the neck or upper extremities, diminished pulses on affected extremity, shortness of breath, hoarseness, dysphagia, or signs of shock may suggest life-threatening impingement of the posteriorly displaced clavicle upon vascular structures in the mediastinum

MECHANISM/DESCRIPTION

- The sternoclavicular joint (SCJ) can dislocate in the anterior or posterior direction
- It is among the least frequently dislocated joints in the body
- Due primarily to trauma from vehicular or athletic injuries; congenital dislocations are extremely rare
- *Anterior dislocation* is much more common
  - —Caused by an anterolateral force compressing the shoulder followed by backward rolling
- *Posterior dislocation* is caused either from a direct anterior-to-posterior blow to the medial clavicle or from a posterolateral force compressing the shoulder followed by forward rolling
- *Posterior dislocation is a surgical emergency*
  - —Compression of trachea, esophagus, and great vessels in the mediastinum demand immediate reduction

PEDIATRIC CONSIDERATIONS

- The medial physeal growth plates of the clavicles fuse between ages 22 and 25
- True dislocations of the SCJ are extremely rare in children because of the strong ligamentous attachments about the medial physis
- Fractures through the medial physis mimic SCJ dislocations
- In patients less than 25 years of age, SCJ dislocations are classified as Salter-Harris Type I or II fractures

Pre-Hospital

CAUTIONS

- Vital signs and an initial neurovascular exam of the affected extremity are mandatory
- The affected arm should be splinted in the position of most comfort prior to transport to the hospital

Diagnosis

ESSENTIAL WORKUP

- Careful history to elicit mechanism of injury, time from the injury, and initial symptoms
- Respiratory, neurologic, and vascular assessments mandatory
- Appropriate analgesia for patient comfort

IMAGING/SPECIAL TESTS

- Rockwood view: x-ray beam aimed at manubrium in a 40° caudal tilt
- Plain chest radiograph is needed to rule out possible pneumothorax in patients with posterior dislocation
- CT scan is the best study to evaluate the SCJ
  - —Useful in the ED when plain films are inconclusive
  - —Accurately differentiate fractures from dislocations
  - —Demonstrates the position of the medial end of the clavicle in relation to the structures in the mediastinum
  - —Shows detailed anatomy of the structures of the thoracic outlet and mediastinum

DIFFERENTIAL DIAGNOSIS

- Sternoclavicular sprain/subluxation
- Medial clavicle fracture
- Septic joint
- Osteoarthritis

Treatment

INITIAL STABILIZATION

- Patients in respiratory distress require endotracheal intubation and immediate reduction
- Emergent reduction is also needed in patients with hoarseness, dysphagia, or neurovascular compromise (upper extremity weakness, paresthesia, diminished pulses, signs of shock)
- *Patients with posterior dislocations represent true orthopedic and surgical emergencies* and appropriate consults should be obtained promptly
- Appropriate analgesia (e.g., narcotics or NSAIDs) necessary for pain control

ED TREATMENT

- *Anterior dislocations* may be reduced in the ED
- Conscious sedation is necessary for pain control and muscle relaxation
- A rolled towel is placed between the shoulder blades in the supine position
  —Longitudinal traction is applied to the ipsilateral arm in the extended position with the shoulder abducted at 90°
  —An assistant can maintain gentle inward pressure over the displaced medical end of the clavicle
  —After reduction, immobilization is achieved using a well-padded figure-eight dressing
  —Many anterior dislocations remain unstable after reduction; however, open reduction and internal fixation is rarely indicated as the deformity is mainly cosmetic without functional loss
  —*Posterior dislocations* require prompt reduction, best achieved in the OR under general anesthesia
  —If an appropriate surgeon is not immediately available to reduce a posterior dislocation in the OR, reduction may be attempted in the ED to relieve serious airway, neurologic, or vascular compromise
  —After adequate sedation, a small incision is made directly over the medial head of the clavicle
  —A sterile towel clamp can carefully be used to encircle the medial clavicular head and gentle anterior traction applied to reduce the dislocation
  —A surgical consultant should subsequently evaluate the patient

PEDIATRIC CONSIDERATIONS

- During childhood, the medial physeal growth plate of the clavicle provides 80% of longitudinal bone growth
- Fractures in the medial clavicle have tremendous capability for healing and remodeling
- Nonunion and significant malunion rarely occur
- Anteriorly displaced fractures of the medial clavicle that mimic SCJ dislocation can be placed in a figure-eight splint without reduction
- Posteriorly displaced fractures uniformly require reduction and should be considered a surgical and orthopedic emergency

MEDICATIONS

- Patients may require oral analgesics upon discharge
  —Acetaminophen: 500–1000 mg q 6 hrs PRN
  —Ibuprofen: 400–800 mg q 6 hrs PRN with meals
  —Acetaminophen 300 mg with codeine: 30 mg q 6 hrs PRN

Disposition

ADMISSION CRITERIA

- All posterior dislocations of the SCJ require admission for prompt reduction in the operating room and evaluation for potential intrathoracic complications

DISCHARGE CRITERIA

- Anterior dislocations of the SCJ that can be reduced and splinted, in the absence of neurovascular compromise, may be discharged with appropriate orthopedic follow-up

Miscellaneous

ICD9: 810.01

CORE CONTENT CODE: 18.4.10.5

SUGGESTED READINGS

Cope R. Dislocations of the sternoclavicular joint. Skeletal Radiol 1993;22:233–238.

Cope R, Riddervold HO, Shore JL, et al. Dislocations of the sternoclavicular joint: Anatomic basis, etiologies, and radiologic diagnosis. J Orthop Trauma 1991;5(3): 379–384.

Gardner MH, Bidstrup BP. Intrathoracic great vessel injury resulting from blunt chest trauma associated with posterior dislocation of the sternoclavicular joint. Aust N Z J Surg 1983;53:427–430.

Lewonowski K, Bassett GS. Complete posterior sternoclavicular epiphyseal separation. Clin Orthop 1992;281:84–88.

Winter J, Sterner S, Maurer D, et al. Retrosternal epiphyseal disruption of medial clavicle: Case and review in children. J Emerg Med 1988;7:9–13.

Authors: Robert Chang; Wallace Carter

Stevens-Johnson Syndrome

Clinical Presentation

SIGNS AND SYMPTOMS

- *Prodrome:* fever, headache, malaise, URI symptoms, arthritis, arthralgias, and myalgias
- *Rash:* target lesions, erythematous, or purpuric macules with or without confluence and small blisters or bullae with skin detachment
- *Mucous membrane:* erosions of the mouth, pharynx, trachea, genitalia, or anus, and may have pseudomembrane formation
- *Eye:* mild to severe conjunctivitis with possible formation of pseudomembranes and corneal ulcers

MECHANISM/DESCRIPTION

- Stevens-Johnson syndrome (SJS) is a severe mucocutaneous disease, which has these features
  - —Blistering of less than 10% of the body surface area
  - —Confluent erosions of at least two mucous membranes
  - —Lesions often begin on dorsal surface of hands and feet, extensor surfaces, and spread centrally
  - —Lesions involve entire epidermal layer
- Stevens-Johnson syndrome, erythema multiforme minor, and toxic epidermal necrolysis (TEN) may be considered variations of the same disease. SJS and TEN are also classified as erythema multiforme major

ETIOLOGY

- The most common etiologies include medications and infections. Circulating immune complexes play an important role in the pathogenesis. An immune mechanism is widely accepted but yet unproven
- *Causative medications:* Sulfonamides, antibiotics, anticonvulsants, NSAIDs, and allopurinol have been associated with these severe cutaneous drug reactions
- *Infections:* Mycoplasma pneumonia and herpes simplex are well-recognized causes of erythema multiforme and Stevens-Johnson syndrome

Pre-Hospital

CAUTIONS

- Patients with significant cutaneous involvement may sustain fluid loss and require IV crystalloid replacement

Diagnosis

ESSENTIAL WORKUP

- A complete history and physical examination with careful attention to mucous membranes, percent of blistering, and identification of likely etiology

LABORATORY

- Electrolytes, liver enzymes, complete blood count, urinalysis, and ESR may be useful

IMAGING/SPECIAL TESTS

- Chest radiography if pneumonia is a consideration
- Skin biopsy of lesions and mucous membranes demonstrate necrosis of the entire epidermal layer

DIFFERENTIAL DIAGNOSIS

- Overlapping Stevens-Johnson syndrome-toxic epidermal necrolysis (skin detachment between 10% and 30% of the body surface area plus widespread macules or flat atypical target lesions)
- Toxic epidermal necrolysis (skin detachment greater than 30% of the body surface area plus widespread macules or flat atypical targets)
- Pemphigus vulgaris
- Bullous pemphigoid (a chronic bullous eruption most commonly presenting in the elderly)
- Epidermolysis bullosa

PEDIATRIC CONSIDERATIONS

- Staphylococcal-scalded skin syndrome is in the pediatric differential diagnosis of severe blistering mucocutaneous diseases
- Bullous impetigo

Treatment

INITIAL STABILIZATION

- ABCs
  - —Endotracheal intubation and ventilatory support may be required for impending respiratory failure (more commonly associated with TEN)
  - —Intravenous fluids

ED TREATMENT

- Recognize and treat underlying infections
  - —Sepsis is the primary cause of death frequently from gram negative pneumonia
- Secondarily infected cutaneous lesions can be treated with debridement of blisters, compresses, and systemic antibiotics
- Steroids are controversial
- Prophylactic antibiotics are not indicated
- Mild systemic symptoms may be treated with acetaminophen or NSAIDs, provided that they are not the cause of the mucocutaneous reaction
- Mucous membrane lesions are extremely painful and may require parenteral analgesics
- Large extensive bullae should be debrided, ideally in a burn unit

MEDICATIONS

- Acetaminophen: adult: 650–975 mg PO/PR; peds: 15 mg/kg/dose
- Acyclovir: 5–10 mg/kg IV q 8 hrs (for HSV infections)
- Erythromycin: 4–5 mg/kg IV q 6 hrs
- Ibuprofen: adult: 300–800 mg po; peds: 5–10 mg/kg/dose
- Meperidine: 1–1.8 mg/kg/dose IV
- Morphine sulfate: 0.1 mg/kg/dose IV

Disposition

ADMISSION CRITERIA

- Patients with Stevens-Johnson syndrome should be admitted to the hospital
- Patients with extensive epidermal detachment should be admitted to a burn center

DISCHARGE CRITERIA

- Patients with erythema multiforme minor may be discharged with appropriate follow-up

Miscellaneous

ICD9: 695.1

CORE CONTENT CODE: 3.5.1

SUGGESTED READINGS

Bastujj-Garin S, Rzany B, Stern RS. Clinical classification of cases of toxic epidermal necrolysis, Stevens-Johnson syndrome, and erythema multiforme. Arch Dermatol 1993;129:92–96.

Jorizzo JL. Blood vessel-based inflammatory disorders. In: Moschella, Hurley, eds. Dermatology. 3rd ed. Philadelphia: WB Saunders, 1992:580–583.

Roujeau JC, Kelly JP, Naldi L, et al. Medication use and the risk of Stevens-Johnson syndrome or toxic epidermal necrolysis. N Engl J Med 1995;333:1600–1607.

Authors: James A. Comes; Herbert G. Bivins

Stridor

Clinical Presentation

SIGNS AND SYMPTOMS

- —Grunting or wheezing with inspiration
- —Shortness of breath
- —Effort required to inhale
- —Increased respiratory rate
- —Use of accessory muscles with inspiration
- —Nasal flaring
- —Respiratory distress and fatigue
  - -Cyanosis
  - -Diaphoresis
  - -Agitation
  - -Somnolence
  - -Decreased respiratory rate
- Certain findings can suggest the underlying cause
- Age between 1–4
  - —Foreign body
  - —Croup
  - —Epiglottitis is more common if the child has not received the vaccine for *Hemophilus influenzae*
- Cough
- Rhinorrhea
  - —Croup
  - —Allergy
- Fever
  - —Infection
- Drooling and inability to control oral secretions
  - —Obstruction proximal to glottis

MECHANISM/DESCRIPTION

- A harsh vibrating sound heard during inspiration in cases of obstruction of the upper airway

ETIOLOGY

- Infection
  - —Bacterial tracheitis
  - —Croup
  - —Diphtheria
  - —Epiglottitis
  - —Peritonsillar abscess
  - —Retropharyngeal abscess
  - —Supraglottitis
  - —Uvulitis
- Subglottic stenosis
  - —Radiation therapy
  - —Postoperative scarring after cricothyrotomy
- Angioedema
- Bilateral vocal cord paralysis
  - —Surgical injury
  - —Overinflation of endotracheal tube cuffs or prolonged endotracheal intubation
  - —Thyroid gland malignancies
  - —Mediastinal masses
- Intraluminal obstruction of the trachea
  - —Cyst
  - —Invasive Tumors
    - -Squamous cell carcinomas
    - -Lymphomas
    - -Thyroid carcinomas
    - -These may invade the larynx or trachea and make endotracheal intubation impossible
  - —Laryngeal or tracheal papilloma
  - —Foreign body
- Extrinsic compression
  - —Trauma
  - —Hematoma
  - —Vascular anomalies (rings and slings)

Pre-Hospital

- Maintenance of an adequate airway
- Bag-valve-ventilation if respiratory status deteriorates
- Intubate if bag-valve-mask-ventilation is ineffective
- Rapid transport with ED notification

CAUTIONS

- Avoid agitating children

CONTROVERSIES

- Racemic epinephrine

Diagnosis

ESSENTIAL WORKUP

- Visualization of the upper airway in a safe environment
  - —Often direct visualization in the operating room with a surgeon prepared to perform a tracheostomy is the safest approach

LABORATORY

- Not generally helpful
- Obtaining blood samples from children should be avoided until the airway has been stabilized

IMAGING/SPECIAL TESTS

- Radiograph of lateral neck
  - —Not essential
  - —Should not be obtained if there is risk of acute airway obstruction
- Direct laryngoscopy
  - —Diagnostic study of choice
  - —Should be performed in a setting where rapid surgical airway intervention can be performed

DIFFERENTIAL DIAGNOSIS

- Munchausen
  - —Patient intentionally breaths against a closed glottis
- Bronchospasm

Treatment

INITIAL STABILIZATION

- Supplemental oxygen
  - —100% nonrebreather by face mask
  - —In children, avoid face mask upsetting the child

ED TREATMENT

- Airway management
  - —Stridor defines a difficult airway
    - -Before attempting intubation be prepared to perform a surgical airway
    - -When possible intubation should be attempted in the operating room
    - -Choose a tube 1–2 sizes smaller than expected
  - —Oral awake intubation
    - -Ketamine induction
    - -Patient will continue to ventilate during the procedure
    - -Method of choice if the patient cannot be adequately ventilated by bag-mask
  - —Avoid blind nasotracheal intubation

MEDICATIONS

N/A

Disposition

ADMISSION CRITERIA

- All cases of stridor require admission until the underlying problem is completely resolved

DISCHARGE CRITERIA

N/A

Miscellaneous

ICD9: 786.1

CORE CONTENT CODE: N/A

SUGGESTED READINGS

Lesperance MM: Assessment and management of loryngotracheal stenosis. Pediatr Clin North Am 1996;43:1413–27.

Milam SB: Supraglotlic airway infections. Prim Care 1996;23:741–58.

Author: Richard Wolfe

Subarachnoid Hemorrhage

Clinical Presentation

SIGNS AND SYMPTOMS

- *Sudden onset* ("thunderclap") of severe constant headache
- Often occipital and different than prior headaches ("worst headache ever")
- Vomiting, diaphoresis and meningeal signs may occur
- Classically without focal deficits
  —Arteriovenous malformation (AVM) may present with focal neurologic deficits
- Nuchal rigidity (most common sign)
  —Absence of neck stiffness does not exclude subarachnoid hemorrhage (SAH)
- Sudden, usually transient, loss of consciousness
- Subhyaloid (preretinal) hemorrhages
- Seizures (up to 25%)
- Coma (up to 25%)

ETIOLOGY

- Most cases of SAH result from either rupture of a cerebral aneurysm (most commonly Berry aneurysm at the circle of Willis) or a bleeding AVM
- The majority of hemorrhages occur before the age of 50
- Overall more common in women, but men dominate under age 40
- Rupture of an aneurysm occurs at a time of increased stress or elevated blood pressure

MECHANISM/DESCRIPTION

- Bleeding occurs outside of the brain parenchyma into the CSF
- *Sentinel* hemorrhage results from small amounts of blood leaking from an aneurysm
  —30% will subsequently rupture
- 10–30% of SAH will rebleed within 3 weeks, greatest risk is within first 24 hours

PEDIATRIC CONSIDERATIONS

- In children, AVM is the most common lesion associated with spontaneous SAH

Pre-Hospital

CAUTIONS

- Patients may rapidly progress to unresponsiveness, emergent endotracheal intubation may be necessary to protect the airway and provide mild hyperventilation
- Careful initial neurologic exam is essential including evaluation of level of consciousness, Glasgow Coma Scale and gross focal deficits
- 12% die before receiving medical attention

Diagnosis

- Most important prognostic factor is the clinical condition at time of presentation. Hunt-Hess grading scale is frequently used for evaluation of SAH
  —Grade I: asymptomatic or mild headache
  —Grade II: moderate/severe headache, nuchal rigidity, with or without cranial nerve deficit
  —Grade III: confusion, lethargy, or mild focal symptoms
  —Grade IV: stupor or hemiparesis
  —Grade V: comatose or extensor posturing

ESSENTIAL WORKUP

- Complete neurological examination
- Emergent noncontrast head CT scan will diagnose 90%
- Lumbar puncture is mandatory if CT scan is negative

LABORATORY

- Lumbar puncture
  —Xanthochromia of the supernatant after centrifugation of the CSF is diagnostic of SAH (preferably by spectrophotometry instead of visual inspection)
  —Blood in a nontraumatic tap confirms the diagnosis
  —RBCs that do not clear in later tubes supports the diagnosis
- Electrocardiogram
  —May see broad or inverted T waves, QT prolongation, ST elevation or depression, U waves

IMAGING/SPECIAL TESTS

- CT without contrast is >90% accurate for parenchymal bleeds
- CT is superior to MRI in detecting acute hemorrhage (<12 hours), whereas MRI is superior in detecting infarcts, aneurysms, and AVM
- Angiography is the criterion standard for SAH/aneurysm

DIFFERENTIAL DIAGNOSIS

- Subdural/epidural hematoma
- Carotid dissection after neck trauma
- Migraine and tension headaches
- Meningitis
- Dementia
- Brain tumor/abscess

Treatment

INITIAL STABILIZATION

- ABCs
  - —RSI and mild hyperventilation to PCO_2 of ~35 for suspected increased ICP
  - —Maintain adequate mean arterial pressure with crystalloid infusion to optimize cerebral perfusion pressure
  - —Urgent neurosurgical consultation
  - —Prophylaxis for seizures is controversial but a seizure increases the risk of rebleeding
  - —Calcium channel blockers (nimodipine) to prevent vasospasm

ED TREATMENT

- Risk of rebleed is greatest in the first 24 hours
  - —Severe hypertension must be treated, but antihypertensives in the ED are generally not indicated because compromise of cerebral perfusion pressure has potentially more deleterious effects than lowering of blood pressure
  - —Keeping SBP $<$160 mm Hg while maintaining MAP in 110 mm Hg range has been associated with lower risk of rebleeding
- Rebleeding prevention
  - —Strict bedrest, elevate head of bed 30°
  - —Control pain with mild analgesia but avoid oversedation
  - —Prevent vomiting and straining with antiemetics and stool softeners
- Vasospasm
  - —Typically occurs 3–12 days after SAH, but may be seen in ED with delayed presentation
  - —Begin nimodipine for patient in Hunt-Hess grades I, II, and III
  - —Maintain euvolemia and adequate cerebral perfusion pressure
- Hydrocephalus and increased intracranial pressure
  - —Mild hyperventilation
  - —Mannitol
- Administer anticrilestic medication
  - —Phenytoin

MEDICATIONS

- Antiemetics
  - —Diphenhydramine (benadryl): adult: 25–50 mg PO/IM/IV TID/QID; peds: 5 mg/kg/24hrs q 6 hrs, max 300 mg/24hrs
  - —Prochlorperazine (compazine): adult: 5–10 mg IV/PO q 6 hrs; peds: 0.1 mg/kg/dose IM/IV
  - —Promethazine (phenergan): adult: 25–50 PO/PR/IM q 4 hrs; peds: (phenergan syrup) po ages 2–6: 1.25 cc q 4–6 hrs; ages 6–12: 2.5 cc q 4–6 hrs; age $>$12: 5 cc q 4–6 hrs
- Antivasospasm agents
  - —Nimodipine: 60 mg po q 6 hrs given to all patients with SAH grade I, II, or III
- Seizure prophylaxis
  - —Phenytoin load to prevent rebleed from seizure: adult:1 g IV not to exceed 50 mg/min; peds: 15–20 mg/kg IV max 1000 mg/24hrs
  - —Diazepam: adult: 5–10 mg IV q 10–15 min, max 30 mg; peds: 0.2–0.3 mg/kg q 5–10 min, max 10 mg
  - —Lorazepam: adult: 2–4 mg IV q 15 min PRN; peds: 0.03–0.05 mg/kg/dose, max 4 mg/dose
- Antihypertensives
  - —Esmolol: adult and peds: 1 mg/kg IV load then 100–150 μg/kg/min
  - —Hydralazine: adult: 10–20 mg IV q 30 min; peds: safety not established
  - —Labetalol: adult: 20 mg/min IV bolus, then 20–80 mg q 10 min, max 300 mg; infusion 0.5–2 mg/min
  - —Mannitol: adult and peds: 0.5–1.0 g/kg IV over 30–60 min; repeat doses at 0.25 g/kg
  - —Nitroprusside: adult and peds: 0.25–10 μg/kg/min

Disposition

ADMISSION CRITERIA

- All patients with SAH must be admitted to a monitored setting
- A patient with stupor or coma after subarachnoid hemorrhage requires ICU admission to maintain adequate cerebral perfusion pressure without excess increase in mean arterial pressures that may cause a rebleed

DISCHARGE CRITERIA

- Patients with SAH should not be discharged

Miscellaneous

PROGNOSIS

- 40% of hospitalized patients die within 1 month of the event
- $>$33% of those who survive have major neurologic deficits

ICD9: 430

CORE CONTENT CODE: 11.1.1

SUGGESTED READINGS

Kothari RU, Barson W. Management of stroke. In: Tintinalli JE, et al., eds. Emergency medicine. 4th ed. New York: McGraw Hill 1996:1014–1020.

Miller J, Diringer M. Management of aneurysmal subarachnoid hemorrhage. Neurol Clin 1995;13(3):451–477.

Schievink WI. Intracranial Aneurysms. N Engl J Med 1997;336(1):28–39.

Vermeulen M. Subarachnoid hemorrhage: Diagnosis and treatment. J Neurol 1996;243:496–501.

Authors: N. Taleghani; R. Smith-Coggins

Subdural Hematoma

Clinical Presentation

SIGNS AND SYMPTOMS

Acute Subdural Hematoma

- Altered or deteriorating level of consciousness
- Headache, vomiting, lethargy (>90% with at least 1 of these 3 symptoms)
- Unilateral limb weakness
- Pupillary asymmetry/enlarged pupil (30%) is a late finding
  - —Hematoma will be on same side as dilated pupil in >90% cases
  - —Indicates increased intracranial pressure (ICP)
- A lucid interval may be seen in up to 30% of patients before neurologic symptoms reappear
- Up to 50% patients will be comatose at the scene of injury

Subacute/Chronic Hematoma

- Headaches of frequent and varying severity
  - —Exacerbated by change in position
- Cognitive changes, or personality changes
  - —In the elderly, can be mistaken for dementia
  - —Dementia of rapid onset should raise clinical suspicion for a chronic subdural
- New onset seizure activity
- Mild hemiparesis/weakness

MECHANISM/DESCRIPTION

- May occur from direct trauma or to acceleration/deceleration forces
- Hemorrhage into the subdural space due to tearing of the veins that bridge the cortical surface and the dural sinuses
- Classification
  - —Acute subdural: diagnosis within first 3 days
  - —Subacute subdural: diagnosis between 4 and 21 days after injury
  - —Chronic subdural: diagnosis from 3 weeks to months after injury

ETIOLOGY

- Most common type of intracranial hematoma (66%)
- Estimated mortality 21–40% for isolated hematomas, 60–90% for patients presenting comatose
- Male to female incidence approximately 3:1
- Peak incidence acute subdural 4th decade of life (median age 39), chronic subdural 6th decade
- Motor vehicle accident most common cause in elderly adult population, assault most common in younger adults
- Patients at increased risk for subacute/chronic subdural
  - —Elderly
  - —Alcoholics
  - —Seizure disorder
  - —Bleeding disorder
  - —Patients with ventricular shunts

PEDIATRIC CONSIDERATIONS

- May occur secondary to birth trauma or more commonly from nonaccidental trauma

Pre-Hospital

- Severely injured patients should be transported to regional trauma centers equipped to deal with neurosurgical emergencies

Diagnosis

ESSENTIAL WORKUP

- Obtain directed history if possible
  - —Mechanism of injury-kinetics, direct injury versus acceleration/deceleration
  - —Neurologic status pre- and postinjury
  - —Complicating factors: drugs/ETOH, medical problems, medications, allergies
- Rapid neurologic assessment
  - —Glasgow Coma Scale
  - —Brain stem reflexes: pupillary light reflex/anisocoria, corneal, gag, oculovestibular/cephalic
- Head CT
- All head injured patients should have C-spine x-rays

LABORATORY

- CBC, ABG, electrolytes/glucose, PT/PTT
- Blood ETOH/Drug Screen

IMAGING/SPECIAL TESTS

- Characteristic abnormality on CT is half-moon or crescent-shaped clot overlying the hemispheric convexity
- Additional intracranial lesions are common (66%), e.g., cerebral contusion
- Chronic subdurals will typically appear hypodense (70%) on CT; however, 30% of the time they may appear isodense with the surrounding brain tissue
- MRI scan easily distinguishes chronic subdural hematoma
- If plain skull films are ordered, fractures are associated with high degree of underlying injury and should always warrant follow-up CT scan

DIFFERENTIAL DIAGNOSIS

Acute Subdural

- Cerebral concussion
- Cerebral contusion
- Intracerebral bleed
- Diffuse axonal injury
- Subdural hygroma
- Shaken baby/battered child syndrome

Chronic Subdural

- TIA/CVA
- Brain tumor
- Dementia
- Depression
- Toxic, metabolic, respiratory, or circulatory causes

PEDIATRIC CONSIDERATIONS

- In infants with patent fontanelles, ultrasound can be used to visualize intracerebral structures
- Persistent vomiting, new onset seizures, lethargy, irritability, or a tense or bulging fontanelle in an infant should all suggest a possible hematoma

Treatment

INITIAL STABILIZATION

- ABCs of trauma care
- C-spine precautions
- Rapid sequence intubation and mild hyperventilation for acute subdural with increased ICP
  - —Maintain $PaCO_2$ approximately 35 mm Hg, SaO_2 >95%
- Elevate head of bed 20–30°

ED TREATMENT

- Early neurosurgical intervention (<4 hours) in comatose patients with acute subdural hematoma significantly reduces mortality
  - —Surgical intervention (midline shift >5 mm) *or*
  - —Nonoperative conservative management (hematoma <1 cm, no shift or effacement of ventricles/cisterns, no neurologic deficit)
- Frequent neurologic reassessment every 30–60 minutes
- Place A-line and monitor PO_2, PCO_2, MAP
- Intracranial pressure monitoring
- Foley catheter to monitor urine output/volume status
- IV fluids 0.45%NS at 75% maintenance
  - —Adjust fluids to maintain mean arterial pressure (MAP) at approximately 110 mm Hg. (optimizes cerebral perfusion pressure CPP = MAP−ICP)
  - —Optimal serum osmolarity should be maintained between 295–310 milli-Osmoles
- Osmotic diuresis to induce hyperosmolar state (reduces ICP)
  - —Give mannitol followed by lasix
- Control hypertension
  - —Labetalol
  - —Hydralazine
- Treat and prevent seizures
  - —Diazepam, dilantin
- Aspiration prophylaxis
  - —Place nasogastric tube (contraindicated if basilar skull fracture suspected)
- Prevent pain/posturing/increased respiratory effort (all increase ICP)
  - —Sedation/versed
  - —Neuromuscular blockade/pancuronium or vecuronium
- Steroid therapy is not helpful
- Antibiotic prophylaxis is not necessary
- Factors predictive of worse outcome
  - —Best GCS score of ≤8 in first 24 hours
  - —Pupillary inequality or nonreactivity
  - —Presence of decerebrate/decorticate rigidity
  - —Interval between neurologic deterioration and surgical evacuation of >4 hours
  - —Presence of associated intracranial injuries (contusion, intradural hematoma) or multisystem trauma
  - —Prolonged elevated ICP
  - —Prolonged hypotension
  - —Advanced age

MEDICATIONS

- Diazepam: 5–10 g IV; peds: 0.5–1 mg IV to max dose 5 mg
- Dilantin: load 18 mg/kg at 25–50 mg/min
- Hydralazine: 10 mg/hr IV; peds: safety not established
- Labetalol: 15–30 mg/hr IV; peds: safety not established
- Lasix: 1 mg/kg IV
- Mannitol: 0.5–1.0 g/kg IV q 3–6 hrs
- Pancuronium: 0.1 mg/kg/hr IV
- Vecuronium: 0.1 mg/kg/hr
- Versed: 2–4 mg IV/hr PRN; peds: safety not established

Disposition

ADMISSION CRITERIA

- Acute subdurals should be admitted to the OR or ICU by the neurosurgical service
- Subacute subdurals should be admitted to a monitored setting

DISCHARGE CRITERIA

- Patients with chronic subdural hematomas often can be managed as outpatients with adequate home resources and appropriate follow-up

Miscellaneous

ICD9: 852.20

CORE CONTENT CODE: 18.4.1.4

SUGGESTED READINGS

Boyle MF. Head trauma, in presenting signs and symptoms in the emergency department. Baltimore: Williams & Wilkins, 1993:577–588.

Dent DL, Croce MA, Menke PG, et al. Prognostic factors after acute subdural hematoma. J Trauma 1995;39(1):36–42.

Greenberg J. Evaluation and stabilization of head trauma. Surg Rounds 1992;15(6):535–50.

Seeling J, Becker D, Miller J, et al. Traumatic acute subdural hematoma. N Engl J Med 1981;304(25):1511–1518.

Author: Paul File

Sudden Infant Death Syndrome (SIDS)

Clinical Presentation

SIGNS AND SYMPTOMS

- No signs or symptoms present in infants to forewarn families or caretakers
- Not possible to predict or prevent SIDS
- Usual history
  - —Infant is placed down to sleep and subsequently found dead
    - -Death occurs while the infant is sleeping and occurs rapidly
    - -Typically a silent event—baby does not cry
  - —No spontaneous respirations and no pulse
  - —Infant usually appears to be well developed and well nourished

Apparent Life-Threatening Episode (ALTE)

- Episode characterized by a combination of
  - —Apnea
  - —Color change (usually cyanosis but occasionally erythema)
  - —Marked changes in muscle tone (usually limp)
  - —Choking or gagging
- Severe unexplained apneic episodes during sleep, requiring vigorous stimulation or resuscitation to terminate the event

MECHANISM/DESCRIPTION

- Sudden and unexpected death of an apparently well infant in whom death remains unexplained after the performance of an autopsy, investigation of the scene and circumstances of the death, and exploration of the medical history of the infant and the family
- Number one cause of death in the pediatric population between the ages of 1 week and 1 year with a peak occurrence at 2–4 months of age
- 5000–7000 SIDS cases annually in the United States
- Cause of SIDS
  - —Most likely multifactorial
  - —Not caused by child abuse, suffocation, aspiration or immunization
- ALTE
  - —Evidence to indicate some but only very small overlap with SIDS
  - —Approximately 50% have unidentifiable causes
  - —Some identifiable causes after evaluation of infants with ALTE are
    - -Infection
    - -Airway obstruction
    - -Congenital heart diseases
    - -Seizures, choking
    - -Breath-holding

ETIOLOGY

- A definite cause of SIDS is not known but the leading hypotheses are the following
- *Infant developmental physiology*
  - —There is strong interaction of cardiorespiratory, thermoregulatory, and sleep/arousal mechanisms
  - —In infants, these systems develop in parallel and are developing at a time that is a very vulnerable developmental stage for infants. Problems with this delicate developmental process appear to be connected to the possibility of either permanent or transient blunted arousal or ventilatory responses and delayed arousal due to prior hypoxia
- *Rebreathing asphyxia*
  - —Associated with prone position sleeping, related to carbon dioxide rebreathing and subsequent hypercarbia and lack of arousal from airway obstruction
  - —Sleeping conditions linked to this are soft bedding and gas-trapping objects such as sheepskin blankets, waterbeds, and soft mattresses. Babies should have good air circulation near their face
  - —In 1992, the American Academy of Pediatrics made recommendations that sleep position be changed from prone to supine
    - *-20–50% reduction in SIDS in countries where sleeping position has been changed*
    - -Sleeping on the side has demonstrated similar improved results
  - —Home monitors have not been shown to decrease mortality from SIDS
- *Hyperthermia*
  - —Overheating of infants secondary to heavy clothing or over dressing of infants, including overheating from bedding and room temperature possibly causing an increased metabolic rate
- *High-risk factors*
  - —Maternal postnatal smoking
  - —Low birth weight
  - —Maternal substance abuse
  - —Young maternal age
  - —Short interpregnancy interval
  - —Increased number of SIDS deaths during winter months
  - —Male gender
  - —High birth order

Pre-Hospital

N/A

CAUTIONS

- Initiate Neonatal (NALS) and Pediatric Advanced Life Support (PALS) protocols at the scene and continued en route to the emergency department

Diagnosis

ESSENTIAL WORKUP

- Diagnosis of exclusion
- Before making the diagnosis of SIDS, the following must be included in the workup
  - —*Investigation of the scene of death*
    - -Where the baby was
    - -How it was sleeping
    - -Who was with it
    - -What it was doing
  - —*Exploration of the medical history of the infant as well as the family*
    - -Prenatal and perinatal history
    - -Baby's medical history since birth

LABORATORY

- Investigate possible causes of death
  - —Complete blood count
  - —Electrolytes
  - —Liver function tests
  - —Toxicology screen
  - —Blood cultures
  - —Other cultures for sepsis workup
  - —Urinalysis, tests for inborn errors of metabolism
  - —EKG
  - —Radiological skeletal survey

IMAGING/SPECIAL TESTS

- Autopsy
  - —Should be done
  - —Helps parents through their grieving process and helps them to understand that there was nothing that they could have done to prevent the death of their child
  - —Several states require a postmortem examination in all SIDS cases
  - —Some previous postmortem findings
    - -Congenital cardiomyopathies
    - -Cardiac rhabdomyomas
    - -Tuberous sclerosis
    - -Rare genetic diseases
    - -Viral myocarditis
    - -Intracranial arteriovenous malformations
  - —Nonspecific postmortem findings used to establish the diagnosis of SIDS
    - -Retention of periadrenal fat
    - -Hepatic erythropoiesis
    - -Brain stem gliosis

DIFFERENTIAL DIAGNOSIS

- Cardiovascular
  —Myocarditis
  —Tuberous sclerosis
  —Cardiomyopathy
  —Congenital heart disease
- Respiratory
  —Asphyxiation
  —Bronchopneumonia
  —Bronchiolitis
  —Drowning
  —Respiratory syncytial virus
  —Pertussis
  —Tracheobronchitis
- Central nervous system
  —Cerebral edema
  —Subdural hematoma
  —Meningitis
  —Encephalitis
  —Arteriovenous malformation
- Gastrointestinal
  —Enterocolitis with diarrhea
  —Dehydration and subsequent fluid and electrolyte imbalance
- Pancreas
  —Cystic fibrosis
  —Islet cell hyperplasia
  —Hypertrophy or neoplasm
- Endocrine
  —Congenital adrenal hyper- or hypoplasia
- Systemic
  —Dehydration
  —Sepsis
  —Intoxication
  —Overheating

Treatment

INITIAL STABILIZATION

- Assess for airway, breathing, circulation, and accucheck
- Begin resuscitation unless rigor mortis or livedo reticularis are present
- Establish intravenous, intraosseous, or central venous access; use an endotracheal tube for medications that are appropriate for this administration route if access is unsuccessful
- Monitor for blood pressure, heart rate, oxygen saturation, and respirations
- Initiate parenteral hydration and fluid challenges where appropriate and according to NALS and PALS guidelines
- Execute a very thorough physical examination and look for obvious as well as not so obvious signs of trauma (intentional and accidental)
- Investigate for toxic ingestions

ED TREATMENT

- If the resuscitation is unsuccessful and no obvious diagnosis is found at the termination of the resuscitation, parents should *not* be told that the cause of death is SIDS
  —It is appropriate to include it among the possible causes when speaking with them but it is a diagnosis of exclusion; until an autopsy, investigation of the scene and circumstances of death, and exploration of medical history of the infant and family are completed, a diagnosis of SIDS cannot and should not be made

Family Support

- If the infant is unable to be resuscitated, the family should become the immediate focus of attention
- All family members are affected including parents, siblings, grandparents, and caregivers
- They experience feelings of grief, guilt, failure, hurt, and inadequacy
- Some parents want to spend quiet time and hold their infants after an unsuccessful resuscitation
- Allow the family to grieve
- Offer support and assure them that there was nothing that they could have done
- Supply them with support resources

Emergency Personnel Support

- A debriefing should be done in the emergency department for nurses, emergency medical service personnel, physicians, and all who were involved in the child's care there. This is important to allow people to express their feelings
- Inform the primary care pediatrician

Disposition

ADMISSION CRITERIA

- Admit all infants who have ALTE for evaluation and monitoring after initial stabilization and resuscitation

DISCHARGE CRITERIA

None

Miscellaneous

ICD9: 798.0

CORE CONTENT CODE: 13.14

SUGGESTED READINGS

Altemeier WA. A pediatrician's view: Crib death and managed care. Pediatr Ann 1995;24(7):345–346.

Centers for Disease Control. U.S. Department of Health and Human Services, Public Health Services. MMWR 1996;45(No. RR-10):526–530.

Dwyer T, Ponsonby A. SIDS epidemiology and incidence. Pediatr Ann 1995;24(7):350–352.

McClain ME, Shafer S. Supporting families after sudden infant death. Pediatr Ann 1995;24(7):373–378.

Valdes-Dapena M. The postmortem examination. Pediatr Ann 1995;24(7):365–372.

Willinger M. SIDS prevention. Pediatr Ann 1995;24(7):358–364.

Author: Thea L. James

Suicide, Risk Evaluation

Clinical Presentation

SIGNS AND SYMPTOMS

- General appearance often downcast, hopeless, helpless, resolved
- May show signs of alcohol intoxication or drug influence

MECHANISM/DESCRIPTION

- *Suicide gestures:* attention-getting behavior not intended to cause death
- *Suicide:* act of taking one's own life intentionally and voluntarily

ETIOLOGY

- Third most important contribution to life years lost (after coronary artery disease and cancer)
- Tenth leading cause of death in U.S.
- Two peaks in age group most at risk for suicide
  - —15–34-year-olds and the elderly
  - —40–50% of patients who complete suicide had contact with physician in month prior to death

Risk Factors

- Social: recent loss or humiliating event
- Mind set: hopelessness or anger
- Those who complete suicide
  - —Older, male (3:1), firearms, hanging, lacerations
- Those who attempt suicide
  - —Younger, female (3:1), overdose

Population at Highest Risk for Completing Suicide

- Depressive disorder-especially the psychotic depression subtype
- Panic disorder
- Alcohol intoxication
- Drug-using patients
- Schizophrenia
- Adolescents

Others at Risk for Completing Suicide

- Patient recently discharged from psychiatric facility
- Separated, widowed, or divorced (i.e. poor support system)
- Family history of suicide
- Serious physical illness or handicap
  - —Present in 25–75% of all suicide victims
- Prisoners
- Doctors
  - —Female physicians increased risk (41 per 100,000) as well as all psychiatrists
- Victims of violence
- Persons expecting secondary gain

Decreased Risk of Suicide

- Patient on lithium or antidepressants
- Patient who has received electroconvulsive therapy

Pre-Hospital

CONTROVERSIES

- Restraining the patient who is potentially danger to self or others despite refusal for transport
  - —Involve police early as they can hold patients against their will for protection
- Risk to medics on the scene in cases of firearms or other weapons
- Know state and local laws, availability of mobile crisis units, when to involve the police department

Diagnosis

ESSENTIAL WORKUP

- To assess patient risk, obtain history
  - —Intent: reasons, goal
  - —Plan: immediate risk for self-injury?
  - —Other psychiatric or physical illness present?
  - —Alcohol or drug abuse present?
  - —Does patient have support network?
  - —Is patient willing to seek help?
  - —Will the patient agree to immediately seek help if suicidal ideation recurs?

LABORATORY

- Blood alcohol level
- Urine drug screen
  - —Many psychiatric facilities require a screen before placement
- ECG, aspirin, acetaminophen, other appropriate levels if suspect ingestion

IMAGING/SPECIAL TESTS

Not routinely indicated but may see radiopaque pills in stomach

DIFFERENTIAL DIAGNOSIS

- Normal despondency
- Bereavement
- Adjustment disorder with depressed mood
- Bipolar disorder
- Organic affective mood disorder (bipolar affective disorder)
- Organic mental disorder
- Major depressive disorder
- Alcoholism
- Schizophrenia
- Drug abuse
- Antisocial personality

PEDIATRIC/ADOLESCENT SPECIAL CONSIDERATIONS

- Suicide is third leading cause of death among young people 15–24 years of age
- More than 5,000 adolescents commit suicide every year
- Less evidence available to link suicide in youth to overt psychiatric illness
- Stresses
  - —Prior attempts
  - —Family disruption
  - —History of psychiatric disorder
  - —Depression
  - —Disciplinary crisis
  - —Broken romance
  - —School difficulties
  - —Bereavement
  - —Rejection
  - —History of physical or sexual abuse
- Early warning signs
  - —Progressive declining school work
  - —Multiple physical complaints
  - —Drug abuse
  - —Disrupted family relations

GERIATRIC CONSIDERATIONS

- Increased risk due to increased means to use more lethal methods
- Increased risk during certain life events
  - —Death of family/friends
  - —Anniversaries
  - —Change in personal status (retirement)

Treatment

INITIAL STABILIZATION

- Manage medical issues first (ABCs)
- Never leave patient unattended
- Take away sharp objects, belts, and other articles that patient could use for self-injury
- Consider physical or chemical restraints as necessary

ED TREATMENT

- Involuntary admission
  —Patient has psychiatric disorder
  —Patient is dangerous to self or others
  —Patient is unable to care for self
  —Patient has extremely poor judgment or refuses to accept appropriate psychiatric care

MEDICATIONS

- Instituted by psychiatric consultation

Disposition

ADMISSION CRITERIA

"SAD PERSONS"

- Mnemonic: used to score patient's suicide risk factors
- score >9) requires emergent hospitalization
- score = 6–8) and good support requires emergent psychiatric evaluation
- score <5) discharge with family or care of competent person
- score = 1) but overwhelmingly lethal potential = emergent psychiatric intervention
- Ultimately if judged to be a real danger to self, others, or if gravely disabled, patient should be admitted for protection

DISCHARGE CRITERIA

- SAD PERSONS score <5
- Patient agrees to return to ED immediately or seek psychiatric help if suicidal ideation recurs
- Good support network or placement in appropriate crisis housing available
- Appropriate outpatient psychiatric follow-up assured

Miscellaneous

ICD9: 300.9

CORE CONTENT CODE: 22.1.39

SUGGESTED READINGS

Garrison C, et al. Aggression, substance use, and suicidal behaviors in high school students. Am J Pub Health 1993;83(2):179–84.

Gunnell D, Frankel S. Prevention of suicide: aspirations and evidence. Brit Med J 1994;308:1227–31.

Hockberger RS, Rothstein RJ. Assessment of suicide potential by nonpsychiatrists using the SAD PERSONS score. J Emerg Med 1988;99:6.

Hoffman D, et al. Depression and suicide assessment. Emerg Med Clin North Am 1991;9(1).

Author: Michelle Gill

MNEMONIC	CHARACTERISTIC	SCORE
Sex	Male	1
Age	<19 or >45	1
Depression or hopelessness	Admits to depression or decreased appetite, sleep, libido, etc.	2
Previous attempt, psychiatric care	Previous psychiatric care	1
Excessive alcohol, drug use	Chronic addiction, frequent use	1
Rational thinking loss	Organic brain syndrome; psychosis	2
Separated, widowed, divorced		1
Organized, serious attempt	Well thought out or "life-threatening" presentation	2
No social supports	No close family, friends, job, etc.	1
Stated future intent	Determined to repeat; ambivalent	2

Supraventricular Tachycardia

Clinical Presentation

SIGNS AND SYMPTOMS

- Palpitations
- Lightheadedness
- Dyspnea
- Diaphoresis
- Dizziness
- Weakness
- Chest discomfort
- Angina
- Syncope
- Prominent neck veins
- Signs of instability
  - —Mental status changes
  - —Chest pain
  - —Acute pulmonary edema
  - —Hypotension

MECHANISM/DESCRIPTION

- A narrow complex rhythm that originates ectopically above the His bundle
- Rate is greater than 140 beats/minute
- Irregular narrow complex SVT
  - —Atrial fibrillation
    - -Most common form of SVT seen in the emergency department
  - —Atrial flutter
  - —Multifocal atrial tachycardia
- Regular narrow complex SVT
  - —Reentrant mechanisms
    - -AV nodal reentry (the most common regular SVT)
    - -AV reentry
    - -Accessory pathways
- Wide complex SVT
  - —Aberrant conduction or a bundle branch block is present
  - —Conduction is outside of the normal His-Purkinje system
  - —More common in younger patients without structural disease
  - —Always suspect a ventricular rhythm with a wide complex rhythm

PEDIATRIC CONSIDERATIONS

- SVT is the most common dysrhythmia seen in young adults and children without underlying heart disease
- Aberrant conduction WPW and AVNRT are the two most common forms of SVT seen in children

ETIOLOGY

Atrial Tachycardia

- Precipitated by a premature atrial or ventricular contraction
- Electrolyte disturbances
- Drug toxicity
- Hypoxia

Junctional Tachycardia

- AV nodal reentry
- Myocardial ischemia
- Structural heart disease
- Preexcitation syndromes
- Drug and alcohol toxicity

Atrial Fibrillation

- Hypertension
- Coronary artery disease
- Hypothyroidism
- Heavy alcohol intake
- Mitral valve disease
- Chronic pulmonary disease
- Pulmonary embolus
- Wolf-Parkinson-White syndrome
- Hypoxia
- Digoxin toxicity
- Chronic pericarditis
- Idiopathic atrial fibrillation

Atrial Flutter

- Ischemic heart disease
- Valvular heart diseases
- Congestive heart failure
- Myocarditis
- Cardiomyopathies
- Pulmonary embolus
- Other pulmonary disease
  - —Electrolyte abnormalities
  - —Postoperative following cardiac surgery

Multifocal Atrial Tachycardia

- Hypoxic effects of chronic lung disease
- Theophylline toxicity

Pre-Hospital

- Supplemental oxygen
- Intravenous access
- Monitor

CAUTIONS

- Cardioversion must be carried out in unstable patients

CONTROVERSIES

- Vagal maneuvers
- Adenosine
  - —Depends on EMS capabilities and field protocols

Diagnosis

ESSENTIAL WORKUP

- Rapid assessment of hemodynamic stability
- A detailed history
  - —Current symptoms
  - —Previous episodes
  - —Cardiac history
  - —Drug use
    - -Illicit, prescription, over-the-counter, and dietary
- 12-lead ECG and rhythm strip determines management
  - —Determine if the rhythm is regular or irregular
  - —Determine if the QRS complexes are narrow or wide

LABORATORY

- Studies are indicated when underlying metabolic abnormalities or ischemia is considered
  - —CBC
  - —Electrolytes
  - —Cardiac enzymes

IMAGING/SPECIAL TESTS

EKG

- Atrial flutter
  - —Regular atrial rate between 250 and 350
  - —Beat to beat uniformity of cycle length, polarity, and amplitude
  - —Sawtooth flutter waves directed superiorly and most visible in leads II, III, aVF
  - —AV block, usually 2:1, but occasionally greater or irregular
- Multifocal atrial tachycardia
  - —Three distinctly different P waves with varying PR intervals
- Atrial tachycardia
  - —Rate of 100–200 beats/minute
  - —P wave precedes QRS and is morphologically different from the sinus P-wave
- Junctional tachycardia
  - —There is usually 1:1 conduction, with ventricular rates equaling the atrial rate
  - —May be either paroxysmal or sustained
  - —Ventricular rates faster than 200/min in an adult suggest an accessory pathway syndrome such as WPW
  - —Absence of preceding P waves
  - —Often retrograde P waves buried in the QRS
  - —Paroxysmal junctional tachycardia rates range from 120–200 beats/minute
  - —Nonparoxysmal junctional tachycardia rates rarely exceed 130 beats/minute

Electrophysiologic Testing

- Not indicated during emergency management
- Diagnostic and determines therapy for accessory pathways

DIFFERENTIAL DIAGNOSIS

- Sinus tachycardia
  - —Sepsis
  - —Hypovolemia
  - —Pericardial tamponade
  - —Acute myocardial infarction
  - —Drug intoxication
  - —Infection
- Wide complex tachycardias
  - —distinguish between supraventricular or ventricular origins

Treatment

INITIAL STABILIZATION

- Intravenous access
- Monitor
- Determination of unstable versus stable patient made by determining whether the patient has organ perfusion
  - —When a supraventricular rhythm causes inadequate organ perfusion, cardioversion must be carried out

ED TREATMENT

- If it is irregular most likely diagnosis is AF and rate control is a priority
  - —Rate control is achieved via β-blockers or calcium-channel blockers
    - -Once this is achieved the separate issue of cardioversion can be addressed
  - —Cardioversion in stable patients should not be attempted unless the arrhythmia is known to be acute (<24 hours in duration), otherwise anticoagulation is the first step
- In regular narrow complex SVTs
  - —The AV node forms a necessary part of the mechanism sustaining the arrhythmia
  - —Vagal maneuvers are often employed initially and occasionally terminate the arrhythmia
  - —If this is unsuccessful, adenosine is the drug of choice
- Wide complex SVT
  - —Assume that these are ventricular in origin and treat accordingly
  - —Administration of AV nodal-blocking agents may result in ventricular fibrillation
  - —Intravenous procainamide is considered the appropriate treatment

MEDICATIONS

- Adenosine: 6 mg rapid IV; if no response after 1–2 min, then 12 mg
- Diltiazem: 0.25 mg/kg IV over 2 min followed in 15 min by 0.35 mg/kg IV over 2 min
- Esmolol: 0.5 mg/kg over 1 min; maintenance infusion: 0.05 mg/kg/min over 4 min, then 0.1–0.2 mg/kg/min continuously
- Metoprolol: 5–10 mg slow IV push at 5-min intervals to total of 15 mg
- Popranolol: 0.1 mg/kg divided into equal doses at 2-3-min intervals
- Verapamil: 2.5–5.0 mg IV bolus over 2 min; may repeat with 5–10 mg every 15–30 min to max of 20 mg
- Digoxin: 0.5 mg IV initially then 0.25 mg IV q 4 hrs until desired effect
- Procainamide: 6–13 mg/kg IV at 0.2–0.5 mg/kg/min until dysrhythmia controlled; up to a total dose of 1000 mg, then 2–6 mg/min

Disposition

ADMISSION CRITERIA

- Possible cardiac ischemic event
- Persistent supraventricular tachycardia
- Other underlying metabolic abnormalities

DISCHARGE CRITERIA

- Terminated rhythm without organ hypoperfusion

Miscellaneous

ICD9: 427.0; 427.2; 427.3

CORE CONTENT CODE: 2.4.1.4

SUGGESTED READINGS

Alpert MA, et al. Pathogenesis, recognition, and management of common cardiac arrhythmias. Part II: Supraventricular premature beats and tachydysrhythmias. South Med J 1995;88(2):153–74.

Connors S, Dorian P. Management of supraventricular tachycardia in the emergency department. Can J Cardiol 1997;13(Suppl A):19A–24A.

Obel OA, Camm AJ. Supraventricular tachycardia: ECG diagnosis and anatomy. Eur Heart J 1997;18(Suppl C):C2–C11.

Authors: John Dutton; James Adams; Lynn Schrader

Clinical Presentation

SIGNS AND SYMPTOMS

Vital Signs

- Tachycardia
  - —Bradycardia possible for cocaine and some other decongestants
- Increased blood pressure
  - —Severely intoxicated individuals may be hypotensive
- Tachypnea
- Hyperthermia
  - —Often present, may be severe, and is often overlooked

CNS

- Anxiety
- Headache
- Agitation
- Altered mentation
- Diaphoresis
- Seizures
- Stroke

Cardiovascular

- Palpitations
- Chest pain
- Myocardial ischemia or infarction
- Tachydysrhythmias
- Cardiovascular collapse
- Murmur (endocarditis)

Other

- Dilated pupils
- Dry mucous membranes
- Urinary retention may cause enlarged bladder
- Needle trackmarks or abscesses on extremities should be sought
- Increased or decreased bowel sounds
- The presence of diaphoresis and bowel sounds may help to differentiate sympathomimetic toxicity from anticholinergic poisoning

MECHANISM/DESCRIPTION

- Clinical effects result from direct or indirect stimulation of adrenergic receptors in the sympathetic and central nervous systems
- There is often no correlation between dose used and degree of toxicity
- Cocaine may in addition block sodium channels of myocytes, leading to "tricyclic" or class 1a-type dysrhythmias

ETIOLOGY

- Sympathomimetic toxicity can result from the use of any sympathetically active drug, including
  - —Amphetamines and methamphetamines
  - —Cocaine
  - —Phencyclidine (PCP)
  - —Lysergic acid diethylamide (LSD)
  - —Decongestants (rare)
- Drug delivery routes: inhalation, injection, snorting, or ingestion

PEDIATRIC CONSIDERATIONS

- Clinical signs and symptoms of sympathomimetic poisoning in children may present similarly to meningitis or other systemic illness

Pre-Hospital

CONTROVERSIES

- Extreme agitation and violent behavior may require restraints
  - —Overzealous use of restraints in significantly intoxicated sympathomimetic patients has led to airway compromise and difficulty with oxygenation
- Treat cocaine-related cardiac ventricular dysrhythmias similarly to tricyclic antidepressant poisoning using sodium bicarbonate
  - —Lidocaine use may help but should be avoided if possible due to its potential for lowering seizure thresholds and its sodium channel interactions
- Use benzodiazepines to control agitation or seizures, and possibly even tachycardia and dysrhythmias in some cases

Diagnosis

ESSENTIAL WORKUP

- Continously monitor vital signs/cardiac rhythm
- ECG and CXR for chest pain or shortness of breath

LABORATORY

- Electrolytes, BUN/Cr, glucose
- ABG
  - —For severe signs or symptoms
  - —Acidosis may precipitate dysrhythmias or renal dysfunction in rhabdomyolysis
- Urine dip for myoglobin
- CPK when rhabdomyolysis suspected
- Urine toxicology
  - —Of limited utility in adults because tests can be positive for 3 or more days after use
  - —Some sympathomimetic compounds used for weight reduction or narcolepsy can cross-react with assays for amphetamines
  - —LSD will not show up on most urine toxicology screens
- Blood toxicology testing is of no value
- Cardiac enzymes
  - —For ECG abnormalities and in those admitted for chest pain

IMAGING/SPECIAL TESTS

- Cranial CT scanning for abnormal neurologic examinations or seizures

DIFFERENTIAL DIAGNOSIS

- Meningitis
- Hypertensive encephalopathy
- Anticholinergic poisoning
- Alcohol or sedative-hypnotic withdrawal
- Organic psychosis
- Heatstroke
- Sepsis
- Thyroid storm
- Hypoglycemia

PEDIATRIC CONSIDERATIONS

- Urine toxicology screening may be the only way to discover sympathomimetic poisoning in children presenting with altered mental status
- Ritalin and other sympathomimetics used for attention deficit disorder (ADD) may cross-react with the assay for amphetamines

Treatment

INITIAL STABILIZATION

- ABCs
- IV 0.9%NS
  - —Administer at least 2 L of crystalloid to hypotensive individuals
- Monitor cardiovascular function
- Treat seizures, acute agitation, or severe hypertension with *liberal* IV benzodiazepines
- Treat ECG changes or histories consistent with myocardial ischemia with aspirin, nitrates, anticoagulant, or thrombolytics as indicated

ED TREATMENT

Elimination

- Administer activated charcoal orally if exposure was through ingestion or body packing
- Whole-bowel irrigation with polyethylene glycol solution for body packers

Cardiovascular

- Treat severe hypertension with nitroprusside, phentolamine, labetolol, or other related antihypertensive therapies
  - —The use of β-receptor antagonists alone may result in worsening hypertension from unopposed α stimulation (labetolol has some α-receptor antagonistic activity)
- Benzodiazepines may aid in controlling dysrhythmias and hypertension
- Administer sodium bicarbonate as the treatment of choice for ventricular dysrhythmias and heart blocks indicative of sodium channel blocking effects with cocaine poisoning
- Use lidocaine for ventricular dysrhythmias refractory to alkalinization, benzodiazepines, and supportive care
- Use β-receptor antagonists (especially esmolol) for ventricular tachydysrhythmias

Other

- Administer butyrophenones such as haloperidol or droperidol *with caution* to manage agitation
  - —May lower seizure thresholds
- Treat hyperthermia aggressively
- Alkalinize urine for rhabdomyolysis

MEDICATIONS

- Activated charcoal: 1 g/kg
- Diazepam: 5–10 mg IV (peds: po 0.2–0.3 mg/kg IV or 0.5 mg/kg PR) as needed
- Droperidol: 1.25–5 mg (peds: 0.088–0.165 mg/kg) IV/IM
- Esmolol: 50–200 μg/kg/min IV infusion
- Haloperidol: 2.5–10 mg IV/IM
- Labetalol: 20 mg IV q 10 min up to 300 mg
- Lidocaine: 1–2 mg/kg IV followed by infusion of 1–3 mg/min as needed
- Lorazepam: 1–2 mg (peds: 0.05–0.15 mg/kg) IV or IM as needed
- Nitroprusside: 0.5–10 μg/kg/min IV infusion
- Phentolamine: 0.05–0.1 mg/kg/dose to max 5 mg IV
- Sodium bicarbonate: 1–2 amps (peds: 1 μg/kg) IV bolus; infusion may be indicated for rhabdomyolysis

Disposition

ADMISSION CRITERIA

- Body packers or stuffers
- Admit severe manifestations of toxicity (seizures, dysrhythmias, hyperthermia, rhabdomyolysis, severe hypertension, or severely altered mental status) to a monitored bed
- Ischemic chest pain

DISCHARGE CRITERIA

- Mildly intoxicated patients can be observed and treated in the ED until resolution of altered mentation and other clinical manifestations

Miscellaneous

ICD9: 971.2

CORE CONTENT CODE: 17.2.43

SUGGESTED READINGS

Callaway CW, Clark RF. Hyperthermia in psychostimulant overdose. Ann Emerg Med 1994;24:68–76.

Chiang WK, Goldfrank LR. Amphetamines. In: Goldfrank LR, Flomenbaum NE, Lewin NA, et al., eds. Toxicologic emergencies. 5th ed. Norwalk, CT: Appleton & Lange, 1994:863.

Derlet RW, Albertson TE. Emergency department presentation of cocaine intoxication. Ann Emerg Med 1989;18:182–186.

McCarron M, Schulze BW, Thompson GA, et al. Acute phencyclidine intoxication: Incidence of clinical findings in 1000 cases. Ann Emerg Med 1981;10:237–242.

Richard CF, Clark RF, Holbrook T, Hoyt DB. The effects of cocaine and amphetamines on vital signs in trauma patients. J Emerg Med 1995;13:59–63.

Authors: Rick Clark; Sean P. Nordt

Syncope

Clinical Presentation

SIGNS AND SYMPTOMS

- Transient loss of consciousness that usually lasts seconds
- Sweating, nausea, weakness, palpitations, or lightheadedness before the event
- Oriented after the event

MECHANISM/DESCRIPTION

- Sudden, transient loss of consciousness and postural tone that spontaneously resolves
- Accounts for 3% of emergency room visits
- Patients older than 65 years suffer syncopal episodes at an annual rate of 6%
- 38–42% of patients with syncope remain undiagnosed
- Syncope during physical activity associated with structural cardiac abnormality (aortic stenosis, coronary artery disease, hypertrophic cardiomyopathy)
- Concurrent neurologic symptoms of vertebral basilar ischemia such as vertigo and diplopia with syncope suggest TIA

ETIOLOGY

- Syncope generally results from a reduction of cerebral blood flow due to one of three causes
  - —Vasomotor instability associated with a decrease in systemic vascular resistance, or venous capacitance, or both, such as in volume depletion or reflex-related syncope
  - —Decrease in cardiac output owing to obstruction of blood flow within either the heart or pulmonary circulation or owing to arrhythmias
  - —Focal or generalized cerebral hypoperfusion leading to transient ischemia of CNS structures responsible for consciousness
- Vasovagal syncope or neurocardiogenic syncope occur when the patient is upright for long periods of time, during a rapid change from supine to standing, or during times of emotional stress
- Unexplained syncope is most often due to vasovagal syncope

Pre-Hospital

CAUTIONS

- Place on cardiac monitor
- Oxygen
- Establish IV access with 0.9%NS

Diagnosis

ESSENTIAL WORKUP

- Careful history
  - —Differentiate from seizure
    - -Urinary incontinence may occur in both syncope and seizure
    - -Tongue biting or significant trauma is more common with seizures
    - -Syncope usually lasts seconds, whereas seizures generally last minutes
- Physical examination
  - —Orthostatic vital signs
  - —Detailed cardiovascular examination for dysrhythmias, murmur, bruits
  - —Differences in blood pressure in the two arms are suggestive of aortic dissection or subclavian steal syndrome
  - —Stool guaiac
  - —Detailed neurologic examination

LABORATORY

- CBC
- Electrolytes, BUN, Cr, glucose
- Pregnancy test
- Cardiac enzymes if cardiac ischemia suspected
- Oxygen saturation
- ABG if pulmonary embolus suspected

IMAGING/SPECIAL TESTS

- ECG/cardiac monitor looking for
  - —Cardiac ischemia
  - —Wolff-Parkinson-White syndrome
  - —Prolonged QT interval
  - —PVCs
  - —Unsustained ventricular tachycardia
- CT head if new onset seizure or abnormal neurologic examination
- Echocardiogram if structural heart defect suggested
- CXR
  - —For aortic dissection, CHF or massive pulmonary embolus

DIFFERENTIAL DIAGNOSIS

- Seizures
- Breath-holding spells
- Metabolic disorders causing global CNS dysfunction
  - —Hypoglycemia
  - —Hypoxemia
  - —Toxicologic disorders
  - —Subarachnoid hemorrhage
  - —Heat illness
  - —Leaking abdominal aortic aneurysm
  - —Pulmonary embolism
  - —Addisonian crisis
  - —Ruptured ectopic pregnancy
  - —Anaphylaxis
  - —Stroke

Treatment

INITIAL STABILIZATION

- Initiate ACLS intervention for unstable cardiac patient
- Place cardiac monitor
- IV access with 0.9%NS
  —500 cc fluid bolus (peds: 20 cc/kg) for suspected hypovolemia
- Dextrose (or accucheck), naloxone, and thiamine for altered mental status

ED TREATMENT

- Treat dysrhythmias in standard fashion according to ACLS guidelines
- Initiate standard therapy for acute myocardial infarction
- Transfuse/IV rehydration/nasogastric tube placement for significant GI bleed

MEDICATIONS

- Dextrose: D50W 1 amp (50 ml or 25 g) (peds: D25W 2–4 ml/kg) IV
- Naloxone (narcan): 2 mg (peds: 0.1 mg/kg) IV or IM initial dose
- Thiamine (vitamin B_1): 100 mg (peds: 50 mg) IV or IM

Disposition

ADMISSION CRITERIA

- Admitted suspected cardiac syncope to monitored bed
- GI bleed

DISCHARGE CRITERIA

- Reflex syncope (e.g, carotid sinus hypersensitivity, cough, micturition, swallowing, defecation) patient may be evaluated as an outpatient to determine the extent of the hemodynamic consequences of these maneuvers
- Hypovolemia-, hypoxia-, anemia-, or hypoglycemia-based syncope patient should be admitted or discharged depending on the severity of the specific underlying diseases

Miscellaneous

ICD9: 780.2

CORE CONTENT CODE: 22.1.40

SUGGESTED READINGS

Gilman JK. Syncope in the emergency department. A cardiologist's perspective. Emerg Med Clin North Am 1995;13:955–971.

Kapoor WN. Workup and management of patients with syncope. Med Clin North Am 1995;79:1153–1170.

Lempert T. Recognizing syncope: pitfalls and surprises. J R Soc Med 1996;89:372–375.

Author: Chuck Seamens

Syndrome of Inappropriate Antidiuretic Hormone Secretion (SIADH)

Clinical Presentation

SIGNS AND SYMPTOMS

- Serum sodium <130 mmol/L
  - —Weakness
  - —Lethargy
  - —Weight gain
  - —Headache
  - —Anorexia
- Sodium serum <115 mmol/L
  - —Mental status change
  - —Seizure
  - —Coma
- Chronic hyponatremia: 50% asymptomatic
- High mortality when hyponatremia develops acutely

MECHANISM/DESCRIPTION

Normal Regulation of Water Balance

- Antidiuretic hormone (ADH)
  - —Integral part of the homeostatic mechanism that controls water balance
  - —Increases water permeability of the kidney collecting tubules resulting in water reabsorption
  - —Released when hypothalamic osmoreceptors, left atrial stretch receptors and carotid baroreceptors detect water deprivation

Definition of SIADH

- ADH secretion in absence of hyperosmolality or hypovolemia
- Criteria for definition
  - —Hyponatremia
  - —Hyposmolality of the plasma
  - —Continued renal excretion of sodium in absence of diuretics
  - —No clinical evidence of volume depletion
  - —Urine osmolality greater than appropriate in respect to plasma osmolality
  - —Normal renal, adrenal, and thyroid function
- Inappropriate ADH secretion can originate from the hypothalamus or extrahypothalmic tissue

Pre-Hospital

N/A

Diagnosis

ESSENTIAL WORKUP

- Electrolytes, BUN/Cr, glucose
  - —Hyponatremia (serum sodium <135 mmol/L)
  - —Serum hyposmolality (serum osmolality <280 mosm/kg)
- Urine osmolality
  - —Inability to excrete a dilute urine
  - —Urine osmolality >100 mosm/kg
- Urine sodium
  - —Continued urinary excretion of sodium
  - —Urinary sodium >20 mEq/L
- Exclude other causes of hyponatremia

LABORATORY

- Serum protein
- Lipid levels
- Serum osmolality
- Liver and thyroid function test
- Morning cortisol level

IMAGING/SPECIAL TESTS

- Chest x-ray and CT head to screen for pathology causing SIADH

DIFFERENTIAL DIAGNOSIS

Causes of Hyponatremia

- Increased Extracellular Fluid
  - —Renal Failure
  - —Cardiac Failure
  - —Liver Cirrohsis
- Normal Extracellular Fluid
  - —SIADH
  - —Physical and Emotional Stress
  - —Myxedema
  - —Sheehan's Syndrome
  - —Reset Osmostat Syndromes
- Decreased Extracellular Fluid
  - —Excessive sweating
  - —Vomitting
  - —Diarrhea
  - —Third-space sequestration
  - —Diuretics
  - —Aldosterone deficiency (Addison's Disease)
  - —Salt losing nephropathies (renal tubular acidosis)
- Pseudohyponatremia
  - —Hyperproteinemia
  - —Hyperlipidemia
  - —Hyperglycemia

Common Causes of SIADH

ADH-PRODUCING TUMORS	PULMONARY DISEASE	CNS DISORDERS	COMMON DRUGS
Carcinomas	Asthma	Meningitis	Fluoxetine (prozac)
Bronchogenic	Pneumonia	CVA	Tricyclic antidepressant
Pancreatic	Tuberculosis	Intracranial hemorrhage	Antipsychotics
Prostatic		Head Trauma	Carbamazepine
Duodenal		Vascilitis (Lupus)	Chlorpropamide
Thymoma			
Lymphoma			

Treatment

INITIAL STABILIZATION

- Severe symptomatic hyponatremia with CNS manifestations
  - —Endotracheal intubation for patients in need of airway protection
  - —Intravenous access
  - —Naloxone, thiamine, dextrose (or Accucheck)
  - —Treat seizures with benzodiazepines
  - —Proceed to hyponatremia treatment

ED TREATMENT

- Most effective treatment—successful eradication of the underlying cause
- Acute life-threatening hyponatremia
  - —Manifestations
    - -Serum sodium <120 mEq/L
    - -Developing rapidly (0.5 mEq/L/hr decrease in serum sodium)
    - -Associated with seizures or coma
  - —Goal: raise the serum sodium level by no more than 0.5–1.0 mEq/L/hr
    - -Administer 3% hypertonic saline
    - -IV lasix to induce a negative fluid balance
- Chronic hyponatremia/minimal symptoms
  - —Fluid restriction to <500 cc/day alone or in conjunction with
    - -0.9%NS infusion
    - -IV lasix
  - —Correct serum sodium by no more than 0.5 mEq/L/hr
  - —Too rapid correction of serum sodium levels can induce central pontine myelinolysis, associated with development of
    - -Bulbar palsy
    - -Quadriplegia
    - -Coma
    - -Death
- Asymptotic hyponatremia
  - —Fluid restriction to <500 cc/day
  - —Drugs that inhibit the secretion or the renal effect of ADH
    - -Indicated when SIADH not self-limited and cause cannot be removed
    - -Demeclocycline (blocks renal effect of ADH)

MEDICATIONS

- Demeclocycline: 300 mg orally bid
- Hypertonic saline solution (3% NaCl): 25–100 cc/ hr
  - —Limit rate in rise of serum sodium to 0.5–1.0 mEq/L/hr
  - —Discontinue when a resolution in hyponatremic seizure is obtained
  - —Rise in serum sodium by 4–6 mEq/L usually sufficient to stop seizures
- Isotonic saline solution (0.9%NS): standard maintenance rates
- Lasix: 1 mg/kg up to 20–40 IVP

Disposition

ADMISSION CRITERIA

- Severe life-threatening hyponatremia
- Symptomatic hyponatremia
- Serum sodium <120 mEq/L regardless of symptoms
- New onset SIADH in which underlying cause must be diagnosed and treated
- Complications secondary to the underlying cause of SIADH
- Patient's compliance an issue

DISCHARGE CRITERIA

- Asymptomatic chronic hyponatremia
  - —Serum sodium >120 mEq/L
  - —Known diagnosis of SIADH

Miscellaneous

ICD9: 253.6

CORE CONTENT CODE: 4.3.8

SUGGESTED READINGS

Kazal LA, et al. Fluoxetine-induced SIADH a geriatric occurrence? J Fam Pract 1993;36(3):341–343.

Sorensen JB, Anderson MK, Hansen HH. Syndrome of inappropriate secretion of antidiuretic hormone (SIADH) in malignant disease. J Intern Med 1995;238(2):97–110.

Spigset O, Hedenmalm K. Hyponatremia and the syndrome of inappropriate antidiuretic hormone secretion (SIADH) induced by psychotropic drugs. Drug Saf 1995;12(3);209–225.

Author: John McCourt

Synovitis, Toxic

Clinical Presentation

SIGNS AND SYMPTOMS

- Unilateral hip pain acute onset
- Painful limp
- Limitation of hip medial rotation and abduction
- Pain in anteromedial thigh and knee
- Refusal or inability to bear weight
- Preferred external rotation, abduction, and flexion
- Pain over anterior portion of hip with palpation
- Low-grade fever
- Possible upper respiratory infection recent or current

MECHANISM/DESCRIPTION

- Acute inflammation of the hip joint in children associated with joint effusion
- Disease process is self-limiting
- Number one cause of hip pain in children less than ten years of age
- Also referred to as transient synovitis and irritable hip syndrome
- Age group most affected is 3–6 years
- 3:1 male predominance
- Right hip is affected more than the left

ETIOLOGY

- Cause of toxic synovitis is unknown
- Although an infectious etiology is suspected because there is a preceding upper respiratory illness in a large number of cases

Pre-Hospital

N/A

Diagnosis

ESSENTIAL WORKUP

- CBC/ESR
  - —Normal or elevated
  - —An elevated CBC or ESR does not differentiate toxic synovitis from septic arthritis or osteomyelitis
  - —However, if both CBC and ESR are normal, more serious causes of hip pain are less likely especially in less serious clinical presentations
- Plain hip films
  - —Usually normal
  - —May detect an effusion or other causes of hip pain
- Ultrasound to rule out joint effusion if high suspicion for septic arthritis
  - —If a joint effusion is present, an ultrasound-guided joint aspiration should be performed to rule out septic arthritis

IMAGING/SPECIAL TESTS

- Joint aspiration
  - —Not necessary if the patient is afebrile with a normal CBC and ESR
    - -Patients with septic arthritis rarely present without one of these elevated values
- MRI
  - —Very useful in diagnosing Legg-Calvé-Perthes disease
  - —Can detect abnormalities in toxic synovitis and may represent the diagnostic modality of the future for toxic synovitis
- Bone scan
  - —Used to differentiate Legg-Calvé-Perthes disease from toxic synovitis
  - —Can detect osteomyelitis
  - —Due to the increased radiation is usually reserved for recurrent cases or cases where the diagnosis is still in question

DIFFERENTIAL DIAGNOSIS

- Septic arthritis
- Osteomyelitis
- Soft tissue infection
- Legg-Calvé-Perthes disease
- Slipped capitol femoral epiphysis
- Juvenile rheumatoid arthritis
- Rheumatic fever
- Chondrolysis
- Gaucher's disease
- Osteosarcoma
- Ewing's sarcoma
- Osteoid osteoma
- Leukemia
- Tuberculosis of the hip

PEDIATRIC CONSIDERATIONS

- Association of toxic synovitis with Legg-Calvé-Perthes disease
  - 2–10% of patients with toxic synovitis will later develop Legg-Calvé-Perthes disease
  - Suggested that synovitis may represent an early reversible stage of Legg-Calvé-Perthes disease, or that synovitis is causative for Legg-Calvé-Perthes disease, or that synovitis is part of the early spectrum of Legg-Calvé-Perthes disease

Treatment

ED TREATMENT

- Conservative treatment
- Bed rest
- Initiate nonsteroidal anti-inflammatory medications
- Antibiotics and steroids are not indicated
- Some authors recommend nonweight-bearing for 7–10 days following improvement and return of normal hip function citing increased risk of recurrence
- Close followup essential

MEDICATIONS

- Ibuprofen: 200–600 mg (peds >6 months old: 5–10 mg/kg) po q 6 hrs

Disposition

ADMISSION CRITERIA

- Patients with severe joint pain or a large effusion may require hospitalization for bed rest and analgesics

DISCHARGE CRITERIA

- All patients that have been excluded for more serious diagnosis of hip pain and diagnosed with toxic synovitis can be discharged from the hospital with good followup

Miscellaneous

ICD9: 727.00

CORE CONTENT CODE: 13.6.5

SUGGESTED READINGS

Adams JA. Transient synovitis of the hip joint in children. J Bone Joint Surg 1963;45B:471.

Hoffer FA, Zawin JK, Rand FF, Teele RL. Joint effusion in children with an irritable hip: US diagnosis and aspiration. Radiology 1993;187:459–463.

Jacobs BW. Synovitis of the hip in children and its significance. Pediatrics 1971;47:558.

Spock A. Transient synovitis of the hip joint in children. Pediatrics 1959;24:1042.

Tachidjian MS. Acute transient synovitis of the hip. In: Tachidjian MS, ed. Pediatric Orthopedics. Philadelphia: WB Saunders, 1990:1461–1465.

Author: Dick Kuo

Syphilis

Clinical Presentation

SIGNS AND SYMPTOMS

Primary

- Small papule
  - —At site of inoculation
  - —10–90 days postexposure
  - —Becomes a *painless* chancre with indurated borders
  - —Commonly found on penis, vulva, and rectum
  - —Usually heals spontaneously in 4–5 days but may last up to 6 weeks
- Rubbery, nontender inguinal adenopathy
  - —May occur 4 weeks postexposure
- Rectal chancre
  - —Painful or painless
  - —Rectal irritation/discharge
  - —Painless enlargement of lymph nodes

Secondary

- Rash
  - —Dull maculopapular, symmetric rash
  - —Classically involving the palms and soles
  - —Starts on the trunk and on flexor surfaces
  - —Appears 6–20 weeks postexposure
  - —May mimic virtually any dermatologic condition
- Fever
- Chills
- Lethargy
- Lymphadenopathy
- Condylomata lata
  - —Flat rectal warts found at this stage
- Patchy alopecia
- Loss of the lateral third of the eyebrows

Tertiary (Latent)

- Occurs years after the initial infection
- Neurosyphilis
  - —Asymptomatic
    - -CSF abnormalities in absence of clinical symptoms
    - -CSF pleocytosis, protein elevation, reactive VDRL
  - —Meningitis
    - -Aseptic
    - -Involves the base of brain
    - -Unilateral/bilateral cranial nerve palsies
  - —General paresis
    - -Progressive dementia
    - -Loss of cortical function
  - —Tabes dorsalis (neuropathy)
    - -Degeneration of posterior columns/posterior roots of spinal cord
    - -Progressive loss of reflexes, vibratory/position sensation
    - -Progressive ataxia
    - -Argyll Robertson pupils
    - -Urinary incontinence
- Cardiovascular
  - —Thoracic aneurysm (ascending most common)
  - —Aortic insufficiency

MECHANISM/DESCRIPTION

- Sexually transmitted disease
- Enters the body through mucous membranes and nonintact skin
- Focal endarteritis
  - —Primary pathologic lesion
- Granulomatous reaction occurs in secondary and tertiary syphilis

ETIOLOGY

- *Treponema pallidum*
  - —Causative agent
  - —Spirochete bacteria
- Increased prevalence in the last 10 years secondary to sexual behavior associated with drug use

Pre-Hospital

N/A

Diagnosis

ESSENTIAL WORKUP

- Serologic tests
  - —Nontreponemal tests: RPR (rapid plasma reagin) and VDRL (Venereal Disease Research Laboratories)
    - -Usually positive 2–4 weeks after the chancre appears
    - -Many early false-negatives
    - -Repeat negative tests in 2 weeks
    - -2% false-positive rate
  - —Treponemal antibody test: FTA-ABS
    - -More sensitive and specific than nontreponemal tests
    - -Used as confirmatory test
    - -More costly and harder to perform

LABORATORY

- Dark-field microscopy
  - —Used to identify treponemes from samples of primary and secondary lesions
  - —Ointments and creams applied to lesions may lead to a false-negative microscopy
- CSF analysis
  - —For tertiary syphilis
  - —Positive VDRL
  - —>5 lymphocytes/ml
  - —Protein >45

DIFFERENTIAL DIAGNOSIS

Genital Ulcer

- Chancroid
- Genital herpes
  - —Vesicles
  - —Multiple
- Lymphogranuloma venereum
- Granuloma inguinale
- Superficial fungal infection
- Carcinoma

Secondary Syphilis

- Pityriasis rosea
- Drug rash
- Acute febrile exanthems
- Psoriasis
- Lichen planus
- Scabies
- Infectious mononucleosis

Treatment

INITIAL STABILIZATION

- Lower blood pressure/IV access for aortic dissection

ED TREATMENT

- Early primary, secondary, latent <1 year antibiotic options
  - —Benzathine penicillin G 2.4 million units IM (best)
  - —Doxycycline 100 mg po bid × 14 days
  - —Tetracycline 500 mg po qid × 14 days
  - —Erythromycin 500 mg qid × 30 days
    - -If above regimes contraindicated
    - -Associated with increased relapse rate
- Latent: >1 year duration (except neurosyphilis) antibiotic options
  - —Benzathine penicillin G 2.4 million units IM q week × 3 weeks (best)
  - —Tetracycline 500 mg po qid × 4 weeks
  - —Doxycycline 100 mg po bid × 4 weeks
- Neurosyphilis
  - —Penicillin G 2–4 million units IV q 4 hrs × 10–14 days
- Pregnancy
  - —Treat with penicillin as above for stage/latency
  - —Admit women allergic to penicillin to desensitize prior to penicillin administration
- Jarish-Herxheimer reaction
  - —Transient febrile reaction to therapy
  - —May be due to liberation of antigens from spirochetes or activation of complement cascade
  - —Occurs in the first few hours with a peak at 8 hours and resolution in 24 hours
  - —Symptoms include
    - -Fever
    - -Myalgia
    - -Headache
    - -Malaise
    - -Worsening of syphilitic rash
  - —Treat with salicylates
  - —No serious sequelae
- Recommend testing
  - —Of sexual partners
  - —For concomitant sexually transmitted diseases including HIV

Disposition

ADMISSION CRITERIA

- Neurosyphilis requiring IV antibiotic therapy
- Pregnant women allergic to penicillin requiring desensitization prior to initiation of penicillin

DISCHARGE CRITERIA

- Follow-up care
  - —Measure for falling titers 1 year posttherapy
  - —Tertiary/latent (>1 year) needs serology at 3, 6, 12, and 24 months posttreatment to measure for falling titers

Miscellaneous

ICD9: 97.9

CORE CONTENT CODE: 9.1.10.3

SUGGESTED READINGS

Adimora AA, Hamilton H, Holmes KK, Sparling PF. Sexually transmitted diseases—Companion handbook. New York: McGraw Hill, 1994.

Berger RE. Sexually transmitted diseases. Adv Urol 1997;2:97.

Centers for Disease Control and Prevention. 1993 Sexually transmitted disease treatment guidelines. MMWR 1993;42:1–102.

Author: David Levine

Systemic Lupus Erythematosus

Clinical Presentation

SIGNS AND SYMPTOMS

- Lupus is a heterogeneous disease with multiple presentations including
  —Fatigue, fever, weight loss
  —Joint pain, chest pain, abdominal pain
  —Dyspnea
  —Psychosis, altered mental status
  —Polyarthritis, symmetrical or migratory
  —Malar rash, discoid rash, oral ulcers
  —Pleural or pericardial rub
- Multisystem involvement including
  —*Skin:* malar rash (butterfly facial), discoid rash (raised red patches), photosensitivity rash (subacute cutaneous lupus), painless oral ulcers
  —*Kidneys:* glomerulonephritis, renal failure
  —*Nervous system:* psychosis, depression, headache, seizures, peripheral neuropathies, hemiplegia, and cranial nerve deficits
  —*Arthritis:* defined as two or more peripheral joints with warmth, tenderness or effusion
  —*Heart:* pericarditis with or without effusion, valve dysfunction, endocarditis, myocarditis, congestive heart failure, conduction abnormalities, and myocardial infarction
  —*Hematological:* Leukopenia, thrombocytopenia, and hemolytic anemia
    -Venous and arterial thrombosis is seen in association with the Antiphospholipid syndrome, and these patients, paradoxically, may have a positive lupus anticoagulant
  —*Lungs:* pleural effusion (usually exudative), pneumonitis, pulmonary hemorrhage, pulmonary embolism, pneumonia, pleuritis, pulmonary edema, and pulmonary hypertension
  —*Gastrointestinal:* peritonitis, mesenteric vasculitis and ischemia, pancreatitis

MECHANISM/DESCRIPTION

- More common in females than males (ratio: 9:1) and more common in African Americans
- Peak onset is between ages 15 and 25

ETIOLOGY

- Autoantibody production against cell nucleus and cytoplasmic structures leading to inflammatory changes, vasculitis, and immune complex deposition in multiple organ systems
- Lupus may be associated with the genetic markers HLA-DR2 and HLA-DR3
- A significant percentage of patients have an associated antiphospholipid syndrome, characterized by antibodies against cellular phospholipid components. These patients tend to have recurrent vascular thrombosis
- Lupus is a chronic disease with exacerbations, which may be brought on by infection, sun exposure, trauma, medications, stress, and possibly pregnancy
- Drug-induced lupus is caused most commonly by chlorpromazine, methyldopa, procainamide, hydralazine and isoniazid

Pre-Hospital

CAUTIONS

- The lupus patient may have multiple presentations, ranging from mild constitutional symptoms, to acute psychosis, to respiratory and cardiovascular collapse
- Do not mistakenly categorize these patients as purely psychiatric or nonemergent

Diagnosis

ESSENTIAL WORKUP

- History and physical examination
- Four of the eleven criteria from the following list are needed to make the diagnosis
  —Malar rash
  —Discoid rash
  —Photosensitivity rash
  —Oral ulcers
  —Arthritis
  —Serositis
  —Neurologic disorders
  —Hematologic disorders
  —Immunologic disorders
  —Renal disorders
  —Antinuclear antibodies

ESSENTIAL WORKUP FOR MAJOR FLARE-UPS

- CBC, electrolytes, Bun/Cr, glucose, U/A, ESR
- CXR, EKG and pulse oximetry for cardiorespiratory symptoms

LABORATORY

- Degree of anemia, thrombocytopenia, and leukopenia suggests degree of disease activity
- The ESR may be elevated during acute exacerbations but this test tends to remain high months after a flare-up has ceased
- PTT may be elevated due to lupus anticoagulant
- Urinalysis for protein, casts, hematuria, and WBCs
- Positive stool guaiac suggests mesenteric ischemia, amylase is elevated in mesenteric ischemia and pancreatitis
- Send ANA or FANA, RF, ASO titer if diagnosis unclear
- Anti-Sm and Anti-dsDNA are diagnostic,
- A false-positive VDRL is supportive of the diagnosis
- Joint aspirate typically shows fluid with less than 3000 WBCs

IMAGING/SPECIAL TESTS

- CXR: pneumonitis, pneumonias, effusions, heart size
- EKG: pericarditis, cardiomegaly
- Echocardiogram: effusions, valvular disorders

DIFFERENTIAL DIAGNOSIS

- Hypotension may be due to shock secondary to a major flare-up or secondary to acute steroid withdrawal in the known lupus patient
- Other autoimmune diseases, rheumatic fever, rheumatoid arthritis, dermatomyositis, overlap syndromes
- Skin changes may mimic urticaria, erythema multiforme
- Depending on presentation, ITP, MS, epilepsy are in the differential

Treatment

INITIAL STABILIZATION
- ABCs

ED TREATMENT
- Mainstays include NSAIDs, antimalarials, corticosteroids, and immunosuppressive drugs
- Special attention must be given to CNS and renal involvement as these are the main determinants of morbidity and mortality
- *Mild flare-ups:* arthralgias, myalgias, and fatigue, rash
  —NSAIDs, ASA, topical steroids for rash, sunscreen
  —If not sufficient, begin low-dose prednisone
- *Major flare-ups:* life- or organ-threatening
  —Methylprednisolone
  —Anticoagulation for thrombosis, give blood products early if needed
  —Psychotropics for neuropsychiatric symptoms
  —Anticonvulsants for seizures
  —If poor response, consult rheumatology before starting cytotoxic medications such as azathioprine or cyclophosphamide
- *Chronically*
  —Prednisone taper
  —NSAIDs
  —Antimalarials: a rheumatologist should initiate quinacrine, chloroquine

MEDICATIONS
- Adult dosages (for pediatric medications consult rheumatologist)
  —Methylprednisolone: 15 mg/kg/day IV up to 1 g
  —NSAIDs dose varies per agent
  —Prednisone: <0.5 mg/kg/day po for minor flare
- Pediatric dosages
  —Ibuprofen: 5–10 mg/kg/dose divided q 6 hrs
  —Prednisone: 0.5 mg/kg/day divided qd or bid

Disposition

ADMISSION CRITERIA
- Patients who have end organ disease such as renal or CNS involvement, pericarditis, pancreatitis, or gastrointestinal symptoms should be admitted
- Those with severe end organ or life-threatening manifestations should be admitted to the ICU
- Patients with lupus should be treated as immunocompromised and suspected or diagnosed infections should be treated aggressively

DISCHARGE CRITERIA
- Patients may be discharged home with mild flare-ups if afebrile, well hydrated, and not ill-appearing
- ESR should not be used as a disposition criteria as it may be elevated long after a flare-up has subsided
- Lupus is a chronic disease and patients must be followed adequately by a rheumatologist or a capable primary care physician

Miscellaneous

ICD9: 710.0

CORE CONTENT CODE: 8.5.2.6

SUGGESTED READINGS

Boumpas DT, Austin HA 3rd. Systemic lupus erythematosus: Emerging concepts. Part 1: Renal, neuropsychiatric, cardiovascular, pulmonary, and hematologic disease. Ann Intern Med 1995;122(12):940–950.

Boumpas DT, Fessler BJ. Systemic lupus erythematosus: emerging concepts. Part 2: Dermatologic and joint disease, the antiphospholipid antibody syndrome, pregnancy and hormonal therapy, morbidity and mortality, and pathogenesis. Ann Intern Med 1995;123(1):42–53.

Hahn BH. Management of systemic lupus erythematosus. In: Kelley WN, et al., eds. Textbook of rheumatology. 5th ed. Philadelphia: WB Saunders, 1997: 1040–1056.

Lahita RG. Clinical presentation of systemic lupus erythematosus. In: Kelley WN, et al., eds. Textbook of rheumatology. 5th ed. Philadelphia: WB Saunders, 1997: 1028–1039.

Lehman TJ. A practical guide to systemic lupus erythematosus. Pediatr Clin North Am 1995;42(5):1223–1238.

Authors: Steven Furer; John Lafleur

Tachydysrhythmias

Clinical Presentation

SIGNS AND SYMPTOMS

- Asymptomatic
  - —Frequent with supraventricular tachycardia
  - —Rare with sustained ventricular tachycardia
- Palpitations
- Lightheadedness
- Dyspnea
- Diaphoresis
- Dizziness
- Weakness
- Chest discomfort
- Angina
- Syncope
- Prominent neck veins
- Ventricular tachycardia
  - —Splitting of heart sounds
  - —Gallop rhythm
- Ventricular fibrillation
  - —Sudden loss of consciousness
  - —Absent pulse, heart rate, and blood pressure
- Signs of instability
  - —Hypotension
  - —Pulmonary edema
  - —Chest pain
  - —Mental status changes

MECHANISM/DESCRIPTION

- Any disturbance of the heart's rhythm resulting in a rate greater than 100 beats per minute
- Caused by disorders of impulse formation or conduction

Sinus Tachycardia

- —Narrow complex regular rhythm at a rate of 100–150 beats/minute
- —Infants and young children can obtain rates of 170–225 beats/minute
- —Functional response to physiologic stress
- —Caused by increased catecholamine tone or decreased vagal stimulation

Supraventricular Tachycardias (SVT)

- A narrow complex tachycardia that originates above the His bundle
- One of the most frequent cardiac disturbances evaluated in the emergency department
  - —Most common dysrhythmia seen in young adults and children without underlying heart disease
- Wide complex tachycardias can be supraventricular in origin
- Irregular
  - —Atrial fibrillation
  - —Atrial flutter
  - —Multifocal atrial tachycardia
- Regular
  - —Atrial tachycardia
    - -Any rapid dysrhythmia from a nonsinus focus above the AV node
  - —Junctional tachycardia
    - -Regular tachycardia without preceding depolarization waves

Ventricular Tachycardia

- Three or more consecutive ventricular ectopic beats at a rate of 100 beats per minute
- Most common initiating rhythm in sudden death in patients with previous myocardial infarction
- Always suspect a ventricular rhythm with a wide complex rhythm, especially in the older patient

Torsades de Pointes

- Paroxysmal form of ventricular tachycardia meeting specific clinical criteria
- Secondary to either congenital or acquired abnormalities of ventricular repolarization
- Often the result of drug therapy or electrolyte disturbances

Ventricular Fibrillation

- ECG shows oscillations without evidence of discrete QRST morphology
- Accounts for 80–85% of sudden cardiac deaths
- Frequently results from degeneration of sustained ventricular tachycardia

ETIOLOGY

- Sinus tachycardia
  - —Acute myocardial infarction
  - —Anemia
  - —Anxiety
  - —Congestive heart failure
  - —Drug intoxication
  - —Hyperthyroidism
  - —Hypovolemia
  - —Hypoxia
  - —Infection
  - —Pain
  - —Pericardial tamponade
  - —Pulmonary embolism
- Atrial tachycardia
  - —Precipitated by a premature atrial or ventricular contraction
  - —Electrolyte disturbances
  - —Drug toxicity
  - —Hypoxia
- Junctional tachycardia
  - —AV nodal reentry
  - —Myocardial ischemia
  - —Structural heart disease
  - —Preexcitation syndromes
  - —Drug and alcohol toxicity
- Irregular narrow complex supraventricular tachycardias
  - —Atrial fibrillation
    - -Hypertension
    - -Coronary artery disease
    - -Hypothyroidism
    - -Heavy alcohol intake
    - -Mitral valve disease
    - -Chronic pulmonary disease
    - -Pulmonary embolus
    - -Wolf-Parkinson-White syndrome
    - -Hypoxia
    - -Digoxin toxicity
    - -Chronic pericarditis
    - -Idiopathic atrial fibrillation
  - —Atrial flutter
    - -Ischemic heart disease
    - -Valvular heart disease
    - -Congestive heart failure
    - -Myocarditis
    - -Cardiomyopathies
    - -Pulmonary embolus
    - -Other pulmonary disease
    - -Electrolyte abnormalities
    - -Postoperative following cardiac surgery
  - —Multifocal atrial tachycardia
    - -Hypoxic effects of chronic lung disease
    - -Theophylline toxicity
- Ventricular tachycardias
  - —Dilated cardiomyopathy
- Torsades de pointes
  - —Drug toxicity (Class IA and IC agents)
  - —Hypokalemia
  - —Hypomagnesemia
  - —Congenital QT prolongation
- Ventricular fibrillation
  - —Acute myocardial infarction (most common)
  - —Chronic ischemic heart disease
  - —Hypoxia
  - —Acidosis
  - —Anaphylaxis
  - —Electrocution
  - —Shock
  - —Hypokalemia
  - —Initiation of quinidine therapy
  - —Massive hemorrhage

Pre-Hospital

- Supplemental oxygen
- Intravenous access
- Monitor

CAUTIONS

- Cardioversion must be carried out in unstable patients with supraventricular or ventricular tachydysrhythmias

CONTROVERSIES

- Vagal maneuvers
- Adenosine
  —Depends on EMS capabilities and field protocols

Diagnosis

ESSENTIAL WORKUP

- Determination of unstable versus stable patient
- A detailed history
  —Current symptoms
  —Previous episodes
  —Cardiac history
  —Drug use
- 12-lead ECG and rhythm strip to categorize the tachycardia
  —Determine if the rhythm is regular or irregular
  —Determine if the complexes are narrow or wide

LABORATORY

- Studies are indicated when underlying metabolic abnormalities or ischemia is considered
  —CBC
  —Electrolytes
  —Cardiac enzymes
  —Thyroid function tests

IMAGING/SPECIAL TESTS

ECG

- Atrial flutter
  —Regular atrial rate between 250 and 350
  —Beat to beat uniformity of cycle length, polarity, and amplitude
  —Sawtooth flutter waves directed superiorly and most visible in leads II, III, aVF
  —AV block, usually 2:1, but occasionally greater or irregular
- Multifocal atrial tachycardia
  —Three distinctly different P waves with varying PR intervals
- Atrial tachycardia
  —Rate of 100–200 beats/minute
  —P wave precedes QRS and is morphologically different from the sinus P-wave
- Ventricular tachycardia
  —QRS is usually 0.12 seconds and often 0.14 seconds
- Torsades de pointes
  —Ventricular rate greater than 200 beats/minute
  —QRS structure displays an undulating axis, with the polarity of the complexes appearing to shift around the baseline
  —Occurrence is often in short episodes of less than 90 seconds
- Ventricular fibrillation
  —ECG shows oscillations without evidence of discrete QRST morphology
  —Oscillations are usually irregular and occur at a rate of 150–300 per minute
    -When the amplitude of most oscillations is 1 mm, the term "coarse" is used
    -"Fine" VF is used for oscillations <1 mm

Electrophysiologic Testing

- Diagnostic but not required emergently
- Determines therapy for accessory pathways

DIFFERENTIAL DIAGNOSIS

- See Etiology

Tachydysrhythmias

Treatment

INITIAL STABILIZATION

- Intravenous access
- Monitor
- Basic life support in patients with loss of consciousness or sudden death
- Cardioversion/defibrillation
  - —Unstable patients with narrow complex tachycardia
    - -Cardioversion with 50–360 J
    - -Sedation when possible
    - -In most patients, it can be accomplished with 25–100 J
  - —Ventricular fibrillation
    - -Asynchronous DC defibrillation at 200 J
    - -If this fails, 200 J or 300 J should be applied, then 360 J if still no response
    - -Intubation and IV access need to be secured if no response to three attempts at defibrillation
    - -Epinephrine 1 mg should then be administered followed by 360 J defibrillation
    - -If VF persists, an IV bolus of lidocaine should be infused followed by another defibrillation attempt at 360 J
    - -If this fails, bretylium is infused
    - -Epinephrine 1 mg should continue to be used at 10-minute intervals
    - -Coarse VF is more responsive to defibrillation than fine VF
  - —Sustained ventricular tachycardia with transient loss of consciousness or sudden death
    - -Immediate DC cardioversion (200 J, increasing to 300 J and 360 J if necessary)
    - -Administration of lidocaine
    - -If lidocaine fails, then bretylium or procainamide infusion

ED TREATMENT

- Irregular narrow complex
  - —Rate control
  - —β-Blockers or calcium-channel blockers
  - —Anticoagulation if onset is greater than 24 hours
  - —Cardioversion
    - -Unstable patients
    - -Once rate control has been achieved, the patient must be anticoagulated if onset of dysrhythmia is greater than 24 hours
- Regular narrow complex tachydysrhythmia
  - —Vagal maneuvers are often employed initially and occasionally terminate the dysrhythmia
  - —Adenosine
    - -Rapid onset and short half-life
    - -90% effective in terminating SVTs
    - -May be diagnostic by slowing the rate and revealing an underlying atrial tachycardia
- Stable wide complex tachycardia
  - —Should be assumed to be ventricular in origin, especially in the elderly or those with CAD
  - —Lidocaine is the drug of choice
  - —If ventricular tachycardia is refractory to lidocaine, procainamide or bretylium are second-line agents
  - —In patients with WPW
    - -Administration of AV nodal-blocking agents may result in ventricular fibrillation
    - -Procainamide is the agent of choice
- Torsades de pointes
  - —Immediate DC cardioversion is indicated with LOC
  - —IV infusion of magnesium or potassium, or β-blocker may prevent recurrence

MEDICATIONS

- Adenosine: 6 mg rapid IV, if no response after 1–2 min then 12 mg
- Digoxin: load 0.25 mg IV q 6 hrs to 1 mg
- Procainamide: 100 mg IV q 10 min
- Quinidine: 324 mg po bid/tid
- Lidocaine: 1 mg/kg push, 1–4 mg/min infusion
- Bretylium: 5 mg/kg push; 10 mg/kg in 20–30 min if no response
- Epinephrine: 1 mg bolus administration

Disposition

ADMISSION CRITERIA

- Ventricular tachycardia
- Possible cardiac ischemic event
- Persistent supraventricular tachycardia
- Other underlying metabolic abnormalities

DISCHARGE CRITERIA

- Terminated supraventricular rhythm without organ hypoperfusion

Miscellaneous

ICD9: 427.0; 427.1; 427.2

CORE CONTENT CODE: 2.4.1.4; 2.4.1.6

SUGGESTED READINGS

Alpert MA, et al. Pathogenesis, recognition, and management of common cardiac arrhythmias. Part I: Ventricular premature beats and tachydysrhythmias. South Med J 1995;88:1–21.

Alpert MA, et al. Pathogenesis, recognition, and management of common cardiac arrhythmias. Part II: Supraventricular premature beats and tachydysrhythmias. South Med J 1995;88:153–74.

Connors S, Dorian P. Management of supraventricular tachycardia in the emergency department. Can J Cardiol 1997;13(Suppl A):19A–24A.

Obel OA, Camm AJ. Supraventricular tachycardia: ECG diagnosis and anatomy. Eur Heart J 1997;18(Suppl C):C2–C11.

Authors: Lynn Schrader; John Dutton; James Adams

Tarsal Injuries

Clinical Presentation

Tarsal bone fractures or dislocations are significant injuries, frequently resulting in prolonged impairment and disability. The anatomy, blood supply and basic foot function (weight support and locomotion) contribute to the morbidity of these injuries. Significant force is required to produce these injuries; often motor vehicle accidents or falls from heights. Frequently multiple fractures and/or dislocations coexist. Many times these are open fractures. Acute and chronic morbidity (specifically stress fractures) can result from overuse

SIGNS AND SYMPTOMS

- A history of trauma or overuse
- Pain
- Deformity
- Soft tissue swelling or discoloration (either ecchymosis or blanching of skin)
- Neurovascular compromise
- Diminished range of motion

MECHANISM/DESCRIPTION

Anatomy

- The foot is divided into three anatomic areas: the hind-, mid- and forefoot
- There are seven tarsal bones. The calcaneus and talus form the hindfoot; the navicular, cuboid, and three cuneiforms comprise the midfoot
- The talonavicular and calcaneocuboidal surfaces are referred to as "Chopart's" joint
- The articular interface of the cuneiforms and navicular bones with the base of the five metatarsal bones is collectively referred to as "Lisfranc's" joint
- The talus is the only bone of the foot to articulate with the tibia and fibula, allowing plantar and dorsiflexion of the foot, and transferring body weight to the foot. In addition, the subtalar joint (talonavicular and talocalcaneal surfaces) provides some rotation, allowing the foot to accommodate uneven walking surfaces
- There are many inconsistent accessory bones in the foot that can obfuscate the diagnosis of acute bony injury
- Fractures involving articular surfaces have a poorer functional outcome
- Fracture, subluxation, or dislocation may occur with any of the tarsal bones. Multiple injuries are usual
- The talus is second only to the calcaneus in the frequency of injury of the tarsal bones
- Because the talus is largely covered with articular surfaces and has no tendon or muscle insertions, its blood supply is tenuous and easily disrupted by fracture or dislocation, potentially resulting in avascular necrosis and long term morbidity
- Chronic illness, particularly diabetes mellitus and peripheral vascular disease, may delay healing

Mechanism of Injury

- Injury results from forced dorsiflexion, axial load, inversion or eversion of the foot, or direct trauma (crush) injury
- Most result from high-speed motor vehicle accidents, falls, or industrial accidents
- Young males are at the highest risk of injury
- Identification of one injury should prompt close scrutiny to rule out associated injuries
- Repetitive stress injuries are most common in athletes
- Although stress fractures of the foot are most common in the calcaneous and second metatarsal, any tarsal bone may be affected

PEDIATRIC CONSIDERATIONS

- Tarsal bone fractures are rare in children, but may be underreported
- Foot injury should be considered in any toddler with a limp
- Delay in diagnosis is the rule in children

Pre-Hospital

- Immobilize to reduce pain, bleeding, and further injury
- Soft splinting is appropriate for many patients
- Cover with clean, sterile cloth if open injuries occur
- Reduction or relocation should not be attempted in the pre-hospital setting

Diagnosis

ESSENTIAL WORKUP

- Plain film radiography with standard anteroposterior, lateral, and oblique films of the foot
  - —These views may be difficult to obtain if much deformity is present
  - —Films may be difficult to interpret, because of multiple, overlying bone shadows and the presence of accessory bones. Images of the contralateral, normal foot may be helpful

IMAGING/SPECIAL TESTS

- Tomograms, CAT scan, or bone scanning may be necessary to further define injuries
- Dislocations should be reduced as soon as possible to limit soft tissue injury and reduce the risk of avascular necrosis
- Diagnosis of occult injuries without displacement can be deferred beyond the immediate ED stay
- Stress fractures are often only visible by CAT or bone scanning

DIFFERENTIAL DIAGNOSIS

- Sprain and soft tissue injury can mimic acute bony injury to the foot. These are diagnoses of exclusion, and should be made only after a thorough search for fracture, dislocation, and subluxation has been completed

Treatment

INITIAL STABILIZATION

- Immobilization of all injuries is mandatory
  —Bulky splint is preferable
- Pain control is essential

ED TREATMENT

- Immediate consultation with an orthopedic specialist is needed
- Precise anatomical reduction is necessary to improve chances of functional recovery
- Reduction of dislocations is attempted in a closed fashion. These frequently require conscious sedation or general anesthesia. Inability to accomplish closed reduction suggests a soft tissue or bone fragment interposition, and mandates open reduction
- All open injuries must be taken to the operating room for debridement and reduction. Most open injuries will be left open until immediate risk of infection has passed
- Suspected injuries should be treated with non-weight bearing until a definitive diagnosis can be established
- Documented injuries should all be treated with non-weight bearing

MEDICATIONS

- Morphine sulfate: 2–10 mg IV/IM titrated to pain control; peds: 0.1 mg/kg IV
- Fentanyl: 50–250 μg IV titrated to pain control
- Meperidine: 25–100 mg IV/IM titrated to pain control

Disposition

ADMISSION CRITERIA

- Admission is often necessary based on concomitant injury
- All open injuries must be admitted for debridement and antibiotic prophylaxis
- All injuries requiring open reduction should be admitted

DISCHARGE CRITERIA

- Repetitive stress injuries may be discharged with outpatient follow-up
- Sprains and soft tissue injuries may also be discharged. Early outpatient follow-up is necessary to continue the search for occult injury should symptoms persist

Miscellaneous

ICD9: 825.29, 838.0

CORE CONTENT CODE: 18.4.13.1.3

SUGGESTED READINGS

Heckman JD. Fractures and dislocations of the foot. In: Rockwood CA, Green DP, Bucholz RW, Heckman JD, eds. Rockwood and Green's fractures in adults. 4th ed. New York: Lippincott-Raven, 1996:2267–2405.

Sangeorzan BJ, Mayo KA, Hansen ST. Intraarticular fractures of the foot. Talus and lesser tarsals. Clin Orthop 1993;292:135–141.

Waeckerle JF, Steele MT. Foot Injuries. In: Tintinalli JE, Ruiz E, Krome RL, eds. Emergency medicine: A comprehensive study guide. 4th ed. New York: McGraw Hill, 1996:1271–1276.

Author: Mara McErlean

Temporal Arteritis

Clinical Presentation

SIGNS AND SYMPTOMS

- Although presentation may be acute, most patients have symptoms for weeks to months before the diagnosis is made. Constitutional symptoms such as fatigue, anorexia, weight loss, low-grade fever, weakness and arthralgias are common, and often appear early
- Headache is the single most frequent symptom, and is often boring or lancinating in quality. In addition, patients may complain of musculoskeletal pain, sore throat, dysphagia, or, tongue or jaw claudication
- Visual findings include diplopia, ptosis, extraocular muscle weakness, scotomata, blurred vision, amaurosis fugax, or blindness
- Visual loss in one or both eyes may be the presenting complaint, but more often visual complaints develop weeks to months after the onset of other symptoms. In patients presenting with unilateral blindness, blindness in the other eye will occur in three-quarters of patients in less than a month if treatment is not instituted
- Although symptoms may initially fluctuate, visual impairment does not usually improve over time, even with treatment
- Scalp tenderness, especially over the temporal artery, is seen in many patients, and rarely patients may present with avascular necrosis of scalp, extremity, or tongue. Decreased pulsations over temporal artery are a common finding. Erythema, warmth, swelling, or nodules over scalp arteries are also seen
- Patients sometimes have bruits or decreased pulses over large arteries. Rarely presentation will feature respiratory symptoms, ischemic chest pain, or congestive heart failure
- Neurologic problems occur in up to one-third of patients, and include neuropathies, transient ischemic attacks, and cerebral vascular accidents
- Temporal arteritis is frequently associated with polymyalgia rheumatica (up to 50%), which may cause stiffness and aching pain in the proximal muscles, worse in the morning and decreasing with exercise. There is often an associated synovitis, especially in the knees

MECHANISM/DESCRIPTION

- Temporal arteritis most commonly causes inflammation of arteries originating from the arch of the aorta, though other vessels, including veins, are sometimes involved
- Though usually clinically silent, involvement of the thoracic aorta occurs in a significant minority of patients and aortic aneurysm may result
- Thoracic aortic aneurysm is a late manifestation with an incidence 17 times those without temporal arteritis
- Abdominal aortic aneurysm is about twice as common in those with temporal arteritis
- Pathologic specimens feature patchy granulomatous inflammation resulting in a markedly thickened intima and occlusion of the vessel lumen
- Occlusive arteritis may involve thrombosis of the ophthalmic artery resulting in ischemic optic neuritis and visual loss
- Similarly, inflammation of arteries supplying the muscles of mastication results in jaw claudication
- Hepatic involvement is seen in about 25% of cases and responds promptly to steroid therapy

ETIOLOGY

- Women affected up to four times more often than men
- Rare in patients <50 years old, >90% are over 60 years old
- Rare in African American patients
- The inciting event is not known with certainty, however, viral infections have been implicated
- Genetic predisposition is linked to HLA-DR4
- There is a strong association with polymyalgia rheumatica

Pre-Hospital

CAUTIONS

- Symptoms may be confused with stroke. Initiate appropriate monitoring, and oxygen
- Patients may be hypotensive from one of the rare sequelae (aortic dissection, abdominal aortic aneurysm, or myocardial infarction)

Diagnosis

- The presence of any 3 or more of the following in patients with vasculitis is sensitive and specific for temporal arteritis
  - —Erythrocyte sedimentation rate greater than 50
  - —Age greater than 50 years
    - -New onset of headache, or change in quality of headache
    - -Tenderness or decreased pulsation of temporal artery
    - -Abnormal artery biopsy
  - —Presence of jaw claudication or neck pain greatly increases the odds of positive temporal biopsy in patients suspected of having temporal arteritis

ESSENTIAL WORKUP

- Erythrocyte sedimentation rate is often >50 mm/hr
- Focused physical exam with emphasis on temporal artery and scalp abnormalities, complete neurological exam, eye exam must including visual acuity, and visual field testing
- Funduscopy is often initially normal, though iritis and fine vitreous opacities may be early findings
  - —Optic nerve edema, hyperemia of the disk, pallor, hemorrhage, scattered cotton wool spots, vessel engorgement, and exudates are seen later
- Any pulse differences in extremities or bruits over large arteries should be noted

LABORATORY

- C-reactive protein above 2.45 mg/dl
- A mild normochromic anemia is typical; platelets tend to be elevated, while white cell count and differential are usually normal
- Liver function tests and PT may be elevated. CPK, tests of renal function, and urinalysis are generally normal

IMAGING/SPECIAL TESTS

- Temporal artery biopsy
- Doppler ultrasound showing decreased blood flow in temporal, facial, and ophthalmic arteries is supportive of the diagnosis
- Angiogram reveals smooth tapered occlusions or stenosis

DIFFERENTIAL DIAGNOSIS

- Vasculitides such as Polyarteritis nodosa, hypersensitivity vasculitis, SLE, Takayasu's arteritis, or Wegener's granulomatosis
- Thrombosis of retinal, ophthalmic, or temporal arteries
- Lyme disease

Treatment

INITIAL STABILIZATION

- Though rare, patients may present with vascular catastrophe such as aortic dissection, or myocardial infarction and need appropriate aggressive early management of ABCs

ED TREATMENT

- Begin steroids for moderate to high suspicion prior to temporal artery biopsy
  —Early treatment significantly reduces the frequency of blindness
  —Steroids effectively control systemic and local symptoms within days to weeks
- Symptomatic pain management with NSAIDs, or salicylates
- Referral to rheumatology
- Treatment with prednisone may continue for years depending on symptoms and lab tests
- Sustained steroid therapy may accelerate osteopenia, cause cataracts, and potentiate hyperglycemia and hypertension

MEDICATIONS

- NSAIDs, such as ibuprofen: 400 mg po every 4 hrs
- Prednisone: 60–100 mg po per day
- Salicylates: 650 mg every 4 hrs
- Solumedrol: 125 mg IV

Disposition

ADMISSION CRITERIA

- Patients with impending vascular complications
- Patients with associated acute visual loss

DISCHARGE CRITERIA

- Less symptomatic patients without evidence of end organ involvement
- Temporal artery biopsy should be performed within 24–48 hours

Miscellaneous

ICD9: 446.5

CORE CONTENT CODE: 2.5.1.3

SUGGESTED READINGS

Hayreh SS, Podhajsky PA, Raman R, Zimmerman B. Giant cell arteritis: Validity and reliability of various diagnostic criteria. Am J Ophthalmol 1997;123:285–296.

Hunder GG. Giant cell arteritis and polymyalgia rheumatica. Med Clin North Am 1997;81(1):195–219.

Nordberg E, Nordberg C, Malmvall B, Anderrson R, Bengtsson B. Giant cell arteritis. Rheum Dis Clin North Am 1995;21(4): 1013–1026.

Swannell AJ. Polymyalgia rheumatica and temporal arteritis: Diagnosis and management. BMJ 1997;314:1329–1332.

Author: John Munyak

Temporomandibular Joint Injury

Clinical Presentation

SIGNS AND SYMPTOMS

- Dull, aching unilateral jaw, ear, or head pain
  - —Exacerbated by opening the mouth
- A "popping" or "clicking" sensation may be noted with chewing
- Limited range of motion of the mandible
- Symptoms more conspicuous in the evening and less prominent upon awakening
- Pain may refer to a variety of locations on the ipsilateral hemicranium and supraclavicular region
- Dentoskeletal malocclusion
- Mandibular deviation with opening and closing of the mouth
- Temporomandibular joint (TMJ) capsule tenderness
- Tenderness over the muscles of mastication
- A palpable click can often be palpated with opening and closing of the mouth

MECHANISM/DESCRIPTION

- The cause of temporomandibular pain dysfunction syndrome (TMPDS) is unknown
- May be related to an abnormality in neuromuscular mechanics
  - —Trauma, dentoskeletal malocclusion, and bruxism are important contributors
- 10–20 million adults suffer TMPDS
- Patients present in fourth decade of life
- Females to male ratio of 2:1

Pre-Hospital

N/A

Diagnosis

ESSENTIAL WORKUP

- Diagnosis based on clinical presentation above
- Exclude other causes of unilateral facial or head pain

LABORATORY

- No specific laboratory tests are indicated

IMAGING/SPECIAL TESTS

- Plain radiographs are of little value
- Tomograms, bone scintigraphy, CT scan, and MRI are not necessary during the initial evaluation of TMPDS in the emergency department

DIFFERENTIAL DIAGNOSIS

- Myocardial ischemia
- Carotid or vertebral artery dissection
- Intracranial hemorrhage (subarachnoid hemorrhage)
- Temporal arteritis
- Multiple sclerosis may present with pain similar to trigeminal neuralgia
- Trigeminal or glossopharyngeal neuralgia
- Vascular headache
- Dental abnormalities
- Herpes zoster
- Salivary gland disorder, otitis media, external otitis, and sinusitis
- Elongated styloid process pain often precipitated by swallowing or turning the head

Treatment

INITIAL STABILIZATION

N/A

ED TREATMENT

- Refer to dentist or oral-maxillofacial surgeon for occlusal splints
- Additional therapeutic options include
  —Tricyclic antidepressants
  —Vapocoolant spray with physiotherapy
  —Behavior modification
  —Intra-articular and local injections of anesthetics or steroids

MEDICATIONS

- Oral or parenteral analgesics
- Muscle relaxants

Disposition

ADMISSION CRITERIA

- None

DISCHARGE CRITERIA

- Treat as outpatients with pain medication, muscle relaxants and warm compresses

Miscellaneous

ICD9: 524.60

CORE CONTENT CODE: 6.3.14

SUGGESTED READINGS

Marbach JJ. Temporomandibular pain dysfunction syndrome. History, physical examination and treatment. Rheum Dis Clin North Am 22(3):477–98.

Author: Timothy J. Mader

Tendon Lacerations

Clinical Presentation

SIGNS AND SYMPTOMS

- Suspect tendon injury when the function appears normal, but the patient complains of pain or weakness with movement or against resistance. Also suspect when the resting position of the hand or fingers has abnormal flexion or extension compared to the uninjured hand
- Flexor tendon injury
  - —Flexor digitorum profundus injury: inability to flex the distal phalanx
  - —Flexor digitorum superficialis: inability to flex the PIP joint
  - —Forearm and wrist flexors: inability to flex ulnar or radial side of wrist or to flex the wrist while opposing the thumb to the little finger
- Extensor tendon injury
- Pain or weakness with extension of the tips of the finger against resistance indicates injury
- Have patient place the palm on flat surface and extend the fingers individually. Palpate each tendon. Loss of normal tension is a clue to injury

ETIOLOGY

- Both flexor and extensor tendon injuries may result from lacerations and crush or avulsion injuries
- Extension injuries are more likely to be due to a closed injury than a flexor injury, especially in the digits

PEDIATRIC CONSIDERATIONS

- Tendon injuries in children have the same characteristics as those in adults. Children may not cooperate with the examination as readily as adults

Pre-Hospital

- No specific considerations

Diagnosis

ESSENTIAL WORKUP

- Tendon injuries are diagnosed from history and physical examination

History

- Include mechanism and circumstances of injury to evaluate potential for foreign bodies and contamination
- Time of injury
- Position of hand during injury
- Dominant hand
- Drug allergies and tetanus status
- Medications and medical history

Physical examination

- Perform neurovascular exam prior to anaesthetizing wound
- Wound must be explored after anesthesia (1% lidocaine or 0.5% bupivacaine) in a bloodless field with good light
- Wound *must* be explored through *complete range of motion* for that digit or hand to uncover injury that is proximal or distal to skin wound
- Each digit must be tested separately from the others. Inactivate the remaining digits by holding them down during the exam

LABORATORY

Wounds presenting more than 12 hours after onset or with signs of infection may be cultured but this is not needed for fresh wounds

IMAGING/SPECIAL TESTS

- X-rays are necessary when foreign bodies (glass, metal) or fractures are suspected
- Ultrasound, CT, or fluoroscopy may be used to evaluate suspected radiolucent foreign bodies

DIFFERENTIAL DIAGNOSIS

- Partial tendon lacerations are more common than complete lacerations and may have intact function
- Consider partial lacerations when there is pain or weakness with movement or movement against resistance
  - —Alteration of the normal resting position of the hand may also indicate a partial laceration
- Lacerations over the MCP joint are considered to be human bite wounds until proven otherwise and frequently have associated extensor tendon injuries
- Lacerations over the PIP joint may involve the lateral bands or the central slip of the extensor mechanism. If not repaired properly, this results in a *boutonniere deformity*
- Avulsion of the flexor digitorum profundus tendon may be present with or without an associated avulsion fracture
  - —Suspect when a grasping finger is hit by a speeding object (e.g., sports injury)
- *Mallet finger deformities* result from disruption of the extensor tendon distal to the central slip

Treatment

INITIAL STABILIZATION

- ABCs
- Do not remove foreign bodies in the field
- Elevate extremity and control hemorrhage with direct pressure
- Remove jewelry or constricting bands

ED TREATMENT

- Tetanus toxoid if needed
- Broad-spectrum antibiotics such as first generation cephalosporin should be given for all tendon lacerations, e.g., cefazolin
- Copiously irrigate using 1 L NS or NS mixed with 50:1 betadine solution. Remove all foreign bodies and débride avascular tissue
- Partial tendon lacerations that involve more than 10% of the cross-sectional area of the tendon must be repaired
- All suspected flexor tendon lacerations require consultation and repair by a hand surgeon, ideally within 12 hours
  —If a surgeon isn't promptly available: after irrigation the skin may be closed without tendon repair and immobilize the hand in a bulky volar splint with the wrists at 20–30° of flexion, the MCP joint at 60–70° flexion, and the IP joints at 10–15° of flexion
- Simple extensor tendon lacerations may be repaired in the ED
  —Use 4-0 or 5-0 nonabsorbable suture in a figure eight or a modified Kessler stitch. Repair the skin as usual
- Tendon lacerations over the PIP joint may result in boutonniere deformities and should be referred to a hand surgeon
- Tendon lacerations at the wrist and distal forearm require repair by a hand surgeon due to retraction of the proximal end
- Multiple tendon lacerations, as well as those associated with fractures, will require referral for operative repair
- All tendon lacerations associated with human bites must be copiously irrigated and given Penicillin G and broad-spectrum antibiotics, immobilized, and elevated

MEDICATIONS

- Cefazolin: 1 g IVPB; peds: 100 mg/kg/day IM or IV divided q 6 hrs followed by 40 mg/kg/day po divided q 6 hrs for 5–7 days
- Penicillin G: 2 million IU IVPB; peds: 100,000–300,000 IU/kg IM or IV followed by 40 mg/kg/day po divided q 6 hrs for 5–7 days
- Tetanus toxoid: 0.5 cc IM; peds: <7 years old: DPT preferred; >7 years old: TD if immunization series not completed; TIG required 250 IU IM

Disposition

ADMISSION CRITERIA

- Any tendon laceration that is infected must be admitted for operative debridement
- Any extensor tendon injury that is due to a human bite wound must be admitted for operative debridement and IV antibiotics
- Any significant flexor tendon laceration must be admitted for timely operative repair or transferred to the nearest hand surgeon

DISCHARGE CRITERIA

- Any extensor tendon laceration that is not infected, nor associated with other significant injury or underlying fracture, and that is repaired by the ED physician and that is properly splinted may be discharged with appropriate timely follow-up arranged with the hand surgeon
- Any tendon laceration that has been repaired in the ED by the hand surgeon may be properly splinted and discharged to his care
- Any extensor tendon laceration that will need surgeon referral for repair (wrist, forearm, PIP joint) and that has been properly treated and splinted and has antibiotics prescribed may be discharged for timely follow-up with the hand surgeon

Miscellaneous

ICD9: 848.9

CORE CONTENT CODE: 18.4.14.1

SUGGESTED READINGS

Hart RG, Kutz JE. Flexor tendon injuries of the hand. Emerg Med Clin North Am 1993;11(3):621–636.

Hart RG, Uenara DT, Kutz JE. Extensor tendon injuries of the hand. Emerg Med Clin North Am 1993;11(3):637–649.

Newmeyer WL. Extensor tendon injury in the hand and wrist. In: Roberts J, et al., eds. Clinical procedure in emergency medicine. 2d ed. Philadelphia: WB Saunders, 1991:752–761.

Authors: Toni Tubb; Robert Galli

Tendinitis

Clinical Presentation

SIGNS AND SYMPTOMS

- Pain—localized over involved tendon, worse with active contraction and passive stretching of involved muscle-tendon unit
- Tenderness—localized along course of tendon, sometimes associated with crepitation or with a rubbery grating feeling on palpation during motion
- Inflammation—usually only mild swelling, erythema, or increased warmth. (Marked swelling, erythema, and warmth suggests possibility of suppurative tenosynovitis)
- Triggering—a snapping on motion usually involving a flexor digitorum tendon, sometimes the finger will lock in flexion requiring manual traction to restore extension

MECHANISM/DESCRIPTION

Tendinitis involves inflammation and/or edema of the tendon or of the tendon sheath. The inflammation is thought to result from microtrauma, response to crystal or lipid deposition, or is an autoimmune response. Calcific tendinitis involves calcium crystal deposition in the area of the tendon

- Areas commonly affected by tendinitis include
  - —Flexor tendons of the digits in the palm
  - —Abductor pollices longus and extensor pollices brevis tendons at the wrist (de Quervain's disease)
  - —One or more extensor tendons over distal one-third or forearm
  - —Origin of extensor tendons at elbow (lateral epicondylitis or tennis elbow)
  - —Origin of flexor tendons at elbow (medial epicondylitis or golfer's elbow)
  - —Biceps tendon at shoulder
  - —Supraspinatus tendon in rotator cuff of shoulder
  - —Achilles tendon at ankle
  - —One or more tendons at ankle including tibialis posterior, tibialis anterior, extensor digitorum, peroneal tendons
  - —Quadriceps or patellar tendon at knee
  - —Hamstring tendons in the popliteal fossa

ETIOLOGY

- Overuse and repetitive motion: this can be from occupational, recreational, or athletic activity
- Trauma: direct blunt trauma
- Thermal injury
- Rheumatoid arthritis
- Lupus erythematosus
- Sarcoidosis
- Gout and other crystal deposition diseases
- Diabetes mellitus
- Lipid deposition disease
- Drug reaction: achilles tendinitis associated with fluoroquinolones

PEDIATRIC CONSIDERATIONS

- Apophysitis occurs in children at an ossification center subject to traction; at the medial epicondyle it is called Little League elbow, and at the tibial tubercle it is Osgood-Schlatter syndrome

Pre-Hospital

N/A

Diagnosis

ESSENTIAL WORKUP

- History
  - —Evaluate for systemic disease, trauma, medications
  - —Uncover the activity that may be perpetuating the tendinitis
- Physical Examination
  - —Complete neurosensory exam of the involved extremity
  - —Examine for skin changes and lymphadenopathy
  - —Assess for local tenderness along tendon
  - —Pain on active or isometric contraction of involved muscles
  - —Pain on passive stretch of involved muscles (e.g., Finkelstein's test for de Quervain's disease produces passive stretch of the abductor pollices longus and extensor pollices brevis muscles)

LABORATORY

- Not indicated except in search of systemic disease

IMAGING/SPECIAL TESTS

- Usually not helpful, may find calcium deposition particularly in supraspinatus tendinitis, but this will not affect initial management
- Obtain plain x-rays to rule out fracture or other bony abnormality in equivocal cases

PEDIATRIC CONSIDERATIONS

- More frequently need x-rays to rule out fracture, avascular necrosis, osteochondritis dissecans, or bony tumor

DIFFERENTIAL DIAGNOSIS

- Suppurative tenosynovitis: physical findings of marked erythema, fusiform swelling and warmth, and a history of proximate penetrating trauma demands workup for infection either by aspiration or surgical exploration
- Indolent infection: history or physical exam suggesting tuberculosis, or gonococcal disease, demands workup for systemic infection. Local aspiration or surgical biopsy may be indicated but it is difficult to culture gonococcus from synovial samples
- Arthritis: pain on any motion of the joint and a joint effusion may help distinguish arthritis. In equivocal cases, do joint fluid examination
- Bursitis: careful physical exam helps to define pathology but may be difficult to isolate bursitis from tendinitis in some cases

- Osteomyelitis or suppurative myositis: if suggested by history and physical, demands workup including plain films, and bone scan or CT-scan as needed
- Phlebitis/DVT
- Myositis: workup including ESR, CPK, and renal function as indicated by history and physical
- Avascular necrosis (Kienböck's disease is necrosis of lunate, diagnosis by x-ray)

PEDIATRIC CONSIDERATIONS

- Avascular necrosis presenting as pain and swelling around a joint can occur in pediatric patients at various locations. Well-recognized sites of avascular necrosis are the capitellum of the humerus, the head of the femur, the tarsal navicular, and the metatarsal head. The diagnosis is made by plain radiograph

Treatment

INITIAL STABILIZATION

- None necessary

ED TREATMENT

- Splint in comfortable position of function
- Instructions to avoid activity or motion thought to be perpetuating problem
- Nonsteroidal anti-inflammatory agents, aspirin, or acetaminophen

MEDICATIONS

- Nonsteroidal anti-inflammatory agents (there are many choices; a few are listed below)
  —Diclofenac: 50 mg po bid tid
  —Ibuprofen: adult: 600 mg po q 6 hrs; peds: 5–10 mg/kg po q 6 hrs
  —Ketorolac: 30 mg IV/IM q 6 hrs, or 10 mg po q 4–6 hrs
  —Piroxicam: 20 mg po q day

Disposition

ADMISSION CRITERIA

- None unless surgical intervention is required (e.g., tenosynovitis)

DISCHARGE CRITERIA

- Discharge home to follow-up within 1–2 weeks with primary physician or occupational medicine

Miscellaneous

ICD9: 726.90

CORE CONTENT CODE: 10.4.1

SUGGESTED READINGS

Hutton C. Regional problems of the arm and leg in adults. In: Maddison PJ, et al., eds. Oxford textbook of rheumatology. Vol. 1. New York: Oxford University Press, 1993 pp 70–79.

Ribard P, Audisio F, Kahn, et al. Seven achilles tendinitis including three complicated by rupture during fluoroquinolone therapy. J Rheumatol 1992;19:1479–1481.

White PH. Regional problems of the arm and leg in children. In: Maddison PJ, et al., eds. Oxford textbook of rheumatology. Vol. 1. New York: Oxford University Press, 1993 pp 80–84.

Author: Joel Pasternack

Tenosynovitis

Clinical Presentation

SIGNS AND SYMPTOMS

- Four cardinal signs of Kanavel
  - —Tenderness to palpation over the flexor tendon sheath
  - —Symmetric edema of the finger ("sausage digit")
  - —Finger is held in flexion at rest
  - —Excruciating pain on passive extension of the finger (most sensitive sign and should be performed by lifting the nail of the affected digit)
- Infection of the tendon sheath of the thumb may spread to the radial bursa, with associated pain and edema of the thenar eminence, hand is held in flexion and radial deviation
- Infection of the tendon sheath of the little finger may spread to the ulnar bursa, with associated dorsal hand edema, other fingers held slightly flexed, and are painful on passive extension
- If the infection communicates between the radial and ulnar bursa, a "horseshoe abscess" results

MECHANISM/DESCRIPTION

Flexor tenosynovitis (FTS) is a closed space infection involving the flexor tendon sheath, and can be one of the most devastating hand infections encountered in the emergency department. If not recognized and treated early, adhesions and tendon necrosis may occur, resulting permanent loss of function

- Penetrating injury, especially at the proximal and distal flexion creases of the finger (where the tendon sheaths are most superficial) is the most common mechanism
- Thumb, index, and middle finger are most commonly involved
- Direct extension from nearby infection, hematogenous, and lymphatic seeding are other less common mechanisms
- High pressure "injection" injuries to the hands and fingers (air tools, paint sprayers, hydraulic equipment) may appear minor on the surface, but are associated with a high incidence of FTS

ETIOLOGY

Most cases of FTS from penetrating injury are caused by polymicrobial infections with Gram positive aerobic (Group A *Streptococcus, Staphylococcus*), and mixed anaerobic organisms (anaerobic *Streptococcus,* Enterobacteriaceae, *Cl. perfringens, Cl. tetani*). Other, less common organisms

- *N. gonorrhea:* if signs of pelvic inflammatory disease, cervicitis, urethritis (hematogenous seeding)
- *Pseudomonas:* in patients with diabetes or water-associated injury
- Gram-negative and fungal organisms: in immunocompromised or diabetic patients

Pre-Hospital

CAUTIONS

- Delay to definitive treatment leads to significantly increased morbidity and loss of function
- Elevation and immobilization of the affected hand or digit should be performed in the pre-hospital setting

Diagnosis

ESSENTIAL WORKUP

- Careful history and physical exam ("Kanavel's signs") are the key to early recognition of FTS, and excluding other less serious hand infections (e.g., cellulitis)
- History should include mechanism of injury (e.g., puncture wound, soil or water exposure, high pressure/compressed air injury), onset, and progression of symptoms
- High pressure injection injury mandates emergent evaluation by a hand surgeon, regardless of how minor the injury may appear on the surface
- Determine tetanus status, and assess other risk factors (diabetes, immunosuppression)
- Identify signs and symptoms of systemic illness (fever, septic appearing), and other potential sites of infection (other septic joints, urethral discharge, PID)

LABORATORY

- CBC and blood cultures are indicated if there are signs of systemic illness
- Urethral or endocervical cultures for *Neisseria gonorrhoeae* are indicated if signs of urethritis or pelvic inflammatory disease are present

IMAGING/SPECIAL TESTS

- Radiographs of the affected digit are indicated to identify foreign body and osteomyelitis
- Ultrasound to detect fluid in the synovial sheath is less sensitive than physical exam for identifying early FTS, and is not helpful

DIFFERENTIAL DIAGNOSIS

- Cellulitis
- Paronychia
- Felon
- Septic arthritis
- Osteomyelitis
- Palmar space infection

Treatment

INITIAL STABILIZATION

- ABCs (especially if patient is septic appearing, hypotensive)
- Elevation and immobilization of the affected digit
- IV access
- Confirm tetanus status

ED TREATMENT

- Intravenous antibiotics: Initial antimicrobial coverage should be broad spectrum and cover both Gram-positive aerobic (staph, strep) and anaerobic bacteria. Penicillin G, Ancef, or clindamycin are recommended initially. Cefotetan and cefoxitin are second-generation cephalosporins which cover staph and strep, have good Gram-negative and anaerobic coverage, and can be used as well
- If the patient is immunocompromised, diabetic, or water related injury, Gram-negative and *Pseudomonas* coverage should be added. Timentin (ticarcillin + clavulanate) or Zosyn (piperacillin + tazobactam) are recommended. An aminoglycoside (e.g., tobramycin) may be added for double coverage
- If suspect *N. gonorrhoeae,* ceftriaxone should be given
- Pain control with parenteral narcotics is appropriate as this is an *extremely* painful condition
- Administer tetanus booster if indicated
- Immediate consultation with a hand surgeon

MEDICATIONS

- Cefazolin: 1–2 g IV q 8 hrs; peds: 50–100 mg/kg/day IV divided q 8 hrs
- Cefotetan: 1–2 g IV q 12 hrs; peds: 50–100 mg/kg/day IV divided q 12 hrs
- Cefoxitin: 1–2 g IV q 8 hrs; peds: 80–160 mg/kg/day IV divided q 6–8 hrs
- Ceftriaxone: 1–2 g IV q 12 hrs; peds: 50–100 mg/kg/day IV divided q 12 hrs
- Clindamycin: 600–900 mg IV q 8 hrs; peds: 20–40 mg/kg/day divided q 8 hrs
- Penicillin G: 12–24 million IU IV divided q 4–6 hrs; peds: 100,000–400,000 IU/kg/day IV divided q 4–6 hrs
- Timentin: 3.1 g IV q 6 hrs; peds: safety not established
- Tobramycin: 1 mg/kg IV q 8 hrs *or* 5 mg/kg IV q 24 hrs; peds: 2–2.5 mg/kg IV q 8 hrs
- Zosyn: 3.375 g IV q 6 hrs; peds: safety not established

Disposition

- All patients suspected of having FTS require admission to the hospital and immediate consultation with a hand surgeon
- If the patient presents more than 48 hours after the onset of symptoms, surgical drainage in the operating suite is required
- If the patient presents within the first 24–48 hours, conservative treatment with continued immobilization and elevation, intravenous antibiotics, and close observation may be attempted
  - —Surgical drainage is indicated if the patient is not markedly improved in 24 hours or if physical findings are not resolved within 2 days
  - —The hand surgeon may opt for continuous catheter irrigation of the tendon sheath instead of formal drainage procedures

DISCHARGE CRITERIA

- It is not appropriate to discharge patients from the ED unless formal evaluation by a hand surgeon has been obtained

Miscellaneous

ICD9: 727.00

CORE CONTENT CODE: 10.6.5

SUGGESTED READINGS

Antosia RE. The hand. In: Rosen P, et al., eds. Emergency medicine: Concepts and clinical practice. 4th ed. St. Louis: CV Mosby, 1998:625–668.

Carter PR. Common hand injuries and infections. Philadelphia: WB Saunders, 1983:17.

Hausman MR, Lisser SP. Hand infections. Orthop Clin North Am 1992;23(1):171–185.

Siegel DB, Gelberman RH. Infections of the hand. Orthop Clin North Am 1988;19(4):779–789.

Author: James Schmitt

Testicular Torsion

Clinical Presentation

SIGNS AND SYMPTOMS

- Sudden onset of unilateral testicular pain and tenderness followed by scrotal swelling and erythema
- Less commonly, torsion may present with pain in the inguinal or lower abdominal area
- Up to 40% of patients may describe previous similar episodes of testicular pain that remitted spontaneously, representing spontaneous torsion and detorsion
- The affected testicle may be found to lie transversely as opposed to the normal vertical lie
- Nausea and vomiting occur in 50% of cases, and low-grade fever occurs in 25%
- There is a bimodal distribution with peak incidences in infancy and adolescence
  —Torsion is rare after age 30
- Symptoms of urinary infection (dysuria, frequency, and urgency) are absent
- In distinguishing torsion from epididymitis, localization of tenderness is helpful early in the course. However, once significant scrotal swelling occurs the anatomy becomes indistinct and some form of testicular flow study or surgical exploration is required
- The cremasteric reflex is frequently absent with testicular torsion
- The classic Prehn's sign, which consists of relief of pain on elevation of the testicle in epididymitis and worsening or no change in the pain with torsion, is considered unreliable

ETIOLOGY

- Most patients have a congenital abnormality of the genitalia with a high insertion of the tunica vaginalis on the spermatic cord and a redundant mesorchium that permit increased mobility and twisting of the testicle on its vascular pedicle
- The anatomic abnormality is generally bilateral, so that both testicles are susceptible to torsion

MECHANISM/DESCRIPTION

- Rotation generally occurs medially and ranges from incomplete (e.g., 90–180°) to complete (540–720°) torsion
- Depending on the degree of torsion, vascular occlusion occurs and the result is infarction of the testicle after 6 hours
- Testicular infarction leads to atrophy and may ultimately decrease fertility

PEDIATRIC CONSIDERATIONS

- Testicular torsion has been described in utero and in virtually every pediatric age group
- The peak incidence occurs in late childhood and adolescence (mode: 13-years old) with a smaller peak in infancy

Pre-Hospital

CAUTIONS

- There is no definitive treatment that can be rendered in the field. However, pre-hospital personnel need to recognize the urgency of acute testicular pain in young patients
- These patients should be transported to the ED immediately as the outcome is time-dependent

Diagnosis

ESSENTIAL WORKUP

- The presentation of an "acute scrotum" in a child or adolescent requires rapid assessment and immediate consultation with an urologist
- These patients will require noninvasive flow studies or surgical exploration to detect torsion
- 25–30% of these patients will ultimately prove to have testicular torsion

LABORATORY

- Urinalysis is usually normal, but up to 20% of cases of torsion have pyuria
- Elevated WBC count with a left shift is present in 50% of cases
- There are no laboratory tests specific for testicular torsion

IMAGING/SPECIAL TESTS

- The criterion standard imaging modality has traditionally been ^{99m}TC-pertechnetate radionuclide scans which shows decreased flow in the torsed testicle compared to the unaffected side
  —Epididymitis will reveal increased flow due to inflammation
  —This technique has an overall sensitivity and specificity of 98% and 100% respectively
- Because of the frequent time delays in obtaining nuclear scans, use of Doppler ultrasound to assess testicular blood flow has increasingly replaced nuclear scanning as a less invasive, more readily available test with comparable accuracy
  —Several modalities are available including color flow Doppler, power Doppler, and pulsed Doppler with mechanical sector scanning, although none of these modalities has demonstrated superiority
  —Color-flow Doppler is the most commonly available
  —Use of Doppler contrast material may soon become available and should enhance the accuracy of this modality
  —Overall sensitivity and specificity for color flow Doppler ranges from 86–100% and 97–100% respectively, although the accuracy tends to be lower in infants
- There are limitations of all flow studies in that they reflect only the current state of perfusion. Consequently, a spontaneously detorsed testicle may show normal or even increased flow and yet still be at high risk for recurrent torsion

DIFFERENTIAL DIAGNOSIS

- Epididymitis/orchitis
- Torsion of the appendix testis
- Testicular trauma or rupture of the testicle
- Incarcerated inguinal hernia

- Testicular tumor
- Acute hydrocele
- Henoch-Schönlein purpura
- Other intra-abdominal conditions (appendicitis, pancreatitis, renal colic may rarely present with testicular pain)

PEDIATRIC CONSIDERATIONS

- All imaging techniques designed to evaluate testicular blood flow have technical limitations when applied to infants because the testicular vessels are very small and the amount of blood flow to the testicle under normal conditions is minimal
- Scrotal exploration may be required

Treatment

INITIAL STABILIZATION

- Intravenous fluid, analgesics as appropriate

ED TREATMENT

- Establish the diagnosis and mobilize appropriate urologic care
- In situations in which definitive care is likely to be delayed beyond 4–5 hours since the onset of torsion, manual detorsion may be attempted
  —This is accomplished by externally rotating the affected testicle (opposite the usual medial direction of torsion) until pain is relieved or normal anatomy is restored. All patients who undergo manual detorsion must be surgically explored

Disposition

ADMISSION CRITERIA

- Any patient with confirmed testicular torsion must be admitted for scrotal exploration and bilateral orchiopexy
- Flow studies that are inconclusive or technical failures mandate further investigation by surgical exploration of the scrotum
- Admission for urgent surgical exploration of an acute scrotum is mandatory if there will be any potential delay in obtaining a flow study

DISCHARGE CRITERIA

- Patients with negative scrotal exploration, or normal flow studies can be discharged with appropriate urologic follow-up
- Appropriate parameters for return to ED must be discussed because of the possibility of intermittent torsion
- Patients with an obvious diagnosis other than testicular torsion (e.g., a nonincarcerated inguinal hernia) can be referred for elective care

Miscellaneous

ICD9: 608.2

CORE CONTENT CODE: 19.2.2.4, 13.13.3.1

SUGGESTED READINGS

Al Mufti RA, Ogedegbe AK, Laferty K. The use of Doppler ultrasound in the clinical management of acute testicular pain. Br J Urol 1995;76:625–627.

Coley BD, Frush DP, Babcock DS, et al. Acute testicular torsion: Comparison of unenhanced and contrast enhanced power Doppler US, color Doppler US, and radionuclide imaging. Radiol 1996;199:441–446.

Patriquin HB, Yazbeck S, Trinh B, et al. Testicular torsion in infants and children: Diagnosis with Doppler sonography. Radiol 1993;188:781–785.

Rabinowitz R, Hulbert WC Jr. Acute scrotal swelling. Urol Clin North Am 1995;22:101–105.

Schul MW, Keating MA. The acute pediatric scrotum. J Emerg Med 1993;11:565–577.

Author: Ed Newton

Tetanus

Clinical Presentation

SIGNS AND SYMPTOMS

Local

- Persistent rigidity of the muscles in proximity to a wound
  - —May be mild
  - —May persist for months and resolve
  - —May evolve to generalized form

Generalized

Initial Presentation

- Trismus (initial)
- Irritability
- Restlessness
- Diaphoresis
- Dysphagia

Later Manifestations

- Muscle group rigidity
  - —Sudden burst of tonic contractions of muscle groups causing
    - -Opisthotonus
    - -Flexion and adduction of the arms
    - -Clenching of fists
    - -Extension of the lower extremities
  - —Diaphragmatic spasm or paralysis
    - -May compromise respiration
- Hypersympathetic state
  - —Begins in the second week
  - —Prominent cause of mortality
  - —Dysrhythmias
  - —Blood pressure changes
  - —Diaphoresis
  - —Hyperthermia
  - —Rhabdomyolysis
  - —Laryngeal spasm

Cephalic

- Uncommon variant
- Follows head injury or otitis media
- Spasm of lower cranial and facial muscles
  - —Cranial nerve VII most common
- May progress to generalized tetanus

Neonatal

- Irritability
- Poor suck
- Facial grimacing
- Muscle spasms with touch
- A form of generalized tetanus resulting from traditional practices of putting dirt or dirty rags on umbilical stump
- Very high mortality
- Incubation period 1–2 weeks

MECHANISM/DESCRIPTION

- Rare disease in the U.S.
- Incubation period
  - —Inoculation to the appearance of the first symptoms
    - -48 hours to 3 or more weeks
    - -<7 days—poor prognosis
  - —Period of onset
    - -Poor prognosis if <48 hours from first symptom to first reflex spasm
- Type of injury associated with poor prognosis
  - —Burns
  - —Compound fractures
  - —Surgical wounds
- Neonatal tetanus
  - —Due to infected umbilical stump
  - —Symptom onset in second week of life when maternal antibodies decrease
- Admission signs associated with poor prognosis
  - —Fever
  - —Tachycardia

ETIOLOGY

- *Clostridium tetani*
  - —Slender, motile, anaerobic Gram-positive rod with a terminal spherical spore
- Spore characteristics
  - —Resistant to oxygen, moisture, temperature extremes
  - —Can survive indefinitely
- When inoculated into a wound, the spores germinate, and if the oxygen tension is low, proliferate and produce toxins
- Toxins
  - —Tetanolysin
    - -Damages tissue
    - -Reduces oxidation-reduction potential
    - -Allowing greater logarithmic growth of organisms
  - —Tetanospasmin
    - -Responsible for the clinical manifestations
    - -Released by manipulation of wound

Pre-Hospital

CAUTIONS

- Careful airway management required
  - —Endotracheal intubation complicated by
    - -Trismus
    - -Vocal cord paralysis
    - -Facial/neck muscle rigidity
- Excessive stimulation may provoke tetany of musculature

Diagnosis

ESSENTIAL WORKUP

- Clinical diagnosis
  - —Suspected in all cases of trismus
  - —No wound recalled in one-fifth of cases
  - —Full tetanus immunization almost eliminates diagnosis

LABORATORY

- CBC
- Electrolytes, BUN/Cr, glucose
  - —For hypocalcemia
- ABG/pulse oximetry
  - —For oxygenation status
- Wound culture for *C. tetani*
  - —Positive in one-third
- *C. tetani* titers
  - —Will only be useful after the fact

IMAGING/SPECIAL TESTS

- CSF analysis
  - —Normal with tetanus
  - —For meningitis
- CT brain for altered mental status
  - —Normal

DIFFERENTIAL DIAGNOSIS

- Strychnine poisoning
- Dystonic reaction to dopamine blockade
- Meningitis
- Rabies
- Encephalitis
- Peritonitis
- Alveolar abscess
- Tetany/hyperventilation syndrome
- Hysteria
- Dislocated mandible/TMJ syndrome

Treatment

INITIAL STABILIZATION

- ABCs
  - —Prophylactic intubation
  - —Require neuromuscular blockade due to trismus
  - —Establish IV 0.9%NS
  - —Monitor BP and cardiac rhythm (autonomic instability)

ED TREATMENT

- Administer benztropine or diphenhydramine to rule out dystonic reaction
- Tetanus immune globulin (TIG)
  - —3000–6000 IU IM, or 250 IU intrathecal (experimental)
  - —Administer *before* debridement of wound
  - —Neutralizes toxins that have not yet entered neurons
    - -No effect on toxin already bound in CNS
- Surgical debridement of the wound
  - —Delay until several hours after the administration of TIG
- Antibiotics to eliminate remaining bacteria
  - —Penicillin G potassium
  - —Metronidazole
  - —In penicillin allergy, use erythromycin, tetracycline, or chloramphenicol
- Supportive care
  - —Treat muscle spasms with diazepam, chlorpromazine, or meprobamate
  - —Nondepolarizing neuromuscular blockage may be required
  - —Meticulous airway support to prevent aspiration/pneumonia
- Autonomic instability therapy
  - —Occurs during the second or third week
  - —Tachydysrhythmia and hypertension
    - -Treat with β blockade
    - -Labetalol more titratable but less effective than propranolol
  - —Hypotension
    - -Rule out septicemia and hypovolemia
    - -Initiate dopamine or dobutamine when low cardiac output
  - —Bradycardia
    - -Temporary pacemaker more effective than atropine

Prophylaxis

- TIG (tetanus immune globulin)
  - —250 IU IM
  - —Separate site from Td
  - —Unimmunized or incompletely immunized in presence of wound
- Tetanus-diphtheria toxoid (Td), 0.5 ml IM
  - —Unimmunized or incompletely immunized
    - -DPT for children under 7
  - —>5 years since booster

PEDIATRIC CONSIDERATIONS

- For prophylaxis, use DPT instead of TD in children under 7 years
- For treatment, base dose of TIG on weight

MEDICATIONS

- Benztropine: 1–2 mg IV
- Chloramphenicol: 1.0 g (peds: 50–100 mg/kg/24hrs) IV q 6 hrs
- Chlorpromazine: 10–50 mg IM
- Diazepam (benzodiazepine): 5–10 mg (peds: 0.2–0.4 mg/kg) IV
- Diphenhydramine: 50 mg IV
- Dobutamine: 2.5–15 μg/kg/min IV
- Dopamine: 2–20 μg/kg/min IV
- Doxycycline: 100 mg IV q 12 hrs
- Erythromycin: 500 mg IV q 6 hrs
- Labetalol: 20 mg (peds: 0.3–1 mg/kg/dose) IV q 10 min up to 300 mg PRN—start infusion 2 mg/min (peds: 0.4–1 mg/kg/hr, max 3 mg/kg/hr) as needed
- Meprobamate: 400 mg po tid
- Metronidazole: 1.0 g (peds: 15 mg/kg) load, followed by 500 mg (7.5 mg/kg) IV q 6 hrs
- Penicillin G potassium: 1.2 million IU (peds: 100,000 IU/kg/24hrs) IV q 6 hrs for 10 days
- Propranolol: 0.5–1 mg (peds: 0.01–0.1 mg/kg) IV

Disposition

ADMISSION CRITERIA

- All patients should be admitted, usually to intensive care settings

DISCHARGE CRITERIA

- None

Miscellaneous

ICD9: 37.0

CORE CONTENT CODE: 9.1.8

SUGGESTED READINGS

Bleck TP. Pharmacology of tetanus. Clin Neuropharmacol 1986;9(2):103–120.

Bleck TP. Tetanus: pathophysiology, management, and prophylaxis. Dis Mon 1991:37:545–603.

Olsen KM, Hiller FC. Management of tetanus. Clin Pharmacol 1987;6:570–574.

Authors: Constance Greene; Gordon Chew

Guidelines for Tetanus Prophylaxis for Wounds

NUMBER OF DOSES OF TETANUS TOXOID	TD	TIG
Unknown or <3	Yes	Yes
3 or more	Yes if >5 years since last dose	No

Clinical Presentation

SIGNS AND SYMPTOMS

Cardiovascular

- Sinus or supraventricular tachycardias
  - —Multifocal atrial tachycardia
  - —Caused by β_1 receptor stimulation
- Hypotension
  - —In acute or acute-on-chronic ingestions only
  - —Associated with theophylline >35 mg/L
  - —Caused by β_2 receptor stimulation
  - —May be refractory to fluids, positioning, and conventional vasopressors

Central Nervous System

- Tremor
- Mental status changes
- Seizures with theophylline level
  - —>100 mg/L in acute overdose
  - —>30 mg/L in acute-on-chronic intoxication
  - —As low as 20 mg/L in chronic intoxication
  - —Usually refractory to and may be enhanced by phenytoin

Gastrointestinal

- Nausea/vomiting
  - —Protracted and refractory to usual anti-emetics at usual doses
- Abdominal pain
- Pharmacobezoar
  - —From sustained-release dosage forms in acute ingestions
  - —Delays peak concentrations

Miscellaneous

- Hypokalemia
  - —As low as 1.5 mEq/L
- Hyperglycemia
- Leukocytosis
- Hypercalcemia, hypophosphatemia, hypomagnesemia

MECHANISM/DESCRIPTION

- Acute overdose
  - —Ingestion within an 8 hour interval in a patient in whom no detectable theophylline would be found
- Acute-on-chronic overdose
  - —Single excessive dose in a patient receiving usual therapeutic doses for ≥24 hours prior
- Chronic intoxication
  - —Accumulation of theophylline >20 mg/L associated with therapeutic use for ≥24 hours secondary to
    - -Drug:drug, drug:diet or drug:disease interactions
    - -Due to use of serial excessive doses
- Electrolyte shifts and hypotensive effects only occur in acute overdoses
  - —Tachyphylaxis to these effects occurs with maintenance therapy
  - —Due to cellular shifts between extra and intracellular fluids

ETIOLOGY

- Acute ingestions require larger concentrations to achieve specific toxic effects than acute-on-chronic or chronic overdoses due to the absence of baseline target organ concentrations
- Drug/drug interactions
  - —Inhibiting theophylline metabolism
    - -H2 receptor antagonists
    - -Macrolide antibiotics
    - -Fluoroquinolones
    - -Allopurinol
    - -Influenza vaccine
    - -Interferons
  - —Enhances theophylline metabolism (lead to toxicity when discontinued)
    - -Carbamazepine
    - -Barbiturates
    - -Smoking
    - -Rifampin
- Chronic theophylline accumulation
  - —New onset uncontrolled congestive heart failure
  - —Liver disease (cirrhosis or severe hepatitis)
  - —Acute viral infections

Pre-Hospital

CAUTIONS

- Bring pill bottles/pill samples in suspected overdose

Diagnosis

ESSENTIAL WORKUP

- Serum theophylline concentration
  - —≥20 mg/L confirms diagnosis
- Detailed history to differentiate acute from acute-on-chronic from chronic intoxication

LABORATORY

- Theophylline level
  - —Repeat every 2 hours until declining to confirm if immediate absorption is complete and "peak" value has occurred
  - —Serious morbidity in acute overdose if ≥100 mg/L
  - —Massive caffeine concentrations can yield detectable and or "toxic" theophylline determinations with conventional laboratory testing
- CBC
- Electrolytes
  - —Transient hypokalemia
- Serum acetaminophen level

IMAGING/SPECIAL TESTS

- KUB
  - —Undissolved sustained-release tablets or pharmacobezoars appear as radiopacities
  - —Bead-filled capsules may appear as radiolucencies
- Ultrasound of the stomach may detect intact sustained-release dosage forms

DIFFERENTIAL DIAGNOSIS

- Caffeine/β-agonist bronchodilator overdose
- Amphetamines
- Sympathomimetic
- Anticholinergic
- Drug withdrawal
- Pheochromocytoma
- Thyroid storm

Treatment

INITIAL STABILIZATION

- ABCs
  - —Cardiac monitor
  - —0.9%NS IV fluid rehydration
- Naloxone, thiamine and D50W (or Accucheck) for altered mental status

Cardiovascular

- Initiate β-blockers or calcium channel blockers for rate control with supraventricular tachyarrhythmias
  - —Theophylline is refractory to adenosine
- 0.9%NS IV fluid resuscitation for hypotension
  - —With treatment failure consider β-blocker to reverse theophylline-induced β_2 receptor stimulated vasodilatation
- Treat ventricular dysrhythmias conventionally

Seizures

- Administer benzodiazepines
- Phenytoin contraindicated

ED TREATMENT

Decontamination

- Perform gastric lavage for severe (≥50 mg/kg) acute overdoses presenting within one hour of ingestion.
- Administer activated charcoal
- Administer cathartics (sorbitol) with the first dose of activated charcoal
- Multi-dose charcoal
  - —Especially with sustained-release products
  - —Binds theophylline which through back-diffusion can return to the small intestine
  - —For mild to moderate toxicity
  - —10–25 g q 1–2 hrs until theophylline level ≤20 mg/L
- Initiate whole bowel irrigation with sustained-release products
  - —Administer until a clear colorless rectal effluent or serum theophylline <20 mg/L
- Treat protracted vomiting with metoclopramide or $5HT^3$-receptor antagonists (ondansetron)
- Avoid ipecac

Electrolyte Disturbances

- Treat hypokalemia in acute ingestions cautiously
  - —Not pathophysiologic: due to β-receptor mediated intracellular shift of extracellular potassium
  - —Aggressive correction leads to symptomatic hyperkalemia as theophylline concentrations decrease
- Most electrolyte imbalances respond to β-blocker therapy
  - —Generally not indicated due to the absence of associated morbidity and the potential for β-blocker induced bronchospasm in pulmonary patients

Extracorporeal Elimination

- Hemoperfusion—more efficacious
- Hemodialysis—faster availability
- Initiate hemodialysis or hemoperfusion if theophylline level
  - —≥100 mg/L in acute ingestions
  - —≥60 mg/L in acute-on-chronic or chronic intoxications

MEDICATIONS

- Activated charcoal: 1 g/kg po
- Diazepam: 0.1 mg/kg IV q 5–10 minutes until seizures abate up to 30 mg
- Diltiazem: 0.25 mg/kg IV bolus, can repeat after 15 min, then 5–15 mg/hr infusion
- Esmolol: 500 μg/kg IV bolus followed by 50 μg/kg/min infusion, increase by 50 μg/kg/min increments to maximum of 200 μg/kg/min
- Metoclopramide: 10 mg IV bolus can repeat to maximum of 1 mg/kg
- Ondansetron: 0.15 mg/kg IV bolus up to maximum of 32 mg total
- Polyethylene glycol (high molecular weight): 1–2 L/hr via NGT

Disposition

ADMISSION CRITERIA

- Acute overdoses with serum theophylline concentrations >100 mg/L
- Acute-on-chronic or chronic theophylline with either a serum concentration >60 mg/L or >60 years old
- Seizures, or fluid and vasopressor refractory hypotension in a patient with serum theophylline concentration >30 mg/L
- Serial unchanged or rising serum theophylline concentrations (2 or more) >30 mg/L an acute or acute-on-chronic ingestion of sustained-release theophylline

DISCHARGE CRITERIA

- Two consecutive (2 or more hours apart) declining serum theophylline concentrations with the most recent concentration <30 mg/L
- Mildly symptomatic patient without comorbid illness or evidence of intention to do self-harm with theophylline level <30 mg/L

Miscellaneous

ICD9: 974.1

CORE CONTENT CODE: 17.2.11.3

SUGGESTED READINGS

Henderson A, Wright DM, Pond SM. Management of theophylline overdose patients in the intensive care unit. Anaesth Intensive Care 1992;20:56–62.

Minton NA, Henry JA. Treatment of theophylline overdose. Am J Emerg Med 1996;14:606–612.

Shannon M. Predictors of major toxicity after theophylline overdose. Ann Intern Med 1993;119:1161–1167.

Stork CM, Howland MA, Goldfrank LR. Concepts and controversies of bronchodilator overdose. Emerg Med Clin N Am 1994;12:415–36.

Author: Frank Paloucek

Thoracic Outlet Syndrome

Clinical Presentation

SIGNS AND SYMPTOMS

Vascular Compression

- Ischemic symptoms
  - —Cool
  - —Claudication
  - —Color changes
- Diminished pulse
- Venous engorgement
- Edema

Neurogenic

- True neurogenic
  - —Pain
  - —Paresthesias
  - —Numbness
  - —Weakness of the arm and hand
    - -Usually in C8/T1 nerve distribution
  - —Vasomotor symptoms
- Disputed neurogenic
  - —Includes above symptoms but not in a neuroanatomical distribution
  - —Protean of other complaints of the shoulder, neck, head, and chest

General

- Symptoms
  - —May be exacerbated by repetitive use or positional (i.e., working overhead)
  - —Usually insidious in onset and progressive
  - —Can occur or worsen suddenly after trauma
- Supraclavicular tenderness
- May have a bruit in supraclavicular area

MECHANISM/DESCRIPTION

- Encompassing diagnosis for a variety of chronic complaints of the upper extremity, shoulder, and neck unified by the underlying pathophysiology of neurovascular compression
- Prevalence is higher in females
- Right extremity is more commonly affected
- Bilateral involvement is not uncommon
- Neurologic symptoms, ischemia or edema of the upper extremity
- Vascular compression thoracic outlet syndrome (TOS) occurs in about 5% of patients
- Neurogenic TOS
  - —About 95% of patients
  - —True (1–3%)—those with objective findings
  - —Disputed (90%)—those with no or limited objective findings

ETIOLOGY

- Compression of the neurovascular components (brachial plexus, subclavian artery, and vein) of the upper extremity as they pass through the thoracic outlet
- Compression results from cervical ribs and other congenital anomalies, trauma, or abnormal tone of the shoulder suspensory musculature

Pre-Hospital

N/A

Diagnosis

ESSENTIAL WORKUP

- Rule out cardiac ischemia
  - —ECG
- Test for diminished strength and or sensation
  - —Adson's test
    - -Arm down, patient rotates head towards extremity, looks up, and inhales
  - —Reverse Adson's
    - -Rotate head away from extremity
  - —Wright's (hyperabduction) test
    - -Shoulders hyperabducted and externally rotated
  - —Roo's—"military surrender" position
    - -Flex and extend fingers for up to 3 minutes
  - —Halsted
    - -Exaggerated military attention position
- During testing
  - —Check for pulse diminution
  - —Reproduction/exacerbation of symptoms
- None of these tests are very sensitive or specific

LABORATORY

N/A

IMAGING/SPECIAL TESTS

- Perform as outpatient except in case of limb threatening ischemia
- CSR
- C-spine series
- Vascular TOS
  - —Vascular noninvasive studies
  - —Arteriograms
- Neurogenic TOS
  - —No "gold standard" test thus diagnosis remains mostly clinical
  - —Nerve conduction studies helpful in confirming the clinical diagnosis and in identifying other disorders in the differential diagnosis

DIFFERENTIAL DIAGNOSIS

- Cardiac ischemia
- Cervical spondylosis or disc disease
- Carpal tunnel syndrome or nerve entrapments
- Pancoast tumor; other neck/mediastinum malignancies
- Neuritis
- Myositis
- Raynaud's disease
- MS or degenerative spinal cord disease
- Shoulder inflammatory diseases—arthritis, rotator cuff injury, bicipital tendonitis
- Atherosclerotic or thromboembolic disease

Treatment

INITIAL STABILIZATION

N/A

ED TREATMENT

- Symptomatic relief
  - —NSAID
  - —Steroids
  - —Muscle relaxants
    - -Cyclobenzaprine
    - -Methocarbamol
    - -Diazepam
  - —Soothing liniments or ointments
- Initial management
  - —Usually conservative involving physical therapy and medications
- Surgery for failure of medical therapy
  - —70–90% of patients experience some to complete relief postoperatively

MEDICATIONS

- Cyclobenzaprine (flexeril): 10 mg po tid
- Diazepam: 5 mg po tid
- Ibuprofen: 800 mg po tid
- Methocarbamol (robaxin): 1000–1500 mg po tid

Disposition

ADMISSION CRITERIA

- Limb-threatening ischemia

DISCHARGE CRITERIA

- Follow-up arranged with a neurologist, thoracic surgeon, or orthopedist

Miscellaneous

ICD9: 353.0

CORE CONTENT CODE: 16.11

SUGGESTED READINGS

Atasoy E. Thoracic outlet compression syndrome. Orthop Clin North Am 1996;27:265–303.

Author: Chris Moore

Thoracic Spine Injury

Clinical Presentation

SIGNS AND SYMPTOMS

- Significant force is required to produce thoracic vertebral fractures, so other injuries may obscure those directly related to thoracic fractures
- Primary symptoms of thoracic vertebral fracture occur from pain at the fracture site or impingement of nearby structures by bone fragments
- Common signs and symptoms
  —Localized soft tissue defect
  —Pain or tenderness
    -Localized—pain and tenderness over spinous process
    -Referred—paraspinal, anterior chest or abdomen
  —Paraspinal muscle spasm
  —Paresthesia or dysesthesia
  —Weakness (focal or global)
  —Distal areflexia, flaccid plegia
  —Bowel or bladder incontinence
  —Priapism
  —Loss of temperature control
  —Spinal shock—hypotension with bradycardia

ETIOLOGY

- The thoracic spine is very rigid due to the rib cage and the costovertebral articulations. The spinal canal is narrowest in the thoracic spine
- Since traumatic thoracic spine fractures require enormous forces, motor vehicle accidents or falls from height account for the majority of fractures
  —A small percentage is caused by penetrating injuries and will be covered in a separate section
  —50% of all spinal fractures and 40% of all spinal cord injuries occur at the thoracolumbar junction (T11-L2)

MECHANISM/DESCRIPTION

- The following forces account for most thoracic fractures
  —Axial compression
  —Flexion-rotation
  —Shear
  —Flexion-distraction
  —Extension
- The spinal column can be divided into three anatomically distinct columns. If two of the three columns are disrupted, then the spinal column is unstable
  —Posterior column: posterior bony arch and interconnecting ligamentous structures
  —Middle column: posterior aspects of the vertebral bodies, posterior annulus fibrosis, and the posterior longitudinal ligament
  —Anterior column: anterior longitudinal ligament, anterior anulus fibrosis, and anterior vertebral body
- Major vs. minor fractures
  —Minor
    -Isolated articular fracture
    -Transverse process fracture
    -Spinous process fracture
    -Pars interarticularis fracture
  —Major
    -Compression fracture
    -Burst fracture
    -Seat belt injury
    -Fracture dislocation
- Compression fracture (anterior or lateral flexion)
  —Fracture of anterior portion of vertebral body with intact middle column of spine
  —May be posterior column disruption
  —Type A: fracture through both endplates
  —Type B: fracture through superior endplate
  —Type C: fracture through inferior endplate
  —Type D: both endplates intact
- Burst fracture (axial loading)
  —Fracture through middle column of spine
  —May have spreading of posterior elements and lamina fractures
  —Type A: fracture through both endplates
  —Type B: fracture through superior endplate
  —Type C: fracture through inferior endplate
  —Type D: burst in middle column with rotational injury leading to subluxation
  —Type E: burst in middle column with asymmetric compression of anterior column
- Seat belt injury (flexion distraction)
  —Distraction of posterior and middle columns with anterior column intact
  —Typically caused by lap belts used without shoulder harness
  —Type A: through bone
  —Type B: primarily ligamentous
  —Type C: disruption of bone through middle column
  —Type D: through ligaments and disk with no middle column fracture
- Fracture dislocations
  —Failure of all three columns following compression, tension, rotation, or shear forces
  —Type A: flexion rotation; fall from height
  —Type B: shear—violent force across long axis of trunk
  —Type C: flexion distraction; bilateral facet dislocation

Pre-Hospital

CAUTIONS

- If the patient's positioning initially prevents placement of a long spinal board, then a short board should be placed until the patient is fully extricated
- Patients with neurologic deficit should be transported directly to a trauma center

Diagnosis

ESSENTIAL WORKUP

- Rapid evaluation of airway, breathing and circulation
- Primary and secondary trauma survey
- Detailed neurologic exam with specific attention to evidence of spinal cord injury, including rectal tone
- Thorough spine exam noting any deformity or tenderness
- Any midline tenderness elicited on examination, distracting injury, or intoxication mandates plain film spine radiography
- If fracture is present, determine if it is stable or unstable, as defined by descriptions of columns above

IMAGING/SPECIAL TESTS

- Pain or tenderness, severe motor vehicle accident, or falls from height are indications for AP and lateral plain film views of the spine
- Thin-cut CT scanning is indicated in any patient with evidence of spinal fracture or ligamentous injury on plain films to assess spinal canal integrity or in patients with normal plain films and significant pain or tenderness and mechanism for severe injury

DIFFERENTIAL DIAGNOSIS

- Arthritis (degenerative and rheumatoid)
- Ankylosing spondylitis
- Spina bifida
- Congenital malformation
- Neoplasm
- Pathologic fracture

Treatment

INITIAL STABILIZATION

- Follow the ABCs of trauma resuscitation
- Airway intervention should be done with in-line cervical immobilization
- Preserve residual spinal cord function and prevent further injury by stabilizing the spine

ED TREATMENT

- Perform all needed resuscitation and diagnostic tests with the patient in full spinal immobilization
- If spinal cord injury is suspected, administer high dose steroids and consult a neurosurgeon
- If spinal fracture or ligamentous injury is suspected without neurologic impairment, arrange CT or MRI scanning while simultaneously consulting neurosurgery or orthopaedic surgery
- Pain control should be administered as soon as possible. NSAIDs, opiates, and benzodiazepines are the mainstays of treatment

MEDICATIONS

- High-dose steroid protocol
  —Solumedrol: 30 mg/kg IV bolus within 8 hours of injury, followed immediately by an infusion of 5.4 mg/kg/hr for the next 23 hours

Disposition

- Patients with significant spinal cord or column injury should be treated in a regional trauma center

ADMISSION CRITERIA

- Unstable spinal column injury
- Cord or root injury
- Ileus
- Pain control
- Concomitant traumatic injury

DISCHARGE CRITERIA

- Stable minor fractures after orthopaedic or neurosurgical evaluation

Miscellaneous

ICD9: 952.10

CORE CONTENT CODE: 18.4.3.1.2

SUGGESTED READINGS

Block BE, et al. Thoracic and lumbar spine injuries in children. Contemporary orthopedics 1994;29(4):253–60.

Chiles BW 3rd, Cooper PR. Acute spinal injury. N Engl J Med 1996;334(8):514–520.

El-Khoury GY, Whitten CG. Trauma to the upper thoracic spine: Anatomy, biomechanics, and unique imaging features. Am J Roentgenol 1993;160:95–102.

Kinashita H. Pathology of spinal cord injuries due to fracture-dislocations of the thoracic and lumber spine. Paraplegia. 1996;34(1):1–7.

Author: Richard D. Zane

Thrombolytic Therapy

Clinical Presentation

SIGNS AND SYMPTOMS

- See "Myocardial Infarction"

MECHANISM/DESCRIPTION

- Thrombolytic agents ("clot-busters") dissolve thrombus formation
  - —Decrease infarct size
  - —Reduce morbidity and mortality in acute myocardial infarction (AMI)
  - —Maximum gains occur when treatment is initiated in the first hour following AMI
- Therapy may be beneficial when started as late as 12
- A significant complication of treatment is CNS hemorrhage

Pre-Hospital

CAUTIONS

- Only administer thrombolytics in the field if specific protocols exist
- Administer under physician's direction
- Capability for field 12-lead ECG verification of AMI

Diagnosis

ESSENTIAL WORKUP

- ECG
- Rapid (typically portable) chest x-ray
- Must evaluate for aortic dissection as cause of chest pain
- Heme test stool
- Inclusion criteria for thrombolytic therapy
  - —Continuous AMI symptoms lasting 30 minutes
  - —ECG changes suggestive of AMI
  - —New onset ST-segment elevation (1 mm (0.1 mV)) in two contiguous limb leads
  - —New ST-segment elevation (2 mm) in two contiguous precordial leads
  - —New left bundle branch block
  - —Obtain a prior baseline ECG for comparison if possible
- Exclusion criteria
  - —Absolute contraindications
    - -Active internal bleeding
    - -Altered consciousness
    - -CVA in past 6 months
    - -Any history of hemorrhagic CVA
    - -Intracranial or intraspinal surgery in the last 2 months
    - -Intracranial or intraspinal neoplasm, aneurysm, AVM
    - -Known bleeding disorder
    - -Persistent hypertension
    - -Pregnancy
    - -Head trauma within 1 month
    - -Trauma or surgery within the last 2 weeks that could result in a closed space bleed
    - -Age is not a contraindication
  - —Relative contraindications
    - -Active peptic ulcer disease
    - -Extended CPR
    - -Current use of oral anticoagulants
    - -Hemorrhagic ophthalmic conditions
    - -Chronic uncontrolled hypertension
    - -History of ischemic embolic disease
    - -CVA >6 months ago
    - -Significant trauma or major surgery >2 weeks but <2 months ago
    - -Subclavian or internal venous cannulation
    - -Patients with a contraindication should be evaluated for emergent cardiac catheterization and reperfusion therapy

DIFFERENTIAL DIAGNOSIS

- Aortic dissection
- Pericarditis
- Other causes of chest pain (see "Chest Pain")

Treatment

INITIAL STABILIZATION

- Standard AMI protocol (see "Myocardial Infarction")

ED TREATMENT

- Patients eligible for thrombolytics should receive treatment within 30 minutes of arrival
- The choice of agent is less important than early administration
- Streptokinase (SK) and anisoylated plasminogen streptokinase-activated complex (APSAC) can cause allergic reactions
  - —May have decreased effectiveness if administered within 12 months of either a streptococcal infection or previous therapy with SK or APSAC
  - —Tissue plasminogen activators (tPA) are preferred in patients who have been previously administered SK or APSAC
- All agents may cause hypotension necessitating a slower rate of infusion
- Lytic therapy requires placement of two peripheral intravenous lines at compressible sites

MEDICATIONS

- Urokinase: 1.5 IU IV over 2 min. then 1.5 IU IV over next 90 min
- APSAC: 30 mg IV over 2–5 min. (Patients should also receive methylprednisolone 250 mg IV.)
- Reteplase (r-tPA): 10 MU IV bolus, and again after 30 min 10 MU IV bolus. (Patients should also receive heparin 5,000 IU IV bolus then, infuse 1,000 IU per hour for 48 hours keeping aPTT = 1.5–2.5.)
- Streptokinase: 1.5 MU over 60 min. (Patients should also receive methylprednisolone 250 mg IV.)
- tPA: 15 mg IV bolus, then 0.75 mg/kg (max 50 mg) over 30 min., then 0.5 mg/kg (max. 35 mg) over 60 min. (Patients should also receive heparin 5,000 IU IV bolus then, infuse 1,000 IU per hour for 48 hours keeping aPTT = 1.5–2.5.)

Disposition

ADMISSION CRITERIA

- Patients receiving thrombolytics should be admitted to a cardiac care unit

DISCHARGE CRITERIA

- None

Miscellaneous

ICD9: N/A

CORE CONTENT CODE: 2.11.1

SUGGESTED READINGS

Collins R, Peto R, Baigent C, et al. Aspirin, heparin, and fibrinolytic therapy in suspected acute myocardial infarction. N Engl J Med 1997;336:847–60.

Mengert TJ, Eisenberg MS. Pre-hospital and emergency department thrombolytic therapy. In: Tintinalli JE, et al, eds. Emergency medicine: A comprehensive study guide. 4th ed. New York: McGraw-Hill, 1996.

Noble S, McTavish D. Reteplase: a review of its pharmacological properties and clinical efficacy in the management of acute myocardial infarction. Drugs 1996;52(4):589–605.

Saltissi S, Mushahwar, . The management of acute myocardial infarction. Postgrad Med 1995;71:534–541.

Selig MB. Early management of acute myocardial infarction: thrombolysis, angioplasty, and adjunctive therapies. Am J Emerg Med 1996;14:209–17.

Authors: Walter N. Simmons; Bert Woolard

Thrombophlebitis

Clinical Presentation

SIGNS AND SYMPTOMS

- Extremity pain, swelling and fullness
  - —Greater than a 1–2-cm circumferential difference in legs
  - —Tenderness on compression of the calf
  - —Warmth
  - —Palpation of a venous "cord."

MECHANISM/DESCRIPTION

- Roughly 2 million cases of thrombophlebitis occur in the U.S. annually
- Part of a systemic process better known as venous thromboembolism
  - —Most significant complication is pulmonary embolism (PE) from which an estimated 60,000 Americans die annually
- Lower extremity deep venous thrombosis (DVT) is divided into distal (to the popliteal vein) or proximal
- DVT also occurs in pelvic and upper extremity veins

ETIOLOGY

- Risk factors
  - —Hypercoagulable states
    - -Cancer
    - -Nephrotic syndrome
    - -Sepsis
    - -Inflammatory conditions such as ulcerative colitis
    - -Increased estrogen (pregnancy, oral contraceptives)
    - -Various protein (S, C, and antithrombin 3) deficiencies
  - —Stasis
    - -Prolonged bed rest
    - -Immobility from a cast, long travel rides
    - -Neurologic disorders with paralysis
    - -Congestive heart failure
    - -Obesity
  - —Vascular damage
    - -Trauma
    - -Surgery
    - -Central lines
  - —Advancing age
  - —Prior thromboembolism
  - —Family history of DVT

Pre-Hospital

N/A

Diagnosis

ESSENTIAL WORKUP

- Doppler ultrasound (duplex scanning)of extremity

LABORATORY

- No blood test diagnoses or excludes DVT with certainty
  - —The absence of D-dimer (ELISA technique) suggests DVT is not present
  - —CBC, PT/PTT baseline measurements

IMAGING/SPECIAL TESTS

- Duplex scanning (combination of color Doppler and B-mode ultrasound)
  - —Rapid, inexpensive, and highly accurate in detecting proximal DVT
- Impedance plethysmography (IPG)
  - —Nearly as accurate as duplex scanning
  - —Not as routinely available as US
- Venography is the historic gold standard
  - —Accurate but invasive
  - —Associated with dye reactions
  - —Can precipitate phlebitis

DIFFERENTIAL DIAGNOSIS

- Superficial thrombophlebitis
- Cellulitis
- Torn muscles and ligaments
- Ruptured Baker's cyst
- Bilateral edema (seen with heart, kidney, or liver disease) is rarely caused by DVT
- Prior DVT and postphlebitic syndrome

Treatment

INITIAL STABILIZATION

- Patients with DVT rarely require immediate stabilization
  —Phlegmasia alba dolens (painful white leg) or phlegmasia cerulea dolens (painful blue leg)
    -Hypoperfusion with blanching and cyanosis
    -May require fluid resuscitation, immediate anticoagulation, and thrombolysis or thrombectomy

ED TREATMENT

- Anticoagulation
  —Contraindications
    -Active internal bleeding
    -Uncontrolled hypertension
    -Significant recent trauma or surgery
    -CNS tumor
    -Initiate in the ED
- Recurrent thromboembolism despite documented adequate anticoagulation (defined as a aPTT of <1.5 times control for heparinized patients and an INR of <2 for warfarinized patients) requires vena caval interruption
- Low molecular-weight heparin (LMWH) is treatment of choice if cost is less important or outpatient management is considered
  —Enoxaparin
  —Does not require laboratory monitoring
  —May be administered as an outpatient
  —Initiate oral warfarin therapy same day

MEDICATIONS

- Enoxaparin: 1 mg/kg SQ bid
- Heparin: 80 IU/kg bolus followed by a drip of 18 IU/kg/hr (aPTT should be checked in 6 hours and tile infusion rate adjusted accordingly)
- Warfarin: 10 mg po, then 5 mg po q day, monitor PT

Disposition

ADMISSION CRITERIA

- Severely ill patients
- Patients with significant comorbid conditions
- Patients without the means for appropriate home administration of LMWH

DISCHARGE CRITERIA

- Isolated DVT
- No significant comorbid conditions
- Resources available for home administration of LMWH
- Appropriate followup assured

Miscellaneous

ICD9: 451.9

CORE CONTENT CODE: 2.5.2.3

SUGGESTED READINGS

Hirsh J, Hoak J. Management of DVT and PE. Circulation 1996;93:2212–245.

Levine M, et al. A comparison of LMWH administered primarily at home with unfractionated heparin administered in the hospital for proximal DVT. N Engl J Med 1996;334:677–81.

Pearson SP, et al. A critical pathway to evaluate suspected DVT. Arch Int Med 1995;155:1773–778.

Author: J. Edlow

Thrombotic Thrombocytopenic Purpura

Clinical Presentation

SIGNS AND SYMPTOMS

Five Major Clinical Features

- Thrombocytopenia
  - —Platelet count <20,000/mm^3
    - -Hemorrhage
    - -Easy bruising
    - -Purpura
    - -Epistaxis
    - -Menorrhagia
    - -GI bleeding
    - -Spontaneous intracranial hemorrhage
- Microangiopathic and hemolytic anemia
  - —Hb <10 g/dl (<6 g/dl in 40%)
- Neurologic symptoms
  - —Typically fluctuating
  - —Occur in 90%
    - -Presenting complaint in 60%
  - —Headache
  - —Altered mentation (confusion)
  - —Behavioral or personality changes
  - —Focal sensory or motor deficits
  - —Aphasia
  - —Seizures
  - —Stupor
  - —Coma
- Renal insufficiency
  - —Usually mild
  - —Creatinine <3.0 mg/dl
- Fever
  - —Occurs in acute episodes and prodromal syndromes

Symptoms

- Weakness
- Fatigue
- Fever
- Malaise
- GI complaints
  - —Nausea
  - —Anorexia
  - —Diarrhea
  - —Abdominal pain

Signs

- Jaundice
- Abnormalities of cardiac conduction
- Pulmonary infiltrates and edema
- GI hemorrhage
- Alteration of vision due to retinal hemorrhage or detachment

Classic Course

- Acute onset
- Fulminant course lasting days to a few months
- Nearly always fatal outcome without treatment
  - —10% mortality with treatment

MECHANISM/DESCRIPTION

- Platelet aggregation and fibrin deposition
  - —From uncertain stimulation
  - —Occurs in the arterioles and capillaries leading to microthrombi and obstruction to blood flow
- Platelet aggregation leads to
  - —Consumption of platelets in excess of the bone marrow's ability to respond producing thrombocytopenia
  - —Widespread microvascular hyaline thrombotic lesions
- Microvasculature obstruction with platelet aggregates leads to
  - —Red cell hemolysis
  - —Accumulation of heme breakdown products
  - —Anemia
- End organ ischemia results from the diffuse thrombosis in small vessels
  - —Most common in heart, brain, kidney, pancreas, and adrenal glands
  - —Lungs and liver relatively spared

ETIOLOGY

- Unknown
- More common in the 3rd to 6th decades
- Uncommon in the pediatric or geriatric populations
- Women affected about twice as frequently as men

Pre-Hospital

N/A

Diagnosis

ESSENTIAL WORKUP

- Clinical diagnosis
- Comprehensive history and physical exam targeted at identification of the major symptoms and signs as identified above

LABORATORY

- CBC/platelet count/reticulocyte count
  - —Anemia: Hb <10 g/dl
  - —Thrombocytopenia <20,000/mm^3
  - —Increased reticulocyte count
- Coagulation studies
  - —Normal
- Peripheral blood smear
  - —Macroangiopathic changes
  - —Schistocytes
  - —Helmet cells
  - —Nucleated RBCs
- Coombs's test
  - —Negative direct Coombs's test
- Electrolytes, BUN/Cr, glucose
  - —Mild elevation of BUN/Cr
  - —Hyperkalemia due to RBC lysis
- LDH
  - —Elevated 5–10 times
- Bilirubin
  - —Increased unconjugated bilirubin
- Urinalysis
  - —Hematuria (microscopic to gross)

IMAGING/SPECIAL TESTS

- Biopsy
  - —Confirms diagnosis
  - —Reveals hyaline lesions in small vessels
  - —Contraindicated during fulminant presentation (hemorrhage risk)
- Bone marrow aspiration
  - —Erythroid and megakaryocyte hyperplasia
  - —Contraindicated during fulminant presentation (hemorrhage risk)
- CT head
  - —For altered mental status

DIFFERENTIAL DIAGNOSIS

- Hemolytic uremic syndrome
  - —Triad of thrombocytopenia, schistocytosis, and renal dysfunction
  - —Neurologic symptoms unusual
- Disseminated intravascular coagulation
  - —Causes the deposition of fibrin in microvasculature and not hyaline
  - —Coagulation studies abnormal
- Idiopathic thrombocytopenic purpura (ITP)
  - —No evidence of hemolysis
  - —LDH and bilirubin normal
- Pregnancy related
  - —Preeclampsia/eclampsia
  - —Pregnancy-associated hemolysis
  - —HELLP
- Evans's syndrome
  - —Autoimmune hemolytic anemia

—Prominence of microsphereocytes rather than schistocytes
—Positive direct Coombs's test
- Malignant hypertension
- Bacterial sepsis
- Subacute bacterial endocarditis
- Prosthetic valves or severely calcified aortic stenosis

Treatment

INITIAL STABILIZATION

- ABCs
- 0.9%NS IV fluid resuscitation for hypotension/GI hemorrhage
- RBC transfusions
  —For significant anemia or bleeding complications
- Platelet transfusions
  —Reserve for life-threatening hemorrhage (e.g., CNS bleeds)
  —May conversely aggravate the thrombotic, microvascular obstructive process and worsen the hemorrhage and outcome

ED TREATMENT

- Fresh frozen plasma (FFP) or fresh unfrozen plasma
  —Initiated as bridge to exchange transfusions upon diagnosis of thrombotic thrombocytopenic purpura (TTP)
  —Success rate approaching 64%
  —Provides a platelet antiaggregating factor absent or diminished in the patients own serum
  —Used prophylactically to prevent recurrence in the chronic relapsing variant
- Plasma exchange transfusions
  —Combination of plasmapheresis and infusion of FFP
  —Plasmapheresis removes
    -Immune complexes responsible for endothelial damage and initiation of TTP
    -Circulating proaggregation factors promoting platelet aggregation
  —Perform daily until
    -After neurologic symptoms improve
    -Renal function improves
    -LDH normalizes
  —Complications include
    -Allergy
    -Secondary infection
    -Hypotension
- Corticosteroids
  —Unproven therapeutic benefit
    -May limit immunologically mediated endothelial damage that could trigger TTP and decrease splenic sequestration of platelets and damaged RBCs
  —Supportive benefit if adrenal glands involved
- Splenectomy
  —Reserved for cases unresponsive to plasma exchange transfusions
- Antiplatelet or immunosuppressive drugs
  —Aspirin, dipyridamole, sulfapyrazine, vincristine, and dextran
    -Utilized with variable effectiveness
  —Vincristine and/or dextran in combination with corticosteroids and splenectomy
    -Alternatives in resistant cases
  —Aspirin
    -Used in resistant cases
    -Can worsen bleeding complications
  —Heparin—ineffective
- Dialysis
  —For renal failure

MEDICATIONS

- Aspirin: 325–650 mg po q 4–6 hrs
- Corticosteroids
  —Methylprednisolone: 0.75 mg/kg q 12 hrs
  —Prednisone: 1–2 mg/kg/day (high dose up to 200 mg/day)
- Fresh frozen plasma (FFP)
  —Plasma infusion: 30 ml/kg/day (75–100 ml/hr)
  —Plasma exchange transfusion: 3–4 L/day
- Vincristine: 2 mg IV q 4–7 days ×4 doses

Disposition

ADMISSION CRITERIA

- Newly diagnosed serious platelet disorder especially with bleeding complications
- ICU admission for TTP with bleeding or neurologic findings
  —Transport to a tertiary care center with appropriate specialty care facilities

DISCHARGE CRITERIA

- None

Miscellaneous

ICD9: 446.6

CORE CONTENT CODE: 7.1.3.2

SUGGESTED READINGS

George JN, El-Harake M. Thrombocytopenia due to enhanced platelet destruction by nonimmunologic mechanisms. In: Beutler E, et al., eds. Williams hematology. 5th ed. New York: McGraw Hill, 1995:1290–1303.

Hayward CPM, et al. Treatment outcomes in patients with adult thrombotic thrombocytopenic purpura—hemolytic uremic syndrome. Arch Intern Med 1994;154:982–987.

Moake JL. Thrombotic thrombocytopenic purpura and the hemolytic uremic syndrome. In: Hoffman R, et al., eds. Hematology, basic principles and practice. 2d ed. New York: Churchill Livingstone, 1995: 1879–1888.

Onundddarson PT, Rowe JM, Heal JM, Francis CW. Response to plasma exchange and splenectomy in thrombotic thrombocytopenic purpura: A 10-year experience at a single institution. Arch Intern Med 1992;152:791–796.

Thompson CE, et al. Thrombotic microangiopathies in the 1980s: Clinical features, response to treatment, and the impact of the human immunodeficiency virus epidemic. Blood 1992;15(80):1890–1895.

Author: Timothy Pavek

Thumb Fractures

Clinical Presentation

SIGNS AND SYMPTOMS

- Pain, swelling and deformity at the base of the thumb metacarpal
- The base of the thumb may appear radially deviated to the rest of the hand in the resting position
- Occasionally, there may be damage to the thumb digital nerves

MECHANISM/DESCRIPTION

- Axial loading of the thumb with the metacarpal phalangeal joint flexed, hand closed or the thumb metacarpal phalangeal joint otherwise stabilized
- *Bennett's fracture* is an oblique intra-articular fracture of the ulnar aspect of the base of the thumb metacarpal with the larger distal fragment displaced
  —The oblique fracture involves the ulnar surface and the metacarpal-carpal joint. The ulnar fragment is maintained in its anatomic position and the larger distal fragment is pulled radially and proximally by its tendon insertions
- *Rolando's fracture* is a comminuted Y- or V-shaped intra-articular fracture of the ulnar base of the thumb metacarpal with the large distal fragment displaced

Pre-Hospital

CAUTIONS

- Consider other injuries
- Dress open wounds
- Immobilization in neutral position
- Elevation, cold to reduce swelling
- Age appropriate social management

Diagnosis

ESSENTIAL WORKUP

IMAGING/SPECIAL TESTS

- Avoid stress-testing of thumb metacarpal-phalangeal joint until radiography is completed

DIFFERENTIAL DIAGNOSIS

- Extra-articular fracture of the base of the thumb metacarpal
- Scaphoid fracture
- Gamekeeper's thumb

PEDIATRIC CONSIDERATIONS

N/A

Treatment

INITIAL STABILIZATION

- Immobilize thumb pending definitive evaluation

ED TREATMENT

- Thumb spica splint with the thumb in neutral position (as if holding a soda can)
- Splint instructions provided to patient
- 72-hour orthopedic referral
- Counsel patient that there is a high likelihood of the need for operative repair

MEDICATIONS

- Pain control with oral analgesic preparations

Disposition

ADMISSION CRITERIA

- Open fracture, presence of multiple trauma, or other more serious injuries

DISCHARGE CRITERIA

- Closed injuries, 72-hour orthopedic follow-up with frequent need for operative fixation

Miscellaneous

ICD9: 816.00

CORE CONTENT CODE: 18.4.12.1

SUGGESTED READINGS

American Society for Surgery of the Hand. The hand: Examination and diagnosis. 2d ed. New York: Churchill Livingston, 1983.

American Society for Surgery of the Hand. The hand: Primary care of common problems. 2d ed. New York: Churchill Livingston, 1990.

Antosia RE, Lyn E. The Hand. In: Rosen P, et al., eds. Emergency medicine: Concepts and clinical practice. 4th ed. St. Louis: Mosby-Year Book, 1998:625–668.

Uehara DT. The hand in emergency medicine. Emerg Clin North Am 1993;11(3):585–600.

Author: Matthew Walsh

Tibial/Fibular Shaft Fracture

Clinical Presentation

SIGNS AND SYMPTOMS

- Pain: usually immediate, severe, and well localized to the fracture site
- Deformity: visible or palpable at the fracture site
- Inability to bear weight if tibia involved; may be able to walk if isolated fibula fracture
- Significant soft tissue damage with high energy trauma
- Edema and ecchymosis surrounding fracture site
- Compartment syndrome of leg particularly anterior compartment
- Possible foot drop on affected leg from perineal nerve injury as it wraps around fibular head

MECHANISM/DESCRIPTION

- Indirect force
- Torsion/rotational force
  - —External rotation produces proximal spiral fracture
  - —Internal rotation produces distal fibula fracture
- Bending force producing oblique, transverse or butterfly fractures, e.g., motor vehicle accident
- Direct force: high-energy trauma producing soft tissue and bony injury, e.g., pedestrian struck, crush injury, high velocity weapons, shotgun

Fracture Description

Tibia

- Extent of soft tissue damage
  - —Open versus closed fracture
  - —Gustilo-Anderson classification of open fractures
    - -Type I: wound <1 cm; little soft tissue damage; no crush injury
    - -Type II: wound >1 cm; moderate soft tissue damage; little or no devitalized soft tissue
    - -Type III: severe soft tissue injury; A—adequate soft tissue coverage of bone; B—tissue loss/periosteal stripping; C—neurovascular injury requiring surgical repair
- Anatomic location
  - —Proximal, middle, or distal third
  - —Articular extension
- Configuration
  - —Spiral
  - —Transverse
  - —Comminuted with butterfly fragment
  - —Comminuted with multiple fragments
- Displacement and angulation

Fibula

- Proximal: associated with peroneal nerve injury
- Middle
- Distal
- Articular extension
  - —*Maisonneuve fracture* is a fracture of the fibular head in association with disruption of the medial (deltoid) ligament of the ankle. The fracture plane extends from the ankle, up the intraosseous membrane, and exits the fibular head

PEDIATRIC CONSIDERATIONS

- Rely on parents for historical information
- May be able to bear weight with a limp if incomplete fracture (greenstick)
- Absence of deformity of extremity: only local swelling or tenderness
- *Bicycle spoke injury:* usually occurs in child riding on handlebars or rear fender and foot gets caught between frame and wheel spoke. Crush injury with damage to soft tissues is the primary problem. Initially, the foot may appear normal or have only minor skin abrasion
- *Toddler's fracture:* spiral fracture involving the distal third of the tibia with intact fibula secondary to rotational force (turning on planted foot). Age range is 9 months to 6 years, most often when learning to walk
  - —Fractures in midshaft or more transverse are suspicious of abuse
- Plastic/bowing deformity of fibula may occur with complete tibia fracture

Pre-Hospital

CAUTIONS

- Look for associated injuries in high energy mechanisms
- Assess for foot drop and other neurologic or vascular compromise
- Adequate immobilization is essential to prevent further injury

Diagnosis

ESSENTIAL WORKUP

- Careful neurovascular examination
  - —Anterior compartment
    - -Dorsalis pedis artery (anterior tibial artery)
    - -Sensation of first web space (deep peroneal nerve)
    - -Ankle and toe dorsiflexion (deep peroneal nerve)
    - -Eversion of the foot (superficial peroneal)
    - -Lateral aspect and sole of foot (superficial peroneal)
- Radiography
  - —Anteroposterior and lateral views of the leg including knee and ankle

IMAGING/SPECIAL TESTS

- Angiogram if vascular compromise suspected
- Compartment pressures if suspected by presence of pain with passive stretch, pain distal to fracture site, abnormality of pulses, paresthesias
  - —Pressures >30 mm Hg are an indication for fasciotomy

DIFFERENTIAL DIAGNOSIS

- Adults
  - —Sprain
  - —Stress Fracture
  - —Compartment syndrome
  - —Pathologic fracture
- Children
  - —Sarcoma
  - —Osteomyelitis
  - —Child abuse

PEDIATRIC CONSIDERATIONS

- Radiographs in internal rotation to better visualize oblique fractures, especially with torsion injury

Treatment

INITIAL STABILIZATION

- ABCs/ATLS protocol for multiple trauma victim
- Elevate extremity
- Apply ice
- Long-leg splint

ED TREATMENT

- Minimally or nondisplaced fractures
  - —IV sedation/analgesia
  - —Closed reduction: 10° angulation in AP plane, 5° in varus/valgus plane and no more than 1.5-cm shortening are acceptable
  - —Long leg cast with slight knee flexion
  - —Crutches
- Open fracture
  - —Remove contaminants
  - —Apply moist sterile dressing
  - —Address tetanus immunity status
  - —Antibiotics
  - —Analgesia
  - —Orthopedic consult
- Isolated fibula fracture
  - —Padded splint, elevate, ice, nonweight-bearing until swelling is resolved, *or* if minimal pain, elastic bandage from knee to toes
  - —Short-leg cast, or cam walker with weight-bearing is definitive treatment
  - —Crutches if nonweight-bearing

MEDICATIONS

- Cefazolin for open fractures: adult: 2 g IV loading dose; peds: 50 mg/kg
- Gentamycin *if* Gustilo-Anderson type III: adult: 1.5–2 mg/kg IV loading dose; peds: 2.5 mg/kg
- Penicillin G *if* farming accident: adult: 10 million IU IV loading dose; peds: 75,000 IU/kg
- Vancomycin *if* penicillin allergy: 1 g IV loading dose; peds: 10mg/kg

Disposition

ADMISSION CRITERIA

- Multiple trauma
  - —Unstable fracture
    - -Extensive soft tissue damage
    - -Articular involvement
    - -Complete displacement
    - -Transverse fracture
    - -Comminution greater than 50% of circumference
    - -Open fracture
- Neurovascular compromise
- Pain control

DISCHARGE CRITERIA

- Adequate reduction
- Adequate pain control
- Reliable patient
- Orthopedic follow-up

Miscellaneous

ICD9: 823.80, 823.81

CORE CONTENT CODE: 18.4.13.1.5.2

SUGGESTED READINGS

Gustilo RB, Merkow RL, Templeman D, et al. The management of open fractures. J Bone Joint Surg 1990;72A(2):229–304.

Manaster BJ, Andrews CL. Fractures and dislocations of the knee and proximal tibia and fibula. Semin Roentgenol 1994;29(2):113–133.

Russel TA. Fractures of the tibia and fibula. In: Rockwood CA, Green DP, Bucholz RW, Heckman JD, eds. Rockwood and Green's fractures in adults. 4th ed. Philadelphia: Lippincott-Raven, 1996. pp 1593–1652.

Authors: Beverly Davison; Stacy Nunberg

Tibial Plateau Fracture

Clinical Presentation

SIGNS AND SYMPTOMS

- Painful, swollen knee
- Inability to bear weight on the injured leg
- Knee effusion (hemarthrosis)
- Decreased (both active and passive) range of motion of the knee
- Tenderness along the proximal tibia
- Possible varus or valgus deformity of the knee
- Possible joint instability due to associated ligamentous injury

MECHANISM/DESCRIPTION

- Fracture or depression of the proximal tibial articulating surface
- Also referred to as tibial condylar fractures
- Valgus or varus force applied in combination with axial loading
  - —The pedestrian struck by an auto (fender fracture where the bumper of a vehicle strikes the lateral aspect of the proximal tibia) is the most common mechanism of injury
    - -This usually results in splitting or depression of the *lateral* plateau
    - -The younger the patient the more resistant the plateau is to depression
    - -Elderly patients present more often with depression type fractures
  - —Fall from a height causing femoral condyles to impact on tibial surface
  - —Violent twisting force, e.g., skiing
- *Medial* plateau fractures are much less common and require significant force to occur
  - —Associated injuries include ligamentous damage (lateral collateral, posterior cruciate, and medial meniscus) and neurovascular injury (peroneal nerve and popliteal vessels) to that knee

PEDIATRIC CONSIDERATIONS

- Tibial plateau fractures are rare in children because of the dense cancellous bone of the tibial plateau

SCHATZKER CLASSIFICATION SYSTEM

- *Type 1* is a split-off fracture of the *lateral* tibial plateau without compression of the plateau
  - —Occurs in younger patients where the plateau resists depression
  - —Usually occurs from a valgus force to the knee in combination with axial load
- *Type 2* is a combination of a split fracture and depression of all or a portion of the remaining *lateral* plateau
  - —The mechanism is similar to the above but these patients tend to be older and have weaker bones; the plateau can be depressed by the femoral condyle
- *Type 3* is a local depression of the articulating surface of the *lateral* plateau
- *Type 4* is a fracture/depression of the *medial* plateau
  - —It requires much more force for this injury to occur
  - —Be suspicious for other injuries
  - —Damage to the popliteal artery, peroneal nerve, lateral collateral ligament, medial meniscus, and cruciate ligaments must be suspected
- *Type 5* is a bicondylar fracture
  - —High-impact injury associated with popliteal vessel injury, peroneal nerve injury, and development of compartment syndrome
- *Type 6* is a bicondylar, grossly comminuted fracture involving both the plateau and the metaphysis
  - —Occurs from a violent force, usually a fall from a height, with associated neurovascular compromise and compartment syndrome

Pre-Hospital

CAUTIONS

- In high energy mechanisms, associated major life-threatening injuries take precedence
- Immobilize to prevent further neurologic or vascular injury

Diagnosis

ESSENTIAL WORKUP

- Neurovascular examination
  - —High energy mechanism (medial plateau or bicondylar fractures) carry risk of neurovascular damage and compartment syndrome
  - —Check popliteal, posterior tibial, and dorsalis pedis arterial pulses
  - —Check integrity of peroneal nerve; ankle and toe dorsiflexion and sensation in webspace between great and second toes
- Plain radiography
  - —Anteroposterior and lateral views of the knee and proximal tibia
  - —Cross-table lateral view may demonstrate lipohemarthrosis (fat-fluid level)
  - —Pay attention to areas of ligamentous attachment where avulsion fractures may take place; i.e., medial and lateral femoral condyles, intercondylar eminence, and fibular head

IMAGING/SPECIAL TESTS

- Oblique views may identify fracture not apparent on other films
- Tibial plateau view-AP view with the knee in 10–15° flexion helps visualize depressions
- Arthrocentesis to look for fat globules if mechanism strongly suggests fracture and effusion present without x-ray findings
- MRI can be used to better elucidate soft tissue injuries
- Angiography indicated if
  - —High energy mechanism
  - —Schatzker type 4, 5, or 6 fracture
  - —Alteration in distal pulses
  - —Expanding hematoma
  - —Bruit
  - —Injury to anatomically related nerves
- Compartment pressures if suspected compartment syndrome
  - —Pain not over fracture site
  - —Pain on passive stretch
  - —Paresthesias
  - —Abnormality of pulses
  - —Pressures greater than 30 mm Hg are an indication for fasciotomy

DIFFERENTIAL DIAGNOSIS

- Knee dislocation
- Cruciate ligament tears
- Meniscal tears

PEDIATRIC CONSIDERATIONS

- Include oblique views as part of routine radiography

Treatment

INITIAL STABILIZATION

- ABCs/ATLS protocol in multiple trauma victim
- Long-leg splint
- Ice
- Elevation

ED TREATMENT

- Nonweight-bearing
- Pain control
- Nondisplaced fractures or minimally displaced *lateral* plateau fractures without ligamentous injury
  —Aspiration of hemarthrosis and injection of local anesthetic
  —Examination for ligamentous instability
  —If knee is stable
    -Compressive dressing
    -Ice and elevation for 48 hours
    -Nonweight-bearing/crutches
  —Early orthopedic follow-up if knee not stable
- Open fractures
  —Remove contaminants
  —Apply moist sterile dressing
  —Assess tetanus immunity
  —Antibiotics
  —Emergent orthopedic consultation

MEDICATIONS

- For open fractures
  —Cefazolin: 2 g IV loading dose (50 mg/kg in children)
  —Gentamycin: 1.5–2 mg/kg IV loading dose (2.5 mg/kg pediatric dose) *if* Gustilo-Anderson type III
  —Vancomycin: 1 g IV loading dose (10 mg/kg in children) *if* penicillin allergy

Disposition

ADMISSION CRITERIA

- Open fractures for débridement, irrigation, and intravenous antibiotics
- Comminuted, bicondylar fractures for traction
- High energy mechanism for observation of neurovascular status
- Pain control

DISCHARGE CRITERIA

- Nondisplaced fractures
- Minimally displaced, stable fractures of the *lateral* plateau

Miscellaneous

ICD9: 823.00

CORE CONTENT CODE: 18.4.13.1.5.1

SUGGESTED READINGS

Rang M. Children's fractures. 2d ed. Philadelphia: JB Lippincott, 1984.

Simon RR, Koenigsknecht SJ. The proximal Tibia & Fibula. In: Simon RR, Koenigsknecht eds. Emergency Orthopedics. Norwalk CT, Appleton and Lange. pp 273–286.

Torrey SB. Lower extrem and pelvis trauma. In: Barkin ed. Pediatric Emergency Medicine. St. Louis: CV Mosby 1992. pp. 357–365.

Wiss DA, Watson JT, Johnson EE. Fractures of the knee. In: Rockwood CA, Green DP, Bucholz RW, Heckman JD, eds. Rockwood and Green's fractures in adults. 4th ed. Philadelphia: Lippincott-Raven, 1996. pp 1593–1652.

Author: Stacy Nunberg

Tinea Infections, Cutaneous

Clinical Presentation

SIGNS AND SYMPTOMS

- Tinea capitis
  - —Disease of children spread through hand to scalp contact
  - —Alopecia
  - —May manifest as a kerion—a boggy inflammatory mass that exudes pus
  - —"Black dots" from infected hairs broken off at the scalp
- Tinea corporis ("ringworm")
  - —Arms, legs, and trunk
  - —Sharply marginated, annular lesion with raised margins and central clearing
  - —Hair follicle involvement may produce indurated papules and pustules
  - —Lesions may be single, multiple, or concentric
  - —Pets are often a vector
- Tinea cruris ("jock itch")
  - —Erythematous, scaly, marginated patches involving the perineum, thighs, and buttocks
  - —Associated with heat, humidity, perspiration, and tight fitting undergarments
  - —The scrotum and penis spared
- Tinea pedis ("athlete's foot")
  - —Scaling, maceration, or fissuring between the toes
  - —Initially third, fourth, or fifth web space, may involve plantar surfaces
  - —Risk factors include the elderly, immunocompromised, hot humid climates, or infrequent changes of socks
  - —Foul odor may indicate secondary bacterial infection
  - —More common in adults than children
  - —"Trichophytid" reaction: vesicular eruption remote from the infection involving hands, mimics dyshidrotic eczema
- Tinea unguium, (onychomycosis)
  - —Yellow or brown discoloration with thickening and debris under the nails
  - —Onycholysis: loosening of the nail from its bed
  - —May involve the plantar surface of the foot
- Tinea versicolor
  - —Most common in warm months
  - —Round or oval superficial brown, yellow, or hypopigmented macules that may coalesce
  - —Upper trunk, arms, and neck
  - —Facial involvement is common in children

MECHANISM/DESCRIPTION

- Superficial fungal infections of the hair, skin, or nails which rarely invade below the stratum corneum

ETIOLOGY

- Most common organisms are dermatophytes (microsporum, trichophyton, and epidermophyton)
  - —Malassezia furfur, a yeast, is the etiologic agent of tinea versicolor
- Trauma or maceration of the skin may allow fungal entry into skin

PEDIATRIC CONSIDERATIONS

- Fungi can be spread from toys and hair care items
- Tinea unguium is rare in children, and is associated with Down's syndrome, immunosuppression, tinea pedis or capitis

Pre-Hospital

N/A

Diagnosis

ESSENTIAL WORKUP

- Diagnose by clinical exam
- Wood's lamp is insensitive as not all fungi fluoresce
  - —Trichophyton does not fluoresce
  - —Microsporum fluoresces bright yellow-green
  - —Malassezia (tinea versicolor) fluoresces yellow-orange
  - —Erythrasma (nontinea corynebacterial infection) will fluoresce coral red
- Microscopy
  - —Cleanse area with 70% ethanol and scrape active margin of lesion with #10 or #15 scalpel blade
  - —Place scrapings on a glass slide, add a drop of 10%–20% potassium hydroxide solution and cover with a coverslip
  - —The presence of budding yeast or hyphae confirms the diagnosis
- Fungal cultures are of limited value in that they may take up to 6 weeks to grow

DIFFERENTIAL DIAGNOSIS

- Tinea capitis: impetigo, pediculosis, alopecia areata, seborrheic dermatitis, and psoriasis
- Tinea corporis: impetigo, herpes simplex, Lyme disease, verruca vulgaris, psoriasis, discoid eczema, herald patch of pityriasis rosea, erythema multiforme, urticaria, seborrheic dermatitis, and secondary syphilis
- Tinea cruris: impetigo, seborrheic dermatitis, psoriasis, candidal infection, irritant and allergic contact dermatitis, and erythrasma
- Tinea pedis: scabies, erythrasma, candida, allergic and contact dermatitis, psoriasis, and bacterial interdigital infection
- Tinea unguium: psoriasis, dermatitis, lichen planus, and congenital nail dystrophy
- Tinea versicolor: vitiligo, secondary syphilis

PEDIATRIC CONSIDERATIONS

- Brushing the hair with a toothbrush or rolling a moistened cotton swab may be easier, less traumatic ways to obtain fungal elements for culture or microscopy

Treatment

INITIAL STABILIZATION

- None required except in immunocompromised patients

ED TREATMENT

- Tinea capitis
  - —Oral griseofulvin is first line treatment
  - —Oral ketoconazole, itraconazole, and terbinafine are alternatives
  - —Selenium sulfide shampoo, once per day, may enhance the elimination of spores
  - —Kerion may respond more rapidly with addition of prednisone
- Tinea corporis
  - —Topical antifungal therapy with clotrimazole, miconazole, or other topical antifungal for 4–6 weeks
  - —Alternative therapy is ketoconazole
- Tinea cruris
  - —Topical antifungal therapy (see tinea corporis)
  - —Area should be kept dry with loose undergarments, and fragrance-free talcum powder
  - —Pruritus can additionally be treated with a low-potency corticosteroid such as topical hydrocortisone
  - —Resistant disease may be treated with oral ketoconazole
- Tinea pedis
  - —Topical antifungals for mild cases
  - —Oral fluconazole is alternative
  - —Acute vesicular tinea pedis may respond to drying agents (Burrow's), or topical corticosteroids
  - —Prevention includes drying between toes, and using talcum or antifungal powders
- Tinea unguium
  - —Itraconazole or fluconazole are first line treatments
  - —Nail removal may be necessary
  - —Does not respond to topical therapy
- Tinea versicolor
  - —2.5% selenium sulfide solution is first-line therapy
  - —Topical antifungals or oral ketoconazole
  - —Alternatives are fluconazole and itraconazole
- Immunocompromised patients may require systemic antifungals for any cutaneous fungal infection

MEDICATIONS

- Clotrimazole: adults: apply cream to affected area 2–3 applications/day for 1–3 wks; peds: same
- Fluconazole: T. unguium: adults: 150 mg po q wk for 3–6 months fingers, 6–12 months toes; T. corporis, cruris, and pedis: 150 mg po q wk for 1–4 weeks; T. versicolor: 400 mg po single dose; peds: none (may cause hepatotoxicity)
- Griseofulvin: T. capitis: adults: 500 mg po qd for 4–6 weeks; peds: 11 mg/kg up to 500 mg po qd until hair regrows (usually 6–8 wks)
- Itraconazole: T. capitis: adults/peds: 3–5 mg/kg po qd; T. unguium: 200 mg po qd for 3 months; T. versicolor: 400 mg po qd for 3 days; peds: none (contraindicated with terfenadine)
- Ketoconazole: T. capitis, corporis: adults 200 mg po qd for 4 wks; peds: 3.3–6.6 mg/kg po qd for 4 wks (contraindicated with terfenadine and astemizole)
- Miconazole: adults: apply cream to affected area 2–3 applications per day for 1–3 wks; peds: same
- Prednisone: adults: none; peds: 1 mg/kg po qd for 2 wks
- Selenium sulfide: adults: 2.5% shampoo to affected area for 10–15 minutes for 1–2 wks, peds: same
- Tolnaftate: adults: apply cream to affected area 2–3 applications per day for 1–3 wks; peds: same

PEDIATRIC CONSIDERATIONS

- Topical preparations are preferred

Disposition

ADMISSION CRITERIA

- Invasive disease in the immunocompromised host
- Kerion with secondary bacterial infection

DISCHARGE CRITERIA

- Most patients may be managed as outpatients
- Children may returned to school once appropriate treatment has been initiated

Miscellaneous

ICD9: 110.9

CORE CONTENT CODE: 3.2.2.2

SUGGESTED READINGS

Bergus GR, Johnson JS. Superficial tinea infections. Am Fam Physician 1993;48:259–268.

Elewski BE. Cutaneous mycoses in children. Br J Dermatol 1996;134(Suppl 46):7–11.

Rezabek GH, Friedman AD. Superficial fungal infections of the skin. Drugs 1992;43(5):674–682.

Wargon, O. Tinea of the skin, hair and nails. Med J Aust 1996;164:552–556.

Authors: Mark G. Richmond; Steven M. Green

Toluene, Poisoning

Clinical Presentation

SIGNS AND SYMPTOMS

Acute

- Neurologic
  - —Depression
  - —Euphoria
  - —Ataxia
  - —Seizures
- Cardiac
  - —Fatal arrhythmias
- Pulmonary
  - —Chemical pneumonitis
- Gastrointestinal
  - —Abdominal pain
  - —Nausea, vomiting
  - —Hematemesis
- Renal
  - —Distal renal tubular acidosis
  - —Hematuria
  - —Proteinuria
- Musculoskeletal
  - —Diffuse weakness

Chronic

- Neurologic
  - —Peripheral neuropathies
  - —Encephalopathy
  - —Optic atrophy
  - —Clonus
- Cardiac
  - —Congestive heart failure
  - —Cardiomyopathy
- Renal
  - —Distal renal tubular acidosis
  - —Renal failure
- Musculoskeletal
  - —Rhabdomyolysis

MECHANISM/DESCRIPTION

- Rapidly absorbed by inhalation
- Readily crossing the blood-brain barrier reaching high concentrations in the brain
- Alveolar excretion and liver metabolism
- Methods of intoxication
  - —"Sniffing"—simple inhalation of substance directly from container
  - —"Huffing"—vapors inhaled through cloth saturated with substance
  - —"Bagging"—inhaling vapors from bag containing substance
- Toxic range
  - —100 ppm—impairment of psychomotor and perceptual performance
  - —500–800 ppm—HA, drowsiness, nausea, weakness, and confusion
  - —>800 ppm—convulsions, ataxia, staggering gait for several days
  - —10,000–30,000 ppm—anesthesia within 1 minute

ETIOLOGY

- Volatile hydrocarbon
- Abused for its euphoric effect
- Used as an organic solvent—found in
  - —Glue
  - —Coolants
  - —Paints and paint thinners
  - —Petroleum products
  - —Aerosolized household products
  - —Correction fluid

PEDIATRIC CONSIDERATIONS

- Prevalent in the adolescent age group
  - —Inexpensive "high" with readily available sources
  - —Many psychosocial problems
  - —Develop chronic neurologic dysfunction

Pre-Hospital

CONTROVERSIES

- Forced emesis usually not indicated
  - —Aspiration due to decreased level of consciousness

CAUTIONS

- Rapid onset of toxicity
- Death possible with sudden cardiac dysrhythmias

Diagnosis

ESSENTIAL WORKUP

- Physical clues to diagnosis
  - —Presence of agent on lips, nose, or clothes
  - —Odor of agents

LABORATORY

- ABG
  - —Acidosis
  - —Hypoxia if chemical pneumonitis
- Electrolytes, BUN, Cr, glucose
  - —Hypokalemia
  - —Normal or high anion gap metabolic acidosis
  - —Hyperchloremia
  - —Impaired renal function
- Calcium and phosphorus
  - —Severe hypocalcemia/hypophosphatemia common
- Urinalysis
  - —Check for myoglobin (rhabdomyolysis)
  - —Hematuria and protein often present
- Creatinine kinase if suspect rhabdomyolysis
- Alcohol level—often a coingestant
- Liver enzymes, PT/PTT if hepatic dysfunction suspected

IMAGING/SPECIAL TESTS

- EKG—atrial and ventricular dysrhythmias
- CXR
  - —Indicated if dyspnea or low oxygen saturation
  - —Chemical pneumonitis
- Urine for hippuric acid (metabolite of toluene)
- CT
  - —For altered mental status/chronic exposure
  - —Cerebral/cerebellar atrophy

DIFFERENTIAL DIAGNOSIS

- Alcohol intoxication
- Methanol
- Ethylene glycol
- Salicylate
- Heavy metal exposure (especially lead)
- Guillain-Barré syndrome
- Metabolic abnormalities

Treatment

INITIAL STABILIZATION

- ABCs
- Cardiac monitor
- 0.9%NS IV access
- Naloxone, thiamine, and check glucose if altered mental status

ED TREATMENT

- Treat cardiac dysrhythmias in a standard fashion
- Correct metabolic abnormalities
  - —Potassium
  - —Calcium
  - —Phosphate
- Acidosis resolves with IV fluids
- If rhabdomyolysis
  - —Maintain high urine output
  - —Alkalinize urine
  - —Consider mannitol
- Gastric decontamination for oral ingestion
  - —Charcoal not been fully studied, other hydrocarbons well absorbed

MEDICATIONS

- Activated charcoal: 1–2 g/kg po
- Dextrose: D50W 1 amp (50 ml or 25 g) (peds: D25W 2–4 ml/kg) IV
- Naloxone (narcan): 2 mg (peds: 0.1 mg/kg) IV or IM initial dose
- Thiamine (vitamin B_1): 100 mg (peds: 50 mg) IV or IM

Disposition

ADMISSION CRITERIA

- Altered mental status
- Dysrhythmias
- Hepatic dysfunction
- Renal failure
- Rhabdomyolysis
- Severe metabolic derangements

DISCHARGE CRITERIA

- After 4–6 hours observation
  - —Mental status at baseline
  - —No evidence of cardiac, metabolic, or neurologic derangement

Miscellaneous

ICD9: 982.0

CORE CONTENT CODE: 17.2.26

SUGGESTED READINGS

Ellenhorn M, et al., eds. Inhalant abuse. In: Medical toxicology: Diagnosis and treatment of human poisoning. 2d ed. Baltimore: Williams & Wilkins, 1997.

Hussain TF, Heidenreich PA, et al. Recurrent non-Q-wave myocardial infarction associated with toluene abuse. Am Heart J 1996;131(3):615–616.

Kamijima M, Nakazawa Y, et al. Metabolic acidosis and renal tubular injury due to pure toluene inhalation. Arch Environ Health 1994;49(5):410–413.

Author: Chris Ervin

Toothache

Clinical Presentation

SIGNS AND SYMPTOMS

- Tooth pain
  - —May be referred to jaw, ear, face, eye, and neck
  - —Pain often associated with chewing, changes in temperature and recumbency
- Malodorous breath
- Fever and chills
- Foul taste in mouth
- Dental caries
- Pain on percussion/palpation of tooth and gums
- Facial swelling or erythema
- Cervical adenopathy
- Trismus
  - —Decreased maximal interincisal opening
  - —Normal 35–50 mm
  - —Abscess

Pre-Hospital

- Maintain patent airway in patients with severe facial swelling or trismus
- The patient should sit up if possible

Diagnosis

ESSENTIAL WORKUP

- Medical and dental history
- Assess need for predental procedure antibiotic prophylaxis
  - —Rheumatic fever
  - —Cardiac valve replacements
  - —Orthopedic joint replacements
  - —Mitral valve prolapse or valvular heart disease
- The oral examination should include
  - —Inspection and palpation of lips, salivary glands, floor of the mouth
  - —Identify periodontal abscess
  - —Evaluate for deep-space infection
  - —Teeth should be percussed for tenderness and mobility
  - —Dental numeric system used in adults
    - -Maxillary: right to left 1–16; mandibular: left to right 17–32

LABORATORY

- None needed except for signs of systemic toxicity or deep fascial space infections

IMAGING/SPECIAL TESTS

- Periapical x-rays and panorex if deeper abscess suspected
- CT scan of the orofacial area and neck if deep fascial space infection suspected

DIFFERENTIAL DIAGNOSIS

- Dental
  - —Dental caries (demineralized hard structures by bacteria)
  - —Pulpitis (inflamed pulp secondary to infection)
  - —Periapical abscess (necrotic pulp and subsequent abscess)
  - —Postextraction pain (dry socket, infection)
- Periodontal Disease
  - —Gingivitis and periodontitis
  - —Periodontal abscess (gum boil)
  - —Pericoronitis (gingival inflammation from malerupted tooth)
  - —Acute narcotizing ulcerative gingivitis (Vincent's gingivitis, trench mouth)
  - —Aphthous ulcers (canker sores)
  - —Denture stomatitis
  - —Herpetic gingivostomatitis
- Nonodontogenic
  - —Sinusitis
  - —Otitis media
  - —Pharyngitis
  - —Peritonsillar abscess
  - —TMJ syndrome (usually present with pain around the ear)
  - —Trigeminal neuralgia
  - —Vascular headache
  - —Herpes zoster
  - —Myocardial infarction

PEDIATRIC CONSIDERATIONS

- Tooth eruption in an infant or child may cause oral pain, irritability, low-grade fevers, diarrhea, and decreased food intake

Treatment

INITIAL STABILIZATION

- Airway management for deep-space infection and airway compromise
- Early pain management as indicated

ED TREATMENT

- Appropriate analgesia
- Dental anesthetic field block
  —Injected along the buccal surface of the affected tooth
  —Specific nerve block for multiple teeth
- Antibiotics if dental infection is present
  —Penicillin is the antibiotic of choice
  —Clindamycin or metronidazole when there is a predominance of anaerobes
- Localized periapical and periodontal abscesses should be incised, drained, and irrigated
- Saline rinses at home four times a day and dental referral in 24 hours

MEDICATIONS

- Antibiotics
  —Cephalexin: adults: 250–500 mg po q 6 hrs; peds: 25–50 mg kg/24 hrs q 6 hrs
  —Clindamycin: adults: 150–450 mg po q 6 hrs; peds: 25–30 mg/kg/24 hrs (max 2 g) q 6 hrs
  —Erythromycin: adults: 500 mg po q 6 hrs; peds: 30–50 mg/kg/24 hrs (max 2 g) q 6 hrs
  —Metronidazole: adults: 500 mg po q 8 hrs; peds: not recommended
  —Penicillin VK: adults: 500 mg po q 6 hrs; peds: 25–50 mg/kg/24 hrs (max 3 g) q 6 hrs
- Analgesics
- Acetaminophen: adults: 650–1000mg po q 4 hrs; peds: 15 mg/kg/dose q 4 hrs
- Ibuprofen: adults: 400–800 mg po q 8 hrs; peds: 10 mg/kg po q 6 hrs
- Acetaminophen and codeine #3: adults: 1–2 tabs po q 4–6 hrs; peds: elixir: codeine 12 mg/5ml
- Acetaminophen and oxycodone: adults: 1–2 tab po q 6 hrs; peds: 0.05–0.15 mg/kg/dose (max 10 mg)
- Ketorolac: adults: 30 mg IV, 60 mg IM q 6 hrs; peds: 1 mg/kg/dose IM
- Morphine sulfate: adults: 2–8 mg SQ/IV q 2 hrs; peds: 0.1 mg/kg/dose SQ/IV q 2 hrs

PEDIATRIC CONSIDERATION

- Teething infants may be helped by over the counter topical anesthetics

Disposition

ADMISSION CRITERIA

- Severe facial swelling
- Suspicion of deep fascial space infections (e.g., Ludwig's angina, retropharyngeal)
- Facial cellulitis proximal to the eye
- Extensive trismus
- Dehydration
- Evidence of systemic toxicity

DISCHARGE CRITERIA

- Toothaches and localized dental infections can be discharged from the ED

Miscellaneous

ICD9: 525.9

CORE CONTENT CODE: 22.2.22

SUGGESTED READINGS

Amsterdam JT. Dental disorders. In: Rosen P, et al., eds. Emergency medicine: Concepts and clinical practice. St. Louis: Mosby-Year Book, 1992:2381–391.

Heir GM. Facial pain of dental origin: a review for physicians. Headache 1987;27(10):540–547.

Smith RG. Toothache and common periodontal problems. In: Harwood-Nuss A, ed. The clinical practice of emergency medicine. Philadelphia: Lippincott-Raven 1996:65–75.

Authors: Marc J. Shapiro; Keith Yattaw

Torticollis

Clinical Presentation

SIGNS AND SYMPTOMS

- Head is rotated and twisted to one direction
- Pure flexion (anterocollis) or extension (retrocollis) is *rare*
  - —Represents symmetrical involvement of muscles
- Intermittent painful spasms of sternocleidomastoid (SCM), trapezius, and other neck muscles
- Neck movements vary from jerky to smooth
- Symptoms usually aggravated by standing, walking, or stressful situations
- Usually does not occur with sleep
- Congenital form
  - —First sign may be a firm, nontender, enlargement of the SCM muscle visible at birth
- Psychological factors (e.g., depression, anxiety, etc.) may play a role

MECHANISM/DESCRIPTION

- "Twisted neck"
- A fixed or dynamic posturing of the head and neck in tilt, rotation, and flexion

ETIOLOGY

Local

- Acute wry neck
  - —Develops overnight without provocation
  - —Most prevalent
  - —Self-limited, symptoms resolve in 1–2 weeks
- Cervical spine
  - —Fracture
  - —Dislocation, subluxation
  - —Infections
  - —Spondylosis
  - —Tumor
  - —Scar tissue producing injuries
  - —Ligamentous laxity in atlantoaxial region
- Inflammatory disease causing muscular damage
  - —Myositis
  - —Lymphadenitis
  - —Tuberculosis
- Infections of surrounding soft tissues
  - —Nasopharyngeal abscess
  - —*Retropharyngeal abscess*
  - —Cervical adenitis
  - —Tonsillitis
  - —Mastoiditis
  - —Sinusitis
  - —Posttrauma

Compensatory

- Tilt with essential head tremor (patient tilts head to suppress *tremor*)
- Ocular muscle palsy

Central

- Idiopathic spasmodic torticollis
  - —Female > Male
  - —Onset 31–60 years old
- Dystonias
  - —Torsion dystonia
  - —Generalized tardive dystonia
  - —Wilson's disease
  - —L-dopa therapy
  - —Acute (neuroleptic drugs)

SPECIAL PEDIATRIC CONSIDERATIONS

Local

- Congenital
  - —Odontoid hypoplasia
  - —Hemivertebrae
  - —Spina bifida
  - —Arnold-Chiari syndrome
  - —Pseudotumor of infancy
  - —Hypertrophy or absence of cervical musculature
- Otolaryngologic
  - —Vestibular dysfunction
  - —Otitis media
  - —Cervical adenitis
  - —Pharyngitis
  - —Retropharyngeal abscess
  - —Pharyngitis
  - —Mastoiditis
- Esophageal reflux
- Syrinx with spinal cord tumor
- Trauma
  - —Cervical fracture/dislocation
  - —Clavicular fractures
- Juvenile rheumatoid arthritis

Compensatory

- Strabismus (fourth cranial nerve paresis)
- Congenital nystagmus
- Posterior fossa tumor

Central

- Dystonias
  - —Torsion dystonia
  - —Drug induced
  - —*Cerebral* palsy

Pre-Hospital

- Ensure patent airway
- Cervical spine precautions for any history of trauma
- Support head

Diagnosis

ESSENTIAL WORKUP

- Geared toward diagnosing life threatening etiologies above
- Distinguish torticollis from other causes of neck stiffness (meningismus)
- Good medication/ingestion history
- *Cervical spine films* to evaluate for fracture except patients with chronic paroxysmal episodes

LABORATORY

- No specific tests helpful

IMAGING/SPECIAL TESTS

- CT or MRI of cervical spine diagnostic of retropharyngeal abscess, tumor

DIFFERENTIAL DIAGNOSIS

- CNS infections
- Tumors of soft tissue or bone
- Basal ganglia disease
- Abscess of cervical glands
- Myositis of cervical muscles
- Cervical disk lesions

Treatment

INITIAL STABILIZATION

- Cervical spine immobilization if fracture is suspected
- If airway management is necessary, RSI/paralytics is procedure of choice

ED TREATMENT

- Drug (e.g., phenothiazine) induced
  —Diphenhydramine or benztropine
- Acquired
  —If less than 1 week in duration, recommend soft collar and rest
  —If less than 1 month in duration, consult orthopedics for possible traction
- Miscellaneous
  —Physical therapy
  —Massage
  —Local heat
  —Analgesics
  —Sensory biofeedback
  —TENS
  —Surgery

MEDICATIONS

- Benztropine (for drug-related dystonia): 1–2 mg IM or slow IV, followed by 3–5 days po
- Botulinum toxin-A (used for failed drug therapy): 50–200 IU IM
- Clonazepam (second-line drug): 0.5 mg po tid
- Diphenhydramine (for drug-related dystonia): adults: 25–50 mg IV/IM, followed by 3–5 days po; peds: 5 mg/kg/24 hrs div q 6 hrs IV/IM/PO
- Trihexyphenidyl (a first-line drug): 2–5 mg po per day, advance to 30 mg/day.Valium: adults: 2–5 mg IV, 2–10 mg po tid; peds: 0.1–0.2 mg/kg/dose IV/PO q 6 hrs

SPECIAL PEDIATRIC CONSIDERATIONS

- Congenital
  —Operative division of involved muscle if physical therapy (e.g., passive stretching) is unsuccessful by 1 year of age

Disposition

ADMISSION CRITERIA

- Cervical spine fracture
- Diagnosis is in doubt
- Infectious causes
- Toxic appearance
- Unable to maintain adequate fluid intake
- No support system

DISCHARGE CRITERIA

- None of the above and symptoms adequately controlled with oral meds

Miscellaneous

ICD9: 723.5

CORE CONTENT CODE: 22.2.23

SUGGESTED READINGS

Duane DD. Spasmodic torticollis. Adv Neurol 1988;49:135–50.

Kahn ML, Davidson R, Drummond DS. Acquired torticollis in children. Orthop Rev 1991;20:667–74.

Smith DL, DeMario MC. Spasmodic torticollis: a case report and review of therapies. J Am Board Fam Pract 1996;9:435–41.

Author: Andrew Chang

Torus Fracture

Clinical Presentation

SIGNS AND SYMPTOMS

- May be subtle or minimal since fracture is incomplete
- Loss of function/mobility
- Decreased limb movement, "pseudoparalysis"
- Localized tenderness, swelling
- Deformity
- Crepitus
- Ecchymoses
- Compartment syndrome rare

MECHANISM/DESCRIPTION

- Long bones are elastic and resilient
- Incomplete fracture at the junction of metaphysis and diaphysis
- Bone angulates beyond bending limit
  - —Side with tension bends
  - —Compression side buckle
- Common in children 5–11 years of age
- Usually involves radius or ulna

ETIOLOGY

- Fall exerting a longitudinal or axial compression force
  - —Fall on a dorsiflexed hand

Pre-Hospital

- Splint involved extremity

Diagnosis

ESSENTIAL WORKUP

- Exclude concurrent injuries
- Assure history consistent with injury
- AP and lateral radiograph of the involved limb, including the joint above and below the fracture
  - —Assess for distal or proximal intra-articular involvement, dislocation, subluxation

LABORATORY

- Required only if concomitant injuries

DIFFERENTIAL DIAGNOSIS

- Other fractures
- Infection
- Tumor

Treatment

INITIAL STABILIZATION

- Resuscitation for concurrent injuries

ED TREATMENT

- Immobilize in long-arm splint (i.e., sugar tong) for 4–6 weeks to prevent angulation during healing
- Refer to orthopedist if angulation >15° in children or >30° in infants
- If suspicious, immobilize and repeat radiograph in 2–3 weeks

Disposition

ADMISSION CRITERIA

- Concurrent injuries requiring admission
- Suspected child abuse

DISCHARGE CRITERIA

- Normally followed as outpatient

Miscellaneous

ICD9: 829.0

CORE CONTENT CODE: 18.6.7.2

SUGGESTED READINGS

Ogden J. Skeletal injury in the child. 2d ed. Philadelphia: WB Saunders, 1990

Author: Leslie Milne

Toxic Epidermal Necrolysis

Clinical Presentation

SIGNS AND SYMPTOMS

- Prodrome: 2–3 days of fever, cutaneous tenderness, malaise, myalgias, arthralgias, conjunctival burning or itching, pharyngitis, dysuria, vomiting, and diarrhea
- Rash: painful generalized urticarial plaques progressing to large, palm-sized, flaccid bullae and vesicles that coalesce and subsequently slough in large sheets yielding an underlying dark red, oozing dermis
- Areas involved: all surface areas including the conjunctival, buccal, pharyngeal, anal, urethral, and vaginal mucosa, but often spares the scalp
- *Nikolsky's sign:* the separation of the epidermis from the dermis caused by shear forces on the skin in areas of erythema

MECHANISM/DESCRIPTION

- One of the most fulminant and potentially fatal of all dermatologic disorders
- Causes a dramatic sloughing of the epidermis that can affect up to 100% of the total body surface area in addition to the mucosa
- The cleavage plane is at the basement membrane of the epidermis (dermal-epidermal junction), so that even the basal cell layer is lost
- Epithelium of the gastrointestinal, renal, and pulmonary systems may be involved
- Ocular involvement including pseudomembranous conjunctival erosions, ulcerations, and synechiae may result in blindness if not aggressively treated
- Skin healing occurs, but often with much scarring
- Toxic epidermal necrolysis (TEN) and Stevens-Johnson syndrome are variants of the same disease
- More than half of all deaths occurring in TEN are due to delayed sepsis
- Mortality rates using modern medical and surgical management range from 11% to 33%

ETIOLOGY

- TEN most often represents an idiosyncratic, drug-induced, dose-independent reaction and is thought to be an immune-mediated process
- Frequently implicated drugs include sulfonamides, NSAIDs, anticonvulsants, penicillins, and allopurinol
  - —The time period between the first dose of the drug and the onset of cutaneous manifestations of TEN is often 1–3 weeks
  - —It is often difficult to determine a single precipitating drug
- Immunizations, viral infections, and neoplasia have also been implicated as causative factors of TEN

Pre-Hospital

CAUTIONS

- Care must be taken to prevent shear forces on the skin during transport
- Intravenous lines need not be started for short transports in hemodynamically stable patients
- Intravenous lines placed through friable skin in the pre-hospital environment should be changed early in the hospital course to avoid infectious complications
  - —Be careful of taping because hard to stabilize sloughing

Diagnosis

ESSENTIAL WORKUP

- TEN is diagnosed clinically based upon identifying the characteristic painful denuding bullous skin lesions or the preceding erythroderma
- Careful ophthalmologic evaluation including visual acuity and fluorescein staining, as well as early ophthalmologic consultation for removal of pseudomembranes and adhesions, is essential in preventing blindness and other sequelae

LABORATORY

- There are no pathognomonic laboratory findings in TEN
- Neutropenia, anemia, and thrombocytopenia may be present
- Serum electrolytes may be abnormal due to fluid imbalances
- Erythrocyte sedimentation rate is typically elevated
- Hematuria due to erosion of the distal urethra mucous membrane may be present

IMAGING/SPECIAL TESTS

- Definitive diagnosis is made by a punch skin biopsy, the results of which will not be readily available to the emergency physician
- Electrocardiogram in appropriate patients to rule out concurrent ischemic damage or electrolyte abnormalities resulting from rapid fluid shifts
- Chest x-ray to rule out pneumonitis

DIFFERENTIAL DIAGNOSIS

- Staphylococcal scalded skin syndrome (SSSS)
- Differentiate TEN from SSSS
  - —*Mucous membranes:* erosions of the mucous membrane which are typically seen in TEN are usually absent in SSSS
  - —*Skin cleavage:* in TEN, occurs at the basement membrane (dermal-epidermal junction); in SSSS, occurs intraepidermally
  - —*Pain of lesion:* the rash of TEN is painful; the rash of SSSS is not
  - —*Age of patient:* TEN may occur in children but is generally a disease of adults; SSSS primarily affects children
  - —*Etiology:* TEN most often represents an idiosyncratic, drug-induced, dose-independent reaction and does not require antibiotics; SSSS is the result of an infection and requires antibiotics
- Stevens-Johnson syndrome
  - —TEN affects >30% of the total body surface area; Stevens-Johnson syndrome affects <10%
- Sunburn
- Scarlet Fever
- Toxic shock syndrome
- Kawasaki disease

Treatment

INITIAL STABILIZATION

- ABCs
- If intubation is required, soft tubes and gentle technique will minimize mucosal damage
- Peripheral intravenous catheter access, cardiac monitor, pulse oximetry, nasogastric tube, frequent core temperature evaluation
- Sterile techniques are paramount
- Patient warming measures
- Foley catheters may produce pain and exacerbate urethral and meatal erosion

ED TREATMENT

- Identify and stop all medications prescribed or bought over-the-counter within the recent 2 months
- Fluid resuscitation with lactated ringers at two-thirds to three-fourths the volume needed for burns covering the same area as estimated using the Parkland formula
  - —4 ml crystalloid/kg body weight/percent body surface area involvement per 24 hours
  - —Give half of total calculated fluid in first 8 hours, remainder in the next 16 hours
  - —Adjust fluids to keep urine output greater than 0.5 ml/kg/hr
- Patients with ocular involvement should receive topical nonsulfa-containing ophthalmic antibiotics
- Warm, air-fluidized bed for prolonged emergency department stay
- Plasmapheresis and hyperbaric oxygen treatment may be considered
- Biobrane or tissue grafting are often used in the burn unit to control heat and fluid losses, to reduce pain, and, in the case of tissue grafting, to promote epithelialization
- Emotional support must be provided to the patient and relatives

MEDICATIONS

- Corticosteroids are controversial and in most reports not effective
- Emergency department use of antibiotics active against staphylococci and streptococci may be considered if the diagnosis of TEN is not known; however, the prophylactic routine use of broad spectrum antibiotics is discouraged
- Silver sulfadiazine and mafenide acetate may cause TEN and should be avoided

Disposition

ADMISSION CRITERIA

- All patients with suspected TEN should be admitted
- Patients should be transferred to a burn center if the diagnosis of TEN is suspected
- Early dermatologic and ophthalmologic consultation is encouraged

DISCHARGE CRITERIA

- Patients with suspected TEN should not be discharged from the ED

Miscellaneous

ASSOCIATED CONDITIONS

- Sepsis
- Disseminated intravascular coagulation
- Pneumonia
- Acute tubular necrosis

SYNONYMS

- Fixed drug necrolysis

ICD9: 695.1

CORE CONTENT CODE: 3.6.3

SUGGESTED READINGS

Avakian R, et al. Toxic epidermal necrolysis: A review. J Am Acad Dermatol 1991;25:69–79.

Parsons JM. Toxic epidermal necrolysis. Int J Dermatol 1992;11(31):749–768.

Rohrer TE, Razzaque AA. Toxic epidermal necrolysis. Int J Dermatol 1991;7(30):457–466.

Roujeau J-C. Drug-induced toxic epidermal necrolysis. Clin Dermatol 1993;11:493–500.

Authors: Richard C. Winters; Theresa M. Schwab

Toxic Shock Syndrome

Clinical Presentation

SIGNS AND SYMPTOMS

Criteria for Diagnosis

- Fever >38.9°C
- Hypotension (systolic BP <90 mm Hg) or shock
- Diffuse, blanching nonpruritic macular erythroderma rash with subsequent desquamation 5–12 days after the resolution of rash (painless "sunburn")
- Clinical involvement of *at least three* of the following
  - —Renal
    - -Increase in BUN and Cr 2× normal or
    - -Sterile pyuria without evidence of infection
  - —Hepatic
    - -Total BR, SGOT, SGPT elevated to >2× normal values
  - —Hematologic
    - -Thrombocytopenia <100,000/mm^3
  - —Gastrointestinal
    - -Profuse diarrhea or
    - -Vomiting
  - —Musculoskeletal
    - -Severe myalgias or
    - -Twofold increase in CPK
  - —Mucosal inflammation
    - -Conjunctival, vaginal, or pharyngeal hyperemia
  - —CNS
    - -Disorientation, confusion, or hallucinations

Other

- Tachycardia
- Hyperemic mucous membranes
- Pharyngitis/conjunctivitis
- Can rapidly progress to multisystem dysfunction
- Associated with tampon use in menstruating females usually between the 3rd and 5th day of menses
- Fatality rate: 2.7 %

MECHANISM/DESCRIPTION

- Severe acute life-threatening illness caused by toxin-producing strains of *Staphyloccus aureus*
- Exotoxin, toxic shock syndrome toxin (TSST-1)
  - —Produced by 20% of *S. aureus* isolates
  - —Significant factor in the production of symptoms associated with TSS
- Biological properties of TSST-1 include the ability to
  - —Induce fever directly on the hypothalmus or indirectly via interleukin-1 (IL-1), and tumor necrosis factor (TNF) production
  - —Promote T-lymphocyte superantigenization and overstimulation
  - —Induce interferon production
  - —Enhance delayed hypersensitivity
  - —Suppress neutrophil migration and immunoglobulin
  - —Enhance host susceptibility to endotoxins
- Massive vasodilation occurs
  - -Causes rapid movement of serum proteins and fluids from the intravascular to the extravascular space

ETIOLOGY

- Initially a disease of young, healthy menstruating females
- 25% of nonmenstruating toxic shock syndrome associated with postpartum *S. aureus* vaginal infections
- Males constitute one-third of patients with TSS
- *S. aureus* enters the body in TSS in a variety of clinical settings
  - -Nasal packing (nasal tampons)
  - -Surgical wounds and infected abrasions
  - -20–40% of the adult population carries *S. aureus* in the nasal vestibule

Pre-Hospital

CAUTIONS

- Fluid resuscitation as for hypovolemia or septic shock

Diagnosis

ESSENTIAL WORKUP

- Clinical diagnosis using diagnostic criteria with the absence of other causes of illness

LABORATORY

- CBC
- Electrolytes, BUN, Cr, glucose
- Calcium, magnesium
  - —Hypocalcemia/hypomagnesemia often present
- Urinalysis
- ABG
- CPK, SGOT, SGPT
- PT, PTT, platelets
- Blood, urine, throat, and CSF cultures as indicated

IMAGING/SPECIAL TESTS

- CXR
- Investigation of other etiologies
  - —Serology for RMSF, rubeola, and leptospirosis
  - —VDRL
  - —Monospot
  - —Antinuclear antibody
  - —Hepatitis B surface antigen

DIFFERENTIAL DIAGNOSIS

- Staphylococcal scalded skin syndrome
  - —In children <5 years old
  - —Initial macular rash followed by the formation of ill-defined bullae that can be rubbed off revealing a shiny, moist, glistening epidermis (Nikolsky's sign)
- Scarlet fever
  - —Preceding streptococcal pharyngitis
  - —Rash begins on the upper chest, neck and back spreading to the remainder of the trunk, sparing the palms and soles
  - —Hypotension absent
- Kawasaki disease
  - —Fever, conjunctival hyperemia, and erythema of the mucous membranes
  - —Not associated with renal failure, hypotension, or thrombocytopenia
- Stevens-Johnson syndrome
  - —Severe, multisystem involvement
  - —Mucosal involvement prominent with involvement of the mouth, conjunctivae, vagina, anus, and urethral meatus
- Leptospirosis
  - —Transmitted through contact with infected animals
  - —Fever, headache, severe myalgias, and conjunctivitis
  - —Truncal rash that only desquamates in children
- Rocky Mountain Spotted Fever
  - —Rash is pink and macular, beginning on the wrists, palms, ankles, and soles of the feet spreading to the trunk and face
  - —Petechiae appear after 4 days

Treatment

INITIAL STABILIZATION

- ABCs
  - —ARDS may complicate TSS and require mechanical ventilation with positive end-expiratory pressure
- Aggressive management of circulatory shock with IV fluids and pressors

ED TREATMENT

- Management depends on severity

Hypotension

- Aggressive fluid replacement
  - —During the first 24 hours may require 4–20 L of crystalloid and fresh frozen plasma (colloid)
  - —*Caution:* large amounts of IV fluids and pressor agents used to treat refractory hypotension can result in the rapid onset of pulmonary edema
  - —Pressors (dopamine) if fluid correction fails to restore normal arterial pressure

Infection Management

- Search for and treat the focus of infection
- Remove the source of infection (e.g., tampon, nasal, or wound packing)
- Some authorities recommend women with tampon-related TSS to have vaginal irrigation with saline or povidone-iodine solution
- Early surgical/gynecologic consultation if drainage or debridement of infectious sites necessary
- Antibiotics
  - —Recommended but have not been shown to not alter the course
  - —Antibiotic choices: β-lactamase-resistant penicillins (nafcillin or oxacillin), clindamycin, cefazolin, or vancomycin

MEDICATIONS

- Cefazolin (ancef): 1 g (peds: 50–100 mg/kg/24hrs) IV q 6 hrs
- Clindamycin: 600–900 mg (peds: 20–40mg/kg/24hrs) IV q 6–8 hrs
- Dopamine: 2–20 μg/kg/min IV titrate to BP
- Nafcillin: 1.5 g (peds: 100 mg/kg/24hrs) IV q 4 hrs
- Oxacillin: 1–2 g (peds: 50–100 mg/kg/24hrs) IV q 4 hrs
- Vancomycin: 500 mg (peds: 10 mg/kg) IV q 6 hrs

Disposition

ADMISSION CRITERIA

- ICU admission for critically ill/shock

DISCHARGE CRITERIA

- None

Miscellaneous

ICD9: 785.5, 785.59

CORE CONTENT CODE: 9.1.9

SUGGESTED READINGS

Callaham ML, Barton CW, Schumaker HM. Decision making in emergency medicine. Philadelphia: BC Decker, 1990.

Harwood-Nuss A, Luten RC. Handbook of emergency medicine. Philadelphia: JB Lippincott, 1995.

May HL, Aghababian RV, Fleisher GR. Emergency medicine. 2d ed. Boston: Little, Brown and Company, 1992.

Tintinalli JE, Ruiz E, Krome RL. Emergency medicine. A comprehensive study guide. 4th ed. New York: McGraw Hill, 1996.

Author: Lawrence Heiskell

Toxoplasmosis

Clinical Presentation

SIGNS AND SYMPTOMS

- Four types of infection

Immunocompromised Host

CNS

- Subacute presentation (90%)
- Encephalitis
- Headache
- Altered mental status
- Fever
- Seizures
- Cranial nerve palsies
- Cerebellar signs
- Meningitis-like symptoms
- Movement disorders
- Neuropsychological symptoms
  - —Psychosis
  - —Paranoia
  - —Dementia
  - —Anxiety
  - —Agitation

Pulmonary

- Pneumonitis
- Prolonged febrile illness
- Nonproductive cough
- Dyspnea

Immunocompetent Host

- 10% with symptoms
- Lymphadenopathy
- Fever
- Malaise
- Headache
- Sore throat
- Night sweats
- Maculopapular rash
- Urticaria
- Self-limited process; resolves in 2–12 months
- Rarely presents with pneumonitis or encephalitis

Ocular Toxoplasmosis

- Blurred vision
- Scotoma
- Pain
- Photophobia
- Retina
  - —Small clusters of yellow-white, cottonlike patches

Congenital Toxoplasmosis

- Results from an asymptomatic acute infection during pregnancy
- First trimester
  - —Spontaneous abortion
  - —Stillbirth
  - —Severe disease up to 25% of the time
- Second or third trimester
  - —50–60% chance of acquiring congenital toxoplasmosis
  - —2% fatal
- Most asymptomatic at birth
- Delayed onset
  - -CNS disease
  - -Ocular disease (blindness months–years later)
  - -Lymphadenopathy
  - -Hepatosplenomegaly

MECHANISM/DESCRIPTION

- *Toxoplasma gondii*—intracellular protozoan parasite
  - —Three forms
    - -Tachyzoite: asexual invasive form
    - -Tissue cyst: persists in tissues of infected hosts during chronic phase
    - -Oocyst: contains sporozoites and produced during sexual cycle in cat intestine
- Transmission
  - —Ingesting tissue cysts or oocysts
    - -Ingesting undercooked meat
    - -Vegetables contaminated with oocysts
    - -Contact with cat feces
  - —Transplacental
  - —Blood product
  - —Organ transplant

ETIOLOGY

- 70% of adults seropositive
- Asymptomatic in the majority of immunocompetent patients
- Chorioretinitis
  - —Usually secondary to congenital transmission
  - —Does not become symptomatic until 20–30 years of age

Pre-Hospital

N/A

Diagnosis

ESSENTIAL WORKUP

- Diagnose via
  - —Isolation of organism
    - -Blood
    - -CSF for encephalitis
    - -Bronchoalveolar lavage for pneumonitis
    - -Amniotic fluid
    - -Aqueous humor
  - —Detection of tachyzoites in tissues or body fluids
  - —Demonstrating characteristic lymph node pathology
- Thorough ocular examination
  - —Retinal examination
  - —Visual acuity

LABORATORY

- CBC
  - —Atypical lymphocytes
- ABG/pulse oximetry for pulmonary symptoms

IMAGING/SPECIAL TESTS

- CXR for pulmonary symptoms
- CT head with contrast
  - —Multiple bilateral hypodense ring enhancing lesions
- MRI brain
  - —High signal abnormalities on T_2-weighted images
- IgM antibodies
  - —Absence excludes diagnosis in immunocompetent host
  - —Diagnoses acute infection
  - —Appear in 5 days
  - —Disappear in weeks–months
  - —Neonatal testing differentiates from maternal infection
- IgG antibodies
  - —High number of false-positives/negatives
  - —Common tests
    - -Sabin-Feldman dye test
    - -Indirect fluorescent antibody
    - -Agglutination
    - -ELISA test
- Brain biopsy for encephalitis-definitive diagnosis

DIFFERENTIAL DIAGNOSIS

- Cryptococcal meningitis
- CNS lymphoma
- Pneumocystis pneumonia
- Cytomegalovirus retinitis

Treatment

INITIAL STABILIZATION

- Treat seizures in standard fashion with diazepam and phenytoin
- Initiate oxygen if hypoxia due to pneumonitis

ED TREATMENT

Immunocompetent

- Toxoplasmic lymphadenitis
  - —No antibiotics unless symptoms severe and persistent
- Treat symptomatic patients with
  - —Pyrimethamine and folinic acid plus sulfadiazine or clindamycin for 2–4 weeks
  - —Reassess to determine if longer therapy needed

Immunocompromised

- Confirmed acute infection by serology/symptoms
  - —Treat with pyrimethamine and folinic acid plus sulfadiazine or clindamycin for 4–6 weeks after resolution of symptoms
  - —Alternative medications
    - -Trimethaphan/sulfamethoxazole
    - -Pyrimethamine and folinic acid plus dapsone
- CNS symptoms plus a lesion on CT or MRI
  - —Treat empirically with pyrimethamine and folinic acid plus sulfadiazine or clindamycin
  - —Brain biopsy or CSF confirm diagnosis
  - —Administer anticonvulsants only if confirmed prior seizures
    - -Poorer outcome for patients on anticonvulsants
- Chronic asymptomatic infection
  - —No therapy required
  - —Prophylaxis options for toxoplasmosis in AIDS patients
    - -Trimethoprim-sulfamethoxazole 1 tablet q day or 2 tablets twice a week
    - -Pyrimethamine (75 mg/week) and dapsone (200 mg/week)
    - -Fansidar (pyrimethamine-sulfadoxine) 3 tablets q 2 weeks

Ocular

- Treat with pyrimethamine and sulfadiazine for 1 month
  - —May add clindamycin
- Administer systemic steroids with macula or optic nerve involvement

Acute Acquired Infection in Pregnancy

- Initially treat with spiramycin pending confirmatory tests
- After the infection documented, initiate treatment with
  - —Sulfadiazine in the first 16 weeks
  - —Pyrimethamine and sulfadiazine after 16 weeks
- Treat congenital infection with sulfadiazine, pyrimethamine, and folinic acid for 12 months

MEDICATIONS

- Clindamycin
  - —600 mg (peds: 20–40 mg/kg/24hrs) IV q 6 hrs
  - —300 mg (peds: 8–20 mg/kg/24hrs) po q 6 hrs
- Dapsone: 100 mg po q day
- Folinic acid: 5–10 mg po q day in conjunction with pyrimethamine
- Pyrimethamine: 100 mg bid on first day loading-dose then 25–50 mg po q day (peds: 1 mg/kg/24hrs po bid for 1–2 days then 0.5 mg/kg/24hrs)
- Sulfadiazine: 500 mg–2 g (peds: 100–200 mg/kg/24hrs) po q 6 hrs
- Trimethaphan/sulfamethoxazole: 5 mg/kg of trimethoprim component IV or po q 6 hrs

Disposition

ADMISSION CRITERIA

- Acute infection with severe systemic symptoms
- Immunocompromised patients with
  - —Toxoplasmosis encephalitis
  - —Pneumonitis
  - —Sepsis

DISCHARGE CRITERIA

- Immunocompetent patients with
  - —Mild symptoms
  - —Ocular
- Maternal/congenital infection with mild symptoms

Miscellaneous

ICD9: 130.9

CORE CONTENT CODE: 9.3.2

SUGGESTED READINGS

Chang HR. The potential role of azithromycin in the treatment of prophylaxis of toxoplasmosis. Int J STD AIDS 1996;Suppl 1:18–22.

Fung HB, Kirschenbaum HL. Treatment regimens for patients with toxoplasmic encephalitis. Clin Ther 1996;18:1037–1056.

Ramsey RG, Bean AD. Neuroimaging of AIDS. I: Central nervous system toxoplasmosis. Neuroimaging Clin N Am 1997;7:171–186.

Rodriguez JC, Martinez MM, et al. Evaluation of different techniques in the diagnosis of toxoplasma encephalitis. J Med Microbiol 1997;46:597–601.

Subauste CS, Remington JS. In: Bennet JC, Plum F, eds. Cecil's textbook of medicine. Philadelphia: WB Saunders, 1996:1907.

Author: Kathryn Brinsfield

Transesophageal Fistula

Clinical Presentation

SIGNS AND SYMPTOMS

- Tracheoesophageal fistula
  - —Children
    - -Coughing, choking, cyanosis, or respiratory difficulty with feeding
    - -Increased secretions in the oropharynx
    - -Fine frothy bubbles of mucus at the lips or nostrils
    - -"Rattling" respirations
    - -Aspiration
    - -Perceived difficulty sucking
  - —Adults
    - -Recurrent bouts of choking and coughing after oral intake (especially fluids)
    - -Hemoptysis
    - -Recurrent lung infection
    - -Dysphagia
    - -Fever
    - -Recurrent aspiration
- Cervical esophageal fistula
  - —Pain
  - —Fever
  - —Cervical crepitus
  - —Leakage of fluid from the neck
- Esophagopleural fistula
  - —Epigastric pain
  - —Back pain
  - —Chest pain
  - —Dysphagia
  - —Localized empyema
  - —Subcutaneous air
- Aortoesophageal fistula
  - —Chest pain
  - —GI bleeding
    - -Symptoms of chronic blood loss
    - -Hypotension
- Esophagocardiac fistula
  - —Hematemesis
  - —Chronic dysphagia
  - —CNS changes secondary to brain embolization of esophageal contents
  - —Chest pain
  - —Dyspnea

MECHANISM/DESCRIPTION

- A transesophageal fistula (TEF) is defined as an abnormal communication between tile esophagus and any surrounding structure
- Congenital TEF occur in association with esophageal atresia
  - —Diagnosed at birth or early in the neonatal period
- Acquired TEF
  - —Complication of esophageal instrumentation
  - —Following mediastinal, pulmonary, or neck surgery
  - —Trauma
  - —Foreign body ingestion
  - —Chemical ingestion
  - —Infection
  - —Neoplasm
  - —Radiation therapy
  - —Diverticula
  - —Peptic ulcer disease
  - —Complication of intubation

Pre-Hospital

- Airway management is paramount
- Blood loss may be significant if erosion occurs into the aorta

Diagnosis

ESSENTIAL WORKUP

- Chest x-ray
- Esophageal contrast studies
  - —Barium should be used instead of water-soluble contrast material when lung involvement is suspected because there will be less toxicity if aspirated

LABORATORY TESTS

- Generally not helpful in the diagnosis of TEF
- WBC may be increased if infection present
- Hemoglobin may be decreased if bleeding present

IMAGING/SPECIAL TESTS

- Children
  - —Failure to fully pass a nasogastric catheter into tile stomach
    - -To confirm the diagnosis, x-rays can be taken after contrast is injected through this catheter
- Adults
  - —Endoscopy
  - —Bronchoscopy
  - —CT may be helpful if aortoesophageal fistula is suspected

DIFFERENTIAL DIAGNOSIS

- Diseases of the esophagus
  - —Diverticula
  - —Achalasia
  - —Esophagitis
  - —Stricture
  - —Malignancy
  - —GERD
- Pneumonia
- Tracheobronchitis
- Epiglottitis
- Pulmonary embolus
- GI bleeding
- Pericarditis or cardiac tamponade

Treatment

INITIAL STABILIZATION

- Assure adequate airway
- Volume resuscitation if hemorrhage or sepsis suspected

ED TREATMENT

- Complications of TEF such as hemorrhage, infection, and sepsis should be treated accordingly
- Surgical consultation is necessary and should be emergent if sepsis or life-threatening hemorrhage is present
- Prevent aspiration with frequent suctioning
- Place nasogastric tube to suction
- Maintain NPO

MEDICATIONS

- No specific medications

Disposition

ADMISSION CRITERIA

- Patients with any signs of respiratory difficulty, bleeding, or infection require admission
- All children should be admitted
- Any patient with airway concerns, bleeding, or sepsis mandate an ICU bed

DISCHARGE CRITERIA

- Adults with chronic symptoms of TEF and without signs of serious complication may be discharged with prompt surgical follow up

Miscellaneous

ICD9: 530.84

CORE CONTENT CODE: 13.1.4.1

SUGGESTED READINGS

Azoulay D, Regnard JF, Levasseur P, et al. Congenital respirato-esophageal fistula in the adult. J Thorac Cardiovasc Surg 1992;104(2):381–84.

Dartevelle P, Macchiarini P. Management of acquired tracheoesophageal fistula. Chest Surg Clin N Am 1996;6(4):819–36.

Fernando I IC, Benfield IR. Surgical management and treatment of esophageal fistula. Surg Clin North Am 1996;76(5):1132–135.

Ginsberg RJ, Cooper ID. Esophageal fistula. World J Surg 1983;7(4):455–62.

Author: David J. Istvan

Transfusion Complications

Clinical Presentation

SIGNS AND SYMPTOMS

General
- Fever
- Chills
- Burning at infusion site
- Urticaria/pruritus/skin erythema
- Anaphylaxis—occurs in 1/20,000 transfusions

Pulmonary
- Dyspnea
- Bronchospasm
- Respiratory distress/failure

Cardiovascular
- Tachycardia
- Hypotension
- Substernal chest pain/tightness

GI
- Nausea
- Vomiting
- Diarrhea

Hematologic
- Bleeding
- Hemoglobinuria
- Oozing from surgical wounds
- Jaundice
- DIC

Miscellaneous
- Low back pain
- Renal failure (oliguria/anuria)

MECHANISM/DESCRIPTION

Acute Intravascular Hemolytic Transfusion Reaction
- Mortality and morbidity correlate with the amount of incompatible blood transfused
- Occurs immediately from
  —ABO incompatibility
  —Blood type identification error
  —Incompatible transfused cells immediately destroyed by antibodies
- Intravascular hemolysis causing activation of the coagulation system leading to inflammation, shock, and DIC
- Mediators (cytokines) released during inflammatory response
- Renal failure
  —Cytokines cause local release of endothelin in kidney causing vasoconstriction
  —Leads to parenchymal ischemia and acute renal failure
- Respiratory failure due to pulmonary edema/ARDS
  —Free Hb causes vasoconstriction in pulmonary vasculature

Other Transfusion-Related Complications
- Hemolysis due to Rh incompatibility
  —Mild/self-limiting
  —1/200 units transfused
- Febrile nonhemolytic transfusion reaction
  —Temperature increases at least 1°C, with chills
  —Antigen-antibody reaction to transfused blood components (WBCs, platelets, plasma)
  —Usually mild
  —Occurs with multiple transfusions or multiparous women
- Allergic transfusion reaction
  —Occur in 1% of transfusions
  —Usually seen with IgA deficient patients

Delayed Reactions
- Infection
  —Blood screened for HIV, hepatitis B, hepatitis C
  —Blood treated to inactivate viruses
  —Risk of transmission
    -HIV: 1/150,000 units
    -Hepatitis B: 1/50,000 units
    -Hepatitis C: 1/ 10,000 units
- Delayed extravascular hemolytic reaction
  —Occurs 7–10 days after transfusion
  —Antigen-antibody reaction that develops after transfusion
  —Coombs test is positive
  —Usually asymptomatic
  —Blood bank analysis detects antibody
- Noncardiogenic pulmonary edema
  —1/5000 transfusions
  —Incompatibility of transfused WBC antibodies
  —Reaction develops within 4 hours of transfusion
- Electrolyte imbalance
  —Hypocalcemia: calcium binds to citrate
  —Hypokalemia: citrate metabolized to bicarbonate, which drives potassium intracellular
- Graft versus host disease
  —Usually fatal (>90%)
  —Immunologically competent lymphocytes transfused into immunoincompetent host
  —Host unable to destroy new WBCs
  —Donor WBCs recognize host as foreign and attack host's tissues

Pre-Hospital

N/A

Diagnosis

ESSENTIAL WORKUP
- Recognize clinical findings of transfusion reaction
- Recheck identifying information of blood and patient for compatibility

LABORATORY
- CBC
- Electrolytes, BUN/Cr, glucose
  —For electrolyte abnormalities
- PT/PTT
- Serum calcium
- Fibrinogen, fibrin degradation products
- Bilirubin (direct/indirect)
- Coombs test
- Hemoglobinemia
  —Pink or red supernatant of plasma or serum indicates hemolysis
- Urinalysis
  —Hemoglobinuria: dipstick-positive blood without RBC on micro

Lab Findings Indicating Hemolysis
- Thrombocytopenia (<100,000)
- Fibrinogenopenia (<150 mg/L)
- Fibrin degradation products
- Prolonged aPTT
- Spherocytosis

Lab Findings Indicating Hemolysis Due to Rh Incompatibility
- Coombs test is positive
- Elevated indirect bilirubin
- Posttransfusion Hgb/Hct does not show expected rise

IMAGING/SPECIAL TESTS
- CXR: diffuse patchy infiltrates without cardiomegaly
- ECG for arrhythmia, signs of electrolyte abnormality

DIFFERENTIAL DIAGNOSIS
- Sepsis
- Anaphylaxis/allergic reaction due to medication

Treatment

INITIAL STABILIZATION

- Immediately stop the infusion
  - —Severity of reaction proportional to amount of blood infused
  - —ABCs
  - —Supplemental oxygen—intubation and ventilation if needed
- Recheck blood identifying information—patients bracelet, blood labels, call blood bank

ED TREATMENT

- Hypotension
  - —0.9%NS hydration with 2 large-bore IVs
  - —Trendelenburg position
  - —Dopamine
- Prevention of renal failure
  - —Maintain urine output of 100 ml/hr
  - —Adequate hydration
  - —Furosemide or mannitol if oliguric
  - —Dopamine infusion 2 μg/kg/min
- Febrile reactions
  - —Antipyretics (acetaminophen/NSAID)
  - —Antihistamine (diphenhydramine) IV
  - —Steroids (solumedrol)
- Allergic reactions
  - —Antihistamine (diphenhydramine) IV
  - —Epinephrine for respiratory symptoms
  - —Steroids (solumedrol)
- Redraw blood sample for repeat ABO/Rh typing, direct antiglobulin testing
- Foley catheter to monitor urine output
- Replete calcium if hypocalcemia develops
- Treat DIC

MEDICATIONS

- Epinephrine (1:1000): 0.3–0.5 cc (peds: 0.01 ml/kg) SQ
- Calcium gluconate: 10 cc of 10% (peds: 100 mg/kg/dose) solution slow IVP
- Dopamine: 2–20 μg/kg/min IV
- Diphenhydramine: 25–50 mg (peds: 1.25 mg/kg) IM/IV/PO
- Mannitol: 1–2 g/kg IV
- Solumedrol: 125 mg (peds: 2 mg/kg) IV

Disposition

ADMISSION CRITERIA

- Acute hemolytic transfusion reaction, pulmonary complications, anaphylaxis, sepsis require ICU monitoring
- Delayed hemolytic transfusion reactions for evaluation/treatment

DISCHARGE CRITERIA

- Uncomplicated febrile or allergic reaction

Miscellaneous

ICD9: 999.8

CORE CONTENT CODE: 7.6.2

SUGGESTED READINGS

Braunwald E, Isselbacher K, et al., eds. Harrison's principles of internal medicine. 13th ed. New York: McGraw Hill, 1994.

Capon SM, Goldfinger D. Acute hemolytic transfusion reaction, a paradigm of the systemic inflammatory response: New insights into pathophysiology and treatment. Transfusion 1995;35(6):513–520.

Hoffman R, Benz E, Shattil S, et al., eds. Hematology: Basic principles and practice. New York: Churchill Livingstone, 1991.

Isersion KV. Transfusion reactions and complications. In: Harwood, Nuss A, eds. Clinical practice of emergency medicine. Philadelphia: Lippincott-Raven, 1996:917–920.

Kruskall MS, Mintz PD, Bergin JJ, et al. Transfusion therapy in emergency medicine. Ann Emerg Med 1988;17:327–335.

Storer DI. Blood and blood component therapy. In: Rosen P, Barkin R, eds. Emergency medicine: Concepts and clinical practice. 4th ed. St. Louis: CV Mosby, 1998 p 129–136.

Author: Marc Gelman

Transient Ischemic Attack

Clinical Presentation

SIGNS AND SYMPTOMS

- The neurologic features of the transient episode indicate the territory of the artery involved
- Anterior (carotid) circulation
  - —Contralateral weakness
  - —Amaurosis fugax
  - —Dysphasia
  - —Contralateral neglect
- Posterior (vertebrobasilar) circulation
  - —Vertigo
  - —Diplopia
  - —Dysphasia
  - —Dysarthria
  - —Crossed weakness
  - —Crossed sensory deficit
  - —Altered level of consciousness

MECHANISM/DESCRIPTION

- Transient neurologic deficits with complete resolution within 24 hours (most within 30 minutes)
  - —To be contrasted with reversible ischemic neurologic deficit (RIND), which are focal deficits lasting longer than 24 hours, that subsequently completely resolve
  - —*Stroke in evolution* is the progressive worsening of neurologic deficits over minutes to hours
  - —*Completed stroke* is one in which a deficit persists longer than 3 weeks despite improvement

ETIOLOGY

- Distal embolization by a thrombus from an atherosclerotic plaque in a large vessel is the most common etiology
- Other causes are
  - —Cardiac conditions such as atrial fibrillation and mitral valve prolapse
  - —Vasculopathies such as carotid or vertebral dissection
  - —Hypercoagulable states such as antiphospholipid antibody syndrome and protein C and protein S

PEDIATRIC CONSIDERATIONS

- Moyamoya disease, which is a primary vascular lesion associated with recurrent strokes
  - —Cerebral vasculopathy characterized by diffuse narrowing of multiple cerebral vessels, presenting as repeated TIAs

Pre-Hospital

- The initial pre-hospital responder must ascertain the neurologic deficit, because reversible defects may completely resolve by the time the patient gets to the hospital

CAUTIONS

- Avoid glucose-containing fluids unless clear hypoglycemia is evident

Diagnosis

ESSENTIAL WORKUP

- A brief, accurate neurologic exam must be performed in every patient in whom a transient ischemic attack (TIA) or stroke syndrome is suspected
- Head CT to evaluate for hemorrhage
- Cardiac monitor, ECG to diagnose atrial fibrillation
- Rapid glucose determination

LABORATORY

- CBC: for anemia or elevated hematocrit producing hyperviscosity
- Electrolytes: for high incidence of comorbid conditions
- PT/PTT: as a baseline, in case anticoagulation is an ultimate goal
- ECG: secondary to the comorbidity of atrial fibrillation and acute MIs
- Toxin screen: for cocaine- or amphetamine-induced pathophysiology

IMAGING/SPECIAL TESTS

- Echocardiography: can identify mural thrombus or valvular vegetation in patients with cardioembolic strokes
- Carotid duplex: with crescendo TIAs, or worsening symptoms, or suspected high grade carotid stenosis. Patients may be candidates for emergent carotid endarterectomy or heparinization
- MRI: visualizes ischemic infarcts earlier than CT and is more effective than CT for posterior circulation strokes. (It is, however, less accurate for diffuse ischemia from hemorrhage)
- MRA: allows the demonstration of large vessel occlusion at the base of the skull

DIFFERENTIAL DIAGNOSIS

- Subdural/epidural hematoma
- Air embolism
- Wernicke's encephalopathy
- Carotid dissection after neck trauma
- Migraine headaches
- Todd's paralysis
- Meningitis
- Dementia
- Giant cell arteritis
- Brain tumor/abscess
- Diabetic ketoacidosis/hyperosmolar coma
- Intracranial hemorrhage

PEDIATRIC CONSIDERATIONS

- In the pediatric population the differential diagnosis includes
  - —Moyamoya disease
  - —Todd's paralysis (postseizure)
  - —Acute infantile hemiplegia
  - —Severe dehydration associated with hypernatremia

Treatment

INITIAL STABILIZATION

- ABCs
- Maintain respiratory and cardiovascular status, especially adequate mean arterial blood pressure
- In the event of an ischemic infarct, a precipitous decline in blood pressure can worsen cerebral ischemia

ED TREATMENT

- TIAs are "mini strokes" that should prompt urgent evaluation in an effort to prevent infarction
- Aspirin
- Neurology consult for workup and possible admission
- Heparin may be started in consultation with neurology for patients with recurrent symptoms
- High risk for recurrence: known high-grade lesion, cardioembolic source, crescendo TIA, and TIAs despite antiplatelet therapy
- Patients with progressive symptoms may be candidates for thrombolytic therapy (see chapter: cerebrovascular accident)

MEDICATIONS

- Heparin: 5000 IU SC q 8–12 hrs, or 5000–7500 IU IV bolus; 1000 IU/hr infusion
- Mannitol: 1 g/kg over 20 min if impending herniation is suspected
- Thrombolytics: controversial in TIAs; refer to institutional protocol

SPECIAL CONSIDERATIONS

- Endarterectomy has been shown to decrease the risk of future strokes in patients with anterior circulation TIAs

Disposition

ADMISSION CRITERIA

- Patients with new onset TIA warrant hospital admission for evaluation and workup
- This includes seeking a surgically reversible cause for the TIA and treatment with anticoagulants

DISCHARGE CRITERIA

- Patients with prior history of TIAs who have been extensively worked up and are completely asymptomatic in the ED may be discharged in consult with neurology and if appropriate follow-up can be assured

PEDIATRIC CONSIDERATIONS

- All children with TIA must be admitted to the pediatric intensive care unit for monitoring of blood pressure, fluid status, and neurologic function

Miscellaneous

ICD9: 435.9

CORE CONTENT CODE: 11.1.4

SUGGESTED READINGS

Adams RD, Victor M. Principles of neurology. 4th ed. New York: McGraw Hill, 1989.

Humphrey PRD. Management of transient ischemic attack and stroke. Postgrad Med J 1995;71(840):577–578.

Klebanoff LM, Fink ME, Lennihan L, et al. Management of cerebral vasospasm in the 1990s. Clin Neuropharmacol 1995; 18(2):127–137.

Kothari RU, Barson W. Management of stroke. In: Tintinalli JE, et al., eds. Emergency medicine. 4th ed. New York: McGraw Hill, 1996.

Authors: N. Taleghani; R. Smith-Coggins

Transplant Rejection

Clinical Presentation

SIGNS AND SYMPTOMS

- Signs of infection are blunted by impaired inflammatory response
- Bone marrow transplant rejection
  - —Respiratory insufficiency with pulmonary infiltrates and hypoxia
    - -Acute graft versus host disease (immune attack of donor marrow on lung tissue)
    - -Interstitial pneumonitis from CMV, pneumocystis, aspergillus, mycobacteria, and nocardia infections
  - —Chronic graft versus host disease (incidence 25–50% of patients)
    - -Skin rash, mucositis, keratoconjunctivitis, esophageal strictures, small and large bowel dysfunction, pulmonary insufficiency, chronic liver disease, and generalized wasting
- Solid organ transplants
  - —Highly susceptible to infection from immunosuppressive drugs (see chapter: Immunosuppression)
  - —Bowel obstruction from B-cell lymphoma
  - —CNS infiltration with confusion, headache, fever, and night sweats
  - —Herpes zoster reactivation
  - —Opportunistic infections (aspergillus, candida, coccidioidomycosis, histoplasmosis) present with subacute respiratory complaints, disseminated or miliary infiltrates, and fever
  - —Gastrointestinal complaints
    - -Diverticulitis—perforation is common at diagnosis
    - -Susceptible to salmonellae and listeria

MECHANISM/DESCRIPTION

- Organ-specific transplant complications
  - —Kidney
    - -Pyelonephritis
    - -Early rejection caused by T- and B-lymphocytes, which attack microvasculature and impair graft perfusion
    - -Chronic rejection from progressive nephrosclerosis of renal vessels
    - -Progressive systemic hypertension as the graft fails
    - -Rejection presents as fever, swelling, and tenderness over the allograft, with decreased urine output and a subtle rise in serum creatinine
  - —Heart
    - -Patients complain of fever, shortness of breath, nausea/vomiting, and chest pain
    - -Acute rejection occurs in 75–85% of patients within the first 3 months
    - -Decreased QRS voltage, new S3 or new CHF or atrial arrhythmias suggest rejection
    - -Patients with fever >38°C, CHF, shortness of breath, hypoxia, hypotension, poorly controlled hypertension or new arrhythmia should be suspected of rejection
    - -Chest pain is not related to ischemia, as the heart is denervated
    - -Accelerated atherosclerosis, though, is the hallmark of chronic rejection, and presents as CHF, ventricular dysrhythmias, hypotension, syncope, or sudden death
    - -ECG commonly demonstrates 2 p waves, as the native sinus node is left in place
  - —Lung
    - -Rejection develops early, only 25–40% develop chronic rejection
    - -Presents with cough, dyspnea, fever, rales and rhonchi, hypoxia or hypercapnia
    - -Diffuse infiltrates are seen in early acute rejection, but when rejection occurs >1 month posttransplant, radiographs may be normal or unchanged
    - -Chronic rejection mimics upper respiratory infection or bronchitis
    - -Transplant lungs have impaired mucociliary clearance, depressed cough reflex (as transplanted lungs are denervated), and defective alveolar macrophages, and are susceptible to infection
    - -CMV pneumonia is most common pathogen in transplanted lungs
    - -The most common fungal infection is from aspergillus
  - —Liver
    - -Rejection presents with fever, right upper-quadrant pain, elevated bilirubin and transaminases
    - -Ascending cholangitis can occur as biliary stent is left in place for months after surgery and can be colonized

Pre-Hospital

CAUTIONS

- Avoid aggressive fluid resuscitation; administer what is necessary to maintain baseline state of hydration

Diagnosis

ESSENTIAL WORKUP

- CBC, blood cultures, urinalysis, CXR
- Other laboratory workup dictated by specific presentation and transplanted organ
  - —Kidney: electrolytes, BUN, creatinine, renal ultrasound/CT
  - —Heart: ECG, ABG, echocardiogram
  - —Lung: ABG, pulmonary function tests, bronchoscopy/biopsy
  - —Liver: liver function tests, bilirubin, ultrasound/CT
  - —Immunosuppressive medication levels (i.e., cyclosporine)

IMAGING/SPECIAL TESTS

- In consultation with appropriate specialist

DIFFERENTIAL DIAGNOSIS

- Infectious agents
  - —Exposure before transplantation: tuberculosis, histoplasmosis, coccidioidomycosis, blastomycosis, strongyloides stercoralis, hepatitis B and C, HIV, cytomegalovirus (CMV), Epstein-Barr virus (EBV), varicella zoster, herpes simplex
  - —Community-acquired exposure after transplantation: influenza, primary varicella, salmonellosis, tuberculosis and fungal infections above, legionellosis, nocardiosis, cryptococcosis, CMV, EBV
  - —Nosocomial exposure: aspergillosis, legionellosis

Treatment

INITIAL STABILIZATION

- ABCs
- Shock state treated with IV fluids and pressor agents
- Treat hypertensive crisis like other hypertensive emergencies

ED TREATMENT

- For kidney, heart, lung and liver rejection, administer 500–1000 mg methylprednisolone IV
- Treatment decisions should be made in consultation with the patient's oncologist, transplant surgeon, or organ specialist
- Avoid blood transfusions, as these need special screening to prevent transmission of disease
- Pressors and inotropics work as usual in the transplanted heart
  —Atropine will have no effect on bradycardia as there is no vagal innervation
  —Use dopamine, epinephrine drips, or external pacing to increase heart rate if bradycardia is symptomatic

Disposition

ADMISSION CRITERIA

- Admit all transplant patients with fever, shortness of breath, signs or symptoms of rejection, abdominal pain, or other signs of organ infection
- Admit to the ICU patients that are septic, or with cardiopulmonary compromise

DISCHARGE CRITERIA

- Nontoxic patients in whom rejection or serious infection has been excluded may be discharged with close follow-up

Miscellaneous

DRUGS USED TO PREVENT REJECTION

- A common regimen is cyclosporine, prednisone, and azathioprine
  —Cyclosporine
    -Dose-related nephrotoxicity
    -Monitor drug levels and renal function
    -Severe hypertension from renal arterial spasm
    -Levels increased by drugs that inhibit cytochrome P450
  —Methotrexate
    -Nausea, vomiting, stomatitis, diarrhea, hepatotoxicity, pneumonitis
  —Steroids
    -GI bleeding, glucose intolerance, skeletal myopathy, and adrenal suppression
  —Tacrolimus (FK506)
    -Neurotoxicity: headache, tremors, insomnia, dysarthria, seizures, and coma
    -Also causes glucose intolerance and may require insulin therapy
  —Azathioprine
    -Bone marrow suppression
    -Nausea, vomiting, stomatitis, pancreatitis, and cholestatic hepatitis

ICD9: 996.52

CORE CONTENT CODE: 8.7.1

SUGGESTED READINGS

Bungardner GL, Roberts JP. New immunosuppressive agents. Gastroenterol Clin North Am 1993;22:421–449.

Petri WA Jr. Infections in heart transplant recipients. Clin Infect Dis 1994;18:141.

Sternbach GL, et al. Emergency department presentation and care of heart and heart/lung transplant recipients. Ann Emerg Med 1992;21:1140.

Sweny P, Burroughs AK. Infections in solid organ transplantation. Curr Opin Infect Dis 1994;7:436.

Author: Mark I. Langdorf

Trichomonas

Clinical Presentation

SIGNS AND SYMPTOMS

Female

- Vaginitis
  - —Malodorous, profuse, itchy discharge
    - -Usually white
    - -May be gray, green, or frothy
  - —Inflammation of vaginal walls
- Cervix
  - —Stippled
  - —Punctate hemorrhages with strawberry coloring
- Dysuria (20%)
- Abdominal pain
- Elevated vaginal pH (>5.5)

Male

- Usually asymptomatic
- Urethritis
  - —Scant discharge
  - —Dysuria
  - —20% of nonspecific urethritis in males caused by trichomonas
- Prostatitis
- Epididymitis
- Reversible sterility

MECHANISM/DESCRIPTION

- Sexually transmitted disease
- Causes urogenital infections in males and females
- Prevalence
  - —<1% in all women
  - —15% in women seen in STD clinics

ETIOLOGY

- *Trichomonas vaginalis*
  - —Causative agent
  - —Flagellated protozoan
  - —Most commonly isolated from the urethra, bladder, and Skene's gland

Pre-Hospital

N/A

Diagnosis

ESSENTIAL WORKUP

- Saline wet mount of cervical smears or spun urine
  - —Motile, pear-shaped flagellated trichomonas
    - -Slightly larger than leukocytes
    - -Seen in 60% of females with active infection
  - —Many PMNs

LABORATORY

- Culture
  - —Prostate message prior to collecting culture in males most sensitive

DIFFERENTIAL DIAGNOSIS

- Urinary tract infection
- Gonorrhea
- Chlamydia
- Candida vaginitis
- Nonspecific vaginitis

Treatment

INITIAL STABILIZATION

N/A

ED TREATMENT

- Nonpregnant patients
  —Metronidazole 2-g single dose
  —Resistant infections: metronidozole 500 mg po bid × 7 days
- Pregnant patients
  —In the first trimester: clotrimazole 100-mg vaginal suppository × 7 days
  -70% effective
  —After first trimester: use metronidazole as above
- Avoid concomitant alcohol use with metronidazole
  —May precipitate antabuse reaction
- Recommend testing
  —Of sexual partners
  —For concomitant sexually transmitted diseases including HIV

Disposition

ADMISSION CRITERIA

- None

DISCHARGE CRITERIA

- All patients

Miscellaneous

ICD9: 131.9

CORE CONTENT CODE: N/A

SUGGESTED READINGS

Adimora AA, Hamilton H, Holmes KK, Sparling PF. Sexually transmitted diseases: Companion handbook. New York: McGraw Hill, 1994.

Berger RE. Sexually transmitted diseases. Adv Urol 1997;2:97.

Centers for Disease Control and Prevention. 1993 Sexually transmitted disease treatment guidelines. MMWR 1993;42:1–102.

Author: David Levine

Tricyclic Antidepressant, Poisoning

Clinical Presentation

SIGNS AND SYMPTOMS

- Rapid deterioration may occur
- Classic tricyclic antidepressant (TCA) compounds (imipramine, amitriptyline, nortriptyline)—greatest cardiovascular toxicity
- Newer agents (serotonergic agents)—less overall toxicity in overdose

Central Nervous System (CNS)

- Stimulation or depression
- Stimulation
  —Tremulousness
  —Agitation
  —Fasciculation
  —Seizures (resulting acidemia may lead to worsening cardiovascular toxicity)
- Depression
  —Drowsiness
  —Lethargy
  —Coma

Cardiovascular System

- Hypotension
- Tachycardia (early; due to blockade of norepinephrine reuptake and anticholinergic effects)
- Bradycardia (late; due to catecholamine depletion state)
- ECG changes
  —QRS widening (>100 msec)
  —Rightward shift in terminal 40 msec in frontal plane axis
- Dysrhythmias
  —SVT
  —Ventricular arrhythmias

Anticholinergic Effects (Less Common)

- Dilated pupils
- Decreased bowel sounds
- Urinary retention

MECHANISM/DESCRIPTION

- Primary mechanism of TCA toxicity
  —Sodium channel blocking effect (quinidine-like effect)
  —Inhibition of norepinephrine reuptake
  —α-Blockade
  —Anticholinergic effect
- Selective serotonin reuptake inhibitors (SSRI)
  —Wider margin of safety than TCA
  —Less CNS/cardiovascular toxicity

ETIOLOGY

- Tricyclic antidepressants
  —Amitriptyline
  —Nortriptyline
  —Imipramine
  —Doxepin
- Newer generation antidepressants (nontricyclic)
  —Have different toxic profile than the TCAs
  —Dibenzoxazepines
    -High CNS toxicity
    -Lower cardiovascular toxicity than TCA
    -Amoxapine (ascendin)
- Triazolopyridines: trazodone
- Tetracyclics: maprotiline (ludiomil)
- Selective serotonin reuptake inhibitors
    -Lack anticholinergic effects
    -Fluoxetine (prozac)
    -Sertraline (zoloft)
    -Paroxetine (paxil)

Pre-Hospital

CAUTIONS

- Do not be lulled into false sense of security with a well-appearing patient
  —Rapid onset of altered mental status, seizures, and dysrhythmias occur
- Perform endotracheal intubation if any evidence of compromise
- Secure IV access
- Administer sodium bicarbonate if any evidence of QRS widening (>100 msec)
  —1 ampule in adults
  —1–2 mEq/kg in children
- Ipecac contraindicated (risk of aspiration with development of depressed mental status, or seizure)

Diagnosis

ESSENTIAL WORKUP

- ECG: factors associated with TCA poisoning
  —Sinus tachycardia (almost always present at sometime after poisoning)
  —QRS widening
    ->100 msec associated with seizure
    ->160 msec associated with ventricular dysrhythmia
  —QT prolongation
  —PR prolongation
  —Rightward shifting of the terminal 40 msec QRS axis
  —R wave amplitude in aVR >3 mm
- Continuous cardiac monitor

LABORATORY

- CBC
- Electrolytes, BUN/Cr, glucose
- ABG
- Urine toxicology screen
  —Rule out other toxins

IMAGING/SPECIAL TESTS

- CXR for aspiration pneumonia/pulmonary edema
- TCA levels
  —Not useful
  —Do not correlate well with the degree of toxicity
  —Qualitative screen appropriate to confirm ingestion if necessary

DIFFERENTIAL DIAGNOSIS

Drugs that Cause Coma

- Alcohols
- Alcohol withdrawal
- Anticholinergics
- Lithium
- PCP
- Opioids
- Phenothiazines
- Sedative hypnotics
- Salicylates

Cardiotoxic Drugs

- Antidysrhythmics (category IA)
- Digoxin toxicity
- Sympathomimetics
- Anticholinergics

Drugs that Cause Seizures

- Alcohol withdrawal
- Anticholinergics
- Camphor
- Isoniazid
- Lithium
- Phenothiazines
- Sympathomimetics
- Phenothiazines
- Toxic alcohols

Treatment

INITIAL STABILIZATION

- ABCs
  - —Low threshold to intubate patients with altered mental status
- IV 0.9%NS
- Oxygen
- Cardiac monitor
  - —For wide complex rhythm (QRS >100 msec) bolus sodium bicarbonate
- Naloxone, thiamine, glucose (Accucheck) for altered mental status
- Flumazenil contraindicated in combined TCA/benzodiazepine overdose

ED TREATMENT

Cardiac Toxicity

- QRS widening (>100 msec)
  - —Bolus with 1 amp (peds: 1–2 mEq/kg) of sodium bicarbonate; repeat if sudden increase in QRS width
  - —Maintain arterial pH of 7.45–7.5 with hyperventilation or sodium bicarbonate infusion
- Dysrhythmia
  - —Sinus tachycardia requires no treatment
  - —Bolus 1–2 amps of sodium bicarbonate (1–2 mEq/kg in children) for sudden change in rhythm
  - —Follow ACLS protocol with addition of sodium bicarbonate boluses
    - -Lidocaine is the second-line agent after sodium bicarbonate
  - —Use of class IA (procainamide) and IC agents and physostigmine contraindicated

Hypotension

- 0.9%NS fluid bolus
- Norepinephrine
  - —Preferred pressor (over dopamine)
  - —Counters the α-blockade better
  - —Dopamine requires higher doses

Decontamination

- Gastric lavage
  - —For recent ingestion (<1–2 hours)
  - —Performed when airway has been secured in the lethargic patient
- Administer activated charcoal with sorbitol
- Ipecac contraindicated

Seizure

- Diazepam first-line followed by phenobarbital/phenytoin
- Neuromuscular paralysis with short-acting agent (rocuronium/vecuronium) for refractory seizures (monitor EEG)
- Sodium bicarbonate bolus to prevent acidosis

MEDICATIONS

- Activated charcoal slurry: 1–2 g/kg up to 90 g po
- Dextrose: D50W 1 amp (50 ml or 25 g) (peds: D25W 2–4 ml/kg) IV
- Diazepam (benzodiazepine): 5–10 mg (peds: 0.2–0.5 mg/kg) IV
- Dopamine: 2–20 μg/kg/min IV infusion titrated to desired effect
- Lorazepam (benzodiazepine): 2–6 mg (peds: 0.03–0.05 mg/kg) IV
- Naloxone (narcan): 2 mg (peds: 0.1 mg/kg) IV or IM initial dose
- Norepinephrine: 4–12 μg/min (peds: 0.05–0.1 μg/kg/min) IV infusion titrated to desired effect
- Sodium bicarbonate: 1–2 amps IVP (peds: 1–2 mEq/kg); drip—add 3 amps to 1 L of D5W (efficacy of a drip is unknown)
- Sorbitol: 1–2 g/kg to a max of 150 g (peds: >1-year old: 1–1.5 g/kg as a 35% solution to a max of 50 g) po mixed in the activated charcoal slurry
- Thiamine (vitamin B_1): 100 mg (peds: 50 mg) IV or IM

Disposition

ADMISSION CRITERIA

- Symptomatic patients observed more than 6 hours
- Altered mental status
- Dysrhythmia or conduction delay
- Seizure
- Heart rate >100 bpm 6 hours postingestion
- Coingestion requiring prolonged observation

DISCHARGE CRITERIA

- Asymptomatic after 6 hours observation
- No alteration in mental status
- Normal ECG with heart rate <100 bpm
- Active bowel sounds; tolerated activated charcoal
- Psychiatry clearance if there has been a suicide attempt or gesture

Miscellaneous

ICD9: 969.0

CORE CONTENT CODE: 17.2.7.3

SUGGESTED READINGS

Ellenhorn MJ, Schoonwald S, Ordog G, Wasserberger J. Cyclic antidepressants. In: Ellenhorn MJ, ed. Ellenhorn's medical toxicology. 2d ed. Baltimore: Williams & Wilkins, 1997:624–650.

Ellison DW, Pentel PR. Clinical features and consequences of seizures due to cyclic antidepressant overdose. Am J Emerg Med 1989;7:5.

Gueye P, Hoffman JR, Taboulet P. Empiric use of flumazenil in comatose patients: Limited applicability of criteria to define low risk. Ann Emerg Med 1996;27:730.

Lavoie FW, Gansert GG. Value of Initial ECG findings and plasma drug levels in cyclic antidepressant overdose. Ann Emerg Med 1990;19:696.

Liebelt EL, Francis PD, Woolf AD. ECGT lead aVR versus qrs interval in predicting seizures and arrhythmias in acute tricyclic antidepressant toxicity. Ann Emerg Med 1995;26:195–201.

Pimentel L, Trommer L. Cyclic antidepressant overdoses. Emerg Med Clinic North Am 1994;12:533–549.

Author: Steven Aks

Trigeminal Neuralgia

Clinical Presentation

SIGNS AND SYMPTOMS

- *Brief, intense, lancinating* pain (tic douloureux)
- *Unilateral* in the distribution of a branch of the trigeminal nerve in the face is most common; however, bilateral trigeminal neuralgias do occur
- May occur without provocation or may be initiated by tactile stimulation of a particular area on the face, lips, tongue, or scalp
- Pain seldom lasts more than a few seconds to several minutes
- Occurs almost exclusively in the middle-aged or elderly patient, and is more common in females than males in this age group
- Associated sensory loss in the effected region may be found
- *Paroxysmal pattern* of pain lasting weeks in duration

MECHANISM/DESCRIPTION

- Idiopathic
- Redundant or tortuous blood vessel in the posterior fossa resulting in irritation of the nerve root
- Space-occupying lesion causing direct compression of the nerve
- Bilateral tic douloureux in younger adult can be seen in multiple sclerosis
- Irritation of the nerve during exacerbation of herpes zoster associated with rash in same distribution

ETIOLOGY

- Primary *idiopathic* is most common
- Multiple sclerosis
- Rarely with herpes zoster
- Space-occupying lesions (aneurysm, neurofibroma, meningioma)

PEDIATRIC CONSIDERATIONS

- Not commonly seen in pediatric population

Pre-Hospital

N/A

Diagnosis

ESSENTIAL WORKUP

- Diagnosis is made clinically, history is of primary importance including
  —Onset, duration of pain
  —Associated constitutional symptoms
  —Visual disturbances
  —Associated paraesthesias
  —History of trauma
- Cranial nerve examination for both sensory and motor function is crucial, including visual acuity
- Neurologic examination for focal deficits
- Skin examination for presence of rash or other abnormalities
- Dental and oral examination

LABORATORY

- No specific tests for trigeminal neuralgia

IMAGING/SPECIAL TESTS

- Idiopathic trigeminal neuralgia (tic douloureux) does not require any special imaging
- The presence of focal cranial nerve or neurologic findings suggest possible intracranial etiologies for the patients pain and CT/MRI should be obtained

Treatment

INITIAL STABILIZATION

- Pain management with narcotic medication is often necessary as other treatments require several days before demonstrating efficacy

ED TREATMENT

- Should focus on pain control and patient comfort
- Recurrent or refractory tic douloureux may require surgical intervention

MEDICATIONS

- Carbamazepine is the mainstay of treatment of trigeminal neuralgia
  - —Doses begin with 100 mg twice daily and can be increased to 600 mg twice daily for control of the patients' symptoms
  - —Gastrointestinal intolerance may be seen in up to one-third of patients
- Narcotic analgesia
- Phenytoin is a second-line medical therapy that has been used with varying efficacy
  - —Starting doses should be 300 mg daily and increased to control pain

PEDIATRIC CONSIDERATIONS

- No specific pediatric considerations are relevant

Disposition

ADMISSION CRITERIA

- Trigeminal neuralgia with presence of other focal neurological findings or positive CT/MRI studies require emergent neurological or neurosurgical consultation
- Refractory or recurrent trigeminal neuralgia not responding to outpatient pain management or anticonvulsant therapy may require admission for surgical intervention and ablation of the trigeminal nerve

DISCHARGE CRITERIA

- Patients without any focal neurological findings and improved pain control in the emergency department may be managed as outpatients

Miscellaneous

ICD9: 350.1

CORE CONTENT CODE: 11.2.2

SUGGESTED READINGS

Dalessio DJ. Trigeminal and glossopharyngeal neuralgia. In: Johnson RT, ed. Current therapy in neurologic disease. 2nd ed. Philadelphia: Decker, 1987:62–65.

Henry G, Little N. Neurological emergencies: A symptom oriented approach. New York: McGraw Hill, 1985.

Selby G. Diseases of the fifth cranial nerve. In: Dyck PJ, et al., eds. Peripheral neuropathy. 2nd ed. Philadelphia: WB Saunders, 1984:1244–1265.

Sweet WH. The treatment of trigeminal neuralgia (tic douloureux). N Engl J Med 1986;315:174.

Author: James M. Leaming

Tuberculosis

Clinical Presentation

SIGNS AND SYMPTOMS

Pulmonary Tuberculosis

- Fever
- Malaise
- Weight loss
- Night sweats
- Chronic cough
- Hemoptysis
- Shortness of breath

Extrapulmonary Tuberculosis

- Central nervous system infections
  —Meningeal irritation and cranial nerve defects
  —Malaise
  —Intermittent headache
  —Low grade fever
  —Confusion
  —Meningismus
  —Diplopia
  —Hyponatremia (due to SIADH)
- Pericardial infection
  —Pleuritic chest pain increased with recumbency
- Renal infection
  —Fever
  —Flank pain
  —Sterile pyuria
- Spinal TB (Pott's disease)
  —Back pain/stiffness
  —Fever
  —Point tenderness
  —Decreased range of motion
- Miliary tuberculosis
  —Multiorgan system involvement
  —Diffuse adenopathy
  —Hepatomegaly
  —Splenomegaly
  —Weight loss
  —Fever

MECHANISM/DESCRIPTION

- Infection with *Mycobacterium tuberculosis,* an acid-fast bacillus, resulting in disease
- Most common route of infection is by droplet nuclei inhaled through the respiratory tract
- Primary infection
  —Initial infection with bacilli occurs when organisms enter the alveoli, then spread via regional lymph nodes to the bloodstream
  —Patients are usually asymptomatic
  —Positive reaction to purified protein derivative (PPD) indicates infection
- Reactivation tuberculosis
  —Characterized by a chronic wasting disease
  —Malaise
  —Low-grade fever
  —Weight loss
  —Night sweats
  —Cough

ETIOLOGY

- Tuberculosis affects approximately one-third of the world's population
- Three tuberculosis epidemics
  —Global resurgence
  —HIV-infected patients
  —Multidrug-resistant tuberculosis
- Conditions that predispose the individual to developing tuberculosis include
  —HIV infection and other immunocompromised states
  —Drug and alcohol abuse
  —Poverty
  —Homelessness
  —Institutionalization
  —Immigration from a high-prevalence area

Pre-Hospital

CAUTIONS

- Place a mask on the patient to prevent respiratory spread of the disease
- Initiate treatment with an IV, oxygen, and pulse oximetry
- Endotracheal intubation may be required in patients with severe hemoptysis or respiratory compromise
- Providers should wear submicron-particulate filter masks
- Inform close contacts

Diagnosis

ESSENTIAL WORKUP

- Diagnosis difficult due to the variety of clinical presentations

Chest Radiography

- Most valuable test for diagnosing pulmonary tuberculosis
- In primary disease, parenchymal infiltrates with unilateral hilar adenopathy are the classic findings
- Reactivation tuberculosis typically appears as upperzone cavitary lesions with or without calcification
- Normal or near normal may occur in AIDS patient
- Unilateral pleural effusion in both primary and reactivation tuberculosis
- Tracheal deviation with scarring or atelectasis
- Ghon focus—calcified scar/healed primary focus of infection

Skin Testing

- Inject 0.1 ml of purified protein derivative (PPD) subcutaneous in the forearm
- Positive test indicates prior or current infection with mycobacterium
- Test results read between 48 and 72 hours after administration
- Interpretation of positive
  —>5 mm induration
    -Close contacts with TB
    -Positive CXR
    -HIV
  —>10 mm induration
    -High-risk groups
    -Immigrants from high prevalence countries
    -Immunosuppressed
    -Health care workers
    -Prison inmates
    -Institutionalized
  —>15 mm induration
    -Low-risk individuals

LABORATORY

- CBC
- Electrolytes, BUN, Cr, glucose
- Pulse oximetry/arterial blood gas
- For respiratory symptoms

IMAGING/SPECIAL TESTS

- Sputum staining for acid fast bacilli (Ziehl-Neelsen stain)
  —Provides a quick presumptive diagnosis
- Sputum, CSF, blood, urine, or peritoneal fluid culture
  —Gold standard for diagnosis of tuberculosis
  —Average time for positive culture is 3–6 weeks
- Spinal tap with CSF analysis
  —For suspected tuberculous meningitis
  —WBC range 0–1500/mm^3 with lymphocyte predominance

—Elevated protein
—Low to normal glucose
- Spine radiographs for Pott's disease
  —May be normal
  —Anterior wedging of two involved vertebral bodies and destruction of disc
- Computerized tomography
  —Better define extent of disease

DIFFERENTIAL DIAGNOSIS

- Bacterial or viral pneumonia
- Lung abscess
- Primary lung cancer
- Lymphoma

Treatment

INITIAL STABILIZATION

- ABCs
  —Control airway as needed
  —With severe hemoptysis, endotracheal intubation with a double-lumen tube can be used to confine bleeding to one lung while rapid surgical consult is obtained
  —While preparing for intubation roll patient to the bleeding side to protect the nonbleeding lung
  —Inflate the balloon on the bleeding side and ventilate the nonbleeding side
  —Oxygenate the patient with 100% oxygen
- Isolate patients in negative pressure rooms with at least 6 air exchanges/hour

ED TREATMENT

- Initiate therapy directed toward area of tubercular involvement

Antituberculosis Medications

- Treatment is dependent on the suspicion of multidrug-resistance
- Any regimen must contain multiple drugs to which the tuberculous bacteria is susceptible
- Directly observed therapy may be necessary to ensure compliance in certain populations
- Standard therapy (no suspected resistance)
  —2 months of
    -Isoniazid
    -Rifampin
    -Pyrazinamide
  —Then 4 months of
    -Isoniazid
    -Rifampin
- Suspected/known drug resistance
  —Individualize with infectious disease consult
  —Need at least three susceptible medications to TB
  —Options
    -Isoniazid
    -Rifampin
    -Pyrazinamide
    -Ethambutol or streptomycin
    -Plus at least two additional drugs (paraaminosalicylic acid, ethionamide, cycloserine, capreomycin, kanamycin, thiacetazone)
- Preventative therapy for positive skin test converters
  —Healthy adults: 6 months isoniazid
  —Children: 9 months isoniazid
  —HIV: 12 months isoniazid
  —Isoniazid resistance suspected: 9 months rifampin
  —Multidrug-resistance suspected: 6 months ethambutol/quinolone and pyrazinamide

Disposition

ADMISSION CRITERIA

- Respiratory compromise
- Question of diagnosis
- Inability to comply with outpatient therapy
- Involuntary admission for noncompliant outpatients occurs
  —Be aware of respective state laws concerning involuntary admission

DISCHARGE CRITERIA

- Without respiratory compromise
- Home isolation procedure compliance
- Ability and willingness to comply with long-term therapy
- Notification of the public health authorities is mandatory

Miscellaneous

ICD9: 011.9

CORE CONTENT CODE: 9.1.5.2

SUGGESTED READINGS

American Thoracic Society. Diagnostic standards and classification of tuberculosis. Am Rev Respir Dis 1990;142:725.

American Thoracic Society. Treatment of tuberculosis and tuberculosis infection in adults and children. Am J Respir Crit Care Med 1994;149:1359.

Iseman MD. Treatment of multidrug-resistant tuberculosis. N Engl J Med 1993;329:784.

Iseman MD. Tuberculosis. In: Bennett JC, et al., eds. Cecil's textbook of medicine. 20th ed. Philadelphia: WB Saunders, 1996; 1683–1689.

Neville K, Bromberg A, Bromberg R, et al. Escalating threat from tuberculosis: the third epidemic. Thorax 1995;50(suppl 1):537–542.

Author: Kathleen A. Raftery

Tularemia

Clinical Presentation

SIGNS AND SYMPTOMS

- Abrupt onset
- Fever >101°F
- Chills
- Headache
- Anorexia
- Myalgias
- Vomiting
- Diarrhea
- Abdominal pain
- Ulcer at site of tick
- Regional lymphadenopathy
- Secondary skin rash
- Primary tularemia pneumonia
  - —Substernal burning
  - —Nonproductive cough

MECHANISM/DESCRIPTION

- Inoculated cutaneously from as few as 50 organisms through inapparent skin lesions
- 3–5 day incubation period

Six Forms

- Ulceroglandular
  - —From tick bites or animal contact
  - —Large tender regional lymph nodes
  - —Red painful papule, reactive ulcer
  - —Fever
- Glandular
  - —Tender regional lymphadenopathy with no local lesions
- Ocular glandular
  - —Entry through conjunctiva
  - —Unilateral
  - —Edema, conjunctivitis, injection, chemosis with periauricular, submandibular, or cervical lymphadenopathy
- Pharyngeal
  - —From contaminated food/water
  - —Severe throat pain
  - —Exudative pharyngitis with ulceration
  - —Regional lymph node involvement
- Typhoidal
  - —Inapparent point of entry
  - —Fever
  - —Severe diarrhea
  - —Bowel necrosis
  - —Pulmonary infiltrates
- Pulmonic
  - —Secondary to inhalation especially in sheep shearers, farmers, or lab workers
  - —Fever
  - —Dry cough
  - —Pleuritic chest pain
  - —CXR: lobar infiltrate, hilar adenopathy, pleural effusion, or a miliary pattern

ETIOLOGY

- Transmission
  - —Tick
  - —Skinning, dressing, and eating infected rabbits, muskrat, beaver, squirrels, and birds
  - —Airborne transmission (laboratory workers)

Pre-Hospital

CAUTIONS

- Clusters or disease in unusual areas should raise suspicion of biologic agents
- Universal and respiratory precautions are recommended

Diagnosis

ESSENTIAL WORKUP

- Diagnosis based on clinical manifestations/serologic studies
- Agglutinin titers
  - —Antibody titer >1:160 with skin ulcer for 2 weeks—diagnostic
  - —4-fold rise in second titer obtained 2 weeks later confirms diagnosis

LABORATORY

- Routine lab tests nonspecific
- CBC
  - —Normal WBC in uncomplicated disease
- Sedimentation rate is elevated
- Gram stain or tissue biopsies often negative
  - —Tissue may show caseation necrosis similar to tuberculosis
- Culture
  - —Source
    - -Blood
    - -Pleural fluid
    - -Lymph node
    - -Wound
    - -Sputum
    - -Gastric aspirate
  - —If special media used, inform lab personnel
- ABG/pulse oximetry for suspected pneumonia

IMAGING/SPECIAL TESTS

- ELISA
  - —Antigen prep useful although not positive until the second week of illness
- Tularemia skin test
  - —Delayed hypersensitivity reaction
  - —Positive skin test similar to tuberculin test response
- CXR for pulmonary symptoms
  - —Lobar infiltrate
  - —Hilar adenopathy
  - —Pleural effusion
  - —Miliary pattern

DIFFERENTIAL DIAGNOSIS

- Tuberculosis
- Cat-scratch disease
- Syphilis
- Chancroid
- Lymphogranuloma venereum
- Toxoplasmosis
- Sporotrichosis
- Rat-bite fever
- Anthrax
- Plague
- Herpes simplex infection
- Ocular symptoms
  - —Adenoviral infection

- Pharyngeal symptoms
  - —Diphtheria, bacterial pharyngitis
  - —Infectious mononucleosis
  - —Adenoviral infection
- Typhoidal tularemia mistaken for
  - —Salmonella
  - —Brucellosis
  - —Legionella
  - —Q fever
  - —Malaria
  - —Disseminated fungal or mycobacterial infections
- Pneumonic form mistaken for
  - —Mycoplasma
  - —Legionella
  - —Chlamydia
  - —Tuberculosis

Treatment

INITIAL STABILIZATION

- 0.9%NS IV fluid for hypotension/dehydration
- Supplemental oxygen for hypoxia
- Administer acetaminophen for fever
- Initiate antibiotic therapy

ED TREATMENT

Antibiotic

- First-line agent: streptomycin or gentamicin
- For tularemic meningitis
  - —Add chloramphenicol or third-generation cephalosporin (ceftriaxone)
- Tetracycline
  - —Oral agent
  - —Only bacteriostatic
  - —High level or relapse occur
- Third-generation cephalosporins and flouroquinolones as primary treatment
  - —Frequent failures
- Treat documented exposures, particularly in lab workers, 1 dose streptomycin IM
- Do not treat tick bites prophylactically

MEDICATIONS

- Ceftriaxone: 1–2 g (peds: 50–100 mg/kg/24hrs) q 24 hrs
- Chloramphenicol: 50–100 mg/kg/24hrs IV divided q 6 hrs
- Gentamicin: 3–5 mg/kg/24hrs IV q 8 hrs for 7–14 days
- Streptomycin: 7.5–10 mg/kg (peds: 20–40 mg/kg/24hrs q 12 hrs IM) q 12 hrs IM or IV for 7–14 days

Disposition

ADMISSION CRITERIA

- ICU admission for advanced age, neutropenic, or presenting with typhoidal tularemia
- Isolation not necessary

DISCHARGE CRITERIA

- Mild cases
  - —Treat with IM/oral therapy

Miscellaneous

ICD9: 21.9

CORE CONTENT CODE: 9.0

SUGGESTED READINGS

Cross JT, Jacobs RF. Tularemia: Treatment failures with outpatient use of ceftriaxone. Clin Infect Dis 1993;17:976–980.

Enderlin G, et al. Streptomycin and alternative agents for the treatment of tularemia. Clin Infect Dis 1994;19:42–47.

Fredricks DN, Remington JS. Tularemia presenting as community acquired pneumonia. Arch Intern Med 1996;156:2137–2140.

Spach DH, et al. Tick-borne diseases in the United States. N Engl J Med 1993;329:936–947.

Author: Kathryn Brinsfield

Tumor Compression Syndromes

Clinical Presentation

SIGNS AND SYMPTOMS

Spinal Cord Compression

- May have symptoms for many months prior to acute presentation
- Back pain
  - —Axial
  - —Referred
  - —Radicular
  - —May occur at any level
- Pain aggravated by
  - —Straining
  - —Movement
  - —Straight leg raising
  - —Neck flexion
- Rest may make pain worse (contrary to degenerative joint disease, where rest improves pain)
- Rarely, weakness or ataxia are the presenting complaints
- Progression of symptoms leads to
  - —Paralysis
  - —Sensory disturbances
  - —Incontinence
- Once symptoms do develop, progression is rapid
  - —30% of patients with advanced symptoms are paraplegic in 1 week

Superior Vena Cava (SVC) Obstruction

- Facial plethora and edema
- Periorbital edema
- Conjunctival suffusion
- Facial swelling
- Shortness of breath
- Thoracic and neck vein distention
- Increased intracranial pressure with severe disease
- Headache
- Blurred vision
- Altered mental status
- Coma
- Papilledema

Inferior Vena Cava (IVC) Obstruction

- Edema of the lower limbs
- Evidence of extensive collateral flow

MECHANISM/DESCRIPTION

Spinal Cord Compression

- 5% of all patients dying of cancer will have some degree of spinal cord compression at autopsy, but only 1% of all patients will have this complication diagnosed during life
- The level of compression
  - —Cervical: 10%
  - —Thoracic: 70%
  - —Lumbar: 20%
- Between 10% and 38% of patients may have multiple, noncontiguous levels, especially if associated with breast or prostate cancer
- Anterior or anterolateral aspect of the cord most often affected
- Site of the metastases
  - —Vertebral column (85%)
    - -Body usually, but also pedicle and posterior arch
  - —Paravertebral spaces (10–15%)
  - —Epidural space (rare)

ETIOLOGY

Spinal Cord Compression

- More than 50% of cases are metastases from lung, breast, or prostate cancer
- Other common causes include multiple myeloma, kidney, melanoma, thyroid, lymphoma, and sarcoma
- In children, common causes are sarcoma, neuroblastoma, germ-cell tumors, lymphoma
- Median survival for patients with epidural compression is 7 months, with a 36% probability of a 1-year survival

Superior Vena Caval (SVC) Obstruction

- Most often secondary to bronchogenic carcinoma or postirradiation fibrosis
- Small-cell lung cancer most common cause

Pre-Hospital

N/A

Diagnosis

ESSENTIAL WORKUP

History

- Previous history of malignant disease
- Prolonged history of back pain, worse with rest
- Development of neurological symptoms

Physical Examination

- Careful neurological examination, including sensory testing
- Assessment of rectal tone
- Assessment of maximal area or areas of bony tenderness

LABORATORY

- Required on a case-by-case basis to assess comorbid conditions (anemia)

IMAGING/SPECIAL TESTS

- CXR
  - —For SVC compression
  - —Mass present in 10%
  - —Pleural effusion in 25%
- Plain spinal radiography
  - —Will show 85% of metastases causing compression
  - —A normal spine (or one showing just degenerative changes) on plain radiology does not exclude the diagnosis of possible cord compression
- Computerized tomography
  - —More sensitive and specific than plain radiography and radionucleotide imaging in distinguishing benign from malignant disease in spinal compression syndrome
  - —To identify mass and impingement in vena cava obstruction
- Magnetic resonance imaging
  - —Investigation of choice to assess extension into the epidural space
  - —Indicated in patients with cancer and unexplained back pain, even in the absence of neurological signs and normal (or degenerative changes only) plain radiographs
  - —25% of adult patients and as many as 65% of pediatric patients with a radiculopathy in this setting will be found to have evidence of spinal cord compression
  - —Early diagnosis utilizing MRI may be a cost-effective option in the investigation of patients with possible spinal cord compression
- Myelography for patients unable to undergo MRI (pacemaker, severe claustrophobia)

DIFFERENTIAL DIAGNOSIS

- Intervertebral disc disease
- Osteoporotic vertebral fractures
- Spondylosis
- Spondylitis
- Epidural abscess

- Primary bone tumors
- Arteriovenous malformations
- Neurological diseases
- Multiple sclerosis
- Amyotrophic lateral sclerosis
- Transverse myelitis
- Spinal infarction

Treatment

INITIAL STABILIZATION

- Early diagnosis and treatment is the key to an improved outcome
  - —Level of neurological dysfunction on presentation is a key factor in the prognosis for spinal cord compression
- Avoid IV line placement in upper extremities if severe SVC compression present

ED TREATMENT

Spinal Cord Compression

- Corticosteroids (dexamethasone)
  - —Administer in ED
  - —Higher doses alleviate the pain more rapidly, but studies indicate no significant difference in outcome with regard to sphincter function or ambulation between the dose schedules
- Radiotherapy
  - —Definitive treatment modality
- Pain medication with narcotics
- Oncology, radiotherapy, and neurosurgical consultation for further management of tumor/malignancy

SVC Compression

- Manage the underlying malignancy with either radiotherapy or chemotherapy
- Elevate head
- Diuretics associated with transient symptomatic improvement
- Administer steroids if respiratory compromise
- Use of stents to hold the vein open has been reported to be successful in relieving symptoms
- Urgent oncology referral

MEDICATIONS

- Dexamethasone: 1mg/kg loading dose, followed by 4–24 mg q 6 hrs

Disposition

ADMISSION CRITERIA

- All patients with spinal cord or acute vena caval compression

DISCHARGE CRITERIA

- None

Miscellaneous

ICD9: 336.9

CORE CONTENT CODE: 11.7

SUGGESTED READINGS

Boogerd W, van der Sande JJ. Diagnosis and treatment of spinal cord compression in malignant disease. Cancer Treat Rev 1993;19:129–150.

Byrne TN. Spinal cord compression from epidural metastases. N Engl J Med 1992;327:614–619.

Johnston RA. The management of acute spinal cord compression. J Neurol Neurosurg Psychiatry 1993;56:1046–1054.

Jordan JE, Donaldson SS, Enzmann DR. Cost effectiveness and outcome assessment of magnetic resonance imaging in diagnosing cord compression. Cancer 1995;75:2579–2586.

Stock KW, Jacob AL, Proske M, Bolliger CT, Rochlitz C, Steinbrich W. Treatment of malignant obstruction of the superior vena cava with the self-expanding Wallstent. Thorax 1995;50:1151–1156.

Author: Martin J. Carey

Tympanic Membrane Perforation

Clinical Presentation

SIGNS AND SYMPTOMS

- Ear pain (mild)
- Decreased hearing (partial)
- Severe pain or complete hearing loss in the affected ear suggests additional injuries
- Purulent or bloody discharge from ear canal
- Tinnitus
- Vertigo
- Otorrhea

MECHANISM/DESCRIPTION

- Blunt trauma (slap to the ear)
- Penetrating trauma (Q-tip)
- Rapid pressure change (diving, flying)
- Extreme noise (blast)
- Lightning
- Spontaneous perforation of acute otitis media
- Acute necrotic myringitis

Pre-Hospital

N/A

Diagnosis

ESSENTIAL WORKUP

- Clinical examination
  - —Direct visualization of tympanic membrane with otoscope
  - —Test hearing in both ears
  - —Note any nystagmus with changes of position or pressure on the tragus occluding the canal (fistula sign)

IMAGING/SPECIAL TESTS

- Insufflation via pneumatic otoscope
  - —Will not cause the perforated tympanic membrane to move normally
  - —Holding pressure for 15 seconds (the fistula test) may cause nystagmus or vertigo if the pressure is transmitted through the middle ear and into a labyrinthine fistula
- Weber test (tuning fork on midline bone)
  - —Sound should be equal or louder in the injured ear, consistent with decreased conduction
  - —Sound localizing to the opposite side of injury indicates possible otic nerve injury
- Rinne test
  - —Usually normal (air conduction detected after bone conduction fades) or shows a small conductive loss

DIFFERENTIAL DIAGNOSIS

- Temporal bone fracture
- Serous otitis media
- Infectious otitis media
- Otitis externa
- Cerumen impaction
- Barotrauma
- Acoustic trauma
- Foreign body
- Child abuse

Treatment

INITIAL STABILIZATION

- ABCs of trauma care
  - —Immobilize C-spine and investigate for intracranial injury when indicated

ED TREATMENT

- Clean debris from the ear canal
- Prescribe antibiotics if there is evidence of infection
  - —Antibiotic choices (7–10 days administration)
    - -Amoxicillin
    - -Trimethoprim-sulfamethoxazole
    - -Cefixime
    - -Augmentin
  - —Prophylactic antibiotics not indicated
- Analgesics if needed for pain
- Do not prescribe topical steroids
- Arrange ENT follow up
  - —After detailed examination and formal audiometric tests, most otolaryngologists follow the perforation with monthly examinations
  - —Operative repair reserved for the 10–20% that do not heal spontaneously
- Provide detailed discharge instructions
  - —Occlude the ear canal with cotton coated in petroleum jelly or antibiotic ointment when showering to prevent entry of water into the middle ear, which can be painful
  - —Swim only with fitted earplugs
  - —Avoid forceful blowing of the nose
- Expected outcome
  - —Most perforations heal spontaneously over a few months
  - —A few require operative repair such as a collagen foam splint or a flap from the canal wall
  - —Perforations caused by molten metal or electrical burns are less likely to heal spontaneously
  - —Forceful entry of water, as in a water skiing accident, is more likely to lead to infection
  - —Complications include infection, dislocation of ossicles, perilymph leak, and cholesteatoma

MEDICATIONS

- Amoxicillin: 250–500 mg (peds: 20–40 mg/kg/24 hrs) po tid
- Trimethoprim-sulfamethoxazole (bactrim DS): 1 tablet (peds: 6–12 mg/kg/24 hrs TMP) po bid
- Cefixime: 400 mg (peds: 8 mg/kg/24 hrs) q d
- Augmentin: 250–500 mg (peds: 20–40 mg/kg/24 hrs) po tid

Disposition

ADMISSION CRITERIA

- Associated injuries requiring admission
- Severe vertigo impairing ambulation

DISCHARGE CRITERIA

- Almost all patients will be discharged

Miscellaneous

ICD9: 384.20

CORE CONTENT CODE: 6.1.9

SUGGESTED READINGS

Gladstone HB, Jackler RK, Varav K. Tympanic membrane wound healing: an overview. Otolaryngol Clin North Am 1995;28:913–933.

Kristensen S. Spontaneous healing of traumatic tympanic membrane perforations in man: a century of experience. J Laryngol Otol 1992;106:1037–1050.

Kristensen S, Juul A, Gamelgaard NP, et al. Traumatic tympanic membrane perforations: complications and management. Ear Nose Throat J 1989;68:503–516.

Turbiak T. Ear trauma. Emerg Med Clin North Am 1987;5:243–251.

Author: Thomas Osborne Stair

Ultraviolet Keratitis

Clinical Presentation

SIGNS AND SYMPTOMS

- Foreign body sensation
- Increased lacrimation
- Photophobia
- Severe pain
- Blepharospasm
- Decreased visual acuity
- 6–10-hour latent period between exposure and the onset of symptoms
- Worse symptoms associated with increased exposure time and more intense exposure

Ocular Findings

- Conjunctival injection
- Corneal edema
- Iritis (cell and flare in the anterior chamber or spasm of the pupillary sphincter)
- Punctate uptake of fluorescein in an interpalpebral pattern—pathognomonic
  —Sloughing of large portions of the cornea may obliterate this finding later in severe cases

MECHANISM/DESCRIPTION

- Prolonged exposure to ultraviolet radiation leads to corneal edema and sloughing, followed by secondary inflammation of the iris
- Sources of ultraviolet radiation
  —Sun lamps
  —Welder's arcs
  —Reflected sunlight (water or snow—worse at high altitude)

Pre-Hospital

N/A

Diagnosis

ESSENTIAL WORKUP

- Accurate history including
  —Type of exposure
  —Timing and duration of exposure
- Visual acuity
- Complete ocular exam including
  —Extraocular movements
  —Conjunctiva/sclera/corneas with fluorescein
  —Anterior chambers (checking for cell and flare)
  —Lenses
  —Eversion of the lids to check for foreign bodies

LABORATORY

N/A

IMAGING/SPECIAL TESTS

- Orbit radiographs/ultrasound/CT/MRI for suspected intraocular foreign body

DIFFERENTIAL DIAGNOSIS

- Foreign body of the cornea or eyelids
- Intraocular foreign body
- Corneal abrasion
- Chemical exposures
- Thermal burns

Treatment

INITIAL STABILIZATION

- Topical anesthesia helps to obtain
  - —More accurate documentation of visual acuity
  - —More thorough eye exam and fluorescein staining
  - —Do not prescribe on outpatient basis—interferes with healing and worsens keratitis

ED TREATMENT

- Initiate short-acting cycloplegic for iritis, which usually develops
- Apply topical broad-spectrum antibiotic ointment or drops (less desirable)
- Apply eyepatch in severe cases
  - —Soft double-patching with mild pressure for patient comfort
  - —If both eyes involved, either patch both eyes or the eye that is more severely affected
- Analgesics (acetaminophen/NSAID/codeine/oxycodone)
- Tetanus prophylaxis if needed

MEDICATIONS

- Topical anesthetics
  - —Proparacaine (ophthaine) 0.5% (onset 20–30 seconds; duration 15 minutes)
  - —Tetracaine (pontocaine) 0.5% (onset 30–60 seconds; duration up to 20 minutes)
- Topical antibiotics
  - —Gentamicin, tobramycin
  - —Sulfacetamide
  - —Fluoroquinolones
- Topical cycloplegics
  - —Cyclopentolate 0.5% (onset 30–60 minutes; duration up to 24 hours)
  - —Homatropine 2% (onset 40 minutes to 3–4 hours; duration 24–48 hours)

Disposition

ADMISSION CRITERIA

- Patients requiring bilateral patching with severely decreased visual acuity and whose social circumstances make it impossible for the patient to take care of his or her own needs

DISCHARGE CRITERIA

- Nearly all patients may be discharged from the ED following treatment with cycloplegics, topical antibiotics, and patching
  - —Lesions usually heal completely within 24 hours
- Ophthalmologist referral for patients who have other eye disorders, or for those who fail to improve significantly after 24 hours

Miscellaneous

ICD9: 370.20

CORE CONTENT CODE: 6.4.2.5

SUGGESTED READINGS

Lerman S. Direct and photosensitized ultraviolet radiation. In: Fraunfelder FT, Roy FH, eds. Current ocular therapy. Sec. 16. 3rd ed. Philadelphia: WB Saunders, 1990: 315–320.

Lubeck D, Greene JS. Corneal injuries. Emerg Med Clin North Am 1988;6(1):73.

Newell FW. Injuries caused by radiant energy. In: Newell FW, ed. Ophthalmology: Principles and concepts. Chap. 8. 7th ed. St. Louis: CV Mosby, 1992:184–185.

Author: Jeffrey Ellis

Urethral Trauma

Clinical Presentation

SIGNS AND SYMPTOMS
- Prior history of trauma
- Pelvic pain, inability to void
- Blood at the meatus, high-riding prostate, perineal or genital swelling

MECHANISM/DESCRIPTION
- Females: injuries to the urethra are rare due to the short, unexposed, and mobile urethra
  —Usually occur at the bladder neck
- Males: urethra is divided into sections
  —Posterior urethra
    -Prostatic
    -Membranous
    -Injuries more common
  —Anterior urethra
    -Bulbar
    -Penile
    -Rarely injured due to its mobility
- Posterior injuries are much more common and have the classification system detailed below
- *Classification of posterior urethral injuries*
  —Type I: urethra stretched but not ruptured
  —Type II: prostatic/membranous portions ruptured (either partially or completely); urogenital diaphragm intact
  —Type III: both the prostatic/membranous urethra and urogenital diaphragm are ruptured, frequently with damage to the proximal bulbar urethra

ETIOLOGY
- Females
  —Childbirth or vaginal surgery
  —Straddle injuries
  —Rare with pelvic fracture
- Males
  —Trauma, especially straddle injuries
  —Mutilation injuries
  —Sexual activity
  —Instrumentation
  —Approximately 95% of posterior urethral injuries are caused by pelvic fractures
    -As many as 25% of pelvic fractures have concomitant urethral injuries

POTENTIAL COMPLICATIONS
- Impotence
- Incontinence
- Strictures
- Infection

PEDIATRIC CONSIDERATIONS
- Urethral damage, frequently caused by traumatic mechanisms similar to adults
- Nonaccidental trauma or sexual abuse, especially females, may be contributory
- Majority of posterior urethral injuries are type 1

Pre-Hospital
- Similar considerations as for major trauma victims

Diagnosis

ESSENTIAL WORKUP
- Female
  —A meticulous vaginal examination to exclude vaginal laceration as the bleeding source
  —Radiographic evaluation of the integrity of the urethra should be performed prior to urinary catheter placement if urethral injury is suspected
    -If this is not possible, suprapubic aspiration, or cystostomy should be done
- Male
  —Determine if the prostate is normally positioned (not high-riding) and examine for blood at the external meatus
  —Radiographic evaluation of the integrity of the urethra should be performed prior to urinary catheter placement if urethral injury is suspected
    -If this is not possible, suprapubic aspiration or cystostomy should be done

LABORATORY
- Urinalysis
- Hematocrit
- BUN and Cr

IMAGING/SPECIAL TESTS
- Retrograde urethrography (RUG)
  —Water-soluble contrast is injected via a catheter-tipped syringe at the urethral meatus
  —Extravasation of contrast and its relation to the prevesical space and urogenital diaphragm should be noted
  —Proximity of the extravasation to the meatus and the bladder should be appreciated
  —If the urethral tear is complete, there will be no contrast within the bladder and marked extravasation will occur
  —A partial tear will demonstrate contrast material within the bladder
  —Excretory urethrography to define proximal urethral tears
- Cystography
  —40% of urethral injuries have concomitant bladder injuries

DIFFERENTIAL DIAGNOSIS
- Perineal and vaginal trauma
- Bladder trauma
- Ureter or kidney trauma

PEDIATRIC CONSIDERATIONS
- If an examination of the introitus and perineum cannot easily be performed, examination under anesthesia should occur
- An examination in the OR, in addition to being better tolerated by the patient, allows the physician to rule out sexual abuse and to confirm that the injury is consistent with the history
- The workup of male pediatric patients should also include an examination in the operating room if an adequate ED examination does not occur or if suspicion of abuse exists

Treatment

INITIAL STABILIZATION

- ABCs of trauma care take precedence

ED TREATMENT

- After RUG, the urologist should be contacted
- Urethral contusions, lacerations, and avulsions are best managed by an experienced urologist
- Catheter placement, if appropriate, or suprapubic aspiration/cystostomy followed by laboratory evaluation comprise the ED treatment

MEDICATIONS

- No specific medications for this injury

Disposition

ADMISSION CRITERIA

- Concurrent closed head injury, blunt abdominal trauma, or pelvic fracture
- Need for operative management of urethral, penile, or bladder injuries

DISCHARGE CRITERIA

- Isolated urethral injuries frequently may be managed in the outpatient setting after appropriate urinary catheterization or suprapubic cystostomy with urologic follow-up

Miscellaneous

ICD9: 867.0

CORE CONTENT CODE: 18.4.11.11

SUGGESTED READINGS

Avanoglu A, Ulman I, Herek O, Ozok G, Gokdemir A. Posterior urethral injuries in children. Br J Urol 1996;77:598–600.

Carter CT, Schafer N. Incidence of urethral disruption in females with traumatic pelvic fractures. Am J Emerg Med 1993;11(3):218–20.

Goldman SM, Sandler CM, Corriere JN Jr, McGuire EJ. Blunt urethral trauma: A unified, anatomical mechanical classification. J Urol 1997;157:85–89.

Lynch JM, Gardner MJ, Albanese CT. Blunt urogenital trauma in prepubescent female patients: More than meets the eye. Pediatr Emerg Care 1995;11(6):372–375.

Watnik NF, Coburn M, Goldberger M. Urologic injuries in pelvic ring disruptions. Clin Orthop 1996;329:37–45.

Authors: Kenneth Bramwell; Roscoe Nelson

Urethritis

Clinical Presentation

SIGNS AND SYMPTOMS

- Urethral discharge, dysuria, cloudy first portion of urine
- Pyuria
- Inguinal adenopathy may be present

MECHANISM/DESCRIPTION

- Symptoms usually develop 1–2 weeks after exposure, but can take up to 4–6 weeks
  —Initially minimal or absent in many patients
- Urethritis may develop after exposure to a partner with a sexually transmitted disease, bacterial vaginosis, or a urinary tract infection
- Urethritis may also develop after orogenital contact

ETIOLOGY

- Sexually transmitted diseases
- The most common causes are
  —*Neisseria gonorrhea* (20%)
  —*Chlamydia trachomatis* (30–50%)
  —*Ureaplasma urealyticum* (10–40%)
- Rarer causes include *Trichomonas vaginalis,* candidal species, herpes simplex virus, genital warts, and foreign bodies
- Sometimes no cause is identified

POTENTIAL COMPLICATIONS

- Recurrent infections
- Ascending urinary tract infections including pelvic inflammatory disease and epididymo-orchitis
- Fallopian tube damage and infertility
- Arthritis
- Conjunctivitis, uveitis, and blindness

PEDIATRIC CONSIDERATIONS

- Urethritis in children should arouse suspicion of child abuse

Pre-Hospital

N/A

Diagnosis

ESSENTIAL WORKUP

- Urethral swabs for *N. gonorrhea,* and *Chlamydia* will confirm the diagnosis
- An RPR or VRDL should be drawn because sexually transmitted diseases frequently occur together

LABORATORY

- Gram stain and cultures from urethral swabs should be reviewed when the patient is reevaluated by their physician after treatment
- Urinalysis should be performed after urethral swabs to identify urinary tract infections

IMAGING/SPECIAL TESTS

- No specific tests

DIFFERENTIAL DIAGNOSIS

- Urinary tract infection
- Prostatitis
- Epididymitis
- Orchitis
- Pelvic inflammatory disease
- Reiter's syndrome

PEDIATRIC CONSIDERATIONS

- Because *Neisseria gonorrhea* infects the entire vaginal vault in prepubescents a speculum examination is not required; external examination and cultures are sufficient

Treatment

INITIAL STABILIZATION

- Most patients will not require significant stabilization

ED TREATMENT

- Treatment may be given empirically based on probable etiologic causes
- Patients should be treated for both gonorrhea and chlamydia

MEDICATIONS

- Gonorrhea
  —Ceftriaxone: adult: 125 mg IM or IV; peds: ceftriaxone 25–50 mg/kg IM
  —Cefixime: adult: 400 mg po
- Chlamydia
  —Azithromycin adult: 1 g po; peds: azithromycin 10 mg/kg po day 1, 5 mg/kg po days 2–5
  —Doxycycline: adult: 100 mg po bid × 7 days
  —Erythromycin base: adult: 500 mg po qid × 10 days; peds: erythromycin: 40 mg/kg/day div q 6 hrs for 10 days
- Single-dose oral therapy is preferred
- The quinolones have been reported as equivalents but do not have adequate activity against ureaplasma to treat these infections

Disposition

ADMISSION CRITERIA

- Patients should not require admission for urethritis unless other complaints or infections so mandate

DISCHARGE CRITERIA

- All patients should be discharged with follow-up arranged at an outside clinic or with their physician

PEDIATRIC CONSIDERATIONS

- If child abuse is suspected, child protective services must be involved and the child should be admitted if a safe home situation cannot be assured

Miscellaneous

ICD9: 597.80

CORE CONTENT CODE: 19.1.5.5, 19.2.3.5

SUGGESTED READINGS

Ingram DL. Neisseria gonorrhoeae in children. Pediatr Ann 1994;23(7):341–345.

Ness RB, Markovic N, Carlson CL, Coughlin MT. Do men become infertile after having sexually transmitted urethritis? An epidemiologic examination. Fertil Steril 1997;68(2):205–213.

Nickel P, Naher H. Nongonococcal urethritis. Curr Probl Dermatol 1996;24:97–104.

Authors: Kenneth Bramwell; Roscoe Nelson

Urinary Retention

Clinical Presentation

SIGNS AND SYMPTOMS

- History of chronic voiding hesitancy
  - —Decreased force of urine stream
  - —Difficulty holding or initiating urinary stream
  - —Feeling of incomplete bladder emptying or postvoid residual
  - —Nocturia
  - —Inability to void
- Abdomen
- Lower abdominal pain
- Distended and tender bladder
- GU
  - —Stenosis at urethra meatus
  - —Urethral mass/fistula
- Rectal
  - —Enlarged or tender prostate
  - —Presence or absence of sphincter tone/sensation

MECHANISM/DESCRIPTION

- Normal micturition *sequence*
  - —As the bladder fills, sensory stretch signals are conducted to the sacral cord through the pelvic nerves and then back through the parasympathetics, supplying the body and neck of the bladder
  - —Once the micturition reflex becomes powerful enough, an inhibitory reflex through the somatic pudendal nerves from S2–3 causes relaxation of the external urethral sphincter
  - —Urination occurs if inhibition is more powerful than the voluntary constriction signals
- Acute urinary retention (AUR)
  - —sudden inability to void urine, resulting in bladder distention
- More common in men than women, less common in children
- Atonic bladder
  - —Destruction of sensory nerve fibers from the bladder to spinal cord that prevents transmission of stretch signals and prevents micturition reflex contractions
  - —Loss of bladder control occurs despite intact neurogenic connections to the brain
  - —Bladder fills to capacity and overflows a few drops at a time (overflow incontinence)
- Automatic bladder
  - —From damage of the spinal cord above the level of S2–3
  - —Micturition inhibited due to "spinal shock" from the sudden loss of facilitory impulse from the brain stem and cerebrum
  - —Intermittent straight catheterization facilitates the return of the excitability of the micturition reflex by preventing physical bladder injury
- Neurogenic bladder
  - —From partial damage in the spinal cord or brain stem that interrupts inhibition
  - —Sacral centers are in a constant state of excitation that even a small quantity of urine results in frequent and relatively uncontrollable micturition

ETIOLOGY

- Benign prostatic hypertrophy: most common in men
- Multiple sclerosis and diabetes: most common in women
- Bladder outlet obstruction
  - —Benign prostatic hypertrophy
  - —Prostate
  - —Cancer
  - —Acute prostatitis
  - —Stones
  - —Blood clots
  - —Prostatic congestion
- Detrusor muscle failure
  - —Acute spinal cord injury
  - —Elderly
  - —Sympathomimetics
- Neurological causes
  - —Detrusor hyperactivity with impaired contractility
  - —Multiple sclerosis
  - —Parkinson's
  - —Stroke
  - —Herniated disk
  - —Diabetes melitis
  - —Dementia
  - —Myasthenia gravis
  - —Brain tumor
  - —Landry-Guillain-Barré syndrome
  - —Bladder neck dysfunction
- Urethral stricture
  - —Meatal stenosis
- Gynecological
  - —Posturethropexy
  - —Postvaginal delivery
  - —Infectious
  - —Periurethral abscess
  - —Urinary tract infection
  - —Constipation
  - —Medications that cause AUR
  - —β-Adrenergic stimulation (detrusor relaxation)
- α-Adrenergic stimulation (vesical outlet contraction)
  - —Musculotropic detrusor relaxation

PEDIATRIC CONSIDERATIONS

- AUR uncommon in children
- Cystitis most common cause
- Exclude testicular torsion

Pre-Hospital

N/A

Diagnosis

ESSENTIAL WORKUP

- Thorough history and physical examination
- Urinalysis

LABORATORY

- Electrolytes, BUN/Cr and glucose
- For renal failure
  - —Prostate specific antigen
  - —Urine culture

Treatment

INITIAL STABILIZATION

- Urinary drainage by catheterization
- Caution with history of urethral stricture or traumatic catheter insertion
- Defer catheterization in patient with pelvic fracture, prostate displacement on rectal examination, or blood at the urethral meatus until retrograde urethrogram
- Suprapubic catheter if urethral catheterization contraindicated or impossible
- Palpable bladder essential

ED TREATMENT

- Drain out and monitor urine output
- Place leg Foley bag prior to discharge if Foley is to remain indwelling
- Initiate therapy for underlying cause of AUR
  - —Rapid decompression following catheter placement may result in transient gross hematuria in the chronically distended edematous bladder
- Postobstructive diuresis
  - —Complication of AUR in the catheterized patient
  - —Occurs from osmotic diuresis or interstitial tubular dysfunction
  - —Hypovolemic or hypotensive may result in severe cases
- Observe for 4–6 hours all patients with chronic or insidious obstructive voiding symptoms and urinary retention with particular attention to hourly intake, urinary output, and vital signs

PEDIATRIC CONSIDERATIONS

- Bladder decompression via Foley catheter or suprapubic bladder aspiration (SPA)
- Estimate the expected bladder capacity in ounces by age in years plus 2

MEDICATIONS

- Baclofen (Lioresal) for external sphincter emptying: peds: 2–7 yrs: 10–15 mg/24 hrs divided Q 8 hrs; titrate to max dose 40 mg/24 hrs; peds: >8 yrs: max dose 60 mg/day divided Q 8 hrs; adults: 5 mg po tid, max 80 mg/day
- Belladonna and opium (B and O) suppositories to alleviate the constant urge to urinate secondary to bladder spasm, frequently accompanying an indwelling catheter: adults: 1 po Q 4–6 hrs
- Bethanechol (urecholine) acts on the detrusor to empty the bladder: peds: po 0.6 mg/kg/24 hrs divided Q 6–8 hrs; SC: 0.15–0.2 mg/kg/24 hrs divided Q 6–8 hrs; adults: 10–50 mg po BID/QID; SC: 5 mg
- Dantrolene (dantrium) for external sphincter emptying: peds: (not indicated <5 yrs) >5 yrs: initial: 0.5 mg/kg/dose po bid; increment: increase frequency to TID-QID at 4–7 day intervals, then increase doses by 0.5 mg/kg; adults: initial: 25 mg po QD, increase frequency to TID-QID then increase dose by 25 mg/dose at 4–7 day intervals
- Diazepam (valium) for external sphincter emptying: peds: IM or IV: 0.04–0.2 mg/kg/dose Q 2–4 hrs (max dose: 0.6 mg/kg within an 8-hr period); peds: po: 0.12–0.8 mg/kg/24 hrs divided Q 6–8 hrs; adults: IM or IV: 2–10 mg/dose Q 3–4 hrs PRN, po: 2–10 mg/dose Q 6–8 hrs PRN
- Doxazosin mesylate (cardura) for vesical outlet emptying: adults: initial 1 mg po QD, after 24 hrs, increase to 2 mg po QD then to 4, 8, 16 mg QD
- Meperidine HCL (demerol) for external sphincter relaxation: peds: po, IM, IV: 1.0–1.5 mg/kg/dose Q 3–4 hrs PRN, max. dose: 100 mg; adults: po, IM, IV: 50–150 mg/dose Q 3–4 hrs PRN
- Oxybutynin (ditropan) for storage: adults: 5 mg po BID-TID
- Phenoxybenzamine HCL (dibenzyline) for vesical outlet emptying: adults: 10 mg po, increase dosage every other day, usually to 20–40 mg, BID-TID
- Prazosin HCL (minipress) for vesical outlet emptying: adults: initially 1 mg po BID-TID, slow increase to 20 mg/day in divided doses
- Pseudoephedrine (sudafed) for vesical outlet storage: peds: <12 yr: 4 mg/kg/24 hrs po divided Q 6 hrs; adults: 30–60 mg/dose po Q 6–8 hrs, max dose 240 mg/24 hrs
- Terazosin (hytrin) for vesical outlet emptying: adults: start 1 mg po qhs, max 20 mg/day
- Trimethoprim without sulfa (trimpex or proloprim) for the duration of catheter insertion, if it is to remain indwelling for more than 5 days: adults: 100 mg tablets QD or bid

Disposition

ADMISSION CRITERIA

- Significant postobstructive diuresis requiring IV fluids, electrolyte, and urine output monitoring

DISCHARGE CRITERIA

- Good health with support system
- No clinical or laboratory evidence of infection
- Urology follow up

Miscellaneous

ICD9: 788.20

CORE CONTENT CODE: 22.4.27

SUGGESTED READINGS

Gausehe M. Genitourinary surgical emergencies. Pediatr Ann 1996;25(8):458–64

Peter JR, Steinhardt GF. Acute urinary retention in children. Pediatr Emerg Care 1993;9:205–07.

Samm BJ, Dmochowski RR. Urologic emergencies. Postgrad Med 1996;100(4):177–84.

Author: Hilarie Cranmer

Urinary Tract Fistula

Clinical Presentation

SIGNS AND SYMPTOMS

- Vesicointestinal fistulas
  - —Chronic or recurrent urinary tract infections
    - -Majority of infections are caused by E. coli
    - -Mixed organisms account for one-third of infections
  - —Pneumaturia—60% occurrence rate
  - —Fecaluria—40% occurrence rate
  - —Abdominal pain
    - -Change in bowel habits
- Vesicovaginal, urethrovaginal, and ureterovaginal fistulas
  - —Constant leakage of urine from the vagina; described as watery vaginal discharge
  - —Malodorous urine
  - —Perineal dermatitis and maceration
  - —Severe perineal pain if fistula is a complication of radiation therapy
  - —Ureterovaginal fistula
    - -Abdominal pain
    - -Flank tenderness
    - -Fever
    - -Drainage of urine through the operative site
- Vesicocutaneous fistula
  - —Constant leakage of urine from bladder through fistula to skin
  - —Usually located in perineal region
  - —Perineal dermatitis and maceration at site of leakage

MECHANISM/DESCRIPTION

- Fistula formation can occur between any part of the urinary tract and contiguous structures
- Communications between the urinary tract and gastrointestinal tract, external perineum, and female reproductive organs are most common
- Urinary fistulas
    - -Not the result of primary urologic disease
    - -Due to rather a complication of gynecologic surgery, child birth, and gastrointestinal disorders

ETIOLOGY

- Vesicointestinal fistulas
  - —Complication of a primary gastrointestinal disease
  - —Diverticulitis: 50–60% of cases
  - —Colon cancer: 20–25% of cases
  - —Crohn's disease: 10% of cases
  - —Radiation enteritis: 7% of cases
  - —Pelvic trauma: 5% of cases
  - —Bladder cancer: 4% of cases
  - —Other causes
    - -Appendicitis
    - -Gynecologic cancers
    - -Tuberculosis
- Vesicovaginal, urethrovaginal, and ureterovaginal fistulas
  - —Gynecologic surgery: 80% of cases
    - -Occurs 10–14 days after surgery
  - —Obstetrical complication: 8–10% of cases
  - —Pelvic irradiation: 6% of cases
  - —Pelvic trauma: 4% of cases
- Vesicocutaneous fistula
  - —Cervical or uterine cancer
  - —Bladder cancer
  - —Advanced prostatic cancer

Pre-Hospital

N/A

Diagnosis

ESSENTIAL WORKUP

- Vesicointestinal fistulas
  - —Thorough history points to diagnosis
- Vesicovaginal, urethrovaginal, and ureterovaginal fistulas
  - —Clinical diagnosis
    - -Speculum exam may reveal a small, reddened area of granulomatous tissue at site of fistula opening
    - -If uncertain if vaginal discharge contains urine, give pyridium 200 mg orally, and perform speculum exam 1 hour later
    - -Orange discoloration of discharge confirms fistula
- Vesicocutaneous fistula
  - —Clinical diagnosis with thorough physical examination

LABORATORY

- Urinalysis
  - —Undigested food residue with vesicointestinal fistulas
  - —Bacteria with vesicovaginal, urethrovaginal, and ureterovaginal fistulas
  - —Bacteria and white blood cells with vesicocutaneous fistula
- Urine culture
  - —E. coli major pathogen with vesicointestinal fistulas
  - —One-third infected with multiple organisms
  - —Mixed organisms with vesicovaginal, urethrovaginal, and ureterovaginal fistulas
  - —To exclude infection with vesicocutaneous fistula

IMAGING/SPECIAL TESTS

- Cystoscopy is the most reliable means of diagnosis

DIFFERENTIAL DIAGNOSIS

- Vesicointestinal fistulas
  - —Recurrent urinary tract infection
  - —Other causes of pneumaturia
    - -Urinary tract infection with gas-forming organism such as clostridia
    - -Fermentation of glucose in urine
    - -Recent urinary tract instrumentation
- Vesicovaginal, urethrovaginal, and ureterovaginal fistulas
  - —Urinary incontinence
  - —Copious vaginal discharge
- Vesicocutaneous fistula
  - —Urinary incontinence

Treatment

INITIAL STABILIZATION

- Treat urosepsis with IV fluid bolus and IV antibiotics

ED TREATMENT

- Vesicointestinal fistulas
  - —Investigate the possibility of a urinary tract infection
  - —Rule out complications from patient's primary disease
  - —Obtain cultures if signs of urinary tract infection
  - —Initiate broad spectrum antibiotic if infection found
  - —Antibiotic resistance is common
  - —Most patients have received multiple antibiotics for recurrent or chronic urinary tract infections
  - —Urologic referral for definitive surgical therapy
- Vesicovaginal, urethrovaginal, and ureterovaginal fistulas
  - —Place Foley catheter for any patient suspected of having a genitourinary fistula
  - —Treat perineal dermatitis and skin maceration with
    - -Antifungal creams such as nystatin, clotrimazole or miconazole
    - -Protective ointment applied to protect skin from moisture
  - —Initiate broad spectrum antibiotics if a urinary tract infection is present
    - -Third-generation cephalosporin, fluoroquinolone, or amoxicillin/clavulanate acid
  - —Prompt urology and gynecology referral
- Vesicocutaneous fistula
  - —Place Foley catheter for any patient suspected of having a genitourinary fistula
  - —Treat perineal dermatitis and skin maceration with
    - -Antifungal creams such as nystatin, clotrimazole or miconazole
    - -Protective ointment applied to protect skin from moisture
  - —Initiate broad spectrum antibiotics if a urinary tract infection is present
    - -Third-generation cephalosporin, fluoroquinolone, or amoxicillin/clavulanate acid
  - —Prompt urology referral

MEDICATIONS

- Amoxicillin/clavulanate: 875 mg po bid or 500 mg po tid
- Ampicillin/sulbactam: 3 g IV q 6 hrs
- Cefaclor: 500 mg po tid
- Ceftriaxone: 2 g IV q day
- Cefuroxime: 250 mg po bid
- Ciprofloxacin: 400 mg IV or 500 mg po bid

Disposition

ADMISSION CRITERIA

- Presence of urosepsis or septic shock
- Unable to take oral antibiotics
- Dehydration
- Complications from primary gastrointestinal disease or pelvic malignancies
- Bowel obstruction
- Malnutrition

DISCHARGE CRITERIA

- No evidence of urosepsis or shock
- Able to administer oral antibiotics if urinary tract infections present
- Able to care for Foley catheter

Miscellaneous

ICD9: 599.1

CORE CONTENT CODE: 19.2.2

SUGGESTED READINGS

Lee RA, Symonds RE, Williams TJ. Current status of genitourinary fistula. Obstet Gynecol 1988;72(3):313–19.

McVay KT, Marshall FF. Urinary fistulas. In: Gillenwater J, et al., eds. Adult and pediatric urology. 3rd ed. St. Louis: CV Mosby, 1996.

Moos RL, Ryan JA. Management of enterovesical fistulas. Am J Surg 1990;159:514–17.

Author: Laurie Lawrence

Urinary Tract Infection, Adult

Clinical Presentation

SIGNS AND SYMPTOMS

- Lower tract infection: dysuria, frequency, urgency, hesitancy, suprapubic pain, hematuria
- Upper tract infection: fever, chills, flank pain, CVA tenderness, nausea, vomiting, anorexia
  - —Some studies show that up to 50% of upper tract infections may be silent
  - —Symptom duration of more than 5 days or being homeless are risk factors for upper tract involvement
- Elderly: altered mental status, anorexia, decreased social interaction, abdominal pain, nocturia, incontinence, asymptomatic

MECHANISM/DESCRIPTION

- Colonization of the urine with uropathogens and invasion of the genitourinary tract
- Defined as urinary symptoms with $\geq 10^2$ to 10^5 colonies/ml of a uropathogen and ≥ 10 WBC/mm^3
- *Uncomplicated cystitis* or lower tract infection
  - —Females aged 13 to 50, no history of fever or chills, no history of flank pain or costovertebral angle tenderness (CVAT)
  - —No recent instrumentation, no genitourinary tract anomalies or previous surgery
  - —Not pregnant
  - —Fewer than four UTIs in the past year
  - —Neurologically intact, immunocompetent, temperature $<38°C$
- *Complicated cystitis*
  - —At least one of the above criteria present
- *Uncomplicated pyelonephritis* or upper tract infection
  - —Renal parenchymal infection with flank pain and CVAT
- *Complicated pyelonephritis*
  - —Infection with signs of sepsis, hypotension, temperature $>40°C$, intractable nausea, and vomiting, diabetes, or immunocompromised

ETIOLOGY

- Organisms colonize the periurethral area and subsequently infect the genitourinary tract
- Population at risk: newborn, prepubertal girls, young boys, sexually active young woman, elderly males and females
- Risk factors: bacterial virulence, host susceptibility including anatomic or functional abnormalities, behavior, age, and gender
  - —Behavior: sexual intercourse, spermicides, diaphragms
  - —Elderly females/postmenopausal state due to less efficient bladder emptying, alteration of bladder defenses including increase in vaginal pH, increased contamination secondary to urinary and fecal incontinence, instrumentation
  - —Elderly males due to prostatic hypertrophy and instrumentation
- Organisms
  - —*Escherichia coli* (80%)
  - —*Staphylococcus saprophyticus* (10%)
  - —*Klebsiella, Proteus mirabilis, Enterobacter spp., Pseudomonas aeruginosa,* group D streptococci (10%)

PEDIATRIC CONSIDERATIONS

- See chapter: Urinary Tract Infection, Pediatric

Pre-Hospital

N/A

Diagnosis

ESSENTIAL WORKUP

- Urinalysis (dip test or microscopic)
- Females: pregnancy test
- Males: rule out urethritis or prostatitis and inquire about anal intercourse and HIV status
- Urologic work-up in a young healthy male with first UTI is not recommended

LABORATORY

- Urine dipstick: laboratory urinalysis is unnecessary if pyuria/bacteriuria confirmed
  - —Sensitivity and specificity of the leukocyte esterase test are 75–96% and 94–98%
  - —Nitrite test is 35–85% sensitive and 92–100% specific
  - —Both tests have excellent negative predictive values
- Urinalysis: obtain if urine dipstick is negative
  - —10 WBC/mm^3 from a clean catch midstream urine specimen indicates infection
  - —If bacteria are seen in an unspun specimen, this indicates $>10^5$ CFU/ml
- Indications for urine culture
  - —Complicated UTIs
  - —No pyuria or bacteriuria on initial dipstick or urinalysis
  - —Symptoms persist for more than 2 days after treatment has been started or relapse occurs
  - —Recently hospitalized patients
  - —Pyelonephritis
- Additional labs dictated by clinical setting include CBC, renal function tests, electrolytes, cultures for chlamydia, gonorrhea, or herpes, VDRL, serum, or urine pregnancy test

IMAGING/SPECIAL TESTS

- Indicated for complicated upper tract disease, see chapter: Pyelonephritis

DIFFERENTIAL DIAGNOSIS

- Urethritis
- Vulvovaginitis
- Cervicitis/PID
- Prostatitis/epididymitis

Treatment

INITIAL STABILIZATION

Urosepsis/Septic Shock

- ABCs
  - —IV access, hydration, cardiac monitor, pulse oximetry, vasopressors as needed, cultures
  - —Antibiotics (ampicillin plus gentamicin; ceftazidime; ceftriaxone; quinolones)
- Judge antibiotic efficacy by clinical response, not by results of cultures or other tests
- Symptomatic and asymptomatic bacteriuria in pregnancy requires treatment
- Antibiotics of choice are trimethoprim-sulfamethoxazole, quinolones (ciprofloxacin, norfloxacin, ofloxacin), or nitrofurantoin
- Second- or third-generation oral cephalosporins are reasonable alternates (cefuroxime axetil, cefixime) but require 7-day treatment regimens
- Amoxicillin and first-generation cephalosporins should not be used because of high failure rates
- Nitrofurantoin is the drug of choice during pregnancy except if G6PD-deficient
- Sulfamethoxazole should not be used late in pregnancy because kernicterus can result
- Quinolones are not recommended during pregnancy due to CNS reactions, blood dyscrasias, and effects on collagen formation
- Treatment of upper tract disease: *Rule of 2s*
  - —Administer 2 L of IV fluid, 2 tablets of Tylenol #3, 2 g of ceftriaxone or 2 mg/kg of gentamicin
  - —If fever drops by 2°C and patient can retain 2 glasses of water, then discharge with prescription for trimethoprim-sulfamethoxazole DS, or cipro × 2 weeks, with follow-up in 2 days

MEDICATIONS

- Ampicillin: 1 g IV q 6 hrs
- Cefixime: 400 mg po qd or 200 mg po bid
- Ceftazidime: 1–2 g IV q 8–12 hrs
- Ceftriaxone: 1–2 g IV/IM q 24 hrs
- Cefuroxime: 250–500 mg po bid
- Ciprofloxacin: 250–500 mg po bid
- Gentamicin: 2 mg/kg IV q 8 hrs
- Nitrofurantoin: 100 mg po bid (sustained release)
- Norfloxacin: 400 mg po bid
- Ofloxacin: 200 mg po bid or 400 mg IV q 12 hrs
- TMP/SMX: 160 mg/800 mg po bid

Disposition

ADMISSION CRITERIA

- Pyelonephritis with intractable vomiting, clinically dehydrated and cannot rehydrate, extremes of age, unremitting fever, pregnancy

DISCHARGE CRITERIA

- Complicated UTIs with adequate follow-up and simple UTIs
- Healthy patients with uncomplicated pyelonephritis who respond to treatment according to rule of 2s

PEDIATRIC CONSIDERATIONS

- Admit boys with febrile UTI and most children under age 3 months with UTI

Miscellaneous

ICD9: 599.0

CORE CONTENT CODE: 19.1.5.5, 19.2.3.5, 13.13.4

SUGGESTED READINGS

Hooton T. A simplified approach to urinary tract infection. Hosp Prac 1995;30:23–30.

Kunin C. Urinary tract infections in females. Clin Infect Dis 1994;18:1–12.

Neu H. Urinary tract infections. Am J Med 1992;92(Suppl 4A):63S–70S.

Pappas P. Laboratory in the diagnosis and management of urinary tract infections. Med Clin North Am 1991;75(2):313–325.

Stamm WE, Hooton TM. Management of urinary tract infections in adults. N Engl J Med 1993;329(18):1328–1334.

Zelikovic I. Urinary tract infections in children—An update. West J Med 1992;157: 554–561.

Authors: Barnett Eskin; Paul Szucs

Urinary Tract Infection, Pediatric

Clinical Presentation

SIGNS AND SYMPTOMS

- Neonates
  - —Manifestations of sepsis
  - —Feeding difficulties
  - —Irritability
  - —Hypothermia
  - —Fever
  - —Decreased responsiveness
- 1 month–3 years
  - —Fever
  - —Irritability
  - —Vomiting
  - —Abdominal pain
  - —Meningismus
  - —Failure to thrive
  - —Hematuria
- >3 years
  - —Dysuria
  - —Frequency
  - —Enuresis
  - —Suprapubic pain
  - —Abdominal pain
  - —Fever
  - —Back pain
  - —Hematuria
  - —Malodorous cloudy urine

MECHANISM/DESCRIPTION

- UTI is defined by culture with >10,000 organisms per ml
- In infants 0–3 months old, UTI is associated with a 30% incidence of sepsis

ETIOLOGY

- Urinary tract infection (UTI) found in 4–7% of febrile infants
- Bacterial agents
  - —*E. coli* accounts for 90%
  - —*Klebsiella*
  - —*S. aureus*
  - —*Enterobacter*
  - —*Proteus*
  - —*Pseudomonas*
  - —*Enterococcus*

Pre-Hospital

N/A

Diagnosis

ESSENTIAL WORKUP

- Urinalysis with microscopic RBC and WBC counts, and smear for bacteria
  - —UA alone has low diagnostic sensitivity in infants
- Urine culture
  - —Clean catch urine may be used, otherwise catheter or suprapubic tap required
  - —Bagged urine samples should be used for UA only (70% contamination rate)
- Urine collection method
  - —Clean catch in cooperative male children
  - —Plastic bag collection adequate for UA
    - -Clean the perineum (females) and glans (males) prior to application
    - -Can be used to rule out an infection
    - -Positive culture may need to be confirmed by suprapubic or catheterized specimen
  - —Suprapubic aspiration
    - -Most reliable method
    - -Preferred in <12 months old
    - -Full bladder optimal
  - —Urethral catheterization
    - -Acceptable in all infants
    - -Higher success rate than suprapubic aspiration
    - -Aseptic technique essential

LABORATORY

- CBC and blood culture for young children with fever or nonspecific symptoms and no source on exam
- Electrolytes, BUN/Cr
  - —Check if dehydration or pyelonephritis

IMAGING/SPECIAL TESTS

- Voiding cystoureterogram (VCUG) and ultrasound (if normal VCUG)
  - —UTI is associated with vesicouretero reflux and other GU abnormalities
  - —Obtain studies in children <5 years after resolution of infection

DIFFERENTIAL DIAGNOSIS

- Sexual molestation
- Genitourinary tract trauma
- Vulvovaginitis
- Urethral meatitis
- Diabetes
- Chemical and viral cystitis
- Nephrolithiasis
- Vaginal foreign bodies
- Glomerulonephritis

Treatment

INITIAL STABILIZATION

- Treat infants <3 months old presumptively for sepsis or meningitis until blood and CSF cultures are final
- Airway intervention for septic/acidotic infants with depressed respiratory drive
- 20 cc/kg bolus 0.9%NS for hypotension, dehydration, or sepsis

ED TREATMENT

- Initiate IV antibiotics in all infants <3 months old
  —Ampicillin and gentamicin in neonates
  —Cephalosporins after 4–8 weeks of age
- Outpatient oral antibiotic for 7–10 days for children discharged
  —Amoxicillin
  —Amoxicillin/clavulanate
  —Ampicillin
  —Cephalexin
  —Nitrofurantoin
  —TMP/SMX

MEDICATIONS

- Amoxicillin: 40 mg/kg/24hrs po q 8 hrs
- Amoxicillin/clavulanate: 40 mg/kg/24hrs po q 8 hrs
- Ampicillin: 100 mg/kg/24hrs IV/PO q 6 hrs
- Cefotaxime: 100 mg/kg/24hrs IV/IM q 6–8 hrs
- Ceftriaxone: 50 mg/kg/24hrs q 12–24 hrs
- Cephalexin: 50 mg/kg/24hrs po q 6–12 hrs
- Gentamicin: 2.5 mg/kg/dose IV q 8 hrs if full term and age >7 days; 2.5 mg/kg/dose IV q 12 hrs if full term and age 0–7 days (special dosing regimens in infants <36 weeks postconceptual age)
- Nitrofurantoin: 5–7 mg/kg/24hrs po q 6 hrs
- TMP/SMX (bactrim, septra suspension): 5 ml liquid (of 40/200 per 5 ml) per 10 kg per dose po bid

Disposition

ADMISSION CRITERIA

- Infants <3 months of age
- Dehydration
- Ill appearance/toxicity/sepsis
- Suspected pyelonephritis
- Urinary obstruction
- Male with febrile UTI
- Vomiting
- Immunocompromised patient
- Renal insufficiency

DISCHARGE CRITERIA

- Sufficiently hydrated
- Low risk for sepsis or meningitis
- Able to take oral antibiotics

Miscellaneous

ICD9: 599

CORE CONTENT CODE: 13.13.4

SUGGESTED READINGS

Durbin WA Jr, Peter G. Management of urinary tract infections in infants and children. Pediatr Infect Dis 1984;3(6):564–574.

Harwood-Nuss AL, Etheredge W, McKenna I. Urologic emergencies. In: Rosen P, Barkin R, Danzl D, et al., eds. Emergency medicine: Concepts and clinical practice. 4th ed. St. Louis: CV Mosby, 1998:2227–2261.

Hoberman A, Han-Pu C, Keller DM, et al. Prevalence of urinary tract infection in febrile infants. J Pediatr 1993;123(1):17–23.

Schlager T, Lohr J. Urinary tract infection in outpatient febrile infants and children younger than five years of age. Pediatr Ann 1993;22:505–509.

Authors: David W. Marby; Gregory R. Lockhart

Urticaria

Clinical Presentation

SIGNS AND SYMPTOMS

- Transient, pruritic, well circumscribed, skin eruptions consisting of erythematous, nonpitting plaques (wheal), which may be surrounded by an erythematous ring (flare)
- Lesions are various sizes and shapes, may become confluent
- Wheals usually resolve in 3–4 hours
- New lesions evolve as old ones resolve
- *Acute:* <6 weeks
- *Chronic:* >6 weeks
- May be associated with systemic features—hypotension, flushing, headache, dizziness, respiratory distress
- May be part of *anaphylactic* reaction (respiratory distress and hypotension) or *angioedema* (swelling of face and tongue)

MECHANISM/DESCRIPTION

- Skin mast cell release of inflammatory mediators, primarily histamine, resulting in increased vascular permeability and pruritus

ETIOLOGY

Acute

- Drugs: especially penicillin, sulfa, aspirin, NSAID, ACE inhibitors
- Foods or additives
- Insect bites, stings
- Connective tissue, endocrine, or neoplastic disorders
- Pregnancy, menstrual cycle
- Infections, particularly virus (including hepatitis), bacteria, fungus, parasite
- Inhalant or contact allergen
- Emotional stress
- Physical urticaria: over 20 identified types including
  - —Dermographism: most common form; reaction to skin pressure, linear wheals under tight clothing or on areas scratched with a firm object
  - —Cholinergic: monomorphic wheals 2–3 mm with bright red flare and intense pruritus
    - -A response to elevated core temperature (hot bath, fever, exercise, occlusive dress, or emotional stress)
  - —Other rare forms include cold-induced (may be fatal in cold immersions), delayed pressure, solar, aquagenic, vibratory, and idiopathic

Chronic

- 75% idiopathic
- Often an unrecognized recurring physical urticaria

PEDIATRIC CONSIDERATIONS

- Urticaria is frequently the result of reactions to foods in infants
- Swelling of distal extremities and acrocyanosis may be prominent in infants
- Bullae may form in the center of the wheal, especially on legs and buttocks

Pre-Hospital

CAUTIONS

- Patients with severe allergic reactions can progress rapidly to respiratory failure

Diagnosis

ESSENTIAL WORKUP

- *Complete history and physical exam:* lesion appearance, location, timing, duration, acute versus chronic, associated symptoms, triggers, coexisting diseases, allergies, medications, environment, exposures, and new foods. Characteristics and location of hives, evaluate for sources of infection, and signs of systemic diseases

LABORATORY

- Acute cases: not needed
- Chronic cases: evaluate for subclinical infection or systemic disease (CBC with differential, erythrocyte sedimentation rate, TSH and thyroid functions, urinalysis, liver function tests, hepatitis panel)
- Skin biopsy if urticarial vasculitis suspected (not done in ED)

IMAGING/SPECIAL TESTS

- Acute cases: not needed
- Chronic cases: chest, sinus, or dental radiographs may help identify subclinical infection
- Dermographism: Scratch skin with a tongue blade, observe for linear wheal
- Cholinergic: Exercise challenge to raise core temp
- Solar: Expose to sunlight
- Cold: Place an ice cube on skin for 5 minutes
- Aquagenic: Apply tap water at differing temperatures

DIFFERENTIAL DIAGNOSIS

- Anaphylaxis
- Angioedema
- Insect bites, stings
- Infection
- Contact or allergic dermatitis
- Rash (varicella and other viral exanthems)
- Erythema multiforme
- Vasculitis
- Urticaria pigmentosa
- Systemic lupus erythematosus

Treatment

INITIAL STABILIZATION

- Severe reaction: ABCs, oxygen, parenteral or inhaled β-agonist, IV crystalloid, and vasopressors as needed
- See chapters on treatment of Anaphylaxis and Angioedema

ED TREATMENT

- Treatment largely symptomatic except in severe reactions
- Significant mucosal edema: suspect angioedema (see chapter: Angioedema)
- Prolonged, painful, or nonblanching lesions: suspect vasculitis (see chapter: Vasculitis)
- Avoid offending agent
- β-Agonist (parenteral or inhaled): severe hives, angioedema, or systemic features
- *H_1-receptor antagonist* (first or second generation) is the mainstay of treatment
- *H_2-receptor antagonist:* may be beneficial as adjunct to H_1 blocker when no response to H_1 blocker alone
- *Corticosteroid* (oral): severe or refractory cases
- *Tricyclic antidepressants:* potent histamine blockers
- Avoid aspirin, NSAIDs, and opiates—may exacerbate condition
- Concurrent use of ketoconazole or macrolides alters hepatic metabolism of antihistamine; use with caution
- Chronic urticaria unresponsive to antihistamines may respond to colchicine or dapsone

MEDICATIONS

β-Agonist

- Albuterol (0.5% soln): adult: 0.5 ml nebulized q 20 min PRN; peds: 0.01–0.05 ml/kg/dose (max 0.5 ml/dose) nebulized q 20 min PRN
- Epinephrine (1:1000 solution): adult: 0.1–0.5 mg SC/IM q 10–15 min PRN; peds: 0.01 mg/kg, SC (max single dose not to exceed 0.3 mg) q 15 min PRN
- Terbutaline: adult 0.25 mg SC q 15–30 min PRN (max 0.5 mg q 4 hrs); peds: <12 yrs 0.005–0.01 mg/kg (max 0.4 mg/dose) SC q 15–20 min × 3 PRN

H_1-Receptor Antagonist (First and Second Generation)

- Diphenhydramine hydrochloride (Benadryl): adult: 25–50 mg PO/IV/IM, up to q 6 hrs; peds: 5 mg/kg/24hrs divided qid (max 300 mg/24hrs)
- Hydroxyzine hydrochloride (Atarax): adult: 25–50 mg PO/IM up to qid; peds: 2 mg/kg/24hrs po divided qid or 0.5–1 mg/kg IM q 4–6 hrs PRN
- Loratadine (Claritin): adult: 10 mg po bid
- Terfenadine (Seldane): adult: 60 mg po bid; peds: 3–6 yrs: 15 mg bid; 7–12 yrs: 30 mg bid

H_2-Receptor Antagonist (Suggested Dosage)

- Cimetidine (Tagamet): adult: 300 mg PO/IV/IM bid; peds: infants <1 year 10–20 mg/kg/24hrs PO/IV/IM divided qid; children >1 year 20–40 mg/kg/24hrs PO/IV/IM divided qid
- Famotidine (Pepcid): adult: 20 mg IV q 12 hrs or 20–40 mg po qhs; peds: 0.6–0.8 mg/kg/24hrs IV (max 40 mg/24hra) divided q 8–12 hrs or 1–1.2 mg/kg/24hrs (max 40 mg/24hrs) po divided q 8–12 hrs
- Ranitidine (Zantac): adult: 150 mg po bid; peds: neonate: 2–4 mg/kg/24hrs po divided q 8–12 hrs or 2 mg/kg/24hrs IV divided q 6–8 hrs; infants and children 4–5 mg/kg/24hrs po divided q 8–12 hrs or 2–4 mg/kg/24hrs IV/IM divided q 6–8 hrs

Corticosteroid

- Prednisone: adult: 40 mg po qd or 20 mg po bid × 3–5 days; peds: 1–2 mg/kg/24hrs (max 80 mg/24hrs) divided qd-bid × 3–5 days

Tricyclic Antidepressant

- Doxepin (Sinequan): adult: 10–25 mg po tid; peds: not approved for under 12 yrs of age

Disposition

ADMISSION CRITERIA

- Respiratory distress or failure
- Refractory hypotension or shock
- Severe refractory cases requiring IV medications
- Other systemic disease or infection

DISCHARGE CRITERIA

- Normal ventilation and oxygenation
- Normal blood pressure
- Absence of other condition requiring admission
- Symptoms controlled
- Adequate ability of caregivers at home to monitor for further exacerbations

Miscellaneous

ICD9: 708.9

CORE CONTENT CODE: 3.3.3

SUGGESTED READINGS

Habif TP. Clinical dermatology. St Louis: CV Mosby, 1996:122–145.

Hurwitz S. Clinical pediatric dermatology. Philadelphia: WB Saunders, 1993:516–519.

Mahmood T. Urticaria. Am Fam Physician 1995;51(4):811–816.

Mahmood T. Physical urticarias. Am Fam Physician 1994;49(6):1411–1414.

Sveum RJ. Urticaria. Post Grad Med 1996;100(2):77–84.

Author: Jeffrey Horton

Vaginal Bleeding

Clinical Presentation

SIGNS AND SYMPTOMS

- Vaginal bleeding
  —Variable amounts (pads/hour)
  —Sometimes associated with fetal tissue
- Lightheadedness
- Weakness
- Thirst
- Acute hypotension with mental status
  —With significant pelvic bleeding due to ectopic pregnancy or ruptured ovarian cyst
  —Abdominal distention or tenderness

MECHANISM/DESCRIPTION

- Common presenting complaint in the emergency department
- Most cases are due to benign causes
- Some patients will have occult, but potentially life threatening, conditions
- Most important principles in evaluating women with vaginal bleeding
  —*All women capable of childbearing might be pregnant*
  —Menstrual and sexual history *do not* rule out pregnancy

ETIOLOGY

- Pregnancy related
  —Early pregnancy
    -Ectopic pregnancy
    -Abortion (threatened, incomplete, complete, missed, inevitable, septic)
    -Molar pregnancy
    -Trauma
  —Later pregnancy
    -Placenta previa
    -Placental abruption
    -Molar pregnancy
    -Labor
    -Trauma
  —Immediate postpartum
    -Postpartum hemorrhage
    -Uterine inversion
  —Early postpartum
    -Retained Placenta
    -Endometritis
- Nonpregnant patients
  —Dysfunctional uterine bleeding
  —Structural abnormalities
    -Uterine fibroids
    -Pelvic tumors
  —Very rare for systemic disorders to present with only vaginal bleeding
  —Trauma

Pre-Hospital

CAUTIONS

- Establish IV 0.9%NS with 1-L fluid bolus for significant bleeding or hypotension
- Administer high-flow oxygen in pregnant or unstable patients
- In later pregnancy
  —Uterine contractions may be transiently terminated with terbutaline 0.25 mg SQ
  —Place women in left-lateral decubitus position to prevent occlusion of inferior vena cava by uterus

Diagnosis

ESSENTIAL WORKUP

- Pelvic examination
  —Essential for all women with vaginal bleeding
  —Delay examination pending an ultrasound to rule out placenta previa for vaginal bleeding present in later pregnancy
  —Speculum exam
    -Sterile if pregnant
    -Initial procedure followed by bimanual examination
  —Bimanual examination
    -Sterile gloves if pregnant
    -Deferred if patient is near-term with possible rupture of fetal membranes and without other indications for emergent bimanual examination
- Pregnancy test for all patients with childbearing potential
- Early pregnancy
  —Rh type
  —Ultrasound (US) to rule in intrauterine pregnancy
    -BHCG if ultrasound is nondiagnostic
  —Hct if significant bleeding
  —Type and cross if ectopic pregnancy or low Hct
  —Urinalysis
- Later pregnancy
  —Rh type
  —Ultrasound if
    -No fetal heart tones
    -No documented intrauterine pregnancy
    -Unknown lie of placenta
  —Hct if significant bleeding
  —Type and cross if placenta previa/abruption or low Hct
  —DIC panel of placental abruption—platelets, PT/PTT, fibrinogen, fibrin-split products
- Early postpartum
  —Ultrasound for retained products
  —Hct
  —BHCG if concerned about retained tissue

LABORATORY

- Hct for nonpregnant women with significant bleeding
- Platelet count for suspected thrombocytopenia
- PT/PTT for suspected coagulopathy

IMAGING/SPECIAL TESTS

- Send any passed tissue to pathology
- Endometrial sampling if age greater than 35–40 years old or there are other risk factors for endometrial cancer

Treatment

INITIAL STABILIZATION

- ABCs
- Oxygen for significant bleeding or unstable patient
- Establish 2 large-bore IVs and initiate fluid bolus (1–2 L) for hypotensive patients
  —Transfuse blood if remain hypotensive in spite of fluid bolus
- Cardiac/pulse oximeter monitors

ED TREATMENT

- If unstable with surgical condition, transfer patient to operating room as soon as possible
- RhoGAM for vaginal bleeding, pregnancy and Rh-negative mother
  —RhoGAM 1 vial IM if >13 weeks pregnant
  —MICRhoGAM (50 μg) IM if <13 weeks pregnant

Early Pregnancy

- To rule out ectopic pregnancy
  —US positive for ectopic
    -Definitive treatment with surgery or methotrexate as per the standard at the treating institution
  —US positive for intrauterine pregnancy (IUP) without concerns of rare (1/2600–1/30,000) coexistent ectopic and IUP
    -Discharge patient for OB follow up
  —US indeterminate for IUP or Ectopic with BHCG greater than institutional discriminatory zone (likely 1000–2000 IU)
    -Diagnosis is ectopic pregnancy versus missed abortion
    -Admit for further diagnostic workup of ectopic pregnancy if symptoms not consistent with missed abortion
  —US indeterminate for IUP or ectopic with BHCG less than institutional discriminatory zone (likely 1000–2000 IU)
    -Patient stable with low risk of ectopic, then discharge with repeat BHCG and OB followup in 2 days
    -Patient may still have an ectopic pregnancy
- Abortions
  —Complete
    -Discharge if stable without significant ongoing bleeding
  —Incomplete
    -OB consult
    -D&C versus expectant management
  —Missed
    -Expectant management initially
    -D&C for infection, bleeding, or if no passage during followup
  —Septic
    -IV antibiotics and admission
- Molar pregnancy
    -Chemotherapy, very responsive in early stages of disease

Later Pregnancy

- Placenta previa
  —Usually expectant management
  —OB consult for possible admission
- Placental abruption
  —Induction of labor if large because can lead to fetal/maternal death
  —May require Cesarean section

Immediate Postpartum

- Uterine inversion
  —Prevent by avoiding strong traction on umbilical cord after delivery
  —Replace uterus immediately
  —Occasionally requires operative management
- Postpartum hemorrhage
  —Extraction of placenta if retained
  —Hysterectomy if uncontrolled bleeding

Early Postpartum

- Retained tissue
  —D&C
- Endometritis
  —IV antibiotics

Nonpregnant

- Menses
  —No treatment
- Dysfunctional uterine bleeding
  —<35–40 years of age
    -Provera 10 mg po × 10 days—warn patient of a withdrawal bleed
    -Discharge if stable
    -If unstable, admit for IV hormonal therapy, possible D&C
  —>35–40 years of age
    -Uterine sampling necessary prior to initiation of hormonal treatment to rule out endometrial cancer
    -US for any masses felt on exam
- Structural abnormalities
  —Fibroids or uterine tumors may require D&C for diagnosis/treatment
  —Ultrasound for workup of other pelvic masses
  —Pap smear/biopsy for cervical lesions

Systemic Disorders

- As indicated by primary condition

Disposition

ADMISSION CRITERIA

- Ectopic pregnancy not meeting methotrexate discharge criteria
- Uterine inversion
- Septic abortion
- Placental abruption
- Postpartum hemorrhage
- Endometritis
- Dysfunctional uterine bleeding
  —Unstable
  —Hct <20%
- Newly diagnosed molar pregnancy

DISCHARGE CRITERIA

- Stable vital signs
- Confirmed intrauterine pregnancy if pregnant
- Ectopic pregnancy meeting institutional methotrexate discharge criteria
- Low-risk patient for ectopic pregnancy with pregnancy without findings of IUP on ultrasound with BHCG below discriminatory zone

Miscellaneous

ICD9: 623.8

CORE CONTENT CODE: 22.4.2

SUGGESTED READINGS

American College of Emergency Physicians. Clinical policy for the initial approach to patients presenting with a chief complaint of vaginal bleed. Ann Emerg Med 1997;29:435–458.

Cowan BD, Morrison JC. Management of abnormal genital bleeding in girls and women. N Engl J Med 1991;324:1710–1715.

Kaplan BC, Dart RG, Moskos M, et al. Ectopic pregnancy: prospective study with improved diagnostic accuracy. Ann Emerg Med 1996;28:10–17.

Turner LM. Vaginal bleeding during pregnancy. Emerg Med Clin North Am 1994;12(1):45–54.

Author: Mark Davis

Vaginal Bleeding in Pregnancy

Clinical Presentation

SIGNS AND SYMPTOMS

- Scant spotting or profuse hemorrhage
  - —Dark brown or bright red in color
  - —Watery, mucous, or mixed with clots or tissue
  - —With or without pain
- Bleeding may originate from the vagina, cervix, or uterus/placenta
- Life-threatening processes may produce only mild visible bleeding

Spontaneous Abortion

- Threatened abortion
  - —Os closed
- Inevitable, incomplete
  - —Crampy pain
  - —Open os
  - —Possible passed tissue

Placenta Previa

- Classically painless, bright red bleeding

Abruption

- Classically pain, uterine tenderness, dark red bleeding, +/− coagulopathy

Major Blood Loss

- Tachycardia
- Hypotension
- Altered mentation

MECHANISM/DESCRIPTION

- Obstetric bleeding
  - —Leading cause of maternal death
  - —Major cause of perinatal morbidity and mortality
- Any vaginal bleeding during pregnancy is abnormal and may herald a serious complication
- Incidence of vaginal bleeding in early pregnancy (<20 weeks gestation) is about 30%
  - —Most common cause of first trimester ED visits
- Bleeding in late pregnancy (>20 weeks) is not uncommon
  - —Requires evaluation in 5–10% of these pregnancies

Risk Factors

- Early pregnancy
  - —Advanced maternal age
  - —Previous spontaneous/elective abortion
  - —Previous infertility
  - —Pelvic infection
  - —IUD use
- Late pregnancy
  - —Maternal hypertension
  - —Advanced maternal age
  - —Substance abuse (tobacco, cocaine)
  - —Multiparity, multiple gestation
  - —Trauma

ETIOLOGY

- Early pregnancy (<20 weeks)
  - —Spontaneous abortion (50% of episodes)
  - —Threatened, inevitable, incomplete, missed
  - —Ectopic pregnancy (2–5% of episodes)
  - —Hydatidiform mole (<0.1% of episodes)
  - —Implantation bleed
  - —Postcoital bleeding
  - —Incompetent cervix
  - —Ruptured-hemorrhagic corpus luteum cyst
  - —Cervical/vaginal infection or pathology
  - —Unknown (50% of first trimester episodes)
- Late pregnancy (>20 weeks)
  - —Bloody show (most common)
  - —Abruptio placenta (30% of episodes)
  - —Placenta previa (20% of episodes)
  - —Preterm labor
  - —Uterine rupture (rare)
  - —Incompetent cervix
  - —Postcoital bleeding
  - —Cervical/vaginal infection or pathology

Pre-Hospital

CAUTIONS

- Unstable vital signs warrant aggressive fluid resuscitation in pregnancy age females with vaginal bleeding

Diagnosis

ESSENTIAL WORKUP

- History
  - —Last menstrual period
  - —Parity
  - —Previous ob/gyn complications
  - —Last intercourse
- General physical exam
  - —Vital signs
  - —Abdominal exam: evaluate for tenderness, uterine irritability, estimate fundal height
- Pelvic exam
  - —Early pregnancy
    - -Determine source of bleeding and patency of os
    - -Evaluate uterus and adnexa for size, tenderness, or abnormalities
  - —Late pregnancy
    - -Do not perform pelvic exam with third-trimester bleeding until previa is ruled out or patient is in the operating room
    - -Pelvic exam with placenta previa may precipitate fatal hemorrhage
  - —Listen for fetal heart tones
    - -Detectable at >10 weeks by Doppler
    - -Monitor continuously in late pregnancy

LABORATORY

- CBC
- Quantitative HCG
  - —Abnormal values suggest abnormal gestations
  - —First trimester HCG normally doubles every 48 hours
- Type and screen for Rh; crossmatch blood with severe bleeding
- Coagulation profile and DIC screen in abruption and missed abortion
- BUN, creatinine in abruption
- Urine/blood toxicology helpful in evaluating preterm labor or abruption

IMAGING/SPECIAL TESTS

- Ultrasound
  - —Perform in all first trimester vaginal bleeding to confirm intrauterine pregnancy (excludes ectopic)
  - —Assesses fetus
  - —Identifies free fluid or retained products of conception
  - —Transvaginal detects yolk sac at 5.5 weeks or BHCG = 1500 IU
  - —Nearly 100% sensitive in diagnosing placenta previa in late pregnancy, and should be performed *before* pelvic exam with suspected previa
- Culdocentesis
  - —Identifies free intraperitoneal blood
  - —Limited use now with ultrasound available
- Laparoscopy/laparotomy
  - —Definitive diagnosis and treatment of ectopic pregnancy or intra-abdominal complications

Treatment

INITIAL STABILIZATION

- ABCs
  - —Oxygen
  - —Large-bore IV aggressive volume replacement with normal saline or Ringer's lactate
  - —Transfuse blood if indicated
- In late pregnancy, position patient on her left side
  - —Decreases uterine compression of vena cava

ED TREATMENT

- Administer RhoGAM if patient is Rh-negative
- Oxytocin
  - —Useful in controlling post-abortion bleeding
- Obstetric consultation for all except stable threatened abortion
- Prognosis
  - —*Abortion:* 50% of first trimester bleeding ends in abortion
  - —*Previa:* <1% maternal mortality; 15–25% fetal mortality
  - —*Abruption:* <1% maternal mortality; up to 35% fetal mortality
- Complications
  - —Anemia
  - —Shock
  - —DIC
  - —Renal failure
  - —Death
- Patient education
  - —Threatened abortion
  - —Activity: no strenuous activity; no douching or intercourse while bleeding
  - —Followup: reevaluation by obstetrician within 24–72 hours
  - —Seek medical advice immediately if bleeding or pain worsens, tissue is passed, or fever develops
  - —Bring any passed tissue to the physician
- Grief counseling for fetal loss

MEDICATIONS

- Oxytocin: 10 units in 500cc saline, 120–240cc/hr IV
- RhoGAM: <12 weeks: 50 mg IM; >12 weeks: 300 mg IM

Disposition

ADMISSION CRITERIA

- Early pregnancy
  - —Unstable vital signs or severe bleeding
  - —Ruptured ectopic
  - —High suspicion for ectopic pregnancy
- Late pregnancy
  - —All patients require monitoring in an obstetric unit

DISCHARGE CRITERIA

- Threatened abortion (os closed) with stable exam and labs
- Bleeding from local vaginal/cervical source

Miscellaneous

ICD9: 623.8

CORE CONTENT CODE: 12.3.3 12.3.1 12.3.4, 12.3.3

SUGGESTED READINGS

Herbst AL, Mishell DR, Stenchever MA, Droegemueller W, eds. Comprehensive gynecology. 2d ed. St. Louis: CV Mosby, 1992:161–164.

Pernoll ML. Third-trimester hemorrhage. In: DeCherney AH, Pernoll ML, eds. Current obstetric and gynecologic diagnosis and treatment. 8th ed. Norwalk, CT: Appleton & Lange, 1994:398–409.

Turner LM. Vaginal bleeding during pregnancy. Emerg Med Clin North Am 1994;12:45–54.

Willis D. Bleeding in pregnancy. In: Benrubi GI, ed. Obstetric and gynecologic emergencies. Philadelphia: JB Lippincott, 1994;127–138.

Authors: Shirin Trachiotis; Betty Tso

Vaginal Discharge

Clinical Presentation

SIGNS AND SYMPTOMS

Normal Vaginal Discharge

- Common
- Varies from thin and watery to thick and opaque
- Asymptomatic
- Odorless

Bacterial Vaginosis

- Copious foul "fishy" smelling discharge
- Mild vaginal irritation

Candida Vaginitis—Candida Albicans (90%)

- Predisposing factors
  —Antibiotic use
  —Oral contraceptive use
  —Pregnancy
  —Diabetes
- Complaints
  —Pruritus
  —Burning
  —Irritation
  —Discharge
  —Dysuria
- Exam
  —Erythema
  —Satellite papules

Trichomonas Vaginitis

- Sexually transmitted
- Caused by protozoa *Trichomonas vaginalis*
- Asymptomatic (50%) to intense vaginal discomfort
- Onset during or immediately after menstrual period
- Complaints
  —Pruritus
  —Irritation
  —Dyspareunia
  —Dysuria
  —Discharge
- Exam
  —Diffuse erythema of the vagina
  —Rarely a "strawberry cervix" (5%)

N. Gonorrhoeae

- Mucopurulent cervicitis with vaginal discharge
- May be asymptomatic
- One-third present with dysuria and vaginal discharge
  —Consider pelvic inflammatory disease (PID)
- Exam
  —Edematous, erythematous, and friable endocervix
  —Lower abdominal tenderness
  —Cervical motion tenderness
  —Adnexal tenderness

Chlamydia Trachomatis

- Most common sexually transmitted disease (STD) in the United States
- Majority asymptomatic
- Discharge and dysuria
- Exam: mucopurulent cervicitis

Atrophic Vaginitis

- Lack of estrogen stimulation of the vaginal epithelium leading to thinning and atrophy of tissue
- Vaginal dryness
- Dyspareunia
- Pruritus
- Occasionally discharge

Vaginal Foreign Bodies

- Insertion of objects by children, sexual stimulation, and forgotten tampons or diaphragms
- Foul-smelling discharge, often bloody, which is commonly an infectious process

MECHANISM/DESCRIPTION

- Vaginal Discharge
  —Very common gynecologic complaint with many etiologies
  —Effective therapy depends on correct diagnosis
- Characteristics of *abnormal vaginal discharge* depend on the etiology and require methodical examination for appropriate diagnosis

Pre-Hospital

N/A

Diagnosis

ESSENTIAL WORKUP

- History
  —Type and duration of symptoms
  —Sexual activity
  —Risks for sexually transmitted diseases
  —Use of oral contraceptives
  —Association of symptoms with menses, previous genital infections, and current likelihood of pregnancy
- Physical Examination
  —Inspection of vulva
  —Speculum examination of the vagina and cervix

LABORATORY

- Determine pH of discharge with nitrazine paper (normal is <4.5)
- Gram stain
- Potassium hydroxide (KOH) "whiff test"
  —A few drops added to a sample of discharge
- KOH wet mount examined at 100X objective for signs of pseudohyphae or mycelia
- Saline wet mount examined at 400X objective for trichomonads and clue cells
- Cultures taken during the speculum examination

Features of Vaginal Discharge

- Normal
  —pH 4.5
  —Clear, floccular
  —Negative "whiff" test
  —Microscopic—epithelial cells and lactobacilli
- Bacterial vaginosis
  —pH 4.5
  —Gray or white, homogenous, adherent, occasionally frothy
  —Positive "whiff" test
  —Microscopic—few leukocytes and clue cells (epithelial cells studded with bacteria)
- Candida vaginitis
  —pH 4.5
  —Clumped, curd-like, white, adherent to mucosa
  —Negative "whiff" test
  —Microscopic—on KOH mycelia or pseudohyphae, on Gram stain blastospore and mycelia (more sensitive)
- Trichomonas vaginitis
  —pH 5.0
  —Classically green-yellow and frothy (10%), more commonly gray and homogenous
  —"Whiff" test usually positive
  —Microscopic—leukocytes, pear-shaped motile trichomonads with flagella, slightly larger than the leukocytes
- Gonococcal
  —Often purulent but variable
  —Microscopic—leukocytes and intracellular Gram-negative diplococci; confirm with culture which is the gold standard

- Chlamydial
  - —Purulent or mucopurulent cervical discharge
  - —Variety of immunoassays and antibody tests available for definitive diagnosis
- Atrophic vaginitis
  - —pH >7
  - —Scant, yellow-pink
  - —Microscopic—erythrocytes, leukocytes, and round or oval parabasal cells
- Foreign body
- Variable, depends on presence of infection

Treatment

ED TREATMENT

- Initiate appropriate medications (see below)
  - —Patients treated with metronidazole should not consume alcohol during treatment or for at least 24 hours after treatment
- Expected course/prognosis
  - —Correct diagnosis and treatment combined with compliance to drug therapy, treatment of partners, and patient education will result in complete cure
  - —Recurrences are common
- Complications
  - —Recurrent infections, pelvic inflammatory disease, tubal infertility, chronic pelvic pain, pelvic abscesses, preterm labor, premature rupture of membranes, chorioamnionitis
- Recommendations for partners
  - —For gonorrhea, chlamydia, and trichomoniasis
    - -Partners should be treated and should avoid sex until the full course of therapy is completed and both partners are asymptomatic
  - —For bacterial vaginosis
    - -Partners should have examination for STDs and treated if positive
  - —For candidiasis
    - -Partners should be treated with a candicidal cream if an associated dermatitis is present

MEDICATIONS

- Gonorrhea and chlamydia (treat for both)
  - —Ceftriaxone: 250 mg IM single dose *or*
  - —Cefixime: 400 mg po single dose *or*
  - —Ciprofloxacin: 500 mg po single dose *or*
  - —Ofloxacin: 400 mg po single dose

  Plus
  - —Azithromycin: 1 g po single dose *or*
  - —Doxycycline: 100 mg po bid for 7 days *or*
  - —Tetracycline: 500 mg po qid for 7 days *or*
  - —Erythromycin: 500 mg po qid for 7 days *or*
  - —Ofloxacin: 300 mg po bid for 7 days
  - —In pregnancy, avoid tetracycline; otherwise unchanged
- Bacterial vaginosis
  - —Clindamycin: 300 mg po bid for 7 days *or*
  - —Clindamycin 2% cream: 1 applicator intravaginally q hs for 7 days *or*
  - —Metronidazole: 500 mg po bid for 7 days *or*
  - —Metronidazole: 2 g po single dose *or*
  - —Metronidazole 0.75% gel: 1 applicator intravaginally bid for 5 days
  - —In pregnancy, treat only if symptomatic
    - -1st trimester: Clindamycin 2% vaginal cream
    - -2nd and 3rd trimester: treatment decisions should be made in conjunction with the patient's obstetrician
- Candidal vaginitis
  - —Butaconazole 2% cream: 5 g intravaginally q hs for 3 days *or*
  - —Clortrimazole vaginal suppositories: 2 100-mg tablets intravaginally q hs for 7 days *or*
  - —Clotrimazole 1% vaginal cream: 1 applicator full intravaginally q hs for 7 days *or*
  - —Fluconazole: 150 mg po once (not FDA approved for this use)
  - —Miconazole vaginal suppositories: 200 mg intravaginally q hs for 3 days *or*
  - —Miconazole 2% vaginal cream: 1 applicator full intravaginally q hs for 7 days
  - —All OTC except for butoconazole
  - —In pregnancy, use clotrimazole 1% cream intravaginally
- Trichomonas vaginitis
  - —Metronidazole: 2 g po single dose *or*
  - —Metronidazole: 500 mg po bid for 7 days
  - —In pregnancy
    - -Clotrimazole: 100 mg intravaginally q hs for 7 days
    - -Metronidazole contraindicated
    - -2nd–3rd trimester infections should be treated in conjunction with the patient's obstetrician
- Atrophic vaginitis
  - —Diethylstilbestrol: 0.5 mg intravaginally every 3 days for 3 weeks *or*
  - —Estradiol: 1 mg po q d *or*
  - —Estrogen: 0.625 mg po q d *or*
  - —Estrogen cream (conjugated): 2–4 g per day
  - —Estrogen therapy is contraindicated in patients with a history of breast cancer

Disposition

ADMISSION CRITERIA

- Disseminated gonococcal infection
- Toxic shock secondary to foreign bodies
- Toxicity as a result of pelvic inflammatory disease

DISCHARGE CRITERIA

- Vast majority will be discharged and treated as outpatients

Miscellaneous

ICD9: 616.10

CORE CONTENT CODE: 19.1.2.1

SUGGESTED READINGS

Fox KK, Behets F. Vaginal discharge: how to pinpoint the cause. Postgrad Med 1995;98(3):87–104.

Goode MA, Grouer K, Gums JG. Infectious vaginitis: selecting therapy and preventing recurrence. Postgrad Med 1994;96(6):85–98.

Reed B, Eyler A. Vaginal infections: diagnosis and management. Am Fam Physician 1993;47(8) 1805–1818.

Vandeven AM, Emans SJ. Vulvovaginitis in the child and adolescent. Pediatric Rev 1993;14:141.

Authors: J. Thomas Ahlquist III; Samuel M. Keim

Vaginal/Cervical Infection

Clinical Presentation

SIGNS AND SYMPTOMS

- Abnormal vaginal discharge
- Pruritus
- Irritation
- Dysuria
- Lower abdominal pain
- Odor
- Dyspareunia
- Inflamed, erythematous edematous cervix with purulent discharge from external os (gonorrhea)
- "Strawberry" petechiae on cervix and vaginal mucosa (trichomonas)
- Can be asymptomatic

ETIOLOGY

- *Candida vulvovaginitis*
- *Chlamydiae trachomatis*
- Gardnerella/bacterial vaginosis
- Herpes simplex virus
- *Neisseria gonorrhea*
- *Trichomonas vaginitis*

PEDIATRIC CONSIDERATIONS

- 80% of vaginitis in prepubertal girls is nonspecific
- Look for foreign body or pinworms
- Sexual abuse is a consideration, careful history should be obtained

Pre-Hospital

N/A

Diagnosis

ESSENTIAL WORKUP

- An abnormal vaginal discharge on physical examination indicates vaginitis. Elicit sexual history and history of sexually transmitted infections in patient and partner. Look for evidence of abdominal tenderness and cervical motion tenderness. Examination of vaginal secretions should reveal the etiology

LABORATORY

- Vaginal secretion pH using nitrazine paper. Normal vaginal pH 3.5–4.1, except before menarche and after menopause, when it is 6.0–7.0
- Saline wet preparation looking for clue cells (vaginal squamous cells covered by bacteria), WICs and trichomonads (motile, flagellated organisms.)
- Microscopic examination of vaginal discharge with few drops of 10% potassium hydroxide. Positive findings include budding yeast cells and hyphae, amine (fishy) odor with KOH
- Gram stain of cervical swab for leukocytes and Gram-negative intracellular diplococci consistent with gonorrhea (low sensitivity)
- Endocervical swab for chlamydia culture, fluorescent antibody staining technique, enzyme immunoassay, and DNA probe tests
- Endocervical, vaginal vault, and rectal specimens for *N. gonorrhea* on chocolate agar
- Pap smear or Tzanck preparation for multinucleated giant cells of herpes virus; viral culture
- Clean catch urinalysis; urine Gram stain and culture if indicated
- VDRL serum test to rule out syphilis if sexually transmitted disease suspected. Other blood tests not indicated for simple vaginal and cervical infections
- Urine and/or serum HCG to rule out pregnancy
- HIV serum test if risk factors exist

DIFFERENTIAL DIAGNOSIS

- Vaginal ulcers: syphilis, chancroid, lymphogranuloma venereum
- Urethritis, cystitis, pyelonephritis
- Pelvic inflammatory disease (PID)
- Disseminated gonococcal infection
- Ectopic pregnancy
- Appendicitis

PEDIATRIC CONSIDERATIONS

- Inquire on bubble bath, change in laundry products, nylon underpants, tights, tight jeans
- Ask about possibility of sexual abuse

DIAGNOSIS	LABORATORY TEST	SIGNS AND SYMPTOMS
Candidiasis	KOH prep shows budding yeast and hyphae	White and curdlike discharge, itching
Chlamydia	Leukocytes on Gram stain without organisms	Yellow, mucopurulent discharge, abdominal pain, cervical motion tenderness
Gardnerella	Amine odor with 10% KOH, clue cells (vaginal squamous cells covered with bacteria), pH between 5.0 and 6.0	Homogeneous white discharge, vaginal odor
Gonorrhea	Gram stain of exudate may show typical Gram-negative intracellular diplococci	Thick and creamy discharge, abdominal pain, fever, cervical motion tenderness
Herpes simplex	Tzank prep shows multinucleated giant cells	Multiple painful ulcers or vesicles
Trichomonas	Many WICs and motile-flagellated trichomonads on wet mount, pH 6–7	Frothy, yellow discharge (1/3), vaginal odor, itching

Treatment

INITIAL STABILIZATION

- No specific considerations

ED TREATMENT

- Candidiasis: can be treated intravaginally with 3–7 days of an imidazole drug: clotrimazole, miconazole, terconazole, or butoconazole. Alternative: single oral dose of fluconazole
- Gardnerella/bacterial vaginosis: treat with either single dose or 1 week of metronidazole except in first trimester of pregnancy; vaginal gel for 5 days is another option. Can use clindamycin cream throughout pregnancy
- Trichomonas: metronidazole given as 1 dose po treatment (contraindicated in first trimester of pregnancy) or for 1 week. Can use clotrimazole tablets for 2 weeks in first trimester of pregnancy, but efficacy is poor
- Gonococcal infection
  - —1-dose treatment with ceftriaxone, cefixime, ciprofloxacin, ofloxacin, norfloxacin, or spectinomycin
  - —Should always treat for concurrent chlamydial infection
- Chlamydial infection
  - —1-dose treatment with azithromycin (safe in pregnancy); indicated for uncomplicated cervicitis, not for PID
  - —10–14 day treatments with doxycycline, tetracycline, ofloxacin, or erythromycin base
- Herpes simplex: acyclovir for herpes virus infection for 10 days for initial attack; same dosage for 5 days for symptomatic recurrences; if more than 6 severe recurrences a year, suppressive therapy may be given for up to 1 year
- Always treat sexual partner(s) for chlamydia, gonorrhea, trichomonas. Encourage condom use
- Follow-up assays or cultures in 1 week

MEDICATIONS

- Acyclovir: 400 mg po tid
- Azithromycin: 1 g PO—1 dose
- Butoconazole 2% cream: 5 g intravaginally qhs
- Cefixime: 400 mg PO—1 dose
- Ceftriaxone: 125 mg IM or 250 mg IM
- Ciprofloxacin: 500 mg po (contraindicated in pregnancy, <16 years old)—1 dose
- Clindamycin: 2% vaginal cream qhs
- Clotrimazole: 2 100-mg tablets intravaginally qhs
- Doxycycline: 100 mg po bid (contraindicated in pregnancy)
- Fluconazole: 150 mg po single dose
- Erythromycin base: 500 mg po qid
- Metronidazole: 2 g po (not in 1st trimester pregnancies)—1 dose, or 500 mg po bid, or 0.75% gel intravaginally bid
- Miconazole: 200 mg suppository intravaginally qhs
- Norfloxacin: 800 mg po (contraindicated in pregnancy, <16 years old)—1 dose
- Ofloxacin: 400 mg PO—1 dose; 300 mg po bid (contraindicated in pregnancy, <16 years old)
- Spectinomycin: 2 g IM
- Tetracycline: 500 mg po qid
- Terconazole: 80 mg vaginal suppository qhs

PEDIATRIC CONSIDERATIONS

- Treat nonspecific vaginitis with sitz baths 3 times a day, proper perineal hygiene, white cotton underwear, and 1% hydrocortisone cream 3 times daily

Disposition

ADMISSION CRITERIA

- Fever and peritoneal signs associated with pelvic inflammatory disease
- Severe Herpes simplex vaginitis may require admission for intravenous acyclovir, especially in immunocompromised patients

DISCHARGE CRITERIA

- Most can be discharged with appropriate antibiotics
- Follow up with OB/GYN in 1 week

Miscellaneous

ICD9: 616.10, 616.0

CORE CONTENT CODE: 19.1.5.2, 19.1.5.4

SUGGESTED READINGS

Berg AC, Soman MP. Lower genitourinary infections in women. J Fam Pract 1986;23(1):61–70.

Cullins VE, Huggins GR. Nonmalignant vulvovaginal and cervical disorders. In: Barker LR, ed. Principles of ambulatory medicine. 4th ed. Baltimore: Williams & Wilkins, 1995:1378–1387.

Reed BD, Eyler A. Vaginal infections: Diagnosis and management. Am Fam Physician 1993;47:1805–1818.

Stevenson M, Brooke DS. Vulvovaginitis in the prepubertal child. J Pediatr Health Care 1995;9(5):227–228.

Authors: Alexander Ostrow; Mark Mandell

Valvular Heart Disease

Clinical Presentation

SIGNS AND SYMPTOMS

- Mitral stenosis
  —Exertional dyspnea
  —Fatigue
  —Palpitations
  —Paroxysmal nocturnal dyspnea
  —Orthopnea
  —Hemoptysis
  —Systemic emboli
  —Pulmonary edema
  —Malar flush ("mitral facies")
  —Prominent jugular "a" waves
  —Right ventricular lift
  —Loud S1
  —Opening snap
  —Low-pitched diastolic rumble
- Mitral regurgitation
  —Acute
    -Acute pulmonary edema
    -JVP exhibits cannon "a" waves and giant "v" waves
    -Harsh apical crescendo-decrescendo murmur radiating to the axilla
    -Palpable thrill at apex
    -S3 and S4
  —Chronic
    -Palpitations
    -Atrial fibrillation
    -Dyspnea
    -Orthopnea
    -Nocturnal paroxysmal dyspnea
    -Edema
    -Systemic emboli
    -Normal jugular venous pressure
    -Left ventricular heave
    -Apical high pitched pansystolic murmur
    -Decreased or obscured S1
    -Widely split S2
    -S3
- Aortic stenosis
  —Exertional angina
  —Syncope (during exercise)
  —Congestive heart failure (initially diastolic failure, then systolic)
  —Arrhythmias
  —Harsh crescendo-decrescendo systolic murmur at aortic focus radiating to carotids
  —Absent aortic component of S2
  —Delayed upstroke in peripheral pulse (pulsus parvus et tardus)
  —S4 gallop
  —Ejection click
- Aortic regurgitation
- Fatigue
- Dyspnea
- Paroxysmal nocturnal dyspnea
- Orthopnea
- Chest pain
- Edema
- Acute pulmonary edema
- High-pitched decrescendo diastolic murmur at aortic area
- Wide pulse pressure
- De Musset's sign (head bobbing with systole)
- Quincke's pulse (nail bed pulsations)
- Austin Flint murmur (soft diastolic rumble)

MECHANISM/DESCRIPTION

- Mitral stenosis
  —Obstruction of diastolic blood flow into the left ventricle (LV)
- Mitral regurgitation
  —Inadequate closure of the leaflets allows retrograde blood flow into the left atrium (LA)
  —Acute
    -Pressure overload in LA and pulmonary veins causing acute pulmonary edema
  —Chronic
    -LV volume overload with dilatation & hypertrophy with LA enlargement
- Aortic Stenosis
  —Resistance to ejection and systolic gradients increase
  —Progressive increase in LV systolic pressure
- Aortic regurgitation
  —Acute
    -Acute LV pressure and volume overload leading to left heart failure and pulmonary edema
  —Chronic
    -Chronic volume overload with LV dilatation and hypertrophy

ETIOLOGY

- Mitral stenosis
  —Rheumatic fever
  —Cardiac tumors
  —Rheumatologic disorders (lupus, rheumatoid arthritis)
  —Myxoma
  —Congenital defects
  —Calcification
- Mitral regurgitation (acute)
  —Ruptured papillary muscle (infarction, trauma)
  —Papillary muscle dysfunction (ischemia)
  —Ruptured chordae tendineae (trauma, endocarditis, myxomatous)
  —Valve perforation (endocarditis)
- Aortic stenosis
  —Congenital aortic stenosis (major cause in persons <30 years old)
  —Congenital bicuspid valve
  —Rheumatic aortic stenosis
  —Calcific aortic stenosis
- Aortic regurgitation (acute)
  —Acute
    -Rheumatic fever
    -Infective endocarditis
    -Rupture of sinus of Valsalva
  —Acute aortic dissection
    -Following valve surgery
    -Trauma

Pre-Hospital

CAUTIONS

- Avoid vasodilators in aortic stenosis
- May result in profound and irreversible hypotension

Diagnosis

ESSENTIAL WORKUP

- Thorough cardiopulmonary examination
- Mitral stenosis
  —ECG
    -LA enlargement
    -Right ventricular (RV) hypertrophy
  —CXR
    -Enlarged LA
    -Prominent pulmonary veins
- Mitral regurgitation
  —Acute
    -ECG
    -Q-wave inferior, posterior, or lateral
    -CXR
- Aortic stenosis
  —ECG
    -LVH most common
    -LAE
    -IVCD
    -LAD
  —CXR
    -LVH
    -Aortic calcification
    -Pulmonary congestion
- Aortic regurgitation
  —ECG
    -Acute = LV strain
    -Chronic = LV hypertrophy and strain
  —CXR
    -Acute = normal heart, pulmonary edema
    -Chronic = enlarged LV and dilated aorta
  —Echocardiogram (valvular anatomy, aortic root size, enlarged LV, LV function, estimate of regurgitation, aortic size and intimal flap)

IMAGING/SPECIAL TESTS

- Echocardiogram
- Cardiac catheterization for acute mitral regurgitation/aortic regurgitation
- Spiral CT scan to exclude aortic dissection with acute aortic regurgitation

Treatment

INITIAL STABILIZATION

- IV access, oxygen, monitor, pulse oximetry
- Mitral stenosis
  - —Treat symptoms of congestive heart failure
  - —Rate control if in atrial fibrillation
- Mitral regurgitation
- Differentiate between acute and chronic MR
- Aortic stenosis
  - —Gentle diuresis if CHF
  - —Mild hydration if hypotensive and not in CHF
  - —Avoid nitrates
- Aortic regurgitation
  - —Distinguish cause of pulmonary edema (acute mitral regurgitation vs. acute aortic regurgitation)

ED TREATMENT

- Mitral stenosis
  - —Digoxin
  - —β-Blockers
  - —Heparin (if new onset atrial fibrillation)
  - —Diuretics
  - —Endocarditis prophylaxis/education
- Mitral regurgitation
  - —Acute
    - -Afterload reduction (nitroglycerin, morphine, or sodium nitroprusside)
    - -Diuresis
    - -Intra-aortic balloon pump (temporizing for urgent surgery)
  - —Chronic
    - -Diuresis
    - -Nitrates
    - -Hydralazine
    - -Angiotensin-converting enzyme inhibitor
    - -Digoxin
    - -β-Adrenergic blocker (ventricular rate control)
    - -Calcium antagonist (ventricular rate control)
    - -Heparin (if atrial fibrillation)
    - -Endocarditis prophylaxis
- Aortic stenosis
  - —Limited role once symptomatic
  - —Digoxin
  - —Consideration for valve replacement or valvuloplasty
  - —Intra-aortic balloon pump (temporize for surgery)
  - —Endocarditis prophylaxis education
- Aortic regurgitation
  - —Chronic
    - -Preload and afterload reduction
    - -Digoxin
    - -Diuretics
    - -Endocarditis prophylaxis education
  - —Acute
    - -Preload and afterload reduction
    - -Intra-aortic balloon pump
    - -Urgent surgery

MEDICATIONS

- Bumetanide: 0.5–1.0 mg q 2–3 hrs PRN; infusion 0.08–0.3 mg/hr; po 0.5–2 mg tid qd
- Digoxin: 0.5 mg IV bolus, then 0.25 mg IV q 2 hrs up to 1 mg
- Diltiazem: 0.25 mg/kg IV over 2 min (repeat in 15 min PRN with 0.35 mg/kg) then 5–15 mg/hr
- Enalapril IV: 1.25 mg q 6 hrs; po 2.5–10 mg bid
- Esmolol: 500 μg bolus IV, then 50–400 μg/kg/min
- Furosemide: 20–80 mg IV q 1–2 hrs
- Heparin: 80 IU/kg IV bolus, then 18 IU/kg/hr drip, adjust to maintain PTT 1.5–2× control (INR 2–3)
- Hydralazine: 10–25 mg q 2–4 hrs IV
- Metoprolol: 5 mg IV
- Nitroglycerin: IV start at 20 μg/min and titrate to effect (up to 300 μg/min); SL 0.3–0.6 mg PRN; Topical 1–2 inches of 2% q 6 hrs
- Phentolamine: 5 mg IV bolus, then 1–2 mg/min IV infusion
- Propranolol: 1 mg IV
- Sodium nitroprusside: 0.5 μg/kg/min; increase in increments of 0.5–1.0 μg/kg/min q 5–10 min up to 10 μg/kg/min

Disposition

ADMISSION CRITERIA

- New onset atrial fibrillation
- Congestive heart failure/pulmonary edema
- Hemodynamically unstable
- Acute mitral or aortic regurgitation
- Cardiac ischemia
- Angina
- Syncope
- Arrhythmias

DISCHARGE CRITERIA

- Hemodynamic stability
- Unchanged ECG
- Resolution of CHF symptoms with diuresis
- Chronic mitral regurgitation

Miscellaneous

ICD9: 746.9

CORE CONTENT CODE: 2.2.5

SUGGESTED READINGS

Carabello BA, Crawford FA. Valvular heart disease. N Engl J Med 1997;337:32–41.

Cheitlin MD, Douglas PS, Parmley WW. Task Force 2: Acquired valvular heart disease. J Am Coll Cardiol 1994;24:874–80.

Roldan CA, Shively BK, Crawford MH. Value of the cardiovascular examination for detecting valvular heart disease in asymptomatic subjects. Am J Cardiol 1996;77:1327–331.

Author: Liudvikas Jagminas

Varicella

Clinical Presentation

SIGNS AND SYMPTOMS

- Varicella, commonly known as chicken pox, causes a spectrum of 4 basic disease patterns

Children (2–12 years old)

- Prodrome of low grade fever (100–103°F) and malaise precedes rash by 1–2 days
- Classic exanthem
  - Lesions begin on the trunk and face, spreading to entire body
  - Vesicles, pustules and small scabs on erythematous bases in varying stages of evolution
  - Round or oval and from 0.5 to 1.0 cm in diameter
  - Duration of vesicle formation is 3–5 days
  - Pruritus, anorexia, and listlessness
  - 10–21-day incubation period
  - Infectious from 48 hours prior to vesicle formation until all vesicles are crusted (typically 4–5 days)

Adolescent/Adults

- Extracutaneous manifestations in 5–50%
- Presenting signs and symptoms are similar to disease in children as above but generally of greater severity

Immunocompromised

- More numerous lesions which may have hemorrhagic base
- Absolute neutrophil counts (ANC) and absolute lymphocyte counts (ALC) <500 are the best predictors of complicated disease (i.e., disseminated disease and bacterial secondary infection)
- Healing may take 3 times longer
- Lesions last 3 times as long
- Extracutaneous manifestations, especially pneumonia, are very common in 20–50% of cases

Extracutaneous Manifestations

- Pneumonitis
  - Most common in adult smokers and immunocompromised children
  - Occurs 3–5 days after onset of rash
  - Early signs are continued eruption of new lesions, fever, and new onset cough
  - Tachypnea, dyspnea, cyanosis, pleuritic chest pain, and hemoptysis
  - 50–75% of cases are preceded by 1–2 days of severe abdominal or back pain
- Cerebellar ataxia
  - Cerebellar ataxia may develop 5 days after rash
  - Ataxia, vomiting, slurred speech, fever, vertigo, nystagmus, and tremor
- Cerebritis
  - Develops 3–8 days after appearance of rash; duration approximately 2 weeks
  - Progressive malaise, headache, meningismus, vomiting, fever, delirium, and seizures
- *Reye's syndrome*
  - Vomiting, restlessness, irritability, and progressive deterioration in mental status from cerebral edema
  - Aspirin use may be associated
- Myocarditis, nephritis, bleeding diatheses, and hepatitis

MECHANISM/DESCRIPTION

- 90% of children are infected by age 15
- Adults have a 15 times greater risk of death due to chicken pox than children
- Most common in late winter and early spring

ETIOLOGY

- DNA virus which is characterized by latency in dorsal root ganglia and periodic reactivation
- Virus is transmitted by respiratory route and initially replicates in the nasopharynx or upper respiratory tract with subsequent viremia
- Humans are only known reservoir

PEDIATRIC CONSIDERATIONS

- Classic disease of childhood
- Perinatal disease occurs in the mother from 5 days predelivery to 48 hours postdelivery
  - Has a high neonatal mortality

Pre-Hospital

CAUTIONS

- Nonimmune transport personnel must avoid respiratory or physical contact with patients
- Transport personnel with varicella or herpes zoster should not come in contact with immunocompromised patients

PEDIATRIC CONSIDERATIONS

- Do not use aspirin for treatment of fever

Diagnosis

ESSENTIAL WORKUP

- History and physical are sufficient in uncomplicated cases
- If confirmation necessary, obtain a tissue culture
- Extracutaneous varicella suspected
  - CXR
    - 2–5 mm ill-defined, diffuse nodular densities
    - Lesions are initially peripheral, then coalesce
    - X-ray abnormalities may persist for several weeks
  - Reye's syndrome
    - Ammonia level peaks early, may normalize in 48–72 hours
    - Liver function tests, transaminases will be elevated
    - PT/PTT
  - Cerebritis
    - Lumbar puncture demonstrates lymphocytic pleocytosis and elevated levels of protein

LABORATORY

- Serologic tests for varicella antibodies
  - Latex agglutination most sensitive
  - Enzyme-linked immunosorbent assay (ELISA)

IMAGING/SPECIAL TESTS

- Liver biopsy is definitive test for Reye's syndrome

DIFFERENTIAL DIAGNOSIS

- Impetigo
- Disseminated herpes
- Disseminated coxsackievirus
- Measles
- Rickettsial disease

Treatment

INITIAL STABILIZATION

- ABCs
- Protect airway of the obtunded patient with Reye's syndrome or CNS disease

ED TREATMENT

- Children (2–12 years old)
  - —Treat symptomatically with antipyretics and antipruritics such as diphenhydramine or hydroxyzine
  - —Closely cropped nails and good hygiene help prevent secondary bacterial infections
  - —*Acyclovir*
    - -Controversial, not generally needed for uncomplicated cases
    - -Must be initiated within 24 hours of disease onset to be efficacious
    - -Reduces total lesions by 25%
    - -Adequate immunity still develops
  - —Prophylaxis with varicella-zoster immune globulin (VZIG)
- Adolescents/Adults
  - —Symptomatic with antipyretics and antipruritics
  - —Acyclovir when initiated within 24 hours of rash decreases progression to disseminated disease
  - —Pregnant females exposed to varicella or zoster should be given VZIG
- Immunocompromised patients
  - —Acyclovir recommended
    - -Must be initiated within 72 hours of disease onset
    - -Decreases progression to disseminated disease
  - —Foscarnet for acyclovir resistant disease
  - —Interferon
  - —Prophylaxis with VZIG for the nonimmune immunocompromised patient
- Extracutaneous
  - —Acyclovir IV, or Foscarnet if viral resistance

MEDICATIONS

- Acyclovir
  - —Uncomplicated
    - -Adult: 800 mg po 5 times a day for 7 days; adolescents (13–18): 20 mg/kg per dose qid for 7 days; peds: 20 mg/kg suspension po qid for 5 days (max 800 mg po qid)
  - —Immunocompromised
    - -Adult: 10 mg/kg IV q 8 hrs infused over 1 hr *or* 800 mg po 5 times a day for 7 days; peds: 10–12 mg/kg IV q 8 hrs infused over 1 hr *or* 500 mg/m^2 IV q 8 hrs
- Diphenhydramine: adult: 25–50 mg IV/IM/PO q 4 hrs; peds: 5 mg/kg/d elixir 12.5 mg/5ml
- Foscarnet: adult: 40 mg/kg q 8 hrs over 1 hr for 10 or more days; peds: same
- Hydroxyzine: adult: 25–50 mg IM/PO q 4–6 hrs; peds 0.5 mg/kg q 4–6 hrs suspension 10 and 25 mg/5ml
- Varicella zoster immune globulin (VZIG): adults: 625 IU IM; peds: 1 vial per 10 kg IM to a max dose of 5 vials (each vial contains 125 IU)

PEDIATRIC CONSIDERATIONS

- Avoid treating with salicylates which may produce Reye's syndrome

Disposition

ADMISSION CRITERIA

- Pneumonia with any evidence of respiratory failure should be admitted to an ICU
- Immunocompromised patients: ICU vs. ward depending on severity of illness
- All admitted patients must be kept in isolation

DISCHARGE CRITERIA

- Immunocompetent children without evidence of Reye's syndrome or secondary bacterial infection
- Adults with no evidence of extracutaneous disease

PEDIATRIC CONSIDERATIONS

- Parents need to be cautioned regarding risk of secondary bacterial infection and possible progression to sepsis
- Newborns need to be admitted for IV acyclovir, NICU vs. ward depending on disease severity

Miscellaneous

ICD9: 052.9

CORE CONTENT CODE: 9.5.9, 13.12.4.5

SUGGESTED READINGS

Feldman S. Varicella-zoster virus pneumonitis. Chest 1994;106(Suppl):22S–27S.

Dunkle LM, Balfour HH. A controlled trial of acyclovir for chickenpox in normal children. N Engl J Med 1991;325:1539–1544.

Tucker JR, Linakis JG. Complications of varicella: Varicella-associated cerebritis in a child. Case report and review. J Emerg Med 1993;11:535–538.

Whitley RJ. Therapeutic approaches to varicella-zoster virus infections. J Infect Dis 1992;166(Suppl 1):S51–S57.

Authors: Mark G. Richmond; Steven M. Green

Varices

Clinical Presentation

SIGNS AND SYMPTOMS

General

- Weakness and fatigue
- Tachycardia
- Tachypnea
- Hypotension
- Cool, clammy skin, prolonged capillary refill

Abdominal

- Significant active upper GI bleeding
  —Hematemesis
  —Hematochezia
  —Melena
  —20–40% of total blood volume loss possible
- Abdominal pain
- History of cirrhosis
- Stigmata of severe hepatic dysfunction
  —Jaundice
  —Spider angiomata
  —Palmar erythema
  —Pedal edema
  —Hepatosplenomegaly
  —Ascites

Cardiovascular

- Chest pain/shortness of breath

CNS

- Syncope—common presentation
- Confusion and agitation at initial presentation
- Lethargy and obtundation—later finding

MECHANISM/DESCRIPTION

- Portal-systemic shunts that develop with elevated portal venous pressures caused by cirrhosis of the liver (in adults)
- Bleeding typically occurs when portal pressure exceeds 12–18 mm Hg
- Finding of large varices at endoscopy—important risk factor for bleeding

ETIOLOGY

- Incidence of bleeding from varices
  —25% within the first 2 years after diagnosis
  —50% incidence over the lifetime
- 40–70% of patients with esophageal varices will die secondary to bleeding or subsequent complications
- 35% rebleed with the incidence increasing with the degree of cirrhosis

PEDIATRIC CONSIDERATIONS

- Massive hematemesis—typical initial presentation
  —Hypotension maybe a late finding
- Etiology
  —Intrahepatic obstruction from biliary cirrhosis (most common)
  —α_1-Antitrypsin deficiency
  —Hepatitis
  —Cystic fibrosis

Pre-Hospital

CAUTIONS

- Aggressive airway management
  —Consider intubation early on in transport
- Treat hypotension with 2 large-bore IVs (18-gauge or larger) and 0.9%NS infusion
- Cardiac and pulse oximetry monitoring

CONTROVERSIES

- Normal saline replacement is of concern as adults with cirrhosis also often have significantly impaired renal excretion
- Overhydration can increase venous and portal hypertension leading to increased bleeding and fluid overload

PEDIATRIC CONSIDERATIONS

- In children <6 years, use intraosseous access after 3 peripheral attempts or 90 seconds if patient unstable
- Vital signs changes may be a very late finding in children
  —Subtle changes in mental status, capillary refill, mild tachycardia, or orthostatic changes may indicate significant blood loss
  —Overaggressive correction in infants can very quickly lead to significant electrolyte abnormalities

Diagnosis

ESSENTIAL WORKUP

- Gastric tube placement
  —Determines if actively bleeding
  —Facilitates a better endoscopic exam
  —Will not increase or cause esophageal variceal bleeding
- Emergent endoscopy
  —One-third to one-half of bleeding in cirrhotic patients come from a source other than esophageal varices; treatment regiments differ significantly

LABORATORY

- Arterial blood gas for
  —Acidosis
  —Hypoxemia
- CBC
  —Hct may be inaccurate with rapid bleeding
- Electrolytes, BUN/Cr, glucose
  —Evaluate renal function
  —Increased BUN may be due to blood in GI tract
  —Monitor electrolyte imbalances (sodium and potassium)
- PT, PTT, and platelets
  —Coagulopathy
  —Prolonged bleeding times
  —Thrombocytopenia
  —Type and cross—6–8 units
  —Significant transfusion requirements

IMAGING/SPECIAL TESTS

- CXR (portable) for aspiration/perforation
- Abdominal radiographs if obstruction suspected
- EKG for myocardial ischemia

DIFFERENTIAL DIAGNOSIS

- Bleeding/perforated peptic ulcer
- Erosive gastritis
- Mallory-Weiss syndrome
- Boerhaave's syndrome
- Aortoenteric fistula

Treatment

INITIAL STABILIZATION

- ABCs with aggressive airway control/intubation
  - —Avoid succinylcholine if hyperkalemia
- Insert 2 large-bore IVs and initiate 1–2 L (20 cc/kg) 0.9%NS bolus for hypotension
- Establish central IV access with invasive intravascular monitoring for hypotension not responsive to initial fluid bolus
- Replace blood loss as soon as possible
  - —Initiate with O-negative blood until type specific blood available
    - -10 cc/kg bolus in children
  - —Fresh frozen plasma and platelets may be required
- Place gastric tube (nasally or orally)

ED TREATMENT

- Emergent endoscopic evaluation required—use pharmacological and tamponade devices as temporizing measures

Pharmacologic Measures

- Vasopressin
  - —Dose: 0.3 IU/min increasing to 0.4–0.6 IU/min
  - —Complications: angina, myocardial ischemia, arrhythmia, mesenteric ischemia, ischemia of extremities, CVA, renal insufficiency
  - —Complications increase with dose
  - —Nitroglycerin may help decrease complications at higher doses
- Octreotide: 50 μg bolus + 50 μg/hr infusion (not yet approved)

Balloon Tamponade

- Sengstaken-Blakemore and Minnesota tubes
- Applies direct pressure to the suspected bleed
- Temporary benefit with risk of esophageal ulceration with extended use

Endoscopy

- Procedure of choice of acute esophageal bleeding
- Sclerotherapy—treatment of choice with active bleeding varices
- Esophageal band ligation preferred by some endoscopists
- Variceal ligation used for large, nonactively bleeding varices

PEDIATRIC CONSIDERATIONS

- Most pediatric bleeding stops spontaneously
- Direct medical intervention at patient support and emergent endoscopic evaluation

Disposition

ADMISSION CRITERIA

- ICU admission for actively bleeding varices
- Recent history of variceal bleeding

DISCHARGE CRITERIA

- Nonbleeding varices

Miscellaneous

ICD9: 454.9

CORE CONTENT CODE: 1.1.2.1

SUGGESTED READINGS

Goff JS. Esophageal varices. Gastrointest Endosc Clin N Am 1994;4(4):747–771.

McGuirk TD, Coyle WJ. Upper gastrointestinal tract bleeding. Emerg Med Clin North Am 1996;14:523–545.

Williams S, Westaby D. Management of variceal haemorrhage. Br Med J 1994;308:1213–1217.

Author: David Hale

Vasculitis

Clinical Presentation

SIGNS AND SYMPTOMS

- Although each vasculitis has specific characteristics, all have several common manifestations including fever, fatigue, weight loss, and diffuse aches and pains, as well as other nonspecific constitutional symptoms
  - —Common signs include a nondestructive oligoarthritis and neuropathy

Large Arteries—Takayasu's Arteritis

- There is a strong predilection for the aortic arch and its branches
- Later phase of arterial insufficiency (pulseless phase)
  - —Diminished pulses and bruits over several large arteries
  - —Pulse discrepancy >30 mm Hg between the left and right arms
  - —Cool upper extremities with claudication and ulceration
  - —Posturally dependent visual blurring, diplopia
  - —Severe or resistant HTN (secondary to renal artery stenosis)
  - —Abdominal angina (from mesenteric artery stenosis)
  - —Myocardial ischemia (secondary to coronary artery stenosis), aortic valve dilation, and congestive heart failure can develop
  - —Decreased cerebral blood flow leading to facial or scalp ulcerations, hair loss, stroke, syncope, visual loss, and postural dizziness

Medium and Small Arteries (Systemic Necrotizing Vasculitis)—Polyarteritis Nodosa (PAN)

- Although PAN may involve any organ system, it has a predilection for the renal and visceral arteries
- Palpable purpura (nodules, ulcers, livedo papules)
- 3 of the following 10 criteria are needed to diagnosis PAN
  - —Weight loss >4 kg
  - —Livedo reticularis
  - —Testicular pain or tenderness
  - —Myalgias or weakness
  - —Mono- or polyneuropathy
  - —Diastolic BP >90 mm Hg
  - —Elevated BUN or creatinine
  - —Hepatitis B virus
  - —Arteriography (see Imaging/Special Tests)
  - —Arterial biopsy
- Usually there is neither pulmonary involvement nor rapidly progressive glomerulonephritis
- Churg-Strauss syndrome: variant of PAN which occurs in patients with asthma, allergic rhinitis, and eosinophilia

Small Arteries (Hypersensitivity Vasculitis)—Henoch-Schöenlein Purpura (HSP)

- Primarily affects the arterioles and capillaries
- Palpable purpura (IgA immune complex deposition) seen on dependent body areas, sparing the head, neck, and trunk
- Transient arthralgias (ankles and knees)
- GI symptoms can include abdominal pain or cramping, nausea, and vomiting, diarrhea or constipation (frequently accompanied by the passage of blood or mucus per rectum)
  - —Rarely intussusception, hematuria, proteinuria, mild glomerulitis, and nephrotic syndrome can occur

MECHANISM/DESCRIPTION

- The vasculitides are defined as acute or chronic inflammation and necrosis of blood vessels. The clinical picture depends on the size of blood vessels affected and which organs they supply. Usually there is multiorgan dysfunction; however, single organ systems can be involved
- The vasculitides are a broad range of diseases with many theorized causes; however, current thinking revolves around several immunopathogenic mechanisms, with immune complex-mediated vessel wall damage leading the list
  - —Immune complexes containing activated complement components are deposited on blood vessel walls. The wall's vascular permeability increases and damage occurs through several mechanisms, one being activation of chemotactic factors (C5a). Owing to the similarities between the vasculitides, there has been confusion in the classification scheme. Aside from the entities listed below, other primary vasculitides include temporal arteritis, and Behçet's and Kawasaki's diseases. Secondary causes of vasculitis include connective tissue disorders; malignancy; infectious EBV, CAH, and Lyme disease; serum sickness secondary to drugs

ETIOLOGY

- The incidence for the vasculitides varies with the diseases
- The highest incidence of Takayasu's arteritis is seen in young (ages 10–30) Asian females. Takayasu's has been seen after streptococcal or tuberculous infections
- The incidence of PAN is 0.7/100,000, and it mostly affects middle-aged men
- HSP is a disease of children (ages 4–11) and is seen mostly in the spring following a bacterial or viral infection. Also, HSP may result from an allergic reaction to food, drugs or an insect bite

Pre-Hospital

N/A

Diagnosis

ESSENTIAL WORKUP

- History and examination suggesting one of the above conditions
- CBC, ESR, urinalysis, BUN/Cr

LABORATORY

- Although lab findings are mostly nonspecific, there are some similarities between the vasculitides
  - —A mild leukocytosis may be seen
  - —ESR >20 mm/hr
  - —Anemia of chronic disease with hemoglobin <12
  - —ANA and ANCA titers elevated (elevated ANCA especially sensitive for Wegener's disease)
  - —Positive tissue biopsy
  - —Specifically, with PAN 30% will be positive for hepatitis B, and usually the ANCA is negative (except with Churg-Strauss, where ANCA is positive)

IMAGING/SPECIAL TESTS

- Arteriography of the involved vessels is the standard
  - —Takayasu's arteritis: arteriography shows irregular vessel walls, stenosis, poststenotic dilation, aneurysms, occlusion, and increased collateral circulation
  - —PAN: mesenteric arteriography shows multiple berrylike aneurysms

DIFFERENTIAL DIAGNOSIS

- Because the clinical manifestations vary so widely and depend on the specific syndrome, differential diagnosis will be very broad and include that of renal failure, arthritis, rash, purpura, congestive heart failure, and so forth

Treatment

INITIAL STABILIZATION

- Patients may present with evidence of end organ damage such as congestive heart failure, myocardial infarction, and pulmonary edema. Initial stabilization is directed toward stabilizing these conditions

ED TREATMENT

- Corticosteroids are the mainstay of treatment
- In HSP, glucocorticoids are used when the patient has GI complications. HSP is usually a benign, self-limited disease that resolves over 1–4 months. Those with severe nephritis or nephrosis may require salt restriction, diuretics, and antihypertensives
- Cytotoxic agents such as cyclophosphamide can be used in Takayasu's and PAN if patients fail to respond to steroid treatment. The decision to use these agents should include an appropriate consultant
- Patients with Takayasu's arteritis may present with CHF or hypertension and can be treated with diuretics or an ace-inhibitor such as captopril
- Patients with Takayasu's arteritis may need referral for procedures to revascularize ischemic organs

MEDICATIONS

- Capoten: adult: 12.5–25 mg po tid initially; peds: 0.5–1 mg/kg per day in 3 doses, max 6 mg/kg per day
- Cyclophosphamide: adult: 2 mg/kg/day (up to 4 mg/kg); peds: dose as per consultant
- Furosemide: adult: 40–100 mg IV; peds: 1 mg/kg IV
- Prednisone: adult: 40–60 mg/day; peds: 1–2 mg/kg/day

Disposition

ADMISSION CRITERIA

- Patients with evidence of severe disease and end organ dysfunction should be admitted

DISCHARGE CRITERIA

- Less symptomatic patients without evidence of end organ involvement

Miscellaneous

ICD9: 447.6

CORE CONTENT CODE: 8.5.5

SUGGESTED READINGS

Allen NB, Bressler PB. Diagnosis and treatment of the systemic and cutaneous necrotizing vasculitis syndromes. Med Clin North Am 1997;81(1):243–259.

Hall S, Buchbinder R. Takayasu's arteritis. Rheum Dis Clin North Am 1990;16(2):411–421.

Hunder GG. Giant cell arteritis and polymyalgia rheumatica. Med Clin North Am 1997;81(1):195–215.

Roberti I, Reisman L. Vasculitis in childhood. Pediatr Nephrol 1993;7:479–487.

Sneller MC, Fauci AS. Pathogenesis of vasculitis syndromes. Med Clin North Am 1997;81(1):221–237.

Author: Andrew Milsten

Venous Insufficiency

Clinical Presentation

SIGNS AND SYMPTOMS

- Pigmentation
- Dermatosclerosis (thickened skin)
- Ulceration
- Brawny edema of the lower extremities
- Pain
- Extreme sensitivity of the skin to minor trauma
- Superficial venous varicosity
- Brisk bleeding from a varicosity

MECHANISM/DESCRIPTION

- Chronic, progressive disorder
- Disease occurs mainly
  —In postthrombophlebitis patients, who have occupations that require long periods of standing
  —In the chronically homeless
  —In persons of lower income and economic status

ETIOLOGY

- Pathophysiology
  —Normally, competent venous valves prevent downward blood flow in the leg after muscular contraction
  —Dysfunction of the superficial or perforating venous valves of the legs allows gravity to fill the veins early after a muscular contraction, leading to pooling of blood in the veins, venous hypertension, and, eventually, capillary leakage of plasma, proteins, and RBC
- Eventually leads to varicosities of the superficial veins, cutaneous hyperpigmentation, eczema or dermatitis, and finally, ulceration
- Venous insufficiency can be either primary or secondary
  —Primary venous insufficiency occurs when no clear cause of valvular insufficiency is found
  —Secondary venous insufficiency describes the result of an identifiable event—most frequently a previous episode of deep venous thrombosis

Pre-Hospital

CAUTIONS

- Control bleeding with direct pressure
- Take special note of estimated blood loss on scene

Diagnosis

ESSENTIAL WORKUP

- Careful history and physical confirms diagnosis
  —History of long-standing edema and pigmentation required for diagnosis
- Determine the time course of the edema or ulceration and change in size
- Increasing redness, pain, warmth suggests cellulitis
- Sudden increased swelling suggests deep vein thrombosis (DVT)

LABORATORY

- Hematocrit if prolonged bleeding or significant blood loss noted

IMAGING/SPECIAL TESTS

- Duplex Doppler ultrasonography if DVT suspected

DIFFERENTIAL DIAGNOSIS

- Chronic loss of autonomic tone (as seen in CVA)
- CHF
- Hypothyroidism

Treatment

INITIAL STABILIZATION

- Control bleeding with direct pressure
- Figure of eight suture to control continued varicose vein bleeding

ED TREATMENT

- Goals
  —Healing ulcers
  —Counteracting the transmission of increased venous pressure to the skin
- Mainstays of treatment for venous insufficiency
  —Leg compression
  —Leg elevation
  —Unna boots
  —Nonelastic compression with a gel paste-impregnated gauze containing zinc oxide and calamine
    -Advantage of providing both compression and local wound treatment
  —Arterial occlusive disease relative contraindication to compression/elevation
- Local wound care
  —Topical povidone-iodine (betadine), sodium hypochlorite (Dakin's solution) and acetic acid (Burow's solution)
    -Widely used but effectiveness controversial
  —Systemic antibiotics
    -Not indicated unless local infection is present
  —Antistaphylococcal coverage indicated if infection (cephalexin or dicloxacillin)
  —Topical antibiotics do not help wound healing

MEDICATIONS

- Cephalexin: 500 mg po qid
- Dicloxacillin: 500 mg po qid

Disposition

ADMISSION CRITERIA

- Cellulitis not controlled by outpatient wound care and antibiotics
- Bleeding not controlled with direct pressure
- Inability to comply with conservative measures (homelessness, inability to change dressings)

DISCHARGE CRITERIA

- Most patients with venous insufficiency will be discharged

Miscellaneous

ICD9: 459.81

CORE CONTENT CODE: 2.5.2.1

SUGGESTED READINGS

Angle N, Bergan JJ. Chronic venous ulcer. Br Med J 1997;314:1019–23.

Greenfield LJ: Venous and lymphatic disease. In: Schwartz SI, Shires GT, Spencer FC, eds. Principles of surgery. New York: McGraw-Hill, 1994:1029–35.

Author: Thomas Amaroso

Ventricular Fibrillation

Clinical Presentation

SIGNS AND SYMPTOMS

- Loss of consciousness
- Pulseless
- Apnea
- Cyanosis
- Death

MECHANISM/DESCRIPTION

- Heart stops effective pumping, brain perfusion ceases and the patient loses consciousness
- Ventricular fibrillation (VFib)
  —Totally disorganized depolarization and contraction of small areas of the ventricle, without effective ventricular pumping
- ECG or cardiac monitor
  —Absence of QRS complexes and T waves
  —Presence of low amplitude baseline undulations that are variable in both amplitude and periodicity

ETIOLOGY

- Initial rhythm in approximately 50–70% of patients sustaining sudden cardiac death in the pre-hospital setting
  —Most often a result of acute myocardial ischemia or infarction
  —Complication of a cardiomyopathy
    -Up to 50% of patients with a dilated cardiomyopathy suffer an episode of Vfib
  —In hypertrophic cardiomyopathy, unexpected sudden death occurs with reported frequency of up to 3% per year
- Other less common causes of Vfib
  —Blunt chest trauma
  —Hypothermia
  —Iatrogenic myocardial irritation from pacemaker placement or a pulmonary artery catheter
- Vfib often preceded by ventricular tachycardia (VT)
- Predisposition to VT
- Drug toxicities (cyclic antidepressants, digitalis)
- Hereditary QT prolongation,
- Metabolic abnormalities that prolong the QT interval (hyperkalemia, hypocalcemia)

PEDIATRIC CONSIDERATIONS

- Primary ventricular dysrhythmias extremely rare in children
- VFib usually results from a respiratory arrest, hypothermia, or near drowning

Pre-Hospital

CAUTIONS

- Do not perform defibrillation until the rhythm has been verified by experienced personnel or the evaluation of an automatic defibrillator
- Patients in VT or supraventricular tachycardia may deteriorate rapidly if defibrillated without ECG synchronization
- Do not defibrillate any awake patients

CONTROVERSIES

- Semiautomatic external defibrillators
  —Value has been well-established with both trained and relatively untrained (firefighters, police) personnel

Diagnosis

ESSENTIAL WORKUP

- Cardiac monitor

LABORATORY

- Laboratory tests will not be useful or timely
- If immediate bedside assays available, determine electrolytes to identify hyperkalemia

DIFFERENTIAL DIAGNOSIS

- Asystole
  —Fine VFib may appear to be asystole on a single ECG lead
  —Check one other lead to make sure there are no fine fibrillations present

Treatment

INITIAL STABILIZATION

- Immediate defibrillation
  —200 J first attempt
  —200–300 J second attempt
  —360 J third attempt
- Initiate CPR and airway management with intubation
- Establish IV access
  —Administer epinephrine 1.0 mg IV or via endotracheal tube
- After the epinephrine repeat defibrillation with 360 J
  —If VFib persists, administer lidocaine intravenously and repeat defibrillation at 360 J
- Further rounds of defibrillation may be preceded by bretylium, magnesium, or procainamide
- Consider sodium bicarbonate for patients with prolonged arrest

ED TREATMENT

- If the patient is successfully resuscitated, administer lidocaine 1.5 mg/kg as a bolus followed by a 2 mg/min infusion to reduce the likelihood of the recurrence of fibrillation
- Begin an evaluation for the cause of the Vfib recognizing that the most likely is myocardial ischemia

MEDICATIONS

- Beryllium: 5 mg/kg repeat 10 mg/kg IV
- Epinephrine 1:10,000 concentration: 1 mg IV/ETT, repeat q 3–5 min
- Lidocaine: l mg/kg IV bolus, repeat 0.5 mg/kg
- Lidocaine infusion: 2–4 mg/min
- Lidocaine via ETT: 2.0–2.5 mg in 10 cc NS
- Procainamide: 20 mg/min IV up to 1 g or QRS lengthens by 50%
- Sodium Bicarbonate: 1 mEq/kg IV

Disposition

ADMISSION CRITERIA

- All patients who survive to the coronary care unit

DISCHARGE CRITERIA

- None

Miscellaneous

ICD9: 427.41

CORE CONTENT CODE: 2.4.1.5

SUGGESTED READINGS

Blum FC. Adult medical resuscitation. In: Howell J, et al., eds. Emergency medicine. Philadelphia: WB Saunders, 1997.

Cobb LA, Eliastarn M, et al. Report of the American Heart Association Task Force on the future of cardiopulmonary resuscitation: Special report. Circulation 1992;85.

Cummins RO, ed. Textbook of advanced cardiac life support. Dallas, TX: American Heart Association, 1994.

Author: Ra'ed Hijazi

Ventricular Peritoneal Shunts

Clinical Presentation

SIGNS AND SYMPTOMS

Shunt Obstruction

- *Headache,* nausea, malaise, general weakness, irritability
- Decreased level of consciousness (LOC) or coma
- Increased head size or bulging fontanelle
- New onset seizures, increased seizure frequency
- Autonomic instability, decreased upward gaze
- Apnea/respiratory arrest
- Papilledema: rare

Overdrainage Syndrome

- Severe headache, focal neurologic signs, malaise, seizures, coma
  —signs and symptoms may be postural
- Rapid overdrainage may cause upward shift of the brain stem causing apnea, bradycardia, hypotension, syncope, laryngospasm
- Subdural hygroma or hematoma, chronic overdrainage, pneumocranium

Shunt Infections

- Signs and symptoms of shunt obstruction
- Fever (may be absent), meningeal signs, local signs of infection (erythema, swelling, tenderness), peritonitis
- Infections usually occur soon after shunt placement (~80% within 6 months)

Slit Ventricle Syndrome

- Episodic headache, alternating periods of normal behavior and lethargy, headache, nausea and vomiting

MECHANISM/DESCRIPTION

- *Obstruction:* shunt malfunction produces impaired drainage of CSF and results in increased ICP
  —Rate of ICP increase determines severity
- *Overdrainage syndrome:* assuming upright posture increases CSF outflow and causes decreased ICP and post LP like headache
- *Infection:* a shunt is a foreign body and a conduit between CSF and the peritoneal cavity
  —Staphylococcal epidermidis and other staphylococcal species: ~75% of infections
- *Slit ventricle syndrome:* prolonged overdrainage causes decreased ventricular size and intermittent increases in ICP due to proximal obstruction

PEDIATRIC CONSIDERATIONS

- If cranial sutures are open, CSF may accumulate without much ICP increase, producing relatively nonspecific signs and symptoms

Pre-Hospital

CAUTIONS

- Patients with shunt malfunction are at-risk for apnea and respiratory arrest
- Oxygen should be applied with close monitoring of respiratory status
- If increased ICP suspected, transport with head elevated to 30°

Diagnosis

ESSENTIAL WORKUP

Suspected Shunt Malfunction

- Manipulation of the pumping chamber: chamber should compress easily and refill within 3 seconds. Failure to compress easily implies distal obstruction, failure to fill implies proximal obstruction (up to 40% of malfunctioning shunts compress/fill normally)
- *Shunt series:* radiographs of skull, chest, and abdomen aid diagnosis of disconnection, malposition, or kinking of shunt components

Suspected Infection

- Aspiration of CSF from shunt reservoir (in consult with neurosurgeon)
  —May be performed using sterile technique and 23-gauge butterfly needle
  —Aspirate slowly 5–10 cc CSF for the studies noted below

LABORATORY

- Electrolytes, anticonvulsant levels, renal function, blood count, and glucose aid in the differential diagnosis of seizures and altered mental status

Suspected Infection

- Analysis of CSF from the shunt reservoir for culture, cell count, Gram stain, glucose and protein levels
  —CSF analysis may be normal early, especially with prior antibiotic treatment
- Blood cultures

IMAGING/SPECIAL TESTS

- Cranial CT: catheter position, ventricular size, subdural hematoma or hygroma, other causes of elevated ICP
  —Enlarged ventricles: shunt malfunction
  —Smaller ventricles: overdrainage
- Ultrasound: may be used to assess ventricular size and position of catheter tip
- Shunt manometry: high pressure (>20 cm H_2O) implies distal shunt obstruction

DIFFERENTIAL DIAGNOSIS

- Seizure disorder (idiopathic, toxic, metabolic)
- Infections: nonshunt-related CNS infection, systemic infections
- Metabolic abnormalities: hypoglycemia, hyponatremia, hypoxia
- Intoxication/poisoning
- Head trauma

Treatment

INITIAL STABILIZATION

Signs of Impending Herniation

- Rapid Squence Intubation (see chapter: Conscious sedation/rapid sequence intabation) and mild hyperventilation to PCO_2 ~35
  - —Pretreat with lidocaine (pediatric: + atropine)
  - —Thiopental/etomidate for induction
  - —Paralytic choice is controversial
    - -Depolarizing agents (succinylcholine) may increase ICP a few mm Hg, though this may not be clinically significant
    - -Use pretreatment dose of nondepolarizing agent if depolarizing agent chosen
    - -Nondepolarizing agents (vecuronium, rocuronium) may be preferable
- Forced pumping of shunt chamber
- Flush the device with 1 cc saline to remove distal obstruction
- Slow drainage of CSF from the reservoir to achieve pressure <20 cm H_2O
- IV mannitol to lower ICP
- *Ventricular puncture* is procedure of last resort if above unsuccessful and neurosurgeon unavailable
- *Status epilepticus* is treated with benzodiazepines (lorazepam)

ED TREATMENT

- Early neurosurgeon consultation
- Shunt malfunction
  - —Elevate head of bed to 30°
  - —Medical management with diuretics (mannitol, furosemide) may be appropriate in certain mild cases
- Overdrainage syndrome
  - —Supine position
  - —Correct volume depletion
- Shunt infection
  - —Systemic antibiotics (vancomycin + cefotaxime *or* gentamycin if Gram-negative suspected)

MEDICATIONS

- Atropine: 0.02 mg/kg IV (min 0.1 mg)
- Cefotaxime: 30 mg/kg IV (newborn 50 mg/kg IV)
- Furosemide: 1 mg/kg IV
- Gentamycin: 2–5 mg/kg IV
- Lidocaine: 1 mg/kg IV
- Mannitol: 1.0 mg/kg IV
- Rocuronium: 0.6–1 mg/kg IV
- Succinylcholine: 1.5 mg/kg IV
- Vancomycin: 15 mg/kg IV
- Vecuronium: 0.1–0.3 mg/kg IV

Disposition

ADMISSION CRITERIA

- Patients with shunt complications require neurosurgical consultation and admission to an ICU or other closely monitored setting

DISCHARGE CRITERIA

- If shunt malfunction is ruled out, disposition depends on diagnosis and patient condition

Miscellaneous

ICD9: 996.2

CORE CONTENT CODE: 11.8.3, 13.5.4

SUGGESTED READINGS

Guertin SR. Cerebrospinal fluid shunts: Evaluation, complication, and crisis management. Pediatr Clin North Am 1987;34(1):203–217.

Key CB, Rothrock SG, Falk JL. Cerebrospinal fluid shunt complications: An emergency medicine perspective. Pediatr Emerg Care 1995;11(5):265–273.

Madsen MA. Emergency department management of ventriculoperitoneal cerebrospinal fluid shunts. Ann Emerg Med 1986;15(11):1330–1343.

McLaurin RL, Frame PT. Treatment of cerebrospinal fluid shunts. Rev Infect Dis 1987;9(3):595–603.

Authors: Gregory Christiansen; Richard S. Krause

Ventricular Tachycardia

Clinical Presentation

SIGNS AND SYMPTOMS

- Syncope
- Near syncope
- Lightheadedness
- Shortness of breath
- Palpitations
- Chest pain
- Asymptomatic
- Cannon A waves
- Hypotension
- Congestive heart failure

MECHANISM/DESCRIPTION

- Rapid and regular depolarization of the ventricles independent of the atria and the normal conduction system
- Reentry
  - —Most common mechanism
  - —Seen in dilated cardiomyopathy, ischemia, and infiltrative heart disease
  - —Usually produces a regular and monomorphic rhythm
- Triggered automaticity
  - —Minority of ventricular tachycardia (VT)
  - —Caused by repetitive firing of a ventricular focus
- Torsades de Pointe
  - —Polymorphic form of VT
  - —Usually due to early after-depolarization
- Regardless of the mechanism, all VT may degenerate to ventricular fibrillation (VF)

ETIOLOGY

- Wide complex tachycardias
  - —80% of sustained proven to be VT
  - —20% supraventricular tachycardia with a baseline left bundle branch block or aberrancy
- Wide complex tachycardia and a history of myocardial infarction
  - —95% likelihood of being in VT
- Incidence of nonsustained VT
  - —0–4% in the general population
  - —Up to 60% of patients with dilated cardiomyopathy
- Associated with increased risk of sudden cardiac death (SCD)

PEDIATRIC CONSIDERATIONS

- Primary cardiac arrest and VT are rare in children
- Usually secondary to hypoxia and acidosis
- VT is tolerated for longer periods in children than adults and is less likely to degenerate to VF
- Infants in VT most commonly present with congestive heart failure
- VT in children results from
  - —Cardiomyopathy
  - —Congenital structural heart disease
  - —Congenital prolonged QT syndromes
  - —Coronary artery disease secondary to vasculitis
  - —Intoxicants

Pre-Hospital

CAUTIONS

- Transport stable patients suspected of being in VT without attempting to convert them
- *Synchronized* cardioversion for unstable patients with a pulse
- Defibrillation for pulseless VT

CONTROVERSIES

- Lidocaine
  - —No benefit in the prevention of VT in patients with isolated PVCs, regardless of the frequency
  - —Patients with documented VT that has resolved should be started on a lidocaine infusion to prevent recurrences during transport

Diagnosis

ESSENTIAL WORKUP

- ECG
  - —Most important initial test to differentiate VT from supraventricular tachycardia with aberrancy or LBBB
- VT
  - —Three or more consecutive QRS complexes with a ventricular rate over 100 bpm and a QRS duration >120 msec
  - —Torsades de Pointe
    - -Polymorphic VT that rotates its axis every 10–20 beats
- Criterion to determine VT
  - —AV dissociation (most reliable)
  - —Fusion beats
  - —Uniform morphology (except in the case of Torsades)
  - —Left axis deviation QRS >140 msec
  - —QRS concordance in the precordial leads
  - —Initial r wave of >30 msec
  - —Wide QRS with LBBB in precordium
- Indicators of supraventricular tachycardia with aberrancy include
  - —Normal axis QRS <140 msec
  - —Absence of Q waves
  - —RBBB in V1 with rsR′ triphasic pattern

LABORATORY

- Cardiac enzymes
- Electrolytes, BUN/Cr, glucose
- Magnesium level
- Calcium level
- Digoxin level if toxicity suspected

IMAGING/SPECIAL TESTS

- Esophageal pacing catheters
  - —May be able to detect atrial activity to establish AV dissociation and therefore diagnose VT
  - —Catheters can then be used to overdrive pace if needed

DIFFERENTIAL DIAGNOSIS

- Supraventricular tachycardia with aberrancy or baseline LBBB
- Proarrhythmia secondary to antidysrhythmia medications; suspect if
  - —VT morphology is different than previous episodes of VT
  - —Medications have recently been started or changed
  - —QT interval is prolonged
  - —Torsades de Points
  - —If VT continues to recur after cardioversion

Treatment

INITIAL STABILIZATION

- Pulseless VT: defibrillate immediately and follow the ventricular fibrillation treatment plan

ED TREATMENT

- Unstable patient
  - —Definition
    - -Chest pain
    - -Hypotension
    - -Evidence of worsening heart failure
  - —Initiate immediate synchronized cardioversion with 100 J, quickly progressing to 200 J, 300 J, and 360 J if no response
    - -If the VT is polymorphic, begin cardioversion at 200 J
  - —Sedate the patient before cardioversion if at all possible
  - —If unable to terminate the VT, administer lidocaine and repeat the cardioversion
  - —After successful return of sinus rhythm, begin lidocaine to prevent recurrences
  - —Administer procainamide or bretylium if there is breakthrough VT after lidocaine
- Stable patient
  - —Lidocaine
    - -Administer as a bolus and infusion
    - -Will only affect VT
  - —Adenosine
    - -Administer if there no response to lidocaine and the diagnosis is in question
    - -Converts supraventricular tachycardia with aberrancy
    - -No effect on VT
  - —Procainamide
    - -Converts both VT and supraventricular tachycardia,
    - -Can be used after lidocaine or as a first line medication if the diagnosis is uncertain
  - —Synchronized cardioversion if unsuccessful conversion with medication
  - —Antitachycardia overdrive pacing
    - -Alternate to synchronized cardioversion
- Torsades de Pointe
  - —Unstable
    - -Immediately perform unsynchronized cardioversion at 200 J
    - -Sedate if possible
  - —Stable
    - -Electrical pacing is the treatment of choice
    - -Cardioversion is often unsuccessful or transiently successful
    - -Administer $MgSO_4$
    - -Isoproterenol is used to overdrive the tachycardia if the patient has no history of coronary artery disease

MEDICATIONS

- Adenosine: 6 mg IVP followed by 12 mg IVP if needed in 1–2 min; peds: 1 mg/kg max 6 mg
- Bretylium: 5–10 mg/kg over 8–10 min, repeat in 5 min if needed
- Isoproterenol: 2–10 μg/min; peds: 0.1 μg/kg/min
- Lidocaine: 1–1.5 mg/kg bolus IVP first dose, 0.5–0.75 mg/kg second dose and q 5–10 min for a max of 3 mg/kg; infusion 1–4 mg/min if converted; peds: l mg/kg bolus with infusion 20–50 μg/kg/min
- $MgSO_4$: 2 g over 5–10 min followed by infusion of 2 g over 1 hr
- Procainamide: 20–30 mg/min for a total of 17 mg/kg or until converted

PEDIATRIC CONSIDERATIONS

- Begin cardioversion at 1 J/kg, 2 J/kg, and 4 J/kg as needed

Disposition

ADMISSION CRITERIA

- Admit sustained VT to a critical care setting
- Admit nonsustained VT and a history of MI or dilated cardiomyopathy for electrophysiologic studies

DISCHARGE CRITERIA

- Rare patients with nonsustained VT and a previous evaluation that revealed no structural heart disease can be discharged
  - —At low risk for sudden cardiac death
- Patients with automatic internal cardiac defibrillators that are well functioning can also be discharged

Miscellaneous

ICD9: 427.1

CORE CONTENT CODE: 2.4.1.6

SUGGESTED READINGS

Alpert MA, Mukeiji V, Bikkina M, et al. Pathogenesis, recognition, and management of common cardiac arrhythmias. South Med J 1995;88(1):1–21.

Chakko S, Kessler KM. Recognition and management of cardiac arrhythmias. Curr Prob Cardiol 1995;20(2):53–117.

Hamdan M, Scheinman M. Current approaches in patients with ventricular tachyarrhythmias. Med Clin North Am 1995;79(5):1097–120.

Hsia HH, Buxton AE. Work-up and management of patients with sustained and nonsustained monomorphic ventricular tachycardias. Cardiol Clin 1993;11(1):65–83.

Pires LA, Huang SK. Nonsustained ventricular tachycardia: identification and management of high-risk patients. Am Heart J 1993;126:189–200.

Author: Mary Beth Kurz

Vertigo

Clinical Presentation

SIGNS AND SYMPTOMS

- "Dizzy" describes a variety of experiences, including
  - —Sensations of motion
  - —Weakness, fainting
  - —Lightheadedness
  - —Unsteadiness
  - —Depression
- True vertigo
  - —Sensation of disorientation in space combined with a sensation of motion
  - —Hallucination of movement either of the self or the external environment
- Peripheral vertigo
  - —Sudden onset
  - —Severe symptoms
  - —Intermittent episodes lasting seconds to minutes occasionally hours
  - —Horizontal or horizontorotary nystagmus (also positional, fatigues, and suppressed by fixation)
  - —Normal neurological exam
  - —Presence of auditory symptoms (tinnitus)
  - —Usual severity of symptoms that worsen by position, and associated hearing loss or tinnitus
- Central vertigo
  - —Gradual onset
  - —Mild continuous symptoms
  - —All varieties of nystagmus (horizontal, vertical, rotatory)
  - —Absence of hearing loss
  - —No positional association
  - —Presence of neurological findings
- Nausea/vomiting associated with vertigo
- Ataxia

ETIOLOGY

Peripheral

- Benign paroxysmal positional
  - —Uncertain etiology
  - —Dependent on head position
  - —Fatigues
- Acute labyrinthitis
  - —Associated with hearing deficit
  - —Sudden onset
  - —May be serous, acute suppurative, toxic, or chronic
- Ménière's disease
  - —Episodic vertigo, hearing loss, and tinnitus
- Vestibule neuritis
  - —Severe vertigo and symptoms resolving over days to weeks
  - —No hearing deficits
  - —Highest incidence in 3rd to 5th decade
- Acoustic neuroma
  - —Tumor of Schwann cells enveloping the 8th nerve
  - —Develops into central cause
  - —Unilateral hearing deficits and tinnitus
  - —May also involve CN V, VII, or X
- Trauma
  - —Rupture of tympanic membrane, round window, labyrinthine concussion, or development of perilymphatic fistula can all have severe symptomatology
- Ototoxic drugs
  - —Aminoglycosides
  - —Antimalarials
  - —Erythromycin
  - —Furosemide
- Otitis media and serous otitis with effusion
- Foreign body in ear canal

Central

- Cerebellar hemorrhage
  - —Sudden onset of headache, vertigo, vomiting, and ataxia, visual paralysis to affected side (ipsilateral CN VI paralysis)
- Vertebral basilar artery insufficiency
  - —Dysarthria
  - —Ataxia
  - —Numbness of the face
  - —Hemiparesis, headache
  - —Diplopia/visual
  - —Disturbances may be transient or exacerbated by movement of the neck
- Cerebellar infarction
  - —Nausea
  - —Vomiting
  - —Ipsilateral nystagmus
  - —Ataxia
- Trauma
  - —Postconcussive syndrome or damage to labyrinth or eighth nerve secondary to basilar skull fracture
- Temporal lobe epilepsy
  - —Associated with hallucinations, aphasia, trancelike states, or convulsions
  - —More common in younger patients
- Vertebral basilar migraines
  - —Prodrome of vertigo, dysarthria, ataxia, visual disturbances, or paresthesias followed by headache
  - —Often a family history of migraines or similar attacks
- Tumor
- Multiple sclerosis
  - —Onset between ages 20 and 40
  - —All forms of nystagmus
  - —May have abrupt onset of severe vertigo and vomiting
  - —History of other vague and varying neurologic signs or symptoms
- Subclavian steal syndrome
  - —Exercise of an arm causing shunting of blood from vertebral and basilar arteries into the subclavian artery causing vertigo or syncope
  - —Secondary to a stenotic subclavian artery
  - —Diminished unilateral radial pulse or differential systolic blood pressure between arms

Pre-Hospital

N/A

Diagnosis

ESSENTIAL WORKUP

- Ask patient describe the sensation without using the word "dizzy."
- Determine whether the cause is a peripheral or a central process using patient's clinical presentation (see above)
- Detailed physical exam
  - —Auscultation of the carotid and vertebral arteries for bruits
  - —Pulses and pressures in both arms
  - —Inspection of the ears
  - —Evaluation of hearing (Weber and Rinne tests)
  - —Ocular assessment (pupils, fundi, visual acuity, nystagmus)
  - —Cardiac auscultation
  - —Full neurological inquiry

LABORATORY

- Electrolytes, BUN/Cr, glucose

IMAGING/SPECIAL TESTS

- ECG
- Head CT/MRI for evaluation of suspected tumor, central cause, and posttraumatic
- Angiography for suspected vertebral basilar insufficiency

DIFFERENTIAL DIAGNOSIS

- Diabetes mellitus
- Hypothyroidism
- Drugs (i.e., alcohol, barbiturates, salicylates)
- Hyperventilation
- Cardiac (i.e. arrhythmia, MI, or other etiologies of syncope)
- Peripheral vascular disease (i.e., hypertension, orthostatic hypotension, vasovagal)
- Motion sickness

Treatment

INITIAL STABILIZATION

- ABCs
- IV access for dehydration/vomiting
- Monitor

ED TREATMENT

- Based upon accurate diagnosis
  - —Central etiologies require more aggressive workup than peripheral
  - —Symptomatic treatment for peripheral vertigo with appropriate followup
- Administer medication to control vertiginous symptoms—options
  - —Diphenhydramine
  - —Meclizine
  - —Promethazine
  - —Diazepam
- Initiate IV antibiotics for acute bacterial labyrinthitis

MEDICATIONS

- Diazepam (valium): 2.5–5 mg IV q 8 hrs or 2–10 mg po q 8 hrs
- Diphenhydramine (benadryl): 25–50 mg IV/IM/PO q 6 hrs
- Meclizine (antivert): 25 mg po q 6 hrs PRN
- Promethazine (phenergan): 12.5 mg IV q 6 hrs or 25–50 mg PO/IM/PR q 6 hrs

Disposition

ADMISSION CRITERIA

- Cerebellar infarct/hemorrhage
- Vertebral basilar insufficiency
- Intractable nausea/vomiting
- Inability to ambulate

DISCHARGE CRITERIA

- Patient with peripheral etiology and stable

Miscellaneous

ICD9: 780.4

CORE CONTENT CODE: 22.2.25

SUGGESTED READINGS

Fitzgerald D. Head trauma: hearing loss and dizziness. J Trauma 1996;40:488–495.

Gizzi M, Riley E, Molinari S. The diagnostic value of imaging the patient with dizziness. Arch Neurol 1996;53:1299–1304.

Gomez CR, et al. Isolated vertigo as a manifestation of vertebrobasilar ischemia. Neurology 1996;47:94–97.

Herr R, et al. A directed approach to the dizzy patient. Ann Emerg Med 1989;18:6:664–672.

Olshaker S. "Vertigo." In: Rosen P, et al., eds. Emergency medicine: concepts and clinical practice. St. Louis: CV Mosby, 1992:1806–1814.

Authors: Aryeh J. Pessah; Jonathan S. Olshaker

Violence, Management of

Clinical Presentation

SIGNS AND SYMPTOMS

- Behaviors suggesting impending violence
  - —Provocative behavior
  - —Anger
  - —Pacing
  - —Loud speech
  - —Tense posture
  - —Pounding of fists
  - —Clenched fists

MECHANISM/DESCRIPTION

- ED is clinical area likely to experience violent episodes due to 24-hour access
- First contact of victims and perpetrators of violence
- High prevalence of intoxicated patients and psychiatric patients
- Only reliable predictors
  - —Male gender
  - —Alcohol or drug abuse
- No difference exists in
  - —Ethnicity
  - —Language
  - —Age
  - —Education
  - —Employment status
  - —Medical diagnosis

ETIOLOGY

- Functional
  - —Psychiatric
    - -Schizophrenia
    - -Affective
    - -Antisocial
    - -Borderline
    - -Paranoid
    - -Adjustment disorders
  - —Antisocial behavior (no associated psychiatric or medical explanation)
- Organic
  - —CNS
    - -Delirium
    - -Dementia
    - -Infection
    - -Seizures
    - -Cerebrovascular accident
    - -Head injury
  - —Metabolic
    - -Hypoglycemia
    - -Hypoxia
    - -Hypo or hyperthermia
    - -Endocrine disorders
  - —Drugs
    - -Alcohol and sedatives (withdrawal, intoxication)
    - -Cocaine
    - -LSD
    - -PCP
    - -Anticholinergics
    - -Steroids

Pre-Hospital

CAUTIONS

- Restrain potentially violent patients
- Seek police aid in control of violent/dangerous patients

Diagnosis

ESSENTIAL WORKUP

Predict Violence

- Identify prodromes of violence
  - —Begins with anxiety
  - —Then defensiveness
  - —Then physical aggression
  - —History
    - -Previous threats and violence
    - -Psychiatric history
    - -Substance abuse
    - -Self-mutilation
    - -Verbalized threats
    - -Plans of violence
- Physical
  - —Focus on identifying and distinguishing between associated functional and medical conditions
  - —Attention to the neurological exam, vital signs, and mental status exam
  - —Often cannot be performed until the patient is safely restrained

LABORATORY

- CBC if infectious etiology for behavior
- Electrolytes, BUN/Cr, glucose if metabolic or toxic etiology suspected
- Drug screen if ingestion likely

IMAGING/SPECIAL TESTS

- CT head for altered mental status or head trauma

Treatment

INITIAL STABILIZATION

- Prevention of violence
  - —Deterrence
    - -Signs stating weapons not permitted
    - -Visible security personnel
    - -Metal detectors
    - -Secure single public entrance
  - —Triage to an appropriate assessment room
    - -Sparse, solid walls
    - -Lockable
    - -Visible
    - -Exits clear of obstruction
    - -Equipment free
    - -Panic button
  - —Never underestimate the potential for violence
  - —ED protocols for violent situations
  - —Educate staff on preventing, recognizing, and dealing with potentially violent situations
- Approaching the potentially violent patient
  - —Immediately assess safety
  - —Call security and employ physical or chemical restraint if the patient is violent or threatening, or if there is an immediate perceived danger
  - —Remove any weapons prior to interview
  - —Maintain open exit for patient and physician
  - —Maintain distance of 6–8 feet
  - —Allow patient to ventilate
  - —Develop therapeutic alliance
    - -Be nonjudgmental, peace-offering
  - —Use submissive posture
    - -Avoid eye contact
  - —Leave immediately and initiate seclusion or restraint if there is any destabilization

ED TREATMENT

Verbal De-escalation

- Situation can be verbally controlled particularly if there is an identifiable situational precipitant

Isolation

- Temporarily isolate patient in an appropriate room prior to more definitive restraint, or to prevent elopement

Physical restraints

- Required for patient's safety, the safety of others, and to allow physical examination
- Performed by several trained personnel, by protocol, with clear documentation of indications and rechecks

Chemical restraint

- Least restrictive and potentially therapeutic
- If uncooperative, patients often require physical restraint first
- Neuroleptic agents (haloperidol, droperidol) or benzodiazepines (lorazepam)
  - —May use combination if single agent ineffective
  - —Administer every 30 minutes until desired effect reached
  - —Droperidol is more rapid in onset with a shorter half-life than haloperidol
  - —Side-effects of neuroleptics include
    - -Dystonic reactions (treat with diphenhydramine or benztropine)
    - -Neuroleptic malignant syndrome (rare)

Duty to Warn

- Doctor can owe a duty to warn a third party when that third party is in danger due to the medical or psychological condition of the patient

MEDICATIONS

- Benztropine: 2 mg IM or IV
- Diphenhydramine: 50 mg IV, IM or pO
- Droperidol: 5–10 mg IV or IM
- Haloperidol: 5–10 mg IV or IM; 0.5–2 mg for elderly
- Lorazepam: 1–2 mg IV, IM, or po

Disposition

ADMISSION CRITERIA

- Violence secondary to an associated organic cause that is not temporary or reversible in the ED
- Psychiatric admission
  - —Violent psychiatric patient requires psychiatric consultation
  - —Patient is felt to be a danger to either self or others
  - —Involuntary commitment if uncooperative

DISCHARGE CRITERIA

- Violent behavior was caused by a temporary, reversible organic cause (e.g., drug or alcohol intoxication) and the patient is now deemed to be in control, competent, and not a danger to self or others
  - —Psychiatric consultation prior to discharge recommended
  - —If violent act is due to antisocial behavior, not an organic or psychiatric condition may be discharged into police custody, with the warning that the patient may be a danger to self or others

Miscellaneous

ICD9: N/A

CORE CONTENT CODE: 14.11.4

SUGGESTED READINGS

American Council of Emergency Physicians. Protection from physical violence in the emergency department. ACEP policy statement, approved January 1993.

Dubin WR, Feld JA. Rapid tranquilization of the violent patient. Am J Emerg Med 1989;7:313–20.

Lavoie FW, Carter GL, Danzl DF, Berg RL. Emergency department violence in United States teaching hospitals. Ann Emerg Med 1988;17:1227–231.

McCoy MC. Violence in the emergency department. In: Tintinalli JE, Ruiz E, Krome RL, eds. Emergency medicine: A comprehensive study guide. 4th ed. New York: McGraw-Hill, 1996.

Rice MM, Moore GP. Management of the violent patient: therapeutic and legal considerations. Emerg Med Clin North Am 1991;9:13.

Author: Robert J. Vissers

Visual Loss

Clinical Presentation

SIGNS AND SYMPTOMS

- Flashing lights
- New floaters
- Decreased vision
- Afferent pupillary defect
- Visual field defects
- Eye pain
- Limitation or pain with eye movements
- Conjunctival injection or discharge
- Corneal opacity
- Cataract
- Optic nerve head swelling
- Pale retina with a cherry red spot
- Palpable temporal artery with or without tenderness
- Carotid bruit
- Heart murmur
- Neurologic symptoms consistent with intracranial or vascular processes

MECHANISM/DESCRIPTION

- Categorize visual loss by the properties associated with the decrease in visual function
- Transient (<24 hours)
  - —Seconds
    - -Papilledema usually (bilateral)
  - —Minutes
    - -Transient ischemic attack (amaurosis fugax) (unilateral)
    - -Vertebrobasilar artery insufficiency (bilateral)
  - —Minutes to 1 hour
    - -Migraine
- Persistent (>24 hours)
  - —Sudden and painless
    - -Artery or vein occlusion
    - -Vitreous hemorrhage
    - -Retinal detachment
    - -Optic neuritis
    - -Temporal arteritis
  - —Gradual and painless (weeks to years)
    - -Cataract
    - -Presbyopia
    - -Refraction error
    - -Open-angle glaucoma
    - -Chronic retinal disease
    - -Macular degeneration
    - -Diabetic retinopathy
  - —Painful
    - -Corneal abrasion or ulcer
    - -Angle-closure glaucoma
    - -Optic neuritis
    - -Iritis/uveitis
    - -Keratoconus with hydrops
- Associated with systemic neurological symptoms or visual field defects
  - —CVA (especially posterior and occipital circulation)
  - —Mass lesions
  - —Pituitary adenomas
  - —Aneurysm
  - —Meningioma
- Malingering

ETIOLOGY

- Decrease in visual function, i.e., visual acuity, visual fields, blurry vision
  - —Vision loss has many etiologies and can be caused by multiple body systems
- Visual system causes
  - —Eyelid or tear film abnormality
  - —Anterior segment (cornea, anterior chamber, iris, lens)
  - —Posterior segment (vitreous, retina, optic nerve)
  - —Posterior to the eye (optic nerve, chiasm, radiations)
- Neurological causes
  - —Cerebral (CVA) or intracranial pathology (mass lesion)
- Cardiovascular causes
  - —Embolic
  - —Thrombotic
  - —Ischemic
  - —Hypertensive events
- Immunological causes
  - —Infectious
  - —Autoimmune (e.g., uveitis, temporal arteritis)
- Endocrine causes
  - —Diabetic retinopathy leading to vitreous hemorrhage or glaucoma

Pre-Hospital

N/A

Diagnosis

ESSENTIAL WORKUP

- Thorough physical examination
  - —Ophthalmologic
    - -Visual acuity
    - -Pupil exam
    - -Confrontational visual field exam
    - -Extraocular muscle function
    - -Slit-lamp examination
  - —Funduscopy
    - -Tonometry
  - —Cardiovascular
    - -Murmurs
    - -Carotid bruit
  - —Neurological for lesions that affect the optic chiasm, radiations, or occipital and posterior circulation

LABORATORY

- Serum glucose if diabetes suspected

IMAGING/SPECIAL TESTS

- Direct towards the suspected etiology of visual loss
- Dilated fundus exam to assess for posterior segment disease
- Erythrocyte sedimentation rate and temporal artery biopsy if temporal arteritis suspected
- Head CT, CT angiography, and transcranial Doppler to evaluate neurologic symptoms and vertebral-basilar artery flow
- Cardiac and carotid ultrasound if a retinal artery occlusion diagnosed

DIFFERENTIAL DIAGNOSIS

- Trauma
- Conjunctivitis with discharge
- Neurological lesion

Treatment

INITIAL STABILIZATION

- Two conditions where treatment must begin in minutes
  - —Central retinal artery occlusion
  - —Chemical burn

ED TREATMENT

- Direct medical and surgical treatment at the underlying cause of visual loss
- Ophthalmologic consultation for visual loss with an uncertain diagnosis

Central Retinal Artery Occlusion (CRAO)

- Clinical criteria
  - —Unilateral, painless, acute loss of vision
  - —Afferent pupillary defect
  - —Pale fundus with a cherry red spot
  - —30–60 minutes before irreversible damage
- Therapy
  - —Maneuvers to lower intraocular pressure, allowing the embolus to move to the periphery
  - —Ocular massage
  - —Acetazolamide 500 mg IV or po
  - —Topical β-blocker (timolol or levobunolol 0.5%) bid
  - —Carbogen (95% O_2, 5% CO_2) therapy for 10 minutes every 2 hours
  - —Anterior chamber paracentesis by an ophthalmologist

Chemical Burn

- Clinical criteria
  - —Alkali worse than acids
  - —White eye (vessels already sloughed) worse than red eye (vessels intact)
  - —Treat mace, cements, plasters, solvents
- Therapy
  - —Copious irrigation of the eyes with LR or NS (nonsterile water is acceptable if LR/NS not available) for at least 30 minutes
  - —Do not neutralize acids with alkalis or alkalis with acids
  - —Moist cotton-tip applicator to sweep fornices
  - —Dilate with cycloplegic (mydriacyl, cyclogyl, atropine)
  - —Avoid phenylephrine—will vasoconstrict already ischemic conjunctival blood vessels

Disposition

ADMISSION CRITERIA

- Ruptured globe
- Hyphema (depending on severity)
- Significant cardiac, carotid, or neurologic disease

DISCHARGE CRITERIA

- Diagnosis is certain and the visual loss will not progress

Miscellaneous

ICD9: 369.9

CORE CONTENT CODE: 22.2.13

SUGGESTED READINGS

Cullom R, Chang B. The Wills eye manual: Office and emergency room diagnosis and treatment of eye disease. 2nd ed. Philadelphia: JB Lippincott, 1994.

Juang P, Rosen P. Ocular examination techniques for the emergency department. J Emerg Med 1997;15:793–810.

Author: Pascal S.C. Juang

Vitreous Hemorrhage

Clinical Presentation

SIGNS AND SYMPTOMS

- Sudden painless loss or decrease of vision
- Appearance of dark spots and floaters in visual axis
  - —Sometimes accompanied by flashing lights, which move with eye movement
  - —Secondary to streaks of blood in the vitreous humor
- Blurred vision/decreased visual acuity
- Loss of red light reflex
- Inability to visualize the fundus on direct ophthalmoscopy
- Mild afferent pupillary defect

MECHANISM/DESCRIPTION

- Vitreous hemorrhage is a secondary diagnosis, and the identification of a specific cause is necessary for successful treatment to occur
- Sudden tearing of vessels due to trauma
- Spontaneous bleeding due to neovascularization

ETIOLOGY

- Blunt or penetrating trauma
- Retinal break
- Proliferative retinopathy
- Diabetes mellitus
- Sickle cell disease
- Retinal vein occlusion
- Eales' disease
- Senile macular degeneration
- Retinal angiomatosis
- Retinal telangiectasia
- Peripheral uveitis
- Subarachnoid or subdural hemorrhages (Terson's syndrome)
- Intraocular tumor

Pre-Hospital

N/A

Diagnosis

ESSENTIAL WORKUP

- History with special attention to systemic diseases and possible trauma
- Complete ocular exam including
  - —Slitlamp
  - —Tonometry
  - —Dilated fundus exam by indirect ophthalmoscopy
- In cases of spontaneous hemorrhage
  - —Scleral depression is indicated if retinal view can be obtained
  - —Scleral depression should not be performed in cases of traumatic hemorrhage for 3–4 weeks after the injury

LABORATORY

- CBC
- PT/PTT, coagulation studies if indicated
- Electrolytes, BUN/Cr, glucose

IMAGING/SPECIAL TESTS

- B-scan ultrasound
  - —Indicated when no retinal view is possible
  - —To rule out retinal detachment or intraocular tumor
- Fluorescein angiography
  - —Used to define the cause
  - —Study quality may be limited by the density of the hemorrhage
- CT scan/AP/lat orbit radiographs for suspected penetrating injury with intraocular foreign body

DIFFERENTIAL DIAGNOSIS

- Vitreitis (white blood cells in the vitreous)
- Retinal detachment (without vitreous hemorrhage)

Treatment

INITIAL STABILIZATION

- Bedrest with head of bed elevated
- No lifting, stooping, or heavy exertion

ED TREATMENT

- Urgent ophthalmologic consultation
- Further treatment based on the etiology of the hemorrhage
  —Laser photocoagulation or cryotherapy for proliferative retinal vascular diseases
  —Repair retinal detachments
  —Avoid all nonsteroidal antiinflammatory drugs, aspirin, and other anticlotting agents
- Delayed vitrectomy for blood that does not clear with time

Disposition

ADMISSION CRITERIA

- Admit if the etiology of the vitreous hemorrhage cannot be established and a retinal break and/or retinal detachment cannot be ruled out

DISCHARGE CRITERIA

- Discharge if
  —Retinal break/retinal detachment can be reliably ruled out
  —A cause for the hemorrhage can be found that does not require admission

Miscellaneous

ICD9: 379.23

CORE CONTENT CODE: 6.4.3.6

SUGGESTED READINGS

Sanders RJ, Wilson MR. Diabetes-related eye disorders. J Natl Med Assoc 1993;85:104–108.

Winslow RL, Taylor RC. Spontaneous vitreous hemorrhage: Etiology and management. South Med J 1980;73:1450–1452.

Author: Evan Liu

Volvulus

Clinical Presentation

SIGNS AND SYMPTOMS

- Bowel obstruction
  - —Colicky, cramping abdominal pain
  - —Obstipation
  - —Marked abdominal distention
  - —Nausea/vomiting
- Previous episodes of similar but usually milder symptoms in 40–60%
- Presence of gangrenous bowel
  - —Peritoneal signs: guarding, rebound, rigidity
  - —Fever
- Cecal volvulus
  - —Dramatic presentation
  - —Similar to acute small bowel obstruction
- Sigmoid volvulus
  - —More insidious than a small bowel obstruction
  - —Acute with more distention than large bowel obstruction

MECHANISM/DESCRIPTION

- Axial twist of a portion of the gastrointestinal tract around its mesentery causing partial or complete obstruction of the bowel
- Blood supply compromised due to venous congestion leading to gangrene of the bowel

ETIOLOGY

- Third most common cause of large bowel obstruction (5%) following tumor and diverticular disease
- Locations
  - —Sigmoid
    - -Most common site for large bowel volvulus
    - -Due to a redundant sigmoid colon with a narrow mesocolon base
    - -Most common in elderly/institutionalized/chronic bowel motility disorders
  - —Cecal volvulus
    - -Second most common site for volvulus
    - -Due to a congenital failure of the mesentery to fuse with the posterior abdominal wall creating a freely mobile cecum
    - -Most common in 25–35-year-old age group

PEDIATRIC CONSIDERATIONS

- Midgut volvulus
  - —Entire midgut from the descending duodenum to the transverse colon rotates around its mesenteric stalk including the superior mesenteric artery
  - —Due to congenital *malrotation* in which the midgut fails to rotate properly *in utero* as it enters the abdomen
  - —Occurs in neonatal period (75% $<$1 month old; 6–20% $>$1 year old)
  - —*Bilious vomiting* (97%)—does *not* normally occur in young children
  - —A previous episode of bilious vomiting which resolved spontaneously
  - —Constipation
  - —Depending on the degree of ischemia present; child may or may not appear toxic

Diagnosis

ESSENTIAL WORKUP

- Plain abdominal radiograph
  - —Establishes diagnosis
  - —Sigmoid volvulus
    - -In 80%, diagnostic findings
    - -Dilated colon forms an inverted U-shaped sausagelike loop
    - -Loop projects obliquely toward the right upper-quadrant
    - -"Central stripe" formed by adjacent edematous walls lying in close approximation
  - —Cecal volvulus
    - -Kidney-shaped distended loop located in the midabdomen toward the left
    - -"Coffee bean deformity"

LABORATORY

- Normal laboratory values do not exclude the diagnosis, but may give clues as to the presence of gangrenous bowel
- CBC
  - —Leukocytosis (WBC $>$20,000) suggests strangulation with infection/peritonitis
- Electrolytes, BUN, Cr, glucose
  - —Anion gap acidosis due to lactic acidosis
  - —Prerenal azotemia due to dehydration
- UA
  - —Elevated specific gravity

IMAGING/SPECIAL TESTS

- Barium enema
  - —Bird's beak deformity at the site of torsion for cecal and sigmoid volvulus
  - —Increased risk of perforation—should not perform routinely

DIFFERENTIAL DIAGNOSIS

- Obstruction due to colonic tumor
- Obstruction due to diverticular disease
- Small bowel obstruction
- Ileus
- Intussusception

PEDIATRIC CONSIDERATIONS

- Evaluate any child with bilious vomiting for malrotation, even if they are nontoxic appearing
  - —Delays in diagnosis result in gangrenous bowel necessitating resection and leading to parenteral nutrition and its associated complications
- Diagnosis of midgut volvulus
  - —Established by upper gastrointestinal swallow
  - —Duodenum assumes a characteristic corkscrew appearance and fails to cross the midline to left due to the congenital malrotation
  - —Bird's beak deformity if volvulus and obstruction present

Treatment

INITIAL STABILIZATION
- ABCs
- Aggressive fluid resuscitation with 0.9%NS bolus of 20 cc/kg
- Nasogastric tube
- Foley catheter

ED TREATMENT
- Prepare patient for operating room
- Correct hypovolemia and electrolyte abnormalities
- Preoperative antibiotics

Definitive Therapy
Sigmoid Volvulus
- Nontoxic patient
  —Reduce volvulus nonoperatively with sigmoidoscopy
  —Follow with elective sigmoid resection and primary anastomosis to prevent recurrence of volvulus
- Toxic patient
  —Emergent resection of sigmoid and any gangrenous bowel and placement of colostomy

Cecal Volvulus
- Emergent operative reduction followed by cecectomy and primary anastomosis

MEDICATIONS
- Ampicillin sulbactam (Unasyn): 3 g (peds: 100–200 mg ampicillin/kg/24hrs) q 8 hrs IV
- Cefoxitin (Mefoxin): 1–2 g (peds: 100–160 mg/kg/24hrs) IV q 6 hrs

PEDIATRIC CONSIDERATIONS
- Surgical detorsion of bowel with resection of gangrenous bowel and a Ladd procedure is performed to prevent recurrent volvulus

Disposition

ADMISSION CRITERIA
- All suspected of having a volvulus with surgical consult

DISCHARGE CRITERIA
- None

Miscellaneous

ICD9: 560.2

CORE CONTENT CODE: 1.7.2.2

SUGGESTED READINGS

Bonadio WA, Clarkson T, Naus J. The clinical features of children with malrotation of the intestine. Pediatr Emerg Care 1991;7(6):348–349.

Frizelle EA, Wolff BG. Colonic volvulus. Adv Surg 1996;29:131–139.

Jones DJ. ABC of colorectal diseases. Large bowel volvulus. BMJ 1992;305(6849):358–360.

Torres AM, Ziegler MM. Malrotation of the intestine. World J Surg 1993;17(3):326–331.

Author: Paula Ward

Vomiting, Adult

Clinical Presentation

SIGNS AND SYMPTOMS

- Presaged by nausea
- Diaphoresis
- Pallor
- Tachycardia or bradycardia
- Signs of an underlying cause
  - —Fever
  - —Papilledema
  - —Nuchal rigidity
  - —Chest pain
  - —Respiratory distress
  - —Abdominal pain
  - —Diarrhea
  - —Headache
  - —Nystagmus
  - —Focal deficits

MECHANISM/DESCRIPTION

- Forceful retrograde expulsion of gastric contents up the esophagus and out the mouth
- Coordinated action of many muscles
  - —Breathing is held
  - —The diaphragm descends
  - —The anterior abdominal wall contracts
  - —The pelvic diaphragm is raised
  - —The pylorus is closed
  - —The esophageal sphincter is opened
- Regulated by a specialized area in the medulla
  - —Requires an intact brainstem and functioning striated muscles
  - —Aspiration will not occur immediately

ETIOLOGY

- Gastrointestinal
  - —Any GI pathology
- Metabolic/endocrine
  - —Ketoacidosis
  - —Thyrotoxicosis
  - —Uremia
  - —Metabolic alkalosis
  - —Adrenal insufficiency
  - —Hyperparathyroidism
- Drugs/Toxicologic
  - —Antibiotics
  - —Opioids
  - —NSAIDs
  - —Chemotherapeutic agents
  - —Digoxin
  - —Ethanol
  - —Anticholinergics
- Neurologic
  - —CNS mass
  - —CNS bleeding
  - —Cerebral edema
  - —Hydrocephalus
  - —Meningitis
  - —Encephalitis
  - —Concussion
  - —Vascular headaches
- Vascular
  - —Myocardial infarction or ischemia
  - —Mesenteric ischemia
  - —Ovarian torsion
  - —Testicular torsion
- Ophthalmologic
  - —Glaucoma
  - —Postsurgical
- ENT
  - —Labyrinthitis
  - —Ménière's disease
- Psychiatric
  - —Bulimia
  - —Anorexia Nervosa
  - —Anxiety disorder
- Other
  - —Urolithiasis
  - —Pregnancy
  - —Motion sickness

Pre-Hospital

CAUTIONS

- Identify hemodynamic or airway compromise
- Intravenous access and fluid resuscitation in volume depleted patients
- Position patient to avoid aspiration

Diagnosis

ESSENTIAL WORKUP

- The history and the physical examination suggest possible underlying causes
- Most patients will not require ancillary studies

LABORATORY

- β-HCG
  - —Women of child-bearing age

IMAGING/SPECIAL TESTS

- EKG
  - —Diabetes mellitus
  - —Patients at high risk for coronary artery disease
- Head CT scan if signs of elevated ICP or focal deficits

DIFFERENTIAL DIAGNOSIS

- Regurgitation
- Hemoptysis

Treatment

INITIAL STABILIZATION

- Large-bore intravenous access
- Supplemental oxygen
- Place patient upright or in a lateral decubitus position
- Airway control indicated to prevent aspiration in patients with altered mental status

ED TREATMENT

- Fluid resuscitation
- Isotonic crystalloid in hypovolemic patients
  - —Avoid overhydration
  - —Caution in patients with potential intracranial hypertension
- Decompress stomach with a nasogastric tube if intractable vomiting
- Antiemetics

MEDICATIONS

- Prochlorperazine: 5–10 mg IV/IM or 25 mg PR
- Droperidol: 0.625–2.5 mg IV/IM
- Metoclopramide: 10 mg IV/IM
- Ondansetron: 4–32 mg IV
- Promethazine: 25–50 mg IV/IM/PR
- Trimethobenzamide: 200 mg IM/PR

Disposition

ADMISSION CRITERIA

- Serious underlying etiologies
- Intractable vomiting
- Inability to take po

DISCHARGE CRITERIA

- Response to treatment
- Able to keep fluids down
- Close follow-up arranged, especially in elderly and pediatric patients

Miscellaneous

ICD9: 787.0

CORE CONTENT CODE: N/A

SUGGESTED READINGS

Brown HG. Anatomy of vomiting. Br J Anaesth 1963;35:163.

Mayer S: Vomiting. In: Harwood-Nuss A, et al. eds. The clinical practice of emergency medicine. Philadelphia: J.B. Lippincott, 1995:1015–1016.

Author: Myles Greenberg

Clinical Presentation

SIGNS AND SYMPTOMS

General

- Diaphoresis, pallor, tachycardia
- Dehydration
- Findings associated with underlying condition

Gastrointestinal

- Examine the nature of the vomitus-color, composition, relationship to eating and position, onset, progression, and whether it is projectile (vomiting at the peak of maximal inspiration)
  - —Undigested food suggests an esophageal lesion at or above the cardia
  - —Nonbilious vomitus may result from a lesion proximal to the pylorus
  - —Bile-containing material involves obstruction beyond the ampulla of Vater or it may result from an adynamic ileus found in sepsis/infection; bile turns green on exposure to air
  - —Fecal odor is consistent with peritonitis or lower obstruction
  - —Bloody vomitus involves a lesion proximal to the ligament of Treitz. If it is bright red, there is little contact with gastric juices (site above cardia). Coffee ground vomitus results from alteration by gastric juice
- Following vomiting
  - —Retching, hematemesis
  - —Respiratory distress due to aspiration

Complications

- Mallory Weiss or Boerhaave's syndrome

MECHANISM/DESCRIPTION

- Forceful, retrograde expulsion of gastric contents
- Coordinated action of many muscles regulated by medulla
- Retching—no gastric contents expelled
- Regurgitation—no forceful abdominal contraction

ETIOLOGY

Neonate

- Gastrointestinal: physiologic regurgitation/chalasia, gastroesophageal reflux (GER), congenital abnormalities (stenosis, fistula, malrotation, meconium ileus, Hirschsprung's disease), necrotizing enterocolitis, milk allergy, lactobezoar
- Metabolic/endocrine: inborn error of metabolism (phenylketonuria, galactosemia, etc.), azotemia, congenital adrenal hyperplasia, kernicterus
- Neurologic: CNS bleeding, hydrocephalus, meningitis
- Infectious: sepsis

Infant

- Gastrointestinal: physiologic regurgitation, GER, intussusception, other obstruction (hernia, bezoar, foreign body), gastroenteritis, celiac disease, congenital abnormalities (pyloric stenosis, and as above), paralytic ileus
- Metabolic/endocrine: inborn error of metabolism as above, renal tubular acidosis, azotemia, adrenal insufficiency
- Infectious: sepsis, otitis media, UTI, hepatitis, ascariasis
- Neurologic: meningitis, intracranial tumor, CNS bleeding, hydrocephalus
- Toxicologic: antibiotics, NSAIDs, digoxin, theophylline, etc

Child/Adolescent

- Gastrointestinal: gastroenteritis, GER, obstruction (hernia, intussusception, foreign body, bezoar), peptic ulcer disease, pancreatitis, appendicitis, peritonitis, paralytic ileus
- Metabolic/endocrine: diabetic ketoacidosis, azotemia, adrenal insufficiency, Reye's syndrome
- Infectious: UTI, sinusitis, URI, sepsis, hepatitis
- Neurologic: CNS mass/tumor, CNS bleeding, cerebral edema, meningitis, encephalitis, concussion, migraine
- Toxicologic: as above, plus chemotherapeutic agents, iron, lead, household chemicals

Pre-Hospital

- Resuscitation—ABCs
- Evaluation/treatment for hypovolemia and hypoglycemia

Diagnosis

ESSENTIAL WORKUP

- Resuscitation
- Hydration assessment and treatment
- Metabolic assessment (glucose, electrolytes) and treatment
- Evaluation as indicated by presentation and etiology

LABORATORY

- As indicated by differential considerations; usually none required
- Females of childbearing age should have pregnancy evaluation

IMAGING/SPECIAL TESTS

- As indicated by findings; usually none required

DIFFERENTIAL DIAGNOSIS

- See etiology and signs and symptoms (vomitus description)

Treatment

INITIAL STABILIZATION

- Resuscitation as indicated by presentation
- Airway as indicated by presentation, risk of aspiration (impaired level of consciousness), and possibility of increased intracranial pressure (hyperventilation)
- Fluid resuscitation of hypovolemic patients with isotonic crystalloid; caution if concern about increased intracranial pressure
- Determine serum glucose

ED TREATMENT

- Continue resuscitation
- Decompress stomach with nasogastric or orogastric tube if vomiting persistent or stomach distended
- Evaluate underlying differential diagnoses
- Consider antiemetic medications

MEDICATIONS

- Prochlorperazine: 0.13 mg/kg IV/IM/PR
- Droperidol: 0.625–2.5 mg IV/IM
- Metoclopramide: 0.1 mg/kg/dose up to q 6 hrs po
- Promethazine: 0.25–0.5 mg/kg/dose q 4–6 hrs po, PR, IM

Disposition

ADMISSION CRITERIA

- Unstable
- Serious etiologic condition
- Intractable vomiting or inability to take oral fluids

DISCHARGE CRITERIA

- Stable, taking fluids
- Benign etiology
- Parental understanding of instructions to advance clear liquids slowly and return if any evidence dehydration or other findings

Miscellaneous

ICD9: 787.03

CORE CONTENT CODE: 1.0, 13.1

SUGGESTED READING

Henretig F. Vomiting. In: Fleischer G, Ludwig S, eds. Textbook of pediatric emergency medicine. 3rd ed. Baltimore: Williams and Wilkins, 1993;506–513.

Author: Myles Greenberg

von Willebrand Disease

Clinical Presentation

SIGNS AND SYMPTOMS

- Most common presenting symptom—mucosal bleeding
  - —Recurrent epistaxis
  - —Bruising at multiple sites
  - —Gingival bleeding
  - —Menorrhagia
  - —GI bleeding
  - —Most often in children and adolescents
- Milder forms—mucosal bleeding
- Severe forms—deep-tissue bleeding (similar to hemophilia)
  - —Hemarthrosis
- Great variation in the frequency and severity of symptoms, even within the same family

MECHANISM/DESCRIPTION

- Caused by an abnormality of von Willebrand factor (VWF)
- VWF
  - —Cofactor for platelet adhesion
  - —Facilitates platelet adhesion by interaction of platelet receptor and the subendothelial matrix
  - —Protects Factor VIII procoagulant from proteolytic degradation in the plasma
- von Willebrand disease (VWD) subtype categories
  - —Type I: quantitative defect
    - -Mild to moderate decrease in VWF plasma levels, but normal structure
    - -Proportionate decrease in activity
    - -Most common type (70%)
    - -Genetic transmission: autosomal dominant
  - —Type II: qualitative defect
    - -Lacks high molecular weight multimers
    - -Impaired ability to mediate platelet adhesion
    - -Caused by decreased VWF synthesis or increased destruction
    - -Genetic transmission: autosomal dominant or recessive
  - —Type III: total (or near) absence of VWF
    - -Markedly defective hemostasis
    - -Greatly reduced levels of Factor VIII procoagulant
    - -Absent levels of VWF
    - -1 case/1,000,000 population
    - -Genetic transmission: autosomal recessive

ETIOLOGY

- Most common congenital bleeding disorder (1% of the population)
- VWD may occur secondary to
  - —Hypothyroidism
  - —Wilms' tumor
  - —Congenital heart disease
  - —SLE
  - —Thalassemia
- VWD is associated with sickle cell anemia, hereditary hemorrhagic telangectasia, hemophilia A, thrombocytopenia, platelet dysfunction, Factor XII deficiency

Pre-Hospital

N/A

Diagnosis

ESSENTIAL WORKUP

- Screen for VWD if
  - —Large bruises
  - —Bruises at multiple sites
  - —Positive family history
- PT, PTT, platelet count, bleeding time, and ristocetin test

LABORATORY

- Bleeding time prolongation
  - —50% of Type I
  - —All of Type II and Type III
- PT: normal
- PTT: normal or prolonged if VWD occurs concurrently with Factor II, Factor XII, or Factor VIII procoagulant deficiency
- CBC: platelet count normal

IMAGING/SPECIAL TESTS

- Ristocetin test
  - —Used to measure VWF activity
  - —Causes VWF to bind platelets; degree of agglutination proportional to the concentration of VWF
- VWF plasma concentration
  - —Can be measured directly
  - —Decreased in Types I and III; normal or decreased in Type II

DIFFERENTIAL DIAGNOSIS

- Platelet defects
- Collagen vascular disease
- Medications (aspirin, NSAIDs and antiplatelet agents)
- Normal platelet count rules out thrombocytopenia
- Normal PT and PTT excludes clotting deficiencies

Treatment

INITIAL STABILIZATION

- Use local measures to control bleeding

ED TREATMENT

- Avoid antiplatelet medications
- Use desmopressin (DDAVP) to treat bleeding or in preparation for surgery
- Patient education and coordination between the primary care provider and a potential surgeon is essential
- Desmopressin (DDAVP)
  - —Causes a 2–5 fold increase in plasma VWF or Factor VIII procoagulant levels by release of VWF from endothelial storage sites
  - —IV or intranasally administration
  - —First-line agent for Type I VWD—excellent response to DDAVP
  - —Types II and III—little or no response to DDAVP
- Tranexamic acid (cyklokapron), ϵ-aminocaproic acid (Amicar), or topical thrombin
  - —For dental procedures, epistaxis, and mucous membrane bleeding
  - —If DDAVP fails
- Cryoprecipitate
  - —Contains Factor VIII and von Willebrand factor
  - —Best for Types II and III VWD bleeding
  - —Best if made from known donors
  - —Reduced risk of virus transmission with newer products
- Factor VIII concentrate that contains VWF—useful for non-DDAVP responders
  - —Response variable and cannot be predicted

Intervention Strategy

Mild to Moderate VWD

- DDAVP for most bleeding
- Add amicar or cyclokapron for mouth bleeding or epistaxis

Severe VWD

- Hematoma: cryoprecipitate, FFP, Factor VIII
- Hematuria: FFP, Factor VIII
- Hemarthrosis: cryoprecipitate, FFP, Factor VIII
- Mouth/gum bleeding: FFP, Factor VIII, amicar, cyclokapron
- Epistaxis: α-agonist, FFP, Factor VIII, amicar, cyclokapron
- GI bleeding: cryoprecipitate, FFP, Factor VIII,
- CNS bleeding: cryoprecipitate, FFP, Factor VIII,

MEDICATIONS

- Amicar: 100 mg/kg q 6 hrs
- Cryoprecipitate: 2–3 bags/10 kg q 12 hrs
- Desmopressin (DDAVP): 0.3 μg/kg (up to 20 μg total) IV/SQ/IN
- Factor VIII concentrate: 10–30 IU/kg
- Fresh frozen plasma: 10–20 ml/kg
- Tranexamic acid 25 mg/kg IV q 6 hrs

Disposition

ADMISSION CRITERIA

- Refractory bleeding
- Observe Type III VWD after major trauma, especially trauma to the head or spinal cord, to rule out occult bleeding

DISCHARGE CRITERIA

- No bleeding

Miscellaneous

ICD9: 286.4

CORE CONTENT CODE: 7.2.4

SUGGESTED READINGS

Association of Hemophilia Clinic Directors of Canada. Hemophilia and von Willebrand's disease: 1. Diagnosis, comprehensive care and assessment. Can Med Assoc J 1995;153:19–25.

Association of Hemophilia Clinic Directors of Canada. Hemophilia and von Willebrand's disease: 2. Management. Can Med Assoc J 1995;153:147–157.

Ginsburg D, Bowie EJW. Molecular genetics of von Willebrand disease. Blood 1992;79:2507–2519.

Pfaff JA, Geninatti M. Hemophilia. Emerg Med Clinic North Am 1993;11:337–363.

Sadler JE, Gralnick HR. Commentary: A new classification for von Willebrand disease. Blood 1994;84:676–679.

Werner EJ. von Willebrand disease in children and adolescents. Pediatr Clin North Am 1996;43:683–707.

Author: Nicholas Jouriles

Warts

Clinical Presentation

SIGNS AND SYMPTOMS

Painful Genital Ulcers

- Pedunculated growths, often with cauliflower-like appearance
- Flesh-colored to slightly pigmented or red
- Usually on glans penis, prepuce, labia, vagina, or perianal area
- May extend into urethra, bladder, or rectum

ETIOLOGY

- Human papilloma virus (HPV), usually subtypes 6 and 11

PATHOLOGY

- Self-limiting benign epithelial tumors lasting months to years

TRANSMISSION

- Direct sexual contact
- Contact with contaminated objects
- Autoinnoculation

Pre-Hospital

CAUTIONS

- Maintain universal precautions

Diagnosis

ESSENTIAL WORKUP

- Diagnosis made by characteristic appearance of lesions
- Screen for other sexually transmitted diseases

LABORATORY

- Pregnancy test for females

DIFFERENTIAL DIAGNOSIS

- Condyloma lata (secondary syphilis)
- Herpes simplex
- Prominent glands around head of penis

Treatment

INITIAL STABILIZATION

- None required

ED TREATMENT

- If available may use podophyllin, trichloroacetic acid, 5-fluorouracil cauterization, or alternative
- Therapies listed below
- Provide appropriate referral
- Consider need to visualize rectum or urethra in referral

MEDICATIONS

- Weekly topical application of 10–25% podophyllin in benzoin
  - —Protect surrounding normal tissue with petroleum jelly
  - —Do not use in pregnancy—highly toxic and teratogenic
- Topical 85% trichloroacetic acid
- Topical 5% 5-fluorouracil cauterization
- Alternative treatment
  - —Cryotherapy with liquid nitrogen or dry ice
  - —Surgical excision
  - —Electrodesiccation

Disposition

ADMISSION CRITERIA

- Disseminated cases in immunocompromised patients may require admission

DISCHARGE CRITERIA

- The vast majority of patients may be treated as outpatients

Miscellaneous

ASSOCIATED CONDITIONS

- Linked to carcinoma of the penis, vulva, anus and cervix
- May produce laryngeal papillomatosis in infants from viral exposure at birth

SYNONYMS

- Genital warts
- Condyloma acuminata

ICD9: 078.19

CORE CONTENT CODE: 19.1.5

SUGGESTED READINGS

Braude AL. Medical microbiology and infectious diseases. Philadelphia: WB Saunders, 1981:1695–1698.

Fitzpatrick TB, et al. Dermatology in general medicine. 3rd ed. New York: McGraw Hill, 1987:2355–2363.

Pointer JE. Genital infections. In: Rosen P, et al., eds. Emergency medicine: Concepts and clinical practice. 3rd ed. St. Louis: CV Mosby, 1992:1964–1971.

Authors: Smeeta Verma; Paul Gennis; Glenn Hebel

Wernicke Encephalopathy

Clinical Presentation

SIGNS AND SYMPTOMS

Classic Triad

- *Ataxia*
  —Stance and gait affected predominantly
- *Mental disturbance*
  —Found in 90%
  —Ranges from mild confusion to coma
- *Global confusional-apathetic* state (most common presentation) characterized by
  —Listlessness
  —Inattentiveness
  —Indifference to the surroundings
  —Disorientation
- *Ophthalmoplegia*
  —Weakness or paralysis of abduction (abducens palsy)
  —Horizontal diplopia
  —Strabismus
  —Nystagmus
  —Ptosis

Other Signs

- Combined sensory and motor loss in "glove and stocking" distribution
- Hypothermia
- Papilledema
- Retinal hemorrhage
- Telangiectasis of the face
- Angular stomatitis
- Tachycardia
- Postural hypotension
- Various forms of liver disease

MECHANISM/DESCRIPTION

- Nutritional neurologic disorder of acute onset occurring almost exclusively in chronic alcoholics
- Affects persons between 30 and 70 years of age with a slight male predominance
- Presence of *amnesia* and *confabulation* in addition to the *ocular ataxic* findings constitute changing the name of Wernicke-Korsakoff syndrome
- Potentially lethal if not treated
  —Occurs in 15–20% of hospitalized patients
  —Usually due to hepatic failure or to a complicating infection

ETIOLOGY

- Nutritional deficiency of thiamine (vitamin B_1) secondary to chronic alcohol abuse
- Other causes include
  —Hyperemesis gravidarum
  —Malabsorption syndromes
  —Prolonged intravenous feeding without thiamine supplementation
  —Prolonged nasogastric hyperalimentation without thiamine supplementation
  —Anorexia nervosa
  —Regional enteritis
  —Hemodialysis/peritoneal dialysis
  —Thyrotoxicosis
  —Refeeding after prolonged starvation
  —Gastroplasty

Pre-Hospital

N/A

Diagnosis

ESSENTIAL WORKUP

- Diagnosis based on history of nutritional deficiencies, physical findings (classic triad) and improvement of symptoms after thiamine administration
  —Wernicke's encephalopathy has a time-dependent reversibility
  —Often underdiagnosed in the ED

LABORATORY

- Electrolytes, glucose and calcium
  —Not helpful to make the diagnosis but necessary to rule out other causes of altered mental status
- Magnesium
  —Cofactor for thiamine pyrophosphate
  —Hypomagnesemia at increased risk for developing Wernicke
- Lumber puncture/cerebrospinal fluid (CSF)
  —Normal or may show a modest elevation of protein content

IMAGING/SPECIAL TESTS

- CT of the head rules out other causes of altered mental status

DIFFERENTIAL DIAGNOSIS

- Intracerebral lesions/masses
- Subdural hematoma
- Meningitis
- Toxic ingestions
- Metabolic abnormalities
- Botulism
- Atypical Guillain-Barré syndrome

Treatment

INITIAL STABILIZATION

- ABCs
- Pulse oximetry/supplemental oxygen
- Cardiac monitor
- Intravenous catheter access

ED TREATMENT

- Thiamine
  - —Administer to all patients with altered mental status
  - —Prior to glucose administration
- Magnesium sulfate
- Response to therapy
  - —Extremely slow
  - —May not be appreciated for many hours or days

MEDICATIONS

- Magnesium sulfate: 2 g (50% solution) IVPB or IM
- Thiamine: 100 mg IVP

Disposition

ADMISSION CRITERIA

- Comatose patients
- Hemodynamic compromise
- Pronounced hypothermia
- Confused patients who warrant close observation
- Significant metabolic/nutritional abnormalities

DISCHARGE CRITERIA

- Resolution of symptoms in patients with mild cases who have good support systems

Miscellaneous

ICD9: 256.1

CORE CONTENT CODE: 4.5.1

SUGGESTED READINGS

Lindberg M, Oyler R. Wernicke's encephalopathy. Am Fam Physician 1990;41(4):1205–1209.

Victor M, Martin J. Nutritional and metabolic diseases of the nervous system. In: Isselbacker K, et al., eds. Harrison's principles of internal medicine. Vol. 2. 13th ed. New York: McGraw Hill, 1994:2329–2331.

Author: Isam Nasr

Wilms' Tumor

Clinical Presentation

SIGNS AND SYMPTOMS

General

- Hypertension in 60% of patients due to renal ischemia from tumor pressure on the renal artery
- Congestive heart failure

Renal

- Abdominal mass that is usually smooth and 5–10 cm in size
  —Does not cross midline

Complications

- Postoperative: bowel obstruction, urinary tract infection, pneumonia
- Chemotherapy: neutropenia, renal insufficiency, anemia, thrombocytopenia, renal insufficiency, hepatitis
  —Hepatitis and thrombocytopenia was seen in 1.4% of patients receiving vincristine and actinomycin-D

MECHANISM/DESCRIPTION

- Solid tumor of kidney, accounting for 8% of childhood solid tumors
- Incidence of 7 cases per million children per year
- Mean age at diagnosis: 3.2 years (median: 2.6 years); age range: 3 months to 16 years
- Male predominance 1.3:1
- Unfavorable tumor include anaplastic tumors
- Stages (10-year survival)
  —I: Limited to kidney (94%)
  —II: Spread by direct extension (86%)
  —III: Spread via lymphatic drainage (71%)
  —IV: May undergo hematogenous metastasis (36%)
  —V: Involves both kidneys
  —Note: 10-year survival with unfavorable histology is 36%

ETIOLOGY

- Abnormal proliferation of metanephric blastema without normal differentiation into tubules and glomeruli

Pre-Hospital

N/A

Diagnosis

ESSENTIAL WORKUP

- Urinalysis: hematuria in 25% of patients
- Ultrasound can distinguish cystic from solid tumor

LABORATORY

- Renal function tests

IMAGING/SPECIAL TESTS

- CT or MRI scan of abdomen to diagnose the disease and stage
- Chest x-ray and chest CT scan evaluating for metastases

DIFFERENTIAL DIAGNOSIS

- Infection: urinary tract infection
- Anomaly: urinary tract anomaly, hydronephrosis, renal cyst
- Neoplasm: neuroblastoma, renal cell carcinoma, sarcoma, lymphoma

Treatment

INITIAL STABILIZATION

- Resuscitation as appropriate including management of hypertension and CHF

ED TREATMENT

- Appropriate referral after initiating diagnostic evaluation
- Chemotherapy reflecting type and stage
  —Stage I with favorable histology: vincristine *or* vincristine plus actinomycin-D
  —Stage II with favorable histology: longer courses than Stage I
  —Stages III and IV with favorable histology and any stage with unfavorable histology: radiation and vincristine and actinomycin-D plus doxorubicin

Disposition

ADMISSION CRITERIA

- Hypertension, CHF
- Renal insufficiency
- Significant anemia
- Pulmonary findings
- Poor compliance

DISCHARGE CRITERIA

- No admission criteria

Miscellaneous

ICD9: 189.0

CORE CONTENT CODE: 13.1.12.2

SUGGESTED READINGS

Green MG, Thomas PRM, Shocar S. The treatment of Wilms' tumor. Hematol Oncol Clin North Am 1995;9:1267–1274.

Kov HP, Hansle TW. Molecular biology of Wilms' tumor. Urol Clin North Am 1993;20:323–331.

Pritchard J, Imeson J, Barnes J, et al. Results of the United Kingdom Children's Cancer Study Group's first Wilms' tumor study. J Clin Oncol 1995;13:124–133.

Raine J, Bowman A, Wallendszus K, et al. Hepatopathy-thrombocytopenia syndrome: a complication of dactinomycin therapy for Wilms' tumor. A report from the United Kingdom Children's Cancer Study Group. J Clin Oncol 1991;9:268–273.

Saghlul MS, Hussein MH, Koutbey ME, et al. Wilms' tumor: long-term results from a single institution. J Surg Oncol 1994;56:25–31.

Author: Joseph Kahn

Withdrawal, Alcohol

Clinical Presentation

SIGNS AND SYMPTOMS

- Agitation/tremulous (most common)
- Anxiety
- Depression
- Anorexia
- Nausea/vomiting
- Confusion
- Hallucinations (25% incidence)
  - —Visual (most common)
  - —Auditory
  - —Olfactory
  - —Tactile
- Seizures (5–15% of withdrawing alcohol-dependent patients)
  - —Peak time between 13 and 24 hours after cessation of drinking
  - —Occurs up to 96 hours after cessation
  - —Typically occur singularly
  - —Generalized tonic-clonic activity
  - —Usually self-limited
- Sleep disturbances (insomnia and nightmares)
- Delirium tremens
  - —Severe sympathetic hyperactivity
  - —Temperature
  - —Tachycardia
  - —Tremor
  - —Altered sensorium
    - -Occurs in up to 5% of withdrawing alcoholics
- Physical signs
  - —Diaphoresis
  - —Flushing
  - —Tachycardia
  - —Hypertension
  - —Tachypnea
  - —Fever
  - —Hyperreflexia
  - —Stigmata of chronic alcohol abuse
  - —Spider angiomata
  - —Rhinophyma
  - —Hepatomegaly
  - —Cirrhosis
  - —Ascites
  - —Muscle wasting

MECHANISM/DESCRIPTION

- Withdrawal syndrome primarily affects persons who are habituated (tolerant) to chronic ethanol ingestion who either cease their drinking or markedly reduce their consumption
- Characterized by a hyperadrenergic state that develops in 6–12 hours after the cessation of drinking and may last for up to 5 days
- Symptom severity determined by the amount of endogenous norepinephrine released during withdrawal

ETIOLOGY

- Predisposing factor
- Acute, prolonged and chronic ethanol ingestion
- Malnutrition
- Dose dependence
- Amount and chronicity of alcohol intake related to the severity of the syndrome

Pre-Hospital

CAUTIONS

- Cardiac monitoring
- Blood glucose if abnormal mental status
- Physical or chemical restraints for agitation
- Seizure precautions

Diagnosis

ESSENTIAL WORKUP

- Rapid blood glucose

LABORATORY

- Electrolytes, BUN/Cr, glucose
- Alcohol level
- Breathalyzer or serum sample
- Drug screen if coingestion suspected

IMAGING/SPECIAL TESTS

- CT scan of the brain
  - —Abnormal mental status
  - —Head trauma
  - —First-time seizure
  - —Focal or status seizures
- Lumbar puncture and CSF analysis if meningitis suspected

DIFFERENTIAL DIAGNOSIS

- Withdrawal from sedative-hypnotic drugs
- Head trauma
- Epilepsy
- Encephalopathy
- Hypoglycemia
- Hyperthyroidism
- Sepsis
- Meningitis
- Encephalitis
- Sympathomimetic overdose
- Pheochromocytoma
- Anticholinergic poisoning
- Psychosis
- Electrolyte disorders

Treatment

INITIAL STABILIZATION

- ABCs
- Correct hypoglycemia
- Administer thiamine
- IV fluids
- Initiate tranquilization to prevent the progression of the syndrome to more severe levels and to relieve the symptoms

ED TREATMENT

Tranquilization

- Benzodiazepines
  - —Standard therapy
  - —High doses required due to cross-tolerance with chronic ethanol ingestion
  - —Administer aliquots and follow the patient's response
- Barbiturates
  - —Alternatives to benzodiazepines
- Butyrophenone antipsychotics
  - —Haloperidol or droperidol (low doses)
  - —Indicated as adjuncts in the hallucinating patient
- β-Blockers
  - —Propranolol and atenolol
  - —Used to relieve some of the signs and symptoms
  - —Considered adjunctive therapy
  - —Avoid in patients with contraindications (asthma, bradycardia, or CHF)
- Clonidine
  - —Adjunct to treat the hyperadrenergic signs and symptoms of alcohol withdrawal
  - —Anticonvulsive prophylaxis
  - —Not useful in alcohol-withdrawal patients who do not also have an underlying seizure disorder that is not alcohol related

General Therapy

- Administer glucose for hypoglycemia or alcoholic ketoacidosis
- Treat hypovitaminosis syndromes due to malnutrition with thiamine and folate
- Correct electrolyte abnormalities
- Replete magnesium
  - —25% of chronic alcoholics are total body magnesium depleted due to malnutrition and increased renal losses
  - —Hypomagnesemic state makes replenishment of potassium difficult and may lower patient's seizure threshold

MEDICATIONS

- Clorazepate: 15–30 mg orally every 8–12 hrs
- Chlordiazepoxide: 25–100 mg orally for mild reactions; 25 mg IV in repeated doses as necessary for more severe reactions
- Clonidine: 0.1–0.2 mg orally every 4–6 hrs
- Diazepam: 5–20 mg orally for mild reactions; 5–10 mg IV in repeated doses as necessary for more severe reactions
- Droperidol: 1.25–5.0 mg IV
- Folate: 1 mg IV or orally
- Glucose: 5% solution in IV fluids; 25 g IV bolus in hypoglycemic patients
- Haloperidol: 2–10 mg orally or IV
- Lorazepam: 7 mg orally per day for mild reactions; 2 mg IV in repeated doses as necessary for more severe reactions
- Magnesium sulfate: 2–6 g in IV solutions, except in renal failure
- Pentobarbital: 100 mg IV in repeated doses as necessary for more severe reactions
- Propranolol: 0.5–1 mg IV; 10–40 mg orally
- Thiamine: 100 mg IV

Disposition

ADMISSION CRITERIA

- Moderate to severe symptoms or persistent symptoms should be admitted to a medical facility
- Severe symptoms ("impending DTs") or delirium tremens should be admitted to an intensive care unit

DISCHARGE CRITERIA

- Mild to moderate symptoms that can be controlled with oral medications

Miscellaneous

ICD9: 291.81

CORE CONTENT CODE: 14.8.4.1

SUGGESTED READINGS

Berner J, Silverstein S. Alcohol withdrawal syndrome. In: Honigman B, Rumack BH, Silverstein S, eds. Disease and trauma monograph for acute care. Emergindex System. Vol. 92. Englewood, CO: Micromedex (edition expires 5/31/97).

Erstad BL, Cotugno CL. Management of alcohol withdrawal. Am J Health Syst Pharm 1995;52(7):697–709.

Lohr RH. Treatment of alcohol withdrawal in hospitalized patients. Mayo Clin Proc 1995;70(8):777–82.

Miller NS. Pharmacotherapy in alcoholism. J Addict Dis 1995;14(1):23–46.

Saitz R, O'Malley SS. Pharmacotherapies for alcohol abuse. Withdrawal and treatment. Med Clin North Am 1997;81(4)881–907.

Sanft C, Hannemann L, Striebel HW, Schaffartzik W. Therapy of alcohol withdrawal syndrome in intensive care unit patients following trauma: results of a prospective, randomized trial. Crit Care Med 1996;24(3):414–22.

Author: Lee Shockley

Withdrawal, Drug

Clinical Presentation

SIGNS AND SYMPTOMS

Sedative-Hypnotic

- Anxiety
- Depression
- Agitation
- Tremulous
- Anorexia
- Nausea/vomiting
- Confusion
- Hallucinations
- Seizures
- Sleep disturbances (insomnia and nightmares)
- Physical signs
  - —Diaphoresis
  - —Flushing
  - —Tachycardia
  - —Hypertension
  - —Orthostatic hypotension
  - —Tachypnea
  - —Fever
  - —Hyperreflexia
  - —Seizures, delirium, and autonomic instability
    - -Markers of severe withdrawal

Opiates

- Mild withdrawal
  - —Lacrimation
  - —Rhinorrhea
  - —Yawning
  - —Diaphoresis
  - —Anxiety
  - —Restlessness
  - —Dysphoria
  - —Mydriasis
  - —Piloerection
- More severe withdrawal
  - —Nausea/vomiting
  - —Diarrhea
  - —Abdominal pain
  - —Mild increase in blood pressure, pulse, and respiratory rate

Sympathomimetics

- Three-phase syndrome: the crash, withdrawal, and extinction
  - —Crash
    - -Extreme exhaustion that follows binge usage
  - —Withdrawal
    - -Lethargy
    - -Psychomotor retardation
    - -Increased appetite or anorexia
    - -Sleep disturbances
    - -Muscle twitching
    - -Depression
    - -Fatigue and dysphoria may last 6–18 weeks in the abstinent patient
  - —Extinction
    - -Episodically evoked cravings that can last for months to years after withdrawal

MECHANISM/DESCRIPTION

- Sedative-hypnotic withdrawal
  - —Characterized by a hyper-excitable state
  - —Severe withdrawal can be life-threatening
- Opiate withdrawal
  - —Decrease in the exogenous opioid binding causes a catecholamine release in the locus ceruleus
  - —Syndrome may be temporarily disabling and very uncomfortable
  - —Not life-threatening
- Sympathomimetic withdrawal
  - —Causes tiredness, depression, and dysphoria
  - —Neurotransmitter depletion
  - —No serious metabolic or neurologic complications
  - —May be associated with an increased suicide risk and cravings for the drug, which often result in cycles of binges and transient abstinence

Pre-Hospital

CAUTIONS

- Initiate cardiac monitoring
- Determine blood glucose if abnormal mental status
- Physical or chemical restraints for agitated patients

Diagnosis

ESSENTIAL WORKUP

- Thorough physical examination to determine nature of withdrawal
- Blood glucose

LABORATORY

- Electrolytes, BUN/Cr, glucose
- Drug screens may be useful if polysubstance abuse is suspected

IMAGING/SPECIAL TESTS

- Lumbar puncture and CSF analysis for withdrawal patients in whom meningitis suspected
- CT scan of the brain for
  - —Abnormal mental status
  - —Head trauma
  - —Focal seizures
  - —Status seizures

DIFFERENTIAL DIAGNOSIS

- Sedative-hypnotic
  - —Withdrawal from alcohol
  - —Head trauma
  - —Epilepsy
  - —Encephalopathy
  - —Hypoglycemia
  - —Hyperthyroidism
  - —Sepsis, meningitis
  - —Encephalitis
  - —Sympathomimetic overdose
  - —Pheochromocytoma
  - —Anticholinergic poisoning
  - —Psychosis
  - —Electrolyte disorders
- Opiates
  - —Sedative-hypnotic and ethanol withdrawal
  - —Gastrointestinal diseases
- Sympathomimetics
  - —Alcohol or sedative-hypnotic intoxication
  - —Acute psychiatric disease (depression or psychosis)
  - —Head trauma
  - —CNS infection

Treatment

INITIAL STABILIZATION

- ABCs
- Correct hypoglycemia with glucose
- Initiate IV fluid for dehydration

ED TREATMENT

- Sedative-hypnotic withdrawal
  - —Reinstitution of therapy or the substitution of a sedative-hypnotic drug with a long half-life to facilitate detoxification
  - —β-Blocking agents
    - -Adjuncts to lessen the adrenergically mediated symptoms
- Opiate withdrawal
  - —Phenothiazines and butyrophenones
    - -Lessens the severity of symptoms, especially nausea and vomiting
  - —Clonidine
    - -Reduces the signs and symptoms of opiate withdrawal
    - -Combination therapy with clonidine and the long half-life antagonist naltrexone
    - -May shorten the withdrawal duration by as much as 50% without increasing the severity of symptoms
  - —Benzodiazepines
    - -May help ease some of the symptoms
- Sympathomimetics withdrawal
  - —Supportive therapy

MEDICATIONS

- Chlorazepate: 15–30 mg orally every 8–12 hrs
- Chlordiazepoxide: 25–100 mg orally for mild reactions; 25 mg IV in repeated doses as necessary for more severe reactions
- Clonidine: 0.1–0.2 mg orally every 4–6 hrs
- Diazepam: 5–20 mg orally for mild reactions; 5–10 mg IV in repeated doses as necessary for more severe reactions
- Droperidol: 1.25–5.0 mg IV
- Glucose: 5% solution in IV fluids; 25 g IV bolus in hypoglycemic patients
- Haloperidol: 2–10 mg orally or IV
- Lorazepam: 7 mg orally per day for mild reactions; 2 mg IV in repeated doses as necessary for more severe reactions
- Methadone: 5–20 mg orally per day
- Naltrexone: 50 mg orally per day
- Pentobarbital: 100 mg IV in repeated doses as necessary for more severe reactions
- Propranolol: 0.5–1.0 mg IV; 10–40 mg orally
- Promazine: 25 mg IM every 30 min as needed, up to 125 mg

Disposition

ADMISSION CRITERIA

- Sedative-hypnotic
  - —Moderate severe or persistent symptoms
  - —Seizures
  - —Psychosis during withdrawal
  - —Severe autonomic instability or delirium should be admitted to an intensive care unit
- Opiates
  - —Medical conditions which may complicate withdrawal
  - —Intractable vomiting
- Sympathomimetics
  - —Extremely lethargic or minimally responsive must be admitted
  - —Suicidal patients require psychiatric evaluation and possible admission

DISCHARGE CRITERIA

- Able to tolerate oral solutions
- Not suicidal

Miscellaneous

ICD9: 292.0

CORE CONTENT CODE: 17.1.7

SUGGESTED READINGS

Cadet JL, Bolla KI. Chronic cocaine use as a neuropsychiatric syndrome: a model for debate. Synapse 1996;22(1):28–34.

DeMaria PA Jr, Weinstein SP. Methadone maintenance treatment. When and how to refer patients. Postgrad Med 1995;97(3):836, 912.

Kuhar MJ, Pilotte NS. Neurochemical changes in cocaine withdrawal. Trends Pharmacol Sci 1996;17(7):2604.

Polevoi SK, Lowenstein S. Drug withdrawal syndrome. In: Honigman B, Rumack BH, Silverstein S, eds. Disease and trauma monograph for acute care. Emergindex System. Vol. 92. Englewood, CO: Micromedex (edition expires 5/31/97).

Wax PM. Withdrawal syndromes. In: Harwood-Nuss A, et al., eds. The clinical practice of emergency medicine. 2nd ed. Philadelphia: Lippincott-Raven, 1996:1434–439.

Williams H, Salter M, Ghodse AH. Management of substance misusers on the general hospital ward. Br J Clin Pract 1996;50(2):948.

Woods JH, Winger G. Current benzodiazepine issues. Psychopharmacology (Berl) 1995;118(2):107–15; discussion 118, 1201.

Author: Lee Shockley

Wolff-Parkinson-White (WPW) Syndrome

Clinical Presentation

SIGNS AND SYMPTOMS

- Asymptomatic
- Palpitations
- Dyspnea
- Dizziness
- Nausea
- Abnormal heart rate
  —Rapid and regular (SVT)
  —Irregular (atrial fibrillation)
- Signs of instability
  —Chest pain
  —Hypotension
  —Change in mental status
  —Rales

MECHANISM/DESCRIPTION

- Syndrome caused by ventricular preexcitation via a bundle of Kent
- Type A or orthodromic is the most common (70%)
  —Impulse travels down the A-V node and then up the retrograde pathway
  —A circuit is created that potentiates reentrant tachycardia
- Type B or antidromic
  —Less common than Type A
  —The circuit operates in the opposite direction

ETIOLOGY

N/A

Pre-Hospital

CAUTIONS

- Supplemental oxygen
- Monitor
- Synchronized cardioversion if signs of instability

CONTROVERSIES

- Pre-hospital use of adenosine
  —Stable patients do not require emergent conversion
  —Unstable patients should undergo cardioversion not receive adenosine

Diagnosis

ESSENTIAL WORKUP

- WPW should be considered as the underlying etiology in all cases of tachydysrhythmias
- The diagnosis should be based on the characteristic EKG findings once the patient has converted to a sinus rhythm
- Electrophysiology studies to assess for radioablation or surgery should be performed as an outpatient

LABORATORY

N/A

IMAGING/SPECIAL TESTS

- EKG
  —Short PR $<$0.12 seconds
  —Prolonged QRS $>$0.10 seconds
  —Delta wave
    -Small slurred upstroke at the beginning of the QRS

DIFFERENTIAL DIAGNOSIS

- AV nodal reentry SVT
- Ventricular tachycardia

Treatment

INITIAL STABILIZATION

- Unstable patients
  - —Synchronized cardioversion starting with 50 J/min
  - —Increase incrementally until sinus rhythm is restored

ED TREATMENT

- Stable patients with narrow complex, regular tachycardia
  - —Vagal maneuvers such as a Valsalva
  - —Right carotid artery massage for no more than 10 seconds
    - -Auscultate the artery first for a bruit which would contraindicated this procedure
  - —Fluid replacement and Trendelenburg if the patient has mild hypotension
  - —Pharmacologic conversion if carotid massage fails
    - -Adenosine
- Stable patients with irregular wide complex tachycardia
  - —Procainamide is the drug of choice
  - —Never use calcium channel blockers, β-blockers, or digoxin
    - -These medications block the AV node and lead to conduction occurs exclusively down the faster accessory pathway resulting in fatal ventricular dysrhythmias

MEDICATIONS

- Adenosine: 6 mg rapid IV push; if ineffective repeat with 12 mg; peds: 0.1 mg/kg rapid IV push
- Procainamide: 6–13 mg/kg IV at 0.2–0.5 mg/kg/min until arrhythmia controlled, up to a total dose of 1000 mg, then 2–6 mg/min

Disposition

ADMISSION CRITERIA

- Patients with signs of instability require admission to a monitored bed
- Failure of outpatient therapy for continuous pharmacological control or ablation

DISCHARGE CRITERIA

- The majority of patients will be stable and can be discharged once converted to sinus rhythm
- Follow up should be arranged with a cardiologist

Miscellaneous

ICD9: 426.7

CORE CONTENT CODE: 2.4.1.3

SUGGESTED READINGS

Shah CP. Clinical approach to wide QRS complex tachycardias. Emerg Med Clin North Am 1998;16:331–360.

Xie B, Thakur RK, Shah C, et al. Emergency management of cardiac arrhythmias. Clinical differentiation of narrow QRS complex tachycardias. Emerg Clin North Am 1998;16:295–330.

Zipes DP. Specific arrhythmias: Diagnosis and treatment. In: Braunwald E, ed. Heart disease: A textbook of cardiovascular medicine. 5th ed. Philadelphia: WB Saunders, 1997:667–675.

Author: Richard Wolfe

Wound Ballistics

Clinical Presentation

SIGNS AND SYMPTOMS

- Severe underlying tissue damage and life-threatening injury may occur with even small entrance wounds
- A knowledge of how different kinds of weapons and bullets wound, the trajectory of the bullet through the body, and the effect on different body tissues will allow the physician to carefully evaluate gunshot and stab wounds and their potential morbidity and mortality

MECHANISM/DESCRIPTION

- Wounding potential of a bullet is determined by its mass and velocity
- The type and severity of a wound is determined not only by the wounding potential, but also the construction and shape of the bullet, its orientation upon striking the body, deformity or fragmentation it undergoes, and what tissues the bullet traverses
- The traditional distinction between low and high muzzle *velocity* bullets does not necessarily differentiate the kind and severity of wounding
  - —A civilian hunting rifle or a large caliber handgun with a hollow point bullet may produce a more severe wound than a round with a full metal jacket from a "high velocity" military rifle
- Bullets wound by two main mechanisms: *crush and stretch*
- The sonic pressure wave that precedes the bullet has no role in wounding
- The bullet crushes the tissue it directly passes through, forming the *permanent cavity*
- *Stretch* is produced by the radial energy transferred from the bullet as it slows down in tissue, forming the *temporary cavity*
- A bullet is stabilized in flight from *spin* transmitted by the rifling in the barrel
  - —This spin minimizes *yaw,* which is the angle between the long axis of the bullet and its flight vector
  - —Without spin, a bullet would yaw to its most stable flight configuration, which is base and center of mass forward
  - —This configuration is not aerodynamically efficient
  - —As a bullet enters tissue, the spin of the bullet is reduced and the bullet will yaw
  - —When yaw is 90°, a bullet crushes the maximal amount of tissue, slows down the most, and maximal stretch injury occurs
- Bullets designed to deform in tissue (soft point, hollow point) will expand on impact into a mushroom shape, increasing the amount of crush injury and moving the center of mass of the bullet forward
- Jacketed bullets prevent lead stripping in the barrel that occurs at high muzzle velocities
  - —Jacketed bullets do not deform but may fragment
  - —Fragmentation increases surface area and crush injury
  - —Bullets striking bone often fragment and may cause bone fragments to become secondary projectiles
- Wound severity is also dependent upon *tissue composition and thickness*
  - —Organs consisting of minimally elastic, near water-density tissue (brain, liver) may be greatly injured by the temporary cavity formation, as are fluid-filled (heart, bowel) and dense organs (bone)
  - —More elastic tissue such as lung and skeletal muscle may absorb the energy from temporary cavity formation and sustain minimal damage
  - —Extremities are often not thick enough for the bullet to fully yaw
    - -Temporary cavity formation is minimal and rarely is responsible for significant tissue injury
    - -Most damage is caused by direct crush injury of the bullet, its fragments, or secondary projectiles
  - —Short-range shotgun blasts produce severe wounds with compromise of the blood supply
    - -In short-range shotgun injuries, although the entrance wounds may be close together, the pellets may be greatly scattered in tissue secondary to the pellets striking each other
- Stab wounds with knives and other sharp instruments are low-energy wounds with tissue injury from direct weapon contact

Pre-Hospital

- Field personnel can provide information about weapon type and size, distance and angle between the weapon and victim
- Gunshot and stab wounds to the chest with unstable vital signs warrant a needle thoracostomy in side of the chest with the entrance wound, and if no improvement, then the contralateral hemithorax should have a needle thoracostomy placed to relieve a potential tension pneumothorax
- Impaled objects or projectiles should not be removed; immobilize with tape and gauze and transport
- The patient should be transported to the closest Trauma Center for definitive care
- In some systems, the hypotensive patient may be taken directly to the operating room

Diagnosis

ESSENTIAL WORKUP

- Radiographs taken in the AP and lateral projections help localize the bullet and with placement of a marker at the entrance wound, the trajectory can be estimated
  - —Additionally, any fragments, fractures, pneumothoraces, or hemothoraces will be identified
- Evaluate for entrance and exit wounds
  - —May estimate trajectory and potential for tissue damage
  - —It is not always possible to differentiate entrance from exit wounds
    - -Exit wounds are often stellate and larger than entrance wounds unless energy is dissipated at skin surface by special bullet type (hollow point, etc.)
    - -With high velocity projectiles, exit wound may be much more extensive than entrance wound
    - -Because of the elasticity of the skin, the bullet can often be palpated subcutaneously if it did not exit

IMAGING/SPECIAL TESTS

- The extent of tissue injury is often only apparent on surgical exploration
- See chapters on penetrating chest and abdominal trauma for further diagnostic considerations

Treatment

INITIAL STABILIZATION

- ABCs of trauma care

ED TREATMENT

- Impaled objects or projectiles should be removed only in the operating room
- The care of such patients in the ED includes initial stabilization, estimation of tissue injury based on the above principles, and initiation of appropriate diagnostic work-up
- Wound care includes appropriate exploration, irrigation, and débridement of devitalized tissue
- Early trauma, orthopedic, and vascular surgery consultation is necessary
- For further treatment considerations, see penetrating chest and abdominal trauma chapters

Disposition

ADMISSION CRITERIA

- Patients with neurovascular compromise and extensive tissue damage must be admitted for appropriate surgical intervention
- Patients with injury to the head, neck, torso, or abdomen should be admitted
- Patients with injury from high velocity projectiles or gunshot wounds should be admitted to a monitored setting for observation of neurovascular status

DISCHARGE CRITERIA

- Patients with minor penetrating extremity trauma, or stabbing victims found not to have significant injury may be discharged with appropriate follow-up

Miscellaneous

ICD9: E922.9

CORE CONTENT CODE: 18.3.2.1.1

SUGGESTED READINGS

Hollerman JJ, Fackler ML. Wound ballistics. In: Tintanelli JE, et al. Emergency medicine: A comprehensive study guide. 4th ed. New York: McGraw Hill, 1996:1196–1203.

Hollerman JJ, Fackler ML, Coldwell DM, et al. Gunshot wounds: 1. Bullets, ballistics and mechanisms of injury. AJR Am J Roentgenol 1990;155:685–690.

Hollerman JJ, Fackler ML, Coldwell DM, et al. Gunshot wounds: 2. Radiology. AJR Am J Roentgenol 1990;155:691–702.

Author: Brian Snyder

Zygoma Fracture

Clinical Presentation

SIGNS AND SYMPTOMS

- Malar edema or flattening
- Periorbital ecchymosis, drooping lateral canthus
- Lateral subconjunctival hemorrhage, diplopia
- Infraorbital anesthesia, trismus/open bite

MECHANISM/DESCRIPTION

- Fractures of the zygoma result from blunt trauma to the side of the face
- The most common mechanisms include motor vehicle accidents, falls, and physical assault
- The direction and magnitude of force will determine the fracture type and degree of displacement
  - —A blow to the side of the face directed posteriorly and medially will produce a zygomatic body (tripod) fracture
  - —A lateral blow often results in an isolated zygomatic arch fracture

PEDIATRIC CONSIDERATIONS

- Maxillofacial fractures are rarely seen in the pediatric population
  - —Only 1% of all facial fractures is seen in children under age 6
  - —Children have a comparatively larger cranium than facial skeleton leading to a higher incidence of head trauma
  - —Falls and motor vehicle accidents account for the majority of facial trauma in children
  - —Consider nonaccidental trauma, particularly in children under age 6

Pre-Hospital

CAUTIONS

- Airway compromise may occur with severe maxillofacial injuries
- Assume that the patient with face or head injury has also sustained a C-spine injury until proven otherwise

Diagnosis

ESSENTIAL WORKUP

- If a high velocity or severe blunt force mechanism is suspected, a thorough evaluation for associated injuries (C-spine, head, globe, other maxillofacial bones, etc.) is imperative

Clinical Examination

- Intraoral palpation of the zygomatic body and arch for bony step deformity
- Assess sensation of the inferior orbital area (cheek, upper lip, and gingiva)
- Examine the globe and orbit carefully
  - —Periorbital ecchymosis and lateral subconjunctival hemorrhages are common
  - —Assess visual acuity, pupillary function, and extraocular movements
  - —Inferior displacement of the globe may lead to diplopia and enophthalmos carefully evaluate extraocular movements
- Mandibular movement may be restricted
  - —Trismus may be seen if there is impingement of the mandibular coronoid process by displacement of the zygomatic body
  - —Zygomatic arch fractures may impede the temporalis muscle or coronoid process
  - —Lastly, temporalis muscle contusion or TMJ effusion may cause pain that limits range of motion
- Unilateral epistaxis may be present and typically resolves spontaneously

Radiographs

- The submental vertex (jug-handle) view is used to diagnose fractures of the zygomatic arch
- Plain films are not as useful in the evaluation of zygomatic body fractures
- The Waters' (occipitomental) view shows the inferior orbital rims and possibly layering of blood in the maxillary sinus
- The articulation between the zygoma and frontal bone can be evaluated on the Caldwell view

IMAGING/SPECIAL TESTS

- Computed Tomography is the diagnostic standard for evaluation of zygomatic body fractures
  - —CT is not usually needed for isolated fractures of the zygomatic arch

DIFFERENTIAL DIAGNOSIS

- Facial contusions
- La Forte fractures

PEDIATRIC CONSIDERATIONS

- Sedation may be required to properly examine some children
- If a head injury is suspected, sedation is not recommended
- If circumstances or injuries raise suspicions of child abuse, a comprehensive investigation for previous nonaccidental trauma is essential

Treatment

INITIAL STABILIZATION

- Airway management is particularly important if there are associated maxillofacial or mandibular injuries causing airway compromise
  - —Isolated zygoma fractures do not typically require aggressive airway intervention
- Life-threatening conditions should be treated first, follow ABCs of trauma care

ED TREATMENT

- Assume that the patient with head and maxillofacial trauma has a cervical spine injury.
  - —The neck should be immobilized until radiographic clearance is obtained
- Do not blindly clamp bleeding vessels as this may cause inadvertent damage to the facial nerve, parotid duct, etc.
- Early consultation with oral maxillofacial or plastic surgeon
- Analgesics, antibiotics, and tetanus prophylaxis if open injury

MEDICATIONS

*SEDATIVE/ANALGESICS:**	*ADULT DOSE (MG/KG IV)*	*PEDIATRIC DOSE (MG/KG IV)*
Diazepam	0.1–0.2	0.1–0.2
Fentanyl	2–10 (mcg/kg)	2–3 (mcg/kg)
Ketamine	2	1–2
Meperidine	1–2	1–2
Midazolam	0.1	0.15
Morphine sulfate	0.1–0.2	0.1–0.2

* All of these sedative/analgesics should be titrated to effect.

PEDIATRIC CONSIDERATIONS

- Multiple injuries are often seen in children including head trauma, skull fracture, and orthopedic injuries
- Definitive repair of facial fractures should not be delayed beyond 3 or 4 days
  - —The facial bones heal rapidly in children and delays of more than 3 to 4 days may result in malunion and cosmetic deformity

Disposition

ADMISSION CRITERIA

- Displaced or comminuted zygomatic body fractures require open reduction internal fixation
- Associated head, neck or other traumatic injuries requiring admission

DISCHARGE CRITERIA

- Nondisplaced tripod fracture can be treated conservatively as an outpatient with close follow-up
  - —Delayed fracture displacement, poor cosmetic outcome, and difficulty with mandibular movement are indications for ORIF
  - —Isolated arch fractures are amenable to outpatient treatment. These typically require open reduction of fracture fragments. If the reduction is unstable, internal fixation is then performed

PEDIATRIC CONSIDERATIONS

- Consult social services and local child welfare agency if needed

Miscellaneous

ICD9: 802.4

CORE CONTENT CODE: 18.4.4.7

SUGGESTED READINGS

Colucciello SA, Sternbach G, Walker SB. The treacherous and complex spectrum of maxillofacial trauma: Etiologies, evaluation, and emergency stabilization. Emerg Med Rep 1995;16;7:59–69.

Covington DS, Wainwright DJ, Teichgraeber JF, et al. Changing patterns in the epidemiology and treatment of zygoma fractures: 10-year review. J Trauma 1994; 37:243–248.

Hunter JG. Pediatric maxillofacial trauma. Pediatr Clin North Am 1992;39:1127–1143.

Rumsey C, Sargent LA. Zygomatic fractures. Trauma Q 1992;9:76–85.

Author: Raymond A. Viducich

Commonly Used Drugs in the Emergency Department

- *Acyclovir* (Zovirax): 5–10 mg/kg IV every 8 hrs
  —Genital herpes: first episode: 400 mg po every 8 hrs; prophylaxis: 400 mg po every 12 hrs
  —Zoster: 800 mg po 5 times/day for 10 days
  —Varicella: 20 mg/kg up to 800 mg po every 6 hrs for 5 days
- *Adenosine* (Adenocard): adult: 6 mg IV followed by flush through central line if possible. If no response after 1–2 min then repeat with 12 mg; peds: initial dose 50 μg/kg followed by 100–200 μg/kg if needed
- *Aminophylline:* load 6 mg/kg IV over 20–30 min; infusion 1 g in 250 cc D5W (4 mg/cc) at 0.5–0.7 mg/kg/hr
- *Amoxicillin* (Amoxil): 250–500 mg po every 8 hrs; peds: 40 mg/kg/day divided in 3 doses
- *Atropine:* 0.5–1.0 mg IV/ET; peds: 0.02 mg/kg
- *Azithromycin* (Zithromax): 500 mg IV per day; oral (adult/peds): 10 mg/kg up to 500 mg the first day, then 5 mg/kg up to 250 mg every day for 4 days
  —Chlamydia: 1000 mg po single dose
- *Benzathine Penicillin* (Bicillin LA): 1.2 million IU IM (dose lasts 2–4 weeks); peds: 300,000–600,000 IU if less than 27 kg; 900,000–1.2 million IU if greater than 27 kg
- *Bumetanide* (Bumex): 0.5–1.0 mg IV/IM
- *Bretylium* (Bretylol): initial 5 mg/kg IV, repeat 10 mg/kg if needed. Infusion 500 mg in 50 cc D5W (10 mg/cc) at 1–3 mg/min (7–21 cc/hr)
- *Carbamazepine* (Tegretol): 200–600 mg po every 12 hrs
- *Cephalexin* (Keflex, others): 250–500 mg po every 6 hrs; peds: 25–50 mg/kg/day
- *Cefazolin* (Ancef, others): 0.5–1.5 g IV/IM every 6–8 hrs; peds: 25–50 mg/kg/day divided every 6–8 hrs; may go up to 100 mg/kg/day for severe infections
- *Ceftriaxone* (Rocephin): 1–2 g IV/IM every 24 hrs; peds: 50–75 mg/kg/day (maximum 2 g), 100 mg/kg/day for meningitis
  —For gonorrhea 125 mg/IM single dose (250 mg for pelvic inflammatory disease)
- *Charcoal* (activated): 0.5–1.0 g/kg po as load. Can repeat if needed
- *Chloral Hydrate* (Noctec): 25–50 mg/kg po up to 1000 mg
- *Chlordiazepoxide* (Librium): 5–25 mg po, larger doses may be required for ethanol withdrawal
- *Ciprofloxacin* (Cipro): 200–400 mg IV every 12 hrs; oral: 250–750 mg every 12 hrs
  —Gonorrhea: 250 mg po single dose
- *Cimetidine* (Tagamet): 300 mg IV/IM/PO every 6 hrs, 400 mg po every 12 hrs, or 400–800 mg every night
- *Clarithromycin* (Biaxin): 250–500 mg po every 12 hrs; peds: 7.5 mg/kg po every 12 hrs
- *Clindamycin* (Cleocin): 600–900 mg IV every 8 hrs. IM dosing should be 600 mg or less; oral: 150–450 mg po every 6 hrs; peds: 20–40 mg/kg/day IV divided in 3–4 doses, or 8–20 mg/kg/day po divided in 3–4 doses
- *Clonidine* (Catapres): hypertension: 0.1 mg po every 12 hrs up to 2.4 mg/day (rebound hypertension can follow abrupt withdrawal)
  —Addiction therapy: 0.1 mg po every 8 hrs
- *Codeine:* 0.5 mg/kg up to 15–60 mg po IM every 4–6 hrs
- *Cyclobenzaprine* (Flexeril): 10 mg po every 8 hrs
- *Deferoxamine* (Desferal): iron poisoning: infusion up to 15 mg/kg/hr. Higher doses may be used in serious poisonings. Use for greater than 36 hrs may lead to pulmonary toxicity
- *Digoxin* (Lanoxin): 0.25 mg IV every 6 hrs up to 1 mg for treatment of atrial fibrillation
- *Digoxin-Immune Fab* (Digibind): 2–10 vials IV; may repeat 10 vials if no response (40 mg/vial)
- *Dexamethasone* (Decadron): croup: 0.6 mg/kg IM
  —Acute pharyngitis: Adult:10 mg IM
- *Diazepam* (Valium): 0.2–0.4 mg/kg up to 5–10 mg IV. Alcohol withdrawal treatment may require higher doses
- *Diltiazem* (Cardizem, others): bolus 0.25 mg/kg or 20 mg IV over 2 min. Rebolus 15 min later (if needed) 0.35 mg/kg or 25 mg; infusion 5–15 mg/hr
- *Diphenhydramine* (Benadryl): 25–50 mg IV/IM/PO every 6 hrs; peds: 5mg/kg/day div q 6 hrs
- *Dobutamine* (Dobutrex): 250 mg in 250 cc D5W (1 mg/cc) at 2.5–15 μg/kg/min
- *Dopamine* (Intropin): 400 mg in 250 cc D5W (1600 μg/cc) at 2–20 μg/kg/min
- *Doxycycline* (Vibramycin, Doryx): 200 mg PO/IV initially, then 50–100 mg every 12 hrs
- *Droperidol* (Inapsine): 1.25–2.5 mg IV/IM every 3–6 hrs
- *Epinephrine:* 1 mg IV/ET for cardiac arrest (1:10,000 solution)
  —Anaphylaxis or allergy dose 0.3–0.5 mg SC (1:1000 solution), may repeat in 15–20 min
- *Erythromycins*
  —Erythromycin base (E-Mycin): 250–500 mg po every 6 hrs, 333 mg po every 8 hrs, or 500 mg po every 12 hrs
  —Erythromycin ethyl succinate (EES): 400 mg po every 6 hrs; peds: 30–50 mg/kg/day po divided in 4 doses
  —Erythromycin lactobionate: 15–20 mg/kg/day (max 4 g) IV divided every 6 hrs
- *Esmolol* (Brevibloc): 5 mg in 50 cc (10 mg/cc), load with 500 μg/kg over 1 min, then infuse 50–200 μg/kg/min (for 70 kg patient, load with 35 mg, infuse at 100 μg/kg/min)
- *Etomidate* (Amidate): induction dose 0.3 mg/kg IV over 30–60 sec
- *Famciclovir* (Famvir): Genital herpes: 125 mg po every 12 hours for 5 days
  —Zoster: 500 mg po every 8 hrs for 7 days
- *Famotidine* (Pepcid): 20 mg IV every 12 hrs; oral 20–40 mg every night
- *Fentanyl* (Sublimaze): 2–3 μg/kg up to 50–75 μg IV
- *Fluconazole* (Diflucan): vaginal candidiasis: 150 mg po single dose
  —Candidiasis: 200 IV/PO, then 100–200 mg every day
- *Flumazenil* (Romazicon): 0.2 mg IV every 1–3 min up to 1 mg until benzodiazepine sedation reversed
- *Fosphenytoin* (Cerebyx): load 15–20 mg/kg (phenytoin equivalents) IV/IM no faster than 100–150 mg/min
- *Furosemide* (Lasix): 1 mg/kg up to 20–40 mg IV
- *Gentamicin* (Garamycin): 1–2 mg/kg IV/IM as load and 1 mg IM/IV every 8 hrs
  —Alternative dosing is 5–7 mg/kg once daily
- *Glucagon:* for hypoglycemia, 1 mg IV/IM/SC
- *Glycopyrrolate* (Robinul): 0.1–0.2 mg IV/IM, 1–2 mg po every 6–8 hrs
- *Haloperidol* (Haldol): 2–5 mg IV/IM
- *Heparin:* load 80 IU/kg IV, then mix infusion 25,000 IU in 250 cc D5W (100 IU/cc) and start at 18–20 IU/kg/hr; peds: load 50 IU/kg IV
- *HIV Prophylaxis* (*Triple Therapy*): initiate as soon as possible (ideally <1 hr) after exposure to HIV
  —Zidovudine (AZT, Retrovir): 200 mg po every 8 hrs
  —Lamivudine (3TC, Epivir): 150 mg po every 12 hrs
  —*And either* Indinavir (Crixivan): 800 po every 8 hrs *or* Saquinavir (Invirase): 600 mg po every 8 hrs
- *Hydralazine* (Apresoline): 10–40 mg IV/IM every 4–6 hrs
- *Hydroxyzine* (Vistaril, others): 0.5 mg/kg up to 50–100 mg IM every 4–6 hrs
- *Ibuprofen* (Motrin, others): 200–800 mg po every 6 hrs; peds: for children older than 6 mo: 5–10 mg/kg po every 6 hrs

- *Indomethacin* (Indocin): 25–50 mg po every 8 hrs
- *Insulin* (Humulin, others): maintenance: 0.5–1 unit/kg/day, extremely variable
  —DKA: begin with 0.1 IU regular/kg IV bolus followed by infusion of 0.1 IU regular/kg/hr
  —Extreme hyperkalemia: 5–10 IU regular IV concurrently with glucose
- *Itraconazole* (Sporanox): start 200 mg po every day, max 400 mg/day
- *Ketamine* (Ketalar): 1–2 mg/kg IV over 1–2 min or 4 mg/kg IM
  —Concurrent atropine (0.02 mg/kg) suggested to reduce hypersalivation
- *Ketoralac* (Toradol): 30 mg IV/IM every 6 hrs as needed; first IM dose may be 60 mg
- *Labetalol* (Trandate, Normodyne): 20 mg IV every 10 min to 300 mg
- *Lidocaine* (Xylocaine): load 1–1.5 mg/kg IV, then 0.5 mg/kg every 8–10 min as needed to max of 3 mg/kg; maintenance infusion 2 g in 250 cc D5W (8 mg/cc) at 1–4 mg/min (7–30 cc/hr); peds: 20–50 μg/kg/min
- *Lorazepam* (Ativan): 0.5–2 mg IV/IM/PO every 8 hrs; higher doses may be required for ethanol withdrawal
- *Magnesium Sulfate:* for eclampsia 1–4 g IV over 2–4 min; infusion 5 g in 250 cc D5W (20 mg/cc)
- *Mannitol* (Osmitrol): 1.5–2 g/kg over 30–60 min
- *Meperidine* (Demerol, others): 1–2 mg/kg IV or IM up to 150 mg every 3–4 hrs
- *Methocarbamol* (Robaxin): 1000–1500 mg po every 6 hrs
- *Methylprednisolone* (Solu-Medrol): 10–125 mg IV/IM; peds: 1–2 mg/kg/day div qd or bid
- *Metronidazole* (Flagyl): trichomonas: 2 g po single dose
  —Giardia: 250 mg po every 8 hrs for 5 days
- *Midazolam* (Versed): adult sedation: 1–5 mg IV/IM, usually administered 1 mg every 2–3 min as needed; peds: sedation 6 mo–5 yrs: 0.05–0.1 mg/kg up to 0.6 mg/kg IV; 6–12 yrs: 0.025–0.05 mg/kg up to 0.4 mg/kg IV. May also be administered IM
- *Morphine Sulfate:* 0.1 mg/kg IV or IM up to 15 mg for analgesia every 3–4 hrs 2–4 mg IV for adjunct treatment of congestive heart failure
- *N-Acetylcysteine* or NAC (Mucomyst): Acetaminophen poisoning: load with 140 mg/kg po followed by 70 mg/kg every 4 hrs for 17 doses
- *Nalmefene* (Revex): 0.5 mg/70 kg adult IV or IM for reversal of opioid toxicity
- *Naloxone* (Narcan): 0.01 mg/kg up to 2 mg IM, IV, ET for treatment of opioid toxicity. May require up to 10 mg to reverse some opioids
- *Naproxen* (Naprosyn, others): 250–500 mg po every 12 hrs
- *Nitroglycerin* (intravenous, Tridil): 50 mg in 250 cc D5W (200 μg/cc), begin at 5 μg/min (2 cc/hr), titrate up as needed
- *Nitroprusside Sodium* (Nipride): 50 mg in 250 cc D5W (200 μg/cc), start at 0.3 μg/kg/min (for 70 kg adult 6 cc/hr)
- *Norepinephrine* (Levophed): 4 mg in 500 cc D5W (8 μg/cc) at 2–4 μg/min. 20 cc/hr = 3 μg/min
- *Pancuronium* (Pavulon): 0.1 mg/kg IV
- *Pediazole* (erythromycin ethyl succinate 200 mg and sulfisoxazole 600 mg/5 cc): 50 mg/kg/day (based on EES dose) po every 6 hrs
- *Phenobarbital:* load 15–20 mg/kg IV at 25–50 mg/min
- *Phentolamine* (Regitine): 5 mg bolus for hypertension related to pheochromocytoma; repeat as needed
  —For extravasation: 5–10 mg in 10 cc saline local injection
- *Phenylephrine* (Neo-Synephrine): 50 μg boluses IV, followed by infusion of 20 mg in 250 cc D5W (80 μg/cc) at 40–180 μg/min (35–160 cc/hr)
- *Phenytoin* (Dilantin): load 15–20 mg/kg IV up to 1000 mg no faster than 50 mg/min (mix in NSS)
- *Physostigmine* (Antilirium): reversal of antimuscarinic poisoning: 0.5 mg IV every 5–10 min up to 2.0 mg max; may cause severe bradycardia or seizures
- *Prednisone:* 1–2 mg/kg po every day
- *Procainamide* (Pronestyl): 100 mg IV every 10 min, or infuse at 20 mg/min until either dysrhythmia resolves, QRS widens more than 50% baseline, 1000 mg infused, or patient becomes hypotensive. Mix 2 g in 250 cc D5W (8 mg/cc), maintenance infusion 2–6 mg/min (15–45 cc/hr)
- *Prochlorperazine* (Compazine): 5–10 mg IV/IM (IV should be over 2–5 min)
- *Propofol* (Diprivan): 40 mg IV every 10 sec until sedation (2–2.5 mg/kg)
- *Ranitidine* (Zantac): 50 mg IV every 6–8 hrs; oral: 150 mg every 12 hrs or 300 mg every night
- *RhoGAM* (RHO immune globulin): 1 vial IM within 72 hrs if mother Rh-negative
  —Microdose (MICRhoGAM) if spontaneous abortion at less than 12 weeks gestation
- *Rocuronium* (Zemuron): 0.6 mg/kg IV
- *Sodium Bicarbonate:* 1 mEq/kg up to 50–100 mEq IV
- *Sodium Polystyrene Sulfonate* (Kayexalate): 1 g/kg up to 15–60 g po or 30–50 g retention enema (in sorbitol) every 6 hrs as needed
- *Succinylcholine* (Anectine): 1–1.5 mg/kg up to 150 mg IV; peds: 2 mg/kg IV preceded by atropine 0.02 mg/kg
- *Sumatriptan* (Imitrex): 6 mg SC; may repeat after 1 hr to maximum of 12 mg/day; oral: 25 mg; if no response, may repeat 25–100 mg every 2 hrs to max 300 mg/day
- *Thiopental* (Pentothal): induction dose 3–5 mg/kg IV
- *Thrombolytics*
  —Alteplase (t-PA, Activase): 15 mg IV bolus, then 0.75 mg/kg (maximum 50 mg) over 30 min, then 0.5 mg/kg (max 35 mg) over next 60 min
  —Anistreplase (APSAC, Eminase): 30 IU IV over 2–5 min
  —Reteplase (Retevase): 10.8 IU IV over 2 min repeat in 30 min
  —Streptokinase (Streptase, Kabikinase): 1.5 million IU IV over 60 min
- *Trimethoprim/Sulfamethoxazole* (Bactrim, Septra, Cotrim, others): 1 double-strength tab po every 12 hrs; peds: 5 cc liquid per 10 kg per dose every 12 hrs
- *Vecuronium* (Norcuron): 0.1 mg/kg IV
- *Verapamil* (Isoptin, Calan): 0.1–0.3 mg/kg up to 5–10 mg IV over 2 min for SVT

Coordinated by Richard F. Clark

Index

*Page numbers in *italics* denote figures; those followed by *t* denote tables.

Tachycardia Algorithm

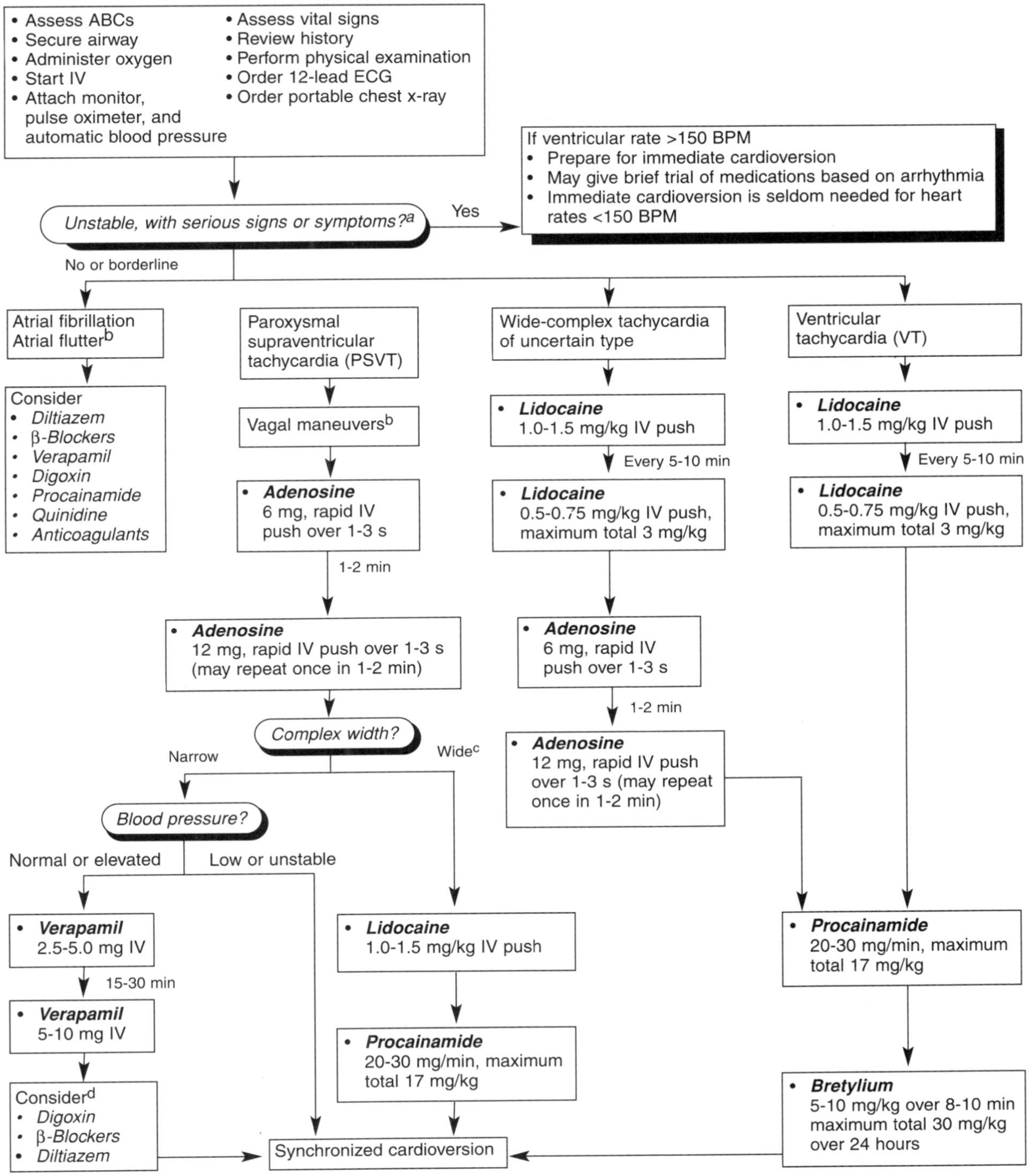

a. Unstable condition must be related to the tachycardia. Signs and symptoms may include chest pain, shortness of breath, decreased level of consciousness, low blood pressure (BP), shock, pulmonary congestion, congestive heart failure, acute myocardial infarction.
b. Carotid sinus pressure is contraindicated in patients with carotid bruits; avoid ice water immersion in patients with ischemic heart disease.
c. If the wide-complex tachycardia is known with certainty to be PSVT and BP is normal/elevated, sequence can include ***verapamil***.
d. Use extreme caution with β-blockers and ***verapamil.***

Ventricular Fibrillation/Pulseless Ventricular Tachycardia (VF/VT) Algorithm

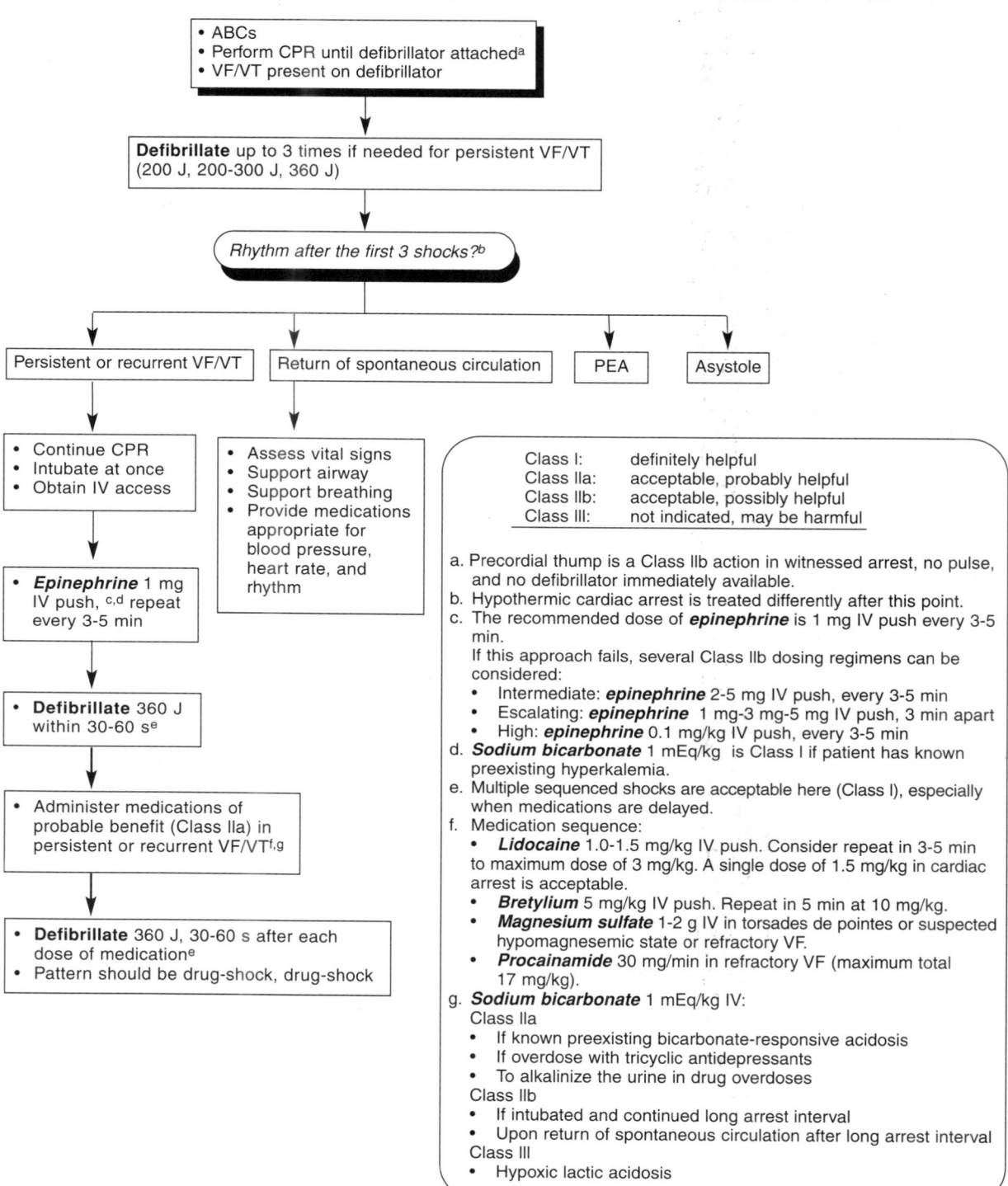

- ABCs
- Perform CPR until defibrillator attached[a]
- VF/VT present on defibrillator

↓

Defibrillate up to 3 times if needed for persistent VF/VT (200 J, 200-300 J, 360 J)

↓

Rhythm after the first 3 shocks?[b]

↓

Persistent or recurrent VF/VT | Return of spontaneous circulation | PEA | Asystole

Persistent or recurrent VF/VT

- Continue CPR
- Intubate at once
- Obtain IV access

↓

- ***Epinephrine*** 1 mg IV push,[c,d] repeat every 3-5 min

↓

- **Defibrillate** 360 J within 30-60 s[e]

↓

- Administer medications of probable benefit (Class IIa) in persistent or recurrent VF/VT[f,g]

↓

- **Defibrillate** 360 J, 30-60 s after each dose of medication[e]
- Pattern should be drug-shock, drug-shock

Return of spontaneous circulation

- Assess vital signs
- Support airway
- Support breathing
- Provide medications appropriate for blood pressure, heart rate, and rhythm

Class I:	definitely helpful
Class IIa:	acceptable, probably helpful
Class IIb:	acceptable, possibly helpful
Class III:	not indicated, may be harmful

a. Precordial thump is a Class IIb action in witnessed arrest, no pulse, and no defibrillator immediately available.

b. Hypothermic cardiac arrest is treated differently after this point.

c. The recommended dose of ***epinephrine*** is 1 mg IV push every 3-5 min.
If this approach fails, several Class IIb dosing regimens can be considered:
- Intermediate: ***epinephrine*** 2-5 mg IV push, every 3-5 min
- Escalating: ***epinephrine*** 1 mg-3 mg-5 mg IV push, 3 min apart
- High: ***epinephrine*** 0.1 mg/kg IV push, every 3-5 min

d. ***Sodium bicarbonate*** 1 mEq/kg is Class I if patient has known preexisting hyperkalemia.

e. Multiple sequenced shocks are acceptable here (Class I), especially when medications are delayed.

f. Medication sequence:
- ***Lidocaine*** 1.0-1.5 mg/kg IV push. Consider repeat in 3-5 min to maximum dose of 3 mg/kg. A single dose of 1.5 mg/kg in cardiac arrest is acceptable.
- ***Bretylium*** 5 mg/kg IV push. Repeat in 5 min at 10 mg/kg.
- ***Magnesium sulfate*** 1-2 g IV in torsades de pointes or suspected hypomagnesemic state or refractory VF.
- ***Procainamide*** 30 mg/min in refractory VF (maximum total 17 mg/kg).

g. ***Sodium bicarbonate*** 1 mEq/kg IV:

Class IIa
- If known preexisting bicarbonate-responsive acidosis
- If overdose with tricyclic antidepressants
- To alkalinize the urine in drug overdoses

Class IIb
- If intubated and continued long arrest interval
- Upon return of spontaneous circulation after long arrest interval

Class III
- Hypoxic lactic acidosis